OXFORD MEDICAL PUBLICATIONS

# Oxford textbook of public health

## Editors

### Walter W. Holland, MD, FRCGP, FRCP, FFCM

Professor of Clinical Epidemiology and Social Medicine,
Department of Community Medicine, and Honorary Director,
Social Medicine and Health Services Research Unit,
St. Thomas's Hospital Medical School (United Medical Schools),
London SE1 7EH, England.

### Roger Detels, MD, MS

Professor of Epidemiology and Dean,
School of Public Health, Center for Health Sciences,
University of California, Los Angeles, CA 90024, USA.

### George Knox, MD, BS, FRCP, FFCM

Professor of Social Medicine, Department of Social Medicine,
Health Services Research Centre,
University of Birmingham Medical School,
Edgbaston, Birmingham B15 2TG, England.

### Ellie Breeze, MSc

Research Assistant, Department of Community Medicine,
St. Thomas's Hospital Medical School,
(United Medical Schools), London SE1 7EH, England.

# Oxford textbook of public health

VOLUME 3

Investigative methods in public health

Edited by

Walter W. Holland, Roger Detels, and
George Knox
with the assistance of
Ellie Breeze

OXFORD  NEW YORK  TORONTO
OXFORD UNIVERSITY PRESS

*Oxford University Press, Walton Street, Oxford OX2 6DP*

*Oxford New York Toronto*
*Delhi Bombay Calcutta Madras Karachi*
*Petaling Jaya Singapore Hong Kong Tokyo*
*Nairobi Dar es Salaam Cape Town*
*Melbourne Auckland*

*and associated companies in*
*Beirut Berlin Ibadan Nicosia*

*Oxford is a trade mark of Oxford University Press*

*First published 1985*
*Reprinted 1986, 1987*

*British Library Cataloguing in Publication Data*
*Oxford textbook of public health.—(Oxford*
*medical publications)*
*1. Public health*
*I. Holland, Walter W.   II. Detels, Roger*
*III. Knox, George   IV. Breeze, Ellie*
*614   RA425*
*ISBN 0–19–261448–7*

*Library of Congress Cataloging in Publication Data*
*Main entry under title:*
*Oxford textbook of public health.*
*(Oxford medical publications)*
*Bibliography: p.*
*Includes index.*
*Contents: v. 3. Investigative methods in public health.*
*1. Public health—Collected works.   I. Holland,*
*Walter W.   II. Series.*
*WA 100 098*
*RA422.509 1985   362.1   84-14717*
*ISBN 0–19–261448–7*

*Printed in Great Britain by Thomson Litho Ltd, East Kilbride, Scotland*

# Preface

It is not an easy task to follow in the footsteps of such a renowned editor as Professor Hobson. We were however very honoured when, on the retirement of Professor Hobson, the Oxford University Press approached us about taking up the challenge of revising Hobson's *Theory and practice of public health*. Since this work first appeared in February 1961, Professor Hobson was responsible for taking it through no less than five editions. Many eminent public health academics and practitioners have contributed to this book and it has been recognized as a standard textbook on the subject. Sadly, Professor Hobson died after a long illness at the end of November 1982. After an early training in public health starting as a medical officer of health and then as a specialist in hygiene and epidemiology in the army, he went on to be Professor for Social Medicine at Sheffield University in 1949. From 1957 until his retirement, he served in a variety of posts at the WHO, where his major responsibilities were always concerned with education and training. His interest in this and in the international aspects of health was well exemplified by the first edition of *Theory and practice of public health*. One of the major strengths of the book has been its international nature and its link to the WHO.

On accepting the daunting task of revising this major work our first step was to look dispassionately at its role within public health, a field which has evolved and changed greatly over the last 25 years. We decided that although this book is held in great esteem in the western world it was appropriate now to introduce major revisions and thus, increase its relevance to the problems facing us as we approach the twenty-first century. A particularly important advance has been the recognition in recent years that the problems in public health facing developing countries are quite different to those facing the developed world. The interests of WHO, quite correctly, have been focused on developing countries. We consider that this book should concentrate on presenting a comprehensive view of public health as it relates to developed countries. (Perhaps there is a place now for a comparable textbook concerned specifically with developing countries.) This is not to say however, that the content will not prove relevant and of interest to the student of public health from a developing country.

The *Oxford textbook of public health* attempts to portray the philosophy and underlying principles of the practice of public health. The methods used for the investigation and the solution of public health problems are described and examples given of how these methods are applied in prac-

tice. It is aimed primarily at postgraduate students and practitioners of public health but most clinicians and others concerned with public health issues will find some chapters relevant to their concerns. It is intended to be a comprehensive textbook present in the library of every institution concerned with the health sciences. The term 'public' is used quite deliberately to portray the dield. Public health is concerned with defining the problems facing communities in the prevention of illness and thus studies of disease aetiology and promotion of health. It covers the investigation, promotion, and evaluation of optimal health services to communites and is concerned with the wider aspects of health within the general context of health and the environment. Other terms in common use, such as community medicine, preventive medicine, social medicine, and population medicine have acquired different meanings according to the country or setting. This gives rise to confusion and we have avoided their use since this book is directed to a worldwide audience. Public health, we believe, is more evocative of the basic philosophy which underlies this book.

The first volume aims to lead the reader through the historical determinants of health to the overall scope and strategies of public health. Through knowledge of historical aspects of the subject we may gain an understanding of what it is possible to achieve now and in the future. Volume 2 of this textbook is concerned with the process of public health promotion. Volume 3 with the investigative methods used in public health, and finally Volume 4 with a description of the specific applications of public health methods of controlling disease processes, and, with tackling the problems of disease in specific client groups.

The development of public health policy is dependent upon a series of scientific methods, and we do not attempt in this book to cover all the methods and their applications. However it is to be hoped that those examples that have been chosen will illustrate to the reader the way in which particular problems can be approached. Each chapter includes a comprehensive list of further reading which should equip the reader with the means of obtaining a deeper knowledge should he or she wish to pursue any theme further.

This is the first of what we hope will be many editions. As each chapter was submitted to the editors we have attempted to identify gaps and areas of overlap. There is no doubt however that some remain. It is only through feedback from readers that we will be able to adapt, modify, and improve further editions. If the book is successful it will be entirely due to the effort of the contributors who undertook with great patience a tremendous amount of work. They were bombarded with instructions, advice, reminders, and modifications and we would like to express our thanks and extend our apologies to all of them. Our gratitude also goes to our secretaries and assistants who coped so admirably with the enormous task of compiling this work. We hope that it will be widely read by all those concerned with the formulation and execution of public health policy and that it will provide a suitable framework for devising approaches to some of the problems challenging public health today.

W.W.H.
R.D.
G.K.

*London*
January, 1985

# Contents

# Contents of Volumes 1, 2, and 4

ix

# Contributors

J.H. Abramson
Professor and Head, Department of Social Medicine, Hadassah Medical Organization and The Hebrew University-Hadassah School of Public Health and Community Medicine, PO Box 1127, Jerusalem, Israel.

Michael Adler, MD, MRCP, FFCM
Professor of Genito-Urinary Medicine, Academic Department of Genito-Urinary Medicine, Middlesex Hospital Medical School, London W1, England.

M.R. Alderson, MD, FFCM
Chief Medical Statistician, Office of Population Censuses and Surveys, St Catherine's House, 10 Kingsway, London WC2B 6JP, England.

M. Ashley-Miller, MA, BM, BCh, D(Obst), RCOG, DPH, FFCM. Director of the Chief Scientist Office, Scottish Home and Health Department, St Andrew's House, Edinburgh EH1 3DE, Scotland.

Mildred Blaxter, MA
Research Fellow, School of Economics and Social Studies, University of East Anglia, Norwich NR4 7TJ, England.

A.P. Brown, BSc, MRCP (UK)
Head of Medical Department, National Radiological Protection Board, Chilton, Didcot, Oxford OX11 0RQ, England.

J.P. Bunker, MD
Director, Division of Health Services Research, Department of Family, Community and Preventive Medicine, Stanford University School of Medicine, CA 94305, USA.

M.L. Burr, MD, MFCM
Epidemiologist, MRC Epidemiology Unit (South Wales), 4 Richmond Road, Cardiff CF2 3AS, Wales.

Marion K. Cooney, PhD
Professor, Department of Pathobiology, University of Washington, Seattle, Washington 98195, USA.

Shan Cretin, PhD, MPH
Associate Professor, Division of Health Services, School of Public Health, University of California, Los Angeles, CA 90024, USA.

Raisa B. Deber, PhD
Associate Professor, Department of Health Administration, Community Health Division, Faculty of Medicine, University of Toronto, Toronto, Ontario, Canada M5S 1A8.

Roger Detels, MD, MS
Professor of Epidemiology and Dean, School of Public Health, Center for Health Sciences, University of California, Los Angeles, California 90024, USA.

M.F. Drummond, BSc, MCom, DPhil
Lecturer in Economics, Health Services Management Centre, University of Birmingham, 40 Edgbaston Park Road, Birmingham B15 2RT, England.

P.C. Elwood, MD
Director, MRC Epidemiology Unit (South Wales), 4 Richmond Road, Cardiff, CF2 3AS, Wales.

F.A. Fairweather, MD
Unilever Research, PO Box 68, Unilever House, Blackfriars, London EC4, England.

John W. Farquhar, MD
Professor of Medicine and Director, Stanford Heart Disease Prevention Program, Stanford University, CA 94305, USA.

Manning Feinleib, MD, DrPh
Director, National Center for Health Statistics, Department of Health and Human Services, Center Building, Room 2-19, 3700 East–West Highway, Hyattsville, MD 20782, USA.

J. Fowles, PhD
Research Associate, Division of Health Services Research, Department of Family, Community and Preventive Medicine, Stanford University School of Medicine, CA 94305, USA.

Michael B. Gregg, MD
Deputy Director for Communications Epidemiology Program Office Centers for Disease Control, Atlanta, GA 30333, USA.

Raymond S. Greenberg, MD, PhD
Assistant Professor, Departments of Community Health and Biometry, Emory University School of Medicine, Atlanta, GA 30322, USA.

Michel A. Ibrahim, MD, PhD
Dean, School of Public Health, University of North Carolina, Chapel Hill, NC 27514, USA.

William H.W. Inman, FRCP, FFCM
Director, Drug Surveillance Research Unit, University of Southampton, North Croft House, Winchester Road, Botley, Hampshire SO3 2BX, England.

George E. Kenny, PhD
Professor and Chairman, Department of Pathobiology, University of Washington, Seattle, WA 98195, USA.

Donald A.B. Lindberg, MD
Director, Information Science Group, and Professor of Pathology, University of Missouri School of Medicine, Columbia, Missouri 65211, USA.

Nathan Maccoby, PhD
Janet M Peck Professor of International Communication Emeritus (Active) and Co-Principal Investigator of

Community Studies, Stanford Heart Disease Prevention Program, Stanford University, CA 94305, USA.

**J.M. McGinnis, MD, MA, MPP**
Deputy Assistant Secretary for Health and Director, US Office of Disease Prevention and Health Promotion, Department of Health and Human Services, Washington DC 20201, USA.

**Robert J. Maxwell, PhD**
Secretary, King Edward's Hospital Fund for London, London, England.

**David C. Morrell**
Department of General Practice, St Thomas's Hospital Medical School, United Medical and Dental Schools, London SE1 7EH, England.

**Jay Moskowitz, PhD**
Associated Director for Scientific Program Operation, National Heart, Lung, and Blood Institute, Bethesda Md 20205, USA.

**Donald L. Patrick, PhD, MSPH**
Associate Professor, Department of Social and Administrative Medicine and Department of Epidemiology, University of North Carolina, Chapel Hill, NC 27514, USA.

**Nancy D. Pearce**
Statistician, Office of Program Planning Evaluation and Co-ordination, National Center for Health Statistics, United States Public Health Service, Hyattsville, Md 20782, USA.

**Pekka Puska, MD**
Professor and Director, Department of Epidemiology, National Public Health Institute, Mannerheimintie 166, 00280 Helsinki 28, Finland.

**J.A. Reissland, BSc, PhD [deceased]**
Head, Physics Department, National Radiological Protection Board, Chilton Didcot, Oxfordshire OX11 0RG, England.

**Dorothy P. Rice, BA DSc(Hon)**
Professor, Ageing Health Policy Center, University of California, San Francisco, CA 90024, USA.

**David M. Robinson, PhD**
Senior Scientific Advisor, National Heart, Lung, and Blood Institute, Bethesda, MD 20205, USA.

**L.L. Roos, PhD**
Professor, Departments of Business Administration and of Social and Preventive Medicine, University of Manitoba, Winnipeg, Manitoba, Canada.

**N.P. Roos, PhD**
Professor, Departments of Social and Preventive Medicine and of Business Administration, University of Manitoba, Winnipeg, Manitoba, Canada.

**A.H. Snaith, MD, FRCPath, DPH, FFCM**
Honorary Consultant, Bristol and Weston Health Authority, Greyfriars, Lewin's Mead, Bristol BS1 2EE, England.

**A.V. Swan**
Deputy Director, Social Medicine and Health Services Research Unit, and Senior Lecturer in Statistics, Department of Community Medicine, St. Thomas's Hospital Medical School (United Medical and Dental Schools), London SE1 7EH, England.

**Paul R. Torrens, MD, MPH**
Professor of Health Services Administration, School of Public Health, University of California, Los Angeles CA, USA.

**M.G.R. Varma, PhD, DrSc, FIBiol**
Professor of Medical Entomology, London School of Hygiene and Tropical Medicine, Gower Street, London WC1E 7HT, England.

**Eugene Vayda, MD, FRCP(C), FACP, FACPM**
Associate Dean, Community Health, and Professor, Departments of Health Administration and of Medicine, Faculty of Medicine, University of Toronto, Toronto, Ontario, Canada M5S 1A8.

**M. van der Venne, DrSc**
Principal Administrator, Commission of the European Communities, L 2920, Luxembourg.

**Robert E. Waller, BSc**
Toxicology and Environmental Protection, Department of Health and Social Security, Hannibal House, Elephant and Castle, London SE1 6TE, England.

**Sir Andrew Watt-Kay, MD, DSc, ChM, FRSE**
Emeritus Professor of Surgery, University of Glasgow and from 1973–81 Chief Scientist, Scottish Home and Health Department, St Andrew's House, Edinburgh EH1 3DE, Scotland.

**H.E. Webb, DM, FRCP**
Consultant Physician, Department of Neurology, and Director, Neurovirology Unit, Rayne Institute, St Thomas' Hospital, London SE1 7EH, England.

**Peter D. Wood, DSc**
Professor of Medicine (Research), and Deputy Director, Stanford Heart Disease Prevention Program, Stanford University, CA 94305, USA.

# Abbreviations

| | | | |
|---|---|---|---|
| ABS | Chromosome abnormalities | DES | Diethylstilbesterol |
| ADAMHA | Alcohol, Drug Abuse, and Mental Health Administration | DHA | District Health Authority |
| | | DHC | District Health Council |
| ADE | Antibody-dependent enhancement | DHEW | Department of Health, Education, and Welfare |
| ADM | Assistant Deputy Minister | | |
| ADR | Adverse drug reaction | DHHS | Department of Health and Human Services |
| AFP | Alpha-fetoprotein | DHSS | Department of Health and Social Security |
| AHA | Area Health Authority | DIMDI | Deutsches Institut fur Medizinische Dekumentation und Information |
| AIDS | Acquired immune deficiency syndrome | | |
| ALI | Annual limit on intake | DMT | District Medical Team |
| ALT | Alanine aminotransferase | DNA | Deoxyribonucleic acid |
| AMA | American Medical Association | DOD | Department of Defence |
| AMO | Area medical officer | DRG | Division of Research Grants, National Institutes of Health |
| ARAMIS | American Rheumatology Association Medical Information System | | |
| | | DSRU | Drug Surveillance Research Unit, Southampton University |
| ARP | Attributable risk population | | |
| BCG | Bacillus Calmette—Geurin | EB virus | Epstein–Barr virus |
| BEIR | Committee on Biological Effects of Low Levels of Ionizing Radiation | ECHO virus | Enteric cytopathic human orphan virus |
| | | EDTA | European Dialysis and Transplantation Association |
| BL | Blood lead | | |
| BMA | British Medical Association | ELISA | Enzyme-linked immunosorbent assay |
| BOND | Business-Oriented New Development Plan | EPA | Environmental Protection Agency |
| BSI | British Standards Institute | EPH | Elderly person's housing |
| CAT | Computerized axial tomography | ERL | Emergency reference level |
| CCPDS | Centralized Cancer Patient Data System | FDA | Food and Drug Administration |
| CDC | Centers for Disease Control | FEP | Free erythrocyte protoporphyrin |
| CDSC | Communicable Disease Surveillance Centre | FES | Food Expenditure Survey |
| CF | Complement fixation | FEV | Forced expiratory volume in one second |
| CHAD | Community Syndrome of Hypertension, Atherosclerosis, and Diabetes Study | FPC | Family Practitioner Committee |
| | | FVC | Forced vital capacity |
| CHD | Coronary heart disease | GHS | General Household Survey |
| CI | Confidence interval | GMENAC | Graduate Medical Education National Advisory Committee |
| CMV | Cytomegalovirus | | |
| CNS | Central nervous system | GNP | Gross National Product |
| COHb | Carboxyhaemoglobin | GP | General Practitioner |
| CPI | Consumer Price Index | GRO | General Registers Office |
| CPM | Critical path method | GSD | Genetically significant dose |
| CSD | Committee on Safety of Drugs | HAA | Hospital Activity Analysis |
| CSM | Committee on Safety of Medicines | Hb | Haemoglobin |
| CSO | Chief Scientist Organization | HCFA | Health Care Financing Administration |
| CUPE | Canadian Union of Public Employees | HDFP | Hypertension Detection and Follow-up Program |
| DAC | Derived air concentration | | |
| DAWN | Drug Abuse Warning Network | HDS | Hospital Discharge Service |
| DDST | Denver Developmental Screening Test | HES | Health Examination Survey |

| | |
|---|---|
| HI | Haemagglutination inhibition |
| HIPE | Hospital In-patient Enquiry |
| HPF | High powered field |
| HRA | Health Resources Administration |
| HRSA | Health Resources and Services Administration |
| HSA | Health Services Administration |
| HSC | Health and Safety Committee |
| ICAS | International Computer Access Service |
| ICD | International Classification of Diseases |
| ICHPCC | International Classifiation of Health Problems in Primary Care |
| ICRP | International Commission on Radiological Protection |
| IEA | International Epidemiological Association |
| IEC | International Electronics Commission |
| IFAT | Indirect fluorescent antibody test |
| IHCE | Institute for Health Care Evaluation |
| IM | Infectious mononucleosis |
| INH | Isoniazid |
| IPS | International Passenger Survey |
| IQ | Intelligence quotient |
| ISO | International Standards Office |
| JICST | Japanese Information Center of Science and Technology |
| $LD_{50}$ | Median lethal dose |
| LET | Linear energy transfer |
| MBA | Master of Business Administration |
| MHE | Mental Health Enquiry |
| MI | Myocardial infarction |
| MOEH | Medical Officer of Environmental Health |
| MOH | Medical Officer of Health |
| MPH | Master of Public Health |
| MRC | Medical Research Council |
| MS | Mean square |
| MYR | Man years at risk |
| NAMCS | National Ambulatory Care Survey |
| NANB | Non-A, Non-B hepatitis virus |
| NAS | National Academy of Science |
| NCHCT | National Center for Health Care Technology |
| NCHS | National Center for Health Statistics |
| NCI | National Cancer Institute |
| NCP | National Cancer Programme |
| NDP | Canadian New Democratic Party |
| NEISS | National Electronic Injuries Survey |
| NGU | Non-gonococcal urethritis |
| NHANES | National Health and Nutritional Examination Survey |
| NHBPERP | National High Blood Pressure Education Research Program |
| NHDS | National Hospital Discharge Survey |
| NHI | National Heart Institute |
| NHIS | National Health Interview Survey |
| NHLBI | National Heart, Lung, and Blood Institute |
| NHS | National Health Service |
| NHSCR | National Health Service Central Register |
| NIDA | National Institute of Drug Abuse |
| NIH | National Institutes of Health |
| NIL | Noise immission level |
| NINCDS | National Institute of Neurological and Communicative Disorders and Strokes |
| NIOSH | National Institute of Occupational Safety and Health |
| NLM | National Library of Medicine |
| NMCUES | National Medical Care Utilization and Expenditure Survey |
| NMFI | National Master Facility Inventory |
| NNHS | National Nursing Home Survey |
| NRPB | National Radiological Protection Board |
| NSAI | Non-steroidal anti-inflammatory agent |
| NSF | National Science Foundation |
| NSU | Non-specific urethritis |
| OC | Oral contraceptive |
| OECD | Organization for Economic Co-operation and Development |
| OHA | Ontario Hospital Association |
| OHIP | Ontario Health Insurance Plan |
| OPCS | Office of Population Censuses and Surveys |
| OR | Odds ratio |
| OSHA | Occupational Safety and Health Association |
| PAH | Polynuclear aromatic hydrocarbons |
| PAHO | Pan American Health Organization |
| PAN | Peroxyacetylnitrate |
| PARP | Population attributable risk proportion |
| PC | Canadian Progressive Conservative Party |
| PCB | Polychlorinated biphenyl |
| PEFR | Peak expiratory flow rate |
| PEM | Prescription event monitoring |
| PERT | Program evaluation and review technique |
| PHLS | Public Health Laboratory Service |
| PHS | Public Health Service |
| PID | Pelvic inflammatory disease |
| PMS | Post-marketing surveillance |
| PPA | Prescription Pricing Authority |
| PRNT | Plaque reduction neutralization test |
| PSRO | Professional Standards Review Organization |
| RADS | Retrospective assessment of drug safety |
| RAWP | Resource Allocation Working Party |
| RCGP | Royal College of General Practitioners |
| RCP | Royal College of Practitioners |
| RCT | Randomized controlled trial |
| RHA | Regional Health Authority |
| RLF | Retrolental fibroplasia |
| RMS | Root mean squares |
| RNA | Ribonucleic acid |
| RR | Relative risk |

| SAQC | Statistical Analysis and Quality Control Center |
| SAS | Statistical Analysis System |
| SBP | Systolic blood pressure |
| sd | Standard deviation |
| se | Standard error |
| SEER | Surveillance, Epidemiology and End Result Program |
| SMON | Subacute myelo-optic neuropathy |
| SMR | Standardized mortality ratio |
| STD | Sexually transmitted disease |
| TRIMIS | TriService Medical Information System |
| TSP | Total suspended particulates |
| UHDDS | Uniform Hospital Discharge Data Set |
| UNSCEAR | United Nations Scientific Committee on the Effects of Atomic Radiation |
| UTI | Urinary tract infection |
| VA | Veterans Administration |
| WHO | World Health Organization |

# Introduction

George Knox

## THE NATURE OF PUBLIC HEALTH INVESTIGATION

Analogies between investigations of the health of individuals, and of populations, have many times been drawn. As in clinical medicine, a public health practitioner can become involved in such investigations through the demands of an acute episode (for example, an epidemic of food poisoning) or through attention having been drawn to a more insidious or chronic problem (for example, a high case fatality from breast cancer, or a rise in perinatal mortality among mature infants). Alternatively, a proactive as opposed to reactive role may be adopted with the public health practitioner seeking out problems on his own initiative. An example might be the potential threat of a declining acceptance rate for pertussis vaccine, or a rising proportion of smokers among pregnant women.

In each case the parallels with normal clinical practice are clear, and they extend to the public health practitioner's subsequent executive behaviour regarding 'investigation' and 'treatment'. Thus, once the problem has been identified, he will undertake a series of goal-directed special enquiries leading to the administrative and planning analogies of diagnosis, prognosis, explanation, advice, and treatment.

These analogies and parallels carry the appeal of a respectable professional image, and conform with the traditions of orthodox professional practice. They are courted at least as much for this reason as for any practical utility. But, although we can continue to accept and even promote them, it may be more valuable in the pragmatic field of public health investigation, to pay more attention to the differences rather than to the similarities between clinical and public health practice.

## TECHNICAL SUPPORT SYSTEMS

The first of the differences between clinical and public health investigation relates to the kinds of technical support system appropriate to each. The great burden of clinical medicine springs from complaints generated by patients who are either already ill or believe themselves to be ill, and the approach expected of the practitioner is therapeutic—that is, curing and caring. In so far as physical treatment is necessary or useful, the practitioner's problem is to modify the internal environment in a manner which will retard or arrest the disease process, or ameliorate its effects. His diagnosis is therefore pathological (including biochemical,

microbiological, and other aspects), and the necessary investigations relate the patient's internal pathological processes. They depend upon the well-developed resources of the clinical investigative departments to be found in any major hospital. The support staff are either medical or laboratory scientists, in turn supported by laboratory technicians, and the whole system serves the unambiguous priority of one professional group.

The technical support systems appropriate to public health investigation are of quite a different nature. They are concerned with processes taking place outside the individual. They include the mechanics of transmission of infectious organisms from one person to another, directly or through intermediate stages, the exposure of people to physical and chemical hazards and the effects of protective procedures: also human responses to social, economic, educational, and work environments, as well as to health education activities. They are concerned in addition with the social and administrative services and processes which bring medical, nursing, and other health services into effective contact with those in need of them.

The investigation of these problems is conducted only in part by doctors and laboratory scientists. The others involved include statisticians, information scientists and computer staff, sociologists, economists, educationists and health educationists, systems analysts, operational research scientists, and management scientists. They also include a range of technical and engineering experts competent in the maintenance of wholesome food, water, and air, and in the protection of the population from the ill effects of noise, radiation, the harmful effects of drugs, inadequate housing, and a wide range of social hazards. The professional identifications of these scientists, engineers, and technicians are not uniquely related to medicine, and many are employed in organizations with indirect or partial responsibilities for health matters. The tight hierarchical structure of the hospitals does not exist and there may be little unified control of staffing, standards, or investment. Joint operations and investigations must be conducted from a basis of professional consensus and agreement, rather than a basis of requisition.

It is an open question whether a dispersed and informally organized investigative resource such as this is more or less effective than a more closely controlled arrangement, and it is not our purpose to discuss this point here. It would however be foolish not to recognize the *de facto* social and professional differences, as well as the technical differences, between the clinical and public health investigative processes.

### Data acquisition and data analysis

The professional autonomies and specializations described above have led, *inter alia*, to a substantial division between data processing and analysis on the one hand, together with health service management and activity information, and the acquisition of information relating to the health of the population, on the other. These divisions are reflected in the headings and sub-headings which we employ in this volume, and our first section is concerned entirely with information systems. It attempts to display both the complexity of the arrangements which have evolved in different countries, and to describe the interactions between the evolution of this complexity, and the advent and development of computer-based processing. Our second section describes in more detail a range of analytical approaches usually associated with the discipline of epidemiology. Our third section describes or exemplifies the contributions to public health of several other professional disciplines.

In the fourth section we describe field investigations concerned with the control of biological, physical, and chemical hazards. These monitoring and data acquisition processes constitute the traditional materials of public health practice. Although they have perhaps been overshadowed in recent years by the growth of those information and scientific processes which have become necessary for the provision and maintenance of comprehensive health care services, their crucial importance remains. Indeed, as our contributors show, improvements in expected and accepted standards of health, combined with technical developments in monitoring and in the theory and practice of defending people from such exposures, are generating renewed momentum in these fields.

### THE MODEL BASES OF PUBLIC HEALTH

The overwhelming concern of the clinical practitioner with the control of the *milieu interieure* has over the years generated a vast range of pathological models. They provide the chief theoretical basis of clinical practice. In so far as they describe the 'causes' of disease, they do so in the sense of describing the mechanisms by which underlying processes produce the clinical phenomena of illness. In other words, the clinician's concern with cause is in the sense of 'pathogenesis'. Although clinicians will nowadays often rely upon empirically investigated measures of the efficacy of therapies, in the majority of their day-to-day decisions they probably rely chiefly upon this pathological, biochemical, or pharmacological theory which has accumulated over the years. It is for this reason that its study constitutes so large a part of the scientific training of doctors.

By contrast, the public health practitioner is concerned more with causes which *precede* illness, and his concern to control them stems from his traditional prior concern with prevention, rather than with treatment. In so far as he relies upon a knowledge of causal processes in the pursuit of these aims, he is concerned with cause in the sense of 'aetiology'. He wishes to know what *precedes* the disease, and how the disease itself is determined by interruptable environmental processes. We have to admit, however, that the body of validated theory available to the public health practitioner is no where so detailed and pervasive as that available to the clinician.

Traditional public health practice was based to a very large extent upon a single causal model. It consisted of an invasive noxious agent—physical, chemical, or biological. Apart from the fact that many of these agents can now be identified, it did not differ in any substantial way from the model represented in the episode of the Gadarene swine. The idea was in the course of time modified by the identification of the noxious agents, and by expunging magical mechanisms of transfer, and more recently by the recognition and development of the notions of non-sufficiency and non-necessity. It was recognized that exposure to tuberculosis and inhalation of tuberculosis bacilli, was not a 'sufficient' cause of developing the disease, and that other events and circumstances combined to determine the outcome. It was also recognized that some disorders may be determined through alternative pathways, so that no *particular* nominated cause always (i.e. necessarily) precedes the disease. In death by firing squad, each bullet may be sufficient, but none individually is necessary! In many aetiological mechanisms it was recognized that the causes were neither necessary nor sufficient, and they were sometimes described as an 'agent–host–environment' interaction in which the causal pathway could best be represented as a network.

### Conceptual evolution

The notion of a causal network of (mainly) non-sufficient and non-necessary causes led to the introduction of 'probabilistic' ideas. The probability of a sequence of necessary events occurring was the product of their individual frequencies, while parallel/alternative causal streams were handled in an additive manner. These ideas had some value, but they were also unfortunately a source of muddle.

The centre of the problem was a confusion between predictive and causal models, and even a lack of appreciation that any specific choice of model was necessary for interpretating measurements of risk or of relative risk. The term 'risk-factor' is still often used without commitment as to whether it represents the strength of a prediction or the strength of a cause. The unfortunate consequence has been a dissociation between the relatively precise idea of 'cause', and the non-commital notions enshrined in 'contributory factor'. Thus, it is not infrequent to hear clinicians, and others concerned with health care at the individual level, deny that low birthweight is a cause of death or handicap, or that dietary patterns are a cause of colon cancer, or that cigarette smoking is a cause of ischaemic heart disease. predisposing factors, yes; but causes, no. And from this denial there follows an attitude of preventive nihlism.

A further limitation of traditional models springs from

their exclusive relevance to diseases which can be defined in qualitative pathological terms. The starting point of studies depending upon such models is a precise taxonomy. This produced an almost specific diversion of the public health approach away from those disorders which could not be so defined. They include psychiatric illnesses, behavioural deviances, and a wide range of disabilities which were definable more in the nature and degree of the impairment which they inflicted upon their owners (blindness, deafness, dementia, mental retardation, arthritis, back pain) rather than in specific pathological terms.

In the last two or three decades, however, we have seen the beginnings of a conceptual liberation, and an extension of the repertoire of models on which public health investigative approaches are based.

First, although effective epidemiological investigation continues to depend very largely upon effective taxonomies (e.g. the differentiation of senile dementia into atherosclerotic and Alzheimer's dementia), there has been a considerable growth of enquiries based upon quantitative models. An example would be the investigation of intelligence, scholastic attainment, physical growth, and emotional development among pre-school and school-children. Each can be expressed as a quantifiable attribute, with a range extending across the whole population. This frees the investigator from the need to define 'diseased' subclasses. He can, nevertheless, relate performance in these respects to the events and circumstances of pregnancy, of delivery, and of early nutritional, toxic, and infective exposures. He can propose and test the hypothesis that the two might be causally related.

Second, the vague notion of a genetic or familial 'predisposition', which was almost devoid of predictive or preventive value, is nowadays being replaced by the development and validation of more specific genetic models. In an earlier section, one contributor describes our improved understanding of immune processes and of their genetic determination (Chapter 3, Volume 1). The study of interactions between such processes, and environmental exposures of different kinds, is now one of the fastest growing points of medical science.

Third, the processes of disease diffusion are being quantified. The mathematical modelling of epidemic processes, is becoming progressively and usefully connected with the problems of real life. This is especially so in the fields of planning vaccination programmes, and predicting the consequences of alternative vaccination policies. Predicting the long-term consequences of chronic exposures to noxious agents with long and variable latent intervals, producing their effects in competition with other causes of illness and death, is also proving susceptible to the newer mathematical and computer simulation approaches.

Fourth, increasing application of the experimental approach, and in particular the technique of the randomized controlled trial, has sharpened up the notion of 'cause' wherever it has been applied. A cause, in this context, is anything which can be manipulated to alter the subsequent prevalence or incidence of a disease, or its consequential effects, or which might modify subsequent physiological or social performance. Thus, cigarette smoking can be seen quite starkly as a cause of perinatal death, so soon as it is demonstrated that mean birth weight and perinatal mortality rate, can be altered through specific health educational methods, or through specific social policy decisions (e.g. taxation).

A fifth major departure has been in the attention given to the behavioural elements of disease causation. Thus, it is not sufficient to say that smoking causes lung cancer; we have to look for more proximate causes, and to study the causes of smoking. We enter here into the provinces of advertising and commercial economics, of education, and of health education, of peer group pressures, addiction, and so on.

A sixth development has been the increased attention given in recent years to behavioural/environmental interactions determining the pattern of use of health services by sick people. These models are not purely behavioural, and include physical and operational elements. We develop this area below.

## Health services research

The investigation of health services, with the evaluation of their effectiveness, appropriateness, accessibility, resource requirements, costs, and benefits, can be seen as a direct extension of the host–agent–environmental model. In the case of iatrogenic disease, the service is seen as the agent. In the case of effective care or prevention, the service is seen as a modifying environment. The rapid growth of this area of research in recent years sprang from the recognition that the disparity between demand and supply of health care services was universal, and would probably be with us for ever. This would apply whatever the arrangements for the provision of resources, so that a choice of priorities and of alternative deployments would also be needed at the service-provision level, as indeed it is at the clinical level. Scientific investigation was necessary to guide these choices. As it developed, health services research came to demand investigative methods which differed in their technical emphases and organization, from those demanded by more traditional public health approaches.

First, there was an increased emphasis upon large data-acquisition systems, managed on a routine basis, with the aim of monitoring performance in continuing and quantitative terms, rather than necessarily addressed to answering qualitative biological questions.

Second, the design of investigations was more often problem-led, than dictated by the availability of data and of developed technique. More insistently than previously, an accommodation was necessary between operational relevance and timeliness, on the one hand, and scientific elegance on the other. Often, the work was so intimately linked with planning and policy processes, as to trouble the consciences of the scientific investigators. Problem-led is one thing; problem-dominated, to the extent of possibly influencing the results, is another. Epidemiologists have often felt uncomfortable with the notion of 'action research', in which the research process is indissolubly linked with the process of advocating and promoting change, in the manner formulated originally by Cherns. Sociologists are more familiar with these problems and necessities; but some epidemiologists have declined to be drawn into health services research, in any shape or form.

Third, 'evaluation' was recognized eventually to have at least two quite different meanings. The first depends upon measuring the performance of services which already exist. In the traditional scientific manner, analysis is based upon collected facts. The problem is that facts are grammatically and syntactically located in the past, while planners and policy-makers are concerned with the future. *Their* need is for prediction. So the second necessary type of evaluation relates to proposals for future services. Facts have no relevance in this process unless some kind of extrapolation can be made. Frequently, the extrapolation must be from one place to another, and from one circumstance to another (e.g. scientific enquiry to service application), as well as from one time to another. The construction and use of predictive and extrapolative models is a thoroughly respectable part of the scientific process, but it is not one which had been very much used in traditional public health contexts. Substantial new development was necessary. Furthermore, the theoretical and model building developments necessary for planning purposes, required a joint consideration of social, operational, and biological processes. The combination was novel. As a result, model-based predictive methods are only now beginning to find their proper place.

Fourth, as health services research developed, its threatening nature emerged. It was not simply that it threatened clinical autonomy, as any management-linked process must, but it also threatened traditional views that social policy and management decisions were the sole prerogative of senior people whose status in this respect was acquired through processes other than special training or special skill in population-investigative methods.

For all these reasons, health services research introduced

a new level of social, political, and technical complexity to the investigative processes associated with responsibilities for the public health. We have therefore included within this third volume a short section on applications and problems arising in this field and have tried to develop the notions of 'complexity' and of 'interactivity' as features with which we will have to contend, and whose nature we might as well begin to try to understand.

## TERMINOLOGY

It is necessary finally to comment upon terminology: and even upon spelling. Our contributors work in a variety of different cultures and we thought it inappropriate to pretend otherwise. The meanings of terms used by one, are not necessarily congruent with the meanings used by another. Terms such as efficiency, efficacy, and effectiveness are given different meanings in different working contexts. Operational research in the UK is operations research in the USA. Cohort study does not mean the same thing to one worker as it does to another. Incidence rate in one context is the same as attack rate in another. And so on.

We have tried, editorially, to ensure that meanings are clear within their contexts and there should be little risk of misunderstanding if a little care is taken.

International dictionaries have of course been constructed (J.M. Last, (1983). *A dictionary of epidemiology*) and have made contributions both towards uniformity and clarity, but we felt that in their present stage of evolution their main function was to supply a descriptive exposition of the manner in which terms were actually used, rather than to provide an authoritative statement of the manner in which they *should* be used. This balance will no doubt change as the processes of validation and consensus proceed, but we did not feel that we were yet at this stage.

# Information systems and routine monitoring

## Health information resources

# 1 Health information resources: United States – health and social factors

Nancy D. Pearce

## INTRODUCTION

This chapter reviews health information systems that provide data for routine monitoring of the health of the population of the US. Since it is possible to discuss only a few of the existing systems, the material in this chapter represents a sampling of the total universe of data systems. Several criteria were applied in the selection of the systems to be included. Each system must be: (i) national in coverage, or representative of the situation in the country as a whole; (ii) currently operational, although it may be periodic in its collection of data (e.g. conducted biennially rather than continuously); (iii) operated by either the federal government or the private sector; and (iv) produce primary data rather than a secondary compilation of data from other sources. Systems excluded are those that provide data for specific programmes, with the exception of the Medicare programme statistical system which has been included because it covers virtually the entire population age 65 years and older. Also excluded are those programmes that operate at the state level, provide data only for the state and some or all of its subdivisions, and important and highly useful compendia that contain highlights from a number of primary data sources. Examples of secondary data sources in the health area are the *Statistical Abstract of the United States,* published annually by the Bureau of the Census and *Health, United States,* the annual report to Congress from the Secretary of the Department of Health and Human Services, prepared annually by the National Center for Health Statistics and the National Center for Health Services Research.

To provide a framework for the organization of these diverse data sources, they are presented in three broad groupings: health status, including morbidity and mortality; health care resources and their utilization; and health economics. Placement of individual data sources in these categories is somewhat arbitrary, but every effort was made to ensure that the placement is as logical as possible. For example, while the National Health Interview Survey produces information on both the utilization and financing of health care services its primary purpose is provision of information on morbidity and so it is located in the section on health status.

The relative paucity of information on health care professionals is noteworthy. Numerous *ad hoc* studies have been conducted for several health occupations but they have typically been limited to the membership of a particular national professional organization and conducted on an irregular basis. Anyone interested in the most current data for any particular health occupation should contact the national professional association.

There are limited sources that meet the criteria for inclusion for health economics data because most health economics studies use secondary data, involve secondary analysis of data from various sources, or are based on 'single-time' studies.

For each data system the material is typically divided into two sections. The first section describes the purpose and scope of the system; the second section provides an overview of the data collection procedures and data items. At the end of each description a reference is given to one or two sources for additional information about each system. The references also frequently identify other data collection programmes of the respective organizations.

## HEALTH STATUS

### National morbidity and mortality reporting systems

*Purpose and scope*

The Centers for Disease Control (CDC) maintain national surveillance programmes for selected diseases, with the co-operation of state and local health departments. Over the years the surveillance systems maintained by these centres have expanded, and emphasis has shifted as certain diseases have lower incidence rates and other diseases have taken on new aspects. The data are used to identify outbreaks of communicable diseases and to monitor trends in those diseases.

In 1878 an act of Congress authorized the collection of morbidity reports by the Public Health Service for use in connection with quarantine measures against pestilential diseases such as cholera, smallpox, plague, and yellow fever. The following year a specific appropriation was made for the collection and publication of reports of notifiable disease, principally from foreign ports; in 1893 an act provided for the collection each week from state and municipal authorities throughout the US. To secure uniformity for the registration of these morbidity statistics Congress enacted a law in 1902 directing the Surgeon General of the Public Health Service to provide forms for the collection, compilation, and publication of such data.

*Data collection procedures and data items*

Reports on notifiable diseases were received from very few states and cities prior to 1900, but gradually more states submitted monthly and annual summaries. In 1913 the state and territorial health authorities recommended weekly tele-graphic reporting by states for a few diseases, but it was not until after 1925 that all states reported regularly. In 1950 the Association of State and Territorial Health Officers author-ized a Conference of State and Territorial Epidemiologists, for the purpose of determining the diseases that should be reported by the states to the Public Health Service. Following approval of the list of diseases by the Association of State and Territorial Health Officers the first manual on reporting procedures was issued; since then recommendations and revisions made by this conference have been incorporated into the *Manual of Procedures for National Morbidity Reporting and Surveillance of Communicable Diseases.*

The following notifiable diseases have been agreed upon by the state and territorial epidemiologists and approved by state and territorial health departments: anthrax, aseptic meningitis, botulism, brucellosis, chickenpox, diphtheria, encephalitis, hepatitis, leprosy, leptospirosis, malaria, measles (rubeola), meningococcal infections, mumps, pertussis, poliomyelitis, psittacosis-ornithosis, rabies in animals and in man, rubella (German measles), rubella congenital syndrome, tetanus, trichinosis, tuberculosis, tularemia, typhoid fever, typhus, and venereal diseases. Physicians report cases of these diseases to their local city, county, or state health departments. Although notification of a case of one of the quarantinable diseases may have been made by telephone to CDC, each case of cholera, plague, smallpox, and yellow fever is reported by the state epidemiologist to CDC in the weekly morbidity report.

Completeness of reporting varies greatly, since not all cases receive medical care and not all treated conditions are reported by physicians. Thus, the data should be interpreted with caution. Some diseases, such as plague and rabies, that cause severe clinical illness and are associated with serious consequences are probably reported quite accurately. How-ever, diseases such as salmonellosis and mumps that are clinically mild and infrequently associated with serious conse-quences are less likely to be reported. Estimates of under-reporting were made several years ago by CDC for two diseases – measles and viral hepatitits. At that time, prior to the institution of the Measles Elimination Program in 1978, it was generally accepted that about 10–15 per cent of all cases of measles and about 15–20 per cent of all cases of viral hep-atitis occurring in the US were reported to CDC. The degree of completeness of reporting is also influenced by the diag-nostic facilities available, the control measures in effect, and the interests and priorities of state and local officials respon-sible for disease control and surveillance. Finally, factors such as the introduction of new diagnostic tests (e.g. for hepa-titis B) and the discovery of new disease entities (e.g. infant botulism and legionellosis) may cause changes in disease reporting independent of the true incidence of disease.

In addition to the weekly report of notifiable diseases, a weekly mortality report is made to CDC by City Health Officers or Vital Statistics Registrars from 121 major cities.

This report is in the form of a table in which total deaths by age categories are cross-classified by number of deaths assigned to pneumonia and influenza. An annual summary of the reported incidence of each listed nationally notifiable disease is also submitted by each State and Territorial Health Department to CDC for the previous calendar year.

Reference: Centers for Disease Control (Weekly).

## Drug Abuse Warning Network

*Purpose and scope*

The Drug Abuse Warning Network (DAWN) is operated by the National Institute on Drug Abuse (NIDA) to monitor drug abuse trends and patterns, identify licit and illicit drugs and new substances associated with drug abuse morbidity and mortality, and provide data for national, state and local drug abuse policy and programme planning. DAWN was initiated in 1972 by the Drug Enforcement Administration under authori-zation of the Comprehensive Drug Abuse Prevention and Controlled Substance Act of 1970. Responsibility for the system was transferred to NIDA in 1981.

*Data collection procedures and data items*

DAWN collects drug abuse information from panels of hospital emergency rooms and medical examiners located primarily in 26 metropolitan statistical areas throughout the continental US. The areas selected were those for which the most valuable information could be obtained to meet the objectives of the system. Geographical location was also taken into consideration to maintain representative regional coverage across the country. Abuse information is also col-lected from a randomly selected sample of emergency rooms drawn from the remaining emergency room population segment outside these 26 areas, but data are not collected from medical examiners outside the selected areas.

Separate forms are completed by emergency rooms and by medical examiners. The data items collected concern specific drugs being abused, the magnitude of the abuse, abuse problems unique to certain specific geographical areas, the source of the abused substance, the form (for example, tablet, capsule, powder) of the abused substance, and the age, race, sex, and employment status of abusers. No patient identifiers or names are ever transcribed on DAWN data-collection forms. Data-collection forms are completed for all drug related events.

Eligible emergency rooms are defined as those which are open 24 hours a day, located in non-federal, short-stay general hospitals, and which have at least 1000 patient visits to the emergency room per year; eligibility is determined primarily from information in the American Hospital Association's *Guide to the Health Care Field*, and is updated with each new annual edition. All medical examiners in the 26 metropolitan statistical areas are considered eligible for participation; infor-mation on medical examiners is compiled from medical-professional society organization membership lists and other available sources.

Reference: National Institute on Drug Abuse (Quarterly).

## National Health Interview Survey

### Purpose and scope

The National Health Interview Survey (NHIS) conducted by the National Center for Health Statistics (NCHS) is a principal source of information on the health of the population of the US. The survey was initiated in July 1957 in response to the National Health Survey Act of 1956 which provided for a continuing survey and special studies to secure on a voluntary basis accurate and current statistical information on the amount, distribution, and effects of illness and disability in the US and the services rendered for or because of such conditions.

The purpose of the survey is to provide national data on the incidence of acute illness and accidental injuries, the prevalence of chronic conditions and impairments, the extent of disability, the utilization of health care services, and other health-related topics. Data collected over the period of a year form the basis for the development of annual estimates of the health characteristics of the population and for the analysis of trends in those characteristics.

The survey covers the non-institutionalized, civilian population of the US living at the time of the interview. Persons excluded are: patients in long-term care facilities (data are obtained on patients in some of these facilities through the National Nursing Home Survey conducted by the NCHS); persons on active duty with the Armed Forces (though their dependants are included); US nationals living in foreign countries; and persons who have died during the calendar year preceding interview.

### Data collection procedures and data items

NHIS is a cross-sectional household interview survey which consists of continuous sampling and interviewing of the population. The sampling plan follows a multistage probability design which yields national estimates, although some estimates are obtained for the four geographical regions. Currently, the first stage consists of a sample of 376 primary sampling units drawn from approximately 1900 geographically defined primary sampling units that cover the 50 states and the District of Columbia. A primary sampling unit consists of a county, a small group of contiguous counties, or a metropolitan statistical area; within primary sampling units, smaller units called segments are defined in such a manner that each segment contains an expected four households.

Households selected for interview each week are a probability sample representative of the target population. Each calendar year, data are collected from approximately 40 000 households including about 110 000 persons. The annual response rate is usually at least 95 per cent of the eligible households in the sample; the 5 per cent who do not respond is divided equally between refusals and households where no eligible respondent could be found at home after repeated calls.

Data are collected through a personal household interview conducted by interviewers employed and trained by the Bureau of the Census according to procedures specified by NCHS. All adult members of the household 17 years of age and older who are at home at the time of the interview are invited to participate and to respond for themselves; the mother is usually the respondent for children. For individuals not at home during the interview, information is provided by a responsible adult family member (age 19 years or older) residing in the household. On some occasions, a random subsample of adult household members is selected to respond to questions on selected topics. Follow-up supplements are sometimes completed for either the entire household or for individuals identified as having particular health problems. As required, these supplements are either left for the appropriate person to complete and return by mail, or the interviewer calls again in person or by telephone to secure the information directly.

On average, the interviews require about 45 minutes in the household. The questionnaire consists of two basic parts: (i) a 'core' set of health, socio-economic, and demographic items; and (ii) one or more sets of 'supplementary' health items. The core items constitute approximately 70 per cent of the questionnaire and are repeated each year. The arrangement of core items complemented by rotating as well as single-time supplements allows the survey to respond to changing needs for data and to cover a wider variety of topics, while providing continuous information on fundamental topics.

The questionnaire includes the following types of 'core' questions: the basic demographic characteristics of household members, including age, sex, race, education, and family income; disability days, including restricted activity and bed days, and work- and school-loss days occurring during the two-week period prior to the week of interview; the physician visits occurring during the same two-week period; the acute and chronic conditions responsible for these days and visits; long-term limitation of activity resulting from chronic disease or impairment and the chronic conditions associated with the disability; short-stay hospitalization data, including the number of persons with hospital episodes during the past year and the number of discharges from short-stay hospitals; and the interval since the last visit by a doctor. The questionnaire also includes six lists of chronic conditions; each concentrates on a group of chronic conditions involving a specific system of the body (e.g. digestive, circulatory, respiratory).

Supplements to the questionnaire change in response to current interest in special health topics. For example, throughout 1981 a child health supplement was included, and in 1982 there were supplements on health insurance coverage and on use of selected preventive care services.

Suggestions and requests for special supplements are solicited and received from many sources, including university-based researchers, administrators of national organizations and programmes in the private and public health sectors, and other parts of the Department of Health and Human Services. A lead time of at least one year is required to develop and pretest questions for new topics to be included as special supplements.

References: National Center for Health Statistics (1981 *a,b*).

## NATIONAL HEALTH AND NUTRITION EXAMINATION SURVEY

### Purpose and scope

The first National Health and Nutrition Examination Survey,

referred to as the NHANES I, was initiated by the NCHS in 1970, with data collection beginning in April 1971. NHANES I was a modification and expansion of the earlier Health Examination Survey (HES) which had been initiated a decade earlier and had carried out three separate programmes. The restructuring and modification of the HES reflected the assignment to the NCHS of an additional specific responsibility – the measurement of the nutritional status of the population and the subsequent monitoring of changes in that status over time. A second National Health and Nutrition Examination Survey (NHANES II) began in February 1976 and ended in February 1980.

NHANES is designed to collect data which can be obtained best, or only, by direct physical examination, clinical and laboratory tests, and related measurement procedures. This information is of two kinds: (i) prevalence data for specifically defined diseases or conditions of ill health; and (ii) normative health-related measurement data which show distributions of the total population with respect to particular parameters such as blood pressure, visual acuity, or serum cholesterol level.

Successive surveys in the HES and NHANES programmes have been directed to different segments of the population and have had different sets of target conditions. The first HES 'cycle' involved examining a sample of adults with the focus primarily on selected chronic diseases. The second and third cycles of the HES were directed respectively to children between the ages of 6 and 11 years and youths between the ages of 12 and 17 years; both of these surveys emphasized growth and development data and sensory defects. The nutrition component of the first NHANES programme was directed to a probability sample of the broad age range 1–74 years, while the detailed health examination component focused on the population between ages 25 and 74 years. NHANES II was again directed to a broad population aged 6 months to 74 years, and the nutritional data collected will be used in conjunction with the earlier NHANES I data to monitor changes in nutritional status over time. A special health and nutrition examination survey directed to persons in families having one or more members of Hispanic origin or descent who live in areas with a high concentration of Hispanics was conducted in 1983 and 1984.

### Data collection procedures and data items

The samples for all of the HES and NHANES programmes have been multistage, highly clustered probability samples, stratified by broad geographical region and by population density grouping. Within strata the sampling stages employed have been the primary sampling unit, the census enumeration district, the segment, the household, and lastly the individual person. Until the household stage is reached, all sampling is carried out centrally.

The final stage of the sampling is conducted in the field in the particular chosen area. It involves interviewer visits and questionnaire completion at each one of the selected households, with the final selection of individuals included in the sample being dependent upon information elicited by the household interview questionnaire. The size of the sample in the survey programme has varied. In each of the three HES programmes the sample size was approximately 7500 persons.

In NHANES I the sample selected for the major nutrition components of the examination contained approximately 28 000 persons, of whom 21 000 were examined. A comparable sized sample for NHANES II again yielded approximately 21 000 examined persons.

Data collection teams consist of specially trained interviewers and examiners including physicians, nurses, dentists, dietitians, and medical, laboratory, and X-ray technicians. The examinations take place in the survey's specially constructed mobile examination centres, each consisting of three truck-drawn trailers which are interconnected and which provide a standardized environment and equipment for the performance of specific parts of the examination. This standardized environment is necessary, for example, for such components of the examination as audiometry, which requires hearing chambers within which the ambient noise level conforms to the American Speech Association standards for accoustical measurements.

The general pattern of data collection has meant that each survey has been conducted over a period of three or four years. This is due to the constraints which limit the number of persons examined in a given time span (e.g. the number of field teams and the number of sample areas). This imposes a limitation on the kinds of data to be collected by this mechanism, since conditions which might show marked year-to-year variation or seasonal patterns cannot be included. However, many important chronic diseases and health-related measurements are not subject to such changes in prevalence within short-run periods.

In the HES and NHANES programmes there has been and continues to be much attention devoted to the question of the response rate, which is the proportion of sample persons who are actually examined. Both NHANES programmes succeeded in obtaining household interview data on about 99 per cent of the sample population. More detailed health data appear in the medical history questionnaires; these were completed for 88 per cent of the selected sample persons in NHANES I and for 91 per cent of the selected sample persons in NHANES II. In NHANES I, 74 per cent of the sample persons selected for the nutrition component and 70 per cent of the persons for the detailed health component were given the standard examinations and tests; in NHANES II the overall response rate for the examination component was 73 per cent. There is considerable ancillary information on most of the non-examined persons in the sample population, and it is possible to make use of that data in the process of imputation and analysis of non-response bias. There is, moreover, some evidence that data obtained through examinations, tests, and measurements such as used in these surveys are less susceptible to potential bias from a given rate of non-response than data provided by the individuals themselves.

The kinds of information collected in the NHANES and other examination surveys are so varied and extensive that they are only illustrated here. With respect to nutrition, four types of data are included: (i) information concerning dietary intake – the mechanisms used have included 24-hour recall interviews and food frequency questionnaires, both administered by an interviewer who is a trained dietitian; (ii) haematological and biochemical tests – a sizeable battery of such tests has been performed, with processing at the mobile examination centres where necessary, but for the most part at a central nutrition laboratory established at CDC; (iii) body measurements – the battery used is especially important in connection with infants, children, and youths where growth may be affected by nutritional deficiencies; and (iv) various signs of high risk of nutritional deficiency, based on clinical examinations.

The health component of the NHANES programme includes detailed examinations, tests, and questionnaires, which have been developed to obtain a measure of prevalence levels of specific diseases and conditions. These vary with the particular programme and have included such conditions as chronic rheumatoid arthritis and hypertensive heart disease. Important normative health-related measurements, such as height, weight, and blood pressure are also obtained.

References: National Center for Health Statistics (1981 *a,b*).

## National Electronic Injury Surveillance System

### Purpose and scope

The Consumer Product Safety Commission, an independent regulatory agency established under the Consumer Product Safety Act of 1972 and activated in May 1973, is responsible to protect the public against unreasonable risk of injury or illness associated with consumer products, to assist consumers in evaluating the comparative safety of consumer products, to develop uniform safety standards for consumer products and to minimize conflicting state and local regulations, and to promote research and investigation into causes and prevention of product-related deaths, illnesses, and injuries. While the Commission relies on a number of sources to meet its data needs, its primary source of injury data is the National Electronic Injury Surveillance System (NEISS) which became operational in 1972 under the auspices of the Bureau of Product Safety of the Food and Drug Administration, which became the nucleus of the Consumer Product Safety Comision.

### Data collection procedures and data items

NEISS operates at two levels and is designed and maintained as an intelligence-gathering system which provides decision-making data. The first level of the system, surveillance, is comprised of 74 hospital emergency rooms, a statistical sample representative of all 50 states and US territories. The sample design is composed of five strata, four based on hospital size, as measured by the annual number of emergency room visits, and a fifth stratum including those hospitals with some type of specialized burn-care unit. In order to ensure reasonable geographic distribution in the selection process, the hospitals were order by zip code within each stratum of the hospital frame.

Each hospital participating in the system is expected to report all injuries treated  within its emergency room that involved a consumer product in any way. It is the usual procedure in most emergency rooms to provide a brief description of the accident within the medical record; i.e., 'amputated finger on lawn mower'. However, the emergency room staff of each participating hospital is urged to provide an adequate description of any product involved. Daily, all emergency room records are reviewed and a coded record is generated for those cases involving a consumer product. This record includes the following data: age of victim; sex of victim; up to two products involved in the accident; whether a third product was involved in the accident; type of injury – a simple 31 element coding scheme in which the injury is described in broad lay terms; body part injured; disposition of the patient after emergency room treatment; accident locale; fire/motor vehicle involvement; comments – space to provide a brief narrative description of the accident or other pertinent information such as product brand name; and other supplementary data – a section of the record set aside to allow for coding specific information for defined accident types.

At the end of each day's coding, the coded data are typed into a teletypewriter installed for this purpose. Simultaneously, a perforated paper tape is automatically punched with complete data on each case. This perforated tape is then loaded in a special 'reader' on the machine.

During late night hours of low telephone traffic, a special switching device attached to the headquarters computer in Rockville, Maryland, automatically polls each of the hospital-based terminals. This device turns on each remote teletype machine and reads the perforated paper tape at high speed, edits the data for accuracy and completeness, and records the data in the computer. The central computer then prepares a daily summary register and detailed case print-outs for headquarters review each morning. The computer also selects cases for follow-up, based on pre-established criteria.

This leads up to the second level of the system – investigation. When possible, effort is made to select cases representative of the NEISS surveillance data. Most cases assigned for investigation are selected to provide data for directing regulatory action, for monitoring existing standards, or for providing a basis for response to petitions submitted to the Consumer Product Safety Commission. Accident investigations are based on personal contact (on-site or telephone interviews) and provide information on the accident sequence, ways in which the product is being used, environmental circumstances related to the accident, and behaviour of the person or persons involved. Whenever possible, investigators document the product brand name, indicate the involvement of the product or its component parts in the accident, and include photographs and diagrams. Police, fire, and coroners' reports may be included as supplementary data. Abbreviated cases, generally conducted by telephone, contain most but not all of these items. None of the investigations include identifying information on the victims or other respondents.

Reference: Haase (1980).

## Annual Survey of Occupational Injuries and Illnesses

### Purpose and scope

The Annual Survey of Occupational Injuries and Illnesses is conducted by the Bureau of Labor Statistics in response to the requirements of the 1970 Occupational Safety and Health

Act for the collection, compilation, and analysis of occupational safety and health statistics. The survey builds upon a record-keeping system, also mandated under the Act, which requires virtually all employers to keep records on all work-related deaths and illnesses and those injuries which result in one or more of the following: loss of consciousness, restriction of work or motion, transfer to another job, or medical treatment beyond first aid.

The present annual survey produces data to reflect the job-related injury and illness experience of the work force as a whole. Survey data are solicited from a sample of employers having 11 employees or more in agriculture, forestry, and fishing; and from all employers in oil and gas extraction; construction; manufacturing; transportation and public utilities; whoelsale trade; retail trade; finance, insurance, and real estate; and services industries. The sample is selected to represent private industries in the states and territories. Data for employees covered by other federal safety and health legislation are provided by the Mining Enforcement and Safety Administration of the Department of the Interior and the Federal Railroad Administration of the Department of Transportation. The Occupational Safety and Health Administration is responsible for the collection and compilation of comparable data for federal agencies; state and local government agencies are not surveyed for national estimates. Self-employed persons are excluded because they are not considered to be 'employees' under the Act.

### Data collection procedures and data items

The universe frame of employers is first stratified into industries and then into employment-size groups. Because the survey is a federal-state co-operative programme and the data must also meet the needs of participating state agencies, the universe is further stratified by state prior to sample selection. The Bureau of Labor Statistics designs and identifies the survey sample for each state, and through its regional offices validates the survey results and provides technical assistance to the state agencies on a continuing basis. In each state participating in the survey on an operational basis, an agency collects and processes the data, prepares state estimates, and provides the data from which the Bureau produces national results.

The national sample for the survey consists of approximately 340 000 sample units in private industry. About 200 000 of the sample units are necessary to produce national estimates. The additional 140 000 units are selected so that states participating in the programme will have sufficient information to generate state estimates.

State agencies mail report forms to selected employers in February of each year to cover the previous calendar year's experience. Each employer completes a single report form which is then used for national and state estimates. Information for the illness and injury portion of the report form is copied directly from the Log and Summary of Occupational Injuries and Illnesses, which is required record-keeping by each employer under the Act. Recorded on the Log is information for each recordable case on the number of lost work days following the day of injury or onset of illness. The days are recorded as either days away from work or days of restricted work activity (days when the employee is assigned to another job on a temporary basis, works at a permanent job less than full-time, or works at a permanently assigned job but cannot perform all duties normally connected with it). The form also contains questions about the number of employee hours worked (needed in calculation of incidence rates), the reporting unit's principal products or activity, and average employment, to ensure that the establishment is classified in the correct industry and employment-size class.

Using a weighting procedure, sample units are made to represent all units in their size class for a particular industry. Data are further adjusted to reflect the actual employment in an industry during the survey year. Since the universe file which provides the sample frame is not current to the reference year of the survey, it is necessary to 'benchmark' the data to reflect current employment levels.

Although the reported data are carefully edited and reviewed it is recognized that there are undoubtedly errors of interpretations of record-keeping definitions by employers that are not uncovered. Therefore a quality assurance programme is conducted to evaluate the extent of this type of error in the records. A sample of establishments which have participated in the annual survey is visited and federal and state survey personnel compare entries on the log with supplementary records and other available information to evaluate the reliability of the log entries which provide the basic data for the reporting system.

Despite progress in identification, recording, and reporting of illnesses there are some known limitations inherent in the system. These include the fact that cases are recorded only in the year in which they are diagnosed and recognized as work related. Many occupational illnesses may develop years after an employee has left the firm where he or she contracted the illness, and many illnesses which may be of occupational origin are not as yet commonly recognized as such.

Reference: Bureau of Labor Statistics (1978).

## Basic vital statistics

### Purpose and scope

Basic vital statistics provided through the registration system come from records of live births, deaths, fetal deaths, and induced terminations of pregnancy. Registration of these events is a local and state function, but uniform registration practices and use of the records for national statistics have been established over the years through co-operative agreements between the states and the NCHS and its predecessor agencies.

The purpose of the basic vital statistics programme is to formulate and maintain a co-operative and co-ordinated vital records and vital statistics system, promoting high standards of performance. The programme is nationwide in scope covering the entire population of the US.

### Data collection procedures and data items.

Both provisional and final vital statistics are derived from the registration system. The provisional data are obtained from counts of vital records registered without reference to the date the event occurred and the final data are obtained from the record and its contents, processed by date of occurrence of the event.

The civil laws of every state provide for a continuous and permanent birth, death, and fetal death registration system. In general, the local registrar of a town, city, county, or other geographical place collects the records of births and deaths occurring in the area, inspects, queries, and corrects if necessary, maintains a local copy, register, or index, and transmits them to the state health department. There the vital statistics office inspects the records for promptness of filing and for completeness and consistency of information; queries if necessary; numbers, indexes, and processes the statistical information for state and local use; and binds the records for permanent reference and safe keeping. Microfilm copies of the individual records or machine-readable data are transmitted to NCHS for use in compiling the final annual national vital statistics volumes.

Provisional vital statistics are collected and published monthly and summarized annually. They are derived from monthly reports from the states to the NCHS giving the number of certificates accepted by the state for filing between two dates a month apart, without regard to actual date of occurrence. These reports to NCHS are to be mailed on or before the 25th of the month following the data month. They are the source of the provisional vital statistics published in the *Monthly Vital Statistics Report* and the annual summary of the monthly reports. Provisional data also include a 10 per cent sample of death certificates, the *Current Mortality Sample,* which provides provisional cause-of-death data on a monthly basis. This sample is selected by NCHS from the regular data file of deaths for those states submitting their entire month's file by the end of the following month. Otherwise the state is asked to provide a sample of records on a current basis. The sample is selected by including each record with a given last digit in the certificate number.

To promote uniformity in the statistical information collected from states and local areas for national statistical purposes, NCHS recommends standard certificates or reports for birth, death, fetal death, and induced termination of pregnancy. The standard certificates and reports are developed co-operatively with the states and local areas taking into account the needs and problems expressed by the major providers and users of the data. They are reviewed about every ten years to assure that they meet, to the fullest extent feasible, current needs as legal records and as sources of vital and health statistics.

Although the use of standard certificates and reports by states is voluntary and their form and content may vary according to the laws and practices of each state, the certificates and reports in most states closely follow the standard. The birth certificate includes information on the child's birth date and place of birth; the parents' state of birth, age, race, educational attainment; previous pregnancy history of the mother; information about the mother's prenatal care, any complications of pregnancy and labour, and any congenital malformations or anomalies noticed at birth. Items on the death certificate include the deceased's date and place of birth and of death, place of residence, usual occupation, and immediate and underlying cause of death.

References: National Center for Health Statistics (1981 *a,b*).

## Vital statistics followback surveys

### Purpose and scope

National natality and mortality surveys are periodic data collections based on samples of registered deaths and births occurring during a calendar year. Mortality surveys were conducted by NCHS annually from 1961 to 1968, and natality surveys from 1963 to 1969 and again in 1972. A National Infant Mortality Survey was also conducted from 1964 to 1966. For 1980, a National Natality Survey was conducted that was expanded to include fetal mortality.

The national followback surveys extend for statistical purposes the range of items which are normally included on the vital records. They provide national estimates of births and deaths by characteristics not available from the vital registration system. They also serve as a basis for evaluating the quality of information reported on the vital records.

### Data collection procedures and data items

The birth or death record serves as the sampling unit, and samples of these units are selected from a frame of records representing births or deaths registered during a given period, usually a calendar year. The sampling frame for the National Mortality Survey is the current mortality sample, the 10 per cent systematic sample of death certificates received each month by NCHS from the registration areas in the US. The sample for the National Mortality Survey is sub-selected monthly from the current mortality sample. The sampling frame for the National Natality Survey is the file of birth certificates from each of the registration areas of the US. Each registration area assigns a file number to each birth certificate; these file numbers run consecutively from the first to the last birth occurring in that area during that year. The survey samples are based on a probability design that makes use of these certificate numbers.

Data for all the followback surveys are collected primarily by mail. In the natality surveys, from addresses given on the birth certificates, questionnaires are sent to the mother, the physician who delivered the baby, and the medical facility where the baby was born. In addition, the 1980 surveys obtained data from the medical sources the woman had named as having given her radiation treatment or examination in the year prior to the delivery.

In the mortality surveys, a questionnaire is sent to the person who provided the funeral director with the decedent's personal information for recording on the certificate. This questionnaire requests socio-economic information about the decedent as well as the names and addresses of hospitals and institutions which might have provided care to the decedent at any time during his last year of life. If the death occurred in a hospital or institution, a hospital questionnaire is sent directly to the hospital or institution asking for information about the care provided and for the names and addresses of other medical facilities providing care.

The questionnaires for national mortality surveys have contained questions concerning the patient's last year of life. The surveys have included questions on hospital utilization, diagnoses, operations performed, institutions in which hospitalized, income, whether working or retired during most of the last year of life, household composition, education, health insurance, and the smoking habits of the deceased.

The questionnaire for the 1964–66 National Infant Mortality Survey included questions on hospitalization of the infant who died, information about other children of the mother, household composition, income, employment of mother, education of mother and father, and health insurance.

The national natality surveys collect information from mothers who had live births during a given year. They have gathered information on the medical and dental care and radiological treatment of the mother, employment and education of mother and father, family income, pregnancy history of the mother, expectations of having more children, household composition, income, whether this was a first or later marriage, whether mother was employed and when during her pregnancy she stopped working, and health insurance coverage.

The 1980 national natality survey was broadened to include fetal mortality and included many of the same or similar questions as previous surveys to allow trend studies in the areas of smoking habits, marriage and pregnancy history, education, income, health status of mother and infant, sterilization, radiological treatment, employment, childbearing expectations, and breast-feeding. Many new areas of study were added such as alcohol consumption, electronic fetal monitoring, amniocentesis, additional maternal and infant health indicators, occupation of mother and father, and ethnicity. Furthermore, there was an oversampling of low-birth-weight infants in the natality survey which will enable more in-depth study of this high risk group.

References: National Center for Health Statistics (1981 a,b).

## HEALTH CARE RESOURCES AND THEIR UTILIZATION

### National Master Facility Inventory

#### Purpose and scope

The National Master Facility Inventory (NMFI), compiled and updated regularly by NCHS, is a comprehensive file of information on virtually all (about 33 000) health facilities in the US. Health facilities are those that provide medical, nursing, personal, or custodial care to groups of unrelated persons on an 'in'-patient' (at least overnight) basis. Facilities in the NMFI are categorized into three broad classes: hospitals, both short- and long-stay; nursing homes, including all types of nursing, personal, and domiciliary care facilities, not just those certified by Medicare or Medicaid; and other facilities of a remedial or custodial nature, such as homes or resident schools for the deaf, blind, mentally retarded, and emotionally disturbed, resident treatment centres for alcohol and drug abusers, and homes for unmarried mothers.

NMFI is the only comprehensive source of information on the nation's in-patient health facilities. Its major purpose is to provide data for the analysis of the supply, distribution, and utilization of health resources.

#### Data collection procedures and data items

NMFI was initiated in 1962–63 by combining the lists of health facilities maintained by four federal agencies, directories of

health facilities prepared by various national associations and organizations, and files from state licensure agencies. At present, NMFI produces hospital data annually and data for nursing homes and other health facilities on a less frequent basis. Generally, the data are collected by mail. The administrator of the facility is sent a questionnaire and asked to complete and return it by mail.

Two mechanisms are used to keep the data in NMFI as current as possible. For all facilities except hospitals, NCHS conducts a series of mail surveys to: (i) insure that the data on file on the basic characteristics of the facilities are accurate, and (ii) identify and then delete those facilities that have gone out of business or are no longer eligible for inclusion. In addition, at regular intervals state licensure agencies, national voluntary associations, and other appropriate sources send to the NCHS their most recent directories or lists of new facilities. These lists are then clerically matched with the most current NMFI file and facilities not already included are added.

For hospitals, data were gathered annually in a joint survey of the American Hospital Association and NCHS. The contractual arrangement which in effect merged the hospital portion of NMFI with the American Hospital Association's annual survey of hospitals began in 1968. Through 1975, the Association performed the data collection (during October–January each year) for its member hospitals, while NCHS performed the data collection for the approximately 400 hospitals not registered with the Association. Both portions of the survey were edited and processed to the same specifications by the Association, which delivered to NCHS two edited tapes, one for Association hospitals and one for non-member hospitals. In 1976 and 1977, the Association surveyed all hospitals as part of its annual survey. The contractual relationship with the Association ceased in 1978; since that time NCHS has purchased hospital data tapes annually from the American Hospital Association, which are solely for NCHS's internal statistical use.

NMFI contains the following types of data for the three categories of facilities:

**Hospitals:** Ownership; major type of service offered; whether various facilities and services are offered; number of beds, admissions, in-patient days of care, and discharges; patient census; number of bassinets, live births, and newborn days of care; out-patient utilization; number of surgical operations; revenue, expenses, and assets; and staffing.

**Nursing homes:** Ownership; major type of service; licensed and staffed beds; beds certified for Medicare and Medicaid, admission policy with regard to age, sex, and various conditions; patient census by age and sex; in-patient days of care; number of admissions, discharges, and deaths; staffing; who is in charge of nursing care; number of patients receiving nursing care; services routinely provided; basic monthly charge; and operating expenses.

**Other facilities:** Ownership; major type of service; licensed and staffed beds; beds certified as intermediate care beds; admission policy regarding age and sex; patient census by age and sex; in-patient days of care; number of admissions, discharges, and deaths; staffing; basic monthly charge; and operating expenses.

References: National Center for Health Statistics (1981 a,b).

## Annual Survey of Hospitals

### Purpose and scope

The Annual Survey of Hospitals is conducted by the American Hospital Association. The primary purpose of the survey, which has been conducted since 1946, is to provide a cross-sectional view of the hospital industry and to make it possible to monitor hospital performance over time; it also provides a sampling frame for other Association surveys and special studies. Information is gathered from a universe of over 7000 hospitals in the country and includes information on the availability of services, utilization, personnel, finances, and governance.

### Data collection procedures and data items

The questionnaire for the annual survey is mailed to both American Hospital Association registered and non-registered hospitals in the US and its associated areas (i.e. American Samoa, Guam, the Marshall Islands, Puerto Rico, and the Virgin Islands); US government hospitals located outside the US are not included.

Survey questionnaires are mailed in late October of each year. After follow-up a response rate of about 90 per cent is achieved. Response rates vary between groups of hospitals categorized by size, ownership, service, geographical location, and membership status. For example, the response rate for community hospitals, defined as all non-federal, short-stay general and other special hospitals, is generally higher than that of non-community hospitals, and the response rate for registered hospitals averages about 90 per cent, while the rate for non-registered hospitals averages less than 60 per cent (registered hospitals comprise approximately 98 per cent of the mailing universe).

When a questionnaire is incomplete or when the information provided does not pass specified edits, the individual hospital is contacted for clarification and confirmation. If it is not possible to obtain information from a hospital, estimates for most missing data items are generated on the basis of their values in the previous year, whether those values were actual or estimated, and on the basis of information reported by hospitals similar to the non-respondents in size, type of control, principal medical service provided, and length of stay (long- or short-term).

Since its beginning the survey questionnaire has been kept in the same format in order to provide continuity and to permit important time series and trend analysis. This means that similar definitions have been used, similar arrangement of questions has been followed, and a relatively consistent data set has been collected. In 1980, the survey questionnaire was considerably expanded, however, in response to the termination of funding for the health facilities component of the Cooperative Health Statistics System, which had been functioning under the auspices of NCHS, and the recognition that additional detail was needed on some topics in order to pro-

vide a more adequate profile of the hospital industry. To facilitate response to the items the organization of the 1980 questionnaire was identical to that of previous years. In addition, all data items requested on the 1979 questionnaire were also requested on the new questionnaire and similar definitions were used.

The questionnaires for 1979 and 1980 were both divided into seven sections: reporting period; classification by governance and principal medical service provided; facilities and services available; beds set up and staffed within distinct in-patient service areas of the hospital and utilization of those units in terms of discharges and patient days; total number of beds set up and staffed, admissions, discharges, patient days, discharge days, out-patient utilization, and surgical operations for the entire reporting period; financial data on total patient and non-patient revenue, payroll and non-payroll expenses, restricted and unrestricted assets, and liabilities; hospital personnel. Significant changes in 1980 were: expansion from 44 to 110 specific services, information on the manner in which the services are provided, and a special subsection devoted to ambulatory care and the manner in which ambulatory services are provided; expansion of general utilization items to include a subsection relating to Medicare and Medicaid admissions and patient days; expansion of the financial section to request information about the sources of patient revenues by type of payer and information on capital expenditures and disposals and retirements of capital assets; expansion of the personnel section to obtain information about full- and part-time employees for 35 categories (as opposed to the six categories included in the past) and about the number of budgeted staff vacancies for each category. The 1981–83 questionnaires were essentially the same as that for 1980.

Information gathered from the survey, while it includes many specific services, does not necessarily include all of each hospital's services, and thus the data do not reflect an exhaustive list of all services offered by all hospitals. Similarly, although respondents are asked to provide data for a 12-month period beginning 1 October and ending 30 September of the following year, for example 1980, most of the survey data are not for the calendar year; about one-fourth of the responding hospitals use a reporting period of July through June and about half use a reporting period of October through September.

References: American Hospital Association (Annual); Kralovec and Mullner (1981).

## National Hospital Discharge Survey

### Purpose and scope

The National Hospital Discharge Survey (NHDS) of the NCHS is the principal source of information on in-patient utilization of short-stay hospitals. Data collection began in 1964 and has been continuous since then.

The purpose of NHDS is to produce statistics that are representative of the experience of the US civilian non-institutionalized population discharged from short-term hospitals. Specifically, the survey provides information on the characteristics of patients, the lengths of stay, diagnoses, and surgical operations, and patterns of use of care in hospitals of different sizes and type of ownership in the four geographical regions of the country. The scope of NHDS encompasses discharges from non-federal hospitals in the 50 states and the District of Columbia; only hospitals with six or more beds and an average length of stay for all patients of less than 30 days are included in the sample.

### Data collection procedures and data items

The unit of enumeration in the survey is a hospital discharge. The sampling frame is each hospital's daily listing of discharges. In 1982, the sample consisted of 550 hospitals from a universe of approximately 8000 short-stay hospitals. Of the 497 in-scope hospitals, information was collected from 426 participating hospitals (approximately an 86 per cent response rate) on approximately 214 000 discharges.

Discharge data are collected throughout the year. Sample discharges are systematically selected, usually on the basis of the final digit(s) of the patient's medical record number. For each sample discharge, an abstractor records personal, administrative, diagnostic, and surgical information from the face sheet of the patient's medical record onto a medical abstract form. Data collection frequency depends on the arrangement made with the hospital. In about half of the participating hospitals, a representative of the Bureau of the Census visits the hospital bimonthly, completes the abstract forms for records selected during the previous visit, and selects records for abstracting at the next visit. This allows time for records to be completed and properly filed (or pulled from file) prior to the visit. In about half of the hospitals, the same forms are completed by members of the medical records department. All completed forms are forwarded to one of the Bureau of the Census Regional Offices for review and then to NCHS for coding and data-processing operations.

The medical abstract form contains items relating to the personal characteristics of the patient, including birth date, sex, race, and marital status, but not name and address; administrative information, including admission and discharge dates, discharge status, and medical record number; and medical information, including diagnoses and surgical operations or procedures. It takes an average of five minutes for medical records personnel to sample and complete each form. The contents of the medical abstract form did not change from the inception of the survey until 1977 when modifications were made so that it more nearly paralleled the Uniform Hospital Discharge Data Set. The items added to the abstract at that time were residence of patient (ZIP Code), expected source of payment, disposition of patient, and date of procedures. For 1968–70, actual hospital charges by service and payment by source were recorded on a ledger abstract form for approximately one-third of the sample discharges.

References: National Center for Health Statistics (1981*a, b*).

## National Nursing Home Survey

### Purpose and scope

Between 1963 and 1969, NCHS conducted surveys of nursing homes and their residents on an *ad hoc* basis. With the implementation of the Medicaid and Medicare programmes, the increased utilization of nursing homes, and the projected increases in the aged population, those who set standards for,

plan, provide, and assess long-term care services needed comprehensive national data on a continuing basis. To meet their needs, NNHS was developed in 1972, with the initial survey conducted in 1973–74 and the second in 1977.

This periodic data collection system is a series of nationwide sample surveys of nursing homes, their residents, and staff. The purposes of the surveys are: to collect national baseline data on characteristics of the nursing home, its services, residents, and staff for *all* nursing homes in the nation, regardless of whether or not they are participating in federal programmes such as Medicare or Medicaid; to collect data on the costs incurred by the facility for providing care by major components such as labour, fixed, operating, and miscellaneous costs; to collect data on Medicare and Medicaid certification (such as utilization of certified beds and the health of residents receiving programme benefits) so that all data can be analysed by certification status; and to provide comparable data for valid trend analyses on a variety of topics.

For the initial survey conducted in 1973–74, the universe included only those nursing homes which provided *some level of nursing care*, regardless of whether or not they were participating in the Medicare or Medicaid programmes. Thus, homes providing only personal or domiciliary care were excluded. Beginning with the 1977 survey, the universe was expanded to include *all* nursing, personal care, and domiciliary care homes, regardless of their participation in Medicare or Medicaid. Homes which provide room and board only are excluded. In both surveys, homes in the universe included those which were operated under proprietary, non-profit, and government auspices. The universe included homes which were units of a larger institution (usually a hospital or retirement centre). A 1985 NNHS is planned.

### Data collection procedures and data items

The National Master Facility Inventory (NMFI) is the universe from which the sample homes are selected. The NMFI listing, maintained by NCHS, contains basic information about the home (such as name, address, size, ownership, number of residents, and number of staff) that is needed to design efficient sampling plans.

Resident data are collected by reviewing medical records and questioning the nurse who usually provides care for the resident. Residents are not interviewed directly. Response rates for the surveys differ according to the type of questionnaire, but range between 98 per cent for the resident questionnaires and 81 per cent for staff questionnaires. The initial survey, conducted from August 1973 to April 1974, had a nationally representative sample of 2100 nursing homes, with a subsample of 25 100 staff and 19 400 residents. The second survey, conducted from May to December 1977, had a total sample of 1700 nursing homes, with a subsample of 16 800 staff, 7100 residents, and 5300 discharged residents.

NNHS uses several questionnaires. The facility questionnaire includes questions on number of beds and residents, services provided, certification status, and various utilization measures. The expense questionnaire includes questions on the facility's expenses by major components, such as labour, fixed, operating, and miscellaneous expenses. The staff questionnaire includes questions about the employee's demographic characteristics, work experience, education, and salary. The residents questionnaire includes questions about the resident's demographic characteristics, health status, functional status, participation in social activities, monthly charge, and source of payment. Included in the 1977 survey was the discharged-resident questionnaire which included some of the same questions as the current-resident questionnaire, selected on the basis of their availability in the medical record.

The survey has a number of respondents in a home and is a combination of personal interview and self-administered questionnaires. Facility information is secured through a 20-minute personal interview with the administrator. Expense data are collected on a self-administered questionnaire, requiring about 30 minutes to answer, completed by the facility's accountant under authorization from the administrator or by the administrator. Sampled staff members complete a brief form that requires about five minutes to complete. Information on sample current residents is secured by the interviewer in a personal interview with the nurse who provides care to the resident and who refers to information in the medical record. About 15 minutes is required for each sample resident. For the 1977 survey, information on the sample discharged residents was secured by the interviewer in a personal interview with the nurse who was most familiar with the medical records and who referred to them for replying to all questions.

References: National Center for Health Statistics (1981*a, b*).

## National Ambulatory Medical Care Survey

### Purpose and scope

In May 1973, the National Center for Health Statistics inaugurated the National Ambulatory Medical Care Survey (NAMCS) on a continuing basis to gather and disseminate statistical data about ambulatory medical care provided by office-based physicians to the population of the US.

The purpose of NAMCS is to meet the needs and demands for statistical information about the provision of ambulatory medical care services in the US. Ambulatory services are rendered in a wide variety of settings, including physicians' offices, neighbourhood health centres, and hospital out-patient facilities. It is expected that NAMCS will encompass all of these settings in the future, and appropriate survey instruments and methodologies will be developed as resources permit.

Through 1981, the NAMCS target population consisted of all office visits within the conterminous US made by ambulatory patients to non-federal physicians who were in office-based practice and engaged in direct patient care. Excluded were visits to hospital-based physicians, visits to specialists in anaesthesiology, pathology, and radiology, and visits to physicians who were principally engaged in teaching, research, or administration. Telephone contacts and other non-office visits were also excluded. Since about 70 per cent of all direct ambulatory medical care visits occur in physicians' offices, this office-based NAMCS design provided data on the majority of ambulatory care services. Future data collection under

NAMCS will be conducted periodically, with data to be collected next in 1985. By that time an assessment of the need for and feasibility of including non-office-based ambulatory visits (e.g. hospital-based) in the survey is expected to be completed.

### Data collection procedures and data items

The NAMCS sampling frame is a list of licensed physicians in 'office-based, patient care' practice compiled from files that are classified and maintained by the American Medical Association and the American Osteopathic Association. These files are continuously updated by both Associations, making them as current and correct as possible at the time of sample selection.

The sample has consisted of approximately 3000 office-based physicians per year, with sample physicians randomly distributed across the 52 weeks of the year so that the resulting data reflect seasonal variations. Since the assignment of the reporting week is an integral part of the sample design, each physician is required to report during a predetermined period, and no substitute reporting periods are permitted. Approximately 75 per cent of the eligible physicians in the sample participate in the survey; they provide information on about 50 000 patient-visits per year.

The final stage involves sampling patient visits within a physician's practice. The sampling rate, determined at the time of the interviewer's appointment, is dependent on the number of days during the reporting week that the physician is in practice and the number of patients he or she expects to see. In actual practice, the sampling procedure is handled through the use of a patient log.

Actual data collection for NAMCS is carried out by the participating physician, aided by office assistants when possible. The physician completes a patient record for a sample of patients seen during the assigned reporting week. Sampling procedures are designed so that patient records are completed each day of practice for at most 10 patient visits. Physicians expecting 10 or fewer visits per day record data for all of them, while those expecting more than 10 visits per day record data after every second, or third, or fifth visit, observing the same predetermined sampling interval continuously. Each form requires only one or two minutes to complete.

Two data collection forms are employed by the participating physician – the patient log and the patient record. The patient log is a sequential listing of patients that serves as a sampling frame to indicate for which visits data should be recorded. The patient record contains 14 items of information about the visit: date and duration of the visit; patient's date of birth; sex, race, and problem; whether the patient has been seen for the particular problem before and whether the patient was referred by another physician; length of time since onset of the problem; diagnoses; diagnostic and therapeutic services; seriousness of the condition; and disposition. Periodically, supplementary items are added to the basic patient record to investigate specific health conditions or other aspects of ambulatory care. For example, questions about medications were added for 1980–81 and questions about accident or product-related illnesses were added for 1979.

References: National Center for Health Statistics (1981*a, b*).

**Statistical system of the Medicare Programme**

*Purpose and scope*

The Medicare programme, enacted on 30 July 1965 as Title XVIII of the Social Security Act, became effective on 1 July 1966. The programme, which is administered by the Health Care Financing Administration, makes available two separate but complementary health insurance programmes: (i) hospital insurance, covering nearly all persons age 65 years and over and disabled beneficiaries under age 65 years entitled to benefits for at least 24 consecutive months, and covered workers and their dependants with end-stage renal disease who require renal dialysis or a kidney transplant; and (ii) supplementary medical insurance, covering those persons who voluntarily pay the premiums.

The primary objective of the Medicare statistical system is to provide data to measure and evaluate programme operation and effectiveness. Benefit payment operations furnish information about the amount and kind of hospital and medical care services used by disabled persons and persons aged 65 years and over, as well as the expenditures for such services. Applications by hospitals, skilled nursing facilities, home health agencies, independent laboratories, and suppliers of portable X-ray and out-patient physical therapy services to participate in the programme provide data on the characteristics of such providers of services. The claim number assigned to each individual serves as the link between the services used under Medicare and the demographic characteristics of individual beneficiaries.

*System components and operation*

The statistical system is based on four related computer records: the health insurance master file, the provider record, the hospital insurance (Part A) utilization record, and the medical insurance (Part B) payment record.

The health insurance masterfile identifies each aged and disabled person eligible for health insurance benefits and indicates whether he or she is entitled to hospital insurance benefits, to supplementary medical insurance benefits, or to both. The entitlement record provides the population data for each part of the programme and serves as the base for the computation of a variety of utilization rates. The enrollment file contains demographic data including age, sex, race, state, county, and ZIP Code of residence, and eligibility information for all enrollees. The file also contains information on date of death so that an important health outcome measure can be linked to records on use of services.

Every hospital, skilled nursing facility, home health agency, independent clinical laboratory, and supplier of portable X-ray or out-patient physical therapy services must apply for participation in the Medicare programme; data on the application forms are stored in the central provider record and are updated as facilities are recertified periodically, as new ones apply for participation, and as some leave the programme. When the information in the provider file is combined with utilization data, it relates the characteristics of facilities and agencies that provide care to the kinds and amounts of services used by the persons insured under Medicare. Information in the provider file includes the institution's size, location, and type of control. Just as each enrollee has a unique identification number, each institutional provider also has a unique identification number.

Administration of the hospital insurance programme requires that two things be known about each person at the time of admission to a hospital – the individual's entitlement under the programme and the extent to which he or she has used the benefits available. When a patient is admitted to a hospital, the admission section of the in-patient hospital admission and billing form is completed by the hospital and forwarded through its intermediary to the Health Care Financing Administration (HCFA) central record. As soon as the record is checked, normally in less than 24 hours, the intermediary is informed of the patient's benefit status and of the number of days of in-patient care to which he or she is entitled during the current benefit period.

This information is then forwarded to the hospital. At discharge the hospital completes the billing section of the form and sends it to the intermediary for payment. When payment is approved, the intermediary forwards the claim to the HCFA for inclusion in the central record.

As part of this process, information on diagnoses and surgical procedures is coded for a 20 per cent sample of beneficiaries based on specified combinations of digits in the health insurance claim number. Admission and billing forms are handled in a comparable manner by home health agencies and skilled nursing facilities. The out-patient billing form is also transmitted to HCFA for entry in the central record after the bill is approved for payment by the intermediary.

All information on utilization experience in hospitals and skilled nursing facilities needed to administer the 'benefit period' provision is recorded centrally. This information includes stays in certain non-participating institutions that meet the definition of a hospital or skilled nursing facility under the law and days of care not covered or reimbursable under the programme.

Each admission and billing form contains both the beneficiary's claim number and the provider's identification number. The resulting record can be readily matched to the beneficiary and provider files. By this process, a statistical tape record is created for the sample of insured persons; it contains the information needed for tabulation from the three files related to hospital insurance use.

Payment or reimbursement under the supplementary medical insurance programme is made only after receipt of the carriers' (intermediaries involved in Part B of the Medicare programme) bills with allowed charges in excess of a set amount during a calendar year. For the enrolled population, carriers need to know from a central source the amount of the deductible that has been met; thereafter, during the remainder of the calendar year, the only additional information required from the HCFA for reimbursement or payment purposes is whether the person is still enrolled under the supplementary medical insurance programme.

Administration and operation of the programme requires accurate and complete information on the amounts paid by the carriers for physician services and for other services and supplies under this part of the programme. To meet these needs, carriers furnish a payment record consisting of tape, punched card, or other machine-readable form of each bill paid. A bill is defined as a request for payment from, or on behalf of, a beneficiary as the result of services provided by a single physician or supplier.

As with hospital bills, the bills for Part B services are linked to the information in the enrollment file through the enrollee's Medicare number. At this time no system operates nationally to identify the physician supplying the service. Thus, physician-service data cannot be aggregated on physician characteristics as hospital data can be on hospital characteristics. This is why patient-origin data for Medicare physician services cannot yet be developed at the national level.

Reference: Health Care Financing Administration (1981).

### Physician Masterfile

#### Purpose and scope

A Masterfile of physicians has been maintained by the American Medical Association since 1906. In the early days of its existence, the Masterfile was primarily a listing of physicians maintained as a record-keeping device for membership and mailing purposes.

The AMA Physician Masterfile is the most comprehensive and complete source of physician data in the US. It includes information on every physician in the country and on graduates of American medical schools who are temporarily practising overseas. The file includes members and non-members of the Association, and graduates of foreign medical schools who are in the US and meet US education standards for primary recognition as physicians. Thus, all physicians comprising the total physician manpower pool are included on the AMA Physician Masterfile.

#### Data collection procedures and data items

A file is started on each individual upon entry into medical school or, in the case of foreign and Canadian graduates, upon entry into the US. As a physician's training and career develop, additional information is added to the file – e.g. internship and residency training, licensure, board certification, professional affiliations, and other characteristics. These characteristics, while they may change over time, are not subject to constant change and are included in the historical portion of the Masterfile. There is also a current professional activities portion of each physician's record that identifies current address, professional activity, specialties, and employment status. By definition, this current portion of the file is subject to constant change and is updated regularly.

Prior to 1966, physician classification by specialty, activity, and employment was made through the Classification of Professional Activities system, which was based upon a 'private practice/not in private practice' concept. Data were collected under this system via a short postcard-type questionnaire entitled 'Verification of Physicians' Professional Activities.'

In 1966 the Association began efforts to update, improve, and expand the Masterfile. Upon determination that it was necessary to make major revisions in both the structure of the file and the data collection procedures, a four-year project (the Reclassification of Physicians Project) was initiated to redesign the classification system. Data collection procedures were also revised to correlate with the new classification system.

A new questionnaire, Record of Physicians' Professional Activities, was first used in 1968 in a census survey of 317 000 physicians. A complete census was scheduled to be conducted periodically. However, in order to verify the information gathered in 1968 under the new system, a complete census of 325 000 physicians was made again in 1969. The questionnaire, structurally the same as that of 1969, contained the physician's 1968 response with a column provided for corrections or changes. Analysis of the two sets of data showed that the data collected in 1969 were consistent with that of 1968, confirming that the questionnaire used to gather the data was a reliable survey instrument. Since 1968 three census surveys have been conducted by the American Medical Association. The most recent census of the physician population was conducted in 1981.

Between census years, a computerized weekly updating system keeps the Masterfile current. Each physician's record is dated to reflect the most recent change, which may be signalled by American Medical Association mailings or publications, by addressing company mailings, by physician correspondence, or by hospitals, government agencies, medical schools, medical agencies, medical societies, specialty boards, and licensing agencies. Any indication of a change in professional status or address triggers a questionnaire similar to the one used in the most recent census.

While the data collected from the Record of Physicians' Professional Activities questionnaire represent a major input to the Masterfile, data from other sources are also incorporated. These other data and their sources include: information on year of graduation, place of birth, date of birth, and professional appointments from medical schools; information on interns and residents, place of birth, and foreign medical graduates in training from hospitals; information on physicians in government provided annually by the Department of Defense; data on board certification of physicians from American specialty boards; information on membership in specialty, state, and county societies provided by the societies; and data on foreign medical graduates provided by the Educational Council for Foreign Medical Graduates.

Reference: American Medical Association, Annual).

### Health occupation data from the decennial census of population

#### Purpose and scope

The Constitution of the US provides for an enumeration of the population every 10 years. It was quickly recognized that enumeration offered an opportunity to obtain important information on characteristics of the population. The first census, taken in 1790, therefore included questions on the age and sex of each enumerated individual, and over the years many additional items have been added to the census. Information on occupation was added in 1850 and has been included since. Beginning in 1940 many questions, including occupation, have been asked of only a sample of the households in the total population in order to reduce the burden on the public. The censuses of 1960 and 1970 obtained information on occupation for persons 14 years of age and over in the experienced labour force or in the labour reserve; the census of 1980 obtained information on occupation for each person age 15 years and over in households that fell into the sample.

### Data collection procedures and data items

Like all information on the questionnaire, occupation is self-reported by household members in sample households where a long form of the questionnaire is received. Upon completion of the questionnaires in the households and their return to census field offices, the questionnaires are edited by hand for completeness and consistency. The questionnaires are then transferred to the Bureau of the Census facilities in Jeffersonville, Indiana, where information provided in narrative form, such as information on occupation, is coded by clerks.

Persons queried about their occupation in the 1980 census were asked whether they worked at all the week prior to 1 April, if so how many hours they worked that week at all jobs (if they worked at more than one job); they were also asked at what location they worked that week, and a number of questions about the trip to work. Those who did not work at all in the prior week were asked other questions about their availability for employment that week.

Specific occupation questions were asked of those who had worked the prior week and of those who did not work the past week but had worked for at least a few days in the period 1975–80. If the person had had more than one job activity or business the prior week, the one at which the most hours were worked was to be described; if the person had no job or business that week information given was to pertain to the last job or business since 1975. These questions included the name of the company or employer for whom the person worked, the kind of business or industry, the kind of work they were doing, their most important duties, and whether they were employees of a private company for wages, salary, or commission, of government (federal, state, or local), self-employed in their own business (either incorporated or not incorporated), or working without pay in a family business or farm.

The occupation classification system used in the 1980 census is similar to that used in each decennial census since 1940. However, the changes made for each of the censuses affect comparability of data from one census to another and require care in making such comparisons. There was a major change in the classification system used for coding occupations between the 1970 (441 specific categories) and 1980 (503 specific categories) censuses.

The 1980 census was the first in which the Standard Occupational Classification system was used. Prior to 1980, the Census Bureau used its own occupational classification system, but the Standard Occupational Classification was developed in 1977 for use by all federal agencies to provide greater comparability of occupation data among government agencies.

Analysis of occupational data from the decennial census requires some caution, since the data are self-reported by individuals in response to open-ended questions. Since census data on occupations are based on a sample of the population, there is also sampling error associated with the estimates.

References: Bureau of the Census (1975); National Center for Health Statistics (1975).

## HEALTH ECONOMICS

### National Medical Care Utilization and Expenditure Survey

#### Purpose and scope

The National Medical Care Utilization and Expenditure Survey (NMCUES), conducted by the National Center for Health Statistics, is a unique source of detailed national estimates on the utilization and expenditures for various types of medical care. NMCUES builds on the experience of the former Current Medicare Survey, the National Health Interview Survey, and the National Medical Care Expenditure Survey. The first cycle of the survey was conducted to cover the calendar year 1980. A second cycle of the survey is planned for the late 1980s.

NMCUES is designed to be directly responsive to the continuing need for statistical information on the health care expenditures associated with health services utilization for the entire US population. Cycle I was designed and conducted in collaboration with the Health Care Financing Administration to provide additional utilization and expenditure data for persons in the Medicare and Medicaid populations. NMCUES will produce comparable estimates over time for the evaluation of the impact of legislation and programmes on health status, costs, utilization, and illness-related behaviour in the medical-care delivery system.

#### Data collection procedures and data items

Cycle I was composed of several related surveys. The household portion of the survey consisted of a national survey of the civilian non-institutionalized population and a separate survey of the Medicaid-eligible populations of the States of New York, California, Texas, and Michigan. These two surveys each consisted of five interviews over a period of about 15 months to obtain information on medical care utilization, expenditures, and other health-related information. A third survey, of administrative records, was designed to verify the eligibility status of the household survey respondents for the Medicare and Medicaid programmes. It also checked insurance claims filed with the national Medicare and Medicaid programmes in each of the four States for persons in the sample of Medicaid eligibles.

The national Cycle I household survey comprised persons residing in about 6000 households. The sample for this survey was a multi-stage area probability sample representing the 50 states and the District of Columbia. The state Medicaid household survey sample consisted of about 1000 families in each of the four states; these families were selected with known probability of selection from the state Medicaid enrollment lists. Thus, the total sample for the survey was about 10 000 households.

An overall response rate for the household interviews of 89.4 per cent was achieved in the first interview for both household surveys in Cycle I: for the national survey the response rate was

91.4 per cent and for the state Medicaid survey, the rate was 86.7 per cent. Attrition over the course of interviewing resulted in final response rates of 84.9 per cent for the national household survey and 76.1 per cent for the state Medicaid household survey.

Interviews in Cycle I were conducted with each household at approximately three-month intervals, with interviewing beginnning in February 1980 and ending in March 1981. The first two interviews were conducted by personal visit of the interviewer to the household, the next two were conducted by telephone (if a telephone was available and acceptable to the household), and the final interview was conducted in person. Each round of interviewing asked about the period following the preceding interview, except the first round, which asked about the period of time following 1 January 1980.

Collection of data from the households was facilitated by the use of a calendar and a summary. At the time of the first interview, the household respondent was given a calendar on which to record information about health problems and health services utilization and to assemble physician and other provider bills between interviews. Following each household interview, information about health provider contacts and the payment of charges associated with them was used to generate a computer summary of information provided. This summary was then printed out in a simple format and mailed to the household for their review for accuracy and completeness prior to the next interview. At the subsequent interview, the interviewers reviewed this information with the household respondent to ensure accuracy and to obtain information not available during a previous interview.

The administrative records survey of Cycle I was a check of the eligibility and claims records of persons reported as covered by Medicare or Medicaid. The supplementary and confirmatory data on Medicaid and Medicare enrollees provided information from the administrative records of the programmes for comparison with that reported by the household respondents; the survey was designed specifically to meet the needs of the Health Care Financing Administration for programmatic data that are not otherwise available. For those individuals identified in the household interviews as being enrolled in either the Medicare or Medicaid programmes, identifying information was collected sufficient to allow the Health Care Financing Administration to flag incoming claims for services paid by Medicare, to allow the state Medicaid agencies in the four states in the state Medicaid survey to abstract data from claims, and to permit all state Medicaid agencies to confirm eligibility and type of eligibility under their state Medicaid programme.

Questionnaires for the household surveys were designed to obtain some information on a repeated basis throughout the survey and some information only once. The repetitive core of questions for Cycle I included health insurance coverage, episodes of illness, the number of bed days, restricted activity days, hospital admissions, physician and dental visits, other medical care encounters, and purchases of prescribed medicines. For each contact with the medical care system, data were obtained on the nature of the health conditions, the characteristics of the provider, the services provided, the charges, sources, and amounts of payment. Questions asked

only once included data on access to medical care services, limitation of activites, occupation, income, and other socio-demographic characteristics.

Reference: National Center for Health Statistics (1981b).

## Consumer Price Index

### Purpose and scope

The Consumer Price Index (CPI) is a measure of the average change in prices over time for a fixed 'market basket' of goods and services. It is revised periodically to reflect changes in what Americans buy and in the way they live. The latest revision, effective with the release of January 1978 data, introduced a new CPI for All Urban Consumers (CPI-U), which covers about 80 per cent of the total non-institutional population, and a revised CPI for Urban Wage Earners and Clerical Workers (CPI-W), which represents about half of the population covered by the CPI-U. The CPI-U includes, in addition to wage earners and clerical workers, groups which historically have been excluded from CPI coverage, such as professional, managerial, and technical workers, the self-employed, short-term workers, the unemployed, and retirees and others not in the labour force.

CPI includes an identifiable medical care component. Effective with the 1978 revision, 'medical care' represents a major category and is no longer a sub-listing under 'health and recreation' as it had been. The general definition of 'medical care' continues, however, to include both medical care services and other commodities.

### Data collection procedures and data items

CPI is based on prices of food, clothing, shelter, and fuels, transportation fares, charges for doctors' and dentists' services drugs, and the other goods and services that people buy for day-to-day living. Prices are collected in 85 urban areas across the country from over 18 000 tenants, 18 000 housing units for property taxes, and about 24 000 establishments – grocery and department stores, hospitals, filling stations, and other types of stores and service establishments. All taxes directly associated with the purchase and use of items are included in the index. Prices of food, fuels, and a few other items are obtained every month in all 85 locations. Prices of most goods and services are obtained by personal visits of Census Bureau representatives. Mail questionnaires are used to obtain public utility rates, some fuel prices, and certain other items.

In calculating the index, price changes for the various items in each location are averaged together with weights which represent their importance in the spending of the appropriate population group. Local data are then combined to obtain a US city average. Separate indexes are also published for 28 local areas. Area indexes do not measure differences in the level of prices among cities; they only measure the average change in prices for each area since the base period. The base period for the general-purpose federal index series is revised approximately every 10 years. Base periods are changed in order to facilitate the visual comprehension of rates of change from a base period that is not too distant in time.

Effective with the release of the January 1982 index, the

standard reference base period for both CPI-U and CPI-W became 1977 = 100. An increase of 22 per cent, for example, is shown as 122.0. This change can also be expressed in dollars: the price of a base period 'market basket' of goods and services in the CPI has risen from $10 in 1977 to $12.20. The revision of base period of the CPI does not involve changes in the base period expenditure weights, which continue to relate to 1972–73. The weights were developed from the Consumer Expenditure Survey conducted for the Bureau of Labor Statistics by the Bureau of the Census in 1972 and 1973. The 1972–73 Consumer Expenditure Survey showed smaller consumption weights for the medical care services component than had the most recent previous survey, conducted in 1960–61. Since the weights for physicians' services and for hospital service charges reflect out-of-pocket expenses, the reported prices used in the calculation of this portion of CPI reflect charges for uninsured patients.

For the CPI-U and revised CPI-W, 11 physician service categories are used: general medical practice, paediatrics, obstetrics and gynaecology, allergy, surgery, psychiatry, radiology, orthopaedic, cardiology, ear, nose and throat, and other specialties. The category from which specific services are selected for pricing varies with the specialty of the physician. Within each of the 11 categories are a number of preselected services; 16 services for general medical practice (eight types of visits and eight procedures) and eight for each of the remaining categories. Approximately 750 physicians report 1766 fees for use in the CPI-U and revised CPI-W. Dental services, limited to fillings, extractions, and dentures in the previous CPI-W, have been expanded for the CPI-U and revised CPI-W to also include bridges, caps, cleaning, and other dental services (oral surgery, orthodontics, root canal therapy, X-rays).

Under 'Other professional services', eye care in the unrevised CPI-W included only vision examination and dispensing of eyeglasses. Still under the same heading in the CPI-U and revised CPI-W, eye care now includes 16 types of services covering vision examinations, dispensing contact lenses, and in-office treatments and surgical procedures.

For the CPI-U and revised CPI-W, 12 general hospital service categories have been identified: hospital rooms, anaesthesia, operating room and other treatment centres (labour, delivery, recovery rooms), radiology, pharmacy, laboratory, neurology and cardiology, nuclear medicine, blood bank, physical therapy, inhalation or respiratory therapy, and emergency room service. In each hospital, fees for hospital rooms and for ancillary services are priced by field representatives to determine, through probability methods, the category of ancillary service as well as the specific service to be priced for each hospital. Approximately 325 hospitals of all types, except those where more than 50 per cent of the patients are non-paying, report 2007 prices for the CPI-U and the revised CPI-W. Room rates for nursing and convalescent home care, not included in the unrevised CPI-W, are part of the CPI-U and revised CPI-W.

The expenditure weight for health insurance in CPI reflects only payments that employees or consumer units make toward health insurance premiums. For computing CPI, contributions of employers are treated as income to consumers, not as a consumer expenditure. Changes in the price consumers pay for health insurance are calculated through an indirect method, instead of through direct pricing.

References: Bureau of Labor Statistics (Monthly); Ginzburg (1978).


## ADDENDUM – HEALTH INFORMATION SYSTEMS: AN OVERVIEW

### Dorothy P. Rice

This chapter on health information systems provides an excellent and comprehensive review of national public and private health data systems in the US. The data systems were selected on the basis of several important criteria, including that each system be national in coverage, currently operational, and that it produces primary data rather than secondary compilation of data from other sources. The descriptions of the data systems are clear, concise, and instructive. The picture that emerges is that the American pluralistic health care economy, with its pragmatic mix of public and private organizations, has produced a wide range of data systems that enable us to monitor the health of the nation. The issue for discussion is their adequacy, timeliness, and reliability for this purpose.

The National Center for Health Statistics – the Federal statistical agency that has the responsibility for the collection, analysis, and dissemination of the statistics on the health of the Nation – encompasses a diversified programme of surveys and inventories that draw on a range of information sources: individual people, institutions, and professions that provide health services, and vital records.

The surveys, particularly the National Health Interview Survey, have delineated the differentials in health status and in the level of health care between the poor and non-poor. In the years since Medicare, Medicaid, and other public programmes to equalize access to care were implemented, the surveys have shown the elimination of these income differentials in regard to receipt of care. Survey findings have also demonstrated the importance of targeting efforts for promoting health toward the poor and less educated, because it is among these groups that cigarette smoking and other poor health habits are most prevalent. These data are from cross-sectional surveys that give a 'snapshot' of the health-status of people at a single point in time.

Similarly, the birth and death records have continued to document such major trends as the marked and sustained decline in death rates from heart disease. The surveys and the vital statistics together meet many of the current needs for aggregate national health data.

Still needed, however, are large-scale prospective or longitudinal studies that record in sequence the health events of life, especially for epidemiological studies and surveillance of environmental hazards. Certain environmental effects on health care are immediate, while others are slow-acting and cumulative. Our current information systems are not adequate for identification of environmental hazards, especially when the effects do not become evident for many years. Longitudinal data on the same individuals over an extended time period provides a capacity to determine which were exposed to certain occupational or environmental hazards and to monitor their health.

Owing to the criteria for selection, this chapter on health information systems appropriately excludes programmes that operate at the state and local level. Nevertheless, it is important to understand that state and local agencies have key interests and roles in the collection and use of health statistics, including state and local health agencies, health planning agencies, rate review bodies, mental health agencies, Governors' offices, legislators, and universities. Many of these data systems have been developed with funding assistance from the federal government either directly or indirectly through service delivery grants.

The recent shift from categorical health programmes to block grants, the cutbacks in federal funding, and the lack of federal requirements for accountability will adversely affect our ability to adequately track and monitor the impact of these programmes on the health of the poor and near poor, children and mothers, and the elderly, as well as on institutions serving the poor.

The private health sector includes organizations of health service providers, health professionals, health insurance payers, consumers, industry, and private philanthropy. Several national private data collection systems are described in this chapter. Data are produced by these private organizations, but their quality is variable. There are duplicative and overlapping data systems in the public and private sectors. Hospital discharge data, for example, are collected by the Professional Activity Study and other abstracting organizations, Blue Cross–Blue Shield, Professional Standard Review Organizations, state rate-setting offices, Health Systems agencies. Medicare, Medicaid, and the National Center for Health Statistics. It is recognized that hospital discharge information is necessary to understand, monitor, and evaluate programmes related to hospital-based delivery of health care. The reporting burden on hospitals is great; the recording, storing, abstracting, and processing of medical records is expensive for both the institution and the users.

Several cross-cutting issues in data collection are discussed below.

## Quality and reliability of data

Many organizations, especially federal statistical agencies such as the National Center for Health Statistics, have made and continue to make considerable and commendable efforts to maintain and improve the quality of their major statistical series. The quality and reliability of data in the private sector, however, is uneven and unknown in many ongoing data bases. Survey results are subject to sampling, reporting, processing, and non-response errors, and these must be reported to fully understand and use the data. Standard errors are routinely reported in federal statistical reports on survey results, but are unavailable in most reports emanating from facility and manpower surveys conducted in the private sector. Thus, the improvement of the quality and reliability of health statistics in the private sector is a most urgent need.

## Standardization of data elements, uniform definitions and coding, minimum data sets

Health data are collected by many organizations and by multiple geopolitical levels for a variety of uses. Standardization of data is necessary across programmes to permit comparisons and avoid duplicative efforts. Considerable progress has been made at the federal level in the promulgation of standards for data collection, analysis, and distribution by the Office of Management and Budget. For example, a standard classification for race and ethnicity has been promulgated and implemented by federal agencies in all their data collection activities.

Some progress has been made in the development of uniform minimum data sets under the auspices of the National Committee on Vital and Health Statistics. Three such minimum data sets have been developed: hospital discharge data, ambulatory medical care, and long-term health care.

The International Classification of Diseases, 9th Revision, Clinical Modification is now used throughout the US in the coding of hospital discharges. The coding of surgical procedures, ambulatory care visits, and drugs, however, have not been standardized.

## Privacy, protection, and confidentiality

Issues of confidentiality, freedom of information, and invasion of privacy and their interactions in relation to data collection have received increasing attention in recent years. The conflict between the public's right to know and the right of individuals and institutions to protection of their privacy must be resolved and a balance struck among competing goals and conflicting and strongly held views as they relate to acquisition of specific kinds of data and the users of those data. Even in those programmes where strong legal safeguards and technical procedures protect the confidentiality of the information collected, there remains a persistent fear that this vast complex of information might be used as an instrument of social control. Several recent reports, including the Report of the Privacy Protection Study Commission, have addressed these important issues.

## Data linkage and data sharing

A considerable amount of health data are collected by a variety of organizations. These data could be shared among agencies, often without introducing problems of confidentiality. However, the data often are not compatible. Data integration among current large data collection activities should be carried out to maximize the results of separate efforts. Linkage of data files should be encouraged when there is a good reason to believe that the results of a specific linkage programme will be sufficiently complete for the specific purpose and that biases and limitations of linkage studies will not be so severe as to vitiate results.

To encourage sharing of data, methodologies need to be developed that will increase the capacity to integrate data sets in the future. We must also work toward commonly accepted definitions and uniform minimum data sets as mentioned earlier.

## Conclusion

As former Director of one of the federal statistical agencies, I believe that the *best* way to provide objective high-quality information on the demographic, economic, social, and health characteristics of the US population and trends in those characteristics is through agencies specifically established for that purpose. These agencies have 'no axe to grind', can usually guarantee confidentiality to respondents, and hence are able to produce unbiased, high-quality information acceptable to a wide array of users both within and outside of government. However, even in the best of economic times it is difficult to obtain adequate budgets to support the necessary data collection and analysis activities. Recognizing the philosophy that the federal government should only be in the business of doing things that cannot be adequately done by state and/or the private sector, it may be necessary to reassess the core programmes of the Federal Statistical System.

Regardless of what changes must be made in the core programmes, we must ensure that an information base continues to be available that will provide baseline data, be useful for monitoring trends, and have the ability to quickly detect any changes or aberrations in the economic, social, or health characteristics of the nation. The appropriate federal role in statistics is to produce national-level data useful for those purposes as well as providing norms to which subnational data can be compared. The data must be of high quality, produced in a timely manner, and relevant to issues of the day.

Federal statistical agencies must assume responsibility for activities that cannot reasonably or feasibly be assumed by individual states, local governments, and the private sector. The federal role must include the development and promulgation of standards and procedures for assuring the validity, reliability, comparability, and quality of statistical products and provide technical assistance in these areas. Federal statistical agencies also have to anticipate future needs for information and design today's systems to meet those needs.

In considering future prospects for improved health statistics to meet the nation's needs, we must recognize that resources will not grow parallel to demands for data and services. The demands for health data are greater than our ability to produce them. Budgetary pressures are requiring assessment of current data collection and dissemination procedures. Statistical agencies must make choices between data collection, research and analysis, and among needed data sets.

As we move closer to our objective of a national and systematic approach to meeting the information needs for policy development and programme evaluation, we also need to co-ordinate our data collection activities both within the federal establishment and between government and the private sector. Although considerable progress has been made in co-ordination, we must continue to avoid unnecessary and costly duplication, to encourage comparability of information collected by different systems, and to use the ongoing data collection programmes to provide specific information for many organizations. More effort is needed to provide essential data, yet reduce the burden on individual and institutional respondents.

## REFERENCES

American Hospital Association (Annual). *Hospital statistics.* Chicago, Illinois.

American Medical Association (Annual). *Physician distribution and medical licensure in the U.S.* Chicago, Illinois.

Bureau of Labor Statistics (Monthly). *CPI detailed report.* US Department of Labor and US Government Printing Office, Washington, DC.

Bureau of Labor Statistics (1978). *Occupational safety and health statistics: concepts and methods.* Report 518. US Department of Labor, Washington, DC.

Bureau of the Census (1975). *Historical statistics of the United States, colonial times to 1970,* Part 1, p. 121. US Department of Commerce, Washington, DC.

Centers for Disease Control (Weekly). *Morbidity and mortality weekly report.* US Department of Health and Human Services, Public Health Service, Atlanta, Georgia.

Ginzburg, D. H. (1978). Medical care services in the Consumer Price Index. *Monthly Labor Review* **101**, 35. US Bureau of Labor Statistics, Washington, DC.

Haase, K. (1980). Acute hazards viewed through the emergency room. In *Proceedings of the 18th National Meeting of the Public Health Conference on Records and Statistics.* DHHS pub. No. (PHS) 81–1214. Public Health Service, Hyattsville, Maryland.

Health Care Financing Administration (1981). *Medicare data system.* HCFA pub. No. 03111. Baltimore, Maryland.

Kralovec, P. D. and Mullner, R. (1981). The American Hospital Association's Annual Survey of Hospitals: continuity and change. *Health Serv. Res.* **16**, 351.

National Center for Health Statistics (1981a). *Catalog of publications of the National Center for Health Statistics.* DHHS pub. No. (PHS) 81–1301. Public Health Service, Washington, DC.

National Center for Health Statistics (1981b). Data systems of the National Center for Health Statistics. Vital and Health Statistics. Series 1, No. 16, DHHS pub No. (PHS) 82–1318. Public Health Service, Washington, DC.

National Center for Health Statistics (1975). *Decennial census data for selected health occupations, United States, 1970.* DHEW pub. No. (HRA) 76–1231. Public Health Service, Washington, DC.

National Institute on Drug Abuse (Quarterly). *Data from the Drug Abuse Warning Network.* Series G. Public Health Service, Rockville, Maryland.

# 2 Health information resources: United Kingdom—health and social factors

M.R. Alderson

## INTRODUCTION

This chapter describes various specific sources of information on health and social factors in the UK; for each source, the text sets out the background, the uses, and warnings about validity or possible errors in the data. The official publications available are listed in the Appendix to this chapter. For many of the topics there may be access to additional analyses beyond that presented in the standard publications; this may be via unpublished supplementary tables that have already been produced, or by requesting an *ad hoc* analysis of the national data. Many of the reports indicate whether this facility is available and give an address which may be contacted. In addition, hard copy publications are in some instances being supplemented by microfiche tables of detailed statistics; this is indicated where appropriate.

The contribution is divided into four sections. The first covers mortality statistics – both general mortality and specific contributions on area mortality, occupational mortality, and mortality from linked files. The second section covers a range of morbidity statistics. This section is set out in alphabetical order, covering: abortion, cancer registration, congenital malformation, General Household Survey (GHS), hospital discharge for non-psychiatric patients ('acute' and non-maternity), hospital discharge for psychiatric patients, morbidity statistics from general practice, and notification of infectious disease. The alphabetical ordering of these subsections was utilized as it is not easy to classify the various sources either by contribution to major or minor sources of morbidity or in a logical classification (such as conditions affecting the pregnant women, the new born, and advancing age). Only data that stem from routine statistical systems are utilized, though some of these systems do not generate annual data (for example the morbidity statistics from general practice), whilst the GHS is an annual survey, which has now produced detailed results from its inception in 1971. Obviously, these sources of data are rather different from other routine sources, such as notification of infectious disease or abortion.

The third section sets out in a much more limited way some of the sources of information on the known or suspect factors that contribute to variation in risk of disease. This is, of course, a very different aspect of health, but has been included because of the interest in matching routine data on these factors to variation in incidence or prevalence of disease, or variation in mortality. It begins with brief comments on various social factors and facets of behaviour – particularly those sources of information on diet, smoking, alcohol consumption, and occupation. The section then discusses sources of data on environmental factors that contribute to illness, dealing very briefly with information on climate, environmental pollution, and products from the manufacturing industries.

The fourth section provides a brief comment about the basic population statistics that are required as a denominator in many of the rates for the event data covered in the sections on mortality and morbidity statistics.

This chapter does not cover statistics on health service activity, health service facilities, staff in the health service, or expenditure. These issues of medical care interest are beyond the terms of reference, not contributing to information about the health of the population but only about the health care of the population. Such UK statistics have been fairly recently reviewed, both from the point of view of routine statistics (Alderson and Whitehead 1974), and data derived from health surveys and related studies (Alderson and Dowie 1979).

## MORTALITY STATISTICS

### Background

The system of registration of deaths in England and Wales dates from the Births and Deaths Registration Act of 1836, though this did not become subject to penalty until 1874. The current chief regulations (Statutory Instrument 1968) are for the registration of births, deaths, and marriages. Mortality data are derived from the medical certificate of cause of death issued by the practitioner, together with the information given to the registrar by the informant. The practitioner completes the regulation form which is similar to that recommended by the WHO (1977). The cause of death is given and other items including whether information from a post-mortem examination has been taken into account, or might be available later. The doctor can also indicate whether the death has been reported to the coroner, or whether other information might be available at a later date. If this latter section is completed, a standard enquiry form is sent by the registrar at the time he or she registers the death.

The death certificate has to be delivered to the registrar of the subdistrict in which the death occurred. The informant may be a relative of the deceased, a person present at death, the occupier of the institution in which death occurred or an inmate of that institution, or a person causing disposal of the body. Where death occurs in a public place the informant may be the relative, any person present at death, any person who found the body, any person in charge of the body, or the person causing the disposal of the body (i.e. the chain of responsibility stretches out until a responsible person is identified). The informant is expected to provide information about the deceased, including date and place of birth, occupation and usual address of the deceased, and some other particulars.

A registrar when informed of a death, reports this to the coroner if: (i) the death is in respect of a deceased person not attended during his or her last illness by a medical practitioner; (ii) the registrar has been unable to obtain a certificate of cause of death; (iii) the particulars of the certificate of cause of death indicate that the deceased was seen neither after death nor within 14 days before death by the certifying practitioner; (iv) the cause of death is unknown; (v) the registrar has reason to believe that death was due to an unnatural cause or violence, neglect, abortion, or from suspicious circumstances; (vi) death appears to have occurred from an operation or before recovery from an anaesthetic; or (vii) from the contents of the certificate, it appears that death was due to industrial disease or poisoning. For those unfamiliar with the coroner's functions, this list indicates categories of deaths into which the coroner may inquire. The history of the development of the office of coroner is set out in the Brodrick report (1971), whilst their particular role in regard to suicides has been described by Jennings and Barraclough (1980). The coroner may provide a notification of the cause of death without an inquest, having in some circumstances had a post-mortem carried out. This will depend on the results of preliminary enquiries and decision as to whether death is from natural causes.

Table 2.1 provides some statistics on place of death, and proportion of deaths where an autopsy is performed. The increase in the proportion of autopsies is a reflection of the increasing numbers of deaths reported to the coroner; in 1980, of the 28.6 per cent deaths coming to autopsy, 24.3 per cent were requested by the coroner and only 4.3 per cent for other medical reasons. The majority of deaths referred to the coroner have an autopsy (about 82 per cent for which the coroner provided a cause of death in 1980). Not all deaths referred to the coroner are certified by him; in 1980, just over 10 per cent of the deaths initially referred to the coroner were finally certified by a doctor.

Similar information is collected in Scotland and Northern Ireland, though the death certificates are slightly different from those used in England and Wales. The law differs in Scotland from that in England and Wales. Instead of a coroner, there is a procurator-fiscal, whose responsibility it is to investigate deaths which are sudden, violent, suspicious, or in which the cause is not known. The medical aspects of a death may be investigated by (i) the procurator-fiscal's medical officer, who may certify the cause of death without an autopsy, or (ii) the pathologist, when an autopsy has been performed.

The certifier may indicate that further information is likely to be available at a later date. An enquiry is then forwarded

**Table 2.1.** (a) Percentage of deaths occurring in different places in England and Wales (E and W) 1980, Scotland 1980, and Northern Ireland (NI) 1979

| Place of death | Percentage of deaths | | |
|---|---|---|---|
| | E and W | Scotland | NI |
| Psychiatric hospital | 2.1 | 2.9 | 2.0 |
| Other hospitals/institutions for the care of the sick | 58.2 | 57.6 | 53.7 |
| Other institutions | 5.0 | 2.7 | 2.3 |
| At home | 28.5 | 35.9 | 42.0 |
| In other private house/other place | 6.2 | | |

(b) Percentage of deaths in which an autopsy was performed in England and Wales, and Scotland, 1954–80

| | Percentage of deaths having an autopsy | | | | | |
|---|---|---|---|---|---|---|
| | 1954 | 1960 | 1965 | 1970 | 1975 | 1980 |
| England and Wales | 20.7 | 21.9 | 26.9 | 26.2 | 27.0 | 28.4 |
| Scotland | N/A | N/A | 16.2 | 14.8 | 16.9 | 15.9 |

and, where appropriate, the cause of death details are amended. In 1979 replies were received relating to about 4.5 per cent of the total deaths; about one third of the replies lead to re-assignment of cause of death codes, about equal numbers changed within the same chapter as changed to another chapter. Rather different is the system whereby queries are sent to certifiers where there are difficulties in coding the cause of death; these are sent out for about 3 per cent of all deaths.

For pregnancies that result in a stillbirth a different form has to be completed; the current regulations are as for deaths (i.e. the 1968 regulations). The English, Scottish, and Northern Ireland stillbirth certificates are very similar, though there are minor differences in size and layout. This form has to be completed where a child has been 'completely expelled or extracted from its mother after the 28th week of pregnancy and which did not at any time after such expulsion or extraction breathe or show any other evidence of life'. The wording of the definition varies marginally and though the intent is the same, the interpretation may be subject to considerable variation. The certifier, who may be the usual medical attendant or the midwife, completes the particulars including the cause of the stillbirth, the weight of the fetus and the estimated duration of pregnancy. It should be indicated whether information has been or will be obtained from a post-mortem.

### Validity

Any routine data collection system is liable to inaccuracies; this problem is best discussed by considering the separate steps in the chain leading to the production of mortality statistics, which are:

1. Conversion of basic information about the patients into the diagnosis by the clinician.
2. Completion of the death certificate.
3. Transcription on to the death notification.
4. Classification of underlying cause of the death.
5. Coding.

6. Processing.

7. Analysis and interpretation of the statistics.

A number of studies have examined the accuracy of the diagnostic information available at the time of death; usually this has been compared with data derived from autopsy. A major study was sponsored by the General Register Office (GRO) (Heasman and Lipworth 1966). This provided a useful guide of the difference between clinical and autopsy diagnoses, though it is not possible to assume that the autopsy diagnosis is invariably correct, nor that the differences observed can be extrapolated to certification of persons dying at home. Alderson (1981) has reviewed the literature on this topic, and pointed out that some studies indicate a worrying degree of variation between autopsy and clinical diagnoses. Other recent studies using this approach have been by Busuttil *et al.* (1981) and Cameron and McGoogan (1981). The latter authors have carried out a number of interrelated studies on this topic, basing their results on data obtained in the Edinburgh locality, or Scotland in general.

Another approach has been to use 'dummy' case histories and obtain 'mock' death certificates from clinicians. Reid and Rose (1964) used this technique with the collaboration of physicians from Norway, UK, and US. McGoogan and Cameron (1978) obtained information from clinicians via questionnaires on their attitudes to the value of an autopsy in altering diagnoses. Gau and Diehl (1982) circulated ten case histories to a sample of GPs; 97 (62 per cent) collaborated and provided 'death certificates'. The number of different causes of death varied from 7 to 26 for the same history. The proportion designated 'refer to coroner' also varied widely. Diehl and Gau (1982) circulated 15 fictitious case histories covering a range of clinical conditions to a representative sample of GPs and housemen in four localities in England and Wales with varying standardized mortality ratios (SMRs). Responses from 97 GPs (62 per cent) and 26 housemen (51 per cent) showed no marked regional variation in certification habits and the authors concluded that regional variation in cause-specific mortality could not be ascribed to certification artefact.

Others have compared death certificates with a review of detailed case histories (see for example, Moriyama *et al.* 1958; Alderson 1965; Puffer and Griffith 1967; Alderson and Meade 1967; Pole *et al.* 1977; Clarke and Whitfield 1978).

Other issues to be considered are the impact of certificate and certification practice, and the influence of coding and revisions of the International Classification of Disease (ICD). The Royal College of General Practitioners (RCGP) study of oral contraception involved GPs in submitting a report of the cause of death for women who had died; this information was coded by the research team. Wingrave *et al.* (1981) compared the coding by the RCGP and OPCS/GRO Scotland of the death certificates for 205 deaths. Using the B codes, there was agreement for 150 of the 171 non-violent deaths (88 per cent); discrepancies occurred from using different sources of information, with the GP often considering previous history not recorded on the certificate. There were 10 codes not in accordance with ICD rules.

It is generally accepted that mortality statistics, because of these problems, must be interpreted with caution. Obviously there are some conditions where the medical knowledge and facilities for diagnosis have altered markedly over time, or may vary from place to place. This will have a major impact on the interpretation of the data, as similarly, where there has been major alterations in the ICD with the splitting or amalgamating of various cause groups. It has been suggested that approximately 20 per cent of coded causes of death involve relatively minor errors and 5 per cent major errors (where a major error is a change from one chapter of the ICD to another, which generally implies alteration from one body system to another). As an example of the difficulty of studying a particular condition, a WHO report (EURO 1981) stated that it was not possible to obtain an exact assessment of the extent of acute respiratory illness in Europe. This was because mortality and morbidity data were absent or incomplete in some countries and there were doubts about the comparability of the data.

Because of the importance of coding and classification, the WHO Regional Office in Europe (1966) investigated coding consistency by circulating standard certificates amongst coders in different European vital statistics offices. It was suggested that there was considerable disagreement, both between coders in different countries, and between these countries, coders and the WHO Centre for Classification, in the selection and coding of the underlying cause of death. There was relatively less variation between coders working within the office in each of the participating countries.

Nearly all the national statistics published are based on tabulations of single causes for individual deaths – the underlying cause of death. It has been pointed out a number of times that converting the information on the death certificate to a single cause of death may fail to identify the combination of different diseases that are or are not related, but are thought by the certifier to contribute to death (see for example, Farr 1854; Moriayma 1952; Guralnick 1966; Markush 1968; Cohen and Steinitz 1969; Abramson *et al.* 1971). The published statistics referred to in this contribution are based on underlying-cause coding.

The above points relate to cause of death – from birth onwards. An associated aspect is the cause of stillbirth. Edouard (1982) compared the clinical case notes with the certified cause of death for 200 stillbirths in eight hospitals in 1973–77. Using 14 categories of cause of death, there was concordance for 69 per cent of the stillbirths; the discrepancies were most frequently omission of particulars known at the time of death.

## Publications

From 1840 until 1974 the Registrar General published annual statistics for England and Wales. In recent times this consisted of three parts, with Part I containing Medical Tables, Part II Population Tables, and Part III being a commentary volume. A range of detailed tables were provided, giving particulars of deaths and death rates by cause, sex, age, locality, and a number of other variates.

This series was replaced in 1974 by separate soft cover volumes incorporating subsets of the mortality statistics. The series (known as series DH) came out in five parts: DH1 – Mortality Statistics; DH2 – Mortality Statistics by Cause; DH3 – Mortality Statistics, Childhood and Maternity;

DH4 – Mortality Statistics, Accidents and Violence; and DH5 – Mortality Statistics, Area. The intention was that individual components of this series would be published with the least delay; individuals could acquire the subset of material that was of particular interest to them. The main tables were those appearing in the cause volume, which presented, at ICD 3 and 4 digit level the numbers of deaths by age and sex; more limited analyses providing rates appearing in the general DH1 volumes.

Prior to 1974 the Registrar General had also published a Weekly Return and a Quarterly Return. There were again changes in 1974, with the Weekly Return appearing as a monitor; this is particularly devoted to statistics on infectious disease (see p. 35). The Quarterly Return was replaced by a quarterly journal, *Population Trends,* which includes articles on specific topics and regular tables, with limited analyses on mortality.

The traditional series of publications have continued for Scotland and Northern Ireland. Details of publications for all three countries are given in the Appendix.

## Area mortality

Place of usual residence is one of the variates recorded at death registration and this permits regular analyses of mortality by area. These appear in the Appendix under publications of mortality statistics. In addition, the opportunity is taken following each decennial census to relate the mortality occurring around the period of the census to the figures of the population as enumerated in the census. The purpose of this is to facilitate more detailed examination of the geographical pattern and variation in these statistics than is possible in the annual data published by the Registrar General. This is possible because (i) the census provides a more accurate denominator, and (ii) deaths for several years around the census are aggregated; therefore more valid rates can be produced for the principle causes of death in local areas of England and Wales. The validity of the data depends upon the considerations already voiced on the cause of death, the accuracy of the population figures (which is very high in comparison to the diagnostic data), and the issue of whether internal migration of ill (or healthy) people affect the regional statistics. Fox and Goldblatt (1982) suggest that differential migration of those with varying health is not a major source of bias in these area analyses. The Registrar General's Decennial Supplement for England and Wales 1969–73 – Area Mortality Tables is part of the series of decennial mortality analyses which have been produced for England and Wales since 1851–60 onwards. The material was published in three parts; initially the computer generated tables were produced on microfiche, with a relatively slender guide to these tables (OPCS 1979). Subsequently a commentary volume appeared with selected tables and text relating to the main variations in the microfiche tables (OPCS 1981*a*). Data were made available for 100 causes of death, tabulated down to the level of individual county boroughs and the remainder of counties. Area is also one of the variates used in tables for the Decennial Supplement on Occupational Mortality (see next section). A full list of area mortality supplements is given in the Appendix.

## Occupational mortality

The first publication in the Registrar General's *Decennial Supplement on Occupational Mortality for England and Wales* appeared in 1855, incorporating information from the 1851 census and the mortality returns from that year. Since that time, at approximately ten-yearly intervals tables have been produced showing the various mortality rates by occupation; the one gap in the series being due to the Second World War, as no census was carried out in 1941. Comparable reports in the Scottish series have been appearing intermittently since 1892.

The data for numerator and denominator in the rates are derived from two sources. The denominator is obtained from the record of current occupation inserted on the census schedule; the information from this is used to derive counts of males and females by age and occupation. Single, widowed, or divorced women are classified by their own occupation; married women, if recorded with their husband at census, are classified by the occupation of their husband: retired people under the age of 75 years are recorded as retired, but also classified by their final full-time occupation. The numerator is a count by occupation and cause of death for persons dying around the time of the census. The period on which the rates were based in 1951 was extended to deaths occurring in a five-year period around the time of the census.

The collection of census data is described below (p. 42). The information on the death registration is collected as described in the previous section on mortality statistics.

### Validity

For many years it has been recognized that there are a number of difficulties in the calculation and presentation of occupational mortality rates. The combination of data from two sources creates problems; the occupation recorded at census and at death registration are provided under very different circumstances and are collected in rather different ways. Each of the supplements on occupational mortality provides a careful discussion about the problems of collecting and interpreting this material.

Heasman *et al.* (1958) carried out a study which provided some facts relevant to a discussion of the accuracy of occupational mortality data, though this work was restricted to a survey on the accuracy of job descriptions on records used for the calculation of indexes of occupational mortality and morbidity in the mining industry. These authors comment on errors in the descriptions of occupations used in the numerator and denominator of the occupational mortality rates, including errors introduced by the coding system. Following the 1961 census, a post-enumeration survey was carried out for the first time to check the accuracy of the information collected at the census; results of this are provided in the General Report of the 1961 Census (GRO 1968). Some of the occupation questions were differently phrased, and thus comparisons between the census and the post-enumeration survey are difficult to interpret; however, it did support the earlier suggestion that there was overstatement of the number economically inactive. The second study discussed in the General Report of the 1961 Census concerned the matching of the information recorded at the death registration with the census schedule for a sample of deaths occurring shortly after the census. Out of 2196 males, 63 per cent were assigned to the same occupation unit at death registration and at census, 10 per cent were assigned to different units within the same occupational order, whilst 27 per cent were assigned to different orders.

Alderson (1972) has reported a study amongst a representative sample of males dying in Bristol during 1962–63. A chronological history was obtained of all occupations held since leaving school for each deceased person in the study; this information being obtained by interview with the next of kin. These occupation histories have been coded, and compared with the coding of the occupations recorded at death registration. Comparison showed that there was complete agreement between the two sets of data regarding the final occupation for 79 per cent of the subjects; there were negligible discrepancies for 6 per cent, minor discrepancies at the unit level for 5 per cent, and major discrepancies for 10 per cent of the subjects.

Where an individual has developed a fatal chronic disease (whether or not occupationally induced) and has had to change his or her occupation because of impaired ability, mortality will be shown against the final occupation. Should the change of job have been due to onset of occupationally-induced disease, this will not be reflected in the mortality rate for the principal occupation; there will also be an erroneously high mortality rate for the final occupation.

The possibility that knowledge of an occupational risk might influence certification in workers was discussed by Mole (1982) and Kneale and Stewart (1982) – the former suggesting that doctors near a plant might 'over-certify', and the latter, that doctors further away might 'under-certify' a particular cancer. No hard evidence to support either contention was presented.

A particular problem is the examination of data for women; occupation is not systematically recorded for all married women and the use of husbands' occupation is obviously examining an indicator of 'way-of-life', rather than the environment of those women who go out to work.

*Use of occupational mortality statistics*

The Registrar General (1855) in introducing his analysis of occupational mortality, suggested that 'the professions and occupations of men open a new field of enquiry, on which we are now prepared to enter, not unconscious, however, of peculiar difficulties that beset all enquiries in the mortality of limited, fluctuating and sometimes ill-defined sections of the population'. Schilling (1960) after discussing the problems in the interpretation of these mortality statistics, suggested that the data bring new occupational risks to our notice, and remind us of old ones still present.

Alderson (1972) has reviewed briefly some of the studies of occupational disease that did and did not appear to use these decennial supplements as background information. However, it is difficult to gauge the contribution made by this routine source of data; there does not appear to be any clear cut example of a hazard that has been initially identified in the occupational mortality statistics and then confirmed in an *ad hoc* study (Alderson, 1983a). The primary use appears to be by individuals wishing to cross-check tentative hypotheses derived from other sources. A major review of the contribution

of these English data to the study of the influence of occupation and social class upon cancer mortality for 1851–1971 has been provided by Logan (1982).

*Publications of occupational mortality*

The Registrar General for Northern Ireland arranged for an analysis of occupational mortality for the years 1960–62, using the 1961 Census as the denominator; no official report has been published. Age-standardized mortality ratios were calculated for males aged 15–64 years for 27 occupation orders and social classes for all causes and four broad causes of death. Crude mortality rates were also shown for males and married women for 27 occupation orders. Park (1965–66) published these limited results, but emphasized that detailed tabulations were available upon request. The full list of publications on this topic for England and Wales, and Scotland and Northern Ireland are given in the Appendix.

## Linked mortality records

It has been recognized for many years that some of the limitations of analysis of event data can be overcome by linking records of events occurring to individuals. This has the advantages that (i) instead of calculating rates based upon estimated denominators, the actual occurrence rate in a group of individuals can be determined and tabulated by the specific characteristics of the individuals; and (ii) the range of items available for analysis may be extended. This was foreshadowed by some of the writings of Farr, particularly in relation to estimation of the outcome of care in different hospitals (Farr 1864) and in recommendations for health statistics to be compiled for the Army (Farr 1861). Little further work was done in England and Wales until Heady and Heasman (1959) provided a summary report of a major project examining the social and biological factors affecting stillbirth and infant mortality. The material was obtained by linking data from the birth registrations to appropriate death details for all infants who died having been born in 1949–50. The analyses used information from over a million births and 80 000 deaths. A similar approach was used by Spicer and Lipworth (1966), who investigated regional and social factors influencing infant mortality for infant deaths during the period 1 April 1964–31 March 1965 matched to appropriate birth registrations.

In 1975, the routine linkage of infant deaths to births commenced: the system uses the NHS number, sex, and date of birth as matching factors and by 1979 only 1.2 per cent of infant deaths could not be matched with birth details. The cause of death can be tabulated against: social class; region of residence; country of birth; month of birth; mothers' age, and parity for legitimate children; legitimacy; father's age, occupation and social class (for legitimate children); duration of marriage; place of confinement; whether singleton or multiple birth; birthweight; certification; multiple causes of death, and associated conditions. The linkage extends the range of items, by making available those recorded at birth and those recorded at death. A number of reports have been produced from this activity and annual statistics are now being made available from the infant linked file. (Owing to the high mortality in the early part of the first year of life, the main analyses are carried out on deaths in a calendar year, rather than accumulating all deaths in a birth cohort.)

A major fresh venture began in England and Wales, with the selection of a 1 per cent sample of respondents from the 1971 national census. (Some work also began on this project in Scotland – see Registrar General, Scotland 1973). Arrangements were made to assemble event data for the sample into a cohort file including births to sample parents, cancer registration, psychiatric hospitalization of over two years duration, emigration or deaths. The sample was enhanced by one per cent of identified immigrants as well as one per cent of all births (in addition to the births mentioned above). The outlines of the system were described, before analyses had become available (OPCS 1973a); a major category of analysis that the system permits is tabulation of mortality in relation to the variates recorded at census. A recent report (Fox and Goldblatt 1982) presents a wide range of results from mortality of the cohort over the period 1971–75. Comparisons of mortality for subgroups of the population were presented, each being derived from broad census questions; this permitted examination of mortality in relation to: economic activity (economic position the week prior to the census; alternative methods of classifying women; economic activity and transport to work); household structure (with emphasis on the elderly and those in non-private households); housing characteristics (tenure, density, amenities etc.); marriage and fertility; education; area of residence; internal migration; and imigrants. Particular probes were made of the influence of various forms of health-related selection (e.g. for occupation, housing, migration), of the influence of those 'permanently sick' upon subsequent mortality patterns, and alternative ways of classsifying individuals into non-occupationally derived socio-economic status.

The publications on linked mortality statistics are provided in the Appendix.

## MORBIDITY DATA

This section deals with eight routine sources of morbidity data, which are presented in alphabetical order. The emphasis is on background description of the sources, comments about the validity of the data, and indication of the published material.

### Abortion

#### Background

The Abortion Act 1967 came into force in Great Britain on 27 April 1968, and regulations made under the Act required notifications of termination of pregnancy to be made within seven days on a standard form which is to be sent to the Chief Medical Officer of England, Wales, or Scotland. The purpose was to amend and clarify the law relating to termination of pregnancy by registered medical practitioners; section 2 (i) deals with the Secretaries of State making regulations requiring any registered medical practitioner who terminates a pregnancy to give notice of the termination and such other information relating to the termination as may be so prescribed. The regulations, including designation of the form for notice of termination,

were made in 1968 and subsequently amended in 1969, 1976, and 1980.

Though information is notified to the Chief Medical Officers, provision is made to enable information to be processed in England and Wales by the Registrar General, and in Scotland by the Information Services Division of the Common Services Agency. The purpose of notification of abortion is to ensure that the provisions of the Act are being properly observed. It also enables basic epidemiological and demographic data to be collected about women undergoing terminations, and the Office of Populations, Censuses and Surveys (OPCS) have in the past processed and published monthly, quarterly, and annual statistics.

It is interesting to note that with this system, direct transmission of information was introduced; the particulars are recorded in the Unit at which termination takes place, the forms then being sent straight to central government. There is no system advocated for collating or checking the material at local or regional level, prior to the onward transmission to central government. The OPCS and Common Services Agency act as agents for central government in processing the data and producing the reports.

#### Validity of abortion data

In discussing 1971 data (Chief Medical Officer 1972) it was suggested that the figures might not be comparable with 1970, as there had been doubts about the completeness of notification. An improvement had occurred following action taken in 1971. There has been no published data quantifying the validity of the material.

#### Publications on abortion

The Registrar General's Statistical Review of England and Wales for 1968 included a supplement on abortion. There was no commentary but explanatory notes and 21 statistical tables. The notification form includes the age of the woman, marital status, number of previous live and stillborn children, the length of gestation period, the area of residence, the occupation of the woman (or her husband if she is married), the statutory grounds on which termination is recorded, the type of premises on which this is performed, the main operation carried out, the length of stay, and the date of operation. These items can be utilized in preparing a range of cross-tabulations.

Since 1974 preliminary information has been published quarterly by OPCS in the *Abortion Monitor Series* (reference AB). This provides relatively quick publication, with limited tables on the number of abortions by place of residence, place of termination and women's age; legal abortions by place of termination and residence in the country by statutory grounds, marital status, parity, and gestation; place of termination for residents and non-residents by region in which pregnancy was terminated; abortions by age of women and country of residence.

More detailed statistics are presented for England and Wales in an annual publication on abortions.

Material is published for Scotland in the Scottish Health Statistics and the Annual Report of the Registrar General for Scotland. This provides one table of trend data since 1970, and a series of tables on numbers (or rates) of abortion by: area of residence and treatment; age and residence; age and marital status; marital status and residence; grounds for termination; complications and method of termination or gestation; gestation and residence; parity and residence.

The Appendix sets out the national publications on abortion.

## Cancer registration

### Background

During the nineteenth century a number of authorities pointed out the drawbacks of mortality data in studying malignant disease and at the beginning of the present century attempts were made to collect cancer morbidity data (for example, Dollinger 1907).

The Ministry of Health in England set up a system in 1923 for the follow-up of patients treated with radium, through the national radium commission. This was based on the premise that statistical information about such patients was essential for planning and operating the cancer care services. The introduction of the NHS in 1948 was accompanied by further reaffirmation of this view, and the move towards a national cancer registration scheme was stimulated by the GRO taking over responsibility for cancer records from the Radium Commission in 1947. Subsequently (Ministry of Health and GRO 1967) it was suggested that studies of epidemiology and the cause of cancer should be considered as additional objectives of cancer registration. Despite the desire for national registration at the introduction of the NHS, it was not until 1962 that all regions in England and Wales became incorporated in the national scheme. A national scheme existed in Scotland since the summer of 1958. In these countries the scheme is voluntary and relies upon co-operation at the clinic and hospital level. The data are organized through regional cancer registries which then forward the material to OPCS in England, the Welsh Office in Wales and then to OPCS, and the Information Services Division of the Common Services Agency in Scotland. A cancer registration scheme was started in Northern Ireland in 1959.

### Validity of cancer registration data

There are three quite different aspects to the validity of the national data: (i) is every patient with malignant disease registered; (ii) are the particulars recorded for each individual accurate; (iii) is the mechanism of follow-up and calculation of survival providing valid survival statistics?

Registration is by a voluntary scheme, relying on co-operation at clinic, hospital, and regional level. Since 1971, patients registered with cancer have been traced and flagged on the NHS Central Register. This permits automatic identification of the fact of death and permits calculation of survival statistics; prior to this the regional registries had to carry out *ad hoc* follow-up at hospital level, or write to GPs. Since 1948 the number of registrations in England and Wales has gradually risen and it is difficult to determine what proportion of this rise is due to extension of the scheme, alteration in the efficiency of registration, or variation in the incidence of malignant disease. Benjamin (1968a) suggested that over the country as a whole it was doubtful whether more than two-thirds of all malignant cases were registered. Some studies have utilized mortality data to check the validity of registration for persons dying from malignant disease; Faulkner *et al.* (1967) suggested that 3.1 per cent of individuals dying from a malignant disease were not known to the registry in Bristol. Alderson (1973) used various sources of records (records held by pathologists, the regional files from the Hospital Activity Analysis (HAA), and death certificates issued for persons dying in the region). Accepting that each of these comparisons were with a biased sample of records, an attempt was made to identify the completeness of the cancer registration system and it was concluded that about 10 per cent of patients might not be registered. A comparable result was obtained by Gillis (1971) examining data for the western region of Scotland.

Methods of organizing the system for cancer registration can have an impact on the overall cancer registration rate. West (1973) and Alderson *et al.* (1976) found that a change from the conventional registration system with clerical staff searching for records independently in hospitals to a system predominantly utilizing HAA resulted in an increase in registration rate. Leck *et al.* (1976) used various sources of information, particularly mortality data, to assess the completeness of the register of childhood tumours. This was in the Manchester region where there was great interest in this topic, and yet they identified deficiencies in numbers of children registered.

Turning to the validity of the items recorded, diagnosis is relatively accurate, but errors and omissions of importance occur with items such as date of registration, place of birth, histology, and occupation (Alderson and Whitehead 1974; West 1976). The level of errors were such that interpretation of the data was feasible, and it appears that the major problem is variation in the completeness of registration, rather than abstraction of particulars for patients that have been identified.

As far as survival statistics are concerned, Silman and Evans (1981) commented on the considerable variation in completeness of registration in different regions and suggested that this might be associated with systematic differences in the prognosis of the registered patients. They questioned whether differences in handling notification of cancer deaths could be a factor but did not specifically indicate all the possible variations in practice. They suggested that when analysing survival, the rates based on post-death registrations should be distinguished from other patients and advocated that the national system should record stage of treatment as a classifying variate (this had been deleted from the national scheme in 1971 as a result of the Advisory Committee Report – OPCS 1970). This issue of potential error in survival statistics has been discussed further in a recent publication of the Cancer Research Campaign (1982).

### Use of cancer registration statistics

At its simplest the aim is to achieve a central register of all patients who develop malignancy. This gives no clear indication of the uses to which such a system might be put. These can be summarized as:

1. Epidemiological studies which may be descriptive, or hypothesis testing.

2. Medical care studies.

3. Studies of survival from malignant disease.

Quite different to the applications of the published statistics, there is continuing opportunity for individuals (research workers and others) to request *ad hoc* analyses from the national files – which may be for descriptive or analytic purposes. A very different category of work is the use of the information about individuals developing malignant disease to serve either as a starting point for retrospective studies or the end-point in historical prospective studies (this issue is beyond the scope of this presentation and has been discussed elsewhere – Alderson 1983*b*).

### Publications on cancer registration data

The Appendix lists the various national published statistics from cancer registration for (i) registrations; (ii) survival. Though Northern Ireland has a register, there have been no publications from this.

## Congenital malformations

### Background

Local schemes for collecting information began in Birmingham (Charles 1951) and in Liverpool in 1960 (Smithells 1962). These two pioneering schemes together covered only about 20 000 births each year, but were sufficient to study the more common abnormalities (for example, spina bifida, anencephaly, and neural tube defects occur in about 30 babies in every 10 000 born).

In part stimulated by the thalidomide epidemic in 1960, the Chief Medical Officer at the Ministry of Health contacted Medical Officers of Health (MOHs) during 1963, to discuss a scheme for notifying congenital malformations. This was launched in 1964 with initial data collection from the doctor or midwife notifying a birth; the informant was asked to include particulars about any identifiable congenital abnormality. This information was forwarded to the appropriate MOH, using the scheme locally that suited them. A standard form was completed in respect of every child with an observable malformation that was identified at birth or found within seven days of birth. Appropriate arrangements were made where the mother was resident outside the area. The MOHs forwarded to the GRO data on infants born to mothers resident in their own areas.

With reorganization of the Health Service a change in the notification system was introduced, the material then being channelled via the Area Medical Officer (AMO) to OPCS. (The further reorganization of the NHS in 1982 has again led to changes in the channel of communication.) The speed of transfer of this material has improved and OPCS now receives about 1200 forms monthly for England and Wales; they are despatched from the local areas about four weeks after the last event to which they relate. The scheme has been described by Weatherall (1978).

### Validity of the congenital malformation data

It must be emphasized that as the aim is to detect 'epidemics' by finding changes in reporting, incompleteness does not affect the value of this work. However, it is obviously of importance to know the degree to which malformations are identified, and also whether the diagnoses are appropriately classified. In order to check on the completeness of notification Weatherall (1969) compared the notification of anencephaly with the number of deaths recorded from this condition. She suggested that there was fairly complete notification, with some variation from one locality to another. A report of the Chief Medical Officer at the DHSS (1972) commented that there had been no further check on completeness since this work.

In Exeter and Devon a more thorough investigation of the child population has indicated that the proportion of malformations found and reported in the national scheme varies with the type of malformation. The levels detected for all but a few internal malformations were thought to be sufficient to expose any increase in incidence (Vowles *et al.* 1975). In a case-control study (Greenberg *et al.* 1977) out of 2867 notifications that were originally sampled, further enquiry by the local health authority indicated that 77 were normal babies who should not have been included. Ericson *et al.* (1977) compared the information provided by (i) specific notifications of congenital malformations, identified at birth, and (ii) computer records of routine birth diagnoses for all infants. Both systems appeared to 'lose' about 20 per cent of the malformed infants, but the quality of diagnostic information was better for the specific notification system and the speed of data transmission was greater.

Nevin *et al.* (1978) compared the system for notifying congenital malformation in Northern Ireland with data recorded in the Child Health System. They found that using data from there and other sources (e.g. autopsy records, the regional spina bifida clinic, and the local association counselling clinics for spina bifida and hydrocephalus) 686 infants with neural tube defects had been identified in 1974–76; 83.6 per cent were identified in the notification system, whilst only 63.3 per cent by the Child Health System.

### Use of congenital malformation statistics

It must be emphasized that the main aim of the scheme is to monitor trends in malformations identified in newborn children – and for this purpose a scheme which collects clinically recognized abnormalities at the time or shortly after birth was thought to be desirable. Waiting for definitive diagnosis, or recognition of congenital malformations that required detailed investigation some while later was not thought to be appropriate. The monitoring takes account of two possible variations – either in one locality over time, or in any given locality compared with the remainder of the country at one point in time. The statistical analyses of the material (see below) are designed to tackle these two different issues.

The data collection system has in addition been found useful for other purposes. It has assisted in planning services for severely disabled children, including the need for special hospital units, hospitals or schools for permanently disabled children, or artificial limb facilities. The material has been utilized to check whether there was a relationship between the incidence of Down's syndrome and fluoride levels in drinking waters (Weatherall 1978). Rather different is the use of the material as a starting point for retrospective enquiries, for example, about the influence of drugs or illness in pregnancy (Greenberg *et al.* 1975, 1977).

*Analyses performed*

There are two quite separate aspects to the analyses, the statistical examination of the material to identify variation in reporting, and the tabulation of data in order to generate the published statistics.

Three main analyses are provided from the data: (i) a tabulation of numbers of babies reported and babies with multiple malformations is sent to each department responsible for forwarding forms to OPCS (i.e. the MOH until 1974, then staff in Area or now District Health Authorities); (ii) the observed numbers of a particular malformation are compared with expected numbers based on the rate for that malformation in the month in the whole of the country – testing whether the rate in one locality is atypical compared with the national statistics for the same period; and (iii) the number of babies with each type of malformation reported is compared with the average number of affected children reported from each area and for each malformation month by month – i.e. checking for an increase in a malformation in a locality compared with previous time periods. If an increase in a malformation in a locality is identified from these analyses, the fact is reported to the local responsible medical staff. Once a given malformation has been identified as increased, the level is reviewed monthly for the following eleven months; if the reporting for that condition in the locality remains significantly higher a new warning should be generated within a further three months.

*Publications of congenital malformation statistics*

England and Wales

Monthly analyses are carried out at area level, regional level, and for the whole of England and Wales. Tables giving summarized information are reported quarterly in a monitor series (MB3 series). A brief introductory text is provided with notes on the tables and this is followed by tables of: numbers of notifications of malformed children by eight major categories of abnormality, quarter of occurrence over the period 1973 to date, with rates per 10 000 live plus stillbirths; malformations, by sex, distinguishing live and stillbirth infants; malformations by Regional and Area Health Authorities (RHA and AHA). The content of tables has varied considerably from issue to issue.

A recent innovation in the statistical analysis has been the examination of occupation. About 60 per cent of notifications recorded a father's or mother's occupation in 1974–79; this permitted examination of the malformation ratios by social class, occupation order, and occupation unit (OPCS 1982*a*). There are problems because: this analysis uses data from two sources (birth registration and malformation notification), proportional analysis was required for the examination of some of the data; and the statistics are based on small numbers and chance fluctuation is a major possibility. It was not thought that parents' knowledge of the child's malformation could influence the information recorded, due to the sources of data and timing of recording (the

occupations were in general derived from obstetric notes and would have been recorded during the pregnancy rather than after the birth of the malformed child).

Special studies

In addition to these routine publications, samples of the notifications are used in conjunction with the Committee on Safety of Medicines (CSM) to explore the potential influence of drug consumption during pregnancy on teratogenicity. As it was felt that the original CSM scheme for reporting of congenital malformations was of limited value (there were only about 50 reports a year submitted), it was decided to mount a case-control study. A pilot in 1969 suggested this was feasible and field work on the main study commenced in 1972. Results from this work have been reported by Greenberg *et al.* (1975, 1977).

International statistics

An informal International Clearing House for Birth Defects Monitoring System (1981) exists, to which England and Wales, and Northern Ireland contribute. In 1976, there were five countries contributing and 20 countries by 1980. Quarterly information is submitted on numbers of total births, and numbers born with each of 11 easily diagnosible malformations. The co-ordinator for the scheme prepares a consolidated report giving baseline rates, incidence rates, and observed/expected ratios for each of the malformations for each country for the period concerned, with graphs of five-year trends (March of Dimes 1982).

Scotland

No scheme equivalent to that in England and Wales for notifying congenital malformations exists in Scotland. A recent study covering an appreciable proportion of mainland Scotland has indicated that useable statistics on the major congenital malformations can be derived from (i) hospital discharge data for neonates, plus (ii) stillbirth registrations. This might be one approach to monitoring trends without a separate congenital malformation notification scheme (Cole, in press).

Northern Ireland

Some material has appeared in the Annual Reports of the Registrar General for Northern Ireland, since 1965.

The national publications of statistics on congenital malformations are listed in the Appendix.

## General household survey

*Background*

From 1945 to 1953 a monthly Survey of Sickness was carried out in England and Wales, questioning a sample of people about their health in the preceding 2–3 months. The sample size was initially 2500 persons aged 16–64 years each month, but increased to 4000 with the addition of those over 64 years.

The final report of the survey (Logan and Brooke 1957) had a considerable section devoted to some of the problems of the survey, with a detailed examination of the bias introduced by the memory factor. This was followed by a general critical appraisal which considered the validity and general usefulness of the data that were obtained. One interesting issue is the comment that the tables that were provided became heavily weighted with data on minor and trivial illness and, in particular, that it was unrewarding to examine for time trends. For example, during the severe influenza epidemic in the first quarter of 1951 the level of reported sickness attained 75 per cent, compared with 71 per cent during the epidemic-free corresponding quarter of the previous year; the increase in morbidity has been 'swamped' by the high level of background minor illness. Apart from the number of comments about interpretation of the data it was emphasized that the surveys' positive contribution was to identify the large amount of ill health which people suffer, that does not lead them to seek medical advice. It was concluded that the main contribution of such a survey should not be to provide a permanent operation identifying the total load of ill health; it was more appropriate, as the need arises, to quantify particular items of information on illness and its effects that cannot be readily obtained in a routine way.

A major alteration occurred in the collection of data in Great Britain, with the initiation of a General Household Survey (GHS) in 1971 (OPCS 1973b). The aim of this survey was to provide a substantially improved flow of social statistics to complement the wide range of routine material currently processed by central government, and to develop an instrument to examine the interaction between different policy areas. The intention was to create a survey that was developed in close collaboration with a number of government departments, such that the material collected was closely linked to their needs for information on five main subject areas (population, housing, employment, education, health, and social services). Consideration of the predominant objective of the survey indicated that a very long interview would be required with all respondents; at the same time there were constraints on resources available. These two factors markedly influenced the study design. It was essential that respondents co-operated willingly in order to obtain the detailed answers called for in the interview.

A nationally representative sample was required and it was initially decided to use a three-stage sampling technique; this operated for 1971–74. The current design is a two-stage rotating one, with electoral wards forming the primary sampling units. The frame of wards is stratified by region, type of area, and two economic indicators (the percentage of heads of households who are in the professional and managerial groups, and who are owner-occupiers). Four wards are selected and allocated to a quarter and then a month, with 672 selections in 1980 (apart from the enhancement for Scotland). Initially the sample was rotating on a quarterly basis, but it is now annual, with one-third of the wards from previous years being replaced by new wards from within the same stratum. The samples have been designed to be representative of the adult population living in private households (i.e. persons over 15 years in 1971 and 1972, and over 16 years in subsequent years). The sampling is similar for the whole of Great Britain, but the number of households contacted is doubled for Scotland in order to provide the minimum of precision thought necessary for separate analysis; since 1978 the supplementary sample in

Scotland has only been questioned on the household schedule. The sampling procedure identifies addresses from the electoral register; the interviewer converts the list of addresses to the identification of households. For addresses containing more than one household, set procedures are used to try to ensure that there is the correct probability of selection of multi-households (see OPCS 1982b). The initial report provided considerable detail on the sampling errors of the survey; further detailed consideration of this appears in the report for 1976 (see OPCS 1978).

This Social Survey uses a detailed structured interview which was tested in pilot trials during the development phase; the interviewers have been carefully trained and supervised. The intention was always to change the items included in the study in response to users' requirements; the main changes in content are discussed by Durant (1978), whilst the impact of some of these changes are reflected in Table 2.2.

The minimum response rate (i.e. completely co-operating households) in 1971 was 71 per cent; including all partial response a maximum rate of 85 per cent was achieved. The figures for 1980 were 70 per cent and 84 per cent, and based on a total effective sample of nearly 14 000 households (excluding the supplementary Scottish sample). There appears to be marked stability in the response rate from month to month, but modest variation across the country. (There was a consistently lower rate in the conurbations and higher rate in the rural areas.) Throughout the reports there are comments on the quality of the information provided. The simplest checks that can be carried out on the data are by comparison with other material or by examination of internal consistency of response. Comparison of the 1971 Survey with 1971 Census data suggested that the GHS provides good representation of the population in private households. (However, an appreciable proportion of the morbidity in the total population is amongst residents in institutions.)

The health section initially collected data on activity limitation caused by sickness, consultations with doctors, use of health and personal social services, and visits to hospitals. In 1980, the following aspects of health were covered (with definitions as listed below):

*Acute sickness* (restriction of the level of normal activity, because of illness or injury, at any time during the two weeks before the interview).

*Chronic sickness* (a two-part question was used 'Do you have any long-standing illness, disability or infirmity?' By long-standing is meant anything that has troubled you over a period of time or is likely to effect you over a period of time. If YES, Does this illness or disability limit your activities in any way? Long-standing illness was defined as a positive answer to the first part of the question, and 'Limiting long-standing illness' as a positive answer to both parts of the question).

*Doctor consultations* (visits to the surgery, home visits, or telephone conversations with NHS GPs in the two weeks before the interview).

*Hospital out-patient attendances* (any attendance at a hospital other than for admission, in the three months preceding the interview).

**Table 2.2.** *Major items covered in the health section of the General Household Survey, Great Britain, 1971–80*

| Item | '71 | '72 | '73 | '74 | '75 | '76 | '77 | '78 | '79 | '80 |
|---|---|---|---|---|---|---|---|---|---|---|
| Chronic sickness | × | × | × | × | × | × | – | – | × | × |
| Cause of illness/disability | × | × | × | × | × | – | – | – | – | – |
| Acute sickness in the past two weeks | × | × | × | × | × | × | – | – | × | × |
| Cause of acute sickness | × | × | × | × | × | – | – | – | – | – |
| Health in general in past twelve months | – | – | – | – | – | – | × | × | × | × |
| GP consultation in past two weeks | × | × | × | × | × | × | × | × | × | × |
| Outpatient attendance in past three months | × | × | × | × | × | × | × | × | × | × |
| Inpatient spells in past three months | × | × | × | × | × | × | – | – | – | – |
| Length of time on waiting list | × | × | × | × | × | × | – | – | – | – |
| Use of various health and welfare services in past month | × | × | × | × | × | × | – | – | (×) | – |
| Difficulty with sight | – | – | – | – | – | – | × | × | × | (×) |
| Difficulty with hearing | – | – | – | – | – | – | × | × | × | (×) |
| Medicines taken in past week | – | ×* | × | – | – | – | – | – | – | – |
| Smoking | – | × | × | × | × | × | – | × | – | × |
| Alcohol consumption in past twelve months | – | – | – | – | – | – | – | × | – | × |

*First quarter only.
(×) Only for the elderly.

Questions about eyesight and hearing were only addressed to those aged 65 years and over in 1980.

An important point to emphasize is that the nature of the GHS provides a powerful analytical tool, by virtue of the ability to cross-tabulate the health data against the wide range of 'social' items collected.

### Validity of general household data

All the material is collected by direct questioning – no independent validation of the data occurs (such as by detailed study of a subsample of the respondents, including medical investigations). The influence of memory bias in probing for events in the past has been indicated above. Obviously some of the general points about validity of surveys to record morbidity statistics apply (see Alderson 1977 for review of this topic).

A Scandinavian study of the validity of health-contact data (Brorsson and Smedby 1982) showed false-positive reporting of 12.8 per cent and false-negative reporting of 13.4 per cent. The mis-classification of reported visits varied with age and self-reported state of health. (It is not known whether this applies equally to a study in the UK.)

### Publications from Survey of Sickness and General Household Survey

Publications from both the Survey of Sickness and the GHS are given in the Appendix to the chapter. The GHS has continued annually since 1971 and data collection covers England and Wales, and Scotland. Table 2.2 indicates the major items covered in the different annual reports (this list is restricted to principle items covered in the health section – the non-health items are identified in Table 2.4).

### Hospital discharge statistics: 'acute' and maternity

There are three main sets of statistics for the morbidity aspects of patient care in hospital. Because of differences in the length of stay, data are handled in a separate system for mentally ill and mentally handicapped patients (see below). For the remainder of hospital discharges, different forms are used for maternity and non-maternity patients.

### Background

A leading article in the *Lancet* (1841) pointed out that data collection on hospital in-patients had been advocated in 1732. Limited progress was made in the nineteenth century, by the Statistical Society (1842, 1844, 1862, 1866). Another notable advocate of collecting and utilizing such data was Florence Nightingale (1863).

Limited progress was made in the UK until the period between the two World Wars, when there was a re-awakening in interest of large scale analysis of hospital statistics (Spear and Gould 1936–37). With the advent of the NHS in 1948, the opportunity arose for more extensive hospital morbidity statistics to be collected. The initial plan envisaged the processing of a sample of patients discharged from hospital, with the items including the patient's name and identification numbers, and the medical data obtained directly from a doctor. The scheme has continued in England and Wales up until the present time with the publication of a set of statistics based on 10 per cent of discharges from all NHS hospitals with the exception of those treating exclusively mental illness, mental subnormality, or convalescent patients. This scheme is jointly organized by the DHSS and OPCS and the Welsh Office (it was formerly the responsibility of the Ministry of Health and GRO). With the exception of private and staff patients treated for minor ailments, those patients for whom an in-patient case record has been opened and for whom the usual admission procedure has been completed are liable to be selected for the sample. The sample consists of one in ten such patients. New-born infants, born in hospital, are only included if they are admitted to a special care baby unit. Maternity patients, because of their rather different health care situation, have a different form completed; the data relating to maternity patients is processed and published separately (discussed above).

In the overwhelming majority of cases, the information in the non-maternity system is derived from the Hospital Activity Analysis (HAA), whereby information is collected under agreed national headings, together with items of local interest which are processed on a regional basis to provide management and clinical information for use by health authorities (see Benjamin 1965, for original description of this scheme). The RHAs then generally submit a tape of sample records to OPCS for processing. The data from the maternity system come from three different sources – 20 per cent from the national maternity HAA scheme in selected hospitals, about 20 per cent from other local detailed schemes, and about 60 per cent from submission of forms completed for a 10 per cent sample of patients.

The non-maternity form consists of personal and demographic, administrative, and medical data. The personal and demographic data provides: sex, marital status, date of birth, area of residence, industry and occupation (not submitted centrally), and number of previous pregnancies (for abortion cases only). The administrative particulars include date on the waiting list, date of admission, date of discharge or death (and thus duration of stay), source of admission (waiting list, booked or planned, deferred, immediate), category of patient (NHS, private, convalescent, staff, day case), type of bed, specialty in which care is provided (at admission and discharge), disposal, and for patients who have had an accident, the place of accident. The brief medical particulars include the main condition treated together with other relevant conditions; for those patients having an operation up to four operations are recorded (with the principal one designated), the date of this, and the other operations if performed, and a count of the number of visits to the theatre. It is possible to identify patients who have been transferred between departments in the same hospital, but the material does not provide adequate information for linkage of repeat admissions to the same patient (this issue is discussed further in a later section on linkage of repeat events).

A recent extension has been the inclusion of 'day-case' patients into the system (i.e. patients coming for investigation, treatment, or operation who occupy a bed on a non-resident basis).

### Scottish hospital in-patient statistics

A somewhat different scheme is operated in Scotland, initially by the Home and Health Department and now by the Information Services Division of the Common Services Agency. The principal differences are that: (i) the information is collected nationally on a 100 per cent basis; and (ii) there has been the development of a facility for assembling a linked file of repeat admissions occurring to the same patients (Heasman and Clarke 1979). The issues of linked or linkable files is discussed below.

### Northern Ireland

A scheme of HAA covers over half the admissions to hospitals other than maternity, mental illness, and mental subnormality in Northern Ireland.

### Maternity system

In England and Wales the enquiry covers all NHS hospitals exclusively treating maternity patients (whether consultant obstetric or GP maternity), and consultant obstetric departments or GP maternity departments in other NHS hospitals. It excludes gynaecology and thus normally does not include admissions for abortion or other conditions of early pregnancy (these should be sampled in the non-maternity scheme). It should be comprehensive for all discharges and deaths whether from in-patients or day cases from obstetric departments and GP maternity units. The particulars available again cover patient, administrative, and medical items. The additional items in the maternity system are (i) for the mother: date of last menstrual period, previous pregnancies (live births, stillbirths, and abortions), for diagnoses of both antenatal or general medical conditions, particulars of delivery and its complications, complications during the puerperium, mode of delivery, onset of labour including induction, date of delivery, and delivery or other operative procedures, presentation, analgesia or anaesthesia, episiotomy, sterilization; and (ii) for the infant: sex, birthweight, transfer to special care, outcome of care, diseases or congenital abnormality, infant feeding (with a facility to record separate items if multiple births occur). The items available at local/regional level from HAA or other systems differ slightly from this list.

Comparable material is collected in the Scottish system, which is on a 100 per cent basis. As over 99 per cent of all births in Scotland occur in hospital this provides a virtually complete picture of obstetric work in the country. The maternity system used in England and Wales has been described in greater detail by Ashley (1980) and that for Scotland by Cole (1980).

### Validity of hospital discharge data

Alderson and Meade (1967) compared the accuracy of hospital discharge data with mortality statistics for patients who had died in hospital; they suggested there were appreciable errors in the principal condition treated for about 13 per cent of completed forms. Before studying the seasonal variation in admissions to Scottish hospitals, Dunnigan et al. (1970) examined 1093 records where the discharge diagnosis had been coded to 'heart disease specified as involving coronary arteries'. Sixty five per cent were judged to be unequivocal myocardial infarction and 27 per cent myocardial ischaemia. In the majority of patients their diagnoses had been the primary reason for admission. More recently Lockwood (1971) demonstrated that there was a high degree of accuracy in the Scottish material. Other studies on the accuracy of such data have produced a range of opinions: McNeilly and Moore (1975) observed appreciable errors in diagnosis and operation codes for a small sample of Welsh patients; Patel et al. (1976) suggested there were a considerable proportion of errors in Scottish morbidity data (in contrast to the earlier work of Lockwood), but Parkin et al. (1976) seriously questioned some of the conclusions of Patel and his colleagues; Martini et al. (1976) quantified the errors in demographic and medico-administrative items for patients treated in the Nottingham area and pointed out that the statistics are almost as good as the clinical notes from which they are derived (these results were very similar to those of Lockwood); Cameron et al. (1977) contrasted autopsy findings with data from the medical records and indicated that fresh findings might arise at autopsy that were not incorporated in the Scottish statistical system.

Rees (1982) utilized operation records and ward admission books to identify patients with proximal femoral fracture in five hospitals in the Newcastle region. Comparison with HAA output showed wide variation between the hospitals in the accuracy of HAA, such that between area comparisons of HAA statistics for this condition were quite misleading. It appeared that failure to insert diagnostic information on the form, HMR1, and inaccurate coding led to these errors.

Whates et al. (1982) compared surgical unit and patient records with printouts from HAA for Hope Hospital, Salford. For patients having proctocolectomy or splenectomy there was a higher proportion of errors of coding of the operation – though the medical staff had completed the operation details on the HMR1, and consultants had checked all entries. About 40–50 per cent of the codes were erroneous, indicating the difficulty of using this source of information.

Stimulated by these papers, Hole (1982) and Crawshaw and Moss (1982) both quoted appreciable error rates for HAA operative data; only limited details were provided of their investigations. Crawshaw and Moss indicate that the relative discrepancy between HAA and operation records for fracture of the proximal femur had decreased in the period 1972–80 in Leicester. Butts and Williams (1982) questioned the rather general conclusions reached by both Rees (1982) and Whates et al. (1982). They presented data for East Anglia for resection of the colon and/or rectum, and splenectomy; 70 per cent of the former and 100 per cent of the latter were correctly coded in this HAA system. They stress that the operation index should be used with caution and suggest steps to improve the quality of the data.

A recent paper, produced as a by-product of the review of health services information in England and Wales, 'Converting Data into Information' (Körner Committee 1982) suggests that external audit procedures (of the quality of data) be set up, organized at a regional level, involving personnel from region and districts – other than that being reviewed.

In checking the validity of Scottish maternity data, Cole (1980) identified some clerical misconceptions from internal inconsistency in the computer-held data: some clerks mistook 'admitted in early labour' for premature labour, whilst others were consistently recording induction when mothers had been admitted in labour but had rupture of membranes performed or oxytocics given in labour. In a comparison between the statistical return and research data abstracted from 1000 records there was close agreement (97–98 per cent) on factual items such as past obstetric history, but about 70 per cent of discrepancies on items such as 'certainty of gestation'.

Goldacre (1981) discussed a range of problems and pitfalls in interpreting hospital in-patient statistics. He indicated that it was difficult to gauge the completeness of ascertainment (as the SH3 returns did not provide a perfect benchmark). He identified problems concerning studies of: (i) discharge rates

(errors in the numerator or denominator; age/sex effects; repeat events in individuals; consistency or short-term effects, such as, industrial disputes; patient attitudes to care; availability of resources; variation in disease frequency or clinical practice); (ii) length of stay (coding errors of diagnosis; age/sex effects; transfer facilities; variation in case-mix; fatality rates; availability of resources; clinical practice); (iii) hospital fatality (variation of 'admission' of patients dying shortly after arrival; documentation of records of fatal cases; differences in diagnostic criteria and clinical severity; age/sex differences; transfer policies; length of stay; readmission rates; mortality prior to admission; variation in clinical facilities).

### Use of hospital discharge data

These data can be used for management and planning at local and regional level – which may involve examination of inter-regional transfers, examination of comparisons of statistics for different regions, or special studies requiring large numbers – for example when looking at trends the regional data may be insufficient but aggregation at national level might suffice (see Wall and Cross 1968; McNay 1969; Wall and Wharton 1970; and Kemp et al. 1971).

Another main use of the statistics is for management and planning by central government, an issue that has been described at some length by Ashley (1972), and Rowe and Brewer (1972).

Rather different is the use of the data to monitor the health of the public, where the discharge statistics may be utilized as an 'indicator' of the distribution of disease in the community. This may facilitate examination of variation in the distribution of the disease, by characteristics of the subject, by locality, or over time. Such data are predominantly of value for descriptive studies or hypothesis generation, rather than for analytical and aetiological studies, due to the innate differences between directly measured incidence or prevalence of disease in a community and the indication given by hospital treated disease (this issue is discussed further in Alderson and Dowie 1979).

### Linkage of repeat events

Reference has already been made to the power contributed by record linkage event data (see p. 25); this general concept applies equally to linkage of morbidity records. Acheson (1967) has described the history of medical record linkage and the pioneering efforts in the Oxford Region in assembling a cumulative record of hospital admissions in the population. He indicated the system used, and the medical care and other epidemiological studies that could be facilitated by such work. The only element of linkage that occurs in England and Wales with morbidity records is the tracing of individuals with cancer registered in the NHS Central Register, so as to identify deaths that occur and permit calculation of survival rates (see p. 27).

The medical record linkage facility developed in Scotland has been described by Heasman and Clarke (1979). The objects are: (i) to provide economical collection of events occurring to an individual to permit statistical analysis; (ii) to enable individuals to be followed-up; and (iii) to produce person-based statistics. The Scottish system, which uses unlinked records for health statistics, includes: (i) general hospital discharge records from 1968; (ii) obstetric discharge records from 1970; (iii) mental and mental deficiency hospital admissions and discharges from 1963; (iv) cancer registrations from 1968; (v) school entrant and leaver medical examinations from 1967; (vi) handicapped children's register from 1973; and (vii) death and stillbirth registrations from 1968. An important point is that for any particular project a linked file is created limited to the appropriate records; the system contains linkable records but only assembles a linked file for a particular (restricted) purpose. Examples are given of the uses for epidemiological and health services research, and for follow-up of specific groups of individuals. Though the intention is to facilitate production of person-based statistics, these have yet to be published as a routine; however, it is thought that this would enable examination, for example, of length of stay for either consecutive spells in different hospitals or multiple admissions into the same hospital. The authors stress the importance of considering the issues of privacy and steps taken to ensure confidentiality of the data.

### Publication of hospital discharge data

The Appendix sets out the routine publications that have appeared for patients treated in hospitals in England and Wales, and Scotland, distinguishing (i) 'acute' and (ii) maternity. No equivalent central government data are published by Northern Ireland.

## Hospital in-patients in psychiatric units and hospitals

### Background

From 1949 to 1960, an individual patient return was sent to the GRO for each admission to, departure from, and death in the main designated hospitals for patients with mental disorder. Over the period 1948–60 the Ministry of Health also collected returns from psychiatric hospitals on the number of patients suffering from mental disorder and the services available. Following the Mental Health Act 1959, the Ministry of Health undertook the collection of psychiatric statistics for general planning and administrative purposes on an individual-patient basis. The enquiry conducted by the GRO, which was designed primarily to contribute to medical knowledge and to help medical research workers continued in a modified form. From 1964, the two sets of statistics were combined into the Mental Health Enquiry (MHE) under the responsibility of the Ministry of Health and all NHS psychiatric hospitals and units were brought into the scheme. The entry of data on admission permits analyses of 'hospital residents', which is appropriate for certain aspects of psychiatric care. In Northern Ireland the data are collected as part of the general statistics on hospital in-patients.

### Validity of data on patients in psychiatric hospitals

The general points raised under the discussion on acute hospital in-patients are potentially relevant to the topic of mental health patients. Forster and Mahadevan (1981) checked the validity of 824 records in the north of England against data inserted in the MHE forms. There were discrepancies for:

source of referral (20.5 per cent), diagnosis (14.8 per cent), outcome (10.8 per cent), previous psychiatric care (6.3 per cent); all others (< 3.0 per cent).

A rather different issue is that the aim of the MHE is to link admission and discharges, and facilitate linkage of repeat admissions for individuals by holding named data for discrete events at central level. This issue created concern about confidentiality of patient data, and over the past few years an increasing proportion of psychiatrists or psychiatric hospitals and units have declined to submit named data to the scheme, though continuing to provide anonymized particulars for subjects admitted to hospital.

### Publications of national statistics on hospital in-patients in psychiatric units and hospitals

The available publications are set out in the Appendix.

## Morbidity statistics from general practice

### Background

A pilot study was launched in 1951 to test a method for collecting and analysing medical records kept by a small number of GPs. The interim conclusion from this work (Logan 1953) was that it was possible, without exceptional difficulty, to keep records over a 12 month period that were suitable for analysis. Various methods of recording were favoured by different doctors, but a specially modified NHS continuation card seemed most suitable. This study was extended for a further two years with data being collected from 1952–54. The Royal College of General Practitioners (RCGP) declared an interest in this topic, and in conjunction with the GRO agreed to launch a morbidity study. This occurred from 1955–56, involving 171 doctors and 106 practices in England and Wales. All used a standard method for recording limited particulars for each patient contact including: identification particulars of the individual, date of birth, diagnosis, date of consultation, and date of admission to hospital if this occurred. The results from this work appeared in three volumes (Logan and Cushion 1958; Logan 1960; Research Committee of the RCGP 1962).

A further national study of morbidity statistics from general practice was carried out in 1970–71, with the aim of collecting mobidity data from general practice that was compatible with the 1955–56 study (RCGP et al. 1974). In addition to collecting morbidity information, particulars about use of facilities both in the community and hospital were recorded, and the patients' consultation patterns were identified. For each episode of care, the date of first consultation, the episode type, the name, and date of birth were recorded; up to six face-to-face consultations could be coded on the same line of the record sheet with continuation if required. Referral to other agencies was also identified. Fifty-four practices were initially involved, though one withdrew during the survey. Unlike the previous study, diagnostic and other information was coded at practice level rather than centrally. The RCGP classification was used for coding the morbidity; this was derived initially from the 7th revision of the ICD, but modified to conform to the 8th revision.

A number of other studies from general practice have

collected data on contact with patients; these vary from pioneer efforts where individual doctors or groups of doctors have invested effort to codify material on the patients they see, up to major collaborative studies, such as that carried out by 68 doctors in South Wales in 1965–66 (Williams 1970).

### Validity of the data

A vital element in such studies is the count of the number of individuals on the doctor's NHS practice list, and the age distribution of these subjects; this is required as the denominator in calculating rates. Lees and Cooper (1963) identified problems of definition, inflation, and net change in practice list. The first national morbidity survey had an inflation of 1.1 per cent, though this was reduced to 0.7 per cent on investigation. Other studies have identified variation of 20 per cent (Backett *et al.* 1954), and 14 per cent (Morrell *et al.* 1970). Less extreme variation was found by Fraser (1978), and Fraser and Clayton (1981).

Another issue is the extent to which contact with a GP indicates the prevalence of morbidity in the population. A number of studies have indicated that there is a varying degree of self-care and undetected disease (Horder and Horder 1954; Last 1963; Kessel and Shepherd 1965; Cartwright 1967; Wadsworth *et al.* 1971).

Equally important is the validity of data recording. The accuracy of the analyses depends on the errors in capture, coding, and processing of the material. This has been discussed by Morrell and his colleagues in a series of papers (Morrell 1972; Morrell *et al.* 1970, 1971; Morrell and Kasap 1972; Morrell and Nicholson 1974), Clarke and Bennett (1971), Dawes (1972), Munroe and Ratoff (1973), and Farmer *et al.* (1974). Other aspects of data validity and coding accuracy have been investigated by Kay (1968) and also by Hannay (1972).

In the second morbidity study the validity of the practice registers was checked, indicating a true inflation of about 1.1 per cent (RCGP *et al.* 1974). An attempt was made to check the morbidity data, which indicated some diagnostic problems and variation between the practices; coding errors resulted in only marginal variation in the morbidity that was recorded. It appeared that about 3.5 per cent of consultations and 2.4 per cent of episodes recorded on practice records were not on the computer records, whilst 0.35 per cent of the events on the computer file could not be identified in the practice notes. There was no independent check of the diagnostic labels used as · specific contacts in any of the practices. The effect of different sysems of classification has been examined by Martini *et al.* (1976), who highlighted the contrast between presenting problems and underlying morbidity.

Such studies involve volunteer GPs and it is not known how typical these are, but Crombie (1973) has suggested that the diagnostic patterns and differences in the case-mix that a family doctor draws towards him can have some influence. However, he suggested that provided the number of doctors is sufficiently large, the overall population that is served approximates closely to the general population. A report (RCGP *et al.* 1979) examines some of the characteristics of the practices' participating in the Second Survey and concludes that morbidity rates were likely to vary in relation to the location of the practice, size of partnership, doctors' age, and availability of ancillary staff.

Using census schedules for the enumeration districts that represented the catchment areas of the practices, a computer matching was carried out without access to full names of the subjects in the study (RCGP *et al.* 1982). The non-matches from the age-sex registers were then examined clerically and possible matches added to the computer file. This resulted in about 65–75 per cent initial matches for most practices and up to a further 20 per cent added by the clerical exercise; the number of enumeration districts was extended for the few practices with a low match rate. The final proportion of the practice register population that could be matched was 78 per cent.

This exercise facilitated a check of the representativeness of the study sample. The matched sample showed some deviation from the characteristics of the total study sample: men and women were slightly under-represented in older age groups, and in the widowed and divorced; Social Classes I, II, III non-manual, and those in owner occupied housing were over-represented. It was concluded that these differences were insufficient to introduce bias such that the consultation rates of the census matched sample were appreciably distorted. It must be remembered that among the GPs that volunteered there was a slight excess from practices with more than four principles, large list sizes, and younger doctors, and of those practising from health centres, or with ancillary help.

The second facet of this linkage exercise was to relate census variates to morbidity rates. Tabulations are presented on morbidity in relation to population characteristics (marital status, country of birth, urban/rural residence); social class (for 179 diagnostic groups), 29 occupation orders (for 18 diagnostic groups); housing tenure and household amenities (for 18 diagnostic groups).

### Publications

Publications of mobidity statistics from general practice are given in the Appendix.

## Notification of infectious diseases

### Background

Compulsory notification of infectious disease was first introduced in England and Wales in Huddersfield in 1876; many other towns soon obtained local powers. This applied to London, through the Infectious Diseases Notification Act of 1889. This Act gave a list of diseases which were to be notified and laid down how, when, and by whom they were to be notified. The original object of the Act was to provide powers to combat 'dangerous infectious disorders'. In 1895, the Registrar General first included in his *Weekly Return* the numbers of cases of five infectious diseases which had been admitted to certain London hospitals. Compulsory notification was extended to all sanitary authorities throughout England and Wales in 1899. Prior to 1922, the Ministry of Health compiled an unpublished document based on a weekly summary of returns from sanitary authorities. The Registrar General's *Weekly Return* continued to include information about infectious diseases notified by the Metropolitan Asylum

Board and the London Fever Hospital. In about 1920 proposals were made for publication of the material handled by the Ministry of Health, and the first issue of this was in January 1922. This was based on provisional weekly returns supplied by MOHs; these statistics were subject to amendment and did not show numbers of patients with infectious diseases by sex or age. In 1943, Stocks suggested that the MOH should submit quarterly returns, which would contain the corrected figures grouped by sex and age, although this was not a statutory requirement, the material was provided (Registrar General 1949).

A number of changes have occurred in the system over time, with revision of the documents for submission of the weekly and quarterly data, and revision of the list of notifiable diseases. The following infections are presently notifiable: acute encephalitis, acute meningitis, acute poliomyelitis, anthrax, cholera, diphtheria, dysentery (amoebic or bacillary), food poisoning (all sources), infective jaundice, Lassa fever, leprosy, leptospirosis, malaria, Marburg disease, measles, ophthalmia neonatorum, paratyphoid fever, plague, rabies, relapsing fever, scarlet fever, smallpox, tetanus, tuberculosis, typhoid fever, typhus, viral haemorrhagic fever, whooping cough, and yellow fever. In 1974, the statutory provisions were changed with reorganization of local government and the NHS; Medical Officers of Environmental Health (MOEHs) took over the duty of submitting weekly and quarterly returns. At the same time the formation of a national communicable disease centre was advocated and subsequently resulted in the establishment of the Communicable Disease Surveillance Centre (CDSC) of the Public Health Laboratory Service (PHLS).

The notification of infectious disease forms have recently been altered (OPCS 1981b); in addition to the pooled data for notifiable disease, there is a new form for entering particulars of individual patients by disease code, providing sex, age in years or months if under one, specificity for subgroups of certain diseases, the facility for correction of the data, and supplementary information. The intention is that these weekly log sheets on individual subjects will be processed by computer to provide periodic statistics but still clerically manipulating the pooled data to produce the *Weekly Return*. The MOEHs will continue to submit quarterly correction forms, with details relating to (unnamed) individuals; these will be used to adjust the summed data for the constituent weeks in any quarter.

The RCGP became interested in collecting data from selected practices, including contact with the patients with various infectious diseases and other conditions, in the late 1960s (RCGP 1968). The College's Research Unit runs a surveillance system which consolidates data on a weekly basis of returns from 84 GPs in 41 practices with a population of about 200 000 patients. It is acknowledged that these practices are not evenly spread throughout the country (they are predominantly concentrated in or near large conurbations); the data are based on clinical diagnosis for most of the patients.

Though the legislation is different for Scotland (being based on the Infectious Disease (Notification) Act, 1889), the present list of notifiable diseases is comparable. The differences being that in Scotland continued fever, erysipelas, and puerperal fever are notifiable but not acute encephalitis or tetanus which

are on the list for England and Wales. The Chief Administrative Medical Officers of health boards are responsible for submitting weekly and annual returns. There has been a Communicable Disease Unit in existence since 1969 in Glasgow.

### Validity of notification of infectious diseases

The validity of statistics from notification have periodically been questioned. Stocks (1949) compared notification statistics with data from the Survey of Sickness and various research reports on incidence or cumulative attack rates. He suggested that completeness varied with the illness, from fairly complete notification of acute poliomyelitis to only fractional notification of dysentery. A discussion by Taylor (1965) has indicated that a number of western countries have variable completion of notification of infectious disease, and for some milder infections notification is poor. The statistics he quoted provided estimates of the shortfall in notification, but agreed estimates of this are not regularly published. This issue has also been discussed by Benjamin (1968b).

A study from general practice (Haward 1973) suggested that there was substantial under-reporting of certain infectious diseases.

Lambert (1973) used Hospital Inpatient Enquiry (HIPE) data to cross-check the statistics from notification of meningococcal infection. Assuming that the hospital data provide a fairly reliable estimate of the total number of cases, he suggested that notifications identify about half of the total. Goldacre and Miller (1976) used a variety of sources of information to study notification of acute bacterial meningitis in children in one hospital region in 1969–73. They concluded that only half the cases of meningococcal and less than a quarter of other types of bacterial meningitis had been notified.

Stewart (1980) suggested there was strong circumstantial evidence to question the validity of whooping cough notification, partly due to confusion with infection from various respiratory viruses. He pointed out (Stewart 1981), that 18 per cent of the practitioners in Glasgow notified all the whooping cough cases reported in 1977–79, with over a third of the cases being reported by 2 per cent of the practitioners. In addition, many of the patients admitted to hospital were not notified.

Davies *et al.* (1981) identified a number of problems with notification of tuberculosis, including duplicate notifications, changes in diagnosis, posthumous registration, and definition of respiratory disease. They concluded that the OPCS statistics had an impressive level of accuracy, which they estimated as being within 10 per cent. Possible solutions were discussed for some of the problems.

Though influenza is not one of the notifiable diseases, it is an infection in which there is considerable interest in identifying epidemics. Tillett and Spencer (1981) discussed the surveillance of routine statistics in England and Wales, and as part of their study they indicated that as an epidemic occurred the use of the term influenza in death certification changed. They suggested that initially there was under-certification until it became common knowledge that an epidemic was in progress. As the epidemic waned there still might be a tendency to certify and possibly over-certification occurred. The absolute numbers of deaths ascribed to influenza might be correct, though this was due to initial under-certification and later over-certification. It is plausible that the same type of change in practice may occur with other acute infectious diseases, and thus the rise and fall in reported numbers may be incorrectly timed, though whether the overall reporting approximates to the correct figure is not clear. It is impossible to cross-check this information from laboratory reports, because of the very biased referral for investigation of appropriate specimens. Where the infection is only rarely fatal, there is no chance of cross-checking the statistics from notification and mortality.

When using notification to monitor progress of an epidemic, it must be remembered that Bank Holidays result in a fall in the count of weekly notifications (of 15–30 per cent), which may not be completely made up in the succeeding weeks.

### Use of notifications of infectious disease statistics

A general aspect of notification of infectious disease is that it should enable the identification of trends in the infectious disease. In particular there has been emphasis on 'monitoring' epidemics. The direct notification at local level is used to facilitate control, whilst the aggregation of national statistics is used to identify the health care and manpower problems of epidemics. A particular aspect of this work is the potential for predicting the size of an epidemic as early as possible during the course of an epidemic. For example, Spicer (personal communication, 1982) applied Kermak and McKendrick modelling to influenza mortality in Greater London.

A rather separate activity of examining trends in infectious disease is to evaluate the effectiveness and efficiency of preventive campaigns (by relating the trend in disease to the trend in uptake of preventive measures).

For some diseases, such as tuberculosis, the more detailed study of the material may be used as one facet of the epidemiological examination of the condition (see for example, Joint Tuberculosis Committee of the British Thoracic Association 1982).

### Publications of national statistics on notification of infectious disease

In England and Wales there are three series of publications at present – weekly, quarterly, and annual. The weekly monitor (which is still titled the Registrar General's *Weekly Return for England and Wales* and identified by the serial WR) includes: notifications of 29 infectious diseases and deaths from certain of these for the preceding six weeks in England and Wales; notifications in the current week in England and Wales, standard regions, administrative areas, and health districts; and newly diagnosed episodes of communicable and respiratory disease giving weekly numbers and rates, from returns from 40 general practices. (Sickness absence is discussed in a later section.) These statistics are handled manually and it is presently thought the computing system could not generate the data with adequate speed.

Corrected data are provided in the quarterly report; this also includes data from the CDSC, with four tables on the laboratory identification of various diseases for England and Wales and RHAs.

The annual publication appears in the series '*Communicable Disease Statistics*'; this provides an appreciable number of tables on infectious disease. There is some data on trends for the preceding (11) years, data on notification and deaths for selected causes for the country and various local areas.

An innovation in 1979 was the drafting of the commentary in the annual report by the staff from the CDSC. In addition this Centre also publishes a weekly and a quarterly report on communicable disease, with data obtained from hospital laboratories and the PHLS. The data refer to specific episodes of infection with bacterial confirmation, often providing background discussion of some detail of particular cases of interest.

In Scotland a weekly report, *Communicable Diseases Scotland* is produced by the Communicable Diseases (Scotland) Unit. This contains counts of notifications of infectious diseases and food poisoning by health board area, and 'current notes' on particular topics of interest. Figures also appear in the weekly return of the Registrar General, Scotland. Annual figures appear in the Scottish health statistics.

The statistics published for England and Wales, Scotland and Northern Ireland are listed in the Appendix.

## Occupational disease and injury

There has been in the past a long sequence of reports from the Chief Inspector of Factories, and more recently statistics are published by the Health and Safety Executive. The two main categories of event that are recorded are: industrial poisoning or disease that is notifiable under the Factories Act (1961); and injuries occurring at work. In addition to these two sources of data other particulars are recorded, that are relevant to other legislation: agricultural accidents notifiable under the Agriculture (Safety, Health and Welfare Provisions) Act (1956); the Explosives Act (1875); the Mines and Quarries Act (1954); the Mineral Workings (Offshore Installations) Act (1971); and Railways (Notice of Accidents) Order (1965).

Data on industrial disease or poisoning published recently include: (i) statistics on deaths and notifications of disease from lead poisoning, other poisoning, anthrax, epithelioma, chrome ulceration; (ii) estimates of the deaths and injuries from a 5 per cent sample of all reported industrial injury classified under 25 types; and (iii) the number of injuries by site, whether or not they were severe, place, and reasons for the injury. Other unpublished statistics are available on special request.

### Merchant seamen

The Department of Trade (1982) produces annual statistics on accidents to men in vessels registered in the UK. The main part of the report relates to merchant vessels, but other material are provided for crew on fishing vessels. The data present deaths by cause, and accidents occurring at sea. It should be noted that the deaths of seamen occurring ashore are excluded, even if they follow an accident at sea – because such deaths should be processed by the normal mortality statistics system.

## Publications

The Appendix gives the recent series published by the Health and Safety Executive.

## Sickness absence

### Background

The National Insurance Act of 1946 provided for the compulsory insurance of everybody between school-leaving and retirement age with the exception of married women, and a few other particular categories such as civil servants. This system provided, for the first time, the base for collecting national data on sickness absence. From statistics sheets completed for a sample of insured persons who were incapacitated, particulars have been recorded of the individual (for example, date of birth, sex, marital status), particulars about the spell (whether for sickness or injury), the duration, whether the spell was linked with another period of illness, injury, or unemployment, and the reason for termination of the spell). Limited medical particulars were available on the diagnosis obtained from the final medical certificate, or the nature and site of injury for an industrial injury.

These data are handled by the DHSS, where the central office at Newcastle is responsible for coding and statistical analysis of the material obtained from the individual local offices.

### Validity of sickness absence statistics

Apart from any direct influence of occupation on health it has been suggested (Alderson 1967) that incapacity rates in the current British situation may be influenced by: the place of residence of the worker, the environment and availability of medical care, the multiple processes of selection into and out of occupation, the physical and psychological demands of the job, the financial and social consequences of declared illness, the completeness of notification of incapacity, the unemployment situation, the morale within an industry, and perhaps other little understood factors. In certain circumstances the certifier will deliberately not disclose the disease; for example, there was clear evidence of gross under-certification of malignant disease in contrast to the hospital discharge statistics and mortality for this condition for people of working age.

### Publications of sickness absence statistics

From 1950 the annual reports of the Ministry of Pensions and National Insurance (subsequently the Ministry of Social Security and then the Department of Health and Social Security – DHSS), provided some information about sickness absence in England, Wales, and Scotland. Tabulations were provided for spells of incapacity, spells commencing, spells current, and total days in the period, by sex and by cause. For a number of years this information was amplified periodically by a more detailed digest of statistics which was available from the statistics division of the Ministry of Health. This incorporated a detailed statistical breakdown and was available to research workers and others interested in public health.

This material was based on a sample of the insured popula-

tion (5 per cent at one time and then 2.5 per cent). It provided detailed information about spells of incapacity, with tabulation by cause, age of the individual, and duration of spell. The data were coded to the ICD and an appropriate list used which predominantly gave data by 140 different causes (these being selected in relation to the numbers incapacitated for different causes).

A special enquiry was carried out in 1961–62. For the 5 per cent sample of insured persons involved in the usual statistical sample, a special request was made to the employers asking for details of the occupation carried out by each individual. This information was used to provide occupational denominator data in calculating sickness absence statistics for the matched certificates of these persons having spells of incapacity lasting four days or more. Two reports of this study were published by the Ministry of Pensions and National Insurance (1965, 1966). Over half a million men were included in the sample and 28 per cent recorded incapacity for at least four days during the year. The data were presented by disease group, region of the country, and occupation. For the first time data were thus available for incapacity by 26 causes for 25 different occupation orders. A specific analysis was also carried out on incapacity in relation to measured air pollution; this permitted examination, for example, of bronchitis incapacity in relation to both the smoke and sulphur dioxide content in high density residential areas. The OPCS *Weekly Monitor* provides counts of new claims for (i) sickness and invalidity benefits, and (ii) injury benefit for England and Wales and the standard regions.

In Scotland sickness and invalidity rates for 25 causes of incapacity are tabulated for (i) days of incapacity, and (ii) numbers of spells per 1000 population each year. Some statistics on new claims also appear in the weekly return of the Registrar General, Scotland.

Limited data are available for Northern Ireland. In addition to the annual publications, a special survey on the statistics from the National Insurance Scheme was prepared by Park and Kidd (1958).

These various national publications are given in the Appendix.

## THE DETERMINANTS OF DISEASE

In studying the health of the community it is important to have access to data on various factors that are thought to be associated with variation in the risk of disease. This section discusses a variety of social and behavioural factors, and environmental statistics that relate to such 'risk'. This is not the place to consider the role that the following factors play, but they are provided as an indication of the source of information about the community – information that can be related to variation in incidence, prevalence, or mortality from various diseases. The coverage is restricted to statistics that are available as a routine at national level, or provide estimates of the national situation.

Two series are referred to in several sections below: (i) the Annual Abstract of Statistics, and (ii) Social Trends. These are both prepared by the Central Statistical Office and published by HMSO; they both incorporate statistics from a wide range of primary sources. They deserve study to identify the detail available directly from current volumes; the topics covered include many social and environmental aspects that are relevant to the populations' health. The following notes refer to sections of these publications that are particularly likely to be of interest, indicating where time series are immediately available.

## Social and behavioural factors

### The census

The decennial census collects information about household composition; household amenities; the educational level of all those who have left school; the occupation of those who are presently employed, temporarily out of work, or retired; migration within the UK; birth outside the UK; and other minor aspects such as travel to work. Table 2.3 sets out in slightly greater detail the information that has been collected from each of the decennial censuses.

### General Household Survey (GHS)

The GHS has already been described, because of the information collected in the health section of this survey (see pp. 29–31). However, as explained, the GHS covers many other topics. Table 2.4 sets out the material that has been collected in each of the surveys from 1971–80, by broad category. It will be seen that the topics overlap with material collected at census, including demographic particulars about population, some information about housing, employment, education, and family formation. Other items, such as particulars about income, burglaries, and theft are very different from issues explored in the census.

### Nutrition

There are two main routine sources of information about the nutrition of the population. A National Food Survey is carried out, and also information from the Family Expenditure Survey (FES) is utilized to quantify expenditure on food.

The National Food Survey is derived from records provided by a sample of private households in Great Britain; it aims to collect data on food entering the house for human consumption, but does not cover the consumption of soft drinks, alcohol, chocolate, sugar, or confectionery. It also has the important defect that meals bought outside the house and consumed away from the house are not considered. The survey is based on multistage sampling to provide locations stratified by standard region and electoral density. In 1979 there were 15 226 addresses initially identified, but for various reasons only about 13 700 were suitable for the survey. Information suitable for analysis was obtained from 6832 households (that is 50 per cent of the initial sample or 60 per cent of the contacted sample). Each house was visited and a log book provided; this was used to record the quantity of food entering the household during the survey period, and also the meals served throughout the week and the persons present for each meal. The main analyses cover consumption for 19 items of food intake and give the nutrient values for: region, type of area, income, household, age of housewife, and housing tenure. The statistics are presented per person, as a percentage of recommended intake, and per thousand calories.

**Table 2.3.** *Various items collected in the population censuses in Great Britain, 1801–1981*

| Item | 1801 | 1811 | 1821 | 1831 | 1841 | 1851 | 1861 | 1871 | 1881 | 1891 | 1901 | 1911 | 1921 | 1931 | 1951 | 1961 | 1971 | 1981 |
|---|---|---|---|---|---|---|---|---|---|---|---|---|---|---|---|---|---|---|
| Name | – | – | – | – | GB | GB | GB | GB | GB | GB | GB | GB | GB | GB | GB | GB | GB | GB |
| Age (any) | GB | GB | GB | GB | GB | GB | GB | GB | GB | GB | GB | GB | GB | GB | GB | GB | GB | GB |
| Date of birth | – | – | – | – | – | – | – | – | – | – | – | – | – | – | – | – | GB | GB |
| Marital status | – | – | – | – | – | GB | GB | GB | GB | GB | GB | GB | GB | GB | GB | GB | GB | GB |
| Relationship to head of household | – | – | – | – | – | GB | GB | GB | GB | GB | GB | GB | GB | GB | GB | GB | GB | GB |
| Usual address | – | – | – | – | – | – | – | – | – | – | – | – | – | GB | GB | GB | GB | GB |
| Migration one year ago | – | – | – | – | – | – | – | – | – | – | – | – | – | – | – | GB | GB | GB |
| Country of birth/birthplace | – | – | – | – | GB | GB | GB | GB | GB | GB | GB | GB | GB | GB | GB | GB | GB | GB |
| Nationality[1] | – | – | – | – | GB | GB | GB | GB | GB | GB | GB | GB | GB | GB | GB | GB | – | – |
| Education: scholar/student | – | – | – | – | – | GB | GB | GB | GB | S | S | GB[2] | GB[2] | – | GB[2] | – | – | – |
| Whether in job/unemployed/retired | – | – | – | – | – | GB | GB | GB | GB | GB | GB | GB | GB | GB | GB | GB | GB | GB |
| Employment status | – | – | – | – | – | GB[3] | GB[3] | GB[3] | GB[3] | GB | GB | GB | GB | GB | GB | GB | GB | GB |
| Occupation | GB[4] | – | – | GB[4] | GB | GB | GB | GB | GB | GB | GB | GB | GB | GB | GB | GB | GB | GB |
| Marriage and fertility (any) | – | – | – | – | – | – | – | – | – | – | – | GB | – | – | GB | GB | GB | – |
| Infirmity: deaf/dumb/blind etc. | – | – | – | – | – | GB | GB | GB | GB | GB | GB | GB | – | – | – | – | – | – |
| Number of rooms[5] | – | – | – | – | – | – | S | S | S | GB | GB | GB | GB | GB | GB | GB | GB | GB |
| Household amenities (any) | – | – | – | – | – | – | – | – | – | – | ± | – | – | – | GB | GB | GB | GB |
| Families per house | GB | GB | GB | GB | – | – | – | – | – | – | – | GB | GB | GB | GB | GB | – | – |

[1] 1841: only for persons born in Scotland or Ireland: 1851–91: whether British subject or not.
[2] Also whether full-time or part-time.
[3] Asked of farmers and tradesmen only.
[4] Only distinguishing (a) agriculture, (b) trade, manufacture or handicraft, (c) others.
[5] 1891–1901 only required if under five rooms.
GB = Great Britain.
S = Scotland.

**Table 2.4.** *Topics covered in the various annual General Household Surveys of Geat Britain, 1971–80*

| Item | '71 | '72 | '73 | '74 | '75 | '76 | '77 | '78 | '79 | '80 |
|---|---|---|---|---|---|---|---|---|---|---|
| Population | × | × | × | × | × | × | × | × | × | — |
| Housing | | | | | | | | | | |
| Costs | — | × | × | × | × | × | × | — | × | × |
| Age of building | × | × | × | × | × | × | × | × | × | × |
| Heating system/type | × | × | × | × | × | × | × | × | × | × |
| Burglaries/theft | — | — | × | × | — | — | — | — | × | × |
| Employment | | | | | | | | | | |
| Economic activity | × | × | × | × | × | × | × | × | × | × |
| Labour force | × | × | × | × | × | × | × | × | × | × |
| Job mobility | × | × | × | × | × | × | — | — | × | × |
| Absence from work | × | × | × | × | × | × | × | × | × | × |
| Education | | | | | | | | | | |
| Education and earnings | × | × | × | × | × | × | × | × | × | × |
| Age on leaving full-time education | — | × | × | × | × | × | × | × | × | × |
| Family formation | | | | | | | | | | |
| MS and cohabitation | × | × | × | × | × | × | × | × | × | × |
| Marriage (date of first) | — | — | — | × | × | × | × | × | × | × |
| Fertility | × | × | × | × | × | × | × | × | × | × |
| Separation and divorce | — | — | — | — | — | — | — | — | × | × |
| Whereabouts of children | — | — | — | — | — | — | — | — | × | × |
| Income | × | × | × | × | × | × | × | × | × | × |
| Leisure* | — | — | × | — | — | — | × | — | — | — |
| Leisure activities † | — | — | × | — | — | — | × | — | — | — |

*Holidays away from home, countries visited in UK, length of holiday.
†Types of leisure activities, numbers of days spent, whether on holiday.

All types of private households in the UK should be covered by the FES; in the period 1968–80 a sample of about 11 000 households has been used. These households are visited and asked to collaborate with an interview on incomes and regular payments; detailed records on expenditure are then obtained for a 14-day period. In 1980 an effective sample of 10 400 households was identified, and 67 per cent of these co-operated. The analyses included expenditure on 32 items of food, and three items of alcohol. These data were tabulated by expenditure and gross income; changes in the period 1953–80; various categories of type of household (such as one adult, combinations of two adults, combinations of two adults and varying numbers of children); the occupation of the head of household; and the age of the head of household.

There are various other sources of statistics on agriculture, fisheries, and food production. There are indirectly related to the topic of individual nutritional consumption. The *Annual Abstract of Statistics* (Central Statistical Office, Annual) is a useful source of summary data on this topic and a cross-reference to primary material.

### Smoking and drinking

As already indicated (see pp. 29–31), the GHS has collected some information about the distribution of smoking and drinking in the population. Other data on this topic can be obtained from the FES (discussed above), and is abstracted into various sets of statistics such as the *Annual Abstract of Statistics* and *Social Trends*.

Extensive material was published in the past by the Tobacco Research Council, providing detailed data on the prevalence of smoking in the country, classified by: type of tobacco used; type of cigarette, age, sex, and social class of smoker; and region of residence. This useful source of statistic is no longer published by the Tobacco Research Council (now Tobacco Advisory Council).

### Self-prescribing

The description of the GHS health section indicated that in 1972 and 1973 data had been collected on self-prescribing. There was in addition a major national study on this topic (Dunnell and Cartwright 1972). Various surveys are carried out for the pharmaceutical companies on the use of drugs bought over the counter, but this material is not published in the conventional scientific literature.

### Occupation

The decennial census is one source of statistics on the number of individuals classified by occupation and industry. Other data are now provided from the periodic Labour Force Survey (OPCS 1982c). Surveys held in 1973, 1975, 1977, and 1979 have amongst other things, quantified the number of individuals in employment by industry and occupation. The breakdown varied, but the maximum number of groups tabulated were 27 industry orders and 16 occupational groups (with counts by sex and age-group).

Other statistics on occupation are provided in the *Annual Abstract of Statistics,* in *Economic Trends,* in the *National Income and Expenditure Estimates*, and other subsidiary sources.

## Leisure and tourism

Limited data on leisure are provided from the GHS. Data are also provided in *Social Trends,* and in the Family Expenditure Survey (the latter specifying expenditure on cinema, theatre, sports, other entertainment, television licences, books, newspapers/magazines, musical instruments, and holidays). The articles in *Social Trends* on leisure are a useful source of material, as they pull together data from a variety of disparate sources, acknowledging that there is a relative shortage of relevant statistics. The material covers local radio, television viewing, cinema attendance, books issued, readership of national newspapers, readership of major magazines, attendances at art galleries and historic properties, and various outdoor activities, including spectator sports.

The GHS and *Social Trends* are also an appropriate source for examining information about holidays that are taken by residents in UK; for those travelling abroad, the destination of the adults is tabulated. Conversely, data are provided on visitors to the UK by country of origin.

## Religion

Again *Social Trends* is a source of basic data on this topic, showing the membership of different religions and the church attendances over the past year (though the completeness of the statistics is not known).

## Environment

### House stock

*Social Trends* has a chapter which provides a useful secondary source of information about housing stock for the UK, commenting that there is a problem in accumulating data due to variation in the way material is collected in the individual countries. The chapter provides information on trends in the number of dwellings and households, the stock of dwellings by tenure, the households by region, the number of houses and flats completed in various periods since 1961, the sale and lease of local authority and new town dwellings, the tenure of households by household characteristic, some information on housing standards and housing renovation, and additional particulars on lack of amenities. (This is, of course, a brief summary of a chapter that contains a mass of other data.)

### Climate

The most convenient source of trend data is the *Annual Abstract of Statistics.* This provides eleven year runs of statistics on air temperature, frost, rainfall, and sunshine. These data are provided by month within the year, for various localities within the country, and in certain circumstances showing also a long-term average figure.

### Environmental pollution

There are various indices of environmental pollution, but one convenient source is the recent venture of a *Digest of Environmental and Water Pollution Statistics* (Department of Environment 1982). The first publication was in 1978 and it is now appearing on an annual basis.

This report provides data for the UK for the latest available

year and presents a range of statistics on environmental pollution. This includes long-term trends in smoke emissions, from coal consumption classified by source from 1955; sulphur dioxide emissions from fuel combustion classified by type of fuel from 1969. Data are also presented on radioactivity from worldwide fall-out giving the country-wide average ratios of strontium-90 to calcium in milk and estimated deposition of strontium-90 in fall-out. Statistics are presented on air pollution giving more detailed tabulations for recent material, on water pollution of fresh water and marine water, on radiation exposure of the population from various sources, noise from various sources, and some statistics on waste and water supply. Some tables have been included with heavy metal concentrations and organo-chloride concentrations in fish and shellfish.

In addition, the Department of Environment has published a number of pollution papers via Her Majesty's Stationery Office (HMSO) since 1974. These cover lead, pesticides, chloro-fluorocarbons, oil, airborne sulphur compounds, mercury, lead in drinking water, lead in Birmingham, cadmium. In addition some methods papers are published. This series is supplemented by pollution reports published directly by the Department of Environment, which cover issues of more limited public interest or which are in a form which do not merit publication as a pollution paper. Since 1977 these have covered general method issues and the above series of *Digest of Environmental Pollution Statistics* (No. 1 in 1978, No. 2 in 1980, and No. 3 in 1980). The latest report No. 10 (1981) provides results from a survey of blood levels in the UK, which took place in 1979–80. Local surveys were co-ordinated by a Steering Group, in order to provide benchmark data on blood lead-level distributions in the people studied. This included adults in urban areas who are not exposed to specific sources of lead, together with other categories of individual. Data were provided on major urban areas, adults living near major roads, children living near major roads, children exposed to lead used in works, together with consideration of factors that influence blood lead levels. Detailed statistics on this are provided. They include results from a second campaign carried out in the spring of 1981.

The National Radiological Protection Board now has an environmental radioactivity surveillance programme; data are obtained from samples of airborne dust, rainwater, and milk throughout the UK. The data from the milk samples are used to estimate dose equivalents of a typical diet. Measurements of total body content of caesium-137 and potassium-40 are also made on a sample of the population in southern England. The first report (of a proposed series of publications) provided results for 1980 (Fry *et al.* 1981).

### Industrial productivity

Rather indirect measures of environmental pollution are indicators of production. Again a useful source of secondary material is the *Annual Abstract of Statistics.* This provides a range of material on production in the UK in the following categories: coal supply and demand; coke supply and consumption; gas, showing fuel used and production; electricity production and fuel used; petroleum supply and disposal; through-put of crude and processed oils; iron and steel supplies; non-ferrous metal production; cotton, man-made fibre, and wool production; jute and hemp; wood pulp, paper,

paper making material; timber; fertilizers; synthetic dye-stuffs, colours, paint, varnish, etc.; inorganic chemicals; organic chemicals; synthetic resins; rubber and carbon black; rubber products; mineral; soap, detergent and polishes; a wide range of manufactured goods including those from the engineering industry, merchant ship building, vehicle and aircraft production; clothes and related goods; domestic furniture; toys and related equipment; pens and pencils; tobacco and alcoholic drinks.

Much of this material is tabulated into relatively fine categories of production and in general shows data for an eleven year span in any given publication. The data are based at the national level, and do not show regional variation. Not all these statistics are available for UK as a whole; some relate to Great Britain.

## POPULATION STATISTICS

The 'medical' data discussed in this chapter are of increased value when they are related to appropriate population statistics. Many comparisons can only be made when rates have been calculated, especially rates that take into account variation in the distribution of certain characteristics in the base population from which the event data are derived. This section discusses the national population censuses and the derivation of annual estimates of population.

### National population censuses

#### Background

General descriptions of the development of censuses in England and Wales can be found in OPCS (1980a) and Redfern (1981). Acknowledgement of the need for a count of the numbers of the population led to the introduction of a Bill in Parliament in the middle of the eighteenth century; however, this was allowed to lapse until the first Population Act was passed in 1800. A national census has been held in Great Britain every 10 years since 1801, with the exception of 1941. The newly appointed Registrar General was responsible for this from 1841 onwards (the method involved specially appointed enumerators supervised in each district by the registrar of births and deaths). A standard pattern had evolved by 1901 with: authorization by an Act of Parliament about a year before the census; the Registrars General of England and Wales, Scotland, and Northern Ireland responsible for the conduct of the census; local registrars to organize local arrangements; the head of each household responsible for making the full return for the house; the information designated confidential, with prescribed penalties for disclosure; population figures published for local government areas down to civil parishes.

The Census Act 1920 governs the taking of censuses in England and Wales, and Scotland, though an Order in Council has to be laid before Parliament prior to submission to the Sovereign for each census. Apart from questions named in the 1920 Act, any others must have the purpose of ascertaining the 'social or civil conditions of the population' and be approved by both Houses of Parliament.

The frequency of the census is associated with the rapidity of the change in the population and their social and economic characteristics. The frequency will be a balance of need for data, resources available, other sources of information, and public attitudes. This balance has resulted in a census being carried out every ten years, with an additional 'mid-term' census in 1966 involving a 10 per cent sample of the population.

The vast majority of the population are counted at the census in their (or someone else's) home – usually on a Sunday in April. There are also arrangements for enumerating people present in institutions. The household is the unit to which the census form relates, being defined in 1981 as one or more persons living at the same address with common housekeeping (i.e. sharing at least one meal a day or a common living room). This definition implies that a dwelling may contain one or more households. Information is collected about the accommodation, as well as the individuals in the household. When individuals so choose they may now make personal returns, rather than have their data included on the household schedule. The range of topics on which information is collected was extended from the beginning of the century (see p. 39). The number of questions asked of respondents reached a peak of 30 in 1971, and was reduced to 21 in 1981.

From the point of providing a denominator for calculating rates, the main demographic items are sex, age, and marital status. More extended epidemiological analyses can be performed using the other material and this was discussed earlier (p. 39).

#### Method

In every census in Britain since 1841, each householder has received a census form to be filled in by him or her – with the help of the enumerator if required. The form is delivered to the householder before census day and collected shortly after that day. In 1981 the enumerators listed addresses during an advance round, before delivering the forms.

Sampling was first used in Britain in 1951, to produce advanced tables of results based on 1 per cent of households. In 1961, to reduce coding and processing costs, only 10 per cent of households were asked to complete a full-length questionnaire; this involved 11 additional questions covering topics such as occupation. A shorter form with 14 questions was used in the remaining households. The mid-decade census of 1966 involved a different approach, with lists of all 1961 dwellings and local valuation records of new buildings erected in the period 1961–66 used to draw a 10 per cent sample. In 1971 and 1981 processing of 'hard-to-code' items (occupation and higher education, for example) is predominantly on a 10 per cent sample of census schedules, all of which were fully completed.

The enumerator should identify the majority of missing answers and obtain the information. Some editing at punching now occurs, by checking that values lie in an acceptable range. Further correction occurs with an auto-edit system – by replacing missing or unacceptable values by an acceptable one (from the last processed complete record with similar demographic or other characteristics). This deals with completion errors which occur on form filling for the simpler items; the auto-edit does not apply to hard-to-code items, which are clerically corrected (these items usually involve coding errors, rather than mistakes made by the original person completing the form (as for the 100 per cent topics).

### Validity

In a census some individuals may be missed, and others counted twice. Characteristics such as age or occupation can be wrongly recorded or incorrectly coded. It has now become standard to check the initial coverage, by attempting to repeat the enumeration for a sample of households, shortly after census day using a skilled team of field staff. In 1981, it was estimated that 0.62 per cent of people had been missed, but about 0.17 per cent had been counted twice. This indicates that net underenumeration was less than 0.5 per cent (OPCS 1982d).

In parallel with checks of enumeration, a post-enumeration survey has followed each census since 1961 to assess the validity of answers. The most recent published (Gray and Gee 1972) shows that the 1966 Census had a misclassification rate that varied from 16.7 per cent for the topic 'rooms' (using the 1966 definition) to 0.5 per cent for *de facto* household size. A major improvement had been the substitution of date of birth for the previous census question on age; this had improved the accuracy of much of the age data (though for the very elderly the age was sometimes out by a decade).

## Annual population estimates

### Background

The census publications will provide the main source of detailed statistics suitable for use as denominators in calculating rates. Annual population estimates are then produced, which take account of (i) the increment in age of the population; (ii) the occurrence of births and deaths; and (iii) estimates of migration into and out of the country or locality. These have been prepared for the country and large towns since the nineteenth century, and since 1911 for local authority areas.

The method used in England and Wales is set out briefly in the 1979 publication (OPCS 1980b); the techniques involved in sub-national estimates have been described in two recent articles (Population Statistics Division 1980a, b).

The method involves tuning the adjustment for ageing and incorporation of births and deaths with available data on migration. International migration is estimated by (i) the International Passenger Survey (IPS) for countries outside the British Isles; (ii) the NHS Central Register (NHSCR) for movement to and from Scotland and Northern Ireland; and (iii) comparison of censuses for the Republic of Ireland and Great Britain. The IPS has the difficulty of a sample survey, the NHSCR relies on initiation of action from individuals re-registering with doctors, whilst the census comparisons form a very approximate guide to Irish migration.

None of these sources of information are adequate to provide local estimates of population movement. These have to come from (i) changes in the size of the electoral role; (ii) estimates of movement of those under 18 years from a 10 per

cent sample of registrations recorded at NHSCR; and (iii) cohort comparison of certain education statistics.

### Validity

The validity of the annual estimates will depend on the quality of the census enumeration, which is the base for the estimates, and the precision with which changes in the population can be gauged. There is no cause for concern over births or deaths, but migration can be very difficult to quantify – both for movement across national boundaries and of persons moving from one locality to another. The difference between the population estimates which have been carried forward from the 1971 census and the estimates derived from 1981 census data have been calculated for England and Wales for each local government area. These differences, for seven age groups as well as the total population, have been published in an OPCS Occasional Paper (OPCS 1982e).

For England and Wales as a whole the estimates were 0.2 per cent lower than the census. This overall difference concealed larger errors for the various age groups. The age groups below 25 years were over-estimated and those above were under-estimated. Apart from those aged 0 to 4 years and those aged 25 to 44 years the errors were all around ± 1 per cent.

At the local level there were considerably larger differences because of the inadequate information about people moving between local authority areas. Overall the differences were 5 per cent or more for about 1 in 20 of the 403 districts; were 2.5 per cent or more for 1 in 4; and were 1 per cent or more for just over half. The average of the differences was approximately 1.8 per cent – ten times as large for England and Wales. The larger ones tended to be over-estimated and the smaller ones under-estimated.

The differences for individual age groups were again much larger than the overall difference. The 15–24 year olds and those aged 80 years or more being the worst two groups. The average error for the 15–24 year olds was 8.3 per cent and one-third of all areas had a difference greater than 10 per cent. For the 80 years and over age group the average error was 13.6 per cent and one-fifth of the areas had a difference greater than 20 per cent. These two groups are particularly difficult to deal with. The first comprises young people who tend to be very mobile while the second group is very small and many live in institutions.

## PUBLICATIONS

The Appendix gives the publications of the main census reports that are relevant to use of denominators for calculating mortality and morbidity rates and of national and local annual population estimates. (Table 2.3 has already indicated the span of topics covered in the different censuses.)

An OPCS Monitor (PP1 82/2, OPCS 1982f) reviewed the national data on ethnic minority groups: Periodic Census, and National Dwelling and Housing Survey; Sample Surveys – Labour Force Survey, General Household Survey, International Passenger Survey; Demographic events – birth and death registration. A table demonstrated the area level available for the different sources.

APPENDIX—
OFFICIAL PUBLISHED SOURCES OF HEALTH INFORMATION

*All publications are available from HMSO unless otherwise stated. For each series, the years for which data are included are indicated and the date(s) of publication are given in parentheses.*

## Publications of mortality statistics, 1839–1980

**England and Wales**

| | | |
|---|---|---|
| 1838–1900 | Annual Report of the Registrar General of Births, Deaths and Marriages in England | (1839–1902) |
| 1901–20 | Annual Report of the Registrar General of Births, Deaths and Marriages in England and Wales | (1903–22) |
| 1921–53 | The Registrar General's Statistical Review of England and Wales, Text, Part I Medical Tables | (1923–54) |
| 1954–73 | The Registrar General's Statistical Review of England and Wales, Part I Medical Tables | (1955–75) |
| 1974–79 | Mortality Statistics, England and Wales, Series DH1 | (1977–82) |
| 1974–80 | Mortality Statistics: Cause, England and Wales, Series DH2 | (1977–82) |
| 1974–80 | Mortality Statistics: Childhood and Maternity, England and Wales, Series DH3 | (1977–82) |
| 1974–80 | Mortality Statistics: Accidents and Violence, England and Wales, Series DH4 | (1976–82) |
| 1974–80 | Mortality Statistics: Area, England and Wales, Series DH5 | (1976–81) |
| 1968–78* | Mortality Surveillance 1968–1978, England and Wales | (1980) |

**Scotland**

| | | |
|---|---|---|
| 1855–1910 | Detailed Annual Report of the Registrar General of Births, Deaths and Marriages for Scotland | (1861–1912) |
| 1911–67 | Annual Report of the Registrar General for Scotland | (1914–68) |
| 1968–78 | Annual Report of the Registrar General for Scotland. Part I Mortality Statistics | (1969–80) |
| 1979–80 | Annual Report of the Registrar General for Scotland | (1981–82) |

**Northern Ireland**

| | | |
|---|---|---|
| 1922–44 | The Registrar General's Annual Reports containing general abstracts of Births, Deaths and Marriages in Northern Ireland | (1924–46) |
| 1945–79 | Annual Report of the Registrar General for Northern Ireland | (1946–82) |

*Available from OPCS, London.

## Publications of area mortality statistics, England and Wales 1851–1973

| | | |
|---|---|---|
| 1851–60 | Supplement to the 25th Annual Report of the Registrar General in England | (1864) |
| 1861–70 | Supplement to the 35th Annual Report of the Registrar General in England | (1875) |
| 1871–80 | Supplement to the 45th Annual Report of the Registrar General in England | (1885) |
| 1900–02 | Supplement to the 65th Annual Report of the Registrar General in England | (1908) |
| 1911–20 | The Registrar General's Decennial Supplement for England and Wales, 1921. Part III Estimates of Populations, Statistics of Marriages, Births and Deaths | (1933) |
| 1921–30 | The Registrar General's Decennial Supplement for England and Wales 1931. Part III Estimates of Population, Statistics of Marriages, Births and Deaths | (1952) |
| 1950–53 | The Registrar General's Decennial Supplement for England and Wales, 1951. Area Mortality | (1958) |
| 1959–63 | The Registrar General's Decennial Supplement for England and Wales, 1961. Area Mortality Tables | (1967) |
| 1969–73* | OPCS Area Mortality Tables, Decennial Supplement 1971. Series DS No. 3, England and Wales | (1979) |
| 1969–73 | OPCS Area Mortality Tables, Decennial Supplement, 1969–73. Series DS No. 4. England and Wales | (1981) |

*Available from OPCS, London (with additional microfiche tables).

## Publications on occupational mortality, 1851–1973

**England and Wales 1851–1972**

| | | |
|---|---|---|
| 1851 | 14th Annual Report of the Registrar General, England | (1855) |
| 1860–61 | Supplement to the 25th Annual Report of the Registrar General, England | (1864) |
| 1871 | Supplement to the 35th Annual Report of the Registrar General, England | (1875) |
| 1880–82 | Supplement to the 45th Annual Report of the Registrar General, England | (1885) |
| 1890–92 | Supplement to the 55th Annual Report of the Registrar General, England | (1897) |
| 1900–02 | Supplement to the 65th Annual Report of the Registrar General, England | (1908) |
| 1910–12 | Supplement to the 75th Annual Report of the Registrar General, England. Part IV Mortality of men in certain occupations | (1919) |
| 1921–23 | The Registrar General's Decennial Supplement, England and Wales. Part II Occupational Mortality, Fertility and Infant Mortality | (1927) |
| 1930–32 | The Registrar General's Decennial Supplement, England and Wales. Part IIA Occupational Mortality | (1938) |
| 1949–53 | The Registrar General's Decennial Supplement, England and Wales | |
| | Part I Occupational Mortality | (1954) |
| | Part II Occupational Mortality, Vol. 1, Commentary | (1958) |
| | Part II Occupational Mortality, Vol. 2, Tables | (1957) |
| 1959–63 | The Registrar General's Decennial Supplement, England and Wales. Occupational Mortality, Tables | (1971) |
| 1970–72* | The registrar General's Decennial Supplement, England and Wales, Occupational Mortality. Series DS No. 1 | (1978) |

## Scotland 1890–1973

| 1890–92 | Supplement to the 38th Annual Report of the Registrar-General of Births, Deaths and Marriages in Scotland | (1895) |
| 1900–02 | Supplement to the 48th Annual Report of the Registrar-General of Births, Deaths and Marriages in Scotland | (1905) |
| 1930–32 | Supplement to the 78th Annual Report of the Registrar-General of Births, Deaths and Marriages for Scotland, Part II General Tables | (1936) |
| 1949–53 | Annual Report of the Registrar-General for Scotland, Number 101, 1955 | (1956) |
| 1959–63 | Second Supplement to the 114th Annual Report of the Registrar-General for Scotland | (1970) |
| 1969–73 | 2nd Supplement to the Registrar-General's Annual Report for 1977 | (1981) |

## Northern Ireland 1960–62

| 1960–62 | Occupational Mortality in Northern Ireland | (1965–66) |

*Additional data available on microfiche from OPCS, London.

## Publication of linked mortality statistics, England and Wales 1949–79

### Infant mortality

| 1949–50 | Social and Biological Factors in infant mortality. Heady, J. A. and Heasman, M. A., Studies on Medical and Population Subjects No. 15 | (1959) |
| 1964–65 | Regional and social factors in infant mortality. Spicer, L. C. and Lipworth, L., Studies on Medical and Population Subjects, No. 19 | (1966) |
| 1975–76 | Social and biological factors in infant mortality. Occasional Paper No. 12 | (1978) |
| 1975–77 | Perinatal and infant mortality: social and biological factors. Studies on Medical and Population Subjects, No. 41 | (1980) |
| 1978–79 | Mortality Statistics: perinatal and infant, social and biological factors. Series DH3 No. 7 | (1982) |

### Longitudinal study

| 1971–75 | Longitudinal Study: socio-demographic mortality differentials. Fox, A. J. and Goldblatt, P. O., Series LS No. 1 | (1982) |

## Publications on abortion statistics, 1968–81

### England and Wales 1968–80

| 1968–73 | The Registrar General's Statistical Review. Supplement on Abortion | (1970–74) |
| 1974–80 | Abortion Statistics, England and Wales, Series AB Nos. 1–7 | (1978–82) |

### Scotland 1969–81

| 1969–80 | Scottish Health Statistics | (1974–82) |
| 1969–81 | Annual Report of the Registrar General for Scotland | (1973–82) |

## Publications on cancer registration and survival, 1945–77

### A. REGISTRATIONS

#### England and Wales 1945–77

| 1945–46 | Cancer Registration in England and Wales 3rd year recovery and survival rates. Studies on Medical and Population Subjects, No. 3 | (1952) |
| 1949–51 | Registrar General's Statistical Review of England and Wales. Supplement on General Morbidity, Cancer and Mental Health | (1953–55) |
| 1952–53 1961–70 | Registrar General's Statistical Review of England and Wales. Supplements on Cancer, 1952, 1953, 1961–1970 | (1957–75) |
| 1971 | Cancer Statistics: registrations. England and Wales, Series MB1 No. 1 | (1979) |
| 1972–73 | Cancer Statistics: registrations, England and Wales, Series MB1 No. 2 | (1979) |
| 1974–77 | Cancer Statistics: registrations, England and Wales, Series MB1 Nos. 4, 5, 7, 8 | (1980–82) |

#### Scotland 1959–77

| 1959–61 | Cancer Registration. Scottish Health Service Studies, No. 5 | (1967) |
| 1962–64 | Cancer Registration. Scottish Health Service Studies, No. 8 | (1969) |
| 1965–67 | Five year survival rates, cases registered 1959–1961. Cancer registration cases 1965–1967. L. D. Howitt. Scottish Health Service Studies, No. 26 | (1973) |
| 1963–77* | Cancer Registration and Survival Statistics Scotland. Scottish Cancer Registration Scheme (Information Services Division) | (1981) |

### B. SURVIVAL

#### England and Wales 1945–73

| 1945–46 | Cancer Registration in England and Wales, 3rd year recovery and survival rates. Studies on Medical and Population Subjects, No. 3 | (1952) |
| 1949–55 1960–66 | Limited tables on survival provided in publications listed above in section on registration | |
| 1971–73 | Cancer Statistics: survival, England and Wales, Series MB1 No. 3 | (1980) |
| 1971–75 | Cancer Statistics: survival, England and Wales, Series MB1 No. 9 | (1982) |

#### Scotland 1959–73

| 1959–61 | Five year Survival rates, cases registered 1959–1961. Cancer registration cases registered 1965–1967. L. D. Howitt. Scottish Health Service Studies No. 26 | (1973) |
| 1961–63* 1966–69* 1971–73* | Cancer Registration and Survival Statistics Scotland. Scottish Cancer Registration Scheme (Information Services Division) | (1981) |

*Available from Common Services Agency, Edinburgh.

## Publications on congenital malformation statistics, 1964–81

### England and Wales 1964–81

| 1964–73 | The Registrar General's Quarterly Returns for England and Wales, September 1965–September 1974 | (1965–75) |

| 1974–81* | Congenital Malformations Monitor, Reference MB3 | (1976–82) |
| 1975–80* | Congenital Malformations – Surveillance Programme, Reference MB3 | (1977–81) |
| 1974–79* | Congenital Malformations and Parents' occupations. Monitor reference MB3 | (1982) |

**Northern Ireland 1964–79**

| 1964–75 | 43rd–54th Annual Report of the Registrar General for Northern Ireland | (1965–77) |
| 1974–79 | Health and Personal Social Service Statistics for Northern Ireland | (1978–81) |

*Available from OPCS, London.

## Publications on morbidity statistics collected from population surveys in England and Wales, 1943–53, Great Britain 1971–80

| 1944–47 | Sickness in the population of England and Wales. Studies on Medical and Population Subjects, No. 2 | (1949) |
| 1943–53 | The Survey of Sickness. Logan, W. P. D., and Brooke, E. M. Studies on Medical and Population Subjects, No. 12 | (1957) |
| 1944–52 | Monthly Bulletins of the Ministry of Health and Public Health Laboratory Service | (1944–52) |
| 1971 | The General Household Survey Introductory Report | (1973) |
| 1972–80 | The General Household Survey | (1975–82) |

## 'Acute' and 'Maternity' hospital discharge statistics 1949–80

### A. ACUTE DATA

**England and Wales 1949–79**

| 1949 | Hospital Morbidity Statistics: a preliminary study of in-patient discharges. D. McKay. Studies on Medical and Population Subjects, No. 4 | (1951) |
| 1949 | Registrar General's Statistical Review of England and Wales, 1949. Supplement on Hospital In-Patient Statistics | (1954) |
| 1950–51 | Registrar General's Statistical Review of England and Wales 1950–51. Supplement on Hospital In-Patient Statistics | (1955) |
| 1955 | Registrar General's Statistical Review of England and Wales 1955. Supplement on Hospital In-Patient Statistics | (1959) |
| 1956–57 | Hospital In-Patient Enquiry, England and Wales | (1961) |
| 1958–59 | Hospital In-Patient Enquiry, England and Wales, Part I Preliminary Tables | (1960–61) |
| 1960 | Hospital In-Patient Enquiry, England and Wales. Part II Detailed Tables | (1963) |
| 1961 | Hospital In-Patient Enquiry, England and Wales, Part I Preliminary Tables | (1963) |
| 1962–68 | Hospital In-Patient Enquiry, England and Wales, Part I Tables | (1966–72) |
| 1969–71 | Report on Hospital In-Patient Enquiry, England and Wales, Preliminary Tables | (1972–74) |

| 1972 | Report on Hospital In-Patient Enquiry, Part I Tables | (1974) |
| 1973 | Report on Hospital In-Patient Enquiry, Tables | (1977) |
| 1974–78 | Hospital In-Patient Enquiry, England and Wales, Main Tables. Series MB4 Nos. 2, 5, 7, 10, and 12 | (1978–81) |
| 1979* | Hospital In-Patient Enquiry, England and Wales, Summary Tables. Series MB4 No. 13 | (1982) |
| 1968–78 † | Trends in Morbidity 1968–78 applying surveillance techniques to the Hospital In-patient Enquiry | (1981) |

**Scotland 1961–79**

| 1961–79 ‡ | Scottish Hospital In-Patient Statistics. (Scottish Home and Health Department 1964–73; Information Services Division, Common Services Agency, 1974–80.) | (1964–80) |

### B. MATERNITY DATA

**England and Wales 1968–78**

| | Prior to 1973 limited tables were published in the main series of reports of the Hospital In-Patient Enquiry for 1968–1972. Before 1968 maternity events were included in the tables for all patients, but identified where appropriate by diagnosis | |
| 1973–76 | Hospital In-Patient Enquiry: Maternity Tables. Series MB4 No. 8 | (1980) |
| 1977 † | Maternity Statistics, POCS Monitor, Reference MB4 80/1 | (1980) |
| 1978 † | Maternity Statistics, OPCS Monitor, Reference MB4 81/1 | (1981) |

**Scotland 1975–80**

| | Prior to 1975, limited data appeared within the 'acute' hospital dischage statistics | |
| 1975–80 | Scottish Health Statistics. Scottish Home and Health Department. | (1977–82) |

*Additional data available on microfiche from OPCS, London.
†Available from OPCS, London.
‡Available from Common Services Agency, Edinburgh.

## Psychiatric hospital statistics, 1949–80

**England and Wales 1949–77**

| 1949–51 | The Registrar General's Statistical Review of England and Wales. Supplements on General Morbidity, Cancer and Mental Health | (1953–55) |
| 1952–60 | The Registrar General's Statistical Review of England and Wales. Supplements on Mental Health | (1959–64) |
| 1961–63 | Report of the Ministry of Health – The Health and Welfare Services, 1961–1963 | (1962–64) |
| 1964–69 | Psychiatric Hospitals and Units in England and Wales. In-Patient Statistics from the Mental Health Enquiry. Statistics Research Series Nos. 4, 5, 11, 12 | (1969–71) |
| 1970–77 | In-Patient Statistics from Mental Health Enquiry. Statistics and Research Report Series, Nos. 4, 6, 12, 17, 20, 22, 23 | (1972–80) |

**Scotland 1955–80**

| 1955–59 | Department of Health Annual Report for Scotland | (1956–60) |
| 1959–80 | Scottish Health Statistics | (1960–82) |
| 1974–79* | Scottish Mental Health In-Patient Statistics (Information Services Division, Common Services Agency) | (1974–82) |

*Available from Common Services Agency, Edinburgh.

## Publications on occupational disease and deaths, including injury at work

| 1971–75 | Health and Safety Statistics, 1975 | (1977) |
| 1976 | Health and Safety Statistics, 1976 | (1979) |
| 1977 | Health and Safety Statistics, 1977 | (1980) |
| 1978–79 | Health and Safety Statistics, 1978–1979 | (1981) |

Statistics were previously published in Annual Report of Chief Inspector of Factories.

## Publications on morbidity statistics from general practice from special studies in England and Wales 1955–72

| 1955–56 | Morbidity Statistics from General Practice – Volume I (General). W. P. D. Logan and A. A. Cushion. Studies on Medical and Population Subjects No. 14 | (1958) |
| 1955–56 | Morbidity Statistics from General Practice – Volume II (Occupation). W. P. D. Logan. Studies on Medical and Population Subjects No. 14 | (1960) |
| 1955–56 | Morbidity Statistics from General Practice – Volume III (Diseases in General Practice). Research Committee of the Council of the Committee of General Practitioners. Studies on Medical and Population Subjects, No. 14 | (1962) |
| 1970–71 | Morbidity Statistics from General Practice. 2nd National Study. Studies on Medical and Population Subjects, No. 26 | (1974) |
| 1971–72 | Morbidity Statistics from General Practice. 2nd National Study. Studies on Medical and Population Subjects, No. 36 | (1979) |
| 1970–71 | Morbidity Statistics from General Practice: socio-economic analyses. Studies on Medical and Population Subjects, No. 46 | (1982) |

## Annual publications on notifications of infectious disease statistics, 1912–80

**England and Wales 1912–80**

| 1912–73 | The Registrar General's Statistical Review of England and Wales | (1913–75) |
| 1974–78 | Statistics of Infectious Diseases, England and Wales, Series MB2 Nos. 1–5 | (1975–80) |
| 1979–80 | Communicable Diseases Statistics, England and Wales, Series MB2 Nos. 6–7 | (1981–82) |

**Scotland 1919–80**

| 1919–28 | Scotland Board of Health Annual Report | (1920–29) |

| 1929–64 | Scotland Department of Health Annual Report | (1930–65) |
| 1958–65 | Scotland Department of Health Statistics | (1959–66) |
| 1966–73 | Scottish Home and Health Department, Health Statistics | (1968–75) |
| 1974–80 | Scottish Health Statistics | (1976–82) |

**Northern Ireland 1935–79**

| 1935–76 | Annual Report of the Registrar General for Northern Ireland | (1936–78) |
| 1974–79 | Health and Personal Social Services Statistics for Northern Ireland | (1978–81) |

## Sickness absence statistics, 1948–80

**England and Wales 1948–78**

| 1948–51 | Report of the Ministry of National Insurance 1944–52 | (1950–53) |
| 1952–64 | Ministry of Pensions and National Insurance Reports 1953–65 | (1954–66) |
| 1964–67 | Ministry of Social Security Annual Report 1966–67 | (1967–68) |
| 1968 | Annual Report of the Department of Health and Social Security 1968 | (1969) |
| 1959–69 | Digest of Health Statistics for England and Wales 1969–71 | (1969–71) |
| 1969–78 | Health and Personal Social Security Services Statistics for England and Wales (with summary tables for Great Britain) | (1973–80) |

**Scotland 1956–80**

| 1956–80 | Scottish Health Statistics | (1959–80) |

**Northern Ireland 1950–80**

| 1950–80 | Sample survey of (a) sickness and (b) injury benefit among the insured population of Northern Ireland | (1951–82) |

## Populations by age, sex, and locality

**A. Census publications**

| 1841 | Census of England and Wales 1841. Enumeration Abstract. Part I England and Wales, Part II Scotland | (1843) |
| 1851 | Census of Great Britain 1851. Population Tables II Volume I | (1854) |
| 1861 | Census of England and Wales 1861 Population Tables, Volume II | (1863) |
| 1871 | Census of England and Wales 1871 Volume IV, General Report and Appendix | (1873) |
| 1881 | Census of England and Wales 1881. Volume IV, General Report | (1883) |
| 1891 | Census of England and Wales 1891 General Report | (1893) |
| 1901 | Census of England and Wales 1901. Summary Report | (1903) |
| 1901 | Census of England and Wales 1901. General Report with Appendix | (1904) |
| 1911 | Census of England and Wales 1911. Summary Tables | (1915) |
| 1921 | Census of England and Wales 1921. Summary Tables | (1925) |

| 1931 | Census of England and Wales 1931. General Tables | (1935) |
| 1951 | Census of England and Wales 1951. General Tables | (1956) |
| 1961 | Census of England and Wales 1961. Age, Marital Condition and General Tables | (1964) |
| 1966 | Sample Census United Kingdom 1966. Volume II Parliamentary Constituency Tables | (1969) |
| 1971 | Census of Great Britain 1971. Age, Marital Condition and General Tables | (1974) |

**B. Other publications**

| 1912–14 | 75th–77th Annual Report of the Registrar General of Births, Deaths and Marriages in England and Wales | (1914–16) |
| 1951 | The Registrar General's Statistical Review of England and Wales 1951. Tables Part II Civil | (1953) |
| 1961 | The Registrar General's Statistical Review of England and Wales 1961 Part II Tables Population | (1963) |
| 1971 | The Registrar General's Statistical Review of England and Wales. Part II Tables Population | (1973) |
| 1974–80 | Population Estimates, England and Wales, Series PP1, Nos. 1–5 | (1976–81) |

Comparable material was published in the census reports for Scotland and Northern Ireland.

## REFERENCES

Abramson, J.H., Sacks, M.I., and Cahana, E. (1971). Death certification data as an indication of the presence of certain common diseases at death. *J. Chronic Dis.* **24**, 417.

Acheson, E.D. (1967). *Medical record linkage.* Oxford University Press, London.

Advisory Committee on Cancer Registration (1981). *Cancer Registration in the 1980s.* HMSO, London.

Alderson, M.R. (1965). The accuracy of the certification of death, and the classification of underlying cause of death from the death certificate. MD thesis, London University.

Alderson, M.R. (1967). Data on sickness absence in some recent publications of the Ministry of Pensions and National Insurance. *Br. J. Prev. Soc. Med.* **21**, 1.

Alderson, M.R. (1972). Some sources of error in British occupational mortality data. *Br. J. Ind. Med.* **29**, 245.

Alderson, M.R. (1973). Cancer registration. In *Cancer priorities.* (ed. G. Bennette) p. 101. British Cancer Council, London.

Alderson, M.R. (1979). The role of epidemiology in occupational health. In *Current approaches to occupational medicine* (ed. A.W. Gardner) p. 151. Wright, Bristol.

Alderson, M.R. (1981). *International mortality statistics,* Macmillan, London.

Alderson, M.R. (1983a). Job titles as surrogates for exposure. In *Conference on Job Exposure Matrices, Southampton, April 1982, proceedings.* MRC Environmental Epidemiology Unit, Southampton.

Alderson, M.R. (1983b). *An introduction to epidemiology,* 2nd edn. Macmillan, London.

Alderson, M.R. and Dowie, R. (1979). *Health surveys and related studies.* Pergamon, Oxford.

Alderson, M.R. and Meade, T.W. (1967). Accuracy of diagnosis on death certificates compared with that in hospital records. *Br. J. Prev. Soc. Med.* **21**, 22.

Alderson, M.R. and Whitehead, F. (1974). Central Government routine health statistics, and Social Security statistics. In *Reviews of United Kingdom statistical sources* (ed. W.F. Maunder). Heinemann, London.

Alderson, M.R., Bradley, K., Rushton, L., and Thacker, P. (1976). Cancer registration as a by-product of hospital activity analysis. *Hosp. Health Serv. Rev.* **72**, 118.

Ashley, J.S.A. (1972). Present state of statistics from hospital in-patient data and their uses. *Br. J. Prev. Soc. Med.* **26**, 135.

Ashley, J.S.A. (1980). The maternity hospital in-patients enquiry. In *Perinatal audit and surveillance* (ed. I. Chalmers and G. McIlwaine) p. 61. Journal of Royal College of Obstetricians and Gynaecologists, London.

Backett, E.M., Heady, J.A., and Evans, J.C.G. (1954). Studies of a general practice. The doctor's job in an urban area. *Br. Med. J.* **i**, 109.

Benjamin, B. (1965). Hospital Activity Analysis. *The Hospital* **61**, 221.

Benjamin, B. (1967). Assessment of medical care. *Proc. R. Soc. Med.* **60**, 17.

Benjamin, B. (1968a). *Demographic analysis.* Allen and Unwin, London.

Benjamin, B. (1968b). *Health and vital statistics.* Allen and Unwin, London.

Brodrick, N. (1971). *Report of the committee on death certification and coroners.* Cmnd Paper 4810. HMSO, London.

Brorsson, B. and Smedby, B. (1982). Validity of health survey interview data concerning visits to doctors at Swedish health centre. *Stat Tidskrift* **1**, 31.

Busuttil, A., Kemp, I.W., and Heasman, M.A. (1981). The accuracy of medical certificates of cause of death. *Health Bull.* **39**, 146.

Butts, M.S. and Williams, D.R.R. (1982). Accuracy of Hospital Activity Analysis data. *Br. Med. J.* **285**, 506.

Cameron, H.M., Clarke, J., and Melville, A. (1977). Autopsies and medical records. *Health Bull.* **35**, 113.

Cameron, H.M. and McGooghan, E. (1981). A prospective study of 1152 hospital autopsies. *J. Pathol.* **133**, 273.

Cancer Research Campaign Cancer Statistics Group (1982). *Trends in cancer survival in Great Britain.* Cancer Research Campaign, London.

Cartwright, A. (1967). *Patients and their doctors—a study of general practice.* Routledge Kegan Paul, London.

Charles, E. (1951). Statistical utilisation of maternity and child welfare records. *Br. J. Soc. Med.* **5**, 41.

Chief Medical Officer (1972). *On the state of public health, for the year 1971,* p. 109. HMSO, London.

Clarke, C. and Whitfield, A.G.W. (1978). Death certification and epidemiological research. *Br. Med. J.* **ii**, 1063.

Clarke, M. and Bennett, A.E. (1971). Problems in the measurement of hospital utilisation. *Proc. R. Soc. Med.* **64**, 795.

Cohen, J. and Steinitz, R. (1969). Underlying and contributory causes of death of adult males in two districts. *J. Chronic Dis.* **22**, 17.

Cole, S. (1980). Scottish maternity and neonatal records. In *Perinatal audit and surveillance* (ed. I. Chalmers and G. McIlwaine) p. 39. Royal College of Obstetricians and Gynaecologists, London.

Cole, S.K. (in press). Evaluation of a neonatal discharge record as a monitor of congenital malformations. *J. Community Med.*

Crawshaw, C. and Moss, J.G. (1982). Accuracy of HAA operation codes. *Br. Med. J.* **285**, 210.

Crombie, D.L. (1973). Research and confidentiality in general practice. *J. R. Coll. Gen. Practit.* **23**, 863.

Davies, P.D.O., Darbyshire, J., Nunn, A., *et al.* (1981).

Ambiguities and inaccuracies in the notification system for tuberculosis in England and Wales. *Community Med.* **3**, 108.

Dawes, K.S. (1972). Survey of general practice records. *Br. Med. J.* **iii**, 219.

Department of Environment (1982). *Digest of environmental and pollution and water statistics. No. 4.* HMSO, London.

Department of Trade (1982). *Casualties to vessels and accidents to men: vessels registered in the UK—return for 1980.* HMSO, London.

Diehl, A.K. and Gau, D.W. (1982). Death certification by British doctors: a demographic analysis. *J. Epidemiol. Community Health,* **36**, 146.

Dollinger, J. (1907). *Statistique des personnes attientes de cancer.* Publ. Statist. Hong. Nouv. Ser. 19, Budapest.

Dunnell, K. and Cartwright, A. (1972). *Medicine takers, prescribers and hoarders.* Routledge Kegan Paul, London.

Dunnigan, M.G., Harland, W.A., and Fyfe, T. (1970). Seasonal incidence and mortality of ischaemic heart disease. *Lancet* **ii**, 793.

Durant, M. (1978). The General Household Survey: 1971–1978. *Statist. News* **42**, 3.

Edouard, L. (1982). Validation of the registered underlying cause of stillbirth. *J. Epidemiol. Community Health* **36**, 231.

Ericson, A., Kallen, B., and Winberg, J. (1977). Surveillance of malformations at birth: a comparison of two record systems run in parallel. *Int. J. Epidemiol.* **6**, 35.

EURO Reports and Studies (1981). *Surveillance of acute viral respiratory infections in Europe—report of a WHO symposium.* Regional Office for Europe, WHO, Copenhagen.

Farmer, R.D.T., Knox, E.G., Cross, K.W., and Crombie, D.L. (1974). Executive council lists and general practitioner files. *Br. J. Soc. Prev. Med.* **28**, 49.

Farr, W. (1854). Letter to the Registrar General. In *13th annual report of the Registrar General of Births, Deaths and Marriages, in England,* p. 129. HMSO, London.

Farr, W. (1861). *Report of the Committee on the preparation of army medical statistics, and on the duties to be performed by the statistical branch of the army medical department.* British Parliamentary Papers XXXVII.

Farr, W. (1864). Hospital mortality. *Med. Times Gazette* **i**, 242.

Faulkner, K., Leyland, L., and Wofiden, R.C. (1967). Cancer registration. *Med. Officer* **118**, 147.

Forster, D.F. and Mahadevan, S. (1981). Information sources for planning and evaluating adult psychiatric services. *Community Med.* **3**, 160.

Fox, A.J. and Goldblatt, P.O. (1982). *Longitudinal study: socio-economic mortality differentials, 1971–75 England and Wales.* OPCS, London.

Fraser, R.C. (1978). The reliability and validity of the age-sex register as a population denominator in general practice. *J. R. Coll. Gen. Practit.* **28**, 283.

Fraser, R.C. and Clayton, D.G. (1981). The accuracy of age-sex registers, practice medical records and family practitioner committee registers. *J. R. Coll. Gen. Practit.* **31**, 410.

Fry, F.A., Dodd, N.J., Green, N., Major, R.O., and Wilkins, B.T. (1981). *Environmental radioactivity surveillance programme: results for UK for 1980.* National Radiological Protection Board, Chilton.

Gau, D.W. and Diehl, A.K. (1982). Disagreement among general practitioners regarding cause of death. *Br. Med. J.* **284**, 239.

General Register Office (1968). *Census, 1961—Great Britain, general report.* HMSO, London.

Gillis, R.C. (1971). *9th annual report of the Regional Cancer Committee for 1969.* Western Regional Hospital Cancer Registration Bureau, Glasgow.

Goldacre, M.J. (1981). Hospital in-patient statistics: some aspects of interpretation. *Community Med.* **3**, 60.

Goldacre, M.J. and Miller, D.L. (1976). Completeness of statutory notification for acute bacterial meningitis. *Br. Med. J.* **ii**, 501.

Gray, P. and Gee, F.A. (1972). *A quality check on the 1966 ten per cent sample census of England and Wales.* HMSO, London.

Greenberg, G., Inman, W.H.W., Weatherall, J.A.C., and Adelstein, A.M. (1975). Hormonal pregnancy tests and congenital malformations. *Br. Med. J.* **ii**, 191.

Greenberg, G., Inman, W.H.W., Weatherall, J.A.C., Adelstein, A.M., and Haskey, J.C. (1977). Maternal drug histories and congenital abnormalities. *Br. Med. J.* **ii**, 853.

Guralnick, L. (1966). Some problems in the use of multiple causes of death. *J. Chronic Dis.* **19**, 979.

Hannay, D.R. (1972). Accuracy of health-centre records. *Lancet* **ii**, 371.

Haward, R.A. (1973). Scale of undernotification of infectious diseases by general practitioners. *Lancet* **i**, 873.

Heady, J.A. and Heasman, M.A. (1959). *Social and biological factors in infant mortality.* General Register Office Studies on Medical and Population Subjects No. 15. HMSO, London.

Heasman, M.A. and Clarke, J.A. (1979). Medical record linkage in Scotland. *Health Bull.* **37**, 97.

Heasman, M.A. and Lipworth, L. (1966). *Accuracy of certification of cause of death.* General Register Office Studies of Medical and Population Subjects No. 20. HMSO, London.

Heasman, M.A., Liddell, F.O.K., and Reid, D.D. (1958). The accuracy of occupational vital statistics. *Br. J. Ind. Med.* **15**, 141.

Hole, R. (1982). Accuracy of HAA operation codes. *Br. Med. J.* **285**, 210.

Horder, J. and Horder, E. (1954). Illness in general practice. *Practitioner* **173**, 177.

International Clearing House for Birth Defects (1981). A communication from the International Clearing House for Birth Defects Monitoring Systems. *Int. J. Epidemiol.* **10**, 245.

Jennings, C. and Barraclough, B. (1980). Legal and administrative influences on the English suicide rate since 1900. *Psychol. Med.* **10**, 407.

Joint Tuberculosis Committee of the British Thoracic Association (1982). Notification of tuberculosis: a code of practice for England and Wales. *Br. Med. J.* **284**, 1454.

Kay, C.R. (1968). A comparison of two methods of determining social status. *J. R. Coll. Gen. Practit.* **16**, 162.

Kemp, I.W., Damblen, D.L., and Lindsay, E.D. (1971). A system for collection of orthopaedic clinical data. *Health Bull.* **29**, 88.

Kessel, W.I.N. and Shepherd, M. (1965). The health and attitudes of people who seldom consult a doctor. *Med. Care* **3**, 6.

Kneale, G.W. and Stewart, A.M. (1982). Hanford radiation study. *Br. J. Ind. Med.* **39**, 201.

Körner Committee (1982). *Converting data into information.* King's Fund, London.

Lambert, P.M. (1973). Recent trends in meningococcal infection. *Community Med.* **129**, 279.

*The Lancet* (1841). Hospital physicians and surgeons. *Lancet,* 649.

Last, J.M. (1963). The iceberg: 'completing the clinical picture' in general practice. *Lancet* **ii**, 28.

Leck, I., Birch, J.M., Marsden, H.B., and Steward, J.K. (1976). Methods of classifying and ascertaining children's tumours. *Br. J. Cancer* **34**, 69.

Lees, D.S. and Cooper, M.H. (1963). The work of the general practitioner. *J. Coll. Gen. Practit.* **6**, 408.

Lockwood, E. (1971). Accuracy of Scottish Hospital Morbidity data. *Br. J. Prev. Soc. Med.* **25**, 76.

Logan, W.P.D. (1953). *General practitioners' records.* GRO Studies on Medical and Population Subjects No. 7. HMSO, London.

Logan, W.P.D. (1960). *Mobidity statistics from general practice—Volume II (Occupation)*. GRO Studies on Medical and Population Subjects No. 14. HMSO, London.

Logan, W.P.D. (1982). *Cancer mortality by occupation and social class 1851–1971*. Studies on Medical and Population Subjects No. 44. HMSO, London.

Logan, W.P.D. and Brook, E.M. (1957). *The Survey of Sickness—1943–1952*. General Register Office Studies on Medical and Population Subjects No. 12. HMSO, London.

Logan, W.P.D. and Cushion, A.A. (1958). *Morbidity statistics from general practice—Volume I (General)*. HMSO, London.

McGoogan, E. and Cameron, H.M. (1978). Clinical attitudes to the autopsy. *Scott. Med. J.* **23**, 19.

McNay, R.A. (1969). Hospital Activity Analysis. Experience in the area of the Newcastle Regional Hospital Board. *The Hospital* **65**, 308.

McNeilly, R.H. and Moore, F. (1975). The accuracy of some hospital activity analysis data. *Hosp. Health Serv. Rev.* **71**, 93.

March of Dimes (1982). *Quarterly report of the International Clearing House for Birth Defects Monitoring Systems*. March of Dimes Birth Defects Foundation, New York.

Markush, R.E. (1968). National chronic respiratory disease mortality study. *J. Chronic Dis.* **21**, 129.

Martini, C.J.M., Hughes, A.O., and Patton, V.A. (1976). A study of the validity of the Hospital Activity Analysis. *Br. J. Prev. Soc. Med.* **30**, 180.

Ministry of Health and General Register Office (1967). *Report of the Cancer Registration Working Party 1967*. Ministry of Health, internal report.

Ministry of Pension and National Insurance (1965). *Report on the inquiry into the incidence of incapacity for work 1964–1965*. HMSO, london.

Mole, R.H. (1982). Hanford radiation study. *Br. J. Ind. Med.* **39**, 200.

Moriyama, I.M. (1952). Needed improvements in mortality data. *Public Health Rep.* **67**, 851.

Moriyama, I.M., Baum, W.S., Haenszel, W.M., and Mattison, B.F. (1958). Inquiry into diagnostic evidence supporting medical certifications of death. *Am. J. Public Health* **48**, 1376.

Morrell, D.C. (1972). Symptoms interpretation in general practice. *J. R. Coll. Gen. Practit.* **22**, 297.

Morrell, D.C. and Kasap, H.G. (1972). The effect of an appointment system on demand for medical care. *Int. J. Epidemiol.* **2**, 148.

Morrell, D.C. and Nicholson, S. (1974). Measuring the results of changes in the method of delivering primary medical care – a cautionary tale. *J. R. Coll. Gen. Practit.* **24**, 111.

Morrell, D.C., Gage, H.G., and Robinson, N.A. (1970). Patterns of demand in general practice. *J. R. Coll. Gen. Practit.* **19**, 331.

Morrell, D.C., Gage, H.G., and Robinson, N.A. (1971). Referral to hospital by general practitioners. *J. R. Coll. Gen. Practit.* **103**, 77.

Munro, J.E. and Ratoff, L. (1973). The accuracy of general practice records. *J. R. Coll. Gen. Practit.* **23**, 821.

Nevin, N.C., McDonald, J.R., and Walby, A.L. (1978). A comparison of neural tube defects identified by two independant routine recording systems for congenital malformations in Northern Ireland. *Int. J. Epidemiol.* **7**, 319.

Nightingale, F. (1863). *Notes on hospitals, 3rd edn*. Longman Green, Longman, Roberts and Green, London.

Office of Population Censuses and Surveys (1970). Report of the Advisory Committee on Cancer Registration. OPCS, London.

Office of Population Censuses and Surveys (1973a). *Cohort studies: new developments*. Studies on Medical and Population Subjects No. 25. HMSO, London.

Office of Population Censuses and Surveys (1973b). *General Household Survey: introductory report*. HMSO, London.

Office of Population Censuses and Surveys (1978). *General Household Survey, 1976*. HMSO, London.

Office of Population Censuses and Surveys (1979). *Area mortality tables, decennial supplement, England and Wales 1969–73*. Series DS No. 3., OPCS, London.

Office of Population Censuses and Surveys (1980a). *Population and health statistics in England and Wales*. OPCS, London.

Office of Population Censuses and Surveys (1980b). *Population estimates, England and Wales 1979*. HMSO, London.

Office of Population Censuses and Surveys (1981a). *Area mortality decennial supplement, England and Wales, 1969–1973*. Series DS No. 4., HMSO, London.

Office of Population Censuses and Surveys (1981b). *Weekly and quarterly returns of infectious and other notifiable diseases*. OPCS Circular (STAT) No. 1/1982., OPCS, London.

Office of Population Censuses and Surveys (1982a). *Congenital malformations and parents' occupations*. OPCS Monitor MB3 82/1. OPCS, London.

Office of Population Censuses and Surveys (1982b). *General Household Survey, 1980*. HMSO, London.

Office of Population Census and Surveys (1982c). *Labour Force Survey 1979*. HMSO, London.

Office of Population Censuses and Surveys (1982d). *Evaluation of 1981 Census*. OPCS Monitor CEN 82/3. OPCS, London.

Office of Population Censuses and Surveys (1982e). *A comparison of the Registrar General's annual population estimates for England and Wales compared with the results of the 1981 Census*. Occasional Paper No. 29., OPCS, London.

Office of Population Censuses and Surveys (1982f). *Sources of statistics on ethnic minorities*. OPCS Monitor PP1 82/1. OPCS, London.

Park, A.T. (1965–66). *Occupational mortality in Northern Ireland (1960–62)*. J. Statist. Soc. Inquiry Soc. Ireland, XXI (4).

Park, A.T. and Kidd, C.W. (1958). Morbidity in the insured population of Northern Ireland. *Br. J. Soc. Prev. Med.* **12**, 75.

Parkin, D.M., Clarke, J.A., and Heasman, M.A. (1976). Routine statistical data for the clinician. Review and prospect. *Health Bull.* **34**, 279.

Patel, A.R., Gray, G., Lang, G.D., Baillie, G.G.H., Fleming, L., and Wilson, G.M. (1976). Scottish hospital morbidity data 1: errors in diagnostic returns. *Health Bull.* **34**, 215.

Pole, D.J., McCall, M.G., Reader, R., and Woodings, T. (1977). Incidence and mortality of acute myocardial infarctions in Perth, Western Australia. *J. Chronic Dis.* **30**, 19.

Population Statistics Division (OPCS) (1980a). Estimating the population of local authorities. *Popul. Trends* **20**, 12.

Population Statistics Division (OPCS) (1980b). *Local authority population estimates methodology*. Occasional Paper No. 18, OPCS, London.

Population Statistics Division (OPCS) (1981). *The revised mid-1971 population estimates for local authorities compared with the original estimates*. Occasional Paper No. 22, OPCS, London.

Puffer, R.R. and Griffith, W.G. (1967). *Patterns of urban mortality*. Pan American Health Organization, Washington.

Redfern, P. (1981). Census 1981 – an historical and international perspective. *Popul. Trends* **25**, 3.

Rees, J.L. (1982). Accuracy of hospital activity analysis data in estimating the incidence of proximal femoral fracture. *Br. Med. J.* **284**, 1856.

Registrar General (1855). *14th annual report of the Registrar General of Births, Deaths and Marriages in England*. HMSO, London.

Registrar General (1949). *The Registrar General's statistical review of England and Wales for the six years 1940–45, Text, Volume 1, Medical, statistics of infectious diseases*, p. 85. HMSO, London.

Registrar General, Scotland (1973). *A longitudinal study of a 1% sample of the Scottish population. Quarterly Return of the Registrar General, Scotland*, No. 471. HMSO, Edinburgh.

Reid, D.D. and Rose, G.A. (1964). Assessing the comparability of mortality statistics. *Br. Med. J.* **ii**, 1437.

Research Committee of the Council of the College of General Practitioners (1962). *Morbidity statistics from general practice—Volume III (Diseases in General Practice)*. HMSO, London.

Rowe, R.G. and Brewer, W. (1972). *Hospital activity analysis*. Butterworth, London.

Royal College of General Practitioners (1968). Returns from general practice. *Br. Med. J.* **iv**, 63.

Royal College of General Practitioners, Office of Population Censuses and Surveys, Department of Health and Social Security (1974). *Mobidity statistics from general practice, 2nd national study, 1970–1971*. Studies on Medical and Population Subjects, No. 26. HMSO, London.

Royal College of General Practitioners, Office of Population Censuses and Surveys, Department of Health and Social Security (1979). *Morbidity statistics from general practice 1971–72. Second national study*. Studies on Medical and Population Subjects No. 36. HMSO, London.

Royal College of General Practitioners, Office of Population Censuses and Surveys, Department of Health and Social Security (1982). *Morbidity statistics from general practice 1970–71: socio-economic analyses*. Studies on Medical and Population Subjects No. 46. HMSO, London.

Schilling, R.S.F. (ed.) (1960). *Modern trends in occupational health*. Butterworth, London.

Silman, A.J. and Evans, S.J.W. (1981). Regional differences in survival from cancer. *Community Med.* **3**, 291.

Smithells, R.W. (1962). The Liverpool Congenital Abnormalities Register. *Dev. med. Child Neurol.* **4**, 320.

Spear, B.E. and Gould, C.A. (1936–37). *Mechanical tabulation of hospital records. Proceedings of the Royal Society of Medicine*, XXX, Part I, p. 633. RSM, London.

Spicer, C.C. and Lipworth, L. (1966). *Regional and social factors in infant mortality*. General Register Office Studies on Medical and Population Subjects No. 19. HMSO, London.

Statistical Society (1842). Report of the committee on hospital statistics. *J. Statist. Soc.* **5**, 168.

Statistical Society (1844). Second report of the Committee on Hospital Statistics. *J. Statist. Soc.* **7**, 214.

Statistical Society (1862). Statistics of the general hospitals of London 1861. *J. Statist. Soc.* **25**, 348.

Statistical Society (1866). Statistics of metropolitan and provincial general hospitals for 1865. *J. Statist. Soc.* **29**, 596.

Statutory Instruments (1968). *Regulation of births, deaths, and marriages etc.* SI No. 2049. HMSO, London.

Stewart, G.T. (1980). Whooping cough in the United Kingdom 1977–78. *Br. Med. J.* **ii**, 451.

Stewart, G.T. (1981). Whooping cough in relation to other childhood infections in 1977–79 in the United Kingdom. *J. Epidemiol. Community Health* **35**, 139.

Stocks, P. (1949). *Sickness in the population of England and Wales, 1944–47*. HMSO, London.

Taylor, I. (1965). The notification of infectious disease in various countries. In *Trends in the study of mortality and morbidity*. WHO Public Health papers 27. WHO, Geneva.

Tillett, E. and Spencer, I.-L. (1982). Influenza surveillance in England and Wales using routine statistics. *J. Hygeine* **88**, 33.

Vowles, M., Pethybridge, R.J., and Brimblecombe, F.S.W. (1975). Congenital malformations in Devon, their incidence, age and primary source of detection. In *Bridging in health—Reports on studies for health services in children*, p. 201. Nuffield Provincial Hospital Trust, Oxford.

Wadsworth, M.E.J., Butterfield, W.J.H., and Blaney, R. (1971). *Health and sickness: the choice of treatment*. Tavistock, London.

Wadsworth, M.E.J. and Jarret, R.J. (1974). Incidence of diabetes in the first 26 years of life. *Lancet* **ii**, 1172.

Wall, M. and Cross, K.W. (1968). Recording and analysis of in-patient data on a regional basis. *Hospital* 354.

Wall, M. and Wharton, D.A. (1970). The elderly in hosptial. *Hospital* **66**, 414.

Weatherall, J.A.C. (1969). An assessment of the efficiency of notification of congenital malformations. *Med. Officer* **121**, 65.

Weatherall, J.A.C. (1978). Congenital malformations: surveillance and reporting. *Popul. Trends* **11**, 27.

West, R.R. (1973). Cancer registration by means of Hospital Activity Analysis. *Hosp. Health Ser. Rev.* **69**, 372.

West, R.R. (1976). Accuracy of cancer registration. *Br. J. Prev. Soc. Med.* **30**, 187.

Whates, P.D., Birzgalis, A.R., and Irving, M. (1982). Accuracy of hospital activity analysis operation codes. *Br. Med. J.* **284**, 1857.

Williams, W.O. (1970). *A study of general practitioners' workload in South Wales 1965–66*. Reports from General Practice, No. 12. Royal College of General Practitioners, London.

Wingrave, S.J., Beral, V., Adelstein, A.M., and Kay, C.R. (1981). Comparison of cause of death coding on death certificates with coding in the Royal College of General Practitioners Oral Contraception Study. *J. Epidemiol. Community Health* **35**, 51.

WHO Regional Office for Europe (1966). *Studies on the accuracy and comparability of statistics on causes of death*. Unpublished WHO Document EURO-215. 1/16. WHO Copenhagen.

World Health Organization (1977). *Manual of the international statistical classification of diseases, injuries, and causes of death*. World Health Organization, Geneva.

# Information systems and routine monitoring

## Applications of information to health promotion

# 3 The impact of automated information systems applied to health problems

Donald A. B. Lindberg

## INTRODUCTION

Research methods in public health are quantitative, beginning with the recording of sickness and deaths. One strives for a modelling or analysis in order to gain understanding of causes and prevention of morbidity and premature mortality in populations. Consequently the advent of automated information systems and the growth of information science techniques contribute greatly to the infrastructure which supports public health concepts and methods. One thinks immediately of the statistical methodologies, such as correlation-regression analysis, tests of significance and fit to hypotheses, of formal mathematical models of life processes, and of the wealth of generalized computer routines which provide these services (Dixon 1981; SAS 1982). Yet these familiar manifestations of the computer in modern scientific and industrial enterprises are probably less significant than its more pervasive influences upon our concepts and style of work.

For example, because of the existence of computer database technology, it is possible to create population-based disease registries and to collect and to pool reliable data on even quite rare diseases from any number of physically separate sources. The rapid communication permitted by computer-based electronic networks also supports this capability. As a result, worldwide disease monitoring, geographical pathology, reporting of drug interaction and adverse drug reaction, multi-causality of disease, and monitoring of the environment for adverse health effects have all become commonplace concepts. Of course nowhere are these all done well. Even at best the essential elements are the inquiring mind and the research organization. But without automated information systems such ideas are impractical, and almost unthinkable.

The remainder of this reveiw will describe particular manifestations of such concepts in public health work. It may be useful, however, first to draw attention to a few more general ideas which fundamentally arise from and depend upon automated information systems. One is the concept of the individual health profile which grows out of the 'biochemical individuality' of Roger Williams (1956) and its refinement to 'the chemical fingerprint' by George Williams (1970). Their ideas are simple and compelling: namely that changes in the physiology of individuals normally traverse a numerical range which is about one-tenth the magnitude of the ranges which would be considered normal for a population. This claim has many times been shown to be true. The implication is that careful measurements over an individual's life should be made, recorded, and monitored, and that abnormalities should be detected and remediated as soon as the individual's normal range or normal pattern is exceeded.

A second concept which becomes plausible because of medical information science is the lifelong medical record. Leaving aside the question of population-based studies, even in the case of the individual citizen or patient, the record must be complete and machine-readable in order to be useful. Whether organized by source or by problem or otherwise, and whether carried by the patient on magnetic card or stored by a hospital computer system, the availability of a complete and readily usable lifelong medical record would have major positive effects upon individual patient care.

A third new concept should be mentioned: the general accessibility of medical knowledge. Modern science assumes the printed publication of facts and conclusions. Information science has extended this availability through literature citation and information retrieval systems. Beyond this, however, is the concept of the artificial-intelligence-based expert consultant programs which embody the scientific and heuristic knowledge of the expert (or groups of experts) in a coded form. This offers at least the possibility that all medical scientific knowledge and the heuristics for using that knowledge could be available immediately to each health-care agent as it is needed via a local computer or through communication connections to regional or central machines. The impact of these ideas is just being felt in health care. It is an open question, for instance, how traditional health education systems ought to adapt to such capabilities. The reader is cautioned not to dismiss these propositions as wholly visionary. Artificial-intelligence-based computer systems are already finding application and acceptance in non-medical fields of so worldly a nature as petroleum exploration, computer systems configuration control, manufacturing robotics, and stock market portfolio management. We can identify some immediate – even if attenuated – effects in health systems. Yet it is certain that more pronounced effects will be seen in the future, and that these will be seen in the theoretical fabric of public health goals and objectives, the daily practice patterns, and in the educational requirements.

## HEALTH DATA COLLECTION

### Mortality data

Data on the occurrence and causes of death in populations is the bedrock of public health studies. The completeness and quality of these data will of course vary with the level of development of the country. A description of this problem and such systems is presented more completely in other chapters. For the moment we should merely note that modern arrangements for collection and processing of mortality statistics rely upon computer systems. This is essential simply because of the volume of data involved. It should be remembered that enumeration of the US census in 1890 was itself the stimulus for creation of the punched card by Hollerith and inducement for the attendant sorting, counting, and listing machines which constituted the beginning of modern data processing.

The use of automated information-processing systems in mortality data is reasonable because of an even more important consideration. Such devices enhance the accuracy of the enumerations. Furthermore, the arrangements of systems associated with automated information processing can enhance the goodness of the observations, hence the quality of the data which are collected.

Evidence on this question is also cited in this article under the topic of Clinical Trials Data. In this situation and for mortality data reporting, erroneous observations arise because of ambiguity in the data collection forms, errors in numerical coding of diagnoses, inadequacies of the coding schemes, and individual considerations such as boredom and ignorance. The effect of many of these flaws can be detected by automatic editing and checking of the input data by computer systems. Depending upon the sophistication of the system, a range of considerations is possible: from numerical and alphanumerical field and field-length restrictions up to subtle medical constraints dealing with gender, prevalence restrictions, likelihoods of valid combinations of observations, and the qualifications of the observer. These techniques are fairly widely understood and used in governmental and investigative data collection.

Amazingly, the simplest improvement in technique is not widely applied: namely, on-line data collection. Where patient observations are entered directly into a computing system and the various editing and reasonableness checks are performed immediately and the results displayed back to the person at the source of the observations, errors can more easily be corrected. The more usual alternative of paper forms, batch processing by the computer, and retrospective analysis and discarding of erroneous data is far less effective and desirable. In recent times independent microcomputer systems and communication terminals connected to central systems have made it possible to improve the quality of health data collection by immediate explanation of requirements, editing, and interaction with the observer to eliminate or limit errors in data and missing observations. An intermediate level of technology is also available: hand-held counting and data-recording devices. These generally do not provide interactive editing but do at least solve the problem of accurate counting and provide data which are in machine-processible form.

Autopsy data are a very special category of mortality observation. Here one has the advantage of a complete reconsideration of the patient's illness along with histopathology and microbiological studies which approach being definitive. The autopsy has historically been the touchstone of quality control in clinical medicine and in public health, serving to monitor and test the quality of clinical cause-of-death reporting and also permitting observations of emergent new disease manifestations and complications. Indeed, many prospective and retrospective studies have confirmed the relative unreliability of death certificate diagnostic impressions unless these are controlled and checked by proper post-mortem examinations (Britton 1974; Holler and DeMorgan 1970; Rigdon 1980; Cameron and McCoogan 1981). During the past 20 years the number of death certificate diagnoses based on autopsy observations has declined greatly in some industrialized countries. In the US for instance, Carter *et al.* (1981) report a reduction in the percentage of deaths investigated by autopsy to only 16 per cent of the total occurring in 1978. This decline makes the results of the autopsy even more precious for epidemiology as well as clinical biomedical research. Carter *et al.* (1981) have reported a project in the US to create a computer-based National Autopsy Data Bank so that the original objectives of the autopsy are served at a national level of aggregation.

### Drug toxicity reporting

Despite the many beneficial effects of modern drug therapy, unwanted side-effects of drugs now constitute a substantial threat to the public health. The problem is made more severe by so-called 'polypharmacy', in which patients receive many drugs simultaneously. In hospital, patients frequently receive a dozen drugs at once, and ambulatory patients often as many as half a dozen. The danger of untoward interactions between drugs is multiplied by the practice of administering multiple simultaneous medications. Many hundreds of pair-wise drug interactions have been reported: far too many for the individual practitioner to be aware of without automated assistance. Even in the case of a single drug, especially the ever-increasing list of new drugs and new formulations, the danger of undesirable and even life-threatening side-effects exists.

That this problem is of worldwide dimension is shown by the unfortunate thalidomide-phocomelia story (Taussig 1963; Mintz 1967). Here a soporific drug was shown to cause congenital malformations in fetuses when taken by the mother during the first trimester of pregnancy. Large numbers of persons were affected in Europe and Japan before the cause was detected in West Germany. The US national regulatory agency (Federal Drug Administration) refused to licence the drug for sale. None the less about 20 000 persons in the US also received thalidomide, some on an experimental basis, some through personal purchases in Canada or Europe. Fortunately only 26 cases of phocomelia resulted (Mintz 1967). Great population mobility, especially among the military, causes all such problems to be of international concern. In any event, despite conscientious efforts on the part of governmental regulatory agencies, there is now still no assurance that computer-based or other safeguard systems will prevent another such tragedy. Of course computing systems are used to record drug reaction reporting data and to subject them to appropriate statistical analysis. Indeed, such fragmentary studies are our main protection at present. What is missing is the determination and resources to maintain a population-based prospective drug-effects monitoring system.

It should be noted that ethical drug houses, when they make every effort to comply with the requirements for data collection during drug testing prior to approval for sale of the agents, themselves also encounter serious information-processing problems. These firms have created rather sophisticated information systems to capture and analyse possible drug reaction events in animal and human test populations. Garten *et al.* (1982) described an *Adverse Experience Controlled Vocabulary* system at Burroughs-Wellcome which provides for detailed descriptions of study elements and derived data outside the file containing the actual clinical study data. This approach is meant to permit tracking of each occurrence of a unique adverse effect throughout many years of testing experience. Steger and Enz (1978) describe a system at Hoechst-Roussel in which a data dictionary describing the format and location of data for each study is linked with the general purpose SAS statistical system for data retrieval and analysis.

## Clinical trials data

Prospective clinical trials of new therapeutic regimens, along with suitable control groups and statistical designs, appear still to be the main course of clinical research. This seems true whether the interventions are targeted on the individual patient or upon groups at risk or upon general populations. This methodology is expensive and somewhat ponderous. It has been subject to criticism because of its slowness compared to the speed with which the therapeutic and surgical regimens themselves change and improve, the ethical dilemmas associated with double-blind studies and selection of the controls, and a number of other problems. Alternative strategies have been proposed. It is beyond the scope of this discussion to evaluate these. For the moment most investigators have not been convinced that reliable conclusions as to the worth of new therapeutic and preventive regimens are available by other means. Leaving aside the overall strategy of such studies, the major practical problem is the validity and integrity of the basic patient or subject observations. Here automated information systems come into play.

Computer-based systems for collecting clinical trials data certainly are capable of solving the problems of data loss and inaccurate tallying, and can provide the necessary statistical testing. The emphasis in use of computer systems in recent times has shifted to data quality assurance, consistency and reproducibility of the observations, and in providing positive assistance to the participating research groups in achieving compliance with the agreed upon protocols for treatment and for observation. Two projects in these new domains are especially notable in the US: the Centralized Cancer Patient Data System (CCPDS), and the projects to provide computer assistance in carrying out cancer therapy protocols.

The CCPDS was created by the 21 US Comprehensive Cancer Centers, with the support of the National Cancer Institute, to standardize and integrate the data collected, so as to form a statistical data base to facilitate information exchange among the Centers. Through the use of standardized definitions, centralized training responsibility, the establishment of a central Statistical Analysis and Quality Control Center (SAQC), and automated data collection techniques which included extensive computer-based editing of the input data, the group achieved what it considered to be 'high quality patient data that are comparable among Cancer Centers' (Feigl *et al.* 1981).

Efforts were made to see that the definitions of CCPDS data items and codes were largely compatible with WHO recommendations and other major American cancer data collections (WHO 1976). Feigl *et al.* acknowledged that the data system requirements for the CCPDS work differ from those of both population-based cancer registries and cancer registries in general hospitals. None the less, the initial experience with the CCPDS experiment serves to emphasize that serious efforts are required to establish comparability and reliability for the critical basic patient observations even among specially selected centres of acknowledged high quality. Evidence for this conclusion includes the results of the initial 1979 combined data analysis, in which it was observed that 'major coding disagreements' in the data submitted for pooling existed for the following three key variables: primary site, 6 per cent; histology (cell type), 14 per cent; and stage, 23 per cent.

The state of diffusion of computer technology is such that in these studies the data centre (SAQC) used extensive data-editing computer programs and provided copies of the programs to all participants. In contrast, only some of the participating centres could actually implement computer data editing at their own sites. The point to be noted is not just that pooling clinical data is a difficult problem – these data were undoubtedly better than most – but that automated information systems technology, and a strong commitment to data quality control, made it possible to detect and to correct at least some data errors before they contaminated the central file and the ultimate conclusions.

Reports of these studies acknowledge in passing one of the central problems in using data processing in support of large clinical and epidemiological studies: namely, that data must be coded and entered into the automated system. That is, clinical records in most institutions are not yet directly computer-based or computer readable. The CCPDS acknowledged their need to use rigid coding categories and complicated coding schemes, along with inherent ambiguities with which even medically qualified personnel would experience difficulty. Even so they conclude that their overall experience is that 'well trained non-physician abstractors make fewer errors due to ignorance than busy physicians do because of boredom'. In the next work to be considered, we will see the beginning of automated systems which are designed to assist both groups.

Shortliffe *et al.* (1981) describes ONCOCIN, a knowledge-based computer system which uses artificial intelligence techniques to assist the oncologist at the time cancer patients are actually receiving out-patient treatment. The system is designed to 'know' and, to the extent it is currently possible, to understand all of the dozens of complex treatment protocols (ranging from 20 to 70 pages of text each) which apply to the patients seen at a university clinic. Further, it accepts observations of the patients' current status, integrates these states and trends for a patient, combines these with the options and requirements of the formal treatment protocol, and presents the results to the physician. The major task here is simply to overcome the difficulty of dealing with complex protocols and thereby to enhance the quality of treatment, and of research data by better compliance with the research design. The recording and validation of the actual data items in this system are automatic by-products. Others too, including Lenhard *et al.* (1982), have reported systems aimed at this same problem in various stages of development and deployment. These systems enhance research in clinical trials not at the level of the mechanics of coding and data entry, but rather by organizing and displaying complex clinical records of patients on oncology protocol-based management in such a way as to improve their comprehension by health care and research personnel. The objectives are to improve both patient care and research data.

The spectrum of specialized clinical data systems also includes simple therapeutic/algorithmic systems. These do not support research as a primary objective. Rather they are designed to support standard treatment of common disabilities – even by paramedical personnel. Examples have been described by Sherman *et al.* (1975) and Slack and Slack (1972).

The CCPDS and ONCOCIN examples relate to patient data collection under conditions of large and complex studies. It should be noted that a great many reports exist in which individual research studies and more restricted research data collection projects also have benefited from implementation of automated information systems. The following systems are selected examples. Tuttle *et al.* (1982) describe a successful automated information system for research records of patients being treated for melanoma. Boyd *et al.* (1979) desribe the increased utility of clinical laboratory data records for education and research when these uses are supported by an automated system. At a more general level, the CLINFO automated record system has had extensive use by numerous clinical research centres for support of many protocol studies and also use by individual researchers for collection and analysis of patient, or even animal care data. The CLINFO system is an exceptional example of successful technology transfer, in that it was specified by the US National Institutes of Health Division of Research Resources, designed and built under contract by RAND Corporation, field tested under public support, and ultimately made available to the public for purchase from an independent industrial company. The results of a survey of research users are encouraging (Hopwood *et al.* 1977). Thirty scientific users of CLINFO were surveyed before and after they employed the system in three clinical research centres. After using the system, 100 per cent felt that the system provided greater insight into the relevant relationships of the clinical research data than was possible without the automated system. Eighty-

nine per cent felt the insight came earlier. Ninety-six per cent felt that more questions could be answered from the data available, and the same percentage felt there were fewer data-manipulation errors. In contrast, most did not feel that the system made possible the use of fewer experimental subjects or fewer test samples per subject.

## HEALTH CARE INFORMATION SYSTEMS

### Regional health care systems

#### Registers and registries

Weddell (1973) offers a distinction between register, the book or catalogue in which facts are recorded, and registry, the place where registers are kept. We shall follow Weddell's usage, extending her concept of registry to include the systems and procedures employed for obtaining and using special clinical records.

Many systems exist for registering special classes of patients. At a minimum the systems link unique patient identifying information with a suitable characterization of the disease in question. Additional patient data must be available within the registry or elsewhere. Depending on the nature of the disease and the objectives of the registry, this may include many observations of the illness in individual patients, detailed information about the treatments given, and observations on the outcome obtained. In contrast, registries (especially multi-centre registries) aimed at prevention of disease in large populations may deliberately restrict to very few items the information which is catalogued within the central data store. Manual registries are a possibility, but even in the case of registries with rather restricted data stores, one operator recommends that any registries larger than 500–1000 patients would warrant the use of a computer system (Hook 1976, p. 18).

Traditionally registries have been institutionally based, such as hospital tumour registries (Queram 1977). The rationale for these and broader efforts have been to contribute in a general way to the study of illness (typically neoplasia), to provide a crude measure of the quality of care at the institution concerned, to facilitate service to patients, and in some registry applications to prevent the occurrence of disease or the complications of disease. Weddell (1973) describes registers of various types, largely in Great Britain. The types include preventive, disease specific, treatment, after-care, and at-risk registers, and also registers of skills, resources, and specific information (for example, information centres related to broad classes of disease or medical practice). Amongst the various activities conducted by registries, the follow-up of patients after the initial detection or therapy has in all cases been the critical and most costly task, and the one most often slighted.

Computer contributions to registry operations are usually of a merely data processing nature, for example, storing and retrieving of records, production of printed lists of cases or counts of cases, maintenance of address and telephone numbers, producing notices for mailing or notices of tasks to be performed. Leaving aside the rare moments of inspired data interpretation, this is the bulk of the work of most registries. Certainly it is the bulk of the work to follow-up of cases. The logic for handling such tasks is not complex; the problem is simply to deal with large number of cases with a minimal investment of the time of the personnel of the registry. Brandenburger *et al.* (1980) reported that use of all of these computer functions in assistance of follow-up of survivors of myocardial infarction resulted in greatly enhanced performance of the registry. Indeed they outlined a recommended procedure for future use in which the logical steps of the strategy of follow-up were executed by the computer system itself. For example, textual case histories were designed to be available to the computer system, and a step such as sending the referring physician a computer-generated questionnaire (based on knowledge that the particular physician has responded promptly in the past) would be followed by a three-months wait, after which the system would print a telephone form instruction that a local relative be called, and would assign this form and task to a staff researcher. Brandenburger felt that his group's effective actual follow-up rate (98.4 per cent) with computer assistance could be improved even further at less personnel cost if the computer follow-up management were adopted. Computer systems were used in a similar way for facilitating follow-up of cardiac pacemaker patients in San Francisco (Szurek *et al.* 1979) and in Toronto (Covvey 1980).

Attempts to broaden the population base of work with individual disease or hospital registries, for instance by establishing statewide networks of collaborating registries, have had varying degrees of success. Sometimes, technical difficulties have been encountered, such as data storage and retrieval limitations and the deficiencies of all numerical coding schemes. Computing equipment has usually not been dedicated to registry work. In contrast, most hospitals for the past ten years have had computing systems for business applications, and these have been available only on a batch-processing basis for registry work. Generally, however, the technical problems have been dwarfed by the behavioural deficiencies, that is, lack of area-wide or national planning authority.

Exceptions to this desultory pattern do exist. The Surveillance, Epidemiology, and End Results (SEER) program is an example of a population-based data system (Young *et al.* 1981). Having been started with appropriate national funding and authority, SEER has been able to achieve its basic objective of monitoring tumour incidence in eleven geographical regions of the US. As of June 1981, data have been fully tabulated, analysed, and published for cases occurring between 1973 and 1977. These include 350 220 malignant and 28 992 *in situ* cases of malignancy that occurred among residents of nine continental US regions plus Hawaii and Puerto Rico. Also included is information on 170 375 cancer deaths among these populations. The combined population of the eleven regions studied equals slightly more than 10 per cent of that of the entire US population.

Special attention was directed to quality control of data observations, with extensive use of training sessions, workshops, site visits by central staff for re-abstracting and recoding of sample cases, as well as actual case-finding audits. Confirmation of primary diagnoses and causes of death included examination of primary medical reports by the collaborating centres. Each participating centre and also the National Cancer Institute staff perform computerized edits of all data. The edits included not only checking for legitimate codes in each data field but also checks for relationship of data in related fields, such as site/sex, site/type, and site/extent of disease. Also, inter-record checks were made for patients with more than one primary cancer, in order to be sure that identification and vital data were consistent. All death certificates for area residents were monitored and abstracted. Interviews with the physicians who signed death certificates for study patients were conducted to establish when and how a diagnosis of cancer was made. If the interview or the confirmation could not be made, the case was classified as 'death certificate only'. The National Cancer Institute suggests that one measure of completeness and quality of data is the percentage of 'death-certificate-only' cases. For all areas (excluding Puerto Rico), only 1.4 per cent of the 327 627 malignant cases were reported by death certificate only.

Clearly the achievement of a successful (and on-going) population-based national cancer registry with reliable data and reasonably timely analysis and publication is a proud achievement built primarily upon scientific excellence of the various participants. Yet it is easy to see that automated information systems facilitated the good project design, and perhaps even constituted a necessary element in the project design. Parenthetically, a secondary benefit of this automated approach is that computer tapes containing the data which constitute the thousand page printed report are available at cost to the public and interested scientists.

Computers have been applied successfully to disease registers in renal dialysis and kidney transplantation. The American College of Surgeons/National Institutes of Health Organ Transplant Registry made an important contribution to advances in understanding in this field. For example, data derived from 16 444 kidney transplants were used to identify survivorship, sex and age distributions, and trends, to compare the relative effectiveness of family-related versus cadaveric donor transplants, survivorship as related to the extent of antigenic matching and methods of kidney preservation and pretransplant preparation of the recipients, and the strategies for attempting sequences of related and unrelated donor transplants (American College of Surgeons 1975). Information in this registry was provided by 288 institutions, of which 164 were American. Follow-up data had been received for 14 479 patients.

This is a successful registry and a worthy subject of automated information processing. None the less, even this project suffers from the data errors associated with batch data collection from paper forms. In a study of the question of transplant survivorship as it might be related to the closeness of antigenic matching of tissue type of donor kidney and recipient, it was noted that out of 7905 cases, 435 were eliminated 'because of obvious clerical errors in reporting typing'. This 6 per cent error rate clearly did not prevent success of the study. Yet these were only the detected errors; one must suspect at least an equal number of undetected errors. In any case, if the errors were obvious once the data were examined, then the same logic could have been incorporated in on-line computer editing procedures to detect the errors at the time of data entry, when they could have been corrected at the source. Because of the increasing availability of computer terminals and the current easy access to commercial telecommunication networks, it would not be necessary to provide computer systems to the 288 participating institutions. Rather, allowing each to transmit data input to a central computer at the registry, where editing routines were applied could significantly improve data quality and completeness in a situation of this sort.

A larger parallel effort in computerized case registration is represented by the work of the European Dialysis and Transplantation Association (EDTA). In the (eleventh) *Combined Report* (Jacobs *et al.* 1981) analysis was reported for 107 004 patients, of whom 14 084 had been added in the latest year (1980). The total number of patients alive on treatment was 67 412 of whom 12 394 had a functioning transplant, 48 408 were on a haemodialysis, and 2749 were on peritoneal dialysis. These data derive from 1495 renal disease registries in 32 European and adjacent countries with a total population of 573 million persons. The Association estimates that the percentage of European patients missing from the registry is probably less than 10 per cent. Annual analyses deal with matters important for health care and health planning. These include distributions of patient variables and comparative studies of costs, access to care, and treatment strategies between the various countries. These reveal some interesting differences, for instance a four-fold difference in the number of patients per million population who receive this treatment comparing two European countries. The reader can easily appreciate the importance of this co-operative registry, the great accomplishment it represents from the point of view of voluntary collaboration and technological capability, and the inherent dependency of this venture upon the use of computer-based information processing systems.

None the less, the fundamental conception of this system as a planning and strategy tool, rather than a patient care aid, has inevitably brought some technical disadvantages. For example, input is via paper forms, 'computer analyses of the data are performed twice each year', and the process of continual updating and validation of the patient file naturally results in 'discrepancies between numbers given in different reports for the same year'. EDTA noted that there were 3029 patients last reported as alive on treatment but for whom no up-to-date follow-up information had been received. This would represent a loss of only about 4 per cent; hence while it is a flaw, would leave a remaining 96 per cent follow-up success rate which most individual registries would consider to be commendable. One explanation is thought to be the familiar problem of patients changing location and being registered in more than one centre. This problem is understandably magnified by the international scope of the EDTA registry system. Somewhat less encouraging was the active participation of only 82 per cent of the known European renal centres. Here too it is apparent that the level of participation (already good) is not likely to increase unless the inducement of data services were to extend beyond the central

registry function to reach the level of timely services which would assist in or affect directly the care of individual patients, or at least to substitute for data processing functions at the level of the local renal centre. Such plans, while difficult to carry through, are (barely) within the state of the art. Indeed with respect to possible double reporting, the EDTA states 'the Registry is improving computer software and administrative techniques'.

### Genetic registers, record linkage, and data privacy

Another example of computer-based regional registries should be noted: those related to genetic diseases. Genetic register systems collect and store data on individuals with genetic diseases or on their families. Often in the past the registers have been used to identify those persons in need of health and welfare services engendered by their genetic affliction. Currently there are substantial efforts to use the registers as a means to help trace individuals at risk of having affected children so that they may be offered genetic counselling. In both cases, accurate identification of the persons involved is an essential element in the register's data.

Technically, computer-based genetic register systems work quite well. Meritt *et al.* (1976) described a university medical centre genetics information system in the US which includes 350 000 persons and grows by addition of 45 000 persons per year. The system can handle file maintenance, edit human input to produce machine-generated pedigrees, and calculate genotype probability distributions for a given individual in a pedigree conditioned on known phenotype information from relatives. A computer-based system in Edinburgh is being tested for feasibility and acceptability as a means to detect and alert individuals at high risk of having children affected by single factor genetically determined diseases (Emery 1976). In Belgium, a computerized national genetic registry serves seven regional centres of human genetics (Vlietinck and Vanden Berghe 1976) with estimated annual additions of 6000 referred patients. An extensive multi-centre genetic registry and information system also operates in California (Mitchell *et al.* 1982).

Financial costs of the genetic registries have been broken down into three categories. Hook (1976) estimated the costs for a 4000 person registry to be $29.97 overall cost/case in 1974 US dollars. This is made up of $1.85 for data ascertainment, $3.12 for internal data processing, and $25 for analysis. Interestingly, the major component of cost, namely analysis, is large partly because of the costs of dealing with erroneous and missing observations which escaped detection at the earlier stages of ascertainment and data processing. Hook estimated that 15–20 per cent of the costs of analysis were directly related to this problem. Once again, there appears to be ample opportunity for cost reduction and improvement in data value through early application of on-line computer assistance in data acquisition during the conduct of such registry operations.

In genetic registers we see a clear example of the dilemma created by information technology. Computers are an essential part of the infrastructure of technology which permits medical geneticists to undertake major applications. With computer techniques they can establish quite sizeable patient data bases and systems, with at least the hope of offering significant preventive services to regional and national population groups. On the other hand, even before this is accomplished, many people have recognized the social danger that such systems offer to confidentiality of data and protection of privacy of patients, families, and the public at large. This matter is complicated even further by a practice adopted by some specialized scientific information centres: namely, of serving an international community. Thus data may be stored outside the national territory, are moved across national frontiers, etc. The potential danger that major genetic registries might be used by a political agency to harm selected persons is well recognized and widely discussed (Advisory Committee on Automated Personal Data Systems 1973; Westin 1976; Griesser et al. 1980). Yet a final balance between this danger and the potential health and social value of such systems has not been settled in any very satisfying fashion, nor are there technical means to offer absolute protection against misuse of such systems.

Considerations of data privacy are quite central to acceptance of genetic registries. Consequently the arrangements made to assure data integrity and data confidentiality are not merely technical matters to be left to the computer system operators. These must be uppermost in the consideration of the system scientists and the political sponsors of such systems. The Belgian system uses a scheme which is illustrative of a strategy designed to avoid day-to-day problems of misuse. Vlietinck and Vanden Berghe (1976) note that for reasons of confidentiality the paper input forms are divided into sections, with all personal identifying data entered separately from the medical data. Identifying data are ciphered, coded, and the sequence mixed. Every user of the Belgian national registry must identify himself or herself, and access is permitted only to limited portions of the record. Identification information for the patient is accessible only if two separate persons each give passwords. Furthermore, the program allows only three erroneous attempts to access patient identification. Then it erases the patient data, which must be retrieved through centrally supervised procedures from back-up storage in fire- and magnetic-proof safes. Of course, these kinds of technical protections can only deter the idly curious and give assurance against easy illegal access on a regular basis.

Similar protections are provided by other registries and medical data banks. In the case of registers whose purpose is the gathering of statistical information, the problem is much more easily resolved. The SEER cancer-surveillance system in the US emphasized quality control of the input data (that is, the ascertainment stage). Consequently, it is apparent that personal identification of patients, hospitals, and providers of care is essential at the level of the regional collaborating centre. On the other hand, regional centres (all of which are non-federal organizations) are forbidden by the terms of their contracts with the federal government from providing to SEER any information regarding patient name or name of the hospital at which the diagnosis was made and/or treatment was given.

Beyond technical protection of privacy is the question of integrity of the operators and sponsors of the registry and the propriety of the social setting in which the systems are operated.

In the case of the Belgian national registry, this further assurance takes the form that there will be no link between the genetic disease register and the health insurance registers. It is permitted that the latter can provide the necessary epidemiological information (Vlietinck and Vanden Berghe 1976). This decision is in agreement with advice that serious students of data privacy in the US also endorsed. In the Report of the Advisory Committee on Automated Personal Data Systems (1973) one of five basic principles endorsed was that; 'There must be a way for an individual to prevent information about him that was obtained for one purpose from being used or made available for other purposes without his consent.' The conclusion of this group followed extensive investigation and interviews with (US) federal government scientists and administrators. There was a surprisingly strong consensus that data integrity could not be assured beyond the bounds of a department, and that cross-linking of federal computer files brought with it the dangers of politicization and misuse.

This matter presents a serious problem both on theoretical and practical grounds. First, save for deliberate redundancy for validation purposes, it is counter to all basic good information processing principles to collect data more than once. To do so increases costs and inevitably creates the problem of erroneous and inconsistent information, especially in the area of identification of persons. On the practical grounds at least, one student of genetic information systems also strongly disagrees with the political decision against cross-linking of files. Trimble (1976) recommends that persons at risk of having a defective child be identified by computing system and genetic registers through use of existing computerized population records, including birth, marriage/divorce/death/ files and also health records (for example, hospital discharge files). He points to the work of Newcombe et al. (1959) at the Chalk River Nuclear Laboratories in Canada as demonstration that techniques exist to perform automatic record linkage. Trimble reports studies from the register of handicapped children and adults of the British Columbia Health Surveillance Registry which 'suggest that more than half of all children with disorders of possible interest would be missed by a genetic register that relies solely on voluntary case reporting and does not make full use of the information contained in routinely produced vital and health records.'

The concepts of automatic record linkage using computer systems arose independently of purely medical concerns but now is seen clearly to apply to a wide range of medical information systems functions, of which the genetic register is just one. Serious studies evaluating and assessing such systems for possible use in the UK for a variety of medical therapeutic and public health purposes began in 1962 in the Oxford Record Linkage Project (Acheson 1967). This study concluded that statistical matching schemes, following the ideas of Newcombe et al. (1959), were effective, reasonable, and economical for the purpose of linking together in a machine-readable form an individual's health record. To go beyond this to link together items at the level of families or communities was also feasible but only if information additional to that usually supplied were to be made routinely available. Necessary information included, for example, maiden name for women, information concerning family history, order of birth within the family, and more consistent use of numerical identifiers such as National Health Service number and date of birth. Obviously the strongest single item of identification would be the use of a logical, readily available number, unique to each citizen, which might be issued at birth and be used throughout life. The technical desirability as well as the political dangers of such a system have been commented upon repeatedly for decades. None the less, Sweden does use such a system of unique national identifying numbers (*personnummers*) and with a resultant vast simplification in medical information processing (Fenna *et al.* 1978). The *personnummer* codes date and place of birth, gender, check digit, and a centrally assigned modifier. Elaborations even beyond this are also possible: for example, the use in Norway of a double self-checking digit which can be used not only to detect but to correct errors in transcription of the identifying digits. It should be emphasized that the use or rejection of personal identifying numbers is not basically a technical debate. Modern societies have long ago resorted to personal numbering systems. Acheson (1967) estimated that the average Englishman already would be issued 35 sets of identifying numbers during his lifetime. Unfortunately such a practice stands as an obstacle to linking the records of births, occupational exposures, diseases, deaths, family inheritances, and environmental/community exposures. The use of a single personal identification number would greatly increase the likelihood that such associations could be made, provided that proper resources were devoted to the task. Objections to such an undertaking rest upon political reasoning. Whatever their validity, they cannot be countered by technological arguments.

Thus the reader and society in general are left with the dilemma, how aggressive and intrusive should public health programmes be? Especially the preventive and the computer-based programmes. Certainly the question is not a new one. Furthermore, the issues of data privacy arising in consideration of genetic registries arise also and quite as naturally in consideration of all computer-based medical information systems. The impact of the computer-based information technology serves to accentuate the problem because information science multiplies both the potential for good and for misuse of health information.

### Other regional information services

A great many additional regional automated medical information services exist. Typically these are special-purpose but cost-effective and important. Two will be noted as examples without a detailed presentation of their functions: the clinical laboratories quality control sample services of the College of American Pathologists (Haven *et al.* 1982) and the central Emergency Medical Services ambulance-dispatching services of Tokyo (Saito 1982). These two systems and many others share two critical features. First, they have come into existence because data must be aggregated and compared in order that an individual observation or request can be evaluated. The single laboratory observation must be compared against that of the reference standard and peer laboratories in order that its quality be evaluated; the individual emergency case must be referenced against a pooled data base of available beds and

available transportation. In this sense, such systems deal inherently with the health of populations, even though the direct user represents a single laboratory or a single ill person. Secondly, the diffusion of all such systems will be influenced in a major way by the relative costs of local computing facilities versus the relative costs of telecommunication services to obtain the information processing at central, shared facilities. These relative costs are determined largely by public policies, which regulate telecommunication carrier charges on a local or regional level, and occasionally subsidize them on a national or international level by policies such as those toward the launching of geostationary satellites and their use for transmission of scientific information. In other words, the public health forces which in former days created systems for flow of pure water, sewage, and good health standards and practices must now be brought to bear upon the more recent challenges of the flow of computing capability, information, and telecommunications. Until this is successfully done, the development of such services will remain fragmentary and incomplete in most countries.

### Patient-based data systems

A modern variant of the hospital registry is a new kind of computer system in which data about particular patients with medical conditions of special interest are collected directly along with the process of caring for the patients. In these systems, there is the possibility of the same patients benefiting from the data collection system, although often the benefits are of a research nature and are expected to flow to other or future patients with the same or closely related disorders. None is truly population based; they tend to be based in a single institution or to be built by co-operating institutions whose participation is founded upon recognition of need for the information or knowledge which can only be derived from pooled data. Their interests are focused on assistance in patient care decision-making. Hence, the data which these systems collect tend to be carefully validated, to be medically meaningful, and often to be rather more extensive than that encountered in the more restricted data sets of the registry systems.

An example is ARAMIS, the American Rheumatology Association Medical Information System (McShane and Fries 1978). This data base system was created by Fries at Stanford University with the co-operation of a dozen collaborating institutions. It contains the records of 40 000 rheumatological cases. Each case record may be described by up to 700 standardized descriptors, and multiple visits for each case are allowed for. Trends in the patient descriptors are of special interest. This is emphasized in the data base design and retrieval mechanisms, and the system is styled as a 'time-oriented data base'. On-line and batch input modes are provided. Even with so extensive a file, it is not intended that the computer record replace the entire medical record for the purpose of individual case management. The experience represented by so many cases can, however, provide a general guidance for individual patient care decisions. The retrieval of records of patients' diagnoses, treatments, and outcomes can be applied, if one wishes, to cases limited to the single contributor's institution, thereby eliminating some of the variances which are inevitable in pooled data. This national pool of case information has permitted a large number of research studies to be conducted.

The Duke patient data base on cardiology also provides for extensive computer-based patient record keeping (Rosati *et al.* 1975). In this case, it is intended from the outset that the ever-increasing set of records of diagnostic, therapeutic, and outcome data should be used directly to guide decision-making concerning individual patients. A typical decision concerns whether surgical or medical management of coronary artery disease should be recommended for a particular patient. A typical data-base query is to retrieve the counts and records of similar cases, with a tally of outcomes corresponding to each treatment plan. Because of the close coupling with actual clinical use of this system, the quality of observations and measurements in the data base has been good. The determination of similarity between cases is recognized to be critical and is the subject of an evolving system of logical and statistical definitions.

An automated hospital system for storing and displaying the records of patients being treated with dialysis and/or kidney transplantation was reported by Gordon *et al.* (1981). This presents another example of a patient-oriented system which is used for patient care. This system is based upon a relatively inexpensive microcomputer configuration. It is thought to be capable of dealing with the records of 750 patients over 10 years of treatment, and actually contains the records of 350 patients over seven years of treatment. The system has a number of interesting technical features, including graphical displays, easily learned control features, and a variable time axis. More important, however, are the authors' explanations for the necessity to create such a system and the effects observed upon clinical thinking and the relationship of the hospital to the centralized European registry. Gordon *et al.* stated that the difficulty of dealing with large volumes of data essential to good dialysis and transplantation was the reason for the automated system. With acceptance of the information system, they noted 'clinicians are beginning to read data in a quite new way looking at the shapes and meaning of graphical presentations, instead of working laboriously through columns of figures'. The system has been adapted to three other renal care units, as well as to additional oncology care units. In addition to their contribution to direct patient care, such developments relate to national and international public health studies as well. Gordon's system, for example, prints the patient data return forms for the EDTA European registry, as well as producing a cassette tape of the data which can be sent to EDTA for direct input to the computerized registry.

Automated data systems that are focused on data from individual patients have become important in the management of end stage renal disease patients. Unlike the registries, these systems have a definite emphasis on timeliness of data acquisition and processing, as well as upon substantial accuracy. One such system in the US holds the records of patients awaiting renal transplants in more than 30 institutions in 10 states, as well as the records characterizing available donor kidneys in a wide geographical area (Stulting and Ward 1975). The most important task to be done seems computationally almost trivial: namely, to present listings of matches of the tissue-typing of potential donors and recipients with sets chosen according to varying criteria for goodness of match. The authors point out, however, that this particular computer system went through six major revisions between 1969 and 1975, and that their latest version 'bears only faint resemblance to the original programs'. This evolution occurred not primarily because of the difficulties inherent to the computational process, but because experience proved the need for changes in the possible schemes for the selection of renal transplant recipients. In the end the criteria for selection were a combination of scientific considerations plus the time each recipient had waited for a possible donor kidney. In connection with the question of data privacy and possible misuse of information systems, it is interesting to note that even in this circumstance the authors feel obliged to state 'identification data are used for patient identification and research purposes only and do not affect selection of recipients for available kidneys' (Stulting and Ward 1975). Additional practical matters such as geographic location of the persons, storage time for cadaveric kidneys, availability of perfusion transportation apparatus, and surgical teams are formidable but seem to be well handled by the human decision-makers. The computer system's job is merely to store data, to create listings of potential pairings of donors and recipients, and thereby to enhance the possibility of optimal matching through access to the largest possible population of potential donors. Experience in this field has shown that survivorship of the transplanted kidneys is directly related to the goodness of the tissue match, and that the goodness of the match is practically related to the size of the potential donor population (Patel *et al.* 1969). The social and scientific co-operation which permits institutional pooling of data is the important element, but the information system also makes a critical contribution. Again one finds that such systems dealing with practical problems, closely tied to decision-making concerning individual patients, are successful systems.

A special kind of patient-oriented data system is the statistical survey. While such undertakings were and are entirely possible without computing systems, their magnitude and reliability are so much associated nowadays with automated systems methodology that they perhaps deserve mention. For this purpose two examples will be presented.

The National Head and Spinal Cord Injury Survey was designed to provide statistics that measure the morbidity and economic costs of injury to the head or spinal cord for the population of the contiguous US for the year 1974, including the occurrence of new cases and the frequency of existing cases (Anderson *et al.* 1980). This large-scale survey was undertaken by the National Institute of Neurological and Communicative Disorders and Stroke (NINCDS) as a basis for planning, especially for determining research priorities. A multistage design was used. An initial feasibility trial paid particular attention to the question of whether privacy considerations could be properly safeguarded and sufficient acceptance of the surveys goals be achieved. Probability sampling rather than total enumeration was the method employed, largely to limit the costs and because a large staff for field investigations was not available. For instance 58 primary sampling units were selected from an initial list of 1675 such geographical areas in the US. Subsequent stages selected 305 hospitals from the 1886 hospitals in the sampling units, and 9745 medical records from the 204 122 medical records listed for the hospital sample selected. Subsequently abstracting of the records had to be done, and follow-up of the patients to determine recovery status and economic costs. The further details of the methodology and the conclusions will not be repeated here. It is clear, however, that automatic data-processing techniques lend themselves well to such large-scale studies. It should also be noted that the validity of the conclusions from such studies are by no means guaranteed either by their magnitude nor by the sophistication of the data-processing techniques they employ. Kraus (1980) undertook to compare and to explain the differences in conclusions which followed for this survey and four others which used different experimental designs to study the same question, namely, the extent of the problem of head and spinal-cord injury.

A second survey of spinal-cord injury may be noted, since this too exemplifies a useful modern approach which is essentially dependent upon automatic data-processing methods. Bracken *et al.* (1981) undertook to estimate the national incidence of acute spinal-cord injury over the period 1970–77, using existing data from the National Center for Health Statistics (NCHS) Hospital Discharge Survey (HDS). The authors emphasize that 'this type of analysis has only recently been made possible because of newly developed techniques for interfacing data bases containing millions of records with computer programs powerful enough to manage, statistically describe, and analyse them'. The NCHS file for this period contained over 1.5 million coded discharge diagnoses for randomly selected hospitals. The search by Bracken *et al.* required a complex subsetting depending upon the codes, followed by study according to additional patient characteristics. The interfacing techniques referred to involve the combination of the well known SAS statistical system with the Autogroup routines developed at Yale (Freeman *et al.* 1979).

## Special information services

These systems differ from those just described in that they either provide specialized information storage and retrieval services, or they operate on data to produce derived information. Consequently the conceptual level of generalization is not great, but the value of the services is easily measured.

### Cardiology

The simplest example is interpretation of the patient's electro-cardiographic signal. This service is often centralized or regionalized and provides expert automated interpretation for areas in which human experts are not available. More than 13 per cent of all electrocardiograms in the US are interpreted automatically by computer systems (Little 1976; Drazen 1982, personal communication). Assurance of good care of the patient requires a local health care system, of course, in addition to the interpretation of the physiological waveform. Successful implementation of these systems by the TriService Medical Information System (TRIMIS) office for uniformed services care facilities is typical of this integration into health services delivery (Huffman and Morgan 1980).

Computer systems now facilitate follow-up of patients with cardiac pacemakers. The function of the pacemaker can be verified by much the same methods by which electrocardiogram is usually analysed by computer systems. Pacemaker failure due either to a manufacturing defect or to normal wear is predictable from the analyses. Analysis can be conducted with the patient in the clinic, or via a telephone (Grant and Hanson 1976).

### Radiology

Computerized axial tomography (CAT) systems are now widely installed in the US and elsewhere. Because the logic for performing the scanning is incorporated in a rather rigid fashion in these devices and their built-in computers, advances in the field present a problem to the hospital and physician owners of older systems. A recent innovation in information processing allows CAT scanners to send raw computer records of the patient studies over commercial telephone lines to a specialized computer centre which transforms the records to include advanced image-display techniques which are meaningful for particular medical decision making. Specifically, in their initial applications, CAT studies of the spinal column in scoliosis are transformed and rotated to orthographic views and plots of the facet surfaces which greatly facilitate planning for corrective surgery (Glenn *et al.* 1975; 1982).

### Drug information systems

The use of computer systems to support pharmaceutical therapy is an important application because of the high cost of drug therapy, its potential morbidity, and the rapid increase in the number of new drugs and preparations and information concerning them. Obviously the hoped for contribution of computing systems has been to increase the availability to the pharmacist and physician of information about the drugs in use for a patient, to keep drug profiles for individual patients and to support systematic searches for potentially dangerous improper dosage, for inadvertent overlaps in prescribing, and for drug interactions. Successful applications have been reported for the following aspects of drug information systems: drug interaction (Biejsens and Abcouwer-McCarron 1980), drug control and adverse drug reaction reporting (Johansson and Manell 1980), and in-patient and out-patient hospital testing with label preparation and interface to pill- and capsule-dispensing machines (Trusty and Nazzaro 1980). Braunstein (1982) estimates that in the US, usage of computer technology approaches 75 per cent in pharmacies providing services to nursing homes, 20 per cent in pharmacies providing ambulatory services, and 10 per cent in pharmacies providing service within hospitals. This field presents examples of local computer systems and also of regionalized services. The latter include poison index and the drug interaction data bases, both requiring aggregation and maintenance of information above the level of the individual facility. In some cases, these as well as the local services are provided to user institutions (such as hospitals and chains of retail pharmacies) by commercial time-shared computer services via the voice-grade telephone network. In addition, special purpose drug information services are available from remote central computing facilities, and these too are accessed via the telephone circuits. Examples include automated systems for the optimization of drug regimes through pharmaco-kinetic modelling (Jelliffe *et al.* 1980) and electrolyte and acid-base balance management (Bleich 1972).

The existence of computer-searchable data bases of drug prescribing covering substantial proportions of the population offers opportunities for public health-oriented studies (Braunstein 1976). The study of prescribing patterns from the point of view of improving cost-containment is an example of such an opportunity. Detection of the deliberate or inadvertant use of duplicate prescriptions for controlled substances is another example. This phenomenon becomes immediately apparent as soon as an automated system is implemented, especially when data are pooled from several locations in a region. Not much has been written about these studies because of ambiguity about the legal status of the privacy requirements for such data. Needless to say, the problem is compounded by the circumstance that most of the computing services are (in the US) commercial in nature, with public health authorities having taken little or no part in creating the services, maintaining the information bases, nor in facilitating access to the services. Computer-based studies of drug information handling practices as a means to detect information lack and to identify potential applications for continuing medical education are being done with encouraging results. Braunstein (1982) reports these for pharmacists and Manning *et al.* (1980), for physicians.

*Computer-based consultation systems*

Computer systems which incorporate the cognitive behaviour and judgement of the medical expert in a number of carefully defined domains are important in public health terms because of their objective. This is, to make available to remote populations through long-distance communication systems the expert consultation which would in traditional systems be available only to patients seen at referral centres or leading hospitals. Such systems accept patient findings and advise concerning diagnosis, differential diagnosis, and recommended management procedures, including therapy. A number of such systems have been implemented in test settings. Examples include successful systems reported in the following areas: antibiotic therapy (Shortliffe *et al.* 1973); glaucoma management (Weiss *et al.* 1978); differential diagnosis in internal medicine (Miller *et al.* 1982); rheumatology (Lindberg *et al.* 1980); oncology (Shortliffe *et al.* 1981); digitalis management (Swartout 1977); pulmonary physiology (Kunz *et al.* 1979); anaesthetic management planning (Miller 1982); and haemostasis (Kingsland *et al.* 1982).

Even though these systems have not yet seen wide medical use, they are important milestones even in computational terms. The artificial intelligence principles on which they were built appear to be quite widely applicable throughout medicine

and other expert domains, and this new approach (symbolic reasoning, self-explanation, formal representation of knowledge through information structures, separation of problem-solving heuristics from the knowledge base) appears to circumvent older obstacles to encoding medical expertise. Consequently there has been a rapid increase in the number of artificial intelligence-based medical expert systems under construction, and a decrease in the time required to create the systems. There seems little doubt that this approach will have a major impact on health care delivery, through increasing access to expert knowledge and consultation. The speed with which this will occur and the shape of the ultimate system will be influenced by both behavioural and technical developments. The latter, that is, the technical developments, include the relative success and cost of communication systems to link remote users to the large central computers on which these systems now operate versus the relative success and cost of ever more capable local microcomputers which can (even now to some extent) operate the consulting systems on a local basis.

The most serious limitations upon the development of expert systems are the maturing of medical understanding of disease processes and progress in translating current understanding to forms which are suitable for computer processing. Gordon *et al.* (1981) comment, with some insight, about this limitation upon current computer contributions to the management of patients on dialysis/transplantation regimens. After noting that good management requires consideration of volumes of numerical data, they regret that 'paradoxically, these must be interpreted in the light of experience, and of conceptual models which presently we do not know how to translate into mathematical or computer language'. For this reason, their institution uses the computer to show graphically these numerous patient care data, presenting those which are most relevant to the clinician's line of thought and relying upon the physician to interpret the data. Considering the advanced concepts which their current information system embodies and the extent to which modelling concepts already infuse this field, it seems likely that the expert's cognitive processes will also eventually be incorporated in a useful way into the computer system.

Decision analysis techniques are also being more widely used as an aid to physician and patient decision-making in the medical context (Pauker and Kassirer 1980). This approach resembles the artificial intelligence-based systems in attempting to render explicit the scope and alternatives in diagnosis and management. It differs in relying upon numerical measures and estimates of likelihoods as the basis for selecting alternative decisions.

Even more squarely in the traditional mathematical realm are the computational models of biological and health care processes. The increasing use of mathematical models in public health work should be noted (Bailey 1978). This too frequently requires access to substantial computing facilities. The field is large. Examples include the modelling of chronic diseases such as diabetes (Ackerman *et al.* 1969), the modelling of epidemic disease and immunization strategies (Elveback *et al.* 1976; Bozikov *et al.* 1982; Longini *et al.* 1982), theoretical public health interventions (England and Roberts 1981), cancer treatment plans (Jackson *et al.* 1982), regional nursing services (Bates *et al.* 1982), and geographical mapping of disease (Hopps 1972; Becker *et al.* 1982). As a natural extension, such models are also used for instruction.

## Advances in the technology

Hundreds of commercial systems are available to provide general information storage and retrieval capability, some on microprocessor-based small computers, some on larger systems. Naturally these represent a wide range of capabilities, but many are useful to the individual institution or even as centralized services. In the area of medical applications, systems have been produced which also attempt to offer flexibility and adaptability while providing features thought to be especially appropriate to health care data. Barnett (1976) has created a medical record system for ambulatory patients (COSTAR), generalized and highly flexible, which has been the basis for a large number of specialized and specific applications. Commercial medical systems have also been adapted to a wide range of applications (Hodge 1977; Hicks 1978). Extensive data-mangement and file-handling abilities have been added to some of the widely available general statistical analytic systems, such as the Statistical Analysis System (SAS Institute Inc. 1982).

Beyond the concept of adaptable systems are newer ideas of 'data-base management systems', in which the vendor system provides only the lowest level tools for the file-handling work of information storage and retrieval, and the user identifies to the system a 'schema' or model for the particular record or data structures to be allowed for (Wiederhold 1977). In accord with these ideas, Blum and Brunn (1981) at Johns Hopkins and Wasserman (1980) at California write about techniques for interaction between research scientists and between scientists and the evolving information systems, so that general methods and systems are designed to produce particular medical target systems. For relatively small jobs, it is possible to purchase 'database application design systems'. These are essentially programming systems which build infor-mation retrieval systems. In these the user is kept at a con-siderable intellectual distance from the actual machinery of data processing, and specifies requirements almost solely in terms of his or her own application.

An additional feature of advances in information technology is the increasing capability and utility of electronic telecom-munication networks. Using combinations of commercial and private telephone wire systems, microwave, and geo-stationary earth satellite re-transmission, computers and computer users over a wide geographical area can be inter-connected.

Two large computers, one at Stanford in California and one at Rutgers on the opposite continental coast, are shared among several dozen research groups in many different institutions. One group itself has more than 200 remote collaborators from 63 research institutions. The SUMEX network provides not only special computing services to health-care research projects, thus sharing physical and software resources, but also provides for considerable sharing of computational techniques, codes, and ideas, thereby sharing intellectual resources as well. An important part of the enterprise is to advance the art of remote collaboration and the electronic 'college' (Freiherr 1980). Much larger numbers of computers can be interconnected for exchange of data at high data rates. The US Department of Defense ARPANET is such a system (Newell and Sproull 1982). The effect of the earth satellite systems is almost to ban ground distance as an economic consideration in sharing information and information services (Lindberg 1982). Within a single institution, networks also play an important role in permitting the integration of previously independent information systems. Simborg *et al.* (1982) describe a local area digital network based on optic fibre lines which links four rather different and completely independent computing systems at a medical centre, so that each can interact with and benefit from data processed by the other three.

## MULTIPHASIC HEALTH TESTING

This is an important field in public health, but space permits only a brief consideration of the impact of computer-based information systems per se. Historically, screening efforts in public health examined populations for evidence of, generally, single diseases. As the prevalence of illnesses such as untreated tuberculosis or untreated syphilis fell in the general population, such approaches became relatively more expensive and relatively less effective. The advent of new testing methods and automated multi-channel laboratory biochemical devices in the decade following the Second World War created the opportunity for systematic screening of populations for multiple diseases with a single examination. The addition of computer-based systems to this process, beginning in the early 1960s had a number of important enhancing effects, most of which are inextricably bound to new insights and concepts in health care which were mutually supportive of information processing ideas.

First, simple electronic automation greatly reduced the unit cost of many testing procedures. Serum glucose estimations, for instance, which cost about $6.00 as manual procedures in 1958 had fallen to about 60 cents by 1962. Secondly, the concept of the linking together of many individual (continuous flow) laboratory analysers was shown by Thiers to result, even with hospitalized patients, in a surprisingly large per-centage of unsuspected abnormalities (Bryan *et al.* 1966). This technique was quickly adopted by Collen (1978*a*) and others for use in screening of healthy populations of subscribers to prepaid health plans, with much the same findings. The role of computer systems was important (even essential) in several aspects of these developments: automation of devices, quality control of the new more complex and more high-volume laboratories, automatic evaluation of multichannel laboratory results previous to or independent of evaluation by the physician, and linking the multi-channel results together so as to permit evaluation of patterns of results of the batteries of tests rather than the former stepwise evaluation of single test results.

Next, computers made possible the realization of the medical concepts of evaluation of individual normal ranges (Williams *et al.* 1978). This concept fits well with the increasing emphasis upon examination of healthy persons on a voluntary basis, the emergence of improved medical techniques to correct abnormalities which were detected in an early state, and the emergence of the periodic health examination. All such ideas involve relatively larger amounts of data taken from populations, require follow-up to be sure that each step of multi-part testing is properly completed and correlated with clinical findings, and demand that examinations for patterns of abnormalities and comparison with previous findings be performed thoroughly. Many of the procedures of a multiphasic health examination were found to be properly performed by automation or by automated testing devices plus non-physician health attendants. It can easily be seen that these changes fit well together, and that automated information methods and ideas were central to the new medical concepts and systems. Yasaka (1982) concludes that the automatic multiphasic health testing system (AMHTS) is a field of medicine which 'could not have been established without the aid of computers'. To emphasize the close tie even further he suggests that 'AMHTS is, in a sense, improperly named due to the circumstance under which it was brought into existence. It should be Automated and Informatized Multiphasic Health Testing and Services, so to speak'.

The current concepts in this field view automated multiphasic health testing in quite new ways. Garfield (1982) considers that it offers to comprehensive health care systems, such as Kaiser Permanente, the critical entry point into the system. Thus in his view 'the free market system fails to work because of the high fees involved, and removal of those fees fails to work because of the overwhelming demand and inflationary costs that result'. He sees automated multiphasic health testing as a comprehensive and cost-effective, service for determining who is well and who is sick and for determining the needs of each. He notes that when it includes physical examination by nurse practitioners, it requires very little physician involvement. For these reasons he considers that the use of multiphasic health screening 'to regulate and manage the demand of free users of medical care' to be 'one of the most important functions it can perform'.

The final form that AMHTS will take is unknown, but it is certain that it will include increasing integration into full-service health-care systems and increasing integration with automated information systems for data acquisition and patient record keeping, and likely too for medical inferencing. As of 1975, Collen (1978a) notes there were 325 AMHTS centres in the US, about 40 in Japan, 30 in Europe, and smaller numbers in Australia, Asia, Canada, and Latin America. There is no actual international register of AMHTS. Consequently the number of these units is not known accurately. Suzuki (1982) reports that 73 AMHTS institutions had been officially designated by the Japan Hospital Association. In addition, however, the Human Dry Dock screening project under sponsorship of the Federation of Health Insurance had completed installations in 330 hospitals and had already completed a 20 year follow-up study (1959–80).

The oldest and best known of the AMHTS is probably the original Kaiser-Permanente unit in Oakland, which was established in 1951. Japan too placed an early emphasis on implementation of this technology. The Human Dry Dock

project was established in 1954. Suzuki (1982) notes that since then more than one million persons have been examined annually through it. In Japan, the Human Dry Dock detected laboratory and clinical evidence of numerous organic diseases (for example, abnormal glucose tolerance, hyperlipaemia, obesity, hypertension, arteriosclerosis, impaired renal function, and malignant neoplasm). Decline in the prevalence of these findings over 20 years was attributed in part to health check-ups and health education. In Australia, some initial negative evaluations of AMHTS (Rowe and Larsen 1977) appear to be reversed in subsequent studies (Larsen and Rowe 1982). Final conclusions concerning the ultimate importance of AMHTS in health care and public health will have to await further evaluation. The technology, like many, seems to have grown even faster than the ability to evaluate it thoroughly. Gelman (1971) published an extensive study of the relevant literature on multiphasic health testing including its practice and evaluation. Probably the best and most thorough evaluation studies were reported by Collen and his group (1978b) after prospective cohort studies at Kaiser-Permanente over ten years. Such evaluations are difficult because of crossing over between groups through free choices made by the patients, and because of the confounding effect of changes in medical practice over so long a time. None the less, it was possible to attribute to the use of multiphasic screening a reduction in morbidity in the population of patients served by the system. Results of evaluations from a number of studies in the US and elsewhere are summarized by Friedman (1978). Generally, measures of process of care can be shown to be favourably affected by AMHTS but measures of outcome as reflected by mortality do not seem consistently to be changed.

## MEDICAL INFORMATION SYSTEMS

### Central concept and central importance

A medical information system may be defined as a set of formal arrangements by which facts concerning the health or health care of individual patients are stored and processed in computers (Lindberg 1979a). Essential data elements include the patient's identification (usually name, number, address); hospital or ambulatory care location; demographic information (including sex and age, and sometimes occupation); past hospitalization; diagnosis/diagnoses; linkage information (whatever is needed to link new information transactions in the file to the pre-existing patient record); and time qualifiers. Additional data elements frequently include cost of care; billing information and insurance status; invariant physiological information (for example, blood type, leukocyte antigen types, karyotype); elements of health status provided by the patient; results of measurements or observations performed on the patient; and interpretive information.

In a majority of such systems, the patient information is organized and retrieved according to the source of the data, for example, patient history, doctors' orders, physical examination, clinical laboratory studies, radiological studies, etc. On the other hand, computer-based systems are perfectly capable of supporting an organizational structure which is problem-oriented, as for instance in the PROMIS system of

Weed (Stratmann 1979). There is no fundamental reason a system could not easily support both organizational rationales simultaneously, thus permitting problem-oriented record retrieval for some practitioners and source retrieval for others.

The practical appeal of these systems in hospitals has to do with their ability to facilitate rapid and sensible communication between the numerous hospital services. Laboratory, radiological, and dietary orders, for example, can be transmitted and scheduled virtually as soon as they are entered. In advanced systems, the medical interrelationships between such orders can be coded into the system itself. Thus radiological studies can automatically be scheduled in the appropriate sequence, clinical laboratory studies of iodine can be done before radiological contrast studies, etc. In addition, computer-based medical information systems provide to health care managers an unrivalled ability to obtain an accurate overview of patient care requirements within the institution and of the institution's ability to respond without undue delay. One can see accurately the facilities utilization and redundancy, can schedule personnel based upon exact patient care needs, and can call up exception reports of all sorts as a means to monitor quality of performance of the institution. Cost-control efforts are also well served by such systems. Indeed, studies have shown that the substantial costs of medical information systems can be regained merely through their practical effects in automating clerical functions, increasing hospital personnel efficiency and institutional productivity – without even taking account of the medical advantages (Heard and Thomas 1978; Coffey 1980).

Medically, such information systems are of great importance, and for much the same reasons: namely, bringing together in one system all the clinical information about a patient in a readily retrievable form. Advantages which have been reported include improved legibility and accuracy, elimination of duplicate testing to replace lost records, faster patient work-ups because of more rapid availability of information, and a variety of opportunities for automatic monitoring and enhancement of quality of medical decision-making and patient care (Barnett 1976; McDonald 1976). A number of advanced programs to provide computer assistance directly to the physician for diagnosis and management have already appeared in research or early developmental form. All of these require input of numerous patient findings such as patient complaints, history, results of the physical examination by the physician, and the results of clinical laboratory and radiological examinations.

When there is no medical information system or no connection with existing departmental computer systems, then the physician who wishes to use a computer-based expert consulting system must himself re-enter all of these items into the expert system. Only after this will the expert system be able to reason about the particular patient in question. Re-entry of so many findings is a substantial impediment to use of expert systems. Indeed it means that they tend to be used only for extremely complex cases, or when one is already aware of a serious management dilemma. Availability of at least routine patient care facts in an information system would, amongst other benefits, make consultation by expert systems available

when desired for a broader range of patient cases. Monitoring of quality of care likewise would be more effective and cost-efficient under these circumstances.

Additional, perhaps still theoretical, advantages of medical information systems are the possibility of creating a true lifetime record for a patient (which would be available regardless of where he or she sought care), and the possibility that the pooled records of two or more institutions would form the basis for the discovery of new medical relationships or principles. That these major potential advantages have not been realized may still be explained by the immaturity of the field of medical informatics, and by the still incomplete diffusion of the technological innovation.

## Limitations to the generalizability of medical information system concepts

Medical information systems are subject to all of the practical limitations of other capital intensive and technologically demanding innovations. In addition, however, conceptual limitations specific to these systems would be mentioned. Knowledge and understanding of medical processes – always partial at best – determines in a rather complete fashion the reach of medical record keeping portion of the system. This is the reason that the association of phocomelia with ingestion of thalidomide by mothers during the first trimester of pregnancy was not discovered through computer systems (Taussig 1963; Mintz 1967). The concept of such a possible association was unknown at the time the early medical information systems were designed. Indeed, multi-institutional, prospective data systems at the time had not allowed for recording of such medications (Mellin 1963). Of course, now it is a responsibility of public health workers to be certain that drug effects in early pregnancy are allowed for in modern computer record systems. The discovery of the effects of diethylstilbesterol (DES) treatment of pregnant mothers upon unborn daughters is another example of advancing medical understanding which was not reflected in computer record keeping. This particular effect (increased incidence of adenocarcinoma) is delayed by 20 years, highlighting the need for automated record systems to be lifelong and to reflect family linkages.

Some of the technical and political problems in utilizing automatic medical record linkage were noted briefly in discussing genetic information systems. That there is a general need to include family linkages within all medical information systems can be seen from consideration of the thalidomide and the DES complications. Likewise one can readily appreciate that identification in the information system of the individual patient is essential. How else could the information system ever be useful to warn the endangered patient or daughter? Mintz (1967) cites a single tragic case which illustrates such a need: namely, a woman who, unaware of her danger, took thalidomide medication during two consecutive pregnancies, and bore two children with phocomelia.

A last limitation to medical information system concepts is doubtless obvious to the reader. On a worldwide stage, there clearly is no definitive computer-based information system which is appropriate to each country's major health care needs. It is not a problem to adapt systems to deal with varying incidences of particular diseases or to particular patient groups. These same adaptations must be made within the confines of any single large country. The problem for computer technology is to identify at what point a sufficient health care and technological infrastructure exists to make installation of computer systems the next logical step. Since health care planning in each country is absolutely dependent upon having accurate information about disease incidence, prevalence, location, and character, the general need and utility of some level of automation is probably worldwide. Yet investing in advanced automation before having solved fundamental problems of nutrition, pure water support, sewage disposal, and immunization may be improper. The decision when to introduce data automation and at which level is a difficult one and must be dealt with in each country individually by those who know it best and love it best. Experiments in this field are now much less expensive than in the past because of microprocessor-based computers. One critical feature of automation trials, however, has not changed: the time required for an evaluation to be meaningful. A meaningful cost-benefit evaluation for a major information system will take five years at minimum, and may well require ten years. If a nation cannot see its way through this kind of serious, long-term commitment, then a trial of medical data automation is probably inadvisable.

## ACCESS TO MEDICAL LITERATURE

Health care for both populations and individual patients is inescapably linked to awareness of advances in understanding of health, disease, and treatment. Hence, the means to provide for access to current medical literature is an essential function of systems for public health. Automated information systems provide the capacity to store literature citations and the speed to process standardized periodic as well as individualized search queries for retrieval of pertinent citations. To this technical resource must be added systems of human scholarship to establish and revise the most useful ways to order the publications and to solve the organizational problems of use by a worldwide clientele.

The outstanding example of an energetic and scholarly response to this problem is the work of the National Library of Medicine (NLM) in Bethesda, Maryland. This is a (US) national biomedical resource which includes the library itself, the National Medical Audiovisual Center, and the Lister Hill Center for Biomedical Communications. Its scope and coverage include the basic sciences as they relate to medicine, clinical medicine, the social and behavioural sciences, and more recently, hospital and health administration and health planning. The NLM has four major functions: acquiring the biomedical and health literature, organizing it, extracting from it information to be disseminated through products and services, and the development of networks for bibliographic access and document delivery.

MEDLINE, the on-line computer system for biomedical literature abstracts and citations, is used directly by 1800 health care and educational institutions in the US, and indirectly by the entire health community. Access to the computer searching is via commercial networks and also the ordinary voice-grade telephone system. In the fiscal year 1981, NLM performed more than two million special searches of the literature. In addition monthly versions of several dozen recurring bibliographies on major topics were printed and distributed. Examples include the recurring bibliographies for *Tropical Diseases* and *Acute Diarrheal Diseases*, which are distributed on a worldwide basis in editions of 5500 each. The NLM also continued to provide training programmes for American and other biomedical information search specialists. These specialists serve local user communities, typically in hospitals and medical schools, and formulate at their home institutions the on-line and off-line computer queries which are processed by the NLM computer center.

Thus NLM has already established a biomedical communications network for access to computerized bibliographic data bases. In addition it has formed a regional library network for access to documents as interlibrary loans via the postal service. The obvious third step, namely direct retrieval of full text of documents from computer storage, is so far only possible on an experimental basis within very narrow subject domains.

The long history of NLM as a national institution is presented in book form by Miles (1982). During the past 40 years it has grown to function ever more as an international resource, reflecting the inherent internationality of scientific discovery and the increasingly strong interdependence of all nations. The international aspects of the NLM programme were described by Corning (1980a). Of the 21 000 serials collected by NLM, about 17 per cent are selected for inclusion in the on-line computer file (MEDLINE) and 14 per cent are selected for inclusion in the printed publication (*Index Medicus*). The 2598 serials in the *Index Medicus* come from 73 countries and are written in 30 languages. Of these serials, 59 per cent are in English only and are produced in 49 countries. Collaborative arrangements for access to the computer-based literature citations and contributions to indexing of the literature were initially made with the UK and Sweden in 1964. Subsequently similar arrangements were found practical and mutually beneficial with Australia, Canada, France, Italy, Japan, Mexico, South Africa, Switzerland, and the Federal Republic of Germany. These collaborations have been based on multiple bilateral agreements which arrange for NLM to make available the MEDLINE system, either through tapes or on-line access to the NLM computer, along with system documentation and training. The participating country must meet technical criteria involving personnel, equipment, and fiscal resources and have a user community large enough to justify an extensive computerized service activity. The participating country then provides and/or funds the indexing of journal articles for input to the MEDLINE data base in return for access to the system. In addition to these highly successful *quid pro quo* agreements, NLM participates in projects with international health agencies.

Simultaneous with these events have been the development of independent computer-based scientific literature services such as the Lockheed Dialog system in the US and Exerpta

Medica in Holland. In addition the DIMDI system in the Federal Republic of Germany (FDR) is notable. The Deutsches Institut fur Medizinische Dokumentation und Information (DIMDI) system operates from a central computer in Cologne through a packet-switched telephone network to nine remote nodes and more than 100 terminals. It offers access to the NLM data bases MEDLARS, TOXLINE, and CANCERLINE, and also to independent international data bases such as Psychological Abstracts and Exerpta Medica, and to unique FDR data bases. One of DIMDI's nodes serves as a gateway to the continental network EURONET. More than 100 000 literature search requests per year are processed, most of them via the DIMDI network (Dudeck 1982). In Japan, JICST (Japan Information Center of Science and Technology) provides a parallel service for medicine, including MEDLARS and TOXLINE services, with an additional emphasis on the literature of physics and engineering. Direct use of American and other information retrieval services is also provided in Japan by ICAS (International Computer Access Service) through the national telephone monopoly. In France, NLM data base services are available at clinical research centres. In addition, however, ambitious experiments are being conducted in several regions to provide direct access in French households and physicians' offices to health literature information services via the TELETEL videotex service. This experimental application employs computer-generated graphical displays on household colour television receivers (Puybasset 1982).

A dozen centres worldwide use and distribute the monthly MEDLINE literature citations, recurring bibliographies, and customized searches. Half accomplish this by operating on computer tapes sent abroad from NLM. The other half distribute the services by accessing the NLM data base and computer centre via satellite transmission. The reader should note this example of countries exercising on a global scale the same choice that individuals make with respect to their preference for remote access to centralized information resources, or alternatively, for the decentralized or distributed model of information access. Both approaches are effective for these developed countries, and the choice may be made on the basis of local preferences and overall economic considerations. What is not at all satisfactory nor effective is the incomplete solution of computer access to medical literature in developing countries. In her book, Corning (1980b) describes the continuing co-operation between NLM and the Regional Library of Medicine (BIREME) of the Pan American Health Organization (PAHO), with funding from governments and foundations. Regrettably many libraries in the areas served did not hold suitable collections of the necessary medical journals themselves, thus vitiating the effectiveness of the computer citation searching. Similar and more serious obstacles are described from collaborative work with the World Health Organization project serving 84 developing countries in Africa, South-east Asia, eastern Mediterranean, and western Pacific.

The need to improve the basic holdings in biomedical libraries in developing countries must, of course, be balanced by public health workers against the need for other educational resources, and in some cases against needs in even more

fundamental areas such as nutrition, water supply, sewage disposal, and immunization. While not all users of systems such as MEDLINE are expected to have access to all the serials cited, some minimal subset of scientific serials must be available at the local level, and arrangements must be made to obtain when needed the more unusual holdings through interlibrary loans or by recourse to a national or regional central resource. An interesting experiment was reported by Horowitz and Bleich (1981) in which a local mini-computer system in a single American hospital was used to conduct searches of that subset of the MEDLINE citations which corresponded to the actual holdings of the hospital library. An additional special feature of the experiment was that all searching was done by health care professionals for themselves, with no assistance from library staff or biomedical information specialists. The system provided an extensive thesaurus which permitted the users to formulate searches in their own terms, relying upon the thesaurus to map these onto the standardized indexing system of the NLM. The experiment was judged highly successful, both with respect to the choice of a restricted subset of literature and also with respect to searching being done by medical library users themselves. Thus it may well be a model for smaller medical facilities in general. To extend this approach to non-English speaking areas would demand new thesauruses. It is entirely within the state of the art of information science to construct such adaptations, provided the domain of discourse is limited to strictly formatted queries using scientific terminology.

The possibility that in the future one can have access to the full text of all medical literature directly through electronic means is exciting. Much has been written about future systems which by-pass the printed book or journal (Overhage and Harman 1965; Lancaster and Smith 1980). Such systems are operational for major segments of law (Mead Data Central 1982), using central digital computer storage and electronic network technology. Alternative schemes involve storage of the textual information at the local user locations, as images transformed either into video or digital form. The current costs of such approaches, while falling fast, are still high and far above those for books. Hence the future impact on public health systems and their need for direct access to medical literature will be determined by relative changes in costs for printed literature, for computers, and for telecommunications network technology, and by the relative urgency placed by society upon the need for improving health care.


## EVALUATION OF INFORMATION SYSTEMS

While many sources testify to the strong and wide-ranging effects of computers on modern life in general, the exact effect on particular segments, such as health affairs, is understandably difficult to measure. More often, evaluations are made of particular technological interventions or innovations. In the case of computers and information systems, a substantial body of research exists concerning methods for such evaluations (Goldman 1979; Lindberg 1979b). This section will summarize the major current approaches and then note briefly the factors which informed speculation identifies as likely to be major determinants of the future diffusion of computer technology in medicine.

## Evaluation methods

### Marketplace

This is a default method. The expectation is that what is preferred will prevail in the marketplace, that valuable technology will compete successfully with less valuable offerings. Use of this method is not suggested out of frivolity; it is the one most commonly employed.

Much medical technology has become standard practice simply because of ready acceptance by physicians and the public. Literary examples of *ad hoc* therapy abound, such as Shaw's 'ripe greengages' in *The Doctor's Dilemma* (1909). These are matched by the modern proliferation of diagnostic computerized tomography scanners in the face of determined opposition by health planners (Institute of Medicine 1977). The slightly more acceptable scientific aspect of this phenomenon is sometimes termed 'patient compliance'. For example, we see the ingestion of tranquilizer tablets receiving ready acceptance as a treatment for anxiety. Whereas, in contrast, decades of stern lectures by diabetologists have not resulted in diabetic patients sticking to a rigorous agenda for diet and insulin injections. The current technology of automated implantable insulin pumps is at least in part a result of the marketplace rejection of personal disciplines and acceptance of the passive subject role.

### Operations research

This approach insists on a protocol for evaluation, with an explicit choice of variables to be examined, and an analytic methodology for processing the observations based on statistically valid procedures. Beyond these constraints, operations research methods are empirical; they may use economic measures, measures of personal convenience, systems efficiency, or other measures. The measurement strategy may use pre- and post-observations; it may discriminate sharply between process and outcome measures; it may use matched sites. There will always be phases of quantitative observation, analysis, and conclusion. The fundamental merit of the approach is that it insists that there is always something that can be measured, no matter how complex the process, and tends to assume that decisions will be wiser when based on some quantitative measure than on none.

### Cost-effectiveness analysis

Cost-effectiveness analysis compares the economic efficiency of alternative systems directed at the same objective. Costs are calculated and compared for alternative ways of achieving a specific set of results. Medical methodologies are often compared in this way.

The cost-effectiveness of a method is traditionally measured by comparing it with an alternative method. Given that the tasks accomplished are roughly the same, it is not conceptually difficult to put a relative cost on the two operations. A familiar example is a manual procedure versus an automated procedure. Frequently, automated procedure can be shown to be more cost-effective.

### Cost-benefit analysis

Cost-benefit analysis provides for calculation of the costs of an activity or system and the potential benefits to be derived from operating the system or activity. It is a method for identifying the relative economic merits of a question. Ordinarily it is used as an aid in choosing between two courses of action. Consequently, it is customary first to identify alternative actions or programmes, and then make a quantitative assessment of all costs to be incurred and benefits to be gained. Last, one examines these alternative costs and benefits against some explicitly stated criteria such as rate of return on investment.

Cost-benefit analysis is suitable, and cost-effectiveness analysis unsuitable, if one is attempting to answer the question, should a new technology be employed? It is reasonable to question whether to expend resources on a particular technology or intervention versus some other purpose, even a non-health-related purpose. This is a valid application of cost-benefit analysis. The analysis will, however, require measurement of the costs and benefits of all the schemes being considered, including the non-health-related ones.

### Technology assessment

Technology assessment is a new, as yet not rigorously defined, approach to evaluation that appears especially well suited for decision making involving public policy. The approach was enunciated by Emilio Daddario in 1967 in studies preceding the establishment of the Office of Technology Assessment within the US Congress. He stated:

Technology assessment is a form of policy research which provides a balanced appraisal to the policy maker . . . It identifies policy issues, assesses the impact of alternative courses of action, and presents findings: it is a method of analysis that systematically appraises the nature, significance, status, and merit of the technological program . . . [It] is designed to uncover three types of consequences – desirable, undesirable, and uncertain . . . The focus of Technology Assessment will be on those consequences that can be predicted with a useful degree of probability.

While the scope of these evaluation goals is extremely broad, a large number of such studies actually have been completed (Arnstein 1977), although generally in non-medical areas. Consequently, the analytical tools for technology assessment have improved and become refined. An example of such studies in the health field was conducted by Westin (1976) and by Griesser (1980) dealing with the indirect effects of computerized medical record systems upon the personal rights of privacy of the public. Ultimately, assessment of proposed technological innovations, including health applications of computers, is meant to include effects on the countries' economies, the physical environment, institutions, culture, the social structure, mores, values, and the law.

The costs of such assessment studies can be large. Arnstein and Christakis (1975) define macro-assessments as comprehensive in breadth and depth, costing $300 000 to $600 000. Mini-assessments are comprehensive in one of these respects and cost $30 000–60 000. Micro-assessments are briefer, including structured conferencing, are aimed at a limited aspect of the task or at defining the scope of a more ambitious assessment, with costs falling under $5000.

Advocates of technology assessment do not recommend that each and every technical advance be subjected to exhaustive analysis. They recommend selecting those technological matters which are clearly the subject of public policy decisions. Since programmes in public health are often both expensive and politically prominent, including plans for national or regional health information systems, there is some merit in conducting a full discussion of all of the implications of such a plan through a public forum employing a scientific structure for the considerations.

Such is the virtue of the technology assessment process.

## Evaluation strategy

The most important uses of computers in medicine are to do things that cannot be done in any other way. Examples include the knowledge-based expert consulting models, elucidation of anatomical structures by computerized tomography, worldwide access to scientific literature, and comprehensive medical information systems. In such uses there really is no alternative methodology with which to compare and measure. Evaluation must be against wholly different alternative uses of resources, such as highway construction or cathedrals. Since such judgements must inevitably be determined by public policy and social values, the rigorous evaluation methods are often not relevant.

In circumstances in which scientific measurements of the effects of information systems are thought to be useful, the methods mentioned may be employed. In this connection, the following personal observations may possibly be helpful. Leaving aside the more fundamental question of whether a particular activity should be done, properly carried out automation of the information handling will often be found to contribute to the activity. Frequently, as noted earlier, data collections may be more timely, the observations less error prone and more numerous, and the data collected may be more easily used because of their integration into an information system. These effects are, in other words, dependent upon the quality of the process. Consequently evaluation of process rather than outcome is often appropriate.

Regrettably, the same kind of thing may be said about much of the medical enterprise. That is, since we have extremely poor measures of health-care delivery and only global measures of the ultimate outcome, we often must fall back on measures of effects upon the process of giving care. Similarly, the expectation that automated information systems (or other single technological interventions) will have a measurable effect on reducing total health care expenditures have usually been futile. There have been easily documented reductions in certain individual aspects, such as the clinical laboratory costs for individual tests, reduced average hospital days of stay, or shifts to more efficient mixes of renal transplantation/dialysis combinations. But the expectation that total health costs will decline has been frustrated in all countries by a vast reservoir of unsatisfied demand for health enhancement and by the resultant inflation of costs when this is made a more readily accessible right.

Formal attempts to measure the effectiveness of information systems are not worthwhile unless the system under study is examined in a reasonably complete form. For instance, the importance of a highly integrated concept such as the medical information system cannot be measured satisfactorily by examination of independent parts (such as laboratory, radiology, etc.). Similarly, the worth of information systems in classic epidemiological investigations, may be seriously underestimated if the information processing (as is often the case) is done in an incomplete way, using out of date methodology such as punched cards, data sheets, batch processing, and numerically coded data instruments.

Lastly, the temptation to conclude that health care requirements for information services can be easily satisfied by commercial instruments should be questioned. No doubt, many of the problems of medical computing are shared with other fields. Even so there are some consistent features of typical medical data which make the problem a bit different from the commercial or purely scientific. These include the use of far more complex records (for example, more fields per record), the frequent difficulty of attempting analysis or decision-making in the face of missing data, the generally 'softer' less quantitative nature of the measures, observations, and diagnostic/classificatory conclusions, frequent changes in methodology and unitage, and frequent addition of entirely new measures. In addition, there is the difference that concerns for privacy and data security are frequently not only important but over-riding considerations in medical information systems. These features distinguish medical/health care data systems and tend to make them not so easily comparable with nominally alternative commercial or purely scientific systems.

## FUTURE DEVELOPMENTS

Future development of information science applications in health care will be influenced by non-technological changes as well as technological developments (Lindberg 1979c). Amongst the latter, four seem especially significant: the increasing availability of inexpensive yet powerful microcomputer systems (Noyce 1977), the refinement of existing, long-distance, and local electronic communication networks (Peterson and Isaksson 1982), perfection of the laser-etched video disk systems for storing medical images and textual/literature information (Leveridge 1983), and the continuing maturation of artificial intelligence techniques as they are applied to medical decision-making (Blois 1980).

Non-technical factors include general social adaptation to automated information systems, incorporation of these new ideas into the programmes of medical education, and advances in fundamental understanding of bodily processes and health care management. A number of relatively successful medical and public health applications of automated information systems have been alluded to. Yet in spite of these, one must admit that adaptation to this technology has been even faster in industry, commerce, and military affairs. The health professions have been relatively conservative in their use of computers (Lincoln 1983). In all countries health professionals who are also competent in computer methods are in notably short supply. It seems safe to bet that the rate of future change and the importance of future computer applications will be determined most strongly by the manner in which this field is included in the future in formal medical educational programmes.

## REFERENCES

Acheson, E.D. (1967). *Medical record linkage,* p. xx. Oxford University Press, London.

Ackerman, E., Gatewood, L.C., Rosevear, J.W., and Molnar, G.D. (1969). Blood glucose regulation and diabetes. In *Concepts and models of biomathematics: simulation techniques and methods,* Vol. 1 (ed. F. Heinmets) p. 131. Dekker, New York.

Advisory Committee on Automated Personal Data Systems (1973). *Records, computers, and the rights of citizens.* USDHEW, Washington, DC. (DHEW Publication No. (08) 73-94.)

American College of Surgeons, Advisory Committee on Renal Transplant Registry (1975). The 12th Report of the Human Renal Transplant Registry. *JAMA* **233**, 787.

Anderson, D.W., Kalsbeek, W.D., and Hartwell, T.D. (1980). The national head and spinal cord injury survey: design and methodology. In *Report on the National Head and Spinal Cord Injury Survey* (ed. D.W. Anderson and R.L. McLauren). *J. Neurosurg.* **53**, 11.

Arnstein, S.R. (1977). Technology assessment: opportunities and obstacles. *IEEE Trans. Syst. Man Cybern. SMC,* 7, 572.

Arnstein, S.R. and Christakis, A.N. (1975). Summary of assessors' perspectives. In *Perspectives on technology assessment* (ed. S.R. Arnstein and A.N. Christakis) p. 155. Science and Technology Publishers, Jerusalem, Israel.

Bailey, N.T.J. (1978). The utilization and validation of mathematical models in medicine and public health. In *Lecture notes in medical informatics,* Vol. 16 (ed. D.A.B. Lindberg and P.L. Reichertz) p. 393. Springer, New York.

Barnett, G.O. (1976). *Computer-stored ambulatory record (COSTAR).* USDHEW–NCHSR, Washington, DC. (DHEW Publication No. (HRA)76-3145.)

Bates, T., Dobra, S., and Harding, L. (1982). Regional study of community nursing policy. In *Lecture notes in medical informatics* Vol. 16 (ed. D.A.B. Lindberg and P.L. Reichertz) p. 329. Springer, New York.

Becker, N., Frentzel-Beyme, R., and Wagner, G. (1982). MONITOR. A system for the evaluation of mortality data. In *Lecture notes in medical informatics,* Vol. 16 (ed. D.A.B. Lindberg and P.L. Reichertz) p. 618, Springer, New York.

Beijsens, A.J. and Abcouwer-McCarron, H. (1980). Drug–drug interactions control in the Tilburg hospitals. In *Proceedings of MEDINFO 80* (ed. D.A.B. Lindberg and S. Kaihara) p. 901. North Holland, New York.

Bleich, H.L. (1972). Computer-based consultation: electrolyte and acid-base disorders. *Am. J. Med.* **53**, 285.

Blois, M.S. (1980). Clinical judgment and computers. *N. Engl. J. Med.* **303**, 192.

Blum, B.I. and Brunn, C.W. (1981). Implementing an appointment program with TIDIUM. In *Proceedings of the Fifth Annual Symposium on Computer Applications in Medical Care, Washington, DC* (ed. H. Heffernan) p. 172. IEEE, New York.

Boyd, J.C., Ladenson, J.H., and Lewis, J.W. (1979). Utilization of clinical laboratory information system databases for medical education and research. In *Proceedings of Third Annual Symposium on Computer Appliations in Medical Care, Washington, DC* (ed. R.A. Dunn). IEEE, New York.

Bozikov, J., Dezelic, G., Cvjetanovic, B., and Stampar, A. (1982). Computerized epidemiometric model of shigellosis and its use in assessing potential usefulness of new tools for disease control. In *Lecture notes in medical informatics,* Vol. 16 (ed. D.A.B. Lind-

berg and P.L. Reichertz) p. 611. Springer, New York.

Bracken, M.B., Freeman, D.H., and Hellenbrand, K. (1981). Incidence of acute traumatic hospitalized spinal cord injury in the United States, 1970–1977. *Am. J. Epidemiol.* **113**, 615.

Brandenburger, L.L., Moore, P., Miller, J.P., Thomas, L.J., and Oliver, G.C. (1980). Development of a computer-assisted follow-up methodology for clinical research. In *Proceedings of the Fourth Annual Symposium on Computer Applications in Medical Care, Washington, DC* (ed. J.T. O'Neill) p. 1037. IEEE, New York.

Braunstein, M.L. (1976). The computer in a family practice center: a public utility for patient care, teaching and research. In *Medical data processing* (ed. M. Laudet, J. Anderson, and F. Begon) p. 761. Taylor and Francis, London.

Braunstein, M.L. (1982). Applications of computers in pharmacy: an overview. In *Proceedings of AMIA Congress 82* (ed. D.A.B. Lindberg, M.F. Collen, and E. Van Brunt) p. 7. Masson, New York.

Britton, M. (1974). Diagnostic errors discovered at autopsy. *Acta Med. Scand.* **196**, 203.

Bryan, D.J., Wearne, J.L., Viau, A., Musser, A.W., Schoonmaker, F.W., and Thiers, R.E. (1966). Profile of admission chemical data by multichannel automation: an evaluative experiment. *Clin. Chem.* **12**, 138.

Cameron, H.M. and McCoogan, E. (1981). A prospective study of 1152 hospital autopsies: 1. Inaccuracies in death certification. *J. Pathol.* **133**, 273.

Carter, J.R., Nash, N.P., Cechner, R.L., and Platt, R.D. (1981). Proposal for a national autopsy data bank. *Am. Soc. Clin. Pathol.* **76**, Suppl., 597.

Coffey, R.M. (1980). *How a medical information system affects hospital costs: the El Camino Hospital experience.* USDHEW–NCHSR, Rockville, MD. (DHEW Publication No. (PHS) 80-3265.)

Collen, M.F. (1978*a*). History of multiphasic health testing services. In *Multiphasic health testing services (MHTS)* (ed. M.F. Collen) p. 33. Wiley, New York.

Collen, M.F. (ed.) (1978*b*). *Multiphasic health testing services (MHTS).* Wiley, New York.

Corning, M.E. (1980*a*). Access to medical literature. In *Proceedings of MEDINFO 80* (ed. D.A.B. Lindberg and S. Kaihara) p. 1375. North Holland, New York.

Corning, M.E. (1980*b*). *A review of the US role in international biomedical research and communications: international health and foreign policy.* USDHHS-NLM, Washington, DC. (NIH Publication No. 80-1638.)

Covvey, H.D., McGregor, D.C., Nolde, E.J., Goldman, B.S., and Wigle, E.D. (1980). A computer aided large scale pacemaker surveillance system. In *Proceedings of the Fourth Annual Symposium on Computer Applications in Medical Care, Washington, DC* (ed. J.T. O'Neill) p. 1125. IEEE, New York.

Dixon, W.J. (1981). *BMDP statistical software.* University of California Press, Berkeley, CA.

Dudeck, J. (1982). The state of the art in the Federal Republic of Germany. In *Communication networks in health care* (ed. H.E. Peterson and A.I. Isaksson) p. 131. North Holland, Amsterdam.

Elveback, L.R., Fox, J.P., Ackerman, E., Langworthy, A., Boyd, M., and Gatewood, L. (1976). An influenza simulation model for immunization studies. *Am. J. Epidemiol.* **103**, 152.

Emery, A.E.H. (1976). RAPID: a genetic register system for the ascertainment and prevention of inherited disease. In *Registers for the detection and prevention of genetic disease* (ed. A.E.H. Emery and J.R. Miller) p. 53. Symposia Specialists, Miami, Florida.

England, W.L. and Roberts, S.D. (1981). Immunization to prevent insulin-dependent diabetes mellitus? The economics of genetic screening and vaccination for diabetes. *Ann. Intern. Med.* **94**, 395.

Feigl, P., Breslow, N.E., Laszlo, J., Priore, R.L., and Taylor, W.F. (1981). *U.S. centralized cancer patient data system for uniform communication among cancer centers. J. Natl. Cancer Inst.* **67**, 1017.

Fenna, D., Abrahamsson, S., Loow, S.O., and Peterson, H. (1978). The Stockholm County medical information system. In *Lecture notes in medical informatics,* Vol. 2 (ed. D.A.B. Lindberg and P.L. Reichertz). Springer, New York.

Freeman, D.H. Jr, Bracken, M.B., Elia, R.F. *et al.* (1979). A SAS-AUTOGRP interface for the analysis of hospital discharge data. In *SAS Users Group International, Proceedings of the Fourth Annual Conference,* p. 68. SAS Institute, Cary, NC.

Freiherr, G. (1980). *The seeds of artificial intelligence: SUMEX-AIM.* USDHEW, Bethesda, MD. (NIH Publication No. 80-207.)

Friedman, G.D. (1978). Effects of MHTS on patients. In *Multiphasic health testing services (MHTS)* (ed. M.F. Collen) p. 531. Wiley, New York.

Garfield, S. (1982). New primary care delivery systems. *Med. Inf., Lond.* **7**, 165.

Garten, S., Nissman, E., and Heatherington, D. (1982). *Clinical data processing system adverse experience controlled vocabulary. Subsystem documentation.* Burroughs Wellcome, Research Triangle Park, NC.

Gelman, A.C. (1971). *Multiphasic health testing systems: reviews and annotations.* USDHEW, Washington, DC. (DHEW publication No. (HSRD) 71-1.)

Glenn, W.V., Johnston, R.J., Morton, P.E., and Dwyer, S.J. (1975). Image generation and display techniques for CT scan data: thin transverse and reconstructed coronal and sagittal planes. *Invest Radiol.* **10**, 403.

Glenn, W.V., Rothman, S.L.G., and Rhodes, M.L. (1982). Computed tomography/multiplanar reformatted (CT/MPR) examinations of the lumbar spine. In *Computed tomography of the lumbar spine* (ed. H.K. Ganant, N. Chasetz, and C.A. Helms) p. 87. University of California, San Francisco, CA.

Goldman, J. (1979). Health care technology evaluation: Proceedings. In *Lecture notes in medical informatics,* Vol. 6 (ed. D.A.B. Lindberg and P.L. Reichertz). Springer, New York.

Gordon, M., deWardener, H.E., Venn, C., Webb, J.T., and Adams, H. (1981). An interactive graphic database microcomputer for clinical control in data intensive therapies. In *Proceedings European Dialysis and Transplant Association,* Vol. 18 (ed. B.H.B. Robinson, J.B. Hawkins, and A.M. Davison) p. 690. Pitman, London.

Grant, M.E. and Hanson, J.S. (1976). A totally computerized cardiac pacemaker surveillance system. In *Proceedings of the computers in cardiology conference, St. Louis, Missouri* (ed. H.G. Ostrow) p. 13. IEEE, New York.

Griesser, G.G., Bakker, A., Danielsson, J. *et al.* (eds.) (1980). *Data protection in health information systems.* North Holland, New York.

Haven, G.T., Lawson, N.B., and Ross, J. (1982). Quality control in the 80s. In *Clinical laboratory annual,* Vol. 1 (ed. H.A. Homburger and J.G. Batsakis) p. 209. Appleton-Century-Crofts, New York.

Heard, M.R. and Thomas, J.C. (1978). A hospital information system, its impact on costs, personnel and patients in one department. In *Cost containment, caps, and consumerism within the health care delivery system,* Vol. 2, p. 21. Center for Hospital Management Engineering of the American Hospital Association, Chicago, IL.

Hicks, I.L. (1978). Technicon medical information system (TMIS): the forum. *J. Med. Syst.* **2**, 373.

Hodge, M.H. (1977). *Medical information systems.* Aspen Systems, Germantown, MD.

Holler, J.W. and DeMorgan, H.P. (1970). A retrospective study of 200 post-mortem examinations. *J. Med. Educ.* **45**, 168.

Hook, E.B. (1976). Genetic registers: types, goals, methods and limitations. In *Registers for the detection and prevention of genetic disease* (ed. A.E.H. Emery and J.R. Miller) p. 9. Symposia Specialists, Miami, FL.

Hopps, H.C. (1972). Display of data with emphasis on the map form. *Ann. NY Acad. Sci.* **199**, 325.

Hopwood, M.D., Groner, G.F., Palley, N.A. *et al.* (1977). *An evaluation of the CLINFO data management and analysis system.* Rand Corporation, Santa Monica, CA.

Horowtiz, G.L. and Bleich, H.L. (1981). Paperchase: a computer program to search the medical literature. *N. Engl. J. Med.* **305**, 924.

Huffman, D.G. and Morgan, E.B. (1980). Tri-service medical information systems (TRIMIS) approach to electrocardiography. In *Proceedings of the Fourth Annual Symposium on Computer Applications in Medical Care, Washington, DC* (ed. J.T. O'Neill) p. 1090. IEEE, New York.

Institute of Medicine (1977). *A policy statement: computed tomographic scanning.* National Academy of Sciences, Washington, DC.

Jackson, R., Birkhead, B.G., and Gregory, W.M. (1982). Review of modelling and computing in a cancer treatment centre. In *Lecture notes in medical informatics,* Vol. 16 (ed. D.A.B. Lindberg and P.L. Reichertz) p. 887. Springer, New York.

Jacobs, C., Broyer, M., Brunner, F.P. *et al.* (1981). Combined report on regular dialysis and transplantation in Europe, XI, 1980. In *Proceedings of the European Dialysis and Transplant Association,* Vol. 18 (ed. B.H.B. Robinson, J.B. Hawkins, and A.M. Davison) p. 4. Pitman Press, London.

Jelliffe, R.W., D'Argenio, D.F., Roman, J., and Schumitzky, A. (1980). A time-shared computer program for adaptive control of Lidocaine therapy using an optimal strategy for obtaining serum concentrations. In *Proceedings of the Fourth Annual Symposium on Computer Applications in Medical Care, Washington, DC* (ed. J.T. O'Neill) p. 975. IEEE, New York.

Johansson, S.G. and Manell, P. (1980). Database technology impact on a drug information system. In *Proceedings of MEDINFO 80* (ed. D.A.B. Lindberg and S. Kaihara) p. 910. North Holland, New York.

Kingsland, L.C. III, Gaston, L.W., Vanker, A.D., and Lindberg, D.A.B. (1982). A knowledge-based consultant system for problems in human hemostasis. In *Proceedings of AMIA Congress 82* (ed. D.A.B. Lindberg, M.F. Collen, and E. Van Brunt) p. 325. Masson, New York.

Kraus, J.F. (1980). A comparison of recent studies on the extent of the head and spinal cord injury problem in the U.S. In *Report on the National Head and Spinal Cord Injury Survey* (ed. D.W. Anderson and R.L. McLauren). *J. Neurosurg.* **53**, 35.

Kunz, J.C., Fallat, R.J., McClung, D.H. *et al.* (1979). Automated interpretation of pulmonary function test results. In *Proceedings of the First International Symposium on computers in critical care and pulmonary medicine, Norwalk, Connecticut* (ed. S. Nair) p. 375. Plenum Press, New York.

Lancaster, F.W. and Smith, L.C. (1980). On-line systems in the communication process: projections. *J. Am. Soc. Inf. Sci.* **31**, 193.

Larsen, L.K. and Rowe, I.L. (1982). Patient and doctor evaluation of AMHT. *Med. Inf., Lond.* **31**, 103.

Lenhard, R.E., Blum, B.I., Sunderland, J.M., Braine, H.G., and Saral, R. (1982). The Johns Hopkins oncology clinical information system. In *Proceedings of Sixth Annual Symposium on Computer Applications in Medical Care, Washington, DC* (ed. B.I.

Blum) p. 28, IEEE, New York.

Leveridge, L. (1983). The interactive videodisc. *Mobius* **3**, 68.

Lincoln, T.L. (1983). Medical information science: a joint endeavor. *JAMA* **249**, 610.

Lindberg, D.A.B. (1979a). Definition and means of comparing medical information systems. In *The growth of medical information systems in the United States*, p. 9. Lexington Books, D.C. Heath and Company, Lexington, MA.

Lindberg, D.A.B. (1979b). Evaluating the worth of MISs. In *The growth of medical information systems in the United States*, p. 69. Lexington Books, D.C. Heath and Company, Lexington, MA.

Lindberg, D.A.B. (1979c). Effects of changes in technology on future medical information systems. In *The growth of medical information systems in the United States*, p. 129. Lexington Books, D.C. Heath and Company, Lexington, MA.

Lindberg, D.A.B. (1982). Computer networks within health care: the state of the art in the USA. In *Communication networks in health care: proceedings of the IFIP–IMIA Working Conference on Communication Networks in Health Care, Sweden* (ed. H.E. Peterson and A.I. Isaksson) p. 109. North Holland, New York.

Lindberg, D.A.B., Sharp, G.C., Kingsland, L.C. *et al.* (1980). Computer-based rheumatology consultant. In *Proceedings of MEDINFO 80* (ed. D.A.B. Lindberg and S. Kaihara) p. 1311. North Holland, New York.

Little, A.D. (1976). *Automated electrocardiography in the United States*. USDHEW–NCHSR, Rockville, MD. (NTIS-PB-257-918.)

Longini, I.M., Koopman, J., Monto, A.S., and Fox, J.P. (1982). Estimating household and community transmission parameters for influenza. *Am. J. Epidemiol.* **115**, 736.

McDonald, C.J. (1976). Protocol-based computer reminders: the quality of care and non-perfectability of man. *N. Engl. J. Med.* **295**, 1351.

McShane, D.J. and Fries, J.F. (1978). ARAMIS: the pilot national arthritis data resource. In *3rd USA–Japan Computer Conference Proceedings*, p. 343. AFIPS Press, New York.

Manning, P.R., Lee, P.V., Denson, T.A., and Gilman, N.J. (1980). Determining educational needs in the physician's office. *JAMA* **244**, 1112.

Mead Data Central (1982). *LEXIS: Handbook* (product description). Mead Data Central, Dayton, OH.

Mellin, G.W. (1963). The fetal life study of the Columbia-Presbyterian Medical Center: a prospective epidemiological study of prenatal influences on fetal development and survival. In *Research methodology and needs in perinatal studies* (ed. S.S. Chipman) p. 88. Thomas, Springfield, IL.

Merritt, A.D., Kang, K.W., Conneally, P.M., Gersting, J.M., and Rigo, T. (1976). MEGADATS: a computer system for family data acquisition, storage and analysis. In *Registers for the detection and prevention of genetic disease* (ed. A.E.H. Emery and J.R. Miller) p. 31. Symposia Specialists, Miami, FL.

Miles, W.D. (1982). *A history of the National Library of Medicine: the Nation's treasury of medical knowledge*. USDHHS-NLM, Washington, DC. (NIH publication No. 82-1904.)

Miller, P.L. (1982). ATTENDING: a system which critiques an anesthetic management plan. In *Proceedings of AMIA Congress 82* (ed. D.A.B. Lindberg, M.F. Collen, and E. Van Brunt) p. 36. Masson, New York.

Miller, R.A., Pople, H.E., and Myers, J.D. (1982). INTERNIST-I, an experimental computer-based diagnostic consultant for general internal medicine. *N. Engl. J. Med.* **307**, 468.

Mintz, M. (1967). *By prescription only*. Beacon Press, Boston, MA.

Mitchell, J.A., Loughman, W.D., and Epstein, C.J. (1982). A medical genetics information system. *J. Clin. Comput.* **11**, 1.

Newcombe, H.B., Kennedy, J.M., Axford, S.J., and James, A.P. (1959). Automatic linkage of vital records. *Science* **130**, 954.

Newell, A. and Sproull, R.F. (1982). Computer networks: prospects for scientists. *Science* **215**, 843.

Noyce, R.N. (1977). Microelectronics. *Sci. Am.* **237**, 62.

Overhage, C.F.J. and Harman, R.J. (1965). *INTREX, report of a planning conference on information transfer experiments*. MIT Press, Cambridge, MA.

Patel, R., Glascock, R., and Terasaki, P. (1969). Serotyping for homotransplantation. *JAMA* **207**, 1319.

Pauker, S.C. and Kassirer, J.P. (1980). The threshold approach to clinical decision making. *N. Engl. J. Med.* **302**, 1109.

Peterson, H.E. and Isaksson, A.I. (eds.) (1982). *Communication networks in health care*. North Holland, Amsterdam.

Puybasset, B. (1982). Computer networks within health care. The state of the art in France. In *Communication networks in health care* (ed. H.E. Peterson and A.I. Isaksson) p. 139. North Holland, Amsterdam.

Queram, C.J. (1977). *Cancer registries and reporting systems in the U.S.* Department of Health and Social Services, Bureau of Health Statistics. Division of Health, Madison, WI.

Rigdon, R.H. (1980). Reliability of data from death certificates. (Letter.) *N. Engl. J. Med.* **303**, 1422.

Rosati, R.A., McNeer, F., Starmer, F., Mittler, B.S., Morris, J.J., and Wallace, A.G. (1975). A new information system for medical practice. *Arch. Intern. Med.* **135**, 1017.

Rowe, I. and Larsen, L. (1977). Evaluation of automated multiphasic health testing of referred patients by general practitioners. *Med. J. Austr.* **2**, 214.

Saito, T. (1982). Communication networks for health care in Japan. In *Communication networks in health care* (ed. H.E. Peterson and A.I. Isaksson) p. 121. North Holland, Amsterdam.

Shaw, G.B. (1909). *The doctor's dilemma*. Brentanos, New York.

Sherman, H., Reiffen, B., and Komaroff, A.L. (1975). *Aids to the delivery of ambulatory medical care: a report from the ambulatory care project of the Harvard Medical School Lincoln Laboratory*. Massachusetts Institute of Technology, Boston, MA.

Shortliffe, E.H., Axline, S.G., Buchanan, B.G., and Merigan, T.C. (1973). An artificial intelligence program to advise physicians regarding antimicrobial therapy. *Comput. Biomed. Res.* **6**, 1.

Shortliffe, E.H., Scott, A.C., Bischoff, M.B., Campbell, A.B., Van Melle, W., and Jacobs, C.D. (1981). ONCOCIN: an expert system for oncology protocol management. In *Proceedings of the 7th IJCAI, British Columbia, Vancouver* (ed. A. Drinan) p. 876. American Association for Artificial Intelligence, Menlo Park, CA.

Simborg, D.W., Chadwick, M., Whiting-O'Keefe, Q.E., and Tolchin, S.G. (1982). Early experience with the first use of a local area communication network technology in a hospital. In *Proceedings of AMIA Congress 82* (ed. D.A.B. Lindberg, M.F. Collen, and E. Van Brunt) p. 140. Masson, New York.

Slack, W.V. and Slack, C.W. (1972). Patient–computer dialogue. *N. Engl. J. Med.* **286**, 1304.

Statistical Analysis system (SAS) Institute, Inc. (1982). *SAS users guide*, SAS Institute, Cary, NC.

Steger, D. and Enz, R. (1978). A data dictionary driven data analysis system. In *Proceedings of the Hewlett-Packard General Systems International Users Group, Denver, Colorado, October 30, 1978*. p. 93, HP 3000 Users Group, Los Altos, CA.

Stratmann, W.C. (1979). *A demonstration of PROMIS: the problem-oriented medical information system at the Medical Center Hospital of Vermont*. USDHEW-NCHSR, Rockville, MD. (DHEW publication No. (PHS) 79-3247.)

Stulting, R.O. and Ward, F.E. (1975). A computerized system for the selection of organ transplant recipients. *Transplantation* **19**, 27.

Suzuki, T. (1982). The experience of the human dry dock project, 1954–82. *Med. Inf., Lond.* **7**, 235.

Swartout, W.R. (1977). A digitalis therapy advisor with explanations. *Proceedings of the 5th IJCAI, Cambridge, Massachusetts* (ed. R. Reddy) p. 819. Carnegie-Mellon University, Pittsburg, PA.

Szurek, J.L., Gertz, E.W., and Henley, R.R. (1979). Computer support system for pacemaker surveillance. In *Proceedings of the 9th annual conference of the Society for Computer Medicine, Atlanta, Georgia*, p. 29. Society for Computer Medicine, Altanta, GA.

Taussig, H.B. (1963). The evils of camouflage as illustrated by thalidomide. *N. Engl. J. Med.* **269**, 92.

Trimble, B.K. (1976). Record linkage and genetic registers. In *Registers for the detection and prevention of genetic disease* (ed. A.E.H. Emery and J.R. Miller) p. 87. Symposia Specialists, Miami, FL.

Trusty, R.D. and Mazzaro, J.T. (1980). A Tri-Service regionalized pharmacy information system: test and experience. In *Proceedings of MEDINFO 80* (ed. D.A.B. Lindberg and S. Kahira) p. 921. North Holland, New York.

Tuttle, M.S., Abarbanal, R., Blois, M.S., and Taylor, H. (1982). Use of a relational DBMS to acquire and investigate patient records in a melanoma clinic. In *Proceedings of AMIA 82* (ed. D.A.B. Lindberg, M.F. Collen, and E. Van Brunt) p. 95. Masson, New York.

United States Congress, House. Committee on Science and Astronautics. Subcommittee on Science, Research and Development (1967). *Technology Assessment, Statement of Chairman, Emilio Q. Daddario. 90th Congress, first session: 1967.*

Vlietinck, R.F. and Vanden Berghe, H. (1976). The Belgian national genetic register. In *Registers for the detection and prevention of genetic registers* (ed. A.E.H. Emery and J.R. Miller) p. 65. Symposia Specialists, Miami, FL.

Wasserman, A.I. (1980). Information system design methodology. *J. Am. Soc. Information Sci.* **21**, 5.

Weddell, J.M. (1973). Registers and registries: a review. *Int. J. Epidemiol.* **2**, 221.

Weiss, S., Kulikowski, C.A., and Safir, A. (1978). Glaucoma consultation by computer. *Comput. Biol. Med.* **8**, 25.

Westin, A.F. (1976). *Computers, health records, and citizen rights.* US Dept. of Commerce, Washington, DC. (NBS monograph 157.)

Wiederhold, G. (1977). *Database design*, p. 368. McGraw Hill, New York.

Williams, G.Z., Widdowson, G.M., and Penton, T. (1978). Individual character of variation in time-series studies of healthy people: differences of value for clinical chemical analytes in serum among demographic groups by age and sex. *Clin. Chem.* **24**, 313.

Williams, G.Z., Young, D.S., Stein, M.R., and Cottove, E. (1970). Biological and analytic components of variation in long-term studies of serum constituents in normal subjects: I. objectives, subject selection, laboratory procedures, and estimation of analytic deviation. *Clin. Chem.* **16**, 1016.

Williams, R.J. (1956). *Biochemical individuality: the basis for the genetotrophic concept.* Wiley, New York.

World Health Organization (1976). *WHO handbook for standardized cancer registries.* WHO, Geneva.

Yasaka, T. (1982). Regional differences amongst test results from AMHTS facilities. *Med. Inf., Lond.* **7**, 249.

Young, J.L., Percy, C.L., and Asire, A.J. (eds.) (1981). *Surveillance, epidemiology, and end results: incidence and mortality data, 1973–77.* USDHHS-NCI, Washington, DC. (NIH publication No. 81-2330.)

# 4 Information systems and routine monitoring in the United States and Canada—with examples from surgical practice

J.P. Bunker, L.L. Roos, J. Fowles, and N.P. Roos

## INTRODUCTION

The need for the evaluation of medical technologies is widely recognized (Nightingale 1859; Hey Groves 1908; Codman 1914; Burger, personal communication, 1975; Bunker *et al.* 1982a; Towery and Perry 1981). Optimally, randomized clinical trials (RCTs) should be carried out on all new procedures and on many old ones, diagnostic as well as therapeutic. For practical and ethical reasons, it is not possible to carry out RCTs on every procedure. But short of the perfect experiment, much can be learned from existing population-based data, from other routinely collected data, and from information systems specially designed for the systemic collection of data for specified purposes (for example, registries, data banks, postmarketing surveillance). These routine data may be used both cross-sectionally and longitudinally, permitting many different types of studies. The savings in cost and in researchers' time make feasible many analyses and projects which could not otherwise be done. But while there is much to be gained from these data, there are many pitfalls as well. In this chapter, we will discuss both the potentials and the limitations of non-experimental data for research on public health issues.

## POPULATION-BASED INFORMATION SYSTEMS

### Vital statistics

The current US federal system of vital and other health statistics is described by Rice (Chapter 1). Routinely collected data have the methodological advantage of minimizing surveillance artefacts. When gathered over a period of years, any influences of the data collection itself are likely to be small. Deliberate suppression of data which reflect poor care may exist, but this problem is present for virtually all data collection methods (Webb *et al.* 1981). When population-based data are available for a given geographical unit, bias is further reduced. When data are generated and submitted as a prerequisite for reimbursement (for example, insurance 'claims data'), the likelihood of selective withholding or omission – perhaps by institutions with quality of care problems – is essentially eliminated (but other problems influencing the data's reliability may be created through its linkage to reimbursement, as discussed below).

Shapiro (1981), summarizes the uses of federal statistics for health planning. He suggests, for example, that birth statistics and measures of infant mortality are useful as indicators of broad health status, and that trends in mortality and inter-area comparisons of mortality can be valuable in planning for resource allocation. This theme is further developed by Gittelsohn (1982), who proposes a national, computer-based, mortality surveillance programme to monitor the geographic distribution of cause-specific deaths by race and sex, and as a function of time.

While mortality statistics are of some value in assessing the overall level of health of a population, they do little to explain why large differences in mortality rates are observed among different population groups, and almost nothing to explain the impact of medical care on mortality.

Mortality statistics are, however, of considerable value in generating hypotheses. This role is considerably enhanced at times of rapid change in mortality, particularly when such change occurs in conjunction with a dramatic social event (or natural experiment). Changes in motor vehicle deaths in the US following the implementation of the 55 mile per hour speed limit, or in Britain with the enforcement of mandatory use of seat belts are examples of such natural experiments. Another example is provided by the 1976 five week strike of physicians in Los Angeles County (Roemer and Schwartz 1979) in which almost all elective surgery was suspended. The strike was accompanied by an approximate 30 per cent decline in mortality which began the second week after the start of the strike. There was a sharp increase in mortality when the strike ended and elective surgery resumed, with a return to the pre-strike mortality level by the second week following the end of the strike. From this observation it was hypothesized that the performance of elective surgery is associated with an increase in a population's mortality.

This episode, of course, tells us nothing about any morbidity that may have resulted from a delay of surgery, about sporadic late deaths that may have resulted, or of the impact of the strike on the overall health of the affected population. But the episode supports the thesis that the known risk of death associated with elective surgery may have a substantial immediate impact on a population's mortality (Bunker and Wennberg 1973). This hypothesis has received some additional support by research correlating population mortality with operation rates among small geographical areas (Roos 1984) but is questioned by other investigators (Vayda and Mindell 1982).

## Small area studies

The comparative analysis of vital statistics and data on the use of medical resources by small geographical areas greatly increases the opportunities for hypothesis generation and, indeed, may provide sufficient detail to draw policy conclusions. Data from a variety of sources are available and suitable for this purpose. These studies, called 'small area' analyses, examine differences in utilization among small geographical units. These units may be pre-existing, politically defined entities (such as counties, or standard metropolitan statistical areas), or they may be especially defined according to medical practice and referral patterns (such as hospital service areas). The methodology has been thoroughly described by Wennberg and Gittelsohn (1980) and Barnes (1982).

In their studies of hospital utilization and operation rates as a function of hospital service areas, Wennberg and Gittelsohn used the Uniform Hospital Discharge Data Set (UHDDS), a national set of standard demographic data that includes age, residence, sex, diagnoses, procedures, and length of stay for each patient. These data allow population-based comparisons among areas classified according to their use of hospitals and procedures. Using this methodology, Wennberg and Gittelsohn (1982) have demonstrated that there are twofold, threefold, and greater variations in utilization of medical and surgical services among homogeneous populations within a single larger geographical area, such as a state. In another application of this technique, international comparisons were made of small areas (McPherson *et al.* 1982). For the three regions, New England, England, and Norway, the rank order of variability was consistent for most procedures. From such studies has emerged the hypothesis of provider-initiated utilization of hospital and surgical services. These large variations are also consistent with the notion of idiosyncratic practice styles, particularly when 'best practice' is poorly defined or ambiguous. In larger geographical areas, such idiosyncracies may be no less common among individual physicians, but the differences are averaged out.

A variety of other policy research questions can also be examined once hospital service areas have been defined. For example, Wennberg (1982) has documented the variability in *per caput* expenditures within local hospital markets and has argued that, because insurance premiums do not reflect these differences, there is extensive cross subsidization and price inflation.

## Claims data – organization and reliability

A major strength of small area analyses is the fact that they can be population-based, so that *per caput* rates (of procedures or diagnoses) can be calculated and areas compared to one another. However, developing population-based estimates can be a major task, requiring the definition of local hospital service areas, assigning people to such areas, and relating all their use – in or out of area – to that region. This works reasonably well in rural areas but is more difficult in urban areas with many hospitals and much border crossing.

A population-based approach is in accord with sound epidemiological principle. The growing use of claims data for health services research represents a further extension of this principle. In the US, the federal government, through its Medicare programme, is the major source of health care information from claims. The Health Care Financing Administration's records of in- and out-patient utilization for enrollees provide a complete record of care given to patients aged 65 years and over. However, the lack of diagnostic information, in contrast to the more specific treatment (procedure) reporting, limits the interpretability of the records for medical treatments. While outcome is limited to deaths as recorded by the Social Security Administration, it is possible to relate survival to diagnosis and treatment modality (Wennberg 1982).

The multiplicity of reimbursement sources in the US precludes the reliable use of claims data for estimating utilization in the population younger than 65 years. Indeed, any attempt to do so may give misleading results. Recently, Luft (1981) called attention to the apparent paradox of increasing overall hospital admission rates reported by the American Hospital Association and the National Health Interview Survey and falling rates for subscribers to Blue Cross, which covers half the insured population. Luft provides evidence that about half of the discrepancy is due to duplicate coverage, suggesting that 'existing data provide an inadequate and potentially misleading picture of the most crucial measures of utilization'.

Although claims data for sub-populations do not permit generalizing to the population as a whole, they may be useful for selected purposes. Thus, claims data from the government's Medicaid programme have been used to assess the quality of antibiotic and other medications prescribed for the population served by that programme (Federspiel *et al.* 1976; Lohr *et al.* 1980). In general, while US claims data may be inappropriate for the estimation of population-based rates, they can facilitate research on patterns of services provided to patients who have entered treatment. For example, claims data from Blue Cross have been analysed to document medical expenses in the last six months of life (Gibbs and Newman 1982). For certain analyses, care must be taken to compensate both for lags in claims submissions and for the 'batching' of reimbursement for several visits on a single claims form. Claims data can also be used to study patterns of provider behaviour. Thus, for example, Wennberg and Gittelsohn (1982) could examine the impact of feedback on surgical rates, and L.L. Roos (1983) could evaluate the influence of the migration of 'surgically-active' physicians.

Most of the difficulties encountered in the US when using claims data for research purposes, such as those introduced by duplicate coverage or by non-random sub-populations of subscribers unrepresentative of the population as a whole, can be avoided in Canada. With cost-sharing by the federal government, provincial health insurance plans reimburse physicians on a procedure by procedure basis. While there is considerable provincial variation, essentially all physician visits and hospital stays are at least partially covered. Although hospitals are reimbursed on a global budget basis, extensive information on admissions and major procedures are systematically captured. The systems which provide the information necessary for reimbursement are also a rich source of data for studies of medical care utilization and outcomes.

The province-wide files maintained for payment and control purposes in Manitoba and Saskatchewan have been extensively used for this purpose. In Manitoba, for example, the registration file contains data on the population covered. The medical claims file has all claims submitted by physicians for services rendered to patients, while the hospital file contains dates of admission and discharge, limited information on services rendered, and surgical procedures.

'Each of these files is maintained separately, with no routine record integration. However, since patient identifiers and physician numbers are unique across all files, files can be built on individuals (all instances of care received from various physicians and in various hospitals over time), or physicians (all care rendered over time), or hospitals (all admissions over time)' (Roos et al. 1982).

The use of administrative data for epidemiological research inevitably raises questions about the quality of the data since although 'such information may have been recorded with care, it certainly was not collected with an eye to satisfying tenets of measurement reliability' (Roos et al. 1979). Roos et al. (1982) examined the reliability of the Manitoba health data system against other information recorded independently (for example in doctor's office, vital statistics, and in-hospital files) and by making computerized internal comparisons where checks were available within the data system itself. On the basis of these validity checks, they concluded that: 'Face sheet information and data on the performance of major surgical procedures were found to be reliably recorded in the Manitoba data bank. Collapsing ICD-8 diagnoses from medical claims into several categories proved much better than relying upon individual diagnoses. Problems in working with the data included difficulty in distinguishing between closely related surgical procedures and the under-reporting of in-hospital consultations and nonsurgical procedures.'

Wennberg and Gittelsohn (1980) have extensively analysed the reliability of Medicare data, hospital discharge data, and death certificates, and compared their findings with other studies of data reliability. They conclude that there are three general levels of reliability which can be commonly demonstrated. The most reliable data are those which relate to the hospital episode itself: the occurrence of hospitalization, patient characteristics, dates, and discharge status. These lend themselves to accurate studies of total hospital utilization rates, patient day rates, occupancy, and length of stay. The second level of reliability is found with procedure data. Here, however, there is greater variability in certain hospitals. None the less, statistical indices for surgical procedures can be reasonably accepted. The least reliable information comes from diagnostic codes, where the most consistent information can be derived at the two digit level of the standard four digit codes. In a preliminary study of Medicare patients in northern California receiving total hip replacements (Fowles et al., unpublished data 1983), a comparison of the claims data to the operative report indicated a 6.8 per cent error in procedure code (a confusion among original total hip replace-

ments, revisions, and hemiarthroplasties) and an 8.9 per cent error in diagnosis.

Special note should be made of the potential errors in the use of claims data in studies of new procedures. In their study of reimbursement for such new procedures, Bunker et al. (1982a) observed that:

With increasing scrutiny by third-party payers of bills submitted for new procedures, and with more than occasional denial of payment of such bills, there is a strong incentive to request payment for a standard procedure rather than a new one. Further complicating this problem is the fact that new procedures often have not been assigned a procedure code number for claims processing. Inaccurate claims may simply reflect the honest effort to use whatever code number seems most nearly to approximate the procedure actually performed. The net result, however, is that the identity of the new procedure may be obscured. Indeed, the very fact that an experimental procedure has been carried out may not become apparent to the payer. How frequently this occurs is not known, but there is an approximately 15 per cent error rate in the coding of all procedures in the claims submitted to Blue Shield of California, and it is estimated that at least one per cent . . . is for procedures in which existing codes are used in the absence of new codes.

A related issue arises from the movement toward basing reimbursement on diagnostic related groups. Simborg (1982) has shown how hospitals can increase their reimbursement merely by shifting the order of primary and secondary diagnoses. Even selective alteration of this coding could result in substantial revenue increases. Increased reliance on diagnostic related groups as a basis for reimbursement may further reduce the validity of such data for research.

## Longitudinal research

Among the advantages of population-based data bases are their representativeness (which leads to generalizability), and their potential for use in more than one study, and for better tracking of individuals (Mednick 1981). By permitting the following of individuals through time, data banks facilitate longitudinal studies which both 'increase the precision of treatment contrasts by eliminating inter-individual variation' and permit the examination of 'changes associated with development or aging' (Cook and Ware 1983). Comprehensive data sources can also help deal with research needs, such as verification of data quality, avoidance of major biases in comparison, vigilance in checking for methodological errors, and maintenance of a distinction between data used to generate hypotheses and that used to test such hypotheses (Feinstein and Howitz 1982).

Research on the outcomes of different surgical procedures in the Manitoba studies (Roos 1979; Roos et al. 1982) uses longitudinal histories developed from registry, hospital, and medical files both for individuals having one of nine common surgical procedures and for population controls. Such extensive histories provide valuable information in themselves and as adjuncts to other sources such as interviews and death certificates. Loss to follow-up was examined across several data sets, with the histories giving in-depth data on those individuals leaving the study population. Overall results compared favourably with participation and follow-up rates in other longitudinal studies (Keys 1980).

One study focusing on elective hysterectomies found over 84 per cent of the women were fully covered for the 24 months before and the 24 months after surgery. Age-adjusted comparisons with population controls (80 per cent follow-up) showed few differences in attrition among groups. Various checks using claims data verified the accuracy of the individual identification and coverage decisions.

These data were used to compare before-surgery and after-surgery utilization, and also to assess post-operative complications. The outcome analysis showed significant risks (40 per 1000 cases) of serious post-operative complications (necessitating readmission to hospital) during the two years after hysterectomy and associated repair procedures. Women having surgery also had increased visits for psychological problems, urinary tract infections, and menopausal symptoms (N.P. Roos 1984).

Comprehensive data bases facilitate the development of a broad array of analyses for any single problem. Extensive longitudinal histories permit better controls of patient risk characteristics. For example, the comprehensive information available in population-based research on tonsillectomies facilitated comparisons of operated and control groups at various levels of pre-operative illness (Roos 1979). By way of comparison, a large American randomized clinical trial of tonsillectomy gathered information from only the fraction of the children with a large number of episodes of tonsillitis in the year before surgery (Paradise et al. 1978).

In addition to their comprehensiveness, extended data bases can help with other problems that plague epidemiological research. When the number of cases seems insufficient for a given study, data banks often permit expansion of the sample size, thus avoiding a common problem in randomized clinical trials; that is, a sample size too small to pick up possibly important effects (Freiman et al. 1978). For example, the Manitoba data on the complications following hysterectomy for the original sample of 1813 fully-covered elective hysterectomy patients was insufficient to control adequately for patient factors (age, comorbidity), physician factors (specialty, experience with the procedure), and hospital factors (volume of surgery). Expanding the study from one year's (1974) to three years' (1974–76) data almost tripled the number of cases, greatly facilitating the data analysis for this low incidence outcome.

Data banks containing large numbers of cases over a period of time help both in studying change and in replicating results with data from a different time period. Because data on contacts with the health care system can be organized using different time intervals (monthly, quarterly, annually), the number of measurements can be changed by shortening or lengthening these time intervals. This flexibility may be useful in designing longitudinal studies (Cook and Ware 1983). Moreover, if previous hypothesis-generating research has not been performed, or if multivariate procedures have been used, various techniques designed to test a study's results on comparable data are particularly appropriate. Mosteller and Tukey (1977) have summarized several such techniques which seem suitable for research with data banks.

Good research design involves more than consideration of case numbers and replication. Longitudinal histories from a population-based data bank would have helped rectify serious problems in the evaluation design of the well-known North Karelia Project (Klos and Rosenstock 1982; McAlister et al. 1982). Because the evidence for the effectiveness of the health intervention programme was based on separate samples five years apart, Klos and Rosenstock note that the North Karelia design does not permit distinguishing 'population changes which are due to programme impact from those due to other forces affecting the population'.

Because population-based data banks allow analysis over an extended period of time, they may be particularly suitable for quasi-experimental designs. Such long-term data permit a number of design options, such as adding an extra year before an intervention (Wortman et al. 1978) or generating longer time-series with several comparison groups – one of the strongest non-randomized designs (Cook and Campbell 1979).

One example of such research is the interrupted time series analysis of a natural experiment – a 30 per cent reduction in the Massachusetts Medicaid reimbursement for physician surgical services. Shwartz et al. (1981) organized 44 months (from May 1975 to December 1978) of Medicaid data for eight elective surgical procedures across four of the five Professional Standards Review Organization (PSRO) regions in Massachusetts. The time series before the February 1976 fee cut was statistically compared with that after the change. Shwartz et al. found that 'with the exception of tonsillectomies/adenoidectomies, a very large reduction in the reimbursement fee for Medicaid surgery had only a small impact on the rate at which eight elective surgical procedures were performed'.

The ability to link population-based longitudinal data bases with other data sets opens up a number of possibilities for implementing complex research designs. Providing more information on each individual both permits better measurement and increases the number of possible controls. Thus, the Manitoba Longitudinal Study on Aging (Mossey et al. 1981) included a representative sample of elderly, combining their responses to a needs assessment interview with their 1970–77 history from the claims data bank. This linkage has provided an extensive archive for studying the health and health care use behaviours of older persons.

Such linkages have been facilitated by the development of a centralized source of Canadian mortality information as well as the software for alphabetic and probability matches (Smith and Newcombe 1980, 1982). The Canadian Mortality Data Base acts as an 'information utility', permitting large scale longitudinal follow-up of individuals with a variety of exposures and conditions. A series of checks have shown individuals to be well enough identified to minimize error; typical search generates both dates and recorded causes of death. This Mortality Data Base has made feasible an increasing number of epidemiological studies concerned 'with the long-term consequences of various occupations, medical treatments and diagnostic procedures, and circumstances of other kinds which may contribute to deaths from cancer, cardiovascular disease and other causes' (Smith and Newcombe 1982).

Smith and Newcombe (1982) are particularly interested in

the possibilities for linking information from the Canadian National Dose Registry for radiation workers with the Mortality Data Base. The US established a National Death Index in the early 1980s, and as a consequence an increasing number of American studies using linkages to a mortality data base may be expected.

## INFORMATION SYSTEMS THAT ARE NOT POPULATION-BASED

While mortality data and other indices of health status are often useful for defined populations, their application in the assessment of the effects of therapy, where the population is not defined, invites erroneous conclusions. The pitfalls of studies that are neither population-based nor adequately controlled have been widely documented, most recently in a comprehensive review published by the Office of Technology Assessment of the US Congress (1983). The following well-known example – the rise and fall of portal venous anastamosis or shunt to prevent life threatening haemorrhage from oesophageal varices – serves to illustrate these pitfalls (Bunker *et al.* 1978). Whipple, in 1945, was the first of a number of surgeons to report that haemorrhage from oesophageal varices could be prevented in most patients by the operative anastamosis of the portal of the systemic circulation (Whipple 1945). Operative mortality was high initially, but so also was the mortality of recurrent haemorrhage with medical management. Such, indeed, was the apparent success of surgery that many years passed before the value of the procedure was seriously questioned.

Success was initially measured in terms of short-term survival and absence of haemorrhage. Not until 1954 was it recognized that portal systemic shunt in man is often followed by a severe intermittent encephalopathy that was given the name 'episodic stupor' or postshunt encephalopathy (McDermott and Adams 1954), now known to be related to disordered amine metabolism. This serious and often lethal complication led many clinicians to doubt the value of shunt surgery, but the unquestioned protection shunts provided against haemorrhage presented an argument that seemed difficult to challenge. There was, in fact, little serious debate concerning the appropriateness of shunt surgery in patients who had already bled from oesophageal varices. The debate had become, rather, whether shunt surgery should be performed as a prophylactic procedure in patients with demonstrable portal hypertension and oesophageal varices who had never bled, but who might, perhaps, bleed sometime in the future. Here, there was sufficient professional uncertainty to justify careful randomized clinical trials (RCTs).

The results of these trials revealed no difference in survival between the patients selected at random for medical therapy and those similarly selected for surgery. Very few of the surgical group had subsequent haemorrhage, whereas those under medical treatment often bled to an extent requiring emergency surgery. The surgical patients, on the other hand, suffered a high incidence of progressive hepatic failure and encephalopathy with a subsequent mortality closely approximating that from haemorrhage in the medically treated group.

With the prophylactic shunt discredited, the value of therapeutic shunts (in patients who had already bled from demonstrable oesophageal varices) was re-examined, and randomized controlled trials were finally deemed necessary and appropriate. These trials are now completed and while differences in the statistical evaluation exist, it is now clear that the 'therapeutic' shunt provides no statistically significant survival value (Reynolds *et al.* 1981), although it unquestionably protects against haemorrhage.

In an equally dramatic error, it was reported that patients suffering from benign prostatic hypertrophy were more likely to survive in London's teaching hospitals than in non-teaching hospitals (Lee *et al.* 1957, 1960; Morris 1964). Ashley and Howlett, together with Morris (1971) later discovered that admissions to London's teaching hospitals were made on the basis of their teaching value; patients were particularly likely to be admitted if they were judged to be acceptable candidates for surgery. Patients too sick for surgery were sent to non-teaching hospitals. The mortality following prostatic surgery was, in fact, nearly identical.

The pitfalls of imperfectly controlled studies have been convincingly demonstrated by two independent reviews and classifications of published reports of clinical trials in which each trial was classified according to the quality of the experimental design: well-designed, randomized, controlled studies on the one hand; poorly designed, non-randomized studies on the other (Grace *et al.* 1966; Gilbert *et al.* 1977). An author's enthusiasm for the procedure he or she was evaluating was found to be inversely related to the quality of the experimental design. Poorly designed studies almost always were interpreted as more favourable to the treatment than were well-controlled studies. More recently, Wortman and Yeaton (1983) compared the results of a number of randomized trials with those from controlled, but non-population-based, studies of coronary artery bypass graft surgery. Wortman and Yeaton's synthesis also strongly suggested that non-randomized studies systematically overestimate the effect of the therapy being evaluated. As suggested by the discussion of benign prostatic hypertrophy, evaluations using population-based data can overcome many of the difficulties with non-randomized studies by clarifying differences between experimental and control groups (L.L. Roos 1979).

### Non-population-based data banks

A wide variety of non-population-based information systems can be used with some success, despite the foregoing limitations. Among such information systems, the greatest claims have been made for the clinical data bank; thus it probably deserves the most careful scrutiny. The computerized clinical data bank is:

. . . a highly interactive time-shared system with the capability to process large files with minimal difficulty [which allows] . . . medical researchers to implement small data bases oriented toward their specific needs . . . Clinicians [are able to] develop individualized, highly structured, and clinically satisfactory medical record systems prior to approaching the problems of efficient computer data storage and generalized retrieval capabilities (Henley *et al.* 1975).

Such a data bank is the ultimate refinement in medical

record-keeping, allowing the online recording, storage, and retrieval of patient care information. Among its many useful functions are the monitoring of patient medication, particularly the identification of drug incompatibilities, and the feedback of this and other clinical events that might need corrective action (de Dombal *et al.* 1974; McDonald *et al.* 1980).

As a badly needed reliable record of clinical events, the well-maintained data base is superb. It can also serve important purposes in research, for example, 'as pure descriptive studies, for identification of prognostic factors, as aides in diagnosis, and for determining the feasibility of contemplated randomized trials' (Byar 1980). As a basis for the evaluation of medical therapies, and as an alternative to randomized clinical trials (Rosati *et al.* 1975; Fries 1976), however, there is strong disagreement. Byar (1980) comments that:

In essence the choice between randomized trials or data banks for comparing the efficacy of various treatments reduces to nothing more than the contrast between observation and experimentation.

Among the many problems with treatment comparisons based on information drawn from data banks, Byar lists bias in treatment assignment; non-standard definitions and definitions changing in time; subset definition; missing data; and multiple comparisons. These problems are not found with every data bank, but researchers should be aware of them before undertaking a study. Byar (1980) concludes that:

. . . in the absence of information from randomized clinical trials, data banks could be useful in choosing therapies for individual patients, but this will be so only if the level of sophistication of data banks is considerably greater than that illustrated in the literature I have read. Moreover, relying on the computer for summaries of observational data might eventually lead to the end of the experimental method in medicine and discourage the introduction of new therapies. The great danger seems to me to be that data banks will be seen as a replacement for randomized trials, whereas in fact, the most useful data which could be stored in data banks would be those obtained from randomized studies. . . .

While the clinical data bank may not provide a reliable alternative for the randomized controlled trial in the evaluation of therapeutic efficacy, it can enormously enhance the quality of clinical observations, and therefore their reliability. The application of automated information systems to health problems is explored in greater detail in the previous chapter by Lindberg.

## Registries

The clinical data bank is, almost by definition, hospital or clinic based, although it may incorporate several institutions in a single network with a single protocol. Even the largest multi-institutional data banks, however, cannot be considered representative of the population at large. The diagnostic or procedure registry, by contrast, does provide the theoretical opportunity to include an entire population, or a portion thereof. The reality is that most registries are far from complete in covering a population and present many additional deficiencies as reliable sources of clinical informa-

tion. Goldberg and his associates (1980) have recently reviewed the use of the case registry in epidemiological research. They adopt Bellows' (1949) definition of the registry as 'a system of recording frequently used in the general field of public health which serves as a device for the administration of programs concerned with the long-term care, follow-up or observation of individual cases [with] changes in status of cases . . . recorded over time'. The potential importance of the registry in surveillance of selected procedures and/or diseases is enormous. Their earliest and most successful use has been to record the incidence and to follow the natural history of malignant neoplasms. Their use in infectious diseases, even those for which reporting is mandatory, has been considerably less satisfactory.

The case registry has recently been used in an attempt to gain a complete record of new medical and surgical technologies. For example, national registries to document the use of the intraocular lens and of percutaneous transluminal coronary angioplasty have been established by the Food and Drug Administration, but submission of cases has been voluntary and under-reporting appears to present a widespread and difficult problem. A second pervasive problem has been the validity of such voluntarily submitted data. There are multiple forces at work which increase the likelihood of reporting by academic centres (whose outcomes may be more favourable) while decreasing the probability that isolated cases (whose outcomes may be less successful) will also be reported.

Several suggestions have been proposed to improve the validity and increase the completeness of the reporting of new procedures. Towery and Perry (1981) have endorsed the proposal that 'third-party payers, including Medicare . . . [make] reimbursement to providers contingent on their submitting certain minimal data under a previously agreed on protocol'. Sherman and his colleagues at the Harvard School of Public Health have made a similar proposal and have identified a number of contingencies for reimbursement (Sherman 1980). These proposals address the problem from the perspective of an agency whose principal responsibility is to provide reimbursement and for which the collection of data is by definition a secondary priority. Mandatory submission of data by providers of medical care can also be assumed to be a secondary priority to such providers, and the quality of the resulting information may be poor.

Bunker *et al.* (1982*a*) have suggested the need for a central agency, which might be called the Institute for Health Care Evaluation (IHCE), to collect information on new, as well as routine, procedures. Among other responsibilities, the IHCE could develop guidelines for an instrument, such as, a patient-registration form, that could serve as both a receipt for billing and a method for monitoring resource use and identifying new procedures. Decentralization of data storage at a regional, local, or even health-plan level would help to address the need for confidentiality of the source of information. For example, each plan or locality might store its own standardized data, which could then be made available to IHCE-authorized researchers after information identifying patients and providers had been censored or altered so as to preserve anonymity.

## Post-marketing surveillance of drugs

Registries of procedures or devices, such as the intraocular lens or percutaneous transluminal coronary angioplasty, offer the opportunity to follow the effect of such therapy over time. The need for such longitudinal surveillance of therapies is now widely recognized, especially when the therapy is a drug (Beebe 1983; Crapo and Melmon 1983). In the US, new drugs are subjected to vigorous pre-marketing testing for safety and efficacy, as required by law. However, no amount of pre-marketing testing can be expected to detect all adverse reactions. Adverse reactions that are very rare (such as Guillain-Barré syndrome in association with vaccination), or that occur only after a passage of many years (such as vaginal cancer in daughters of women who have received diethylstilbestrol during pregnancy) are examples of toxic effects that cannot be detected by even the largest or most careful pre-marketing clinical trial.

The need for a comprehensive system of post-marketing surveillance to detect such rare reactions, or adverse effects that develop only over long periods of time, is widely recognized. Experimental programmes of such surveillance, for example, the Boston Collaborative Drug Surveillance Program, have been attempted. The reporting of cases to this and to other post-marketing surveillance programmes is voluntary and, as with diagnostic and procedure registries, plagued by the problem of incomplete data. The recently completed report of the Joint Commission on Prescription Drug Use (1981) proposes a strategy designed to overcome the limitations of post-marketing surveillance as currently practised, but its recommendations remain to be implemented, and their success will take years to determine. (Post Marketing Surveillance is considered in greater detail in Chapter 21.)

## Routine hospital-based data

While non-experimental hospital-based data provide a poor basis for inference of therapeutic effectiveness, such data are of potential value in assessing the quality of medical care provided by institutions or by physicians. When standards of care have been established, by controlled clinical trials or by concensus, adherence to these standards can be assessed by review of the medical record in the so-called 'medical audit'.

The use of hospital chart review as a form of medical audit of individual physicians was suggested by Lembcke (1956) who is generally given credit for instituting the modern medical record audit. Weed (Promis Laboratory 1981) has explored in detail the use of the computerized data bank in facilitating good patient care and clinical research. He describes his 'problem oriented medical information system' as 'a problem solving tool for health care. A single, central, electronic, problem-oriented record for each patient provides the means to coordinate the actions of all providers, who interface directly to the record by making selections on displays at a terminal. Guidance for action and instant access to patient data reduce dependence on memory. The record is generated automatically as the provider follows the guidance of the computer program preserving his logic. Because infor-

mation is structured and coded, it can be interrogated by computer programs and used as audits to improve provider performance . . .' While the hospital-based medical information system has found its widest use for hospital administrative purposes, for example, for billing and accounting and for patient census, it has been only modestly accepted by the medical profession as a clinical adjunct.

Sanazaro (1980) has reviewed the use of the medical audit in quality assurance of medical care, and concludes that 'studies of physician performance have not produced standardized methods of reliably evaluating actual performance in the care of patients'. The recent demise in the US of the Professional Standards Review Organizations (PSROs), while undoubtedly hastened by the Reagan Administration's policies of de-regulation, must also be considered a reflection of the failure to develop effective and efficient methods for measurement of the quality of care provided by individual medical practitioners.

The use of the hospital record to assess the performance of a hospital has been suggested by Florence Nightingale (1859), by Ernest Hey Groves (1908), and by Ernest A. Codman (1914). It holds considerably greater promise than audits for physician performance and has achieved a modestly successful record to date (Stanford Center for Health Care Research 1976; Luft et al. 1979). The basic data for such institutional reviews are the patient population, categorized by age, sex, diagnosis, and procedures performed, coupled with minimal outcomes data, for example, mortality, complications, and length of stay.

Using these basic data, as collected and made available by the Commission on Professional and Hospital Activities in Ann Arbor, Michigan, Luft and his colleagues were able to demonstrate that hospitals in which high volumes of complex surgical procedures, such as coronary artery bypass graft, total hip replacement, and transurethral resection of the prostate are performed, have lower case mortality rates for these procedures than do hospitals with low volumes. Luft et al. (1979) and Bunker et al. (1982b) have explored the policy implications of these observations for regionalization of complex procedures, but there has been relatively little implementation of their recommendations.

The comparison of hospitals on the basis of outcome has been plagued by the problems of case mix: some hospitals have sicker patients than others. In the study by Luft et al. case mix could have confounded the results only if the hospitals with small volumes of cases operated on sicker patients. This was considered unlikely, and, if true, inappropriate. The problem of case mix is, never the less, a difficult one, particularly if comparisons are attempted between individual hospitals. The current flurry of efforts to measure severity of illness (including attempts to classify patients by diagnosis related groups) may offer the opportunity to improve the reliability of inter-hospital comparisons (Fetter et al. 1980; Horn 1983; Horn et al. 1983). Among the obstacles to be overcome are the unreliability of routinely collected hospital data from hospital discharge summaries (Institute of Medicine 1976) and the anticipated distortion of diagnosis related group classification when used as a basis for re-imbursement (Simborg 1982).

## POLICY IMPLICATIONS

We have seen that routine monitoring and information systems can serve as a basis for hypothesis generation, and as the source of data needed for post-marketing surveillance. They can also be used to identify medical problems in need of study, and to assess the quality of care provided by physicians or by hospitals. Routine data can be used to complement experimental research strategies, such as clinical trials, when they are applied carefully with sensitivity to their limits. This chapter has described some of those limitations as well as some of the methods that can be used to mitigate them. But how much effort and money should be invested in the further development of routine data systems?

There is no national or regional programme in the US to collect comprehensive data on medical and surgical procedure rates and outcomes. The National Center for Health Statistics does collect hospital admissions and procedure rates based on a small statistical sample. In addition, the privately owned and operated Commission for Professional and Hospital Activities in Ann Arbor, Michigan, collects and publishes data on procedure rates and associated in-hospital mortality. The sample is a large one (approxiamtely one-fourth of all hospitalized patients and one-third of the hospital discharges in the US), but it is not a probability sample, and represents only the hospitals that subscribe to the service.

The data from the National Center for Health Statistics and the Commission for Professional and Hospital Activities may or may not include new or experimental procedures. Some institutions collect and publish their own individual experiences with new procedures, but such published data clearly do not represent the national experience (see, for example, the data of Chalmers *et al.* (1978) comparing the low mortality in published reports of coronary-artery bypass grafting and the higher unpublished mortality of this procedure in New York state).

The National Center for Health Care Technology (NCHCT), under its enabling legislation, was directed to undertake and support multifaceted assessments of health-care technology, taking into account 'the safety, effectiveness, and cost-effectiveness of, and the social, ethical, and economic impact of health care technologies' (Committee on Interstate and Foreign Commerce on the Health Services Research, Health Statistics, and Health Care Technology Act of 1978). To carry out its mandate NCHCT would have needed, and, with adequate appropriations, could have offered grants and contracts for data banks, registries, and for surveillance of drugs, of devices, and of other procedures. Yet, despite the widely publicised concern of Congress about the costs and effectiveness of medical technology, appropriations for NCHCT, which had never been adequate (only $3.25 million in 1980), were terminated in 1982, and the Center now exists only on paper.

Despite the demise of NCHCT, there is a growing awareness in the US of the need for technology assessment (Frederickson 1980; Relman 1980; Bunker *et al.* 1982*a*). The Institute of Medicine, a non-governmental agency within the National Academy of Sciences, is currently (1984) exploring the feasibility of establishing a 'technology assessment consortium' for this purpose. Such an agency, if it is to succeed, will need a considerably enhanced national capability and investment in medical information systems and routine monitoring. The importance of information systems and monitoring as part of an overall strategy to evaluate the effectiveness of medical procedures is discussed earlier in this chapter. Enhanced information systems and monitoring will also be essential to the policy effort to control the costs of medical care in the US, a country committed to the provision of all effective medical care, and in which cost has been to date only a relatively limiting factor.

While technology assessment is increasingly perceived as essential to the effort to control the costs of medical care in the US, such assessment has been minimal in Canada, where costs have been controlled, with considerable success, by sole-source public funding tightly controlled at the provincial government level (Evans 1982). Ironically, the capability for routine monitoring in Canada, as we have seen in the foregoing, is considerably greater than in the US. Whether or not Canada in the future chooses to take greater advantage of this unique information resource, much can be learned by the US and other countries that face the need for the continued monitoring and evaluation of the medical care they provide.

## ACKNOWLEDGEMENTS

Preparation of this chapter was facilitated by Career Scientist Awards Nos. 6607-1314-48 and 6607-1001-22 (to L.L. Roos and N.P. Roos) and by Grant No. 6607-1156-46 from Research Programs Directorate, Health and Welfare, Canada.

We wish to acknowledge Harold Luft's comprehensive review of an earlier version.

## REFERENCES

Ashley, J.S.A., Howlett, A., and Morris, J.N. (1971). Case fatality of hyperplasia of the prostate in two teaching and three regional-board hospitals. *Lancet* ii, 1308.

Barnes, B.A. (1982). Population-based small unit analysis of health care. In *Regional variations in hospital use* (ed. D.L. Rothberg), p. 187. Lexington Books, Lexington, Mass.

Beebe, G.W. (1983). Long term follow-up is a problem. *Am. J. Public Health* **73**, 245.

Bellows, M.T. (1949). Case registers. *Public Health Rep.* **64**, 1148.

Bunker, J.P., and Wennberg, J.E. (1973). Operation rates, mortality statistics and the quality of life. *N. Engl. J. Med.* **289**, 1251.

Bunker, J.P., Fowles, J., and Schaffarzick, R. (1982*a*). Evaluation of medical technology strategies. *N. Engl. J. Med.* **306**, 620 and **306**, 687.

Bunker, J.P., Hinkley, D., and McDermott, W.V. (1978). Surgical innovation and its evaluation. *Science* **200**, 937.

Bunker, J.P., Luft, H.S., and Enthoven, A.C. (1982*b*). Should surgery be regionalized? *Surg. Clin. N. Am.,* **62**, 657.

Byar, D.P. (1980). Why data bases should not replace randomized clinical trials. *Biometrics* **36**, 337.

Chalmers, T.C., Smith, H., Jr., Ambroz, A., Reitman, D., and Schroeder, B.J. (1978). In defense of the VA randomized control trial of coronary artery surgery. *Clin. Res.* **26**, 230.

Codman, E.A. (1914). The product of a hospital. *Surg. Gynecol. Obstet.* **18**, 491.

Committee on Interstate and Foreign Commerce on the Health Services Research, Health Statistics, and Health Care Technology Act of 1978. *Report no. 95–1190*. US Government Printing Office, Washington, DC.

Cook, N.R. and Ware, J.H. (1983). Design and analysis methods for longitudinal research. *Ann. Rev. Public Health* **4**, 1.

Cook, T.D. and Campbell, D.T. (1979). *Quasi-experimentation.* Rand McNally, Chicago.

Crapo, I.M. and Melmon, K.L. (1983). Optimal therapy for the geriatric patient: the challenge to clinical pharmacology. *J. Chronic. Dis.* **36**, 39.

de Dombal, F.T., Leaper, D.J., Horrocks, J.C., Staniland, J.R., and McCann, A.P. (1974). Human and computer-aided diagnosis of abdominal pain: further report with emphasis on performance of clinicians. *Br. Med. J.* **i**, 376.

Evans, R.G. (1982). The fiscal management of medical technology: the case of Canada. In *Resources for health* (ed. H.D. Banta) p. 178. Praeger Publishers, New York.

Federspiel, C.F., Ray, W.A., and Schaffner, W. (1976). Medicaid records as a valid data source: the Tennessee experience. *Med. Care.* **14**, 166.

Feinstein, A.R. and Horwitz, R.I. (1982). Double standards, scientific methods and epidemiologic research. *N. Engl. J. Med.* **307**, 1611.

Fetter, R.B., Shin, Y., Freeman, J.L., Averill, R.F., and Thompson, J.D. (1980). Case mix definition by diagnosis-related groups. *Med. Care.* **18** No. 2, Suppl., 1.

Frederickson, D.S. (1980). Sorting out the doctor's bag. *Controlled Clin. Trials.* **1**, 263.

Freiman, J.A., Chalmers, T.C., Smith, H., Jr., and Kuebler, R.R. (1978). The importance of beta, the type II error and sample size in the design and interpretation of the randomized control trial. Survey of 71 'negative' trials. *N. Engl. J. Med.* **299**, 690.

Fries, J.F. (1976). A data bank for the clinician? *N. Engl. J. Med.* **294**, 1400.

Gibbs, J.O. and Newman, J.F. (1982). *Study of health services used and costs incurred during the last six months of a terminal illness. Final Report.* Blue Cross and Blue Shield Association, Chicago, Illinois.

Gilbert, J.P., McPeek, B., and Mosteller, F. (1977). Statistics and ethics in surgery and anesthesia. *Science* **198**, 684.

Gittelsohn, A.M. (1982). On the distribution of underlying causes of death. *Am. J. Public Health* **72**, 133.

Goldberg, J., Gelfand, H.M., and Levy, P.S. (1980). Registry evaluation methods: a review and case study. *Epidemiol. Rev.* **2**, 210.

Grace, N.D., Muench, H., and Chalmers, T.C. (1966). The present status of shunts for portal hypertension in cirrhosis. *Gastroenterology* **50**, 684.

Henley, R.R., Wiederhold, G., Dervin, J. *et al.* (1975). *An analysis of automated ambulatory medical record systems.* Technical Report No. 13 (NTIS PB-254-234). Office of Medical Information, University of California, San Francisco.

Hey Groves, E.W., (1908). Surgical statistics, a plea for a uniform registration of operation results. *Br. J. Med.* **ii**, 1008.

Horn, S.D. (1983). Measuring severity of illness: comparisons across institutions. *Am. J. Public Health* **73**, 25.

Horn, S.D., Chachich, B., Clopton, C. (1983). Measuring severity of illness: a reliability study. *Med. Care.* **21**, 705.

Institute of Medicine (1976). *Assessing quality in health care: an evaluation.* National Academy of Sciences, Washington, DC.

Joint Commission on Prescription Drug Use, Inc. (1981). *Final report.* US Government Printing Office, Washington, DC.

Keys, A. (1980). *Seven countries: a multivariate analysis of death and coronary heart disease.* Harvard University Press, Cambridge, Mass.

Klos, D.M., and Rosenstock, I.M. (1982). Some lessons from the

North Karelia Project. *Am. J. Public Health* **72**, 53.

Lee, J.A.H., Morrison, S.L., and Morris, J.N. (1957). Fatality from three common surgical conditions in teaching and non-teaching hospitals. *Lancet* **ii**, 785.

Lee, J.A.H., Morrison, S.L., and Morris, J.N. (1960). Case-fatality in teaching and non-teaching hospitals [Letter]. *Lancet* **i**, 170.

Lembcke, P.A. (1956). Medical auditing by scientific methods: illustrated by major female pelvic surgery. *JAMA*, **162**, 646.

Lohr, K.N., Brook, R.H., and Kaufman, M.A. (1980). Quality of care in the New Mexico Medicaid program. *Med. Care* Suppl. **18**, 1.

Luft, H.S. (1981). Diverging trends in hospitalization: fact or artifact? *Med. Care.* **19**, 979.

Luft, H.S., Bunker, J.P., and Enthoven, A.C. (1979). Should operations be regionalized? The empirical relation between surgical volume and mortality. *N. Engl. J. Med.* **301**, 1364.

McAlister, A., Puska, P., Salonen, J.T., Tuomilehto, J., and Koskela, K. (1982). Theory and action for health promotion: illustrations from the North Karelia Project. *Am. J. Public Health* **72**, 43.

McDermott, W.V., Jr., and Adams, R.D. (1954). Episodic stupor associated with an Eck fistula in the human with particular reference to the metabolism of ammonia. *J. Clin. Invest.* **33**, 1.

McDonald, C.J., Wilson, G.A., and McCabe, G.P., Jr. (1980). Physician response to computer reminders. *JAMA*, **244**, 1579.

McPherson, K., Wennberg, J.E., Hovind, O.R., and Clifford, P. (1982). Small-area variations in the use of common surgical procedures: an international comparison of New England, England, and Norway. *N. Engl. J. Med.* **307**, 1310.

Mednick, S.A. (1981). Methods of prospective, longitudinal research In *Prospective longitudinal research* (ed. S.A. Mednick and A.E. Baert) p. 11. Oxford University Press.

Morris, J.N. (1964). *Uses of epidemiology, 2nd edn.* Livingstone, Edinburgh.

Mossey, J.M., Havens, B., Roos, N.P., and Shapiro, E. (1981). The Manitoba longitudinal study on aging: description and methods. *Gerontologist* **21**, 551.

Mosteller, F. and Tukey, V.W. (1977). *Data analysis and regression: a second course in statistics.* Addison-Wesley, Reading, Massachusetts.

Nightingale, F. (1859). *Notes on hospitals.* John W. Parker, London.

Office of Technology Assessment, Congress of the United States (1983). *The impacts of randomized clinical trials in health policy and medical practice, 1983.* US Government Printing Office, Washington, DC.

Paradise, J.L., Bluestone, C.D., Bachman, R.Z. *et al.* (1978). History of recurrent sore throat as an indication of tonsillectomy. Predictive limitations of histories that are undocumented. *N. Engl. J. Med.* **298**, 409.

Promis Laboratory (1981). *Executive summary. Final Report for Contract HRA 233-78-3011.* Promis Laboratory, Washington, DC.

Relman, A.S. (1980). Assessment of medical practices: a simple proposal. *N. Engl. J. Med.* **303**, 153.

Reynolds, T.B., Donovan, A.J., Mikkelsen, W.P., Redeker, A.G. Turrill, F.L., and Weiner, J.M. (1981). Results of a 12-year randomized trial of portacaval shunt in patients with alcoholic liver disease and bleeding varices. *Gastroenterology* **80**, 1005.

Roemer, M.I. and Schwartz, J.L. (1979). Doctor slowdown: effects on the population of Los Angeles County. *Soc. Sci. Med.* **13C**, 213.

Roos, L.L. (1979). Alternative designs to study outcomes: the tonsillectomy case. *Med. Care* **17**, 1069.

Roos, L.L. (1983). Supply, workload and utilization: a population-based analysis of surgery in rural Manitoba. *Am. J. Public Health* **73**, 414.

Roos, L.L. (1984). Surgical rates and mortality rates: a correlational analysis. *Med. Care* **22**, 586.

Roos, L.L., Nicol, J.P., Johnson, C., and Roos, N.P. (1979).

Using administrative data banks for research and evaluation: a case study. *Eval. Q.* **3**, 236.

Roos, L.L., Roos, N.P., Cageorge, S.M., and Nicol, J.P. (1982). How good are the data? Reliability of one health care data bank. *Med. Care* **20**, 266.

Roos, N.P. (1984). Hysterectomies in one Canadian province. A new look at risks and benefits. *Am. J. Pub. Health* **74**, 39.

Rosati, R.A., McNeer, J.F., Starmer, C.F., Mittler, B.S., Morris, J.J., and Wallace, A.G. (1975). A new information system for medical practice. *Arch. Intern. Med.* **135**, 1017.

Sanazaro, P.J. (1982). Quality assessment and quality assurance in medical care. *Ann. Rev. Public Health* **1**, 37.

Shapiro, S. (1981). Issues in developing routine data sources for health planning. *Public Health Rep.* **96**, 212.

Sherman, H. (ed.) (1980). *Issues raised by third party reimbursement for investigational procedures: options and criteria.* Report to the National Center for Health Care Technology.

Shwartz, M., Martin, S.G., Cooper, D. *et al.* (1981). The effect of a thirty per cent reduction in physician fees on Medicaid surgery rates in Massachusetts. *Am. J. Public Health* **71**, 370.

Simborg, D.W. (1982). DRG creep. A new hospital-acquired disease. *N. Engl. J. Med.* **304**, 1602.

Smith, M.E. and Newcombe, H.B. (1980). Automated follow-up facilities in Canada for monitoring delayed health effects. *Am. J. Public Health* **70**. 1261.

Smith, M.E. and Newcombe, H.B. (1982). Use of the Canadian mortality data base for epidemiological follow-up. *Can. J. Public Health* **73**, 39.

Stanford Center for Health Care Research (1976). Comparison of hospitals with regard to outcomes of surgery. *Health Serv. Res.* **11**, 112.

Towery, O.B. and Perry, S. (1981). The scientific basis for coverage decisions by third-party payers. *JAMA* **245**, 59.

Vayda, E. and Mindell, W.R. (1982). Variations in operative rates: what do they mean? *Surg. Clin. N. Am.* **62**, 627.

Webb, E.J., Campbell, D.T., Schwartz, R.D., Sechrest, L., and Groves, J.B. (1981). *Nonreactive measures in the social sciences,* 2nd edn. Houghton Mifflin, Boston.

Wennberg, J.E. (1982). Should the cost of insurance reflect the cost of use in local hospital markets? *N. Engl. J. Med.* **307**, 1374.

Wennberg, J.E. and Gittelsohn, A. (1980). *A small area approach to the analysis of health system performance.* Health Planning Methods and Technology Series. DHHS Pub. No. (HRA) 80-14012. Washington, DC.

Wennberg, J.E. and Gittelsohn, A. (1982). Variations in medical care among small areas. *Sci. Am.* **246**, 120.

Whipple, A.O. (1945). The problem of portal hypertension in relation to the hepatosplenopathies. *Ann. Surg.* **122**, 449.

Wortman, P.M., Reichardt, C.S., and St. Pierre, R.G. (1978). The first year of the education voucher demonstration: a secondary analysis of student achievement test scores. *Eval. Q.* **2**, 193.

Wortman, P. and Yeaton, W.H. (1983). Synthesis of results in controlled trials of coronary artery bypass graft surgery. In *Evaluation studies review annual,* Vol. 8 (ed. R.J. Light) p. 536. Sage Publications, Beverley Hills, CA.

# Epidemiological techniques and planned investigations

# 5 Cross-sectional studies

J.H. Abramson

## INTRODUCTION

This chapter deals with prevalence and other cross-sectional studies, i.e. with surveys of the situation existing in a given group or population at a given time. These surveys may be concerned with:

1. The presence of disorders, such as diseases, disabilities, and symptoms of ill health.

2. Dimensions of positive health, such as physical fitness.

3. Other attributes relevant to health, such as blood pressure and body measurements.

4. Factors associated with health and disease, such as exposure to specific environmental factors, defined social and behavioural attributes, and demographic characteristics; the correlates may be determinants, predictors, or effects of health and disease states.

Such a study may be descriptive, analytical, or both. At a descriptive level it yields information about a single variable (diabetes, haemoglobin concentration, capacity to work, cigarette smoking, etc.), or about each of a number of separate variables, in a total study population, or in various specific population groups. At an analytical level, it provides information about the presence and strength of associations between variables, permitting the testing of hypotheses concerning such associations.

The distinctive feature of cross-sectional studies is that they essentially collect information relating to a single specified time. They are often extended, however, to include historical information that can easily be collected at the same time.

These studies must be distinguished from incidence and other surveys that require or imply information relating to the state of the individual at two or more points in time. The latter studies, which are discussed in later chapters, measure changes in status, e.g. disease onset, death, growth, changes in blood pressure, etc. or they examine associations between variables with a defined temporal relationship, e.g. between childhood experiences and health in adulthood. The difference between cross-sectional surveys and these surveys is often likened to the difference between snapshots and motion pictures.

The *uses of cross-sectional studies* can be categorized as follows:

1. The study may be used to promote the health of the specific group or population studied, i.e. as a tool in community health care.

2. The study may contribute to the clinical care of individual patients.

3. The study may provide 'new knowledge', in the sense of yielding generalizable inferences that can be applied beyond the specific group or population studied. This new knowledge may relate, for example, to the aetiology of a disease or the value of a type of health care.

These uses are, of course, not mutually exclusive; a single study may fulfill more than one purpose.

This chapter briefly considers the terms *'prevalence'* and *'incidence'* and then reviews the *methods* used in cross-sectional studies, paying special attention to the *statistical measures* commonly used, including prevalence rates of various kinds. The main body of the chapter has three sections, which give separate consideration to each of the three uses of cross-sectional studies (as listed above) and deal with some of the specific features of studies that meet each purpose. The first of these sections, on *uses in community health care*, considers *community diagnosis, surveillance, community education and community involvement,* and the *evaluation of a community's health care.* The subsection on community diagnosis deals with studies of health status, determinants of health and disease, and associations between variables (including the measurement of effect; risk markers; and community syndromes), and with the identification of groups requiring special care. The section on the second function of cross-sectional studies, their *uses in clinical practice,* briefly describes applications in *individual and family care* and then considers the role of these studies in *community-oriented primary care.* The last section, which deals with *studies yielding new knowledge,* reviews *studies of growth and development, studies of aetiology,* and *programme trials.*

### Prevalence and incidence

The term 'prevalence' refers to the number of individuals who have a given disease or other defined attribute at a specified time, as opposed to 'incidence', which refers to the number of events that occur in a given period. The event may be the onset of a new disease or a new disease episode, death, etc. The prevalence of a disease in a population at any point in time depends on the prior incidence of new cases and on the average duration of the disease from onset to recovery or death. This relationship is shown diagrammatically in Fig. 5.1, in which the contents of the container represent prevalence, and the time spent in the container is the duration of the disease.

If incidence and the average duration have remained

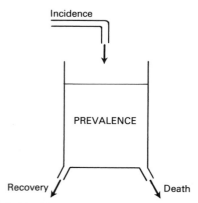

**Fig. 5.1.** Relationship between prevalence and incidence.

constant over a long period (a condition seldom if ever encountered in practice), the point prevalence rate (defined below) is the product of the incidence rate of new cases per time unit $t$ and the average duration of the disease (mean $t$ per case). For a disease that runs an episodic course, the point prevalence rate of active disease is (under certain assumptions) the product of the incidence rate, the average duration of an episode, and the average number of episodes per case (Von Korff and Parker 1980).

## METHODS

Like any other kind of study, a cross-sectional study can yield useful findings only if sound methods are used. At all stages – in the planning phase, during the collection of data, and when the data are processed and interpreted – there is a need for detailed attention to the minutiae of survey technique, so as to ensure that the results will be as accurate as practical constraints permit (Abramson 1984). Care must be taken to minimize bias, and to make allowance for it when it cannot be avoided.

A cross-sectional study may be performed in a total population or other defined group, or in a sample. Simple random sampling or systematic, stratified or cluster sampling may be used (see Volume 3, Chapter 9). In some large-scale studies it may be appropriate to use medical practices as the sampling units (Bevan and Draper 1965; Fraser 1978). If medical visits are sampled, adjustments may be needed to overcome bias caused by the over-representation of patients who pay more frequent visits (Shepard and Neutra 1977). Cross-sectional studies that compare the characteristics of people with and without a given disease are discussed (with other case-control studies) in Volume 3, Chapter 8.

Methods of collecting information may be broadly classified as follows:

1. Clinical examinations, special tests, and other observations.

2. Interviews and questionnaires. The subjects themselves may be questioned, or proxy respondents, e.g. household informants, may be used.

3. Clinical records and other documentary sources. Sources of information on the prevalence of diseases include hospital and other medical records, disease registers (Weddell 1973),

records of routine examinations (e.g. in schools, army induction centres, and health insurance schemes), and published statistics based on these and other records. Health information resources in the US and the UK are described in Volume 3, Chapters 1 and 2.

Each method has its own advantages and limitations and carries its own possible biases. If information on the prevalence of a disease is obtained from hospitals, for example, people with mild disease are especially likely to be under-represented. The degree of bias may vary for different categories of the study population, as a result of variation in the accessibility or use of health services, or differences between clinical services in their diagnostic and recording procedures. Associations observed in a study of hospital or clinic patients may differ from those in the general population ('Berksonian bias') if admission rates to the study population are connected with the variables whose association is studied. A catalogue of biases, most of them applicable to cross-sectional studies, has been published by Sackett (1979).

Some biases can be avoided or measured, others cannot, but must still be taken into account when inferences are drawn from the findings. Sometimes bias can be corrected. Smith and Hill (1974), for example, have suggested a technique for estimating the number of patients with a chronic disorder – the example they use is Buerger's disease – who are missed because their disease is early or mild. Their procedure requires the collection of information on the prior course of the disease.

Studies of disease prevalence may be conducted in two stages, e.g. by using a screening test to identify people who are likely to have a specific disease. These are then subjected to more specific and elaborate tests to determine whether the disease is present.

### Statistical measures

The statistical measures used for summarizing the findings of descriptive cross-sectional studies include means and standard deviations of distributions of quantitative attributes; medians, percentiles, and other quantities; and proportions (including the rates described below). Ratios other than proportions are occasionally used, e.g. the sex ratio (usually the male:female ratio) among people with a specific disease. Separate statistical measures (e.g. sex- and age-specific rates; see below) may be provided for specific sex and age categories, ethnic groups, social classes, regions, etc.

In analytical cross-sectional studies, associations between variables may be measured by correlation and regression coefficients, differences between means, and other statistics. If both variables are dichotomies, the measures of the strength of their association include those listed in Table 5.1. The most commonly-used of these are the *odds ratio, rate ratio* (relative risk), and *rate difference*. If the variables are exposure to some factor and the presence of a disease, an odds ratio of three means that the odds in favour of the disease are three times as high among people exposed to the factor as they are among people not exposed to it. It also means that the odds in favour of exposure are three times as high among people with the disease as they are among people free of the disease. The odds ratio can

**Table 5.1.** *Measures of association between a dichotomous variable and presence of a disease in a cross-sectional study of a population*

|              | Disease present | Disease absent | Total |
|--------------|:---------------:|:--------------:|:-----:|
| Factor present | $a$ | $b$ | $a+b$ |
| Factor absent  | $c$ | $d$ | $c+d$ |
| Total          | $a+c$ | $b+d$ | $N$ |

Odds ratio $= ad/bc$
Rate ratio $= [a/(a+b)]/[c/(c+d)]$

**If the factor is a risk factor:**
Rate difference (excess risk among exposed):
$\quad = a/(a+b) - c/(c+d)$
Population excess risk $= (a+c)/N - c/(c+d)$
Attributable fraction among exposed $= [a/(a+b) - c/(c+d)]/[a/(a+b)]$. Also termed the aetiologic fraction (exposed), the attributable risk (exposed), or, if expressed as a percentage, the attributable risk per cent (exposed).
Attributable fraction in population $= [(a+c)/N - c/(c+d)]/[(a+c)/N]$. Also termed the aetiologic fraction (population), Levin's attributable risk, or, if expressed as a percentage, the population attributable risk per cent.

**If the factor is a protective factor:**
Rate difference (excess risk among unexposed) $= c/(c+d) - a/(a+b)$.
Population excess risk $= (a+c)/N - a/(a+b)$.
Prevented fraction among exposed $= [c/(c+d) - a/(a+b)]/[c/(c+d)]$. This is also the preventable fraction among the unexposed.
Prevented fraction in population $= [c/(c+d) - (a+c)/N]/[c/(c+d)]$.
Preventable fraction in population $= [(a+c)/N - a/(a+b)]/[(a+c)/N]$.

be calculated from the findings in a total population (or a representative sample), or from the findings in representative samples of exposed and non-exposed people, or of diseased and healthy ones. A rate ratio of three means that the prevalence rate of the disease is three times as high among people exposed to the factor, as it is among those not exposed. The rate ratio can be calculated from the findings in a population or in groups of exposed and non-exposed people. If the frequency of the disease in the population is low, the odds ratio is a good estimate of the rate ratio. The rate difference is the absolute difference between the rates in exposed and non-exposed people. This measure, the population excess risk (also an absolute difference) and the attributable and prevented fractions based on them (discussed under 'Measurement of effect', p. 93), are often used to indicate the practical significance of an association in terms of its public health importance. For a fuller explanation of the various measures and their uses, see Fleiss (1981).

In analytical studies that aim to explain associations between variables as well as to describe them, a variety of techniques and measures may be used to control confounding factors and permit appraisal of the modifying effects of other variables on the associations. These procedures range in complexity from stratification and standardization to sophisticated multivariate techniques that permit the simultaneous consideration of a large number of variables and their relationships.

If the data were obtained from a random sample, confidence limits may be calculated in order to obtain an interval that has a high probability of containing the true value of the measure in the total study population. Confidence limits are also often calculated when it is wished to generalize from the findings in a

study population to a broader 'reference' population (e.g. 'White men in the US'), but in this instance the procedure is open to criticism.

*Prevalence rates*

A prevalence rate is used to measure the relative frequency of a disease or other qualitative attribute in a group or population: it is a proportion. It should be noted that this use of the term 'prevalence rate', which conforms with common usage by epidemiologists, is disparaged by some experts who prefer to confine the term 'rate' to measures of the rapidity of change, and therefore use 'prevalence' rather than 'prevalence rate', claiming that 'the term "prevalence" is quite legitimate, but "prevalence rate" is an impossible concept' (Elandt-Johnson 1975).

There are different kinds of prevalence rate. When the term is used without qualification, it usually refers to a *point prevalence rate*, i.e. the prevalence at a specified point of time. The point prevalence rate of a disease per 1000 population, for example, is calculated by the formula:

$$\frac{\text{Number of individuals with the disease at a specified point of time}}{\text{Population at that time}} \times 1000.$$

The numerator of this rate is the total number of people who have the disease at a stated point of time, irrespective of the time of onset of the disease. The denominator is the total population (actual or estimated) at that time, including affected and unaffected people. The multiplier used in this and other rates may be 100, 1000, or any other convenient or conventional multiple of ten.

Like other rates, this rate may express the findings in a specific subgroup of the population; when so used, both the numerator and denominator must refer to the same population category. As an example of a sex- and age-specific rate, the point prevalence rate of a disease per 1000 men aged 45–54 years is calculated by the formula:

$$\frac{\text{Number of men aged 45–54 years with the disease at a specified point of time}}{\text{Total number of men aged 45–54 years in the population at that time}} \times 1000.$$

In a prevalence survey in which interviews or examinations of the study subjects are staggered over a period, so that the point of time at which the presence of the disease (or other attribute) is determined varies for different individuals, the formula is:

$$\frac{\text{Number of individuals with the disease at the time the individual is studied}}{\text{Number of individuals studied}} \times 1000.$$

For a long-term disease, this may be regarded as equivalent to an ordinary point prevalence rate.

Paradoxically, there are some point prevalence rates that can be accurately measured only by a longitudinal study. An example is the rate of congenital anomalies per 100 births. This may be regarded as a point prevalence rate whose 'point of time' is the moment of birth. However, as many anomalies become manifest only weeks, months or years after birth, reasonably full ascertainment of cases requires long-term follow-up.

A *period prevalence rate* measures prevalence not at a single point of time, but during a defined calendar period (usually a year, month or week). The *period prevalence rate (persons)* of a disease during a particular year, for example, is the proportion of the population manifesting the disease at any time during that year. The formula is:

$$\frac{\text{Number of individuals manifesting the disease in the stated time period}}{\text{Population at risk}} \times 1000.$$

The numerator is the number of people with the illness during the specified time period, including those whose illness started before this period. The denominator is the average size of the total population during the specified period. It is often estimated by using the population at the middle of the period, or by averaging the size of the population at the beginning and the end of the period. Other methods may be needed if the change in population size during the given period did not occur at an approximately even rate, especially if this change was large. It is usually more helpful to know the point prevalence rate (e.g. at the beginning of the period) and the incidence rate of new cases during the period, than the period prevalence rate.

The numerator of the little-used *period prevalence rate (spells)* is the number of spells of an illness observed during the specified period, irrespective of their time of onset (the same person may be ill more than once). The denominator is the population at risk. For a short-term disease, this rate is usually similar to the incidence rate (spells).

A *lifetime prevalence rate* is a period prevalence rate in which the period studied is the whole of the subject's prior life. It refers to the presence of a given disorder or of a scar, antibodies, or other evidence that the disorder was present at some time in the past. The formula is:

$$\frac{\text{Number of individuals with evidence of the disorder (past or present)}}{\text{Number of individuals studied}} \times 1000.$$

This rate is usually useful only if it refers to a specific age-group, and if valid information on prior occurrence is available. As an example, a cross-sectional study in Jerusalem revealed that the point prevalence rate of inguinal hernia among men aged 65–74 years was 30 per cent. An additional 10 per cent had scars of hernia repair operations, with no current evidence of hernia. The lifetime prevalence rate for this age-group was thus 40 per cent (Abramson *et al.* 1978). It could be inferred that in this cohort of men the risk of developing this condition by the age of 65–74 years, among men surviving to that age, was 40 per cent. Such information would be of little value if the disorder were one with an important association with survival, such as cancer.

As a further example, the lifetime prevalence rate of definite psychiatric disorder among men aged 60–69 years was 11 per cent, according to the Stirling County Study in Canada, in which diagnoses of disorder were based both on current symptom patterns and on information about previous symptom patterns. If probable psychiatric disorder was added, the lifetime prevalence rate in this age-group rose to 41 per cent (Leighton *et al.* 1963). As historical information was probably not complete, these rates were probably underestimates of the risk.

The lifetime prevalence rate of a disorder among the blood relatives of an index case may be used as a measure of familial risk, especially in genetic studies.

There is also a type of period prevalence rate that refers to a defined period of the individual's life. An example is the prevalence rate of anaemia in pregnant women, expressed as the proportion of a group of pregnant women who have anaemia at any time during their pregnancy.

## USES IN COMMUNITY HEALTH CARE

Cross-sectional studies can fulfil important functions in the health care of a community. They can contribute to the planning of services, to the effective implementation of care, and to decision-making on the continuance and modification of services. In this discussion, 'community' may be taken to refer to any aggregation of people for whose care a physician, health care team, agency or authority is responsible; it may be a nation or region, a local neighbourhood, a list of registered patients, a defined group of schoolchildren or workers, inmates of an institution, etc.

We will give separate attention to the use of cross-sectional studies in community diagnosis, in ongoing surveillance, in community health education and the promotion of community involvement, and in the evaluation of the community's health care.

### Community diagnosis

Cross-sectional studies can provide a major part of the epidemiological foundation for community diagnosis (McGavran 1956; Morris 1975; Kark 1981), i.e. for determining the health status of a community and the factors responsible for producing it. They can supply information on the nature, extent, and impact of health problems, as a basis for the identification of priorities and the planning of intervention. Such studies may relate to a broad spectrum of health states and their correlates, or may be limited in their scope. Even the simplest of information, e.g. about the population's size and its age and sex distribution, may be of help in planning the allocation of resources.

### Health status

Cross-sectional studies may yield useful information on a variety of dimensions of health and disease, including self-appraised health, mental health status, growth and development, physical fitness, the distribution of blood pressures, etc. The following remarks refer only to the prevalence of disorders; the cross-sectional method for the study of growth and development is discussed on page 98.

Information on the prevalence of diseases and disabilities in the community, supplemented by incidence and mortality data, provides a basis for inferences about needs for curative and rehabilitative care, i.e. for secondary and tertiary prevention. It must be remembered that the picture provided by prevalence studies alone, especially by studies of point prevalence, may be incomplete because of the under-representation of conditions with a short duration; these include not only the acute non-fatal diseases that usually provide a considerable load for the health services, and acute episodes of long-term or recurrent diseases, but also severe and rapidly fatal conditions, such as fatal strokes and sudden deaths from coronary heart disease.

The most direct evidence of a need for improved secondary and tertiary prevention, at least for long-term diseases that are not rapidly fatal, is an unduly high prevalence of remediable disease that is undiagnosed, or that is diagnosed but untreated or inadequately treated. Prevalence surveys providing such evidence may be based on examinations, interviews, clinical files or other documentary sources, or a combination of these. An examination survey, for example, may reveal a high prevalence of untreated dental caries, or hypertension that (according to the subjects' statements or their medical files) is not under treatment. An interview survey in which many respondents report that they have been told they have high blood pressure, but say they are not currently receiving care for it, may provide similar if less valid evidence of a need for improved care. Or a review of clinical files may reveal that there are many known hypertensives who are currently not under control or are not receiving treatment.

Needs for primary prevention can be inferred from the presence of disorders known to be preventable, i.e. those whose incidence can be reduced by known preventive measures. These include ischaemic heart disease and lung cancer, which are presently of epidemic proportions in many parts of the world. For this purpose too, the prevalence data should be supplemented by data on incidence and mortality, both because diseases with a high fatality rate will otherwise be under-represented, and because prevalent cases may be long-standing ones and may not reflect present preventive needs. A high prevalence of crippling caused by poliomyelitis, for example, does not necessarily mean that current preventive procedures are ineffective. Information on the recent incidence of new cases is to be preferred for this purpose. If data on prevalence are to be used, it is advisable to seek information (if this can be obtained) on the duration of the disorder, so that the prevalence of disease of recent onset can be measured. For some diseases, information on their stage of activity may fulfil the same purpose. In institutional and other settings where people who develop a disorder are especially likely to remain in the study population, prevalence data may overestimate the need for primary prevention. In a hospital, for example, patients who develop nosocomial infections are for this reason likely to have a longer hospital stay. Such patients may thus be over-represented in a prevalence study of such infections in a hospital, giving an exaggerated idea of the need for primary prevention.

The use of highly valid measures of the presence of a disease often presents practical difficulties, and reliance may be placed on a proxy measure that is of lower validity, but is simple, inexpensive, and acceptable. The result of a screening test may be used for this purpose. If the prevalence of a proxy attribute in the population or a sample is known, methods are available for estimating the confidence limits of the prevalence of the disease itself in the population (Peritz 1971; Rogan and Gladen 1978).

### Determinants of health and disease

Information on modifiable factors that are known to affect health is of obvious relevance to the planning of health care. These may be factors that affect the community's health in a general way, e.g. dietary, infant rearing and family planning practices, and (presumably) the use of health services, and they may be factors that affect the risk of developing specific disorders. They may be *risk factors*, e.g. cigarette smoking or obesity, which increase the risk of ill health, or *protective factors*, e.g. physical activity or specific immunity (natural or acquired) to a pathogenic agent.

To collect information on the current prevalence and distribution of such determinants, there is no substitute for descriptive cross-sectional studies.

### Associations between variables

When associations are investigated in a cross-sectional study in the context of community health care, the dependent variable is usually the presence of a disease or disability (or some other dimension of health). The aim of such analyses is usually to throw light on determinants or predictors. The dependent variable may also be a supposed risk factor or protective factor, as in studies of the determinants of cigarette smoking by schoolchildren, of the use of a health service, or of compliance with medical advice. Attention may also be paid to associations among diseases or other dimensions of health, or among determinants of health.

### Measurement of effect

In the context of community health care, analyses of associations between diseases (or other outcomes) and putative causes are usually undertaken in order to determine what causal factors (of those known to be potentially important) are active in the community studied, and to measure their impact. The primary aim is to obtain information that will be useful in the specific local situation, not to generate new knowledge about aetiology, although this may be a secondary gain. Difficulties that arise when prevalence data, rather than incidence data, are used in the analysis of causal relationships are discussed on page 98.

In a situation where it is believed that an association of a risk factor with the prevalence of a disease expresses a causal relationship, the effect may be measured by the attributable fraction in the population (for formula see Table 5.1). This is the proportion of the disease in the population that can be attributed to exposure to the factor. According to data from a study of workers aged 20–64 years in a population in Jerusalem, for example, in which the association between reported posture at work and varicose veins was examined (Abramson *et al.* 1981*a*), the fraction of the prevalence of varicose veins that could be attributed to work involving much standing was 16 per cent in each sex, after controlling for effects connected with age, region of birth, weight, and height. Such values must always be interpreted with caution, as part or all of the apparent causal effect may be due to other (uncontrolled) factors associated with the apparent causal factor. Use may also be made of the excess risk among the exposed and the attributable fraction among the exposed (see Table 5.1). In the study cited, 31 per cent of the prevalence of varicose veins among men whose work involved much standing could be attributed to their work posture; for women, this fraction was 32 per cent.

For a protective factor, the corresponding measures (Table 5.1) are the excess risk among the unexposed, the prevented fraction in the population, which is the proportion of the hypothetical total prevalence that has been prevented by exposure to the factor, and the preventable fraction, which is the proportion of the observed prevalence that would be or would have been prevented if everyone was exposed to the factor.

Attributable, prevented, and preventable fractions in the population are influenced by the prevalence of the risk or protective factor in the population.

### Risk markers

Interest may not be confined to cause-effect relationships. Any attribute or exposure that is strongly associated with a disease or other disorder, even non-causally, has potential value as a predictor, provided there is reason to believe that it precedes the disease in time. Such predictors may be used as risk markers (Grundy 1973) to identify vulnerable individuals or groups.

A risk marker may be a factor that itself influences the risk, or it may be a precursor or early manifestation of the disorder, or it may be an attribute that is secondarily associated with the disorder as a result of its association with a cause or precursor of the disorder. Risk markers for stroke, for example, may include hypertension (which is a modifiable risk factor), age and ethnic group (non-modifiable determinants of the disorder), and episodes of transient cerebral ischaemia (a precursor condition). Among the elderly, risk markers for early mortality may include impaired memory and inability to work (Abramson et al. 1982a). These are obviously not causes of mortality, but outcomes of underlying disease states that increase the risk of dying.

Risk markers are best identified by longitudinal studies, but can also be detected by cross-sectional studies. A survey of the developmental quotients of two-year-olds in a Jerusalem neighbourhood, for example, revealed that poor development was more prevalent if the mother had little education or if there were many other children in the family, and especially if these factors were present together (Palti et al. 1977). These two attributes and their combination could be used as risk markers for the identification of children requiring special care in their early infancy.

The value of a risk marker, or combination of risk markers, depends on the following considerations:

1. Is its use practical? Questions of cost, resources, acceptability, safety, and convenience must be considered. The most useful risk markers are those whose measurement can be built into ordinary clinical care.

2. Is detection of vulnerability likely to be beneficial? Are resources and techniques for reducing the risk available? Is the anticipated benefit outweighed by the harm that may be caused by intervention, such as toxic side-effects, anxiety, or even iatrogenic chronic invalidism?

3. How prevalent is the risk marker? If over half the children in the community fall into a high-risk group needing special attention, might it not be more efficient and possibly more effective to modify the routine care programme so as to give extra attention to *all* children? A risk marker for a disorder may have a high prevalence because the disorder itself has a high prevalence, or because the marker has a low specificity, i.e. it occurs in a high proportion of people who will not develop the disorder.

4. What proportion of the individuals with the disorder will be identified? That is, what is the sensitivity of the marker as a predictor of the disorder? If the marker can identify only a small minority of the prospective cases, a different approach to the problem may be preferable.

The answers to these questions may vary in different populations, as may the associations between specific factors and diseases. A given risk factor may be useful in one setting but not in another.

### Community syndromes

The term 'community health syndrome' may be used to refer to diseases or other health characteristics found to occur together in a community. Examples described by Kark (1974, 1981) who introduced the community-syndrome concept and has emphasized its potential importance for the development of community medicine programmes, are a syndrome of malnutrition, communicable diseases, and mental ill health in a poor rural community undergoing rapid change, and the syndrome of hypertension, coronary heart disease, and diabetes frequently found in affluent communities characterized by nutritional imbalance and excesses, limited physical activity, and a drive for achievement.

The components of a syndrome may occur together because they possess shared or related causes, or because they are themselves causally interrelated. The syndrome points to a nexus of causal processes in the community. Even if the 'web of causation' (McMahon et al. 1960) is not completely understood, a health programme directed at the syndrome as a whole may be more effective and efficient than an endeavour to deal separately with the individual components.

Associations between diseases or other health states may be detected by observing that they occur together in the same population or population groups. They may also, and more convincingly, be detected by a tendency to affect the same individuals. As an example of the latter approach, an analysis of co-prevalence in a Jerusalem neighbourhood revealed an unexpected cluster of mutually associated disorders – migraine, chronic bronchitis, congestive heart failure, gallbladder disease, and chronic arthritis (Abramson et al. 1982b). The clustering was especially strong when people with clear objective evidence of these diseases were removed from consideration; that is, the clustering was essentially between complaint-based disorders. People with one or more of these common conditions made especially heavy use of the primary care service. These disorders were frequently associated with emotional symptoms and with family disharmony or other stressful situations. The analysis drew attention to the occurrence of a community syndrome that represented a considerable burden of discomfort for the many affected individuals and their families, and for which there was no organized programme in the health service.

### Identification of groups requiring special care

Community diagnosis may focus not only on the community as a whole, but on its component groups. In most cross-sectional studies of health characteristics in a population or population sample it is possible to compare the findings in different population categories – age and sex groups, regions, social classes, ethnic groups, etc. Such comparisons may serve to identify population groups that require special care because of a relatively high prevalence of ill health or of factors predisposing to ill health.

Use may also be made of known risk markers (which need not be causal factors) for this purpose.

A differential approach in community diagnosis is of basic importance for the identification of priorities and the allocation of resources. Simple descriptive findings often suffice for these purposes. It may be enough to know that differences between population groups exist, without endeavouring to explain them. In other circumstances the planning of effective care may be impossible unless the reasons for the differences are better understood. This may require the use of analytical epidemiological techniques.

## Surveillance

Ongoing surveillance permits the identification of changes in health status and its determinants in the community, and updating of the community diagnosis. Both cross-sectional and incidence studies have a role in surveillance. For many purposes, e.g. to detect changes in the community's smoking habits or blood pressure distributions, the only practicable method of surveillance is the performance of repeated cross-sectional studies.

Surveillance of the prevalence of chronic disorders may be based on repeated prevalence studies, or on the use of a case register that is constantly or periodically updated as new cases are found or old ones recover, die, or leave. Changes in the prevalence of chronic disorders may be of importance as an indication of changing needs for curative and rehabilitative care facilities.

Changes in the prevalence of a chronic disease cannot, however, be glibly taken to indicate changes in the risk of developing the disorder; for this purpose, incidence data should be used. There are a number of possible reasons for changes in prevalence. As demonstrated in Fig. 5.1, these changes reflect the interplay of incidence, recovery, and fatality rates. Changes in prevalence may be caused by changes in the demographic characteristics of the population, as a result of ageing or inward or outward migration. Especially in studies of small local communities, prevalence may be influenced by a tendency of affected persons to leave or to enter the neighbourhood, e.g. because of changes in admission and discharge policies of hospitals or other institutions, or in the

availability of these institutions. Often, apparent changes in prevalence are artefacts caused by changes in methods of case identification (e.g. the introduction of a case-finding programme), in the use of medical services, in diagnostic procedures or definitions, or in recording, notification, or registration practices. They may also be caused by incomplete updating of a case register, especially with respect to deaths and departures.

## Community education and community involvement

Community surveys can be used as tools for community health education. This may be done not only by communicating the findings and their implications to the community and its leaders, but also by using the educational potential of the survey situation itself, e.g. by explaining to participants why the collection of specific information is important. If accurate results are required, such explanations should preferably be given after the information has been collected, to minimize bias in the responses.

An example of the use of the survey as an educational tool is provided by the 'Know Your Body' programme, a school health education programme aimed at motivating children to adopt a healthier life-style (Williams *et al.* 1977). An essential component of this programme is a simple set of measurements of chronic disease risk factors. Each child receives a feedback of his or her results on a 'health passport', together with explanations of desirable ranges for each test, in the hope that this may provide a significant motivating force toward behavioural change. Subsequent health education seeks to capitalize on the children's personal knowledge of their own risk factors. Besides their educational use, the survey results provide a picture of the prevalence of risk factors in the schoolchildren studied.

Involvement of key community members in the planning and conduct of a health survey may be a useful way to motivate them to a more active participation in the promotion of their community's health. If community members participate in the performance of the survey, special attention should be paid to the protection of privacy and confidentiality (Wolf 1964).

A community's interest and involvement in its own health care may find expression in the performance of community self-surveys, with or without the participation of professional health workers. Such studies are usually simple descriptive cross-sectional surveys, and do not always collect very accurate or sophisticated information.

## Evaluation of a community's health care

In the context of community health care, the purpose of an evaluative study is to yield a factual basis for decisions concerning the provision of care to a specific community. This kind of evaluative study, the 'programme review', can be contrasted with the 'programme trial' (see pp. 98–9), which aims to provide generalizable inferences about the value of a given type of health programme. In programme reviews, considerable attention is given to evaluation of the 'process' of care (the performance of activities by providers and recipients of care, as well as to measurements of desirable and undesirable effects, especially more immediate outcomes.

Certain findings that are used in the process of community diagnosis as indicators of needs for health care, such as a high prevalence of preventable or remediable disorders, may by the same token be seen as indicators of the value of previous health care. In a few instances, a prevalence survey may reveal more direct evidence of the quality of previous care; the quality of the dental work found in subjects' mouths may be appraised, for example, or the presence of inguinal hernia recurrences may be recorded (one in five operated hernias showed evidence of recurrence in one such study – Abramson *et al.* 1978).

Evaluative judgements that relate to the subjects' prior health care as a whole, however, may be less helpful than those relating to recent or current health care, and especially to a specific health programme or service. Cross-sectional and other studies designed for the latter purpose focus on the performance of specific planned activities and the achievement of specific objectives. They might deal, for example, with compliance with medical advice (what proportion of hypertensives are taking the medicines prescribed for them?), with satisfaction with medical care, or with the immunization status of one-year-olds or two-year-olds in the community.

In these as in other cross-sectional studies, separate attention is usually paid to various population sub-groups. The impact of a health programme often varies with age, sex, social class, and other characteristics.

The demonstration of outcomes usually requires evidence of change. This may be provided not only by incidence and other longitudinal studies but also, for many purposes, by repeated cross-sectional studies. Surveys of the contraceptive practices of postnatal women in a Jerusalem neighbourhood in 1971 and 1977, for example, revealed that during this period the proportion using the pill, an intrauterine device or condom increased from 33 to 62 per cent (Kark 1981). Such information would be of obvious interest to a health service operating a family planning programme in the neighbourhood, even in the absence of rigorous proof that the change was actually an outcome of the programme and not an effect of other influences. It is usually believed that such changes (or their absence) are, at least to some extent, reflections of the effectiveness of the programme. They are hence often used as a basis for decisions on the need for continuation or modification of the programme. At the very least, they may indicate whether there is a need for more detailed evaluative study.

More rigorous proof that it was the programme that produced the change requires a comparison with controls (see pp. 98–9).

## USES IN CLINICAL PRACTICE

Epidemiological studies serve important functions in clinical care. We will consider the role of cross-sectional studies in (i) individual and family care and (ii) community-oriented primary care.

## Individual and family care

As Roberts (1977) explains in detail in his textbook of epidemiology for clinicians, 'a great many routine clinical decisions about individual patient care relating to matters such as the choice of diagnosis and treatment options, and advice on prognosis can only be based upon information from properly designed and executed studies in groups or populations'. He points out that epidemiological considerations are an intrinsic component of the day-to-day practice of clinical medicine.

For the clinician whose decisions are based on epidemiological facts rather than on dogma or impressions, the information required may be derived from any epidemiological studies whose results can validly be generalized to the population in which the clinician works. If information about this specific population is available, it is of course of especial value. Such information (usually largely based on cross-sectional studies) may deal with the prevalence of various diseases and their causes, the frequency distributions of biochemical and other measurements in the population, patterns of child growth, customary practices of significance to health, and so on. This information is, of course, seldom the fruit of the clinician's own labours. Sometimes, however, even a clinician whose sole concern is with the care of individual patients may conduct a small-scale epidemiological survey (usually crosss-sectional). He may, for example, need to survey a patient's contacts for evidence of a specific communicable disease (such as gonorrhoea), if only to reduce the patient's risk of reinfection.

A family physician, whose responsibility extends to the care of the whole family, may need to perform such investigations more often. Whenever a patient is found to have a disease with a known tendency to 'run in families' – e.g. rheumatic heart disease, amoebiasis or diabetes mellitus – this may be seen as a signal that the family as a whole should be surveyed for the disease.

### Family diagnosis

The process of appraising a family's health status and the factors that affect it (Kark and Kark 1962), is an exercise in small-group epidemiology. Its aim is to determine a family's health needs, as a basis for the planning of a family care programme. This involves the elucidation of the health of the family's members and appraisal of relevant features of the family life situation, e.g. the family's structure and composition, the role performance and health-relevant behaviour of its members, relationships, material resources and their use, and the family's social and physical environment. At an analytical level, it involves assessment of the ways in which individuals' health is or may be affected by other family members and by the family life situation.

## Community-oriented primary care

We have previously considered the use of cross-sectional studies in community health care. Separate consideration must be given to their use in community-oriented primary care. The latter term, which was introduced by Kark (1974, 1981), refers to a practice in which a clinician or practice team providing primary clinical care for the individuals in a defined community also undertakes activities concerned with the health of the community as such, by focusing on the community and its subgroups when appraising needs, planning and providing services, and evaluating the effects of care. Defined programmes are undertaken to deal with the community's health problems, in the primary care framework. This integration of individual-oriented and community-oriented functions in a primary care setting carries important implications for the conduct of epidemiological studies.

In such a practice a good deal of the information needed for community diagnosis, ongoing surveillance, and programme evaluation can be obtained in the course of routine clinical care. The collection of data can serve a double function. When a child is weighed or a question is asked about smoking or a diagnosis is determined, the results may be used both in the management of the patient, and as data for subsequent analysis at a group level. Such information may be derived either from routine data collected in the ordinary diagnostic investigation and surveillance of patients, or from questions or tests specially added to clinical procedures for epidemiological purposes. In a practice where periodic health examinations are conducted, these provide an especially useful opportunity for the collection of such information.

This use of clinical data demands careful attention to methods of obtaining, recording, and retrieving data, to ensure that the information will be as accurate and complete as possible. Standardized procedures are required, and definitions and diagnostic criteria should be standardized as rigorously as possible.

The performance of a cross-sectional study in this way may, of course, extend over a considerable span of time. However long the time allotted, there will often be a need for supplementary survey procedures to obtain information about members of the community who have not attended for clinical care. These people may be invited to attend for health examinations, visited at home, or asked to supply information by mail or telephone. In population groups with very high attendance rates (say infants and their mothers, pregnant women, and the elderly) there may be little bias if non-attenders are excluded.

For chronic diseases, a common technique is the maintenance of a register of cases, which is updated as new cases are diagnosed and old ones die or leave. This register, like the other practice records, has a dual purpose. It permits the calculation of point prevalence rates or other epidemiological indices, and it can also be used as a tool for ensuring that specific patients get the care they need.

Information may also be obtained by special surveys. These may be conducted primarily for purposes of community diagnosis or surveillance or to evaluate health programmes. For such purposes (say to measure smoking habits) it may be satisfactory to investigate a representative sample of the population. More usually, surveys in the context of community-oriented primary care aim not only to provide information at a community level, but also to identify individuals who need care. This identification may be based on the presence of disorders, on screening tests that point to a need for further investigation, on the presence of modifiable risk factors, and/or on the presence of risk markers indicative of vulner-

ability and a need for preventive care. In such surveys the use of a sample is clearly unsatisfactory.

A survey that has obvious importance for the community's health may be a useful means of stimulating the community's interest and involvement in their own health care. The purpose of the survey should be explained to the community, and a 'feedback' of results provided to community leaders and to the community at large, using local newsletters and whatever other media may be available.

Sackett and Holland (1975) have contrasted the roles of epidemiological surveys, screening, and 'case-finding' in the detection of diseases. They define epidemiological surveys as studies of carefully selected population samples, aimed at generating new knowledge and implying no health benefits to the participants. Screening involves the testing of apparently healthy people who respond to an invitation to be examined, and it carries an implied promise of benefit. 'Case-finding' is performed among patients who have sought health care, and is concerned with tests to reveal disorders that may be unrelated to their complaints.

In the context of community-oriented primary care, such distinctions become blurred or may vanish. An epidemiological survey may aim to provide information that will benefit individual participants, as well as providing a basis for decisions about care at a community level. The survey may be conducted in a clinical setting. In this form of practice, people are seldom invited to attend solely for screening purposes. Screening tests may be added to the routine procedures for patients who attend for treatment, or incorporated in health examinations that provide an opportunity for appraisal and surveillance of the individual's health status and life situation and for counselling, and that are not concerned solely with screening for disease. Screening tests used in this clinical context should be of high sensitivity; i.e. they should yield few false-negative results.

The collection of information in a care setting – i.e. by the providers of care – carries advantages and disadvantages. On the one hand, if relationships with the community are sound it may be relatively easy to obtain answers to awkward questions, and to achieve a high response rate. On the other hand, possibilities of bias must be recognized. The respondents may be aware of what replies are acceptable to care-providers, and their desire to please may lead to biased responses. Also, care-providers who evaluate the care they themselves provide may tend to make biased observations and inferences. Precautions are needed to reduce these forms of bias, by using objective measures when possible, and by obtaining the assistance of independent observers or investigators.

It is often difficult to obtain satisfactory denominator data, i.e. information about the size and other demographic characteristics of the population that is the target of health care and the denominator for calculating rates and other proportions. Information on age, sex, and other attributes of this population are seldom readily available from census and administrative sources, and the health service may have to devise its own data-gathering mechanism. For this purpose, a 'defined area' (Kark 1966; Kark and Abramson 1983) is sometimes demarcated for the purpose of epidemiological measurement. One approach is to incorporate the collection of demographic data in a broader household health survey. In a practice where voluntary or other community health workers are active, demographic surveillance often becomes one of their functions.

## STUDIES YIELDING 'NEW KNOWLEDGE'

Many cross-sectional studies are performed to expand the horizons of knowledge, rather than solely to promote the health of the specific group or population studied. They aim to yield generalizable inferences that are of broad application, and not relevant only to a specific local situation.

We will briefly consider studies of growth and development, studies of aetiology, and programme trials. Other topics include the natural history of health and disease (usually better investigated by longitudinal studies) and methodological issues. Cross-sectional studies are commonly used to examine the effects of differences in operational definitions or methods of study and to appraise the validity of screening tests and proxy measures. These methodological studies may aim to develop and evaluate diagnostic procedures for use in both community and individual diagnosis.

### Studies of growth and development

Growth and development can be studied cross-sectionally as well as longitudinally. The cross-sectional method compares different age-groups observed at one point of time, whereas the longitudinal method makes repeated observations of a single cohort through various age levels. The cross-sectional method is simpler, but has limitations. At best it can provide information about average changes, not about intra-individual changes or inter-individual differences in change.

The main limitation of the cross-sectional method is that the age-groups that are compared may differ in other respects than that under study, e.g. in demographic characteristics other than age, so that the effects of age and other influences may be confounded. There is always a confounding of age changes with differences between birth cohorts, as the age-groups that are compared must belong to different cohorts. Cohort differences may be negligible, but they may be significant if cohorts were exposed to very different circumstances, e.g. different infant-feeding or child-rearing fashions, changes in economic prosperity, or war. As a result the cross-sectional method may yield a misleading picture. If there has been a secular increase in height, a cross-sectional study may show a decrease in average height throughout adult life; but young adults will be taller because they belong to a more recently-born generation, not because of their youth. Similar confounding has been demonstrated in studies of the development of intelligence during adult life. Cross-sectional studies have indicated an early decline beginning at about 30 years of age, whereas longitudinal studies have shown increases or no change in intellectual performance until the age of 50 or 60 years (Baltes *et al.* 1977). If a series of cross-sectional studies has been done, suitable re-arrangement of the data may permit examination and comparison of the longitudinal changes in different cohorts.

In studies (cross-sectional or longitudinal) that include the middle-aged and elderly, selective survival may be important.

The mean blood pressure may be lower in the very old, not because blood pressure tends to drop with age, but because hypertensives are more likely to have died and thus left the study population. The possibility that the validity of measures may vary with age also requires consideration. The results of a memory test in the elderly may be expressions of hearing ability or of attentiveness, rather than of memory capacity.

### Studies of aetiology

Cross-sectional studies often provide useful clues to aetiological processes. They have two features, however, that often restrict their value for the testing of aetiological hypotheses.

First, any associations they reveal are with the *presence,* not the *appearance,* of the disorder or other variable studied. Transient or rapidly fatal cases of the disorder are inevitably under-represented. The causes that determine the appearance of the disorder are confounded with those that influence its duration, and it may be difficult to draw clear inferences about either set of causes. Such confounding is relatively unimportant if the disorder studied is seldom fatal and if it has a high chronicity or data on lifetime prevalence are used. In such instances the main difficulty is that the causal factors may no longer be apparent because of the time-lag since initiation.

Secondly, in a strictly cross-sectional study the absence of information on time relationships may render it difficult to separate effects *on* a dependent variable from effects *of* the dependent variable. The influence of blood pressure, serum cholesterol, and cigarette smoking on the occurrence of myocardial infarction, for example, may be confounded with changes in these characteristics resulting from the occurrence of the disease. The value of a cross-sectional study in the search for causes and precursors is limited whenever there is a possibility that the disease may change the subject's life-style, bodily functions, or circumstances. To throw light on time sequences, cross-sectional studies are often extended to include relevant historical information on times of disease onset or of other occurrences. Repeated cross-sectional studies of the same population can sometimes provide information on the order of events.

A cross-sectional study may form the first stage of a longitudinal study, for which it provides baseline measurements of dependent and independent variables. If the study is concerned with the incidence of a disease, the prevalence study identifies affected people, who must be excluded from the population at risk of subsequently developing the disease. The affected individuals may be followed up in order to study the natural history of the disease.

### Programme trials

To obtain convincing evidence of the effectiveness of a health programme that aims to modify the distribution of a variable in a population or to reduce the prevalence of a disease, it is necessary to measure the change in the population, and to demonstrate that this can be attributed to the programme and not to other causes. Changes in the population can be appraised by repeated cross-sectional studies. In a Jerusalem population, for example, where the prevalence of anaemia (haemoglobin

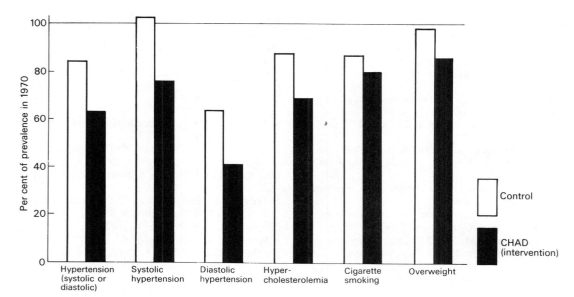

**Fig. 5.2.** Prevalence of risk factors in CHAD (intervention) and control populations in 1975, expressed as per cent of the prevalence in the same population in 1970. Based on age- and sex-standarized rates.

under 10 g/100 ml) in pregnant women was originally 12.0 per cent, the introduction of an intervention programme in 1963 was followed by a progressive drop of prevalence to 8.8 per cent in 1964–66, 3.3 per cent in 1970–71, and 1.6 per cent in 1975–76 (Kark 1981).

The cause-and-effect relationship between a programme and its apparent outcome may be difficult to substantiate without observations of a control population not exposed to the programme. For this purpose, a simple comparison of the changes observed in people who voluntarily participate or do not participate in the programme is seldom justifiable, as the comparison may be confounded by differences between the groups.

In trials of programmes directed at populations it is unfortunately seldom possible to neutralize the effects of confounding variables by using randomization. There is often little or no choice as to *what* population will be exposed to the programme under trial, and a restricted choice concerning a control population. Most programme trials are therefore quasi-experiments, in which the control group or groups are purposely selected so as to be as similar as possible to the intervention group (see Volume 3, Chapter 7).

As an illustration, Fig. 5.2 summarizes some results of a controlled evaluation of the CHAD programme for the control of cardiovascular risk factors in a Jerusalem neighbourhood (Abramson *et al.* 1981*b*). This is a community health programme integrated into primary care, implemented by family physicians and nurses; its name is an acronym representing 'Community syndrome of Hypertension, Atherosclerosis, and Diabetes'. The figure is based on age- and sex-standardized prevalence rates derived from cross-sectional studies of adults aged 35 years in 1970 (before the introduction of the programme) and in 1975, in the intervention ('CHAD') population and a neighbouring control population. It shows

the rates in 1975, expressed as percentages of the initial rate (in the same population) in 1970. For each of the risk factors shown, the decrease in prevalence (or the 'prevented fraction', as defined in Table 5.1) was greater in the CHAD population than in the control population, pointing to the effectiveness of the programme. The fact that the prevalence of some risk factors also declined in the population not exposed to the programme – apparently as a result of changes in the community's and the medical profession's awareness of the importance of preventing heart disease – underlines the need for control groups in such studies.

## REFERENCES

Abramson, J.H. (1984). *Survey methods in community medicine*, 3rd edn. Churchill Livingstone, Edinburgh.

Abramson, J.H., Gofin, R., and Peritz, E. (1982*a*). Risk markers for mortality among elderly men: a community study in Jerusalem. *J. Chronic Dis.* **35**, 656.

Abramson, J.H., Hopp, C., and Epstein, L.M. (1981*a*). The epidemiology of varicose veins. A survey in western Jerusalem. *J. Epidemiol Community Health* **35**, 213.

Abramson, J.H., Gofin, J., Hopp, C., Makler, A., and Epstein, L.M. (1978). The epidemiology of inguinal hernia. *J. Epidemiol. Community Health* **32**, 59.

Abramson, J.H., Gofin, J., Peritz, E., Hopp, C., and Epstein, L.M. (1982*b*). Clustering of chronic disorders – a community study of coprevalence in Jerusalem. *J. Chronic Dis.* **35**, 221.

Abramson, J.H., Gofin, R., Hopp, C., Gofin, J., Donchin, M., and Habib, J. (1981*b*). Evaluation of a community program for the control of cardiovascular risk factors: the CHAD program in Jerusalem. *Isr. J. Med. Sci.* **17**, 201.

Baltes, P.B., Reese, H.W., and Nesselroade, J.R. (1977). *Life-span developmental psychology: introduction to research methods.* Brooks/Cole, Monterey, California.

Bevan, J.M. and Draper, G.J. (1965). Sampling problems in studies of general practice. *Med. Care* **3**, 168.

Elandt-Johnson, R.C. (1975). Definitions of rates: some remarks on their use and misuse. *Am. J. Epidemiol.* **102**, 261.

Fleiss, J.L. (1981). *Statistical methods for rates and proportions*, 2nd edn. Wiley, New York.

Fraser, G.E. (1978). The estimation of disease frequency using a population sample. *Int. J. Epidemiol.* **7**, 277.

Grundy, P.F. (1973). A rational approach to the 'at risk' concept. *Lancet* **ii**, 1489.

Kark, S.L. (1968). An approach to public health. In *Medical care in developing countries* (ed. M. King) p. 5:1. Oxford University Press.

Kark, S.L. (1974). *Epidemiology and community medicine.* Appleton-Century-Crofts, New York.

Kark, S.L. (1981). *The practice of community-oriented primary health care.* Appleton-Century-Crofts, New York.

Kark, S.L. and Abramson, J.H. (1983). Community-oriented primary care: meaning and scope. In *Community-oriented primary care.* Warrenton, Virginia, March 1982. Institute of Medicine (ed. E. Connor and F. Mullan). National Academy Press, Washington, DC.

Kark, S.L. and Kark, E. (1962). In *A practice of social medicine* (ed. S.L. Kark and G.W. Steuart) p. 3. Livingstone, Edinburgh.

Leighton, D.C., Harding, J.S., Macklin, D.B., Macmillan, A.M., and Leighton, A.H. (1963). *The character of danger.* Basic Books, New York.

McGavran, E.G. (1956). Scientific diagnosis and treatment of the community as a patient. *JAMA* **162**, 723.

McMahon, B., Pugh, T.F., and Ipsen, J. (1960). *Epidemiologic methods.* Little Brown, Boston.

Morris, J.N. (1975). *Uses of epidemiology,* 3rd edn. Churchill Livingstone, Edinburgh.

Palti, H., Adler, B., Flug, D., Gitlin, M., Shamir, Z., Tepper, D., and Kark, S.L. (1977). Community diagnosis of psychomotor development in infancy. *Isr. Ann. Psychiatry* **15**, 223.

Peritz, E. (1971). Estimating the ratio of two marginal probabilities in a contingency table. *Biometrics* **27**, 223; correction note in *Biometrics* **27**, 1104.

Roberts, C.J. (1977). *Epidemiology for clinicians.* Pitman Medical, Tunbridge Wells.

Rogan, W.J. and Gladen, B. (1978). Estimating prevalence from the results of a screening test. *Am. J. Epidemiol.* **107**, 71.

Sackett, D.L. (1979). Bias in analytic research. *J. Chronic Dis.* **32**, 51.

Sackett, D.L. and Holland, W.W. (1975). Controversy in the detection of disease. *Lancet* **ii**, 357.

Shepard, D.S. and Neutra, R. (1977). A pitfall in sampling medical visits. *Am. J. Public Health* **67**, 743.

Smith, A.H. and Hill, G.L. (1974). Corrections for sampling bias in the epidemiological survey of a chronic disease. *Int. J. Epidemiol.* **3**, 63.

Von Korff, M. and Parker, R.D. (1980). The dynamics of the prevalence of chronic episodic disease. *J. Chronic Dis.* **33**, 79.

Weddell, J.M. (1973). Registers and registries: a review. *Int. J. Epidemiol.* **2**, 221.

Williams, C.L., Arnold, C.B., and Wynder, E.L. (1977). Primary prevention of chronic disease beginning in childhood. the 'Know Your Body' program: design of study. *Prev. Med.* **6**, 344.

Wolf, E.P. (1964). Some questions about community self-surveys: when amateurs conduct research. *Human Organization* **23**, 85.

# 6  Cohort studies

Manning Feinleib and Roger Detels

## INTRODUCTION

The cohort study is an observational epidemiological study, which after the manner of an experiment, attempts to study the relationship between a purported cause (exposure) and the subsequent risk of developing disease. As in other observational epidemiological studies, and unlike experimental studies, the suspected causal factor or exposure is not randomly assigned to the study population. However, the cohort study follows the same time direction of an experiment in that the suspected exposure is identified as having or not having occurred in the study population before the occurrence of disease is investigated. Thus, certain biases which may occur in other forms of epidemiological studies can be avoided, specifically those concerned with ascertaining the exposure status of the population. Furthermore, because disease occurrence is identified subsequent to enumeration of the exposure groups, this type of study allows direct estimation of the risk of developing disease.

Cohort studies have been called by a variety of names including incidence studies, longitudinal studies, prospective studies, follow-up studies, and panel studies. They are similar to the usual scientific experiment in that they proceed from the suspected cause or aetiological agent to the disease outcome with controls or comparison groups selected on the basis of absence of exposure to the putative cause. As a type of observational study there is no randomization to exposure classes nor is there any attempt to manipulate the exposure. Retrospective studies, on the other hand (also known as case-control studies or case-referent studies), have no counterpart in experimental science since they work from the outcome event back towards the supposed aetiological factor. In this way the cohort studies offer the possibility of studying the full range of effects of the suspected aetiological factor. Frequently the suspected aetiological factor is related not only to the occurrence of the disease of primary interest but may influence the natural history of the disease, and may be related to a variety of other health conditions which may not have been suspected at first. A particularly important aspect of cohort studies is that they provide direct estimates of the risk of disease for each exposure group separately. These separate estimates of risk can then be used to estimate a variety of measures of interest to epidemiologists such as the attributable risk, relative risk, and odds ratios. (These measures of risk are discussed in the analysis section below and in Table 6.3.) Although these risks can often be estimated

from other types of studies when certain assumptions are made or ancillary information is available, cohort studies permit direct estimates of these measures from the data obtained in the study itself.

The disadvantages of cohort studies are primarily logistical and administrative. Often they require the following of relatively large populations for long periods of time, thus entailing considerable expense in terms of funding and professional resources. If the disease outcome of interest is rare the sample sizes required for prospective studies may be prohibitive. If the follow-up period is long, which is often the case for chronic diseases, the problem of attrition of the study group due to loss from follow-up, migration, competing causes of death, or gradual deterioration of interest in participation, may present serious analytical problems which might negate the value of the overall study. Longitudinal follow-up requires careful attention to maintaining standardized diagnostic methods and criteria. And, of course, the longer the study is continued the more difficult it is to maintain a committed investigative team and stable funding for the project.

In the first part of this chapter we will discuss the major methodological aspects of cohort studies: forms of cohort studies, selection of study cohorts, gathering of baseline information, follow-up, and analysis. To illustrate these points we will use examples from two studies: a prospective cohort study of heart disease in Framingham, Massachusetts (Kannel *et al.* 1961; Dawber *et al.* 1963) and a retrospective cohort study of artificial menopause and breast cancer (Feinlieb 1968). The second part of the chapter will present the various types of bias which can confound interpretation of cohort studies and will suggest ways to identify, reduce and/or resolve these biases. In this section examples will be drawn from a wider range of studies.

## FORMS OF COHORT STUDIES

Cohort studies may take a variety of forms. The key distinction that has been established in the past is based primarily on the availability of data. In *prospective cohort studies* data on exposure status and disease outcome are not available at the outset of the study; they must be ascertained through the direct efforts of the investigator in the future. In *ambispective cohort studies* data on exposure status have been collected in the past and are available from existing records while disease outcome is unknown or incompletely known; the investigator is obliged to follow the cohort for subsequent occurrence of the disease. In *retrospective, non-concurrent, historical cohort studies* data on exposure status and disease outcome have been collected in the past and are available from existing records; the investigator's efforts are devoted primarily to linking the relevant data files. Each type of study involves certain basic steps which will be described briefly below. These include the selection of the study and comparison groups; obtaining baseline information with regard to exposure and health status initially; follow-up of the members of the cohort and surveillance for disease outcome; and analysis of the results.

## SELECTION OF THE STUDY COHORTS

### Objective

Selection of representative samples of exposed and non-exposed groups.

There are two approaches to the selection of the groups to be followed in a cohort study:

1. The identification of a *special exposure group* defined because of (a) unusual exposure to a suspected causative (aetiological) factor, or (b) unusual life-style or work experience.
2. Using a *general population sample* in which there will be heterogeneity of exposure to the suspected aetiological factor.

Where the starting point is with a special exposure group it will be necessary to find appropriate comparison groups or the means to make comparisons with the general population. When the general population sample is used as a starting point the various levels of exposure within the study group will provide the basis for internal comparisons. Each approach will also take into consideration various logistical constraints, for example, accessibility and co-operativeness of the study groups, availability of medical and other records, and anticipated completeness and cost of end-point surveillance.

*Example 1 – A retrospective cohort study of the relation between artificial menopause and breast cancer*

Seven case-control studies done between 1926 and 1962 all reported that the occurrence of artificial menopause (surgical removal of the uterus and/or ovaries) occurred significantly less frequently among breast cancer patients than among a variety of controls. Because the case-control studies did not present information about the extent of surgery (the effect of removal of only the uterus versus removal of the ovaries) nor about the effects of the age at which the artificial menopause occurred, it was decided to investigate these issues by means of a cohort study. The disadvantage of using a prospective cohort method in elucidating the relation between artificial menopause and breast cancer is that there is a long period between the gynaecological procedure and the appearance of the disease in appreciable frequency. To abridge this delay it was decided to use the retrospective cohort approach. The

cohorts were selected from the records of two teaching hospitals in the Boston area. The study cohort included all eligible patients seen at these hospitals from 1920 through 1940. Women 55 years of age or younger were eligible for inclusion in the study if they had undergone any of the following procedures as determined from the surgical and pathological records: (i) hysterectomy; (ii) unilateral oophorectomy; (iii) bilateral oophorectomy; (iv) radium or X-ray treatment of the ovaries or uterus; or (v) cholecystectomy. The last group served as a control cohort.

Certain patients were excluded from the study: (i) women who had had a prior mastectomy or a prior breast malignancy or who had undergone castration as part of the treatment for an existing breast tumour; (ii) women treated for pelvic malignancies; (iii) women who had had previous removal of their ovaries or a history of natural menopause before 40 years of age; (iv) women who did not survive their index admission; and (v) all who were not residents of Massachusetts at the time of their index procedure. At the final editing of the study abstract forms and the elimination of duplicate records there were 8387 patients in the study population. They were subdivided into four 'exposure' categories:

1. Natural menopause – 1479 women (including 953 women who underwent cholecystectomy and 526 women who were post-menopausal at the time of the gynaecological procedures for benign conditions).
2. Hysterectomy and bilateral oophorectomy – 3241 women (this constitutes the surgically castrated group who were believed to have no residual ovarian activity).
3. Those undergoing hysterectomy and/or unilateral oophorectomy and who, as far as could be ascertained from the surgical and pathological records, retained at least one intact ovary – 2149 women (referred to as the 'partial surgery' group).
4. Radiation-induced artificial menopause – 1518 women.

The partial surgery group constituted a second control cohort of 'sham operations' with which to contrast the women subjected to hysterectomy and bilateral oophorectomy.

It should be noted that it is not possible to relate the actual cohort studied to a clearly definable population. Although in this case adequate records were available for virtually every woman admitted to these hospitals who was eligible for the study, it is not known from what source population the women using this hospital came. However, it is assumed that the reasons for coming to these particular hospitals were not correlated with both the type of procedure and the subsequent risk of developing breast cancer, that is, they were not confounding factors (see section on 'biases').

*Example 2 – Prospective cohort study of risk factors for heart disease: the Framingham Heart Study*

The Framingham Heart Study is a long-term follow-up study of a sample of adults who lived in the town of Framingham, Massachusetts, in 1950. The first participants were actually examined in 1948 as part of an effort to conduct a demonstration programme in the detection and natural history of cardiovascular diseases. In 1950, however, the Study was reconstituted as a long-term epidemiological investigation of coronary heart disease, hypertension, and other cardio-vascular diseases, and the original voluntary participants were incorporated into a random sample drawn from all adults aged 30–60 years living in the town. Of the eligible random sample of 6507 persons, 4469 (68.7 per cent) participated in the examinations and when this was supplemented with the volunteers, a total cohort of 5209 was obtained. The possible effects of supplementing the cohort to replace the originally selected participants who refused to participate is discussed in Example 9 (p. 109).

Although it was recognized from the outset that the town of Framingham could be considered neither a random nor completely representative sample of the US, the town did have certain characteristics which made it extremely suitable for a long-term epidemiological study. The town was of adequate size (28 000) to provide enough individuals in the desired age range. It was compact enough that the study population could be observed conveniently by means of an examination at a single examining facility, and most of the residents received their hospital care at a single central hospital in the town. Due in part to a relatively stable economy supported by a diversity of employment opportuni-ties, the population was relatively stable so as to enable adequate follow-up for a long period of time. Both the general community and the medical profession of the town were felt to be co-operative. The town was not believed to be 'grossly atypical in any respect that appeared relevant'.

Since only 68.7 per cent of the eligible random sample participated in the examination, it is possible that they might not be representative of the total population. This is a serious concern in all epidemiological studies where participation is voluntary and may be subject to self-selection. In this study it was felt that reasons for not participating were not appreci-ably related simultaneously to both the characteristics to be studied in the investigation and the risk of developing heart disease (see section on 'biases').

## GATHERING OF BASELINE INFORMATION

### Objectives

1. Valid assessment of the exposure status of the members of the cohort groups.

2. Define the individuals 'at risk'; exclude those indivi-duals with known disease at baseline.

3. Establish a basis for follow-up – obtaining identifying data, informed consent, commitment to co-operate in the follow-up (for example permission to contact family members, physicians, and to obtain hospital and employment records).

4. Obtain data on important co-variables (that is, other exposures which may be associated with the risk of acquiring the disease) so that adjustments can be made for their contri-bution to the incidence of disease in analysis (see section on confounding variables).

### Sources of baseline information

#### Existing records

Baseline information about the cohorts can be obtained from a variety of sources such as available records from hospitals or employment records; interviews of the cohort members or other informants; direct medical and other special examina-tions; and indirect measures of exposure estimated from investigations of the environment. The availability of written records such as medical or employment records may provide useful information to select and define the cohort. If high-quality records are available, they may permit the study to begin from the point of the recording of the information thereby adding a considerable period of follow-up time prior to the actual initiation of the investigation. Studies based on such records with follow-up of patients from some prior point in time to the present have been called by special names such as retrospective cohort studies, non-concurrent cohort studies, and historical prospective studies. There are several other advantages for using previously recorded information. The data are apt to be free of certain biases since they are recorded prior to any knowledge of the particular study for which they are used. Written records may provide details that are not fully known to the subject such as details on medical conditions or actual levels of exposure. However, such records may also have certain drawbacks. Records may not be uniformly available for all cohort members. Even when available, the detail and quality of the data in the records are not controllable by the investigator and it will be difficult to verify the accuracy of questionable items.

#### Interviews

One of the more common methods of obtaining information is to interview the cohort members or other informants. A variety of techniques may be used – direct personal inter-views, mailed questionnaires, telephone interviews, and, recently, having the subject complete a questionnaire admini-stered by computer. When approaches are made to individual cohort members there will be varying rates of response to requests to participate in the study. A wide variety of cohort studies have reported response rates of approximately 65–75 per cent for direct interviews. Mail questionnaires, depending on the length of the questionnaire and motivation of the group, often have appreciably lower rates of response. The advantages of interviewing the cohort members include the ability to obtain information on a wide variety of topics. Interviews can provide data on attitudes and permit the asking of quite complex questions with the possibility of probing to insure accurate recording of responses (such as eliciting histories about diet, exercise, or measures of stress). On the other hand, interview data may not always be reliable because the subject may fail to recall information or may not be aware of his or her own habits or history. There is also the possibility that the information may be biased by the subject's knowledge of the aims of the investigation.

#### Examinations

Medical and other special examinations are necessary to obtain information of which the subject cannot be expected to be aware. Direct examination is often necessitated by the nature of the aetiological factor to be investigated and may be the only way to obtain biologically meaningful information. Subjects often appreciate the availability of an examination and this may enhance the response rate to certain types of investigations. On the other hand, special examinations are usually expensive and require attention to standardization of procedures, training of appropriate observers or laboratory personnel, and quality control across observers and over time. It has also been reported that response rates to medical examinations tend to be biased towards subjects who are relatively free of disease. Direct examination can also be used to validate information obtained from interviews. For example, testing for urinary thiocyanate has been a useful adjunct to smoking studies.

### Measure of environment

The fourth type of baseline information is that obtained for each of the groups as a whole, especially when one is dealing with special exposure groups. Thus, it might be appropriate to measure air pollution, exposure to radiation or other toxicological substances, or exposures on the job for an entire group of workers and apply this measure to each of the individuals in the group. Although this type of information is usually quite useful, especially when individual measures of exposure cannot be obtained directly, one should be aware that it essentially constitutes 'ecological data', that is, the measurement of a mean or modal value for a group which may conceal individual variability within the group.

### Example 3 – Artificial menopause and breast cancer

All of the baseline information for this investigation were obtained from the available surgical and pathological records already filed in the record rooms of the two hospitals between 1920 and 1940. The data were felt to be adequate for providing a valid assessment of the exposure status of the members of the cohorts in terms of whether or not they had received the indicated operation. Furthermore, as indicated above, those individuals with known disease could be identified from the available records. In part, the high quality of the records is due to the fact that the hospitals chosen were teaching hospitals for a major medical school and were generally filled out by medical students and interns who provided careful and detailed histories. However, if there was no mention of existing or pre-existing breast cancer, there was no way of confirming this independently of the available records. Likewise, the existence of breast cancer was based solely on the report of the patient to the interviewing physician. Covariables that were available from the hospital records were the age at the time of the index procedure and the parity of women. Other co-variables of possible interest since they could have been related both to the risk of cancer and the risk of gynaecological procedures were not available from the records. These included body weight, history of breastfeeding, and exposure to diagnostic X-rays.

### Example 4 – The Framingham Heart Study

On the basis of an initial examination and detailed interview the sample was characterized according to a variety of 'risk factors', viz. blood cholesterol, blood pressure, cigarette smoking status, body mass index, and the presence of a variety of other diseases and conditions. Two types of exposure variables were used. The first was an external factor, smoking. The second – internal factors – included levels of biochemical characteristics (e.g. cholesterol) and physiological characteristics (e.g. blood pressure).

On the basis of a medical history and examination, electrocardiogram, and other medical tests, it was found that 82 individuals in the base cohort of 5209 had had a cardiovascular event prior to the baseline examination. Thus, the cohort of individuals 'at risk' for the key cardiovascular endpoint of coronary heart disease numbered 5127.

To establish the basis for follow-up 'each of the subjects was advised at the initial interview that it was intended to reexamine him at two-year intervals, and that he would be approached directly at the appropriate time. The names of a relative, a friend, and the family physician were all recorded so that the subject could be traced in case he moved during the interval. An abstract of the initial examination was sent to the family physician and the subject was advised by letter as to whether the physician should be consulted or not. The objective of this procedure was to provide some tangible benefit to the subject other than the knowledge of his contribution to medical science. At the same time, care was taken not to become involved in the medical management of the subjects and to avoid interfering in any way with the relationship between the subject and his physician. This helped to maintain rapport, not only with the subjects themselves, but with the medical community as well' (Dawber 1963).

## FOLLOW-UP

### Objectives

1. Uniform and complete follow-up of all cohort groups.
2. Complete ascertainment of outcome events.
3. Standardized diagnosis of outcome events.

One of the key criteria by which the quality of a longitudinal incidence study can be judged is the extent to which the investigator achieves equally complete ascertainment of outcome events in all exposure classes. A variety of methods are available for follow-up but to ensure uniform ascertainment across all subgroups it is desirable that the follow-up methods be independent of the method used to classify the exposure category. Methods of follow-up include correspondence with the subject and other informants, periodic reexamination of the subjects, and indirect surveillance of hospital records and death certificates. (In the US, the National Death Index is a useful resource for achieving death certificate surveillance for deaths occurring after 1978.) The duration of follow-up will be governed primarily by the natural history of the disease and the length of the incubation period between exposure and the onset of illness. It is important that the criteria for diagnosis of end-points be standardized early in the follow-up period. Although criteria for the end-points may change in the clinical community during the study, it is important that some criteria remain stable over time so that the incidence of cases occurring early in the period of follow-up can be compared to similar cases occurring later on in the observational period. Attention should be paid to criteria to verify the absence as well as the presence of the study end-points (that is, to minimize both false-positive and false-negative diagnoses).

Unequal loss to follow-up across different exposure categories presents serious problems in the analysis and every method possible should be used to assure uniform surveillance of each group. Because of the possibility of ascertainment bias resulting from knowledge of the exposure class it is often desirable to have objective end-point criteria which can be measured by 'blinded' observers. Information used in these criteria should be sought with equal diligence in all exposure classes. This is particularly important when the exposure class is defined by a variable that may lead to different degrees of medical observation, especially medical examinations that are not under the direct control of the study investigators. For example, if in a study of cardiovascular diseases there is a tendency for participants with high cholesterol levels to receive more frequent electrocardiograms or other examinations by cardiologists, there may be a tendency to diagnose more cardiovascular events, especially milder events, in this group than in the group with low cholesterol levels. Repeat examination of the subjects, besides providing standardized information on the illnesses under investigation, can often yield additional information about covariables which may be of importance and also allows studies of longitudinal changes in the exposure status.

### Example 5 – Artificial menopause and breast cancer

All patients in the study were followed from their index admission to 1 December 1961 so that the potential period of observation ranged from 21 to 42 years. The follow-up information was obtained from three sources of which the first was the hospital records. All information relating to a given patient from any and all admissions to either hospital in the study was located and the data for each patient was then combined into a single record. The second source was the death certificates registered at the Massachusetts Division of Vital Statistics from 1 January 1920 to 31 December 1961. Alphabetical listings of the study patients' names were compared with those in the index of vital records. Whenever a possible match was obtained, the death certificate was located and the information on the certificate and the identifying data obtained from the hospital chart were compared according to a prescribed set of criteria designed to minimize false matches. Therefore, there may have been increased risk of discarding acceptable matches due to some discrepancies in the available identifying information. All conditions mentioned on the death certificates were coded according to a uniform system. In addition, the underlying cause of death was coded according to the revision of the International Classification of Diseases in use at the State Division of Vital Statistics at the time of the patient's death. Thus, direct comparison could be made with published mortality statistics. The third source of follow-up information was the Massachusetts Tumor Registry, a unit of the Bureau of Chronic Disease Control of the Massachusetts Department of Public Health. Since 1927 this registry had recorded all patients diagnosed with, or treated for, malignancies at state or state-aided cancer clinics. Possible matches were obtained

according to rules similar to the criteria for death certificate matching. With regard to mortality follow-up, the assumption was made that all patients dying during the study period should be registered at the Division of Vital Statistics. If no death certificate was located then one of three situations may have occurred: (i) the patient was still alive; (ii) before death she had emigrated from the state and was not a resident of Massachusetts at the time of death; or (iii) she had died, but no record could be located because of reporting or matching errors (misspellings, changes of name, failure to file a death certificate, etc.). From the three sources of information the status of 19 per cent of the women was known as of January 1962. It was noted that those receiving pelvic radiation had slightly more complete follow-up to death than those surgically treated – 20 per cent versus 18.9 per cent. This difference was statistically significant but there was no significant difference in completeness of follow-up among the surgically treated groups. The relative success of the follow-up procedure was estimated by comparing the percentages of those in the cohorts known to have died before 1962 with those expected on the basis of published mortality rates and estimated migration rates. It was estimated that the deaths observed comprise 72.8 per cent of the expected number after allowance for migration.

### Example 6 – The Framingham Heart Study

The key method of follow-up in the Framingham Heart Study was through repeated medical examinations on a two-year cycle. The greatest loss due to dropouts occurred between the first and second examinations and those who came in most reluctantly for the initial examination (that is, toward the end of the recruitment period) seemed to have the highest dropout rate during the next 30 years. During the first 14 years of follow-up, more than 85 per cent of the participants who were still alive at any examination cycle came in for their examinations. During the subsequent 12 years the examination rates fell to about 80 per cent of the surviving cohort. The chief reasons for non-examination were believed to be the increasing numbers of people who were physically incapacitated or had migrated from the Framingham area.

Indirect follow-up through secondary sources of information was also pursued. The Framingham Union Hospital, the major source of hospital care for the Framingham community, identified each of the Framingham Study participants and notified the study staff of admissions of participants to the hospital. This is particularly important for allowing standardized examination of stroke cases while symptoms of the disease are still present. Mortality follow-up was maintained through periodical perusal of vital records at the Town Registrar and following up obituary notices in newspapers. Mortality follow-up after 30 years is virtually complete with the vital status of less than 2 per cent of the cohort being unknown.

The criteria for diagnosis of cardiovascular and other end-points investigated in the Framingham Study have been precisely defined and the utility of the various sources of information in providing diagnostic information according to the Study criteria has been investigated. Throughout the follow-up period the core criteria for the major cardio-vascular end-points have remained fixed and all potential cases are reviewed by a trained panel of medical reviewers.

It should be noted that the rate of disease occurrence in this cohort might have been altered by the subjects' continued participation in the biennial series of examinations. Although no direct advice or treatment was offered the participants, they were informed through their physicians of abnormal findings such as high blood pressure. If effective preventive measures were instituted in such subjects, then rates of overt cardiovascular diseases would be lowered and would interfere with estimating the 'true' effects of the risk factors. It was felt that during the early period of the study such treatment was not widely offered in this population.

## ANALYSIS

If a cohort study has been appropriately designed according to the principles given above, if careful attention has been paid to the accurate collection of data, and if biases have been avoided, the analysis of the results is relatively straight-forward. The first step is to enumerate the population at risk if this has not already been done in the design of the study, that is, all cases in existence at the start of the follow-up period (the prevalent cases) are eliminated from the population at risk, from both the study group (henceforth referred to as the 'exposed' group) and from the comparison group (henceforth referred to as the 'non-exposed' group). The second step is to enumerate the new cases of disease occurring during the follow-up period of the study, that is, the incident cases. The risk of disease during the period of follow-up, also referred to as the cumulative incidence, is then the total number of incident cases divided by the total population at risk at the beginning of the follow-up period (Table 6.1, eqn 6.2). If the follow-up period is relatively short and there is no loss to follow-up due to deaths from other conditions this simple estimate of risk will serve satisfactorily. However, if there is appreciable loss in either the exposed or non-exposed groups due to deaths from other causes or due to the occurrence of the illness of interest itself, or if the follow-up period is relatively long so that the risk of disease may differ during different intervals of follow-up, various adjustments are called for. These are indicated in Table 6.1, eqns 6.3 and 6.4.

Losses to follow-up are adjusted for by means of the 'one-half rule', that is, those who withdraw due to deaths from other causes or for other reasons are included in the base population as if they had been there for only half of the follow-up period (eqn 6.3). If the follow-up period is relatively long, it is advantageous if the follow-up period can be divided into several discrete intervals (equals number of intervals) and the risk calculated for each interval (eqn 6.4). This requires that the time of occurrence of each new event and the time of withdrawal from the population at risk are known for each individual. If such data are not available the investigator must make certain simplifying assumptions such as the use of the one-half rule.

The risk of disease, therefore, is the conditional probability for developing the disease during the follow-up period on the assumption that the subject does not succumb to some other cause of death prior to the end of the follow-up period. As a conditional probability it must range in value between zero and one, and is a unitless quantity.

The incidence rate, on the other hand, is a measure of the frequency of the occurrence of disease per unit of time relative to the size of the population at risk. The crude incidence rate is therefore simply the ratio of the risk of disease during an interval to the duration of the interval (Table 6.2, eqn 6.5). The units for the incidence rate are $1/time$ and have no upper limit quantitatively. Although the 'one-half rule' can be used for estimating the average incidence rate for relatively short periods of time (eqn 6.6), for longer periods of follow-up it will usually be necessary to take into account the distribution of follow-up of all individuals (eqn 6.7). The

**Table 6.2.** *Measures of incidence*

| Eqn 6.5 | (Crude) incidence rate | $I = \dfrac{R_{(t_0,\,t)}}{t - t_0}$ |
|---|---|---|
| Eqn 6.6 | For short periods | $I = \dfrac{D}{(N_0 - W/2)\,(t - t_0)}$ |
| Eqn 6.7 | For longer periods, when $t_i$ is the duration of follow-up of the $i$th person in the cohort | $I = \dfrac{D}{\displaystyle\sum_{i=1}^{N_0}(t_i - t_0)}$ |

denominator in eqn 6.7 is seen to be the total duration of follow-up for all of the persons in the cohort and is usually referred to as the 'person-years' of follow-up. If the exact duration of follow-up for each person in the cohort is not known precisely, various methods are available for approximating the person-years of follow-up depending upon the information that is available. Whereas the risk of disease measures the probability of developing disease during the entire period of follow-up, the incidence rate gives an average rate of the chance of developing the disease during any unit of time over the period of follow-up. It has been called by various names including instantaneous risk, hazard rate, and force of morbidity.

Cohort studies enable direct estimation of both the risk of disease and the incidence of disease in the population studied. They also allow for the estimation of various measures of

**Table 6.1.** *Measures of risk*

| Eqn 6.1 | Proportion of cohort developing disease during period of follow-up ($t_0$ to $t$) | $R_{(t_0,\,t)}$ |
|---|---|---|
| Eqn 6.2 | For short period, with no losses to follow-up ($D$ = number of new cases in population at risk; $N_0$ = size of population at risk) | $R_{(t_0,\,t)} = \dfrac{D}{N_0}$ |
| Eqn 6.3 | For short period, with $W$ losses to follow-up | $R_{(t_0,\,t)} = \dfrac{D}{N_0 - W/2}$ |
| Eqn 6.4 | Risk of disease for long period of follow-up | $R_{(t_0,\,t)} = 1 - \prod_{j-1}^{k}[1 - R_{(t_{j-1},\,t_j)}]$ |

association between the exposure of interest and the occurrence of disease. When the incidence rate in the exposed group is compared to the incidence rate in the non-exposed group one obtains the incidence ratio (Table 6.3, eqn 6.8). More commonly, however, epidemiologists prefer to use the ratio of the risk of disease in the exposed group during the period of follow-up to the risk of disease in the non-exposed group; this is referred to as the relative risk or the risk ratio (eqn 6.9). When the risk of disease becomes fairly large, it is useful to use as a measure of association the ratio of the odds of disease in the exposed group to the odds of disease in the unexposed group (eqn 6.10). The odds of developing disease are simply the risk of disease divided by the risk of not getting the disease. If the risk of developing disease is relatively small, the odds ratio will be a good estimate of the risk ratio and this relationship is often used in analysing case-control studies (see Chapter 5). Whereas the measures of the association described by ratios give an estimate of the relative impact of exposure on the occurrence of disease, it is often useful to get an absolute measure of the effect of exposure. The incidence difference, which is the difference between the incidence in the exposed group and the incidence in the non-exposed group, is such a

measure (eqn. 6.11). More frequently, the epidemiologist prefers to contrast the risk in the exposed group to the risk in the unexposed group. The difference between these two quantities is called the risk difference and is also known as attributable risk or excess risk (eqn 6.12).

Data from cohort studies can also be used to measure the potential impact on the removal of a suspected aetiological factor. Potential impact is usually measured in terms of the estimated effect of removal of the exposure upon the incidence of disease in the population. The most direct measure of potential impact is known as the aetiological fraction and is given by eqn 6.13 in Table 6.4. The aetiological fraction represents the proportion of all new cases of disease which can be considered due to exposure. Thus, if the exposure were removed the aetiological fraction represents the proportion of new cases that would be prevented. Eqn 6.14 shows how the aetiological fraction can be represented using the two parameters $P_E$, the proportion of the total population with the exposure, and $IR_E$, the incidence ratio for the exposure.

**Table 6.3.** *Measures of association*

| Eqn 6.8 | Incidence ratio $I_0$ = incidence rate in standard non-exposed group; $I_E$ = incidence rate in exposed group | $IR_E = \dfrac{I_E}{I_0}$ |
|---|---|---|
| Eqn 6.9 | Relative risk (risk ratio) | $RR_E = \dfrac{R_E}{R_0}$ |
| Eqn 6.10 | Odds ratio (relative odds) | $OR_E = \dfrac{\dfrac{R_E}{1-R_E}}{\dfrac{R_0}{1-R_0}}$ $= RR_E \left( \dfrac{1-R_0}{1-R_E} \right)$ |
| Eqn 6.11 | Incidence difference | $ID_E = I_E - I_0$ $= I_0\,(IR_E - 1)$ |
| Eqn 6.12 | Risk difference (attributable risk, excess risk) | $RD_E = R_E - R_0$ $= R_0\,(RR_E - 1)$ |

**Table 6.4.** *Measures of potential impact*

| Eqn 6.13 | Aetiological fraction (proportion of all new cases due to exposure; $I_T$ = incidence rate in total population; $I_0$ = incidence rate in group without exposure) | $AF = \dfrac{I_T - I_0}{I_T}$ |
|---|---|---|
| Eqn 6.14 | If $P_E$ = proportion of population with exposure | $AF = \dfrac{P_E\,(IR_E - 1)}{P_E\,(IR_E - 1) + 1}$ |

### Example 7 – Artificial menopause and breast cancer

A portion of the results of this study are shown in Table 6.5. For the four 'exposure' categories of women who were less than 40 years old at time of admission into the cohort, 37 cases of breast cancer were discovered to have occurred during the follow-up period. Several difficulties in applying the usual estimates for incidence and risk are readily apparent:

1. Because of migration and incompleteness of follow-up, the observed cases are known to be an undercount.

2. The time of onset for each malignancy was not usually known (those ascertained from death certificates did not usually state age at onset).

3. The duration of follow-up for most of the women was not precisely known.

**Table 6.5.** *Breast cancer in patients with and without artificial menapause*

| Exposure group | Number in group | Number of cases | $R_1$ (crude rate) | $R_2$ (adjusted rate) | $RR$ (relative risk) |
|---|---|---|---|---|---|
| Cholecystectomy | 400 | 6 | 0.0150 | 0.0198 | 1.00 |
| Unilateral oophorectomy | 1635 | 20 | 0.0122 | 0.210 | 1.06 |
| Hysterectomy and bilateral oophorectomy | 1278 | 6 | 0.0047 | 0.0054 | 0.27 |
| Radiation | 468 | 5 | 0.0107 | 0.0106 | 0.54 |

However, by making several assumptions it is possible to obtain some reasonable estimates of the association of breast cancer occurrence to the extent of pelvic surgery. The basic assumption is that whatever inadequacies there were in the follow-up procedures, they occurred uniformly in each of the exposure groups, for example, the women with natural menopause were no more likely to have migrated than those with surgical menopause, and any cases of breast cancer were equally likely to be ascertained in each group. Another problem is that during the 21 years of potential admission to the study, the frequency with which the various procedures were performed varied considerably, for example, pelvic irradiation was more frequent in the 1920s than later on. Thus, the women in the radiation group tended to have longer potential periods of follow-up than those in the surgical groups. This was handled by examining the specific dates of entry into the study for each woman.

In Table 6.5, the column labelled $R_1$ gives an estimate of the crude risk of developing breast cancer from eqn 6.2 ($R = D/N_0$). For the reasons given above, this is a very poor estimate. Column $R_2$ gives a somewhat better estimate of the risk of developing breast cancer by adjusting for the different times of entry of the women into the cohorts and for the estimated incompleteness of follow-up. Because of the inadequacies in follow-up mentioned above, it is hazardous to attempt to estimate the incidence of breast cancer in these groups, and no estimates of the incidence rates are given. Estimates of the relative risks of breast cancer are shown in the last column. The cholecystectomy group was considered to be the 'unexposed' or control group. Using eqn 6.9, the relative risk for the women with unilateral oophorectomy is 1.06, not statistically different from the standard group. For the women with hysterectomy and bilateral oophorectomy, the relative risk is 0.27, significantly less than in the standard group. The women receiving irradiation also had a low relative risk for developing breast cancer, 0.54, but because this group is small, the risk is not statistically significant.

Because incidence rates cannot justifiably be estimated for these cohorts, one cannot obtain valid estimates of the aetiological fraction from these data.

### Example 8 – The Framingham Heart Study

During the three decades of its existence, the Framingham Study has generated more than 300 publications. Many have involved quite sophisticated methodological applications which are beyond the scope of this presentation. An example of the relation between the occurrence of coronary heart disease (CHD) and serum cholesterol based on six years of follow-up is shown in Table 6.6. Data are shown for men who were between the ages of 40 and 59 years and were free of CHD at entry. There were 1333 men with measured cholesterol levels and follow-up was complete for six years for nearly all of them. These men were stratified into tertiles on the basis of their initial serum cholesterol levels as shown in the first column of the table. The risk of CHD developing during the six years of follow-up was calculated by eqn 6.2 and is shown in the column labelled $R$. Because withdrawal due to deaths from other causes and loss to follow-up were very small (less than 3 per cent), application of eqn 6.3 will make little difference in the estimates. Dividing $R$ by six years, the duration of follow-up, gives the annual incidence rates shown in column $I$. The relative risk associated with high cholesterol levels are shown in the next column, where the men with cholesterol levels less than 210 mg/100 ml are taken as the standard or unexposed group. Men with cholesterol levels between 210 and 244 mg/100 ml have 1.8 times the risk of developing CHD as do men with lower cholesterol levels, and men with cholesterol levels above 244 mg/100 ml have risks 3.39 times greater. The attributable risks (RD) associated with higher cholesterol levels are shown in the last column.

If men could be prevented from having cholesterol levels above 245 mg/100 ml, the potential impact upon the incidence of CHD can be estimated from the aetiological fraction (eqn 6.13). The combined group of men with cholesterol levels below 245 mg/100 ml is considered to be the unexposed group ($I_0 = (16 + 29)/6 (454 + 455) = 0.0083$). Then $AF = (0.0120 - 0.0083)/0.0120 = 0.31$. That is, the incidence rate of CHD among men could potentially be lowered by 31 per cent if none of the men had cholesterol levels over 245 mg/100 ml. A similar calculation showed that if all the men had cholesterol levels below 210, the aetiological fraction would be 51 per cent, that is, half of the cases of CHD could potentially be prevented.

### TYPES OF BIAS AND THEIR RESOLUTION

In this section the different types of bias that may occur in cohort studies will be presented and discussed. Because all the different types of bias are not necessarily present in the same study we will draw examples from additional studies as well as the two presented earlier.

Factors related to the selection of population, response rate, collection of information, methodologies used, and analytical strategies employed often introduce bias which, if not anticipated, can lead to an incorrect conclusion concerning a possible relationship between an exposure (independent variable) and a disease (outcome variable). Such

**Table 6.6.** *Six-year incidence of coronary heart disease according to initial serum cholesterol in men aged 40–59 years*

| Serum cholesterol (mg/100 ml) | Number in group | Number of cases | R (crude risk) | I (average annual incidence) | RR (relative risk) | RD (attributable risk) |
|---|---|---|---|---|---|---|
| <210 | 454 | 16 | 0.0352 | 0.0059 | 1.00 | 0.0000 |
| 210–244 | 455 | 29 | 0.0637 | 0.0106 | 1.81 | 0.0285 |
| ≥245 | 422 | 51 | 0.1203 | 0.0200 | 3.39 | 0.0851 |
| Total | 1333 | 96 | 0.0720 | 0.0120 | – | – |

biases are inherent in all types of epidemiological studies and are discussed in Chapter 8 for case-control studies, in Chapter 5 for prevalence studies, and in Chapter 7 for experimental studies. In this section we shall confine our discussion to the type of biases which affect cohort studies.

There are five broad categories of bias which are operative in cohort studies. These are selection bias, follow-up bias, information bias, confounding bias, and *post-hoc* bias. Each of these will be discussed separately below. These biases can cause systematic errors which affect the internal validity of a study. This is in contrast to random errors which may not affect the internal validity of the study, but will reduce the probability of observing a true relationship. A true bias, that is, a systematic error which is introduced into one group or subgroup to a greater extent than in other subgroups, will often lead to the observation of a relationship which is not a true relationship, or vice versa, will lead to the conclusion that there is no relationship when, in fact, there is a true relationship between the independent and outcome variables. Random errors occur with equal frequency in all subgroups and, thus, do not usually affect the validity of a relationship. On the other hand, because a certain proportion of all the subgroups will contain an error, the probability of observing a true relationship is diminished.

While internal validity is paramount, it is often important to have external validity in cohort studies as well. External validity refers to the degree to which an association observed in the study populations holds true in the general population as well. In order to insure external validity the population studied must be representative of the general population to which the results of the study will be generalized. In many cohort studies, it is necessary for various reasons to study some subpopulation of the general population. This subpopulation may represent a non-random sample of the general population, such as an occupational group, a group selected from a particular health plan, etc. If such subpopulations are used external validity may be reduced.

## Selection bias

Selection bias may occur when the group actually studied does not reflect the same distribution of factors such as age, smoking, race, etc. as occurs in the general population. This may be because some of the originally selected members of the cohort refuse to participate or in a non-current cohort study because records on some individuals are missing or incomplete. The response rates among the various subgroups invited to participate in the study may, therefore, differ. In some studies particular subgroups may be used for convenience or other reasons which are not representative of the general population.

### Example 9 – Effects of volunteering

An example of selective non-response to recruitment was observed and documented in the Framingham studies cited earlier in this chapter (Example 2). It was found that individuals who agreed to participate in these cohort studies were healthier than individuals who did not agree to participate in the studies. While this would not affect the internal validity

of the study, since the groups to be followed were characterized on the basis of factors present at baseline, it would be likely to reduce the incidence, particularly in the first few years of the study, of the diseases of interest. Thus, the external validity would be diminished, but the internal validity should not be affected for those independent variables defined at baseline. However, because the incidence of disease might be lower in this healthier group which is being followed-up, the probability of finding significant relationships would be somewhat diminished.

A second problem with selection non-response has to do with the extent to which the population which agrees to participate in the study actually represents the true spectrum of the independent variable.

### Example 10 – Representatives of study group

Early studies of the relationship of dietary cholesterol and saturated fats intake to coronary heart disease in the US gave inconclusive results. This may have been due, in part, to the fact that very few Americans have dietary cholesterols and saturated fat intakes in the lower ranges, whereas residents of less affluent countries have a higher proportion of individuals with these low levels of intake. If there exists a threshold level of the independent variable necessary to produce disease and the respondents include only individuals with levels of the independent variable which are above that threshold level, no relationship will be seen between the variable and the disease under study. Thus, some of the comparisons of the incidence of coronary heart disease among Americans with higher levels of cholesterol and fat in the diet may not have shown a relationship because the threshold level of dietary fats was below the levels consumed in the study population. Even in situations where there is no threshold level, inclusion of individuals at only one end of the spectrum of the independent variable will reduce the likelihood that a dose-response relationship will be observed. Thus, non-response or non-inclusion of participants in the cohort who represent one or the other extreme of the independent variable may affect the internal validity of the study and lead to a false observation that there is no relationship.

Another problem of selection bias occurs when individuals who have incipient disease are included in the cohort. Individuals with the disease should be excluded from the study population at the time of recruitment. However, with many chronic diseases which have a long induction period such as cancer and heart disease, it is difficult to identify individuals with incipient disease. Their inclusion in the study population may lead to an observation of associations which are, in fact, a result of the disease process rather than a risk factor for the disease.

### Example 11 – Presence of incipient disease

An association between low cholesterol and risk of cancer has been observed in several cohort studies. The induction period for cancer is probably one or more decades. Individuals who develop cancer in a follow-up period of less than the induction period probably had incipient disease at the time of the formation of the cohort. Thus, a low cholesterol level in these individuals may have been a result of the cancer process rather than a risk factor for it.

A final example of selection bias occurs when the distribution of co-variables which may be related to disease incidence is not equally represented in the study cohorts.

*Example 12 – Distribution of co-variables*

Smoking is related to a number of diseases. In some, it is the probable major cause whereas in others, such as coronary heart disease, it represents only one of several risk factors which increase the probability of developing disease. Thus, if the non-respondents include a higher proportion of smokers than non-smokers, the total incidence of coronary heart disease in the study cohort would be lower than if smokers were appropriately represented in the cohort. The effect, however, would not only be to make the observed incidence of coronary heart disease lower in the study population than in the general population but would also have the effect of leading to a false estimate of the proportion of coronary heart disease that is associated with smoking (the aetiological fraction). Specifically, the incidence of coronary heart disease among the smokers would be correct, but the proportion of the total number of cases which were associated with smoking would be smaller than actually exists because the proportion of smokers in the study population would be lower than in the general population. Thus, any estimates of the aetiological fraction of coronary heart disease due to smoking would be underestimated.

**Follow-up bias**

One of the major problems in cohort studies is to accomplish the successful follow-up of all members of the cohort. If the loss to follow-up occurs equally in the exposed and unexposed groups the internal validity should not be affected assuming, of course, that the rate of disease occurrence is the same among those lost to follow-up as among those not lost to follow-up within each exposure group. If, however, the rate of disease is different among those lost to follow-up, then the internal validity of the study may be affected. That is the relationship between exposure and outcome may be changed.

*Example 13 – Bias resulting from differential incidence in those lost to follow-up*

If the rate of lung cancer is higher in those smokers who are lost to follow-up than in those who remain in the study, the observed incidence of lung cancer in those smokers who remain in the study will be lower than the actual incidence of lung cancer in the entire cohort of smokers. The effect will be to observe a lower association between lung cancer and smoking than actually exists (provided that the incidence of lung cancer is the same in non-smokers who are or are not followed-up). If the lung cancer incidence rate is lower in smokers who are not followed, than in those who are, the reverse effect would occur, that is, the observed association would be greater than the true association.

Usually, the incidence of disease is not known among those lost to follow-up making it difficult to look for this type of bias. If possible, the occurrence and cause of death should be sought in those who are lost to follow-up. This will be easier in the US now that there is a National Death Registry. If the death rate is similar between those lost and not lost to follow-up within each group, the occurrence of a different incidence of disease in the two groups is less likely.

Another strategy is to compare the known characteristics at baseline of those lost and not lost to follow-up. The more similar they are the less likely it is that a different incidence of disease occurred in them.

Neither of these strategies guarantees that the incidence was the same in both those followed and those not followed. Therefore, the best strategy is to reduce the number lost to follow-up to the lowest level possible.

Another possible source of bias may be observed in studies in which the independent variable is being documented concurrently with the development of the outcome variable presenting the opportunity for misclassification resulting from loss to follow-up.

*Example 14 – Bias resulting from loss to follow-up of individuals under observation for the independent variable*

In evaluating the relationship between a decline in lung function test results and concurrent levels of exposure to photochemical oxidants at place of residence, a problem arises in considering how to evaluate individuals who have moved from the study area to other areas. In some instances, they will have moved to areas with lower levels of exposure to photochemical oxidants and in other instances to areas with higher levels. It is not feasible to maintain constant monitoring for levels of photochemical oxidants in all the areas to which these individuals have moved. If there is indeed a relationship between levels of exposure to photochemical oxidants and decreasing lung test performance, the inclusion in analyses of individuals who have moved to a cleaner area, as if they had remained in the area of high exposures, will lead to misclassification bias, and, thus, to an underestimate of the relationship whereas inclusion of individuals who moved to a dirtier area will lead to misclassification bias with the reverse effect.

On the other hand, if the individuals who have moved are excluded from the analysis to avoid misclassification bias, another potential bias is introduced. Individuals who have moved out of the study area may have done so because of the high level of exposure to photochemical oxidants and their awareness of declining respiratory performance. This would result in an observed relationship in those not moving which is lower than the true relationship.

While this type of bias is almost impossible to prevent, there are several pieces of information which can assist the investigator in evaluating the magnitude of the bias that may be introduced. First, the investigator may compare lung function test results among those who remained and those who moved away at baseline. Any differences between those retested and those not retested would provide information about the direction of the bias and possibly about the magnitude of the bias which occurred.

Second, it is often possible to send a mailed questionnaire

to individuals who have moved away from the study area which should include questions regarding reasons for moving. If it is found, for example, that many of the respondents moved because of the development of respiratory symptoms, the probability of potential bias can be recognized. In addition, the ascertainment of *diagnosed* respiratory impairment among those not retested would also indicate the presence of bias.

Although there is no completely satisfactory solution to this problem resulting from loss to follow-up, awareness of the potential for bias will enable the investigator to explore various methods to evaluate its effect.

### Example 15 – Selective bias

The proportion of individuals lost to follow-up is often not equal in all subgroups of the study group. Thus, there may be a tendency for individuals who smoke to be more likely to be lost to follow-up than non-smokers. The impact of this will depend to some extent on the analytical strategies used.

If person years, lifetable analysis, or some other strategy which takes into account number of years of exposure is used an association can be underestimated. This occurs because participants are included in the denominator (person years, etc.) for as many years as they stay in the study, but would not appear in the numerator if they were lost to follow-up before the development of disease. Thus, a smoker who stayed in the study for five of the ten years of the study would account for five person years of exposure. However, if he had a heart attack in the sixth year of the study, he would not appear in the numerator, thus, the relationship between the independent variable, smoking, would be underestimated if this type of analysis is used when there is a greater loss to follow-up among smokers than non-smokers.

Conversely, another form of error may result if there is more intensive follow-up or a greater likelihood of diagnosis being made in one subgroup of the study population than in another.

### Example 16 – Unequal observation

Smoking is associated with a wide range of adverse health outcomes. Any one of these adverse health outcomes is more likely to result in smokers being seen by a physician, thus, increasing the likelihood that the disease of interest may also be diagnosed at that time. That is to say, there would be an earlier diagnosis of disease in the smoking individual than in a comparable non-smoking individual who would be less likely to come under medical care. As a result, there would be an overestimate of the association of the disease of interest with the smoking variable, both when a straight incidence analysis is used (since cohort studies usually have a defined follow-up period) and when an analytical strategy such as person year is used (since the individual would appear as a case after fewer years of follow-up than would normally occur if he were not brought to medical attention earlier as a result of smoking).

### Information bias

Information bias occurs when there is an error in the classification of individuals with respect to the outcome variable. This may result from measurement errors, imprecise measurement, and misdiagnosis for whatever reason. Information bias is also termed misclassification bias. If the misclassification occurs equally in all the subgroups of the study population, the internal validity of the study will not be affected, but the precision or probability of being able to demonstrate a true relationship is reduced.

### Example 17

If the proportion of cases under- or over-reported in a cohort study of the risk of coronary heart disease is equal among smokers and non-smokers, no change in the observed risk ratio for smoking would occur and the internal validity of the study would be unaffected. If, however, the misclassification occurs to a greater extent among either smokers or non-smokers the observed risk will be altered thereby affecting the relative risk and incidence difference and, as a result, the internal validity of the study.

### Confounding bias

Confounding occurs when other factors which are associated with the outcome and exposure variables do not have the same distribution in the exposed and unexposed groups. Two common confounders in cohort studies are smoking and age. The risk of disease varies with age for almost all diseases. Likewise, smoking increases the risk of acquiring a wide range of diseases.

### Example 18

In a cohort study to determine the risk of coronary heart disease among individuals who drink and do not drink, the prevalence of individuals who smoke is likely to be higher among those who drink than those who do not drink. If one does not take into account the prevalence of smoking in the two groups, there will be a higher incidence of coronary heart disease in the drinking group than in the non-drinking group which is, in fact, ascribable to smoking rather than to drinking. A false association or non-association also might be observed if the age distributions were not the same in the drinking and non-drinking groups since the incidence of coronary heart disease increases with age.

Confounding bias can result in either an overestimate or an underestimate of the relative risk of an independent variable with disease. Estimates of the effect of confounding variables in a cohort study usually require primarily the use of the investigator's judgement, although the application of specific statistical procedures can help in reducing the effects of recognized confounders.

### *Post hoc* bias

Another source of potential bias is the use of data from a cohort study to make observations which were not part of the original study intent. Thus, interesting relationships often are observed in cohort studies which were not originally anticipated. These findings should be treated as interesting hypotheses which are an appropriate subject for additional studies. Such fortuitous findings should not be considered to have established the validity of a relationship and in no circumstance should the same data be analysed to test hypotheses arising from that data.

### Resolution of bias

There are various strategies for reducing the presence of bias in cohort studies. Selection bias can be reduced by careful selection of individuals for inclusion in the study, and by making every attempt to characterize differences which may exist between respondents and non-respondents. Although consideration of characteristics which may be more frequent in non-respondents will not eliminate bias, it may permit the investigator to assess the directionality and degree of bias which may have resulted from specific selection procedures. Information bias can be reduced by using well-defined precise measurements and classification criteria for which the sensitivity and specificity have been determined. Follow-up bias can be reduced by intensive follow-up of all study participants and by establishing criteria for follow-up which will assure that all members of the cohort have an equal opportunity for being diagnosed as having the outcome variable. Comparison of the characteristics present at baseline among those lost to follow-up and those successfully followed-up may provide information upon which estimates of the nature and degree of bias that may have been introduced through loss to follow-up may be based.

Confounding bias can be reduced in the analysis stage by careful stratification and/or adjustment procedures. However, controlling for multiple confounders reduces the likelihood of observing a significant difference. Thus, careful consideration should be given to whether specific factors not equally represented in all groups are, in fact, related to the probability of observing the outcome variable. If they are not, it is usually better not to attempt to restrict the selection of participants and/or stratify or adjust during analysis.

The identification and resolution of bias is primarily a matter of epidemiological judgement. Although statistical techniques and analytical strategies can be used to reduce bias, they can only be applied to factors which in the judgement of the investigators are a potential source of bias. We have discussed the major sources of bias in a cohort study. This list, however, is far from exhaustive and additional types of bias will surely be described in the future for which investigators should be alert. A group of references are given at the end of this chapter which will assist individuals requiring a more detailed discussion of the problems of cohort studies.

## SUMMARY

Cohort studies are usually the best type of studies for demonstrating the association between an exposure and a disease because it is possible to derive relative and attributable risks and often incidence measures from them. They are, however, usually expensive to carry out and are unsuitable for rare diseases. In addition, there are very significant problems associated with selection of appropriate groups to be studied and with complete ascertainment of disease occurrence in them. Usually it is necessary to compromise the ideal which then provides the opportunity for various types of bias to occur which can result in incorrect conclusions. The success of a cohort often depends on the care of the investigator in recognizing and correcting for these biases.

## SUGGESTED READING

Dawber, T.R., Kannel, W.B., and Lyell, L.P. (1963). An approach to longitudinal studies in a community: the Framingham Study. *Ann. NY Acad. Sci.* **107**, 539.

Feinleib, M. (1968). Breast cancer and artificial menopause: a cohort study. *J. Natl. Cancer Inst.* **41**, 315.

Kannel, W.B., Dawber, T.R., Kagan, A., Revotskie, N., and Stokes, J. III (1961). Factors of risk in development of coronary heart disease – six-year follow-up experience. The Framingham Study. *Ann. Intern. Med.* **55**, 33.

Kleinbaum, D. G., Kupper, L.L., and Morgenstern, H. (1982). *Epidemiologic research.* Lifetime Learning Publications, Belmont, California.

MacMahon, B. and Pugh, T.F. (1970). *Epidemiology. Principles and methods.* Little Brown, Boston.

Mausner, J.S. and Bahn, A.K. (1974). *Epidemiology. An introductory text.* Saunders, Philadelphia.

# 7 Intervention and experimental studies

Pekka Puska

## INTRODUCTION

There are two major approaches to investigations: observational studies or surveys (the various forms of which have been dealt with in earlier chapters in this volume) and experimental studies. In an experiment the researcher will decide which subjects are to be exposed to or deprived of a particular factor(s) (the 'intervention' or 'experimental' group). If at all feasible, this group will be compared with a control or reference group where again allocation is directed by the researcher. In contrast, in an observational study the investigator has no control over which subjects will be exposed to or deprived of a particular factor.

In applying the experimental method to human populations, it may not be possible, for a variety of reasons, to achieve all the requirements of a true experiment. The researcher may not have absolute power to decide which subjects will be exposed to a factor, it may not be possible to set up a control group, or the two groups—intervention and control—may not be strictly comparable. Study designs to accommodate such problems are often referred to as quasi-experimental. On occasions two or several groups in a population may have different levels of exposures to a factor in their environment. Although commonly referred to as 'natural experiments' and often offering great potential for study, they can only be treated as subjects of an observational study since there is no control over which subjects experience which exposure level and no assurance that the groups are comparable.

The classical application of the experimental design to studies of human populations is the clinical trial of a drug, which usually takes the form of a randomized controlled trial in which patients are randomly allocated to receive the new drug or to receive either the best available therapy or a placebo treatment. The same basic design can be applied to investigate approaches to prevention of disease including both individual measures, such as physical activity as a means of reducing an individual's risk profile for coronary heart disease, and multifactorial population-based preventive programmes to reduce the overall incidence of a disease in a community.

A further application of the experimental study is to the testing of hypotheses about the aetiology of a disease generated from various forms of observational studies. Where it is possible to manipulate exposure to one or more factors, then the natural progression is to an experiment. Any change observed in the intervention group following manipulation of its exposure to a factor or factors under study, while not automatically proving causality, will provide strong evidence for such an association. To confirm causality it must be shown that no confounding exists, that there is a biologically feasible mechanism of action, and that there is supporting evidence from observational and animal studies.

Since the early classical experimental studies conducted by the Medical Research Council (MRC 1948) on prevention of tuberculosis, the effectiveness, efficiency, and acceptability of many public health programmes have been subjected to rigorous controlled experimental trials (Cochrane 1972). Many of the diseases of current public health concern have very complex aetiologies requiring multifactorial preventive programmes often based on a community-wide campaign. The evaluation of such a programme through an experimental study presents unique problems, and will be discussed later in this chapter.

Experimental studies of human populations and as applied to public health, however, follow general rules common to all scientific studies. In the following sections the basic design, planning, and organization of an experimental study are outlined. This is followed by a discussion of the conduct of a specific form of experimental study, the community-based intervention trial, which is of particular relevance to present-day public health problems and will also provide a general discussion of practical issues in applying the experimental design to public health.

## BASIC PRINCIPLES

### General study design

The general principle of an experiment is to achieve, through purposive allocation of subjects—individuals, groups, even whole communities—to two or more groups that are as similar as possible. The factor under study is then manipulated in one group (the intervention group) and the end-points in both groups are compared. Given that the two or more groups are comparable in all aspects other than exposure to the factor under study, it can be concluded that any observed differences in the end-point—for example, mortality from a particular disease—is due to this factor.

The method of choice for achieving comparability between groups is by random allocation, and this should be adopted if at all possible. Assuming that no bias is introduced, following random allocation any initial differences between intervention and control groups will be due to chance. Where random allocation is not possible, great effort must be made to ensure that there is no bias in allocation and that the study and control groups are as comparable as possible. Where the study unit is a whole community it is rarely possible to study a sufficient number to allocate communities randomly. In such situations, it remains only to select a reference community or communities that resemble the intervention community as closely as possible. Whatever method is adopted the comparability of study groups must be checked and described.

Before subjects are recruited to a study, their consent to participate must be obtained. Final recruitment may be proceeded by a screening procedure to achieve a homogeneous group, although for studies to evaluate the performance of a programme in a service mode, a criterion of the study may be to have a heterogeneous group representing a cross-section of the population who would use the service. There may also be a 'run-in' period with repeated visits to check the compliance of subjects, for example monitoring adherence to a drug regimen by undertaking urine analyses. Only those subjects who could comply successfully with the regimen would be included in the actual study and allocated randomly to intervention or control group. Such a procedure would reduce the drop-out rate during the period of the trial. Again, however, for evaluating the success of a programme in practice, the extent to which subjects dropped out would represent an important outcome of the study.

Following allocation of study subjects, the experimental component is applied, usually for a fixed period of time. End-points, for example, morbidity, mortality, blood pressure, etc., are assessed after the experimental period is terminated, and on occasions at intervals throughout the study period. The control group is essentially either deprived of something that may be beneficial, or remain exposed to something that may be harmful to them; thus often the study design will include rules which would allow the termination of the experiment earlier than planned if a significant difference is observed between the groups. There may for example be sequential, that is continuous, analysis of data, with termination of the study once a predetermined difference is obtained.

In certain circumstances, for example, when evaluating a drug whose principal action is symptom relief, a cross-over trial may be performed in which each subject acts as his or her own control. In such a study a patient would be given the test drug for a fixed period of time and the outcome compared with that following a similar period during which he or she received a different or placebo drug. Such a design was adopted in a study of diet and coronary heart disease in a mental hospital in Finland (Mittenen *et al.* 1972).

## Study population

The choice of study population is very important and should be clearly defined and stated. In medical studies the subjects are usually human, although they need not be, and this discussion will be restricted to considerations when selecting human populations. Often the nature of the problem to be studied, for example interest in a particular community or health programme, will dictate and define the population to be studied but in many, it must be purposively selected.

In selecting a study population, the suitability of the population for attaining the objectives of the study must be considered. For example, should the subjects be drawn from a random sample of a whole population or would it be more appropriate to select a specific homogeneous subgroup? A random population sample has the advantage that the results would be applicable to the general population. However, in other cases, for example, when attempting to determine a causal relationship, a more homogeneous population would be more appropriate.

It must also be decided whether to restrict the study population to a particular section of the population defined by for example, age, sex, ethnicity, or occupation. If, for example, the disease under study is associated with a certain age group then the study can be restricted to individuals in that age range. In this way the study size can be reduced since the findings within that age range would not be diluted by those of other age groups who are not affected by the disease. Similarly where a condition is known to be related to a particular occupation it is appropriate to confine the study to that group; and when evaluating a preventive measure only asymptomatic individuals, possibly also from a specific age range, would be included.

Often economic and practical limitations will dictate the selection of the study population, for example, the decision to study a random sample rather than every individual within a community. The study population must be of a manageable size—not too large that it is administratively impossible to handle, but not too small that the findings, even if positive do not reach statistical significance.

## Experimental component and study end-points

The experimental component applied to the intervention group will be determined by the objective of the study which must, as in all investigations, be clearly defined at the planning stage. If the objective is to confirm a causal relationship between a single factor and a specific disease then the experimental component would be to limit exposure of the intervention group to that factor and observe the number of end-points, for example, positive diagnoses of the disease or mortality in each group.

However, the decision is not always so clear cut. There are good indications that many diseases have a multifactorial origin, and in addition some risk factors are synergistic, for example, smoking and asbestos exposure in development of chronic bronchitis. Thus it must be decided whether to concentrate on one or several factors. It may be of interest to demonstrate the role of individual factors but, on the other hand, the potential for preventive actions may only be determined by examining a combination of factors in the environment.

The selection of end-points must also be considered carefully. These must be measureable and selected to complement the stated objectives. Mortality from a particular disease could be the end-point of an experimental study with the objective of assessing the effectiveness of a new therapy for a fatal condition. However, it may not be appropriate to confine the outcome measurement to a single disease. An environmental factor may not be specific to the disease under study. If low serum cholesterol prevents coronary heart disease but also increases the risk of, for example, colon cancer then both these disease outcomes should be considered. A major WHO co-ordinated study (Committee of Principal Investigators 1980) found that while clofibrate reduced risk of coronary heart disease, the overall health outcome in the intervention and control groups was similar because the former group had a greater incidence of a number of other problems, particularly hepatic disorders, perhaps as side-effects of the drug.

To study the natural course of disease it is sufficient to observe the occurrence of disease in experimental and control groups. But from a general and public health point of view a broader approach to outcome assessment should be considered. A drug trial should include adverse side-effects as an end-point and major preventive programmes should attempt to measure the overall impact of intervention on health.

Often age-specific total mortality can be used as the ultimate end-point of a study and this is an outcome indicator applicable to the individual and the community. However, it is very unsensitive and can be used only for a powerful risk factor for a major fatal disease, for example, for the study of the importance of treatment of blood pressure. Elevated blood pressure is a major risk factor for cardiovascular diseases that are responsible for approximately every second death in the middle-aged population of the US for example. A randomized controlled trial in the States involving 10 000 persons with raised blood pressure randomly allocated to systematic treatment or referral to community medical therapy, found a 17 per cent lower total mortality rate in the actively treated group compared with the control group over the five years of the study (HDFP Study Group 1979).

## Sample size and study period

The ultimate objective of an experimental study is to compare predetermined, measureable end-points in the intervention and control groups. Even where strict randomization of subjects has been observed there will always be random variation due to chance and a sufficient number of subjects must therefore be studied such that it is possible to determine that observed differences are statistically significant, that is, that the probability of such a result occurring by chance is small.

It is not always easy to determine how large the study population should be; however, a calculation of the necessary sample size must be attempted at the planning stage. To do this a certain amount of information is required about: the objectives and design of the study including characteristics of each study group; the expected disease rates and the magnitude of the change in disease rate or risk-factor level resulting from intervention; the accuracy of any measurements to be made; and the level of significance required to draw conclusions.

The nature of an intervention study may also result in a change in the control group, for example, improvement in

risk-factor score resulting from a change in behaviour brought about by an awareness of participation in a study. This was observed in the hypertension detection and follow-up study (HDFP) where at the end of five years 78 per cent of subjects in the intervention group were under antihypertensive therapy but there was also an increase in the control group to 58 per cent under therapy (HDFP Study Group 1979). Similarly, another commonly experienced problem is an improvement in outcome in the control group because ethical considerations dictate that they should receive the best possible care. This may also follow from merely keeping the control group under regular observation. All these factors must be considered when planning study sample sizes since they may reduce the difference in end-points between study and control groups and thus necessitate a larger study population to achieve statistical significance.

The length of time over which subjects will be recruited into the study must also be carefully considered. If extended over too long a period, those entering the study early may not be comparable with later recruits owing to changes in other circumstances, such as introduction of new forms of treatment, publicity for a particular programme, etc. However, extending the study period is one means by which the sample size can be increased and where a condition is rare it may be the only practical means of obtaining an appropriate number of subjects.

The time over which the subjects are studied following entry into the experiment is dictated by many practical problems not least the commitment of subjects and investigators to co-operate with the study over long periods of time, and it is rare for experimental studies to extend over more than 5–10 years. Increasing the length of time for observation does, on the other hand, reduce the required sample size since this affords more time for differences between intervention and control groups to show up. And in the case of prevention programmes for chronic diseases, there is often a considerable time lag between the time which is optimal for initiating preventive action and positive diagnosis of disease.

## Methods of intervention

The nature of the factor to be manipulated within the experiment will dictate the method of intervention. Where the study concerns the impact of a drug the intervention is simply the administering of the drug to the intervention group and of a placebo or established treatment to the control group. Appropriate measures should however be taken to ensure that the subjects take the drugs as advised, and these range from counts of pills to assessment of serum drug concentrations.

For environmental and behavioural factors the selection of an approach to intervention is more problematic since individuals have great trouble changing established life-styles such as smoking, diet, and physical activity. Furthermore, in long-term studies, while only a small proportion of the intervention group may achieve the desired change in exposure, an additional small proportion of the control group may make similar changes on their own initiative.

These problems may be so great, for example, where studying chronic disease and weaker risk factors, that it is impossible in practice to conduct a controlled experimental study. The only really successful experimental study of the effect of dietary changes on risk of coronary heart disease was conducted in a psychiatric hospital using a captive population (Mittinen *et al.* 1972).

Thus the choice of intervention technique and the intensity of the intervention may be critical factors in the success or failure of an experimental study. Before answering the question 'Did the intervention prevent the disease?' one must address the question 'Did the intervention procedure succeed in manipulating the factor under study and to what extent?'. In the HDFP study mentioned above, although a drop in diastolic pressure of 17 mm Hg was achieved in the actively treated group, that of the reference group also fell by 12 mm Hg and the net difference after five years was only 5 mm Hg.

### Assessment of end-points

This requires appropriate epidemiological methods for assessing the disease rate, for example, repeated examination of subjects or recording and evaluating disease attacks or deaths of subjects.

It is important that all individuals originally included in the study are followed. Drop-outs should be traced where possible and included in any analysis, because they are often a highly selected group. The assessment of end-points must be identical for the intervention and control group and every effort made to avoid bias. This is best achieved by a double-blind study design, in which neither the subjects nor the investigator knows whether the subject was allocated to an intervention or control group. This is commonly applied to clinical trials of drugs; however, often it is obvious to which group the subject has been allocated either to the investigator (a 'single-blind' experiment), or to both investigator and subject (open study). In such trials it is vital to apply fixed, quantitative criteria against which to assess end-points. Bias from knowledge of allocation may be overcome by having the end-points reviewed by an expert group unaware of the allocation. This would, in particular, exclude false-positive cases in an unbiased way. However, attention should also be paid to the elimination of bias concerning false-negatives, for example, cases that are more likely to remain undetected in the reference or control group.

### COMMUNITY-BASED EXPERIMENTAL STUDIES

The classical experimental trial based on random allocation of individuals to experimental and control groups has limitations for studying certain currently important public health problems that focus on life-styles and chronic diseases where the absolute risk is relatively low. Clinical intervention is expensive to implement on a large scale, treats individuals outside the context of their natural environment, and is unrealistic to consider for nation-wide application. Furthermore, as discussed earlier, where diseases have multifactorial aetiologies and individual factors may affect more than one disease state it is not possible to restrict changes in the intervention group to specific risk factors without considering concurrent changes in other factors and disease outcomes.

A community-based approach overcomes many of these problems. This strategy aims at achieving overall change within the whole community rather than concentrating on individual persons and tests the effects of a comprehensive package of interventions aimed at a whole range of aetiological factors within a natural community setting. Intervention is implemented through existing channels of influence and organizations within the community and takes advantage of natural interactions. Such a strategy may reduce costs significantly; and, in some cases, obviate ethical problems that might otherwise arise. The disadvantage of a community study is that the epidemiological inferences that can be drawn may be more restricted than those of a clinical trial because the use of large units can reduce the statistical power of a comparative study. However, despite this limitation, community studies can contribute significantly to clarifying the causality of chronic disease. Furthermore, a community study often has other aims such as achieving better use of existing health and other community services or providing a demonstration model (see below).

In the fight against the present epidemic of coronary heart disease, research has proceeded from basic and descriptive epidemiological studies to large-scale intervention studies that were started during the 1970s. The first major community-based study was the North Karelia Project in Finland that was launched in response to a petition by the local people for governmental action to counter the extremely high prevalence of heart disease in that region. Recently several community studies have been launched in other countries (see Chapter 12 for further discussion). The following text makes reference to some experiences from this North Karelia Project (Puska *et al.* 1981).

### Community-based intervention—study design

Such a study uses a quasi-experimental design in which one or several communities are allocated to receive the experimental intensified intervention programme and one or several communities are selected to serve as reference areas which represent the 'natural' development in the country. In the intervention community an innovative programme is implemented to apply the best possible approaches to changing the population level of one or more factors in the whole community or in a major segment of it. The reference community is not deprived of any new developments in health care, etc. which might occur other than those represented by the experimental programme.

The observation unit is a community. Several communities may be used to increase the population but it is not realistic to include a sufficient number to use the community as a unit of the statistical analysis. In addition, the use of two or more communities creates interpretational complications in the event of a positive result in one community and a negative one in another. Such a situation may arise through transfer of knowledge and experience between intervention teams.

In all quasi-experimental designs, where the assignment into experimental and control units is not random, there is the possibility of both biased selection of experimental and reference units and biased sampling (selection of study units). In the case of the North Karelia Project the experimental unit was already given before 'sampling'. North Karelia is a mainly rural county in Eastern Finland with approximately 180 000 inhabitants. The only choice for the evaluation was in the selection of a suitable reference unit. Another county in Eastern Finland was chosen as the reference area.

The main design for the assessment of the effect of intervention on risk-factor levels is the 'separate-sampling pre-test–post-test control group' design as presented by Campbell and Stanley (1963). Separate cross-sectional samples are drawn from the same populations, one in the intervention and another in the reference area, before and after the study period. The net reduction in disease and risk-factor levels in the intervention community (the reduction in the intervention area minus the reduction in the reference area) is considered to be the effect of the intervention.

## Selection of intervention and reference communities

The intervention community ideally should be typical of the larger area or the whole country to which the results are to be applied. Often, however, this choice is guided by historical or practical factors, as was the case in the decision to make North Karelia the subject of an intervention trial. In selecting a community it is, however, particularly important that the area chosen does not have exceptionally good resources; North Karelia, for example, had the lowest level of service resources and was the least developed in socio-economic terms of all the counties of Finland. If the intervention is successful in a community of average or below average resources, it can be concluded that the introduction of similar programmes would be feasible in other parts of a country.

It is usually easier to establish an intervention programme in a small community, and the evaluation of the intervention process would also be simpler. However, increasing the community size provides a greater number of disease events and usually provides a setting more typical of the region or nation as a whole for which the intervention programme is ultimately to be applied. Where one intervention and one reference community are to be compared, each community should be large enough to provide a sufficient number of disease events of interest and to enable relatively independent samples at subsequent time points and of sufficient size, so that the significance of the net differences in the disease rates in the two communities can be tested.

Where, for example, a risk factor is very prevalent, change in that risk factors will be the only end-point in assessing the effect of intervention activities and in such cases only a relatively small community would be required. However, where chronic-diseases are included as end-points of the study, considerably larger communities are required. Depending on the disease rates and the length of follow-up, a community of 250 000–500 000 would be necessary for a community intervention study aimed at coronary heart disease (WHO 1981).

A reference community is essential because changes may occur 'spontaneously' as societies change their life-style, for example, through increased popular awareness of the risk factors; technological or fashion changes, or increasing or improved treatment of risk factors by health professionals. In order to separate the effect of intervention from general trends of change, the intervention must be compared with a reference community. If risk-factor levels are decreasing nationally, then the 'net' reduction in the intervention community, that is, the impact of the intervention programme, will be lowered. Where the national trend is for risk-factor levels to increase then there may not be sufficient time to reverse that trend although even a slowing-down of the increase would suggest that the programme had had some positive effect on life-styles.

Changes in an intervention area can be compared with national trends. This, however, may be misleading since often there is considerable within-country variation and the 'natural' trends occurring in an area in the absence of intervention might not coincide with the national pattern. Thus it is preferable to select a reference community that is similar in all aspects to the intervention community.

In the case of the North Karelia project, the reference unit selected was a neighbouring county in Eastern Finland, Kuopio. This was the county that most resembled North Karelia in its cardiovascular disease mortality and morbidity, and in its geographical, occupational, economical, and social features. The reference unit was in this sense 'matched'. Bias in the selection of the control unit if any, was against the study hypothesis, because the reference county was not amongst the most unfavourable in view of its future prospects of improvement in economy, social conditions, living habits of the population, and mortality and morbidity. For example, a new university including a medical school was opened in the reference area in 1972.

The available results from the North Karelia project surveys confirm that North Karelia had slightly higher risk-factor levels than the reference area. The significant net reduction observed during the five-year period was to a great extent due to North Karelia catching up with the reference area. The results might have been due to a saturation effect or to regression towards the mean; but this is not the case for all risk factors. For example, for diastolic blood

**Table 7.1.** *Mean risk-factor levels for men in North Karelia and reference area in 1972 and 1977*

| Risk factor | Area | 1972 | 1977 | $p$† |
|---|---|---|---|---|
| Cholesterol | North Karelia | 269.3 | 259.0 | <0.05 |
| | Reference | 260.4 | 261.1* | |
| Cigarettes/day | North Karelia | 9.9 | 8.1 | <0.001 |
| | Reference | 8.9 | 8.1* | |
| Blood pressure | | | | |
| Systolic | North Karelia | 147.3 | 143.9 | <0.001 |
| | Reference | 145.0 | 146.8* | |
| Diastolic | North Karelia | 90.8 | 88.6 | <0.001 |
| | Reference | 92.4 | 92.8* | |
| Risk-factor score | North Karelia | 5.7 | 4.4 | <0.001 |
| (additive) | Reference | 5.4 | 4.7* | |
| CHD risk estimate | North Karelia | 4.1 | 3.4 | <0.001 |
| | Reference | 3.7 | 3.7* | |

*Significant change.
†The significance tests relate to the net change (i.e. change in North Karelia adjusted for that in the reference area).
Source: Puska *et al.* (1981).

pressure, and also for the overall risk scores North Karelia overtook the reference area (Table 7.1).

There were, however, also some favourable changes in the reference area (for example, reduction of smoking). It is difficult to determine whether these changes represent national trends independent of the intervention, whether the intervention programme contributed to national interest and life-style changes and risk-factor control, or whether there was direct 'spill over' or contamination from North Karelia to the neighbouring county.

## Study period

The length of time over which the intervention study continues is very important since a short study period may not provide sufficient time for permanent changes to occur while a long study period may result in a levelling-off in the differences between areas. Furthermore, different end-points may have different optimum time periods. Changes in health behaviour, for example, can be detected quite quickly, changes in levels of risk factors somewhat later, while changes in incidence and finally mortality will only be detected after a considerably longer time period.

In the North Karelia project, for example, most of the reduction in cigarette smoking took place in the first year of the programme, most hypertensives who brought their blood pressure under control, achieve this by the end of the third year, dietary changes took place gradually over a five-year period, and, as noted earlier, at the end of five years, a net reduction in risk-factor levels was observed. Five years, however, was too short a period of time to detect any net change in mortality. There was a reduction in mortality but this was not significant since mortality rates had also fallen in the reference area. A reduction in incidence of myocardial infarction began to be observed as mortality rates started to fall (Puska *et al.* 1981), but for other classes of disease this might be observed earlier.

## Samples for population surveys

The aim of an intervention programme is to effect changes in risk factors that will in turn lead to changes in disease rates. The success of a programme in achieving such changes is assessed by comparing risk-factor levels and disease rates in a cross-sectional population sample at the outset with the findings for an independent cross-sectional sample at the end of the intervention.

Independent cross-sectional samples are used in preference to a longitudinal follow-up of a cohort because disadvantages of the cohort design severely limit its application to estimating the impact of intervention. Involvement in a survey may in itself affect the behaviour of the subjects and those who participate in the survey preceding implementation of an intervention programme subsequently may be more sensitive to the programme activities. Among this group, any observed change may be due in part to participation in the pre-test survey and not to the intervention. Thus the true magnitude of the effect in the intervention pro-

gramme can be measured only by examining a new random sample of the population at the end of the trial period.

Findings from the North Karelia project confirm that longitudinal follow-up inflates changes compared with the findings from independent cross-sectional surveys. For example, North Karelian men followed-up longitudinally decreased their smoking by 11 per cent from that of the baseline survey over three years, while in an independent representative random sample surveyed three years into the study, a drop of only 7 per cent was recorded.

For these reasons the main assessment of the impact of intervention is based on repeat cross-sectional samples. Longitudinal follow-up of baseline survey samples, however, can provide useful supplementary information, for example, about the characteristics of individuals who change their behaviour and life-styles compared with those who do not. The cohort design also has certain analytical advantages such as adjustment for differences in base-line levels of risk factors and more efficient testing procedures.

The choice of sample size usually depends on the magnitude of changes that are to be detected, the required confidence, and the cross-sectional intra- and interpersonal variation. Change in the reference area must also be taken into consideration. The detection of risk factors per se does not usually need a very large sample size. However, detection of net changes that, while small, are important if in the same direction for all risk factors implies a larger sample size. This is also the case if several sub-groups are to be analysed separately.

The sample age-range is also an important issue. Obviously the whole population is the target of the intervention, but often, as in North Karelia, the intervention programme although comprehensive, emphasizes persons of certain ages because of the nature of the problem.

At the end of the intervention period either a second independent sample of the same age groups is examined, or an independent cross-section of the same birth cohort. Use of the same birth cohort increases the comparabiity of the baseline and terminal measurements because it avoids any possible unrecognized birth cohort effects (for example, due to wars or famines). However, this means that the sample at the end is, for example, five years older which may bias the observed absolute changes (that is, intervention-related changes in risk factors are countered by increases due to ageing). This effect is controlled for when the change in the intervention area is compared with the change in the reference area to describe the net change. Obviously, the analyses can, if necessary, be restricted to the same age group at both time points.

## Survey implementation

The pre- and post-test survey conducted in intervention and reference areas should be strictly comparable. The measurements should be well standardized and tested. Often self-administered and precoded questionnaires are used. The measurements are carried out by personnel (often nurses) who are carefully instructed and trained before the surveys to use standardized and often internationally accepted measurement techniques. Strenuous efforts must be made to use identical procedures in the two areas and in the two surveys. The time of the year should also be considered because of possible seasonal variation.

High participation rates are of vital importance to avoid bias in the results. In the North Karelia project the data quality was strengthened by the high participation rates of both areas in the two surveys (over 90 per cent). The participation rate did vary between the two areas, although, the tendency was small. At the outset the participation was higher in the intervention area, presumably because people were interested in participating in the programme. At the end, however, the response rate was smaller in the intervention area, probably due to a fall off of interest following exposure to the numerous intervention activities organized during the several years of the programme.

Proper laboratory standardization of survey measurement is important if results are to be comparable and ideally samples should be sent to a central laboratory for analysis by technicians who do not know whether samples originated from the intervention or reference area.

### Disease and mortality surveillance

Monitoring disease and mortality rates at the community level has many problems. Examinations of cross-sectional representative samples do not give much information about the incidence of new cases.

A register, even with the most complete coverage and rigorous criteria, is dependent on individuals seeking health services or being identified in other ways. It is possible and even likely that an intensive community intervention stimulates people to seek medical aid more actively and with milder symptoms, which would tend to spuriously increase the incidence rates. In the North Karelia register it was found that incidence of 'definite' acute myocardial infarction decreased more than 'possible' acute myocardial infarction during the intervention. This might have been because, in response to the intervention, persons with milder symptoms were more eager to seek medical help. The actual decrease in the acute myocardial infarction incidence rate in North Karelia may thus have been greater than indicated by the register.

A further problem encountered with a community-based disease register is the maintenance of the same diagnostic criteria and coverage. A blind reclassification of cases may be done after the study period to confirm the consistency of the diagnostic criteria. To ensure the completeness of coverage, death certificates, hospital records, and other available sources of notification should be checked continuously.

The launching of a new permanent disease register in the references area can represent a substantial intervention which may minimize the impact of the programme in the intervention area. And because a better health information system (including registers) can be part of the comprehensive intervention programme its contribution cannot be assessed if a register is also established in the reference area. To avoid contamination due to the introduction of an *ad hoc*

register, the ideal solution would be to monitor disease and mortality rates based on national routine statistics. This is adequate when a comprehensive centralized hospital data system is available. In some countries hospital discharge data achieve complete coverage although the reliability of the diagnostic data is less satisfactory. In other countries, where hospital discharge data are less complete and reliable, it is necessary to establish disease registers both in the intervention and reference area.

The hardest end-point is mortality, although there are limitations with regard to cause-specific mortality, especially in areas where autopsy rates are relatively low. The observed rates are dependent on physician customs of completing the death certificates and these may change along with the programme. Age- and age-specific total mortality rates are, of course, the more reliable indices; however, they lack sensitivity because mortality is the far end-point in the course of the disease and, for example, only part (although a major one) of the total mortality is due to cardiovascular disease.

### Interpreting the results of a community study

If the effect of the intervention programme on a risk-factor level is negative this may be due to two reasons: (i) the effort was not great enough or (ii) the method was ineffective. A major problem is that often the intensity of the intervention is too limited compared with the magnitude of the task and the limited success achievable through curative medicine. It is difficult to separate these two alternative explanations.

In the case of the North Karelia Project, the results indicate that the population risk-factor levels were changed as a consequence of the intervention. Five years was considered a sufficiently long period to conclude that the changes on the individual level were not short-term fluctuations. The community-based disease registers showed in North Karelia a reduction first in the incidence of stroke and, later, in the incidence of acute myocardial infarction and cardiovascular disease. Since this was reflected in all-causes mortality rates it was not due to a shift in diagnostic habits. However, since there was also a reduction of cardiovascular disease and all-cause mortality in the reference area, no final conclusions regarding the effect on mortality could be drawn on the basis of the first five years of observation. There were several possible explanations for this: (i) the risk factors are not causal; (ii) the risk factor changes should be initiated earlier in life; (iii) the risk factor changes were not large enough; or (iv) the risk factor changes should be sustained for a longer time for disease changes to occur.

The evaluation of a community-based intervention can ultimately only assess the effect of the whole package that is applied to the intervention community. The relevant contributions of the different components to the success or failure can be evaluated only to a limited extent; separate study designs would be needed for that. It is therefore important that the whole package be designed for possible application on a larger scale in other areas or the whole country.

The results concerning the effects of community intervention on risk factors are bound by time, place, and situation. However, through careful and comprehensive evaluation, the meaningfulness of the situation as well as the effects of different intervention components can be discussed and interpreted. The results concerning the impact of risk-factor changes on disease rates should be more universal, although even here there may be differences between populations.

In follow-up studies it has been shown that the relative impact of some risk factors can vary in different populations. In this field as in many others, comparing experiences from different community studies in different cultural and community settings is valuable.

## EVALUATION OF A COMMUNITY-BASED INTERVENTION PROGRAMME

As stated earlier, a community-based intervention study can usually be seen from a broader perspective than just an experiment to test the possible relationship between a given exposure (risk factor) and a disease. It aims at assessing to what extent and by what means present knowledge can be applied to the community to tackle a health problem. Thus it is often a demonstration of the effectiveness of a given intervention programme and a prerequisite is a considerable amount of prior epidemiological knowledge about the health problem concerned. The intervention is usually carried out as a systematic programme, often integrated with the community service structure and social organization. Depending on the needs and resources, a broad range of evaluation objectives and principles can be applied to the assessment of a community-based intervention programme.

### General concepts

Evaluation is an essential and integral part of any programme, for example, to determine whether the programme is achieving its objectives and to improve the programme (for decisions concerning its continuation and wider application). The aims and priorities of the particular programme concerned obviously have a great influence on the details of the evaluation.

The intervention aims, through certain inputs and processes in the community (health services and other activities), to achieve certain desired effects, output. The programme involves planning, implementation, and finally evaluation of the results. Often this is an continuous process, with all these activities occurring at the same time, and evaluation results continuously fed back into the planning.

Different kinds of evaluation are needed; the proper balance of which is determined by the nature and priorities of the programme. Some of these different (and overlapping) concepts are listed below:

1. Evaluation concerns whether the programme has reached the stated objectives, while evaluation research involves scientific inference of the basic hypotheses on changes which occur.

2. Formative evaluation is continuously carried out in connection with the different activities in order to formulate and improve the programme during its course. It often takes the form of simple interviews of small groups of people or follow-up of such things as utilization or sales statistics. Summative evaluation is conducted after a set period of the programme, to obtain a summary picture of the programme results.

3. Every programme should include both continuous evaluation and final or periodic evaluation. Continuous evaluation concerns the follow-up of the indicators of different levels of objectives (health services use, habits, risk factors, disease rates, etc.). Monitoring of these trends is a tool of this continuous follow-up. Final or periodic evaluation is carried out after a certain, usually predetermined, period of programme operation. The same data sources as for the continuous evaluation (e.g. disease registers) are normally also used for final evaluation, as are specific terminal surveys, etc.

4. Internal evaluation deals with the simple evaluative measures built into as many of the programme activities as possible and usually carried out by the same people that implement the activities. External evaluation is carried out by a specific evaluation team to assess the overall programme results. The former activity usually deals with easily obtainable forms of information on the activities, while the latter concerns the high-quality data related to the central programme aims.

### Evaluation priorities and components

Intervention programmes aim at the prevention and control of certain diseases in an area. The aims of the programme may have a different emphasis which leads in turn to a different emphasis in the evaluation. Major long-term programmes in larger communities are interested in assessing, in epidemiological terms, whether the programme has influenced the level of risk factors in the target population and whether this in turn has resulted in decreased disease rates and improved health ('experimental' component). Other programmes are restricted only to demonstrating that certain activities lead to such changes in habits, risk factors, or environmental factors that are generally considered beneficial to prevention or control of certain chronic conditions ('demonstration' component). Still other programmes are primarily health-service oriented, that is, the development of better ways to deliver the health services to control these diseases ('health-service operational' component).

If the programme is health-service oriented (for example, better detection and treatment), then the evaluation naturally emphasizes health-service-oriented research. But in programmes of intervention against chronic disease risk factors much of the work goes far beyond the health services (various strategies in promoting life-styles changes in the community, etc.) and evaluation focuses on other aspects, such as, epidemiology, sociology, etc. Even in a health-service-oriented programme in a larger community it is advisable, in the long run, to evaluate performance also in terms of effects on mortality and morbidity.

Since in practice most programmes will combine different aims, the evaluation should accordingly be comprehensive with emphasis dependent upon that of the programme and upon local conditions.

The evaluation of any pilot programme should consider the following related, and on occasions overlapping, evaluation components.

1. *Feasibility.* This is the assessment of whether the planned intervention activities could be implemented and to what extent, and what proportion of the target population was covered or reached by the programme. In feasibility evaluation, the final performance of the programme is compared with the initial list of planned activities, and this forms the basis for understanding the possible effects of the programme. If this part of the evaluation shows that the programme was not feasible under the local conditions it is not necessary then to conduct an effect evaluation.

2. *Effects.* This part of the evaluation is concerned with assessing whether the programme reached its stated objectives. Depending on the local programmes (as mentioned above) this may concern health-related habits, risk factors, and/or health service utilization, plus, possibly, mortality, morbidity, and/or disability rates (representing different levels of objectives).

After definition of the objectives the respective indicators of the objectives have to be defined and appropriate data sources and measurements (mortality statistics, disease registers, random sample surveys, health service utilization data, etc.) selected. A standardized system for comparing changes in these indicators will be required because the changes observed may be due to factors other than the programme ('spontaneous change', 'national development', etc.). For this purpose, a reference community is needed, that is, ideally, matched with the programme community and even decided by randomization. In practice, however, choice of both programme and reference communities are often determined by a number of practical aspects. The changes in the intervention community should also be compared with whatever statistics are available on a regional and national basis. This is important, especially in those cases where a specific reference area is not feasible.

3. *Process.* Process evaluation aims at assessing how the different programme components in the local community (integrated with the local health services and social organization of the community) achieve, with time, the programme objectives. This evaluation concerns both detailed assessment of the different steps and measures in the intervention, and the occurrence of risk factor and disease changes with time. In the latter aspect the systems for monitoring these trends form the evaluation tool. In order to facilitate process evaluation, it is advisable at the planning stage to have a detailed flow-chart to illustrate the plan of action.

4. *Other consequences.* A major intervention in the community is likely to lead to consequence other than those specified in the objectives. These may include health-related, social, or psychological changes, and can be both positive or negative. Such consequences might be, for example, increased side-effects or widespread medication, increased anxiety, or increased feelings of security, satisfaction about the services, and better quality of life. A major pilot programme should pay attention to this part of evaluation because of its implications for more widespread nation-wide application of the programme.

5. *Costs.* Assessment of programme costs in relation to the observed effects, that is the cost-effect ratio of the programme (the efficiency), may be expressed, for instance, as costs per saved life. This information can be used to compare costs of different strategies leading to the same effect or to compare programmes leading to different effects but which cost a similar amount to run. The essence of a cost-benefit analysis is to quantify and value all benefits and costs associated with the programme and to express them in a common denominator.

The first step in the evaluation of costs is to assess the direct costs of the project, that is the extra input (training, materials, co-ordination) that lead to the implementation of the integrated programme in the community. Thereafter, the direct community costs should be assessed. They include the costs of the health services and other activities in the community for prevention and control of the diseases under study. It may, however, be advisable to differentiate between (the usually very large) costs that would have occurred in the absence of a specific programme and the extra costs (or savings) resulting from the intensified system. Comparison with the respective costs in the reference area may be used in such an evaluation.

## Other aspects

The evaluation of a programme draws on a number of different professional skills, preferably in an integrated way, although the emphasis will again be guided by the priorities of the programme. Epidemiological research (disease rates, risk-factors levels, etc.) and health-service research (operations research) are especially important. But attention should also be paid to research concerning nutritional, economical, psychological, social, cultural, and anthropological aspects. In addition to conventional statistical-type studies, other approaches should be considered, such as in-depth, unstructured interviews, participatory observations, and other unobtrusive measurements.

The suitable time period for a summative evaluation depends very much on the nature of the programme and the aims of the evaluation. it is obvious that a long period would be required to assess possible morbidity and mortality changes, while a shorter period would be sufficient for such intermediate objectives as changes in health service use, environmental factors, life-styles, and, possibly, risk factors.

Even if a programme ultimately concerns a whole community, for evaluation purposes practical priority decisions have to be made concerning the age groups to be assessed. Again, these obviously depend on the nature of the programme. A major emphasis on mortality and disease rates, invalidity, health services, and disease-related costs would emphasize older age groups, while a major emphasis on future community development and social processes would stress younger age groups in the community.

Finally, it is important that appropriate decisions be made on the basis of the evaluation results. They may concern either the strengthening and/or continuation of a programme or possible national or other large-scale applications. It is important to realize that evaluations seldom give a straightforward answer to the problems concerned. Thus, it is highly recommended that the programme team, throughout the process of evaluation, stay in close contact with the decision makers for continuous feedback of information and ideas to contribute both to the ongoing evaluation and health policy decision making.

## REFERENCES

Campbell, D.T. and Stanley, J.C. (1963). *Experimental and quasi-experimental designs for research.* Rand McNally, Chicago.

Cochrane, A.L. (1972). *Effectiveness and efficiency. Random reflections on health services.* The Nuffield Provincial Hospitals Trust, Oxford.

Committee of Principal Intestigators (1980). WHO co-operative trial on primary prevention of ischaemic heart disease using clofibrate to lower serum cholesterol: mortality follow-up. *Lancet i*, 379.

Hypertension Detection and Follow-up Program Co-operative Group (1979). Five-year findings of the Hypertension Detection and Follow-up Program. Reduction in mortality of persons with high blood pressure, including mild hypertension. *JAMA* **272**(23), 25.

Medical Research Council (1948). Streptomycin treatment of pulmonary tuberculosis. *Br. Med. J.* **ii**, 769.

Mittinen, M., Turpeinen, O., Karvonen, M., Elosuo, R., and Paavilainen, E. (1972). Effect of cholesterol-lowering diet on mortality from coronary heart disease and other causes: a 12 year clinical trial in men and women. *Lancet* **ii**, 835.

Puska, P., Tuomilehto, J., Salonen, J. *et al.* (1981). *The North Karelia project: evaluation of a comprehensive community programme for control of cardiovascular diseases in North Karelia, Finland 1972–1977.* WHO, Copenhagen.

WHO (1981). *Proposal for the multinational monitoring of trends and determinants in cardiovascular disease and provisional protocol (MONIC project).* WHO, Geneva.

# 8 The case-control study

Raymond S. Greenberg and Michel A. Ibrahim

## INTRODUCTION

The retrospective study provides an economical but not a foolproof method of studying certain types of relations. Its results, like all results in science, must be checked in a variety of other ways before they can be accepted with confidence . . . sweeping condemnation of the retrospective method or uncritical acceptance of the results of single studies are equally to be avoided. The frame of mind which condemns any method that could lead to error under some conceivable set of circumstances, without also considering whether those circumstances have in fact arisen, is unlikely to be satisfied with any result outside the field of pure mathematics (Cornfield and Haenszel 1960).

Although the case-control (retrospective) study design originated in the nineteenth century (Lilienfeld and Lilienfeld 1979) this method was not utilized widely in health research until the 1950s. Even in recent years, the admonition of Cornfield and Haenszel, two pioneers in case-control methodology, has gone largely unheeded. Case-control studies have been subjected to a number of 'sweeping condemnations', and 'uncritical acceptances'. In spite of these criticisms, case-control studies have proven to be an efficient method of investigation, especially for the study of rare and chronic diseases.

The case-control study is used primarily to assess risks and to study causes of disease in general. This chapter is devoted to the latter or aetiological use. There are several terms which are sometimes used in lieu of the case-control study. Terms such as case-referent, case-compeer, and trohoc have been preferred by some investigators. However, the term case-control seems to be preferred by most epidemiologists and, therefore, is the one used throughout this chapter. The nature, setting, design, biases, and analysis of case-control studies will be covered. Finally, some scientific standards and obligations of scientists are proposed. Examples from the literature are cited to illustrate the various concepts and methodological issues.

This chapter is intended for readers who wish to learn about the case-control study or to use it in a particular investigation. For these purposes, the reader should find this chapter self-contained and sufficient. However, supplementary references are provided for more advanced issues of design and analysis.

## THE NATURE OF CASE-CONTROL RESEARCH

As with most epidemiological research, case-control studies involve observations of naturally occurring exposures and disease. In these non-experimental or observational methods, the investigator observes and studies, but does not intervene with, the natural history of disease processes. This contrasts with experimental studies, in which the investigator intervenes to influence the exposure status of subjects.

Within the broad category of observational research, a further subdivision can be made. Certain types of observational studies are 'exploratory' since they are used for the generation of research hypotheses. This type is particularly useful at an early stage of inquiry, when there is relatively little known about the condition under investigation. In these studies, a variety of potential aetiological factors are assessed to identify promising areas for further research. The exploratory approach is typified by the case series (a summary of individuals with a particular disease), the ecological study (a correlation of exposure and disease distributions), or the proportional mortality study (a comparison of cause-specific contributions to total mortality in exposed and unexposed groups). Occasionally, case-control studies are used for exploratory purposes, by evaluating possible associations between a single disease entity and a variety of different exposures. Ideally, exposure-disease associations detected in an exploratory study should be considered tentative until more definitive evidence is obtained.

A research hypothesis concerning a specific cause-and-effect relationship may be tested in an 'explanatory study'. Although such studies focus on a single exposure-disease association, it is usually necessary to collect information on other factors which might distort or modify that relationship. There are three different approaches to observational explanatory research: cross-sectional, cohort (also prospective, follow-up), and case-control studies. These three approaches differ with regard to the sequence of observations on exposure and disease status. In cross-sectional research, both variables are measured simultaneously. A cohort study begins with a measurement of exposure status and then follows the subjects forward in time for subsequent disease outcome. In contrast, a case-control study begins with a determination of disease status and then traces the subjects backward in time for prior exposure history.

Regardless of the sequence of observations in an explanatory study, an observed exposure-disease association does not necessarily imply a causal relationship. Even when chance and known systematic errors are reasonably excluded, it is possible that unrecognized factors influenced the relationship of interest. This problem is somewhat alleviated in experimental studies, where randomization tends to balance the distribution of both known and unrecognized factors between study groups. Therefore, experimental studies are often considered the best evidence of a causal relationship. Unfortunately, many exposure-disease associations cannot be studied with human experimentation, since it would be unethical to expose people intentionally to detrimental agents. In these situations, explanatory observational studies provide the best available assessment of causation.

## THE ANATOMY OF CASE-CONTROL RESEARCH

This study design is portrayed schematically in Fig. 8.1, which shows that subjects enter the study from two separate populations: persons with (cases) and without (controls) the disease. This sampling scheme differs from experiments, as well as cross-sectional and cohort studies, where a single, well-defined population is usually sampled. Since cases and controls are sampled from separate populations, a central assumption of case-control research is that the comparison subjects are drawn from the same candidate population from which the cases arose (Kleinbaum *et al.* 1982).

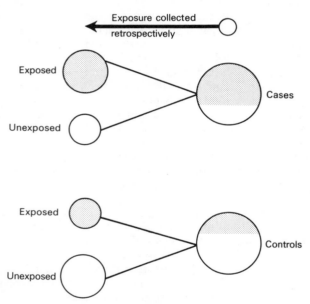

**Fig. 8.1.** The case-control study. Shaded areas represent exposed persons and unshaded areas represent unexposed persons.

The structure of a case-control study affords certain advantages as well as certain limitations (Table 8.1). The most obvious advantage is that the investigator can choose the ratio of cases to controls. Thus, a disease which is rare in the general population can be heavily sampled in the study population. In this manner, uncommon diseases can be studied efficiently, with relatively few subjects and a modest expenditure of resources.

*Example 1—The efficiency of case-control studies for rare diseases.*

As a simple illustration, consider two different approaches to

**Table 8.1.** *Advantages and limitations of case-control studies*

**Advantages**
1. Efficient sampling of rare diseases
2. Rapid evaluation of chronic diseases
3. Economy of expense and personnel
4. May serve either exploratory or explanatory purposes

**Limitations**
1. Not practical for rare exposures
2. Subject sampling prone to systematic errors
3. Historical information often cannot be validated
4. Relevant co-factors may be difficult to control
5. Temporal sequence of exposure and disease may be obscured

the study of leukaemia in children. The crude annual incidence rate of this disease is about 3.4 cases for every 100 000 children under 15 years of age (Silverberg 1982). A cohort study of leukaemia in children would require a year of observations on a million children to identify 34 cases of this disease. In a study that evaluates the association between leukaemia and a proposed aetiological agent, these 34 children with leukaemia would be subdivided into two or more exposure categories. Consider how much easier it would be to identify the 34 leukaemia cases as they are diagnosed and then select an appropriate comparison group of children without leukaemia to evaluate possible aetiological exposures.

The case-control approach is also advantageous when there is a long induction period between the exposure and clinical onset of disease. Rather than waiting years for the prospective accrual of cases, the investigator may 'compress time' by using historical documents to evaluate earlier exposures. Indeed, the case-control approach was first widely utilized for the study of chronic diseases such as cancer and cardiovascular disease.

The limitations of case-control studies are related principally to the sampling scheme and the retrospective sequence of observations. These two features make case-control studies susceptible to errors in the evaluation of exposure-disease relationships. These systematic errors, also termed 'biases', may arise in the selection of subjects, collection of information, or the mixing of multiple effects. While biases may occur in any study design, case-control studies are especially vulnerable to these errors. Later in this chapter, we will present an overview of bias and methods for its containment or elimination.

## THE SETTING OF CASE-CONTROL RESEARCH

Aetiological research is traditionally performed in one of three different contexts: clinical, community, or occupational settings. These research environments differ with regard to the goals and logistics of investigation. Clinically-oriented research is usually directed at the mechanisms of disease causation and modes of management. Typically, the subjects of clinical investigations are patients who seek care at a particular hospital or medical centre. Since the conditions of interest may be relatively uncommon, clinical studies are often necessarily based upon small samples. The 'exposure' under study might be a specific physiological state, a past medical event, a pharmacological agent, or a therapeutic procedure.

In contrast, community-based aetiological research is

usually directed toward public health concerns. The emphasis in community research is on the population health impact of various exposures. This might be a particular life-style, diet, socio-economic status, or place of residence. To evaluate public health consequences of these exposures, it is usually necessary to study relatively large populations. Since public health impact is directly related to exposure prevalence, community studies are often directed at common exposures and diseases.

The major aim of occupational research is to identify associations between certain conditions and chemical, physical, or radiological exposures in the workplace. This information may be used to remove potential hazards and develop epidemiological and environmental surveillance systems. Although common diseases have been considered in occupational studies (e.g. lung cancer), emphasis has generally been on rare conditions (e.g. angiosarcoma of the liver).

A typical progression of study designs employed in clinical research is depicted in Fig. 8.2. In the clinical setting, aetiological research often begins with isolated case reports, followed by a larger case series. These investigations are intended to describe the characteristics of a group of patients with a specific disease. After the cases are described, it is necessary to determine how the cases differ from other persons.

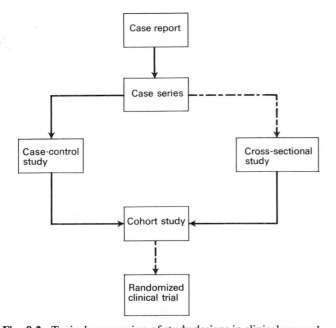

**Fig. 8.2.** Typical progression of study designs in clinical research.

These differences are defined through comparative studies using case-control or cross-sectional methods. If the hypothesized aetiological association is supported, then that relationship may be confirmed by a subsequent case-control (or possibly a cohort) study. Ultimately, logistics and ethics permitting, an intervention study may be undertaken so that the most convincing evidence of causation may be realized, or *in vitro* and/or animal studies are conducted for confirmatory evidence.

*Example 2—The sequence of study designs in clinical research.*
The role of oxygen in retrolental fibroplasia (RLF) among premature infants was shown by a progression of studies beginning in 1941. The first in a series of RLF cases was noted on 14 February of that year by a Boston paediatrician Dr Stewart H. Clifford (Silverman 1980). That case was a premature infant girl suffering from nystagmus and scar tissue behind the lens of the eye. A case-control study was subsequently conducted on 53 RLF children and 298 normal children. In spite of the association between longer hours of oxygen use and RLF, it was postulated that poor health of infants necessitated longer hours of oxygen. That is, poor health, and not oxygen use, 'caused' RLF (Silverman 1980).

The frequency of RLF in a cohort of infants exposed to high oxygen was compared to that in a cohort of infants exposed to moderate oxygen in several international studies. Some studies confirmed the oxygen–RLF association and some did not. These contradictory findings stimulated the initiation of randomized clinical trials. The first was at the Gallinger Municipal Hospital in Washington, DC, and the second was a collaborative multi-centre trial. Although the results of these trials confirmed the role of oxygen in the aetiology of RLF, questions concerning a safe exposure level remain unresolved (Silverman 1980).

Figure 8.3 illustrates a typical progression of study designs utilized in community research. Since data collection in the community setting can be an expensive proposition, one often begins with descriptive data which were collected originally for some other purpose. For example, one may undertake an ecological study to correlate mortality data with aggregate exposure data, such as per caput consumption of dietary ingredients. If a promising exposure-disease correlation is observed, the next step is to conduct a cross-sectional survey of a defined community population. Often, results from a cross-sectional study are used as the baseline observations for a cohort investigation. Alternatively, from the ecological study,

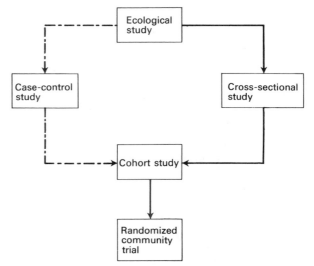

**Fig. 8.3.** Typical progression of study designs in community research.

one may proceed to a case-control study. If the hypothesized relationship is confirmed, the investigator would have some justification to consider undertaking a cohort study. The definitive study design in community aetiological research is an intervention study in the form of a randomized community trial.

*Example 3—The sequence of study designs in community research.*

An analysis of death rates from coronary artery disease according to per caput fat consumption in 20 countries represented an important beginning for the generation of the lipid-atherosclerosis hypothesis (Joliffe and Archer 1959). Cross-sectional studies such as the initial cross-sectional surveys of the Framingham and Evans County heart studies (Dawber *et al.* 1957; Cassel 1971) provided evidence of associations between serum cholesterol levels and coronary artery disease. These findings were confirmed by a number of case-control studies.

Cohort studies, such as the long-term prospective investigations in Framingham, Massachusetts, and in Evans County, Georgia, were the logical next step (Truett *et al.* 1967; Tyroler *et al.* 1971). Coronary artery disease incidence was clearly shown to be related to high levels of cholesterol in these and other studies. Community-based controlled trials of lipid reduction were undertaken and are still in progress (Lipids Research Clinics Program 1979). The major objective of these trials was to find out if reduction of serum cholesterol by dietary or pharmacological means would reduce deaths from coronary artery disease.

Figure 8.4 depicts a typical progression of study designs utilized in occupational research. At the exploratory level, the cause-specific distribution of deaths within an industry may be considered in a proportional mortality study. This type of descriptive study can be performed rapidly, without enumerating the entire workforce or evaluating individuals'

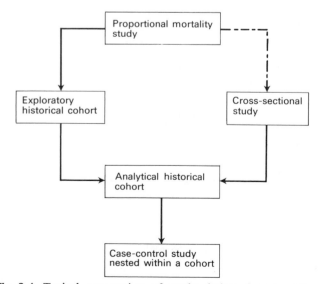

**Fig. 8.4.** Typical progression of study designs in occupational research.

exposures. If a particular cause of death appears elevated, then mortality rates within the industry may be calculated and compared with another industrial group or the general population (viz. standardized mortality ratio). If the mortality excess is confirmed, specific aetiological relationships may be investigated by collection of exposure information on a historical cohort of workers. The relative risk for the hypothesized aetiological factor may be estimated directly in a cohort, or estimated indirectly with a case-control analysis. The latter approach may prove useful when the disease under investigation is uncommon.

*Example 4—The sequence of study designs in occupational research.*

The sequence of study designs in occupational research may be illustrated by studies of cancer in rubber workers. Mancuso (1949) reported a proportional elevation of respiratory, genitourinary, and central nervous system cancer mortality in the rubber industry. A subsequent standardized mortality study revealed excess rates of colon, prostate, and haematopoietic cancers in rubber workers (McMichael *et al.* 1974). Further examination of the haematopoietic cancer deaths indicated that the greatest elevation in risk corresponded to lymphatic leukaemia in middle-aged workers (McMichael *et al.* 1975). This observation led the investigators to conduct a matched case-control study within the industrial cohort. This analysis revealed a consistent association between solvent exposure and lymphatic leukaemia (McMichael *et al.* 1975).

While clinical, community, and occupational research often follow the respective sequences outlined above, many exceptions to these rules could be cited. In practice, the course of scientific inquiry is less predictable than is suggested by Figs. 8.2-8.4. For some associations, such as tampon use and toxic shock syndrome, case-control studies may be viewed as exploratory research (Davis *et al.* 1980). For other associations, such as pre-natal diethylstilbestrol exposure and adenocarcinoma of the vagina, case-control studies may be considered as more definitive research (Herbst *et al.* 1971). However, most case-control studies fulfil an intermediate role between these two extremes and should be viewed as complementary to the other observational research strategies available in epidemiology.

## THE CONDUCT OF CASE-CONTROL RESEARCH

The decision to conduct a case-control study is determined by characteristics of the exposure and disease under investigation, the current state of knowledge about the hypothesized aetiological relationship, the immediate goals of the study, the research setting, and the resources available. Case-control studies are especially useful at a preliminary stage of investigation, for the study of rare and chronic diseases, and when resources are scarce. After the decision to conduct a case-control study is made, the investigator must next consider the methods of subject enrollment, data collection, and analysis.

### Case identification

The first task for the case-control investigator is to define the disease state. In some situations, the designation of a case may be relatively simple and straightforward. For example, the identification of children with cleft palates could be based entirely upon a simple physical examination. In other situations, it may be difficult to decide what constitutes a disease state. For example, should hypertension be defined by systolic, diastolic or mean arterial blood pressure? Even if one decides on the appropriate diagnostic marker, what level of blood pressure should one consider abnormal? In case-control studies, continuous variables, such as blood pressure, must be categorized and this process is apt to be somewhat arbitrary. The process of disease categorization is schematically represented in Fig. 8.5. The most stringent criterion for a disease is likely to misclassify some mild cases as normals. On the other hand, a less stringent criterion may misclassify some normals as diseased. There is no universal rule for balancing these risks of disease misclassification. Either form of misclassification is likely to lead to a biased study result. Cole (1979) has argued for the use of homogeneous case groups, which would support the use of stringent case definitions. However, as Fig. 8.5A illustrates, this may diminish the number of eligible cases of an already rare disease. While homogeneous case groups may be desirable, the investigator may be forced to use more liberal definitions of disease in order to obtain a sufficient number of cases.

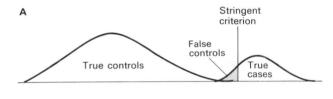

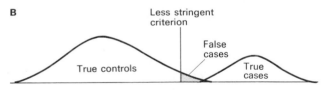

**Fig. 8.5.** Misclassification errors in the dichotomization of a continuous variable.

A variety of methods may be employed alone or in combination to establish the presence of a disease, as depicted in Table 8.2. It is often possible to obtain a direct confirmation of the disease process as in certain forms of cancer, which can be objectively diagnosed by histopathology. Other diseases, such as mental illness, cannot yet be defined in terms of structural alterations. For conditions in which the diagnosis cannot be made with reasonable precision, it may be useful to require several diagnostic procedures obtained by different means before accepting a case into the study.

In addition, the diagnostic criteria established by convention of previous investigators and/or consensus committees may provide a standard for disease classification. The designation of standard diagnostic schemes would be useful in comparing the results of independent studies.

**Table 8.2.** *Methods of disease identification with illustrative examples related to coronary artery disease*

| Method of disease identification | Cardiovascular example |
| --- | --- |
| 1. Report of symptoms | Angina pectoris |
| 2. Physical examination | Hypertension |
| 3. Passive observation of abnormality | Cardiac arrhythmia |
| 4. Induced observation of abnormality | Exercise stress testing |
| 5. Indirect marker of abnormality | Abnormal myocardial enzymes |
| 6. Response to pharmacological agent | Nitroglycerin trial |
| 7. Direct observation of abnormality | Coronary angiography |

It is often recommended that case-control studies should be limited to 'incident' or newly diagnosed cases (Sackett 1979). There are several advantages to the study of incident cases. First, the aetiological exposures in these persons are presumably more recent and therefore more reliably recalled. In addition, it is likely that the aetiological milieu of incident cases is relatively homogeneous. Finally, the exclusion of older, surviving cases may prevent the selection bias which is introduced by factors affecting clinical prognosis.

The procedure for locating cases is largely dictated by the research setting. In the medical care setting it is often convenient to identify potential cases from clinical records, hospital discharge rosters, or institutional registries. In the community, case identification can be a more tedious and time-consuming process. Potential cases may be located from surveillance programmes, employment records, or death certificates. Often, it is necessary to use several sources to identify a sufficient number of cases. Similarly, several sources may be needed to locate cases in occupational studies. In almost all instances where a search for the deceased is required, the investigator must supplement employment records with other data sources, such as state health departments and the social security administration.

## Controls

Perhaps the greatest challenge of case-control research is to identify an appropriate comparison population. In a strict sense, comparison subjects in a retrospective study are not true controls. The term 'control' derives from experimental research, where the treatment and comparison populations originate from the same source population, and thus only differ with regard to the experimental manipulation. The notion of 'control' is that extraneous influences on the outcome have been eliminated by studying two groups which differ only in a randomly allocated treatment.

Since cases and controls are sampled from two different populations, extraneous influences on the outcome cannot be entirely eliminated. It is possible to account for differences in known relevant co-factors, but there is always the uncertainty that other unknown influences were not considered. With the recognition that a comparison group in a retrospective study is not necessarily a true 'control' group, a valid comparison requires that extraneous variables associated with the disease are not differentially distributed between exposure groups (Feinstein 1979). There are two basic approaches to the control of such extraneous variables:

1. Restrict the sampling of subjects to certain levels of relevant co-factors.

2. Sample the comparison population without restriction and perform *post hoc* adjustment.

Restricted sampling of subjects can involve either absolute or partial limitations on subject enrollment. With absolute restriction, all participants are limited to narrowly defined co-factor levels (e.g. White males in the fifth decade of life). Absolute restriction may sacrifice important information and limit generalizability of study results. Partial restriction, also known as matching, involves selecting a comparison group which parallels the relevant co-factor distribution of the case group.

The usual intent of matching in case-control studies is to adjust for the effects of extraneous variables. Perhaps the strongest argument for matching is that it is comparatively simple to execute and understand. In addition, matching may allow for control of extraneous variables which are difficult to accommodate with other adjustment methods. For example, matching on place of residence may provide adequate control for socio-economic status.

Matching may be accomplished in either of two different mechanisms:

1. *Pair-wise matching.* For each case, a specific comparison subject (or subjects), with similar values of the matching factors is (are) selected.

2. *Frequency matching.* The group of comparison subjects is chosen so that the overall distribution of matching factors parallels the distribution in the cases.

Despite apparent differences in subject selection, pair-wise and frequency matching usually achieve the same result, since pairs are typically not unique and could be pooled into larger generic strata (Kupper *et al.* 1981). However, in situations where there are natural unique pairs, such as monozygotic twins, pair matching may be advantageous.

The usually perceived intent of matching is to adjust for the effects of relevant co-factors. In prospective studies, where matching occurs prior to disease onset, known relevant factors may be adequately controlled. However, in case-control studies, where subject selection transpires after disease onset, appropriate adjustment of extraneous variables is not always obtained by matching (Kupper *et al.* 1981). When matching is used in a case-control study, it should be accompanied by an analysis which accounts for the method of subject selection. In particular, a pair-wise matched study should account for the pairings when the data are analyzed.

Perhaps the most common misunderstanding about matching is the erroneous impression that the goal is to make the case and control groups similar in all respects, except for disease status (Cole 1979). An optimal matching scheme involves only those variables which improve statistical efficiency or eliminate bias from the effect of interest. Often it is difficult to predict in advance which variables are appropriate for matching. When prior work is available, independent risk factors for the disease may be identified for matching. In some situations, matching by interviewer or hospital may be used to balance out the effects of interviewer and observer errors. For exploratory studies,

usually it is best to limit matching to basic descriptors, such as age, race, and sex, or not match at all.

Overzealous matching may have two adverse effects: first, matching on a strong correlate of the exposure, which is not an independent risk factor for the outcome (overmatching) may lead to an underestimate of the study effect (Miettinen 1970); second, matching may lead to a false sense of security that a particular variable is adequately controlled. The following example illustrates how overmatching can lead to an underestimate of the study effect.

*Example 5—Overmatching in case-control research.*
Overmatching may be illustrated by a hypothetical study of prenatal exposure to diethylstilbestrol and the occurrence of clear cell adenocarcinoma of the vagina in young women, whose mothers were matched for history of threatened spontaneous abortion. Since the matching factor was the indication for diethylstilbestrol administration, it is a strong correlate of exposure, but is not known to be an independent risk factor for clear cell adenocarcinoma of the vagina. By matching on history of threatened spontaneous abortion, one over-represents diethylstilbestrol exposure in the control group and thereby diminishes any observed exposure-disease association.

Inadequate control of a variable by matching may be illustrated by the treatment of a continuous variable, such as age. To match on age it is usually necessary to categorize the range of possible values into discrete intervals. A common strategy is to employ five-year age spans for matching. In essence, this assumes that the persons within a particular age interval have the same age effect. For certain situations, such as the study of childhood diseases, there may be residual age effects within five-year age intervals. As a result, such matching intervals will not adequately control the effect of age for these diseases.

Ultimately, a decision on whether or not to use matching in a particular study depends upon the circumstances of that investigation. Table 8.3 indicates some of the advantages and

**Table 8.3.** *The advantages and disadvantages of a matched subject selection*

**Advantages**
1. In some situations, there are natural partners for comparison (e.g. identical twins)
2. Matching may account for extraneous variables which are otherwise difficult to control (e.g. neighbourhood matching to adjust for socio-economic status)
3. Matching may improve the statistical precision of study results, especially for studies with small sample sizes and when the matching factors are strong predictors of the outcome
4. Matching may enhance the validity of study results
5. Matched results are often easier to interpret than those obtained with alternative procedures

**Disadvantages**
1. When there are a large number of matching variables, it may be difficult to find suitable matches
2. Unmatched cases and controls cannot be analysed, thereby entailing a loss of potential information
3. Overmatching may lead to an underestimate of the study effect
4. Matching may increase the costs of a study

disadvantages of matching. As a general rule, matching is most beneficial when there are only a few matching factors which otherwise would be difficult to control. Furthermore, the logistics of matching are favoured when there is a limited number of cases and a large pool of eligible controls. In other situations, it may be preferable to obtain unmatched samples and adjust for extraneous effects in the analysis.

The investigator must also decide upon the source of control subjects. Two different types of comparison populations may be utilized: hospital and community controls. A hospital control group often is employed in clinical studies, since it is convenient to sample controls from the institutions which contribute cases. Table 8.4 provides a summary of advantages and disadvantages of a hospital control group.

**Table 8.4.** *The advantages and disadvantages of a hospital control group*

**Advantages**

1. Subjects are easily accessible
2. Patients usually have time to participate in a study
3. Patients are often motivated to co-operate with investigators
4. Controls and cases may be drawn from similar social and geographical environments
5. Differential recall of prior exposure is likely to be minimized

**Disadvantages**

1. Differential hospitalization patterns may introduce selection bias
2. Difficult to blind disease status of cases and controls
3. An underestimate of the study effect may be obtained if control diseases are aetiologically similar to case disease

The term 'community controls' is used as a generic label for comparison groups obtained from non-clinical sources. Within this broad category, several specific types of controls may be recognized. For instance, the cases may be matched to acquaintances, such as co-workers, classmates, friends, or neighbours. These acquaintances may be identified by the cases, by the investigator, or by a third-party, such as an employer. In other situations, it may be preferable to sample the general population, either through a simple random sample, or with a probability sample to adjust for extraneous variables.

The advantages and limitations of community controls are indicated in Table 8.5.

**Table 8.5.** *The advantages and disadvantages of a community control group*

**Advantages**

1. May reduce the opportunity for selection biases
2. Study results may be generalizable to a wider target population
3. For some research questions, a 'natural' community control group will exist
4. May provide convenient control of extraneous variables

**Disadvantages**

1. Usually time-consuming and expensive to obtain
2. May suffer from low participation rates
3. Cases and controls may exhibit differential recall of prior exposures

From the preceding discussion, it should be apparent that the choice of a hospital or community control group depends upon the research question and study setting, as well as logistical considerations. An increasingly popular approach is to collect two separate control populations, one from hospitals and one from the community. For example, Schoenbaum *et al.* (1975) performed a case-control study to evaluate the association between maternal parity and congenital rubella syndrome. These authors utilized a community control group matched from birth certificate registration, as well as a hospital control group matched from discharge records. When the cases were compared separately with each control group, the results indicated that primiparae are at increased risk of congenital rubella syndrome. Although the consistency of these results does not guarantee their validity, it does increase confidence in the reported association. Whenever possible, the use of more than one control population is encouraged to provide an opportunity for replication of study results.

**Information on exposure**

Exposure data may be self-reported (in response to an interview or self-administered questionnaire), obtained either from medical or occupational records, or by the use of a biological marker (e.g. serological determination). Information elicited should pertain to the presence of exposure, its intensity and duration. With self-reported information, problems of inaccuracy and incompleteness may arise. The validity and reliability of self-reported data continues to be an important issue in case-control studies. Validity may be assessed by comparing self-reported data to other suitable records, such as hospital charts. Reliability may be assessed by comparing answers to similar questions which are posed in different forms. For example, the subject may be asked his/her age, as well as his/her date of birth.

Medical records can be more valid and reliable than self-reports but only when events related to medical care are always recorded in hospital charts. Unfortunately, many relevant events are not recorded, and the researcher is often at the mercy of the quality of the medical record. Medical records, even when accurate, may not contain the necessary data in a form required to answer the specific research questions.

The method of obtaining exposure data is an important source of information bias. For example, the numerous studies of the reserpine-breast cancer association employed a variety of methods to determine drug exposure (Labarthe 1979). Some studies of this association relied upon the mere mention of reserpine use, while others required at least six months of reserpine use to be classified as 'exposed'. Similarly, some studies based the drug exposure determination on self-reporting, while other studies used medical records.

In conducting case-control studies the investigator must decide on the best means of data collection. Occasionally, self-reported data may be verified against information in medical records to assess the validity of subject reports. It is incumbent upon the investigator to consider possible deficiencies which may exist in the information. This requires the assurance of proper data collection, standardized definitions of exposure and disease, as well as criteria which minimize misclassification, and conclusions which are tempered by the possible presence of information bias.

## SAMPLE SIZE DETERMINATION

In general, the statistical confidence in study results is strengthened as the sample size increases. This relationship argues for the use of large study populations. At the same time, there are several feasibility considerations which may restrict the number of subjects examined. First, case-control studies are typically undertaken for the investigation of rare diseases. For extremely uncommon conditions, there may be a limited number of cases available for study. Furthermore, there are usually constraints upon the time, personnel, and financial resources which may be devoted to a particular study. Thus, a balance must be achieved between the interest of statistical precision and matters of practicality.

The traditional approach to sample size ($n$) estimation is to perform a calculation based upon:
- The anticipated prevalence of exposure in the control population, $p_0$;
- The magnitude of association between exposure and disease, as measured by the relative risk, $RR$; ($<1$, negative association; $=1$, no association; $>1$, positive association);
- The probability of erroneously finding an exposure-disease association when none exists in reality (Type I error), $\alpha$;
- The probability of erroneously not finding an exposure-disease association, when one exists in reality (Type II error), $\beta$.

For unmatched studies, with equal numbers of cases and controls, the approximate number of subjects required in a group is given by (Schlesselman 1982):

$$n = 2\bar{p}\bar{q}(z_\alpha + z_\beta)^2/(p_1 - p_0)^2 \qquad (8.1)$$

where

$$p_1 = p_0 RR/[1 + p_0(RR - 1)]$$
$$\bar{p} = \tfrac{1}{2}(p_1 + p_0) \qquad \bar{q} = 1 - \bar{p} \qquad q_1 = 1 - p_1$$

and $z_\alpha$ and $z_\beta$ are the values of the standard normal distribution that are exceeded by $\alpha$ (one-sided test) and $\beta$, respectively. Applying eqn 8.1, we can generate sample size estimates for specified values of $p_0$, $RR$, $\alpha$ and $\beta$. In Table 8.6, sample size

**Table 8.6.** *Sample size for each group in an unmatched case-control study with equal numbers of cases and controls* *

| | | | | $p_0$ | | | |
|---|---|---|---|---|---|---|---|
| $RR$ | 0.01 | 0.1 | 0.2 | 0.4 | 0.6 | 0.8 | 0.9 |
| 0.1 | 1420 | 137 | 66 | 31 | 20 | 18 | 23 |
| 0.5 | 6323 | 658 | 347 | 203 | 176 | 229 | 378 |
| 2.0 | 3206 | 378 | 229 | 176 | 203 | 347 | 658 |
| 3.0 | 1074 | 133 | 85 | 71 | 89 | 163 | 319 |
| 4.0 | 599 | 77 | 51 | 46 | 61 | 117 | 232 |
| 5.0 | 406 | 54 | 37 | 35 | 48 | 96 | 194 |
| 10.0 | 150 | 23 | 18 | 20 | 31 | 66 | 137 |
| 20.0 | 66 | 12 | 11 | 14 | 24 | 54 | 115 |

$\alpha = 0.05$ (two-sided), $\beta = 0.10$.

*Adapted from Schlesselman (1982).

calculations are summarized for various levels of $p_0$ and $RR$ using conventional values for the probabilities of Type I and II errors. This table may be used to estimate sample sizes, as indicated in the following illustrative example.

*Example 6—Sample size estimation in case-control research.* Suppose we wish to perform a case-control study of the relationship between cigarette smoking and lung cancer. From previously published work, we anticipate that smokers have a tenfold excess risk ($RR$) of lung cancer (Doll and Hill 1950) and the prevalence of cigarette smoking ($p_0$) is about 0.4 (Schuman 1977). From these values, with an $\alpha = 0.05$ (two-sided) and a $\beta = 0.10$, it would be necessary to study at least 20 cases and 20 controls. Note that this relatively small sample size is possible because of the strength of the cigarette smoking–lung cancer association and the substantial prevalence of smoking.

Several general relationships are apparent in sample size calculations:

1. For a given level of $\alpha$, $\beta$, and $p_0$, the sample size requirement decreases as the strength of the exposure-disease association increases.

2. For a given level of $\alpha$, $\beta$, and $RR$, the sample size requirement is usually minimized at intermediate levels of control exposure prevalence.

3. For a given level of $\beta$, $RR$, and $p_0$, the sample size requirement decreases as the probability of a Type I error increases.

4. For a given level of $\alpha$, $RR$, and $p_0$, the sample size requirement decreases as the probability of the Type II error increases.

When there are a limited number of cases available for study, it may be advantageous to include a larger number of controls. Although the discriminatory power of a study will progressively improve with the addition of more controls, the marginal gain in power is small when the study group sizes are greatly unbalanced. As a rule of thumb, it is often recommended that the case:control ratio should not exceed 1:4 (Ury 1975). A simple modification of eqn 8.1 allows the calculation of sample size for studies with different numbers of cases and controls (Schlesselman 1982).

$$n = (1 + 1/c)\bar{p}'\bar{q}'(z_\alpha + z_\beta)^2/(p_1 - p_0)^2, \qquad (8.2)$$

where   $c =$ number of controls per case

$$\bar{p}' = (p_1 + cp_0)/(1 + c),$$

and   $\bar{q}' = 1 - \bar{p}'$.

For sample size calculations in pair-matched case-control studies, the end point is not the total number of cases, but rather the number of case-control pairs which are discordant with regard to exposure status. The necessary number of discordant pairs ($m$) can be calculated as (Schlesselman 1982):

$$m = [z_\alpha/2 + z_\beta\sqrt{P(1-P)}]^2/(P - \tfrac{1}{2})^2 \qquad (8.3)$$

where

$$P \simeq RR/(1 + RR).$$

From eqn 8.3, one can predict the total number of case-control pairs required if the probability of a discordant pair is known or can be estimated. However, this information is not usually known prior to data collection.

All of the sample size calculations discussed thus far are based upon the assumption of a fixed sample size. That is, the size of the study population is set and maintained prior to the collection of any data. An alternative approach, referred to as group sequential sampling, involves accumulating subjects until there is a sufficient amount of information to accept or reject the null hypothesis at some specified level of $\alpha$ and $\beta$. The group sequential method may be especially useful for surveillance studies in which there is no prior estimate of the magnitude of an exposure-disease association and data collection proceeds in a continuous fashion.

In practice, the group sequential method involves enrolling a subgroup of $K$ cases and an equal number of controls and then testing for statistical significance of an exposure-disease association. If the result is significant at the predetermined $\alpha$ level, data collection is terminated. However, if the observed effect is consistent with no association, another group of $K$ cases and $K$ controls is enrolled. This process is repeated until either the null hypothesis is rejected, or a specified number of subgroups are entered without rejection of the null hypothesis. In light of the repeated statistical significance tests, it is necessary to test for the exposure-disease association at a nominal $\alpha$ level which is smaller than the overall significance level. Pocock (1977) has published a reference table for rapid determination of appropriate nominal significance levels in group sequential studies.

The sample size for a group sequential study may be calculated for specified values of the maximum number of subgroups, $\alpha$, $\beta$, $p_0$, and $RR$. Pasternack and Shore (1981) have published tables of maximum group sequential sample size calculations and the interested reader is referred to their work. It should be remembered that these values represent upper limits of required subjects, since early detection of significant associations may permit a smaller sample.

## ESTIMATION OF RELATIVE RISK IN UNMATCHED CASE-CONTROL RESEARCH

The traditional measure of an exposure-disease association is the relative risk (risk ratio). Relative risk may be defined as the probability of disease development in exposed persons, divided by the probability of disease development in unexposed subjects. As the ratio of two probabilities, the relative risk has a range of possible values from zero to positive infinity. The value of relative risk which corresponds to 'no association' is unity. A relative risk significantly greater than unity implies an excess disease risk in exposed persons, whereas a relative risk significantly less than unity corresponds to a diminished disease risk in exposed persons. While there are no universal rules for the interpretation of relative risks, Table 8.7 may serve as a rough guideline. The probability of disease development conditional upon exposure status, can be estimated directly in prospective cohort studies. However, in case-control studies, the subjects are sampled conditional on disease status, and thus one cannot obtain a direct estimate of relative risk. In the simplest unmatched situation, consider a four-fold table with disease status on one axis and a dichotomous classification of

**Table 8.7.** *Guidelines for the interpretation of a relative risk value, in terms of exposure-disease association*

| Relative risk range | Interpretation |
| --- | --- |
| 0–0.3 | Strong benefit |
| 0.4–0.5 | Moderate benefit |
| 0.6–0.8 | Weak benefit |
| 0.9–1.1 | No effect |
| 1.2–1.6 | Weak hazard |
| 1.7–2.5 | Moderate hazard |
| >2.6 | Strong hazard |

**Table 8.8.** *Simple four-fold table for an unmatched case-control study*

| | | Exposure status | | |
| --- | --- | --- | --- | --- |
| | | Exposed | Unexposed | Total |
| **Disease status** | Case | $a$ | $b$ | $m_1$ |
| | Control | $c$ | $d$ | $m_0$ |
| | Total | $n_1$ | $n_0$ | $t = m_1 + m_0$ |

exposure history on the other axis (Table 8.8). Each subject in the study fits into one and only one of the cells labelled $a$ through $d$. For example, a case with a positive exposure history would be placed into cell $a$, whereas another case with a negative exposure history would be placed in cell $b$. When all of the subjects have been classified in this manner, the table marginal totals ($m_1 + m_0$ or $n_1 + n_0$) may be summed to obtain the value $t$, the total number of study subjects. In the case-control sampling method, subjects enter the study based upon their disease status. Thus, the investigator chooses the ratio of cases-to-controls, and therefore the ratio of $m_1$ to $m_0$ is fixed. Notice the contrast with a prospective cohort study in which the investigator determines the ratio of exposed to unexposed persons (ratio of $n_1$ to $n_0$ fixed).

Although one cannot obtain a direct estimate of relative risk in case-control studies, Cornfield (1951) demonstrated that an indirect estimate may be obtained. This indirect estimate, subsequently termed the (exposure) odds ratio (OR), requires two assumptions:

1. The controls are representative of the candidate population from which the cases arose (Miettinen 1976).

2. The disease under investigation is rare (Cornfield 1951).

The odds ratio is calculated as the simple cross-product of the four-fold table:

$$\widehat{OR} = \frac{ad}{bc} \qquad (8.4)$$

Where $\widehat{OR}$ indicates that the odds ratio is an estimate from the study population. An advantageous property of the odds ratio is that its value does not depend on the underlying research design. This advantage allows direct comparison of odds ratio estimates from cohort, cross-sectional, and case-control studies (Fleiss 1981).

*Example 7—Calculation of odds ratio in unmatched case-control research.*

Suppose a case-control study is performed to test a postulated association between prenatal irradiation and childhood leukaemia. One hundred cases of leukaemia are identified from a tumour registry and then 200 neighbourhood controls are obtained. From interviews with the parents of all subjects it is determined that 30 cases and 45 controls were exposed to intrauterine diagnostic irradiation. These data may be represented in the format shown in Table 8.9. Thus, if the assumptions of the odds ratio calculation hold, we estimate a relative risk of 1.48. This means that children irradiated *in utero* have almost a 50 per cent excess risk of developing leukaemia.

**Table 8.9.** *Data for unmatched case-control study of prenatal irradiation and childhood leukaemia*

|  |  | Prenatal irradiation | | |
|  |  | Exposed | Unexposed | Total |
| --- | --- | --- | --- | --- |
| Childhood leukaemia | Case | 30 | 70 | 100 |
|  | Control | 45 | 155 | 200 |
|  | Total | 75 | 225 | 300 |

## MEASURES OF POPULATION HEALTH IMPACT IN CASE-CONTROL RESEARCH

In aetiological research, the emphasis of analysis is usually on evaluating the strength of an exposure-disease association, as indicated by relative risk. However, for public health concerns, it is often useful to consider measures which address the population impact of an exposure, or the social benefit of curtailing an exposure.

The attributable risk proportion (ARP) may be defined as the proportion of total disease risk in exposed persons which may be attributed to their exposure. Cole and MacMahon (1971) have shown that the ARP may be estimated in case-control studies by:

$$\widehat{ARP} = \frac{\widehat{OR} - 1}{\widehat{OR}} \qquad (8.5)$$

When the $\widehat{OR}$ is $> 1$, the ARP has a range of possible values from zero to unity. In the limiting case when $\widehat{OR}$ is equal to unity (no exposure-disease association), none of the disease risk in exposed persons will be attributed to that exposure ($\widehat{ARP} = O$). At the other extreme, when the $\widehat{OR}$ is very large, much of the total disease risk in exposed persons may result from that exposure.

Another population health impact measure of special note is the population attributable risk proportion (PARP). This measure, also known as the aetiological fraction, corresponds to the proportion of disease risk in all persons which may be attributed to the exposure under investigation. Under the assumption that the exposure histories of controls are typical of the target population, Cole and MacMahon (1971) have demonstrated that the PARP may be estimated in case-control studies by:

$$\widehat{PARP} = \frac{\widehat{p_0}(\widehat{OR} - 1)}{1 + \widehat{p_0}(\widehat{OR} - 1)} \qquad (8.6)$$

where $\widehat{p_0}$ represents the estimated prevalence of exposure in controls (and by inference the exposure prevalence in the target population). Again, when the $\widehat{OR}$ is $> 1$, the limits of this expression are zero to unity. Notice, however, that the PARP is determined by both the frequency of exposure and the strength of association between exposure and disease. Taylor (1977) has shown that the PARP may be simply estimated from case-control studies by:

$$\widehat{PARP} = 1 - \left[ \frac{b(c+d)}{d(a+b)} \right]. \qquad (8.7)$$

*Example 8—Calculation of attributable risk per cent and population attributable risk per cent in case-control research.*

Using the data presented in Example 7, ($\widehat{OR} = 1.48$), we can calculate measures of childhood leukaemia population impact for intrauterine irradiation. First, the ARP is estimated by:

$$\widehat{ARP} = \frac{1.48 - 1}{1.48} = 0.32.$$

Thus, to the extent that the $\widehat{OR}$ provides a valid estimate of the strength of the exposure-disease association, we conclude that about one-third of childhood leukaemia in the irradiated children may be attributed in part to prenatal irradiation. Similarly, we may estimate the PARP with Taylor's formula:

$$\widehat{PARP} = 1 - \left[ \frac{70(45 + 155)}{155(30 + 70)} \right] = 1 - 0.90 = 0.10.$$

Thus, we conclude that about 10 per cent of all childhood leukaemia may be attributed in part to intrauterine irradiation.

## STRATIFIED ANALYSIS OF CASE-CONTROL RESEARCH

Up to this point, the simplest evaluation of an exposure-disease association has been considered. In most research situations, it is also necessary to take into account the influence of other factors, such as age, race, and sex. One approach to the accommodation of these co-variables is to stratify the data into subsets by co-factor level. For example, if we are interested in assessing the relationship between dietary fibre intake and colon cancer risk, we might examine the fibre-colon cancer association separately in four race-sex groups: white males, white females, non-white males, and non-white females. If the association does not vary across the race-sex specific categories, then it may be desirable to obtain a summary measure of this association. This condition of uniformity of an exposure-disease association is termed 'homogeneity' and means in this instance that the effect of dietary fibre on colon cancer risk is not modified by race or sex. For homogeneous data, all of the four race-sex stratum-specific odds ratio estimates would be the same. A statistical test for homogeneity of the natural logarithm of OR is available (Woolf 1955), and may be used to determine whether the strata are sufficiently homogeneous to allow summarization.

The most popular approach to calculating a summary $\widehat{OR}$ was first introduced by Mantel and Haenszel (1959). This measure may be obtained in the following manner:

$$\widehat{OR}_{MH} = \sum_{i=1}^{I} \left( \frac{a_i d_i}{t_i} \right) \bigg/ \sum_{i=1}^{I} \left( \frac{b_i c_i}{t_{i,}} \right) \qquad (8.8)$$

where the subscript MH designates a Mantel-Haenszel estimate, $i$ is an index for covariate-specific strata, $I$ is the total number of summarized strata, and the remaining symbols are the stratum-specific equivalents of those specified in Table 8.8. It can be shown that the $\widehat{OR}_{MH}$ is a weighted average of the stratum-specific values, where the weights are $b_i c_i / t_i$. In this approach, the strata with the most information and hence the greatest statistical precision, receive the most weight (Mantel and Haenszel 1959). Furthermore, this summary measure has the advantage that it can be used without modification when there are 'zero' entries in some of the stratum-specific tables. When there are multiple covariates to accommodate it is likely that the study subjects will become thinly spread over the relevant strata. Thus, the Mantel–Haenszel summary odds ratio is often preferred over alternative approaches on the basis of its precision (Kleinbaum *et al.* 1982).

## HYPOTHESIS TESTING IN UNMATCHED CASE-CONTROL RESEARCH

Once the odds ratio is calculated in a case-control study, the next step is to perform a test of statistical significance. The purpose of a significance test is to assess whether the observed odds ratio is sufficiently different from unity to exclude chance as a likely explanation for the observed exposure-disease association. The hypothesis test is formulated in either a one- or two-sided direction:

*Two-sided alternative hypothesis:*
$H_0$: There is no association between the exposure and disease (OR = 1).
$H_a$: There is an association, either positive or negative, between the exposure and diseases. (OR < 1 or OR > 1).

*One-sided alternative hypothesis:*
$H_0$: There is either a negative or no association between the exposure and disease (OR ≤ 1).
$H_a$: There is a positive association between the exposure and disease (OR > 1).

If the direction of the tested association can be predicted in advance, the use of a one-sided test may be justified. In other circumstances, it is preferable to use the two-sided version.

Mantel and Haenszel (1959) proposed the use of a large sample test statistic based upon the hypergeometric model. This test statistic (without continuity correction) may be calculated with the following formula:

$$\chi^2_{MH} = \left( \sum_{i=1}^{I} \frac{a_i d_i - b_i c_i}{t_i} \right)^2 \bigg/ \left[ \sum_{i=1}^{I} \frac{m_{1i} m_{0i} n_{1i} n_{0i}}{(t_i - 1) t_i^2} \right] \qquad (8.9)$$

The Mantel–Haenszel procedure was shown to have optimal statistical features when the stratum-specific odds ratios are homogeneous (Radhakrishna 1965). Under the large sample assumptions, the Mantel–Haenszel test statistic follows a chi-square distribution with one degree of freedom. It should be noted that the large sample assumption pertains to the total amount of data aggregated over all strata. Mantel and Fleiss (1980) have proposed the following criteria for appropriate use of tabled chi-square distributions with one degree of freedom:

$$\text{and} \quad \left[ \sum_{i=1}^{I} \frac{n_{1i} m_{1i}}{t_i} \right] - \left[ \sum_{i=1}^{I} \max (0, m_{1i} - n_{0i}) \right] \leqslant 5$$

$$\left[ \sum_{i=1}^{I} \min (n_{1i}, m_{1i}) \right] - \left[ \sum_{i=1}^{I} \frac{n_{1i} m_{1i}}{t_i} \right] \geqslant 5$$

When both of these conditions are satisfied, the sample size is considered sufficient to use the large sample calculation.

## CONFIDENCE INTERVAL ESTIMATION IN UNMATCHED CASE-CONTROL RESEARCH

In addition to the point estimate of an odds ratio, it is often useful to calculate a measure of variability of that estimate. The standard approach is to calculate a confidence interval for the odds ratio estimate. A 95 per cent confidence interval is a range of values such that the chances are 95 out of 100 that the true value lies within that range.

Several methods for calculating odds ratio confidence intervals have been proposed. For small sample sizes, it is often recommended that 'exact' type confidence intervals be used (Kleinbaum *et al.* 1982). However, the exact method requires complex calculations, which may become prohibitive for even modest sample sizes. Thomas (1971) has provided a computer algorithm to assist in the determination of exact confidence intervals.

For larger sample sizes, it may be more practical to calculate 'approximate' confidence intervals. Several different approximation methods have been proposed, which may differ with regard to the estimation of the odds ratio variance. A Taylor series approximation yields a $(1 - \alpha)$ 100 per cent confidence interval of the following form (Woolf 1955):

$$\widehat{OR} \exp \left( \pm z_{1-\alpha/2} \sqrt{1/a + 1/b + 1/c + 1/d} \right) \qquad (8.10)$$

Miettinen (1976) proposed an alternative, test-based confidence interval, in which the odds ratio variance may be estimated from the square of the odds ratio divided by the Mantel–Haenszel test statistic. From this approximation it is possible to construct a $(1 - \alpha)$ 100 per cent confidence interval of the following form (Miettinen 1976):

$$\widehat{OR}^{(1 \pm z_{1-\alpha/2} \sqrt{\chi_{MH}})} \qquad (8.11)$$

In general, the test-based confidence intervals tend to be slightly narrower than the Taylor series intervals. Either of these estimation procedures may provide unsatisfactory approximations for small samples (Kleinbaum *et al.* 1982). The test-based procedure has also been shown to introduce a systematic bias as the magnitude of the observed odds ratio increases (Brown 1981). Therefore, this procedure should be used with caution when the odds ratio point estimate is five or more.

*Example 9—Calculation of unmatched summary odds ratio, confidence interval and test statistics.*

Returning to the prenatal irradiation-childhood leukaemia data presented in Table 8.9, let us consider a stratified analysis which accounts for the effect of maternal gravidity. In the simplest situation, we might stratify the crude data into two levels: primigravidae and multigravidae. Table 8.10 demonstrates the gravidity-specific four-fold tables for the association between prenatal irradiation and childhood leukaemia.

**Table 8.10.** *Data for unmatched case-control study of prenatal irradiation and childhood leukaemia, stratified by maternal gravidity*

(a) **Primigravidae**

| | | Prenatal irradiation Exposed | Unexposed | Totals |
|---|---|---|---|---|
| Childhood leukaemia | Case | 23 | 37 | 60 |
| | Control | 22 | 38 | 60 |
| | Total | 45 | 75 | 120 |

(b) **Multigravidae**

| | | Prenatal irradiation Exposed | Unexposed | Total |
|---|---|---|---|---|
| Childhood leukaemia | Case | 7 | 33 | 40 |
| | Control | 23 | 117 | 140 |
| | Total | 30 | 150 | 180 |

As a preliminary assessment of homogeneity of effect between levels of gravidity, stratum-specific odds ratios may be calculated and compared. Using eqn 8.4 we obtain the following measures of effect:

$$\widehat{OR}_{primigravidae} = \frac{(23)(38)}{(37)(22)} = 1.07$$

$$\widehat{OR}_{multigravidae} = \frac{(7)(117)}{(33)(23)} = 1.08$$

Since these stratum-specific effect measures are homogeneous, it is appropriate to determine a summary odds ratio, with corresponding confidence intervals and an associated hypothesis test.

The point estimate of the Mantel–Haenszel summary odds ratio is calculated with eqn 8.8:

$$\widehat{OR}_{MH} = \frac{\left[\dfrac{(23)(38)}{(120)} + \dfrac{(7)(117)}{(180)}\right]}{\left[\dfrac{(37)(22)}{(120)} + \dfrac{(33)(23)}{(180)}\right]} = 1.08$$

This measure may be interpreted to suggest that prenatal irradiation results in an 8 per cent increased risk of childhood leukaemia, after the effect of maternal gravidity is taken into account. Notice that this summary odds ratio is less than the crude odds ratio previously obtained in Example 7. The difference in these measures may be attributed to the confounding effect of maternal gravidity, which exaggerates the apparent effect of prenatal irradiation in the crude data.

The statistical significance of the summary measure may be tested with eqn 8.9:

$$\chi^2_{MH} = \frac{\left[\dfrac{(23)(38)-(37)(22)}{(120)} + \dfrac{(7)(117)-(33)(23)}{(180)}\right]^2}{\left[\dfrac{(60)(60)(45)(75)}{(119)(120)^2} + \dfrac{(40)(140)(30)(150)}{(179)(180)^2}\right]}$$

$$= 0.06, \quad p_{(two-tailed)} > 0.80$$

This test statistic may be interpreted as indicating that the remaining weak association between prenatal irradiation and childhood leukaemia could easily have arisen by chance in these data.

Test-based 95 per cent confidence limits for the summary odds ratio may be calculated with eqn 8.11:

$$95 \text{ per cent CI} = 1.08^{(1 \pm 1.96/\sqrt{0.06})} = (0.58, 2.00)$$

Notice that this confidence interval crosses unity, thereby confirming the lack of statistical significance of the odds ratio point estimate.

## ESTIMATION OF RELATIVE RISK IN PAIR-MATCHED CASE-CONTROL RESEARCH

When matching is used to choose comparison subjects, the matching process should be considered in the analysis. The actual form of analysis depends upon the case-to-control ratio. In this discussion, we present the simplest situation in which one control is individually matched to one case. For the analysis of more complex situations, such as multiple controls per case, the reader is referred to the excellent discussion by Schlesselman (1982).

The analysis of a pair-matched case-control study may be considered as a logical extension of stratified analysis. In the pair-matched situation, each stratum is composed of one case and one control. For any case-control pair there are four possible exposure histories:

    A. Case exposed, control exposed;
    B. Case exposed, control unexposed;
    C. Case unexposed, control exposed;
    D. Case unexposed, control unexposed.

After each case-control pair is classified into one of these exposure categories, a four-fold table may be constructed to summarize all of the pairs (Table 8.11).

**Table 8.11.** *Simple four-fold table for a pair-matched case-control study\**

| | | Control Exposed | Unexposed | Total |
|---|---|---|---|---|
| Case | Exposed | A | B | A+B |
| | Unexposed | C | D | C+D |
| | Total | A+C | B+D | N=A+B+C+D |

*\*Each cell entry in this table represents a pair of subjects, comprised of a case and his/her control.*

Notice that Table 8.11 is different from the previous layout in Table 8.8. For the pair-matched study, each entry into the four-fold table represents a pair of subjects. For example, the cell labelled $A$ includes all pairs in which both the case and control were exposed. The cell labelled $B$ includes all exposed case/unexposed control pairs and so forth. Thus, the total number of entries ($N$) in the table represents the number of case-control pairs, not individual subjects.

When the exposure histories of a case and control are similar, the pair is termed 'concordant'. When the exposure histories of a case and control differ, the pair is termed 'discordant'. Since we are interested in differential exposure histories within each case-control pair, the primary focus is upon the cells in Table 8.11 labelled $B$ and $C$. Kraus (1960) demonstrated that the maximum likelihood estimate of the odds ratio is given by:

$$\hat{OR} = B/C \qquad (8.12)$$

An identical expression for the Mantel–Haenszel odds ratio would be obtained from a stratified analysis, where each stratum consists of a case-control pair (Mantel and Haenszel 1959).

## HYPOTHESIS TESTING IN PAIR-MATCHED CASE-CONTROL RESEARCH

A simple statistical significance test for matched case-control studies can be constructed with a normal approximation to the binomial distribution. This test statistic (without continuity correction) may be calculated with the following formula (Schlesselman 1982):

$$\chi^2_{(1)} = (B-C)^2/(B+C) \qquad (8.13)$$

This statistic is distributed approximately as a chi-square with one degree of freedom for matched studies with large numbers of discordant pairs. If the number of discordant pairs is small, an exact hypothesis test must be performed (Schlesselman 1982).

## CONFIDENCE INTERVAL ESTIMATION IN PAIR-MATCHED CASE-CONTROL RESEARCH

For matched case-control studies with large numbers of discordant pairs, an approximate $(1 - \alpha)\,100$ per cent confidence interval for the odds ratio may be estimated by (Schlesselman 1982):

$$(B/C)\exp[\pm z_{1-\alpha/2}\sqrt{{}^1\!/_B + {}^1\!/_C}]_i \qquad (8.14)$$

If the number of discordant pairs is small, an exact $(1 - \alpha)\,100$ per cent confidence interval may be calculated (Schlesselman 1982).

*Example 10—Calculation of pair-matched summary odds ratio, confidence interval and test statistic.*

Suppose we wish to conduct a matched case-control study of the association between infectious mononucleosis (IM) and the subsequent development of lymphoma. It is decided that

**Table 8.12.** *Data for pair-matched case-control study of infectious mononucleosis (IM) and lymphoma\**

|  |  | Control | | |
|---|---|---|---|---|
|  |  | IM infection | No IM infection | Total |
| **Lymphoma patient** | IM infection | 15 | 60 | 75 |
|  | No IM infection | 35 | 40 | 75 |
|  | Total | 50 | 100 | 150 |

\*Each cell entry in this table represents a pair of subjects, comprised of a case and his/her control.

controls (persons without lymphoma) will be pairwise matched to lymphoma patients by age ($\pm$ five years), race, and sex. After enrollment of cases and controls, histories of prior IM infection are obtained. The resulting data are displayed in Table 8.12. The corresponding maximum likelihood estimate of the odds ratio is calculated with eqn 8.12:

$$\hat{OR} = 60/35 = 1.71.$$

To the extent that this odds ratio is a valid estimate of relative risk, this measure suggests that persons exposed to IM have about a 70 per cent excess risk of lymphoma when compared with persons not exposed to IM.

The statistical significance of this result may be tested with the test statistic in eqn 8.12:

$$\chi^2 = (60-35)^2/(60+35) = 6.58$$

This statistic yields a two-sided $p$-value of about 0.01. Thus, we conclude that the association between IM and lymphoma is unlikely to have occurred by chance alone.

A 95 per cent confidence interval for the estimated odds ratio may be calculated with eqn 8.14:

$$95 \text{ per cent CI} = 1.71 \exp[\pm 1.96\sqrt{(1/60)+(1/35)}]$$
$$= (1.13, 2.59)$$

Notice that the entire range of this confidence interval is greater than unity, thus confirming the statistical significance of the odds ratio point estimate.

## LOGISTIC REGRESSION ANALYSIS OF CASE-CONTROL RESEARCH

In the study of complex aetiological processes, there may be many variables which influence the disease risk. Even relatively direct exposure-disease associations may be affected by variables such as age, race, sex, socio-economic status, as well as other exposures. As already indicated, these relevant co-factors may be accounted for with a stratified analysis. However, as the number of co-factor-specific strata increases, the study sample may be sparsely distributed across each level. For example, suppose we have conducted a case-control study of the relationship between hepatitis infection and subsequent risk of liver cancer. It is determined that the following co-variables require control: age (20–39, 40–59, $\geqslant 60$ years), race (white, non-white), sex (male, female), socio-economic status (high, middle, low), and alcohol consumption (heavy, moderate, occasional). A stratified analysis accounting for these co-factors would require $3 \times 2 \times 2 \times 3 \times 3 = 108$ strata. Even with a relatively large sample size, it is likely that there will be insufficient data in many of these strata. Moreover, if the stratum-specific effects are heterogeneous, then it may be a challenge to summarize and interpret these study results.

For these multivariable situations, it may be desirable to estimate independent and joint effects with a mathematical model. A popular model for analysis of case-control studies is the logistic regression approach (Schlesselman 1982). The theory and appropriate use of logistic analyses require some familiarity with regression techniques. The principles of logistic analysis are briefly summarized in this chapter and the reader who is interested in a more detailed discussion is referred to three advanced textbooks (Breslow and Day 1980; Kleinbaum *et al.* 1982; Schlesselman 1982).

In the logistic model, the conditional probability of disease ($D$) occurrence given exposure ($E$) is represented by a linear function (Kleinbaum *et al.* 1982):

$$\text{logit } P(D|E) = \ln \left[ \frac{P(D|E)}{1 - P(D|E)} \right] = \alpha + \beta E \qquad (8.15)$$

where logit is an abbreviation of logarithmic unit, ln is the natural logarithm, $P(D|E) = $ probability of disease given exposure; $\alpha$, $\beta = $ regression coefficients; and $E$ may be dichotomized: ($0 = $ no exposure, $1 = $ exposure), or expressed as a continuous variable.

From eqn 8.15 it is possible to derive an expression for the odds ratio which reduces to the following form (Kleinbaum *et al.* 1982):

$$\hat{\text{OR}} = e^{\beta} \qquad (8.16)$$

The simple model presented in eqn 8.15 can be extended to account for potential confounders ($V_i$) and effect modifiers ($W_j$) (Kleinbaum *et al.* 1982):

$$\text{logit } (P|E, V_i, W_j) = \ln \left[ \frac{P(D|E, V_i, W_j)}{1 - P(D|E, V_i, W_j)} \right] \qquad (8.17)$$

$$= \alpha + \beta E + \sum_{i=1}^{I} \gamma_i V_i + \sum_{j=1}^{J} \delta_j W_j$$

where $\alpha$ and $\beta$ have their former definitions; $\gamma_i$ and $\delta_j$ are the regression coefficients for the potential confounders and effect modifiers respectively.

From eqn (8.17) the following expression for the odds ratio may be obtained (Prentice 1976):

$$\hat{\text{OR}} = \exp [\beta + \sum_{j=1}^{J} \delta_j W_j]. \qquad (8.18)$$

Thus, the odds ratio can be expressed as the exponential of the sum of the main effect and the effect modifiers. Although the confounders are not explicitly represented in this odds ratio estimate, their inclusion in eqn (8.17) will influence the estimated values of $\alpha$, $\beta$, and $\delta_j$, thereby indirectly influencing the odds ratio estimate. Moreover, a matched study design may be accommodated in logistic analysis.

The coefficients in a logistic analysis may be estimated by either of two approaches: discriminant analysis (Cornfield 1962), or maximum likelihood estimation (Prentice and Pyke 1979). For the usual situation in which the data are not multivariate normally distributed, discriminant analysis can produce misleading results (Press and Wilson 1978). Thus, maximum likelihood estimation is usually the preferred approach to parameter estimation (Schlesselman 1982). The details of maximum likelihood estimation and statistical inference may be found in three advanced textbooks (Breslow and Day 1980; Kleinbaum *et al.* 1982; Schlesselman 1982).

While logistic regression is a powerful analytical method, it should be recognized that there are several potential drawbacks to such modelling procedures. First, the linear model is most useful when disease risk can be expressed as a monotonic function of the independent variables (Gordon 1974). Occasionally, curvilinear exposure-disease relationships will be encountered and alternate models should be employed, such as the use of quadratic independent variables or logarithmic transformation of the independent variables. A second limitation of logistic regression is that it assumes a multiplicative statistical relationship between independent variables (Greenland 1979). In certain situations, the data may fit better with an additive statistical relationship between independent variables. For any particular research application, the appropriateness of a logistic model will depend upon the nature of the exposure-disease and exposure–co-variate relationships.

## BIAS IN CASE-CONTROL RESEARCH

Most of the criticism of case-control research has centered around the possibility of systematic errors in these studies (Hayden *et al.* 1982). It should be emphasized that all types of observational research and even randomized experiments (May *et al.* 1981) are subject to potential systematic errors (*viz.* bias). Nevertheless, some authors have suggested that case-control studies have a special vulnerability to bias because of the retrospective timing of observations. For instance, Horwitz and Feinstein (1979) compiled a list of 17 substantive research topics for which case-control studies yielded discordant results.

While such contradictory findings are of concern, they do not constitute an incontrovertible indictment of case-control studies. Many instances of conflicting study results can be cited from other observational and experimental work. As a single illustration, consider two well-designed and executed randomized, placebo-controlled clinical trials which reached opposite conclusions about the efficacy of sodium nitroprusside in the reduction of mortality from acute myocardial infarction (Durrer *et al.* 1982; Cohn *et al.* 1982). The apparent disagreement between these investigations may be explained in part by differences in the study populations, such as the prevalence of left ventricular failure and the time to initiation of treatment. Thus, such disparate findings do not imply that randomized clinical trials are inherently subject to bias. By the same token, occasional discordant results in case-control studies cannot be construed as evidence that case-control studies are inherently prone to errors.

As Sartwell (1974) suggested, a more prudent attitude

toward epidemiological research is to use 'all contributory methods with discernment and recognition of their weaknesses and through efforts to cope with these weaknesses'. In certain situations, such as the study of uncommon and chronic disease, a case-control approach may be the most feasible research method. The decision to conduct a case-control study should be accompanied by a consideration of potential biases which may distort the research findings. These potential biases can often be minimized or prevented with careful planning of the study design and analysis.

Sackett (1979) provided a catalogue of biases which may occur in analytical research. This serves as a handy reference for the design and conduct of a proposed investigation. In the following sections we present an abbreviated overview of some systematic errors which may occur in case-control studies. We divide these errors into three general categories:

*1. Selection bias:* A distortion in the study effect which results from the manner in which subjects are sampled for investigation.

*2. Misclassification (information) bias:* A distortion in the study effect which results from inaccurate determination of exposure or disease status.

*3. Confounding:* A distortion in the study effect which results from the mixing of the exposure-disease association with the effect(s) of extraneous variable(s).

## Selection bias

Kleinbaum *et al.* (1981) proposed a conceptual framework for the consideration of selection bias. From this model it is possible to define the conditions which give rise to selection bias in the estimation of the odds ratio. In the present context, we emphasize two situations which may result in a biased odds ratio estimate:

*Situation 1:* The odds of selection into the sample conditional on exposure status is different for cases and controls. In case-control studies the outcome variable (exposure) occurs prior to subject selection and consequently exposure status may differentially affect the selection probabilities of cases and controls.

*Situation 2:* The odds of selection into the sample conditional on disease status is different for exposed and unexposed persons.

Potential selection biases may be controlled either in the design or analysis stage of a case-control study. With either approach to bias control, the first step is to recognize the manner in which such errors arise. Toward this end, we present a brief review of some classical selection biases, along with suggestions for avoiding these potential errors.

### Berkson's paradox

In 1946, Berkson constructed a theoretical argument that hospital samples may systematically differ from general populations because of factors which influence the likelihood of hospitalization. As a result, hospital samples may exhibit spurious associations between two variables, even though these variables are independently distributed in the general population. Figure 8.6 provides a schematic representation of

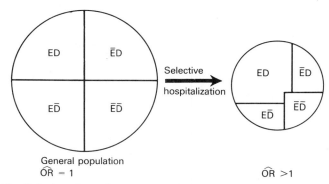

**Fig. 8.6.** A schematic representation of the Berkson paradox creating a spurious association: E = exposed; Ē = unexposed; D = case; D̄ = control.

the Berkson paradox. This type of selection bias was demonstrated empirically by Roberts and co-workers (1978) who studied the associations between several conditions in a hospital sample and in the general population. For example, respiratory and bone diseases were not associated in the general population (ÔR = 1.06), but a strong positive association (ÔR = 4.06) was observed in a hospital sample. The authors also demonstrated that distorted medication-disease associations could arise in hospitalized populations. For instance, laxative use and arthritic disease were only weakly associated (ÔR = 1.48) in the general population, but a strong relationship (ÔR = 5.00) was observed in the hospital sample.

Walter (1980) has specified two particular circumstances for which the Berkson paradox will be negligible:

(a) The exposure under investigation is not a direct cause of hospitalization; and/or

(b) The case and control populations are mutually exclusive.

These two conditions can be used as guidelines for evaluating the potential of a Berkson paradox in any particular hospital-based case-control study.

### Neyman fallacy

In 1955, Neyman proposed that distorted exposure-disease associations could be obtained from the study of prevalent disease cases, if exposure is related to disease prognosis. As an illustration, consider the relationship between sex and risk of colorectal cancer. The incidence rate of colorectal cancer is slightly higher in males than females (Devesa and Silverman 1978). However, the survival from colorectal cancer is significantly longer in females than males (Koch *et al.* 1982). Since the female colorectal cancer patients live longer than males, a sample of prevalent cases will include a higher proportion of women than a corresponding sample of incident cases (Fig. 8.7). To remove the influence of selective survival (or demise), it is often recommended that the cases in a case-control study should be limited to newly diagnosed patients (Schlesselman 1982).

### Selective referral

For investigations of rare diseases, it is often necessary to obtain the study cases from tertiary care centres, or population surveillance programmes. Either of these referral networks can

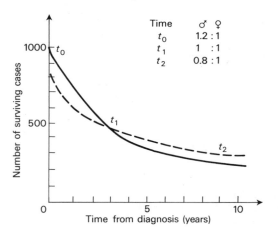

| Time | ♂ : ♀ |
|------|-------|
| $t_0$ | 1.2 : 1 |
| $t_1$ | 1 : 1 |
| $t_2$ | 0.8 : 1 |

**Fig. 8.7.** Sex-specific survival from colorectal cancer as an illustration of selective survival.

introduce a selection bias if cases within the population are differentially reported. It is likely that patients at tertiary care centres tend to have complicated or severe forms of their diseases, which may differ aetiologically from other cases. For example, it is estimated that only one in seven poisoning incidents is officially reported (Illinois Department of Public Health 1975). As a result, studies based upon reported poisonings may under-represent benign and illicit substances (Greenberg and Osterhout 1982).

Even when a concerted effort is made to identify most of the disease cases within a population, selection factors may arise. For instance, in a case-control study of the toxic-shock syndrome, the Wisconsin Division of Health mailed questionnaires to 3500 licensed physicians in that state (Davis *et al.* 1980). The mailing included a description of toxic-shock syndrome and indicated a possible association with menstruation. Of the 38 cases thus identified, 35 occurred during menses. Since studies in other geographic areas have reported a lower proportion of menstruation-related cases (Clayton 1982), it is possible that the information included in the Wisconsin Survey caused preferential reporting of menstrual cases. As a general rule, case surveillance will be most reliable when there are clear definitions of disease, adequate access to medical care, appropriate diagnostic facilities, and uniform reporting practices.

### Detection bias

A non-causal exposure-disease association may occur in observational studies if exposure status influences the likelihood of clinical recognition of the disease. For example, Horwitz and

Feinstein (1978) proposed that the association between use of exogenous oestrogens and endometrial cancer may be partially attributed to the preferential detection of this cancer in exposed women. These authors speculated that oestrogen use may lead to dysfunctional bleeding, thus prompting an intra-endometrial diagnostic examination and diagnosis of an otherwise asymptomatic endometrial cancer. In contrast, women who do not take oestrogens might be less likely to manifest bleeding per vagina, and thus a greater proportion of endometrial cancer cases may be undetected in unexposed women. Note that a premise for this bias is that some cases will never be diagnosed (Fig. 8.8). Hutchison and Rothman (1978) argued that a progressive disease, such as endometrial cancer, would ultimately produce symptoms independent of exposure status. As a result, they suggest that the proportion of detected cases will be comparable in oestrogen-exposed and unexposed women. Indeed, detection bias is more likely to occur in the study of diseases with documented asymptomatic cases, such as 'silent' gallstones (Feinstein 1979). Case-control studies of these diseases should attempt to evaluate the extent to which exposure brings an otherwise asymptomatic case to clinical detection.

### Non-response

Both experimental and observational studies of human populations may suffer from poor subject co-operation. Selection bias may be introduced if enrolled subjects systematically differ from non-participants. In the conduct of a case-control study, there are several stages at which subject enrollment may be impaired. First, some cases may be omitted because of limited access to medical care. Second, some diagnosed persons may be overlooked because of incomplete reporting practices. Third, some diagnosed persons may be excluded because of restricted access to their records. Finally, some patients, or their attending physicians, may decline to participate in a research project.

Many of these selection factors were illustrated by a case-control study of colon cancer (Herrmann *et al.* 1981). In that investigation, over 20 per cent of eligible hospitals denied permission to contact their patients. In addition, 25 per cent of attending physicians placed restrictions on patient contact. The authors noted that the most commonly cited reasons for non-participation were concerns about confidentiality and lack of personal advantage for the patient involved.

Criqui and co-workers (1979) have demonstrated that subjects who participated in a cardiovascular disease survey tended to be a biased subset of the target population. Respondents were characterized as 'worried well' individuals, that is to say, persons with risk factors but without disease. This

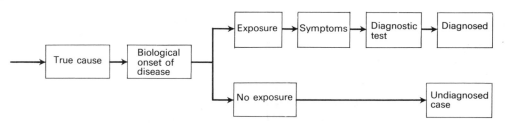

**Fig. 8.8.** Schematic representation of detection bias.

pattern of non-response produced minor to moderate errors in estimated odds ratios between specific risk factors and disease occurrence. However, the authors concluded that larger errors could occur with a similarly biased sample and a lower level of response. These non-response effects can be minimized by repeated attempts at subject enrollment and the collection of auxiliary data to evaluate the comparability of participants and non-participants. In addition, subject response may be increased in studies with protections of confidentiality and demonstrable personal advantage to participation.

## Misclassification bias

The second major source of potential bias in analytical research is referred to as misclassification (information) bias. This type of error may result from inaccurate assignment of either exposure or disease status. Copeland and colleagues (1977) developed a conceptual framework for the consideration of misclassification in outcome variables (exposure status in case-control studies). Other authors (Shy et al. 1978; Gladen and Rogan 1979) have considered the effects of exposure misclassification on risk estimates in environmental studies. In the present context, we note that two types of information error may occur:

### Non-differential misclassification

The errors in classification of one variable (e.g. exposure status) do not depend on the level of the other variable (e.g. disease status). As an example, consider a sphygmomanometer which always reads 10 mm Hg higher than the true blood pressure value. With these erroneous measurements, some normotensive persons will be misclassified as hypertensive, but these errors will not depend on disease status (e.g. myocardial infarction).

### Differential misclassification

The errors in classification of one variable (e.g. exposure status) depend on the level of the other variable (e.g. disease status). As an example of differential misclassification, consider an interviewer who systematically over-reports prior history of hypertension in myocardial infarction cases compared with control subjects.

The distinction between non-differential and differential misclassification may provide information on the anticipated direction of bias. It has been demonstrated that non-differential misclassification errors will tend to decrease the observed odds ratio (Gullen et al. 1968). In this situation, the study will provide an underestimate of the true exposure-disease association. Differential misclassification can produce either an overestimate or an underestimate of the true odds ratio (Copeland et al. 1977).

A variety of errors may result in non-differential misclassification bias. The following two examples illustrate the general considerations of non-differential misclassification of exposure in case-control studies.

### Exposure specification

One source of potential non-differential misclassification of exposure may arise if the exposure under investigation is not accurately assessed. For example, in occupational research it is often impossible to identify or quantify specific exposures to individual workers. As a surrogate of exposure status, a common practice is to classify subjects by job title. Without accurate information on individual exposures, it is possible that these surrogate measures may misrepresent the true odds of exposure in cases and controls. This type of error in case-control studies may be minimized when detailed information on specific exposures is available.

### Unacceptability bias

A second potential source of non-differential misclassification may occur when the exposure under investigation is a behaviour or characteristic which subjects are inclined to under-report. For example, subjects often answer questions about sexual practices, alcohol consumption, or use of illicit drugs with the perceived 'socially acceptable' response. More reliable answers to such sensitive questions may be obtained with self-administered questionnaires and strict guarantees of confidentiality.

A large number of systematic errors may lead to differential misclassification of exposure status in case-control studies. The following examples provide an overview of some common differential misclassification biases.

### Recall (anamnestic) bias

When historical exposure information is collected in case-control studies, it is possible that the subjects' memory of earlier events will be influenced by disease status. Cases are often highly motivated to remember any event which may have contributed to their disease aetiology. In their eagerness to identify possible causal factors, cases may even inadvertently over-report certain exposures. For example, in a case-control study of gestational drug use and adverse pregnancy outcome, the mothers of cases reported more unsubstantiated drug use than mothers of normal neonates (Klemetti and Saxen 1967).

There are several strategies which may be used to minimize the effects of differential recall of exposures. First, subjects and interviewers should not be aware of the specific exposure-disease association under investigation. Second, whenever possible, subject responses should be compared with other data sources, such as employment or medical records. Third, the use of a hospital control group may select comparison subjects who are similarly motivated to report possible aetiological exposures.

### Protopathic bias

Even when accurate historical exposure data are obtained, it is possible that the disease onset may actually precede the exposure. This error, referred to as 'protopathic bias' (Horwitz and Feinstein 1980), may result when the early manifestations of a disease cause a change in the pattern of exposures in cases. In case-control studies, the retrospective sequence of observations makes it difficult to determine whether a particular exposure occurred prior to the disease under investigation. This temporal confusion can produce erroneous conclusions about either suspected protective or deleterious exposures. For instance, physicians may refuse oral contraceptive prescriptions to women with breast ' lumps'. If these women are subsequently studied as breast cancer cases, then the relative lack of oral contraceptive use in these women may be mistakenly interpreted as a protective effect of the medication (Feinstein 1979). On the other hand, a particular exposure may be spuriously labelled as a causal factor if early disease signs or symptoms increase the likelihood of exposure. For example, Feinstein and colleagues (1981) speculated that an erroneous association between coffee consumption and pancreatic cancer could arise if pancreatic cancer cases increased their coffee drinking as a result of anxiety about vague abdominal discomfort.

### Interview bias

A third common source of differential misclassification may arise in case-control studies with exposure status determined by subject interview. In particular, the circumstances under which cases and controls are interviewed should be comparable. This requirement for comparability of data collection procedures includes such features as:

(a) the time from suspected exposure to interview;
(b) the setting of interview (e.g. hospital versus subject's residence);
(c) the format of the interview;
(d) the manner in which questions are phrased;
(e) the amount of interviewer prompting for specific answers;
(f) subject and interviewer knowledge about the research hypothesis.

Examples of potential interview bias abound in the case-control literature. For instance, in a study of tampon use and toxic shock syndrome, Davis *et al.* (1980) conducted personal interviews with cases, but presented controls with self-administered questionnaires. In a study of salicylate use and Reye syndrome (Halpin *et al.* 1982), the time to interview of parents of controls was systematically longer than time to interview parents of cases.

One must also recognize that intentional or inadvertent differential misclassification errors may occur when the interviewers are aware of the research hypothesis and the disease status of individual subjects. To avoid this type of differential misclassification, it is advisable to 'blind' the interviewers to the research hypothesis and, if possible, to the disease status of individual subjects. Similarly, cases and controls should be 'blinded' to the specific exposure-diease hypothesis under investigation.

### Confounding bias

The third major source of potential bias in analytical research is referred to as confounding bias. This relates to the distortion which may occur when the study effect is mixed with another effect. This mixing process may introduce bias if the resulting exposure-disease association is meaningfully altered from its 'uncontaminated' value.

Under the prevailing notion of this bias, a confounder (contaminating variable) in a case-control study must be:

(a) extraneous to the exposure-disease association under investigation; and
(b) predictive of the disease; and
(c) unequally distributed between exposure groups.

These conditions for a confounder are schematically represented in Fig. 8.9.

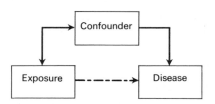

**Fig. 8.9.** Schematic representation of confounding.

Confounding may be illustrated by the data presented in Example 7. In that example, the study exposure was gestational irradiation and the disease was childhood leukaemia. A crude odds ratio of 1.48 indicated a modest positive association between these variables. However, when the effect of maternal gravidity was taken into account (Example 9), the observed irradiation-leukaemia odds ratio was 1.08. The latter value, which may be described as an 'adjusted' measure, indicated little or no association between gestational irradiation and leukaemia. In this situation, we conclude that the apparent irradiation-leukaemia association may be attributed to the confounding effect of maternal gravidity. It can be demonstrated easily with these data that maternal gravidity was associated conditionally both with the exposure and the disease under investigation.

The problem of confounding may become particularly acute in the study of diseases with multiple risk factors. For example, in planning a case-control study of the relationship between oral contraceptive (OC) use and acute myocardial infarction (MI), a list of potential confounders might include: age, race, hypertension, cigarette smoking, alcohol use, sedentary lifestyle, and serum triglycerides. Since all of these variables are known MI risk factors, they should be considered as potential confounders of the association between OC use and MI. However, it should be recognized that those risk factors which are not associated with OC use in the data will not confound the study results. Thus, it may be possible to arrive at a convenient subset of these risk factors which actually confound the association between OC use and MI. In other words, a valid study result will be obtained by controlling for only the confounding risk factors. Controlling for a minimal number of co-variables has the additional appeal of a possible gain in precision (Kleinbaum *et al.* 1982).

The effects of potential confounders may be controlled in the design or analysis of a case-control study. At the design stage, one may select subjects so that the potential confounder is not associated with disease status. For example, if age is an anticipated risk factor, then the cases and controls may be restricted to a narrow age band. As indicated earlier in this chapter, partial restriction (matching) is another mechanism for eliminating co-variable-disease associations. Indeed, matching is frequently employed with the intent of adjusting for potential confounders. However, the risk factor-disease association criterion for confounding relates to unexposed persons. Thus, matching on a covariate does not necessarily guarantee the elimination of confounding by that factor (Kupper *et al.* 1981).

At the analysis stage of investigation, confounding may be controlled by stratification or mathematical modelling. The data in Examples 7 and 9 demonstrate the use of stratification to obtain an adjusted odds ratio. When there are multiple co-variates, an analogous adjusted odds ratio may be obtained from summarization over multiple strata. Alternatively, when there are many potential confounders, a modelling technique such as logistic regression may be preferred. Equation 17 illustrates the manner by which potential confounders may be entered into a logistic model. The reader interested in a more detailed description of mathematical modelling strategies is referred to two excellent textbooks (Breslow and Day 1980; Schlesselman 1982).

In summary, there are a number of approaches which may be employed to adjust for potential confounders. With each method, one must first anticipate which factors might confound the exposure–disease association under study. Then, sufficient data must be collected to evaluate each of these covariates. Finally, the effects of covariates which actually confound the study results should be controlled, either by subject selection or analytical adjustment. Control of non-confounders is discouraged since this may entail a loss of precision.

## CONCLUDING REMARKS

In 1978, the Editors and the publisher of the *Journal of Chronic Diseases* invited thirty scientists to attend a symposium in Bermuda on case-control studies. One of us (MAI) was responsible for moderating the Symposium and editing the proceedings which were published in a special issue of the *Journal* (Ibrahim and Spitzer 1979). The discussions at the Symposium clearly highlighted the controversial issues surrounding the strategies used in case-control studies, the interpretation of these studies, and the policy action to be taken on the basis of such findings. The Symposium took place at a time when several health issues, such as those of reserpine use and breast cancer or oestrogen use and endometrial cancer, were vigorously debated in scientific journals and national meetings. Since the publication of that special issue of the *Journal,* numerous case-control studies on important and controversial issues have been conducted and a book entirely devoted to case-control studies was published (Schlesselman 1982). The question today is not whether case-control studies should be used, but how to conduct one properly.

Several points were made earlier in this chapter concerning the place of case-control studies in epidemiological investigations, the design problems which must be resolved before the study is begun, and the various analytical methods which are currently available. Some important issues are summarized below:

1. Scientists must exercise caution in publicizing the results of preliminary findings of case-control studies. This is especially important when the study is used to generate rather than to test an hypothesis. Investigators should resist the temptation to publicize their results before adequate peer review and appraisal have taken place.

2. It is important that a clear account of the study methods is included in the published article, and a more detailed description is available upon request. The published report should include a description of the cases, choice of controls, methods of collecting exposure data, and analytical technique.

3. Cases must be defined unambiguously and preferably limited to new or incident cases. Criteria and rationales for exclusions must be documented.

4. Whenever possible, two control groups should be included in a given study. Controls may be matched to cases or chosen randomly from the candidate population.

5. The three types of bias – selection, misclassification, and confounding – must be addressed at the inception of the study in order to avoid or minimize them. Biases that could not be avoided by the study design should be considered in the analysis.

6. Inferences from case-control studies and resulting public policies depend on the prevailing climate, feasibility of conducting more elaborate and expensive studies, state of knowledge, and consequences of the actions contemplated. It is reasonable to act on the basis of the results of a number of well-designed case-control studies, especially when cohort or experimental studies are not feasible.

## REFERENCES

Berkson, J. (1946). Limitations of the applications of fourfold table analysis to hospital data. *Biometrics Bull.* **2,** 47.

Breslow, N.E. and Day, N.E. (1980). *Statistical methods in cancer research,* Vol. 1 *The analysis of case-control studies.* IARC Scientific Publications No. 32. International Agency for Research on Cancer, Lyon.

Brown, C.C. (1981). The validity of approximation methods for interval estimation of the odds ratio. *Am. J. Epidemiol.* **113,** 474.

Cassel, J.C. (1971). Review of 1960 through 1962 cardiovascular disease prevalence study. *Arch. Int. Med.* **128,** 890.

Clayton, A.J. (1982). Toxic shock syndrome in Canada. *Ann. Intern. Med.* **96** (Part 2), 881.

Cohn, J.N., Franciosa, J.A., Francis, G.S. *et al.* (1982). Effect of short-term infusion of sodium nitroprusside on mortality rate in acute myocardial infarction complicated by left ventricular failure: Results of a Veterans Administration Cooperative Study. *N. Engl. J. Med.* **306,** 1129.

Cole, P. (1979). The evolving case-control study. *J. Chronic Dis.* **32,** 15.

Cole, P. and MacMahon, B. (1971). Attributable risk percent in case-control studies. *Br. J. Prev. Soc. Med.* **25,** 242.

Copeland, K.T., Checkoway, H., Holbrook, R.H. *et al.* (1977). Bias due to misclassification in the estimate of relative risk. *Am. J. Epidemiol.* **105,** 488.

Cornfield, J. (1951). A method of estimating comparative rates from clinical data: applications to cancer of the lung, breast, and cervix. *J. Natl. Cancer Inst.* **11,** 1269.

Cornfield, J. (1962). Joint dependence of risk of coronary heart disease on serum cholesterol and systolic blood pressure: a discriminant function analysis. *Fed. Proc.* **21,** 58.

Cornfield, J. and Haenszel, W. (1960). Some aspects of retrospective studies. *J. Chronic Dis.* **11**, 523.

Criqui, M.H., Austin, M., and Barrett-Connor, E. (1979). The effect of non-response on risk ratios in a cardiovascular disease study. *J. Chronic Dis.* **32**, 633.

Davis, J.P., Chesney, P.J., Wand, P.J. *et al.* (1980). Toxic-shock syndrome: epidemiologic features, recurrence, risk factors and prevention. *N. Engl. J. Med.* **303**, 1429.

Dawber, T.R., Moore, F.E., and Mann, G.V. (1957). Coronary heart disease in the Framingham Study. *Am. J. Public Health* **47**, 4.

Devesa, S.S. and Silverman, D.T. (1978). Cancer incidence and mortality trends in the United States: 1935–1974. *J. Natl. Cancer Inst.* **60**, 545.

Doll. R. and Hill, A.B. (1950). Smoking and carinoma of the lung: preliminary report. *Br. Med. J.* **ii**, 739.

Durrer, J.D., Lie, K.I., Van Capelle, F.J.L. *et al.* (1982). Effect of sodium nitroprusside on mortality in acute myocardial infarction. *N. Engl. J. Med.* **306**, 1121.

Feinstein, A.R. (1979). Methodologic problems and standards in case-control research. *J. Chronic Dis.* **32**, 35.

Feinstein, A.R., Horwitz, R.I., Spitzer, W.O. *et al.* (1981). Coffee and pancreatic cancer: the problems of etiologic science and epidemiologic case-control research. *JAMA* **246**, 957.

Fleiss, J.L. (1981). *Statistical methods for rates and proportions*, 2nd edn. Wiley, New York.

Gladen, B. and Rogan, W.J. (1979). Misclassification and the design of environmental studies. *Am. J. Epidemiol.* **109**, 607.

Gordon, T. (1974). Hazards in the use of the logistic function with special reference to data from prospective cardiovascular studies. *J. Chronic Dis.* **27**, 97.

Greenberg, R.S. and Osterhout, S.K. (1982). Seasonal trends in reported poisonings. *Am. J. Public Health* **72**, 394.

Greenland, S. (1979). Limitations of the logistic analysis of epidemiologic data. *Am. J. Epidemiol.* **110**, 693.

Gullen, W.H., Bearman, J.E., and Johnson, E.A. (1968). Effects of misclassification in epidemiologic studies. *Public Health Rep.* **53**, 1956.

Halpin, T.J., Holtzhauer, F.J., Campbell, R.J. *et al.* (1982). Reye's syndrome and medication use. *JAMA* **248**, 687.

Hayden, G.F., Kramer, M.S., and Horwitz, R.I. (1982). The case-control study: a practical review for the clinician. *JAMA* **247**, 326.

Herbst, A.L., Ulfelder, H., and Poskanzer, D.C. (1971). Adenocarcinoma of the vagina: association of maternal stilbestrol therapy with tumor appearance in young women. *N. Engl. J. Med.* **284**, 878.

Herrmann, N., Amsel, J., and Lynch, E. (1981). Obtaining hospital and physician participation in a case-control study of colon cancer. *Am. J. Pub. Health* **71**, 1314.

Horwitz, R.I. and Feinstein, A.R. (1978). Alternative analytic methods for case-control studies of estrogens and endometrial cancer. *N. Engl. J. Med.* **299**, 1089.

Horwitz, R.I. and Feinstein, A.R. (1979). Methodologic standards and contradictory results in case-control research. *Am. J. Med.* **66**, 556.

Horwitz, R.I. and Feinstein, A.R. (1980). The problem of 'protopathic bias' in case-control studies. *Am. J. Med.* **111**, 389.

Hutchison, G.B. and Rothman, K.J. (1978). Correcting a bias? *N. Engl. J. Med.* **299**, 1129.

Ibrahim, M.A. and Spitzer, W.O. (1979). The case-control study: The problem and the prospect. *J. Chronic Dis.* **32**, 139.

Illinois Department of Public Health (1975). *Poison Control Program report: 1974.* Released by the State of Illinois, July.

Jolliffe, N. and Archer, M. (1959). Statistical associations between international coronary heart disease death rates and certain environmental factors. *J. Chronic Dis.* **9**, 636.

Kleinbaum, D.G., Kupper, L.L., and Morgenstern, H. (1982). *Epidemiologic research: principles and quantitative methods.* Lifetime Learning Publications, Belmont, California.

Kleinbaum, D.G., Morgenstern, H., and Kupper, L.L. (1981). Selection bias in epidemiologic studies. *Am. J. Epidemiol.* **113**, 452.

Klemetti, A. and Saxen, L. (1967). Prospective versus retrospective approach in the search for environmental causes for malformations. *Am. J. Public Health* **57**, 2071.

Koch, M., McPherson, T.A., and Edgedahl, R.D. (1982). Effect of sex and reproductive history on the survival of patients with colorectal cancer. *J. Chronic Dis.* **35**, 69.

Kraus, A.S. (1960). Comparison of a group with a disease and a control group from the same families, in search for possible etiologic factors. *Am. J. Public health* **50**, 303.

Kupper, L.L., Karon, J.M., Kleinbaum, D.G. *et al.* (1981). Matching in epidemiologic studies: validity and efficiency considerations. *Biometrics* **37**, 271.

Labarthe, D.R. (1979). Methodologic variation in case-control studies of reserpine and breast cancer. *J. Chronic Dis.* **32**, 95.

Lilienfeld, A.M. and Lilienfeld, D.E. (1979). A century of case-control studies: progress? *J. Chronic Dis.* **32**, 5.

Lipids Research Clinics Program (1979). The coronary primary prevention trial: design and implementation. *J. Chronic Dis.* **32**, 609.

McKinley, S.M. (1977). Pair-matching – a reappraisal of a popular technique. *Biometrics* **33**, 725.

McMichael, A.J., Spirtas, R., and Kupper, L.L. (1974). An epidemiologic study of mortality within a cohort of rubber workers, 1964–72. *J. Occup. Med.* **16**, 458.

McMichael, A.J., Spirtas, R., Kupper, L.L. *et al.* (1975). Solvent exposure and leukemia among rubber workers: an epidemiologic study. *J. Occup. Med.* **17**, 234.

Mancuso, T.F. (1949). Occupational cancer survey in Ohio. *Proc. Public Health Cancer Assoc. Am.* **56**.

Mantel, N. and Fleiss, J.L. (1980). Minimum expected cell size requirements for the Mantel–Haenszel one-degree-of-freedom chi-square test and a related rapid procedure. *Am. J. Epidemiol.* **112**, 129.

Mantel, N. and Haenszel, W. (1959). Statistical aspects of the analysis of data from retrospective studies of disease. *J. Natl. Cancer Inst.* **22**, 719.

May, G.S., DeMets, D.L., Friedman, L.M. *et al.* (1981). The randomized clinical trial: bias in analysis. *Circulation* **64**, 669.

Miettinen, O.S. (1970). Matching and design efficiency in retrospective studies. *Am. J. Epidemiol.* **91**, 111.

Miettinen, O.S. (1976). Estimability and estimation in case-referent studies. *Am. J. Epidemiol.* **103**, 226.

Neyman, J. (1955). Statistics – servant of all sciences. *Science* **122**, 401.

Pasternack, B.S. and Shore, R.E. (1981). Sample sizes for group sequential cohort and case-control study designs. *Am. J. Epidemiol.* **113**, 182.

Pocock, S.J. (1977). Group sequential methods in the design and analysis of clinical trials. *Biometrika* **64**, 191.

Prentice, R. (1976). Use of the logistic model in retrospective studies. *Biometrics* **32**, 599.

Prentice, R.L. and Pyke, R. (1979). Logistic disease incidence models and case-control studies. *Biometrika* **66**, 403.

Press, S.J. and Wilson, J. (1978). Choosing between logistic regression and discriminant analysis. *J. Am. Stat. Assoc.* **73**, 699.

Radhakrishna. S. (1965). Combination of results from several $2 \times 2$ contingency tables. *Biometrics* **21**, 86.

Roberts, R.S., Spitzer, W.O., Delmore, T. *et al.* (1978). An empirical demonstration of Berkson's bias. *J. Chronic Dis.* **31**, 119.

Sackett, D.L. (1979). Bias in analytic research. *J. Chronic Dis.* **32**, 51.

Sartwell, P.E. (1974). Retrospective studies: a review for the clinician. *Ann. Intern. Med.* **81**, 381.

Schlesselman, J.J. (1982). *Case-control studies: design, conduct, analysis.* Oxford University Press, New York.

Schoenbaum, S.C., Biano, S., and Mack, T. (1975). Epidemiology of congenital rubella syndrome. *JAMA* **233**, 151.

Schuman, L.M. (1977). Patterns of smoking behavior. In *Research on smoking behavior* (ed. M.E. Jarvik, J.W. Cullen, E.R. Gritz, *et al.*) p. 36. Department of Health, Education, and Welfare. US Government Printing Office, Washington, DC.

Shy, C.M., Kleinbaum, D.G., and Morgenstern, H. (1978). The effect of misclassification of exposure status in epidemiological studies of air pollution health effects. *Bull. N.Y. Acad. Med.* **54**, 1155.

Silverberg, E. (1982). Cancer statistics, 1982. *Ca-A Cancer J. Clinic* **32**, 15.

Silverman, W.A. (1980). *Retrolental fibroplasia: a modern parable.* Grune and Stratton, New York.

Taylor, J.W. (1977). Simple estimation of population attributable risk from case-control studies. *Am. J. Epidemiol.* **106**, 260.

Thomas, D.G. (1971). Exact confidence limits for an odds ratio in a $2 \times 2$ table. *Appl. Stat.* **20**, 105.

Truett, J., Cornfield, J., and Kannel, W. (1967). A multivariate analysis of the risk of coronary heart disease in Framingham. *J. Chronic Dis.* **20**, 511.

Tyroler, H.A., Heyden, S., Bartel, A. *et al.* (1971). Blood pressure and cholesterol as coronary heart disease risk factors. *Arch. Intern. Med.* **128**, 907.

Ury, H.K. (1975). Efficiency of case-control studies with multiple controls per case: continuous or dichotomous data. *Biometrics* **31**, 643.

Walter, S.D. (1980). Berkson's bias and its control in epidemiologic studies. *J. Chronic Dis.* **33**, 721.

Woolf, B. (1955). On estimating the relation between blood group and disease. *Ann. Hum. Genet.* **19**, 251.

Yen, S., Hsieh, C.C., and MacMahon, B. (1982). Consumption of alcohol and tobacco and other risk factors for pancreatitis. *Am. J. Epidemiol.* **116**, 407.

# 9 Statistical methods

A. V. Swan

## INTRODUCTION

Statistical methods are required whenever groups of individuals, not entirely predictable in their characteristics or behaviour, need to be described or compared. A wide range of techniques have been developed and this text cannot cover them all. The most useful are known as regression techniques. This chapter will concentrate on statistical methods that can be considered under that heading. The material on case-control studies is dealt with more fully in a separate chapter.

The chapter is divided into six sections which can be regarded as a course in three parts. The first two sections after this introduction, 'Design and sampling' and 'Practical questions from a statistical point of view', provide a general survey of statistical ideas and practical problems. This is followed by a more advanced discussion of the underlying principles of statistical reasoning under the heading, 'Basic concepts'. The final part discusses in some detail the application of the statistical methods appropriate to the problems presented in the 'Practical questions' under the heading 'Types of analyses'.

The aim of the chapter as a whole is to give a clear picture of the range of problems that can be handled by statistical methods with a general appreciation of the methods and the underlying statistical concepts necessary for analyses using computer packages such as Minitab (Ryan *et al.* 1980) and GLIM (Baker and Nelder 1978). In addition more comprehensive details are provided for the special cases where the problem can be simplified sufficiently for the analysis to be done by hand.

## DESIGN AND SAMPLING

The statistical design of an investigation is determined by the form of analysis appropriate to answering the question of interest, the precision required, and the assumptions that appear justified. The practical question should indicate quite clearly what analyses are necessary. The design is then determined by what is necessary to make these analyses possible and sufficiently precise.

Circumstances and ethics may mean an *observational* study has to be used. That is, a study where subjects exposed to a variety of influences are simply observed. In such cases sampling is restricted to a process of choosing who enters the study. If the investigation is using previously collected data, for example, cardiovascular mortality figures from areas of differing water hardness, there is no sampling involved. If an *experiment* or *clinical trial* is possible then the sampling process also includes allocation to the groups to be compared. A comprehensive discussion of this and other aspects of clinical trials is given by Pocock (1984). Because it is often important to determine the most effective treatment as quickly as possible and minimize the number of patients receiving the other treatments, what are known as sequential trials with special allocation rules may be very useful. The subject is well covered by Armitage (1960).

In general sampling does not need to be complicated. Although it may be awkward in an administrative sense, the process is in principle straightforward. The first necessity is to decide on the population of interest and identify that part of the population that is accessible in practice. The sampling process is then applied to that subgroup of the population with due regard to the possibility that it is not properly representative of the whole. For the sampling process it is usually sufficient in both selection and allocation to use what is known as simple random sampling. This means any technique, such as 'tossing coins', 'drawing names from a hat', 'taking every tenth name on a list assumed to be in random order', etc., that gives every subject an equal chance of selection.

In practice the problem tends to be that of obtaining a list – called a sampling frame – of all the candidates for inclusion. In community health surveys in the UK a commonly used sampling frame is the electoral register.

For complex sampling problems it may be necessary to use random sampling numbers which are included in most sets of statistical tables (Lindley and Miller 1964). They usually consist of sequences of two-digit numbers, for example 87, 31, 47, 55, 56 . . . generated in such a way that in any reasonably long sequence the number of 0s, 1s, 2s, . . . 9s and consequently 00s, 01s, . . . 99s are the same. Each single digit will occur on average once in every ten digits and each double-digit combination once in every hundred pairs. For example, to allocate subjects to three groups in a trial a sequence of digits, ignoring the zeros, would be assigned, one at a time, to each of the subjects. Then taking the digits 1, 2, and 3 to represent group 1; the digits 4, 5, and 6 to represent group 2; and the digits 7, 8, and 9 to represent group 3 determines the allocation. Sometimes particular subgroups (essentially subpopulations) of individuals are of specific interest, for example, sex or age groups. In that case it may be appropriate to identify the individuals belonging to the groups – known as strata – and sample separately within each. This is known as stratified random sampling.

# PRACTICAL QUESTIONS FROM A STATISTICAL POINT OF VIEW

## Trends – routinely collected grouped data

It has been suggested that the 'hardness' of drinking water may affect the risk of an individual developing heart disease. The cardiovascular death rates and some measure of the water 'hardness' in each of a number of geographical areas (for a particular year) might give a picture as in Fig. 9.1. This is known as a scatter diagram.

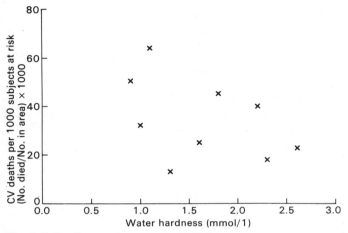

**Fig. 9.1.** Cardiovascular mortality (CV) by water hardness.

The question is: 'Does the risk of cardiovascular disease change according to the 'hardness' of the water you drink?' In terms of the pattern in the diagram the question becomes: 'What is the trend in this sample of points and does it reflect a real trend in all the points from other subjects, other years, and other areas that these points represent?'

The 'truth' were it possible to see it might be as in Fig. 9.2. The analysis is a process of determining which is the most likely 'truth'.

## Trends – individuals in an observational study

In an investigation of blood pressure and salt intake the question could be: 'Does an increase in salt intake increase systolic blood pressure?'

If it were possible to determine salt intake for a sample of individuals a plot of each individual might give a scatter diagram such as Fig. 9.3.

As before the question becomes: 'Is there a trend in these points consistent enough to suggest a real trend in the large population of points that this sample is taken to represent?'.

If data were available from men and women (Fig. 9.4), then the question would be more complicated. The relationship between systolic blood pressure and salt intake, such as it might be, could differ between the sexes. The initial question becomes several separate questions: (i) Are the trends in the populations of men and women represented by these samples different? (ii) Is either one, if they are different, non-horizontal? (iii) What are the trends?

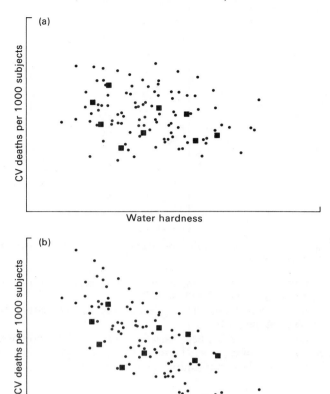

**Fig. 9.2.** Possible population patterns for cardiovascular death rates by water hardness. (a) No trend. (b) A negative trend.

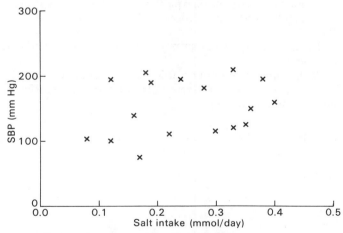

**Fig. 9.3.** Systolic blood pressure (SBP) against salt intake (simulated data).

There is also information with which to answer the questions: (a) At a given salt intake do the male and female populations differ on the systolic blood pressure scale? That is, at a given salt intake are the population points for the males higher or lower, on average, than those of the females? (b) Do the male and female populations differ with respect to salt intake? Or, in

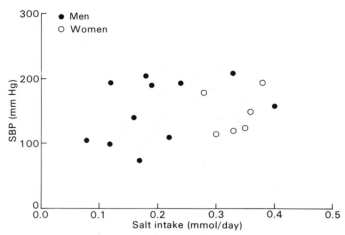

**Fig. 9.4.** Systolic blood pressure against salt intake in men and women (simulated data).

the population are the male and female points positioned differently on the salt intake scale?

Simply introducing another factor, sex, has considerably complicated the problem.

In practice it may be necessary to consider weight, exercise, age, and possibly other factors related to systolic blood pressure, and the complications multiply rapidly.

### Comparing groups of individuals

Investigations of air pollution and respiratory health encounter considerable problems in determining an individual's exposure. Often the design has to be a simple two group comparison of individuals living in an area of high pollution with those living in one of low pollution. Such a study might produce peak expiratory flow rate (PEFR) values from children in high and low pollution areas as shown in Fig. 9.5.

The question is: 'Does air pollution affect lung function in children?'

With some assumptions this can be phrased as: 'Do children in areas with different pollution levels have different lung function values on average?'.

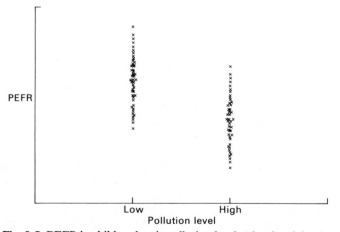

**Fig. 9.5.** PEFR in children by air pollution levels (simulated data).

On the plot this becomes: 'Do the heights of these two samples of points differ enough to suggest a difference between the populations they represent?'.

### Proportions from two categories of outcome

Frequently an all-or-nothing response such as presence or absence of a symptom will be the outcome measure of interest. The appropriate response scale is the proportion with the symptom, that is, the prevalence of the symptom. An investigation of pollution as above may be interested in the prevalence of morning cough in children from areas with different levels of pollution.

The question is: 'Does exposure to pollution increase the risk of a child developing morning cough?'. A plot of the prevalences against pollution level with the points joined by straight lines will generally give a line with a number of bends in it (Fig. 9.6).

The question becomes: 'Do these sample proportions differ enough to suggest that differences would be seen if the populations of all such children exposed to these pollution

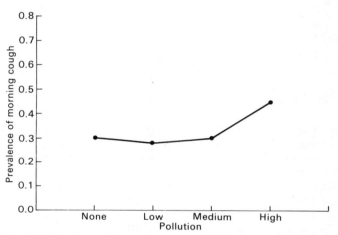

**Fig. 9.6.** Prevalence of morning cough in children against pollution level (simulated data).

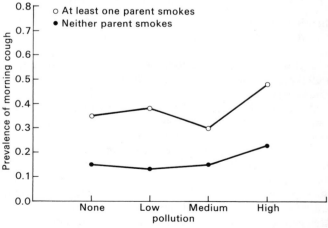

**Fig. 9.7.** Prevalence of morning cough in children against pollution level by parents' cigarette smoking habits (simulated data).

levels could be observed?'. In other words is the equivalent population line horizontal?

Information on parents smoking habits will give a plot of two lines (Fig. 9.7). There are now several questions: (i) Are the differences between the pollution groups in the population the same in the two parental smoking groups? That is, are the population lines parallel to each other? (ii) Are the population differences between the pollution groups non-zero in either parental smoking group? That is, is either population line non-horizontal? (iii) At a fixed pollution level is there a difference between the parental smoking groups in the population? That is, is there a vertical separation between the population lines?

### Proportions – case-control studies

In a study of sudden infant death syndrome various information was collected on all the infants dying this way in a particular area and period of time – these were the cases. The same information was collected on the same number of randomly selected control children born in the same period and still alive. Such studies are known as case-control or retrospective studies. The latter name arises because the study starts after the event of interest and consists of looking back in time at what preceded the event. The data are given in Table 9.1.

**Table 9.1.** *Cases of sudden infant death and controls by mother's age*

|  | Mother's age (years) | | | |
| --- | --- | --- | --- | --- |
|  | <20 | 20– | 25– | 30+ |
| Cases | 17 | 22 | 17 | 5 |
| Controls | 9 | 23 | 16 | 13 |
| Cases and Controls | 26 | 45 | 33 | 18 |
| *P* | 0.65 | 0.49 | 0.52 | 0.28 |

The question here is: 'Does the risk of sudden infant death change with the age of the mother?' It is not possible to obtain a direct estimate of this risk, which is that of an infant becoming a case (risk = no. of cases/no. at risk), because the number at risk is not known. However, with some assumptions – mainly that the sampling fraction for the controls (the proportion the sample is of the population) is the same for all the age groups – it is possible to manage without it. A proxy measure, the proportion, $p$ = cases/(cases + controls), is constructed and used to investigate the patterns in the data. These proportions are given in the last row of Table 9.1.

Plotted against the mid-point of the mothers' age group (Fig. 9.8) these proportions show a slightly negative trend with increasing mother's age.

If the controls were known to be 1 per cent of all possible controls, that is, a sampling fraction of 0.01, then the usual estimates of risk would be:

$$\frac{17}{17+900} \qquad \frac{22}{22+2300} \qquad \frac{17}{17+1600} \qquad \frac{5}{5\times1300}$$

or    0.0185    0.0095    0.0105    0.0038

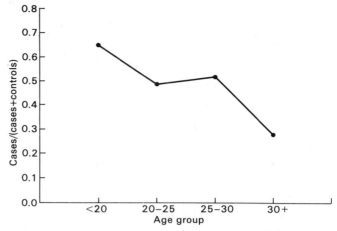

**Fig. 9.8.** Cases of sudden infant death as proportions cases/(cases + controls) by mother's age group.

These are much smaller than the proportions, but plotted give a line with practically the same shape.

The question then becomes: 'Does the line deviate from the horizontal more than could easily arise by chance if the equivalent population line is horizontal?'

### Three or more categories of outcome

A study of illness behaviour in women used, as a measure of depression, the number of positive responses to questions on 'loss of appetite', 'nerves', 'depression or irritability', 'sleeplessness', and 'undue tiredness'.

The numbers in the various depression categories by their marital state are given in Table 9.2. The question is: 'Does the pattern of depression in women differ according to their marital status?'

**Table 9.2.** *Classification of women by marital status and answers to questions related to depression*

| Marital status | No. of positive responses (%) | | | | |
| --- | --- | --- | --- | --- | --- |
|  | 0 | 1 | 2 | 3 or 4 | Total |
| Single | 17 (45) | 12 (32) | 7 (18) | 1 (5) | 38 (100) |
| Married | 51 (58) | 17 (19) | 12 (14) | 8 (9) | 88 (100) |
| Widowed or divorced | 8 (13) | 25 (42) | 11 (18) | 16 (27) | 60 (100) |

Statistically, as a deduction from the sample to the population, the question becomes: 'Is the proportional distribution among the depression categories in the population of all such women the same for each marital status?'.

That is, are the 38 single women distributed among the depression categories in the same proportions, apart from differences which could arise from sampling variation, as the 88 married and the 60 widowed or divorced? The proportional allocation can be seen more easily if the frequencies are expressed as percentages of the total in that particular marital status group (Table 9.2).

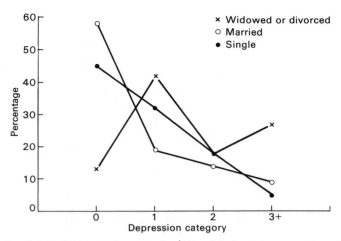

**Fig. 9.9.** Percentage of women in each marital status group plotted against depression category.

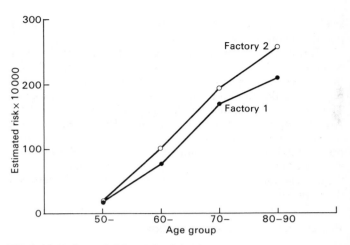

**Fig. 9.10.** Estimated risks of death against age by factory.

**Table 9.3.** *Mortality from all causes and estimated risk of death from any cause per man per year by age group and factory*

| Age at start of study (years) | Factory 1 | | | Factory 2 | | |
|---|---|---|---|---|---|---|
| | Numbers dying | (Man years at risk) | Estimated risk of death | Numbers dying | (Man years at risk) | Estimated risk of death |
| 50–59.9 | 7 | (4045) | 0.0017 | 7 | (3701) | 0.0019 |
| 60–69.9 | 27 | (3571) | 0.0076 | 37 | (3702) | 0.0100 |
| 70–79.9 | 30 | (1771) | 0.0169 | 35 | (1818) | 0.0193 |
| 80–89.9 | 8 | (381) | 0.0210 | 9 | (350) | 0.0257 |

Figure 9.9 gives a plot of the percentage frequencies as a separate line for each marital status group. If the proportional allocation to the depression categories were the same these lines would fall on top of one another.

So the question becomes: 'Are these lines, obtained from a sample, more different than could easily arise by chance if the three equivalent population lines are really identical?'.

### Survival data

This general title is used to cover data which arise when the interest is in the risk of some event occurring. The event may be death, but it need not be, and survival data techniques are appropriate for comparing the chances of remission for patients on different treatments and other such events.

The first example considered annual mortality in relatively large groups of people. The usual analyses for data of that type assume that all subjects were at risk of the event for the whole period. However, if someone dies halfway through the year they have only been at risk for half a year. With large numbers and small risks the numbers observed for only part of the period are small and ignoring the problem does little harm. When the numbers in the groups to be compared are relatively small the times at risk must be taken into account.

If it can be assumed that, within each group of subjects to be compared, each individual is running the same risk throughout the chosen time period this is relatively straightforward. The period of time each individual was observed are summed over all the individuals in the group. If the period of time is a year and the times at risk are expressed as fractions of a year this gives the number of 'man years at risk' (obviously it may at other times be necessary to use 'woman years at risk', 'patient weeks at risk' and so on).

The estimate of the annual risk of death (or other event) is then simply:

The no. of deaths/The no. of man years at risk.

In an occupational health study of cancer, groups of current and ex-workers in two industrial environments were observed for a number of years. The overall mortality is as given in Table 9.3.

The initial question is: 'Is the risk of death from any cause different in the two environments?'.

The estimated risks per man per year are given in Table 9.3 and Fig. 9.10 shows the estimated risks plotted against age.

The question becomes: 'Are these lines surprisingly far apart if the equivalent lines in the population represented by this sample of individuals are identical?'.

The techniques for answering this question are essentially the same as those for the previous examples.

When risks are changing during the period of observation techniques assuming one overall risk are inappropriate. To illustrate survival data of this sort, survival curves are used. These are plots of the percentage in a group still surviving against time elapsed since some defined starting point such as date of entry to the study.

Data of this type arose from a clinical trial comparing radiotherapy with hormone treatment for cancer of the prostate. The question was: 'Which is the better treatment?'

This is not at all a simple question. The treatment giving the greater chance of survival at five years (say) is not necessarily the treatment which gives the longest life expectancy. It is necessary to look at the relative shapes of the survival curves. During the trial 44 patients received radiotherapy and 48 hormone treatment. The survival curves for the two groups are shown in Fig. 9.11.

There is some divergence of the curves and the question becomes: 'Do the curves for the population represented by these samples differ?'.

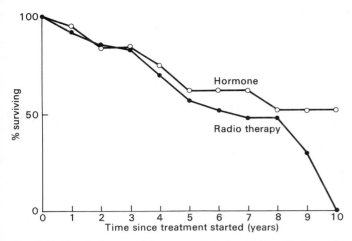

**Fig. 9.11.** Survival curves for cancer of the prostate patients receiving radiotherapy or hormone treatment.

Or in other words: 'Are these sample curves too different to have easily arisen by chance sampling from populations with identical survival curves?'.

## BASIC CONCEPTS

Because individuals subject to biological variation are to some extent unpredictable in their characteristics and behaviour, factual statements concerning them take the form:

Individuals like 'this', treated like 'this', tend to respond like 'this'.

The *individuals* are the items being observed. They may, for example, be patients, tissue samples, rats, or geographical areas. They may even be the same patient observed at different times, for example when a sequence of separate blood samples are taken or results obtained from a repeatedly administered psychiatric test.

The 'individuals like this' make up the *population* in the statistical sense. That is, any strictly defined group of individuals.

The human population of a country may be the statistical population of interest, but it will usually be a sample of the general population of all such humans who might exist now or in the future. Researchers in London will want to be able to generalize their findings beyond Londoners and will generally wish to conclude that the results apply to all such patients in Britain now and possibly in the future.

The population should be defined before the study begins and the sample chosen accordingly. Practical circumstances, however, can have a considerable effect on the sampling. This makes it necessary for the researcher to indicate how and with what qualification results from a sample apply to a particular population. In addition most studies will involve individuals from identifiable subpopulations. For example, studies involving physical characteristics such as lung function which may differ systematically between the sexes require that results are obtained separately for the two samples representing the subpopulations male and female. If that is not done, and the findings in the two samples not shown to be consistent, it is not safe to combine all the data to arrive at a general conclusion.

This implies that if there are two subpopulations which may differ in respects important to the study in question then data must be collected to identify from which subpopulation each individual arose. These subpopulation-defining characteristics or variables, such as sex, age, social class, and so on, are often a nuisance. It is not usually necessary, for example, to study how the sexes differ – this is mostly known. It is necessary in order to confirm that the effects of interest are consistently found in all the subpopulations. If this can be assumed at the beginning, studies can be simplified by restricting them to, for example, one sex or one age group, an option that is always worth considering at the design stage. Generally, however, data must be collected on individuals from a number of subpopulations.

Clinial trials are studies of subjects who have been 'treated' in some way which must be defined and possibly measured, for example, as a dose. In most trials two or more groups receiving different treatments will be compared and so from one individual to another the treatment, type or dosage may vary. The treatment is therefore a variable and will be represented in the data collected during the trial by numerical values identifying either or both the type of treatment and the dosage.

Observational studies of naturally occurring 'experiments' may be concerned with assessing the effect on individuals of some experience or exposure to some aspect of the environment. As for a treatment, it is necessary to define and measure the experience or exposure. Again it must be represented by a variable with numerical values.

To assess the manner in which individuals treated in some way or undergoing some experience 'tend to respond', requires a variable to measure or classify the response. This is the response or outcome variable. Furthermore, because they will vary in a random way even among individuals from a homogeneous population in which all are treated in the same way these variables are known as random variables. The way in which they vary is described by the distribution of their values in the sample and by inference in the populations.

### Types of variables

Which analytical approach to use largely depends on the nature of the response variable. There are two main categories *quantitative* and *qualitative*.

*Quantitative* variables have an obvious associated scale on which distances have a clear interpretation. They can arise in two forms, continuous or discrete. Continuous variables are generally measurements and every value within some sensible range is possible, for example, serum cholesterol or PEFR. Discrete variables are generally counts where only certain values on the scale are possible, such as number of previous heart attacks or number of schistosome eggs in a stool sample.

*Qualitative* variables are those associated with a set of categories. The categories may have a natural ordering as in severity of a condition, category of remission, social class and so on. These are known as ordinal variables and although they have to be treated as categories they are usually interpretable as sections of an underlying scale. Categories such as blood group and type of health services contact do not have an order and are termed nominal variables.

### Functions of variables

The function of response variables is clear. They provide the 'yardstick' on which the effects of treatment or experience are measured. However, variables are also used to identify the subpopulation to which an individual belongs so that an analysis can assess and allow for differences between subpopulations. They are also used to measure or classify treatment or experience.

There is no obvious general term for these last two classes of variables. They are sometimes called 'predictor' variables because studies are often concerned with how well they predict outcome or response. They may also be referred to as independent variables because the analysis is essentially assessing how response or outcome depends on their values. Obviously in this terminology the response variable is known as the dependent variable.

Perhaps the simplest terminology of all, following mathematical conventions, classes the treatment, exposure and subpopulation variables all of which tend to appear on the horizontal axis of graphical plots, as *x*-variables. The response variables generally appear on the vertical axis of such plots and are known as *y*-variables.

### Describing data patterns – models

A model is simply an algebraic formula for describing some pattern or structure in variable data.

Consider the relationship between forced expiratory volume in one second ($FEV_1$) and height in a sample of students (Fig. 9.12). There is a tendency for the taller individuals to have the larger FEVs. If the individuals are grouped on the height scale, for example, all individuals with heights between 62 and 64 are treated as if they were 63 in,

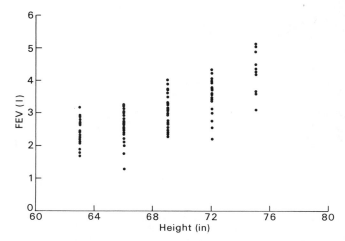

**Fig. 9.13.** FEV (l/min) in young adults by height groups.

those between 65 and 67 as if they were 66 in, and so on, the plot becomes a set of separate groups of points (Fig. 9.13.).

For each height group there is an array or distribution of FEV values. These are known as conditional distributions. They are the distributions of FEV values conditional on the individuals concerned all having the same height (or in this case being in the same height group). It can now be seen that the trend in FEV values is a systematic tendency for these conditional distributions to move up as height increases. The distributions overlap, but their centres are located at a generally higher position in the taller height groups. It is not easy to describe the behaviour of the individual points, but it is possible to be reasonably precise about the relative positioning or location of the conditional distributions. The models to describe this sort of pattern have the form:

Location of distribution = Reference value + Horizontal
position effect

The behaviour of individual points has to be described in terms of the location of their particular distribution and the way in which they are dispersed or spread about that location.

In Fig. 9.13 the data were grouped to show the conditional distributions, but this is wasteful of information. Some method is needed to describe the trend in the raw data.

The simplest model is a straight-line trend. This model assumes that the height or *x*-variable effect is a steady increase (or decrease) in the FEV or *y*-variable distribution locations usually represented by the arithmetic mean defined below. That is to say that for each unit change in height there is the same change in mean FEV at all points on the height axis. The model for this is:

Mean FEV = Reference value + Change/unit ht × Height

This is known as a regression line model. In more general terms it becomes:

$$y = a + bx$$

which is the equation representing a straight line on a plot of *y* against *x* (in this case FEV against height) shown in Fig. 9.14, where *a* is known as the intercept which is the height of the line

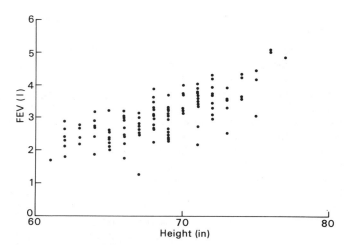

**Fig. 9.12.** Forced expiratory volume (l/min) in young adults by height in inches.

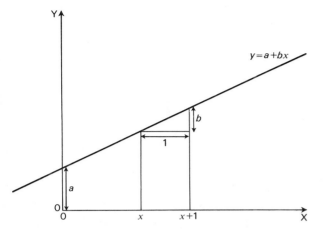

**Fig. 9.14.** Diagrammatic representation of the straight line regression model $y = a + bx$.

when $x = 0$ and $b$ is the slope of the line called the regression coefficient. Force expiratory volume at zero height makes no practical sense but it makes the algebra simpler to represent the regression line by:

$$FEV = Intercept + b \times Height$$

Finding the 'best' straight line to describe a trend means estimating the appropriate intercept and slope and is known as fitting the regression line. The possibilities are infinite. Any value of $a$ and $b$ are, in theory, possible. The problem is to define what is the 'best' line to describe a set of data and then to deduce the values of $a$ and $b$ which give this 'best' line as functions of the data values.

In practice the 'best' fitting line is defined by the 'principle of least squares'. This principle can be illustrated by considering a general line on a scatter diagram with $a$ and $b$ unspecified (Fig. 9.15). Each point deviates from the line (in the $y$ direction) by some amount. The principle of least squares states that, the 'best' line is the one which makes the 'sum of all the deviations squared' as small as possible. This means that $a$ and $b$ must be chosen to make the sum of all the $d^2$s a minimum. Using this principle it is possible to deduce

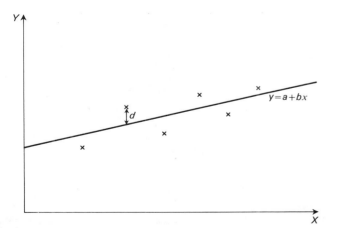

**Fig. 9.15.** Deviations of data points from the model $y = a + bx$.

mathematically how to calculate the appropriate values from the data. The mathematics provides standard formulae with which the appropriate $a$ and $b$ can be calculated for any set of data.

Before further discussion of how models are defined and used it is necessary to consider how to define and measure the important characteristics of the distributions whose relative positioning they are used to describe and test.

**The characteristics of distributions**

The characteristics of the distributions represented by the arrays of points in Fig. 9.13 are not at all clear. Their location can be judged to some extent but how the individuals are dispersed about the central location cannot be seen so easily. Single distributions are better displayed as histograms.

To represent a sample as a histogram the scale is divided into intervals of equal length and the points within an interval drawn on top of one another as shown in Fig. 9.16. Points falling where two intervals join could go in either, but for graphical techniques it does not really matter. Usually they are allocated to the higher interval.

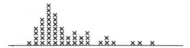

**Fig. 9.16.** Representing a sample of values as a histogram.

The shape is rather 'ragged' but one can see, in addition to its location and spread, that the distribution is rather asymmetrical. There is a longer 'tail' on the high-value or positive side. Such distributions are called skew and since skewness can affect the analysis some method is needed to detect and measure it. There are specific measures of skewness, but they are rarely necessary in practice. Graphical techniques are usually adequate to detect whether it is present to an extent that matters. Location and dispersion on the other hand require precise measures and on occasion a complete numerical specification of the distribution is required for which centiles (sometimes referred to as percentiles) are used.

*Measures of location*

There are three commonly used measures of location:
*The arithmetic mean.* This is the sum of all the values in a distribution or a sample divided by the number of values. It is by far the most useful measure of location and is usually referred to simply as the mean. For a sample it is:

$$Mean = Sum\ of\ all\ values/Number\ of\ values$$

*The median.* This is the variable value such that half the values in a distribution are above it and half below. It is easy to find and useful for simple descriptions of asymmetrical distributions. It is not however very easy to handle in more complex analyses.

*The mode.* This is the value in a distribution that occurs most frequently. It is of occasional use for describing single distributions.

### Measures of dispersion

There are a multitude of these in the literature, but only a few are commonly used.

*The range.* This is the distance, on the scale of measurement, between the highest and lowest values. It is occasionally used for describing the spread of small samples. Obviously, as sample sizes increase the range will automatically increase and, since it depends on the least characteristic pair of individuals in the sample, its usefulness is limited.

*The variance and standard deviation.* The variance is a direct measure of spread about the arithmetic mean. For a sample it is defined as:

Sum for all values of (value −mean value)²/(No. of values − 1).

Notice that 'squaring' the deviations of values from their mean ensures that negative deviations from low values do not cancel out with those from high values.

For the population, usually defined so generally that the size is infinite, the variance cannot be calculated in this way. It is defined as the value approached by the calculated value as the sample size increases indefinitely.

Because the variance is an average squared deviation it is not in the original units of the variable in question. For this reason its square root the standard deviation (sd) is frequently more useful. This gives quite an accurate measure of how far from the mean individuals are likely to occur in a given distribution. Unless a distribution is very asymmetrical, individuals more than three sds from the mean will only occur very rarely and most (approximately 95 per cent) of individuals will fall within two sds of the mean.

### Centiles

These are points on the variable scale that exceed a specified percentage of the distribution. Consider a sample of 10 systolic blood pressure values with the distribution in Table 9.4. Ten per cent (one value) of the sample is below 110 mm Hg and that is therefore the 10th centile. Seven values (70 per cent) are below 130 mm Hg so that is the 70th centile and so on. However, this approach only gives the centiles that occur at the ends of the intervals. Considering the sample as a representative of a much larger population it is possible to go a bit further by plotting the cumulative frequency, as a percentage, against the upper ends of the intervals (Fig. 9.17). It is far from smooth, but various centiles may be deduced by estimating where the 'curve' reaches the equivalent height on the per cent cumulative frequency scale. This method estimates the 50th centile, which is the median, as 125 mm

**Table 9.4.** *Frequency distribution of a sample of 10 adult males according to their systolic blood pressures*

| Systolic blood pressure (mm Hg) | Frequency of values | Cumulative total |
|---|---|---|
| from 100 to just under 110 | 1 | 1 |
| from 110 to just under 120 | 2 | 3 |
| from 120 to just under 130 | 4 | 6 |
| from 130 to just under 140 | 2 | 9 |
| from 140 to just under 150 | 0 | 9 |
| from 160 to just under 170 | 1 | 10 |

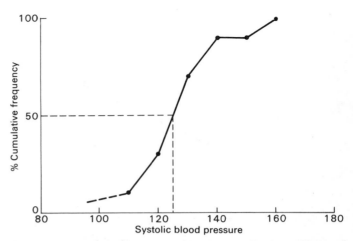

**Fig. 9.17.** Cumulative frequency plot of a sample of systolic blood pressure values.

Hg. For more precise estimates a smooth curve could be drawn through the points. Alternatively, assumptions about the shape of the population curve may be made and the appropriate estimates deduced mathematically. To understand that process it is necessary to consider in detail how sample distributions and their characteristics relate to those of the population.

### Inferring the truth – sample to population

#### Distributions

Consider a sequence of histograms obtained from larger and larger samples of an infinite population (Fig. 9.18). As the sample size increases the distributions becomes smoother with a more clearly defined shape. As the sample size is increased indefinitely (with the vertical scale reduced appropriately) the shape tends to a smooth curve. For many biological variables this will be close to a symmetrical 'bell-shaped' distribution known as the normal distribution which can be defined in precise mathematical terms.

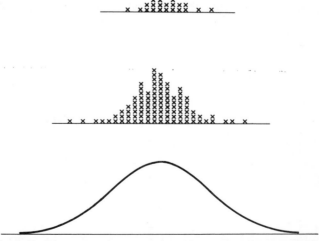

**Fig. 9.18.** Histograms from samples of increasing size approaching a smooth population curve.

## Probabilities

In the sample of 10 systolic blood pressures (Table 9.4), two out of 10 were in the range 110 to 120 mm Hg. The proportion of the sample between 110 and 120 mm Hg is therefore /10, that is 0.2. If the names of the 10 individuals were written on pieces of paper, mixed up in a 'hat' and then one picked at random the probability that it was an individual in the range 110 to 120 would be 2/10 (0.2). There are two of the sort required and 10 in total.

The probability of selecting an individual with a systolic blood pressure less than 100 mm Hg from this 'hat' is 0/10, that is, zero or impossible. The probability of one with a pressure less than 180 is 10/10, that is 1.0 or certain. Notice that 120 is the 30th centile and the probability of an individual below 120 is 0.3 or 30 per cent. The probability of an individual below the 15th centile is 0.15 or 15 per cent and so on.

From the probability of selecting an individual below a particular point it is possible to deduce the probability of an individual on or above that point. There are three of the 10 individuals below 120 which gives the probability of such an individual as 0.3. There are seven of the 10 equal to or greater than 120, that is a probability of 0.7. Thus probability (value > 120) is:

$$\frac{\text{No.} \geqslant 120}{\text{Total no.}} = \frac{10 - \text{No.} < 120}{\text{Total no.}} = \frac{10 - 3}{10} = 7/10 \text{ or } (10 - 3)/10.$$

The probability of an individual being greater than or equal to some value is one minus the probability of being less than that value:

$$p(\text{value} \geqslant 120) = 1 - p(\text{value} < 120)$$

For example:

$$p(<110) = 1/10 = 0.1.$$
$$p(\geqslant 110) = 9/10 = 1 - p(<110) = 0.9$$

and so on.

As sample sizes increase and the histogram approaches the smooth population curve, the numbers become indefinitely large. However, the area above an interval and beneath the curve is in the same ratio to the total area as the number in that interval to the total number. In practice, population distributions are scaled so the curve encloses an area exactly equal to one. This means that the area above any interval is the proportion of individuals with values in that interval. This in turn is the probability that an individual picked at random has a value in that particular interval. So, if the area of the population distribution between two values 110 and 120 is 0.15 then the probability of an individual picked at random from this population having a systolic blood pressure between 110 and 120 is 0.15 (Fig. 9.19).

The probability that an individual selected at random has a value >150 is the area A under the curve from 150 upwards. Since A is 0.1 it means that 10 per cent of the population will have systolic blood pressures of 150 or above.

The area below 150 is 1 − A so the probability of an individual below 150 is 1 − A or 0.9. This means that the remaining 90 per cent of individuals have systolic blood pressures

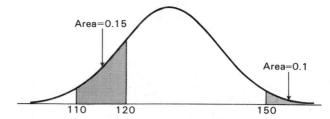

**Fig. 9.19.** Areas of the population distribution as probabilities.

below 150. Consequently 150 is the 90th centile of the population distribution.

The centiles of the population can be obtained as long as there is some way of obtaining the areas under the population distribution curve. Representing the tenth centile of the variable $y$ as $y_{0.1}$ the area below $y_{0.1}$ is 0.1, the area below $y_{0.2}$ is 0.2 and so on.

## The normal distribution

For various reasons random variables that appear to follow this distribution are common in nature – for example, human height, haemoglobin levels, systolic blood pressure. Others can be made to follow a normal distribution by a transformation of their scale. Possibly even more important is the fact that for all but the smallest samples averages are themselves variables from approximately normal distributions whatever the distributions of the original values. Because of this and its amiable mathematical nature the normal distribution holds a central place in statistical theory and practice.

The theoretical normal distribution is completely specified by its mean and variance. The distribution is symmetrical about the mean and areas beneath the curve can be obtained mathematically. It is known for example that if the variable is $y$ then the 2.5 centile:

$$y_{0.025} = \text{mean} - 1.96 \text{ sd}$$

This implies that in a normal distribution only 2.5 per cent of the individuals will be more than 1.96 sds below the mean. Similarly only 2.5 per cent will be more than 1.96 sds above it. Combining these it further implies that the range of values:

$$\text{mean} - 1.96 \text{ sd to mean} + 1.96 \text{ sd}$$

will include 95 per cent of individuals in the population and exclude only 5 per cent.

The normal distribution is so useful that the percentage cumulative frequencies for the standard distribution, which has mean = 0 and variance = 1 have been widely tabulated (Lindley and Miller 1964). From these the equivalent values for a normal variable with any mean and variance can be deduced.

The tabled values are the areas under the mathematically defined population distribution curve below the given values of the standard normal variable $u$ (say) as in Fig. 9.20.

The area $P_0$, in Fig. 9.20, is the percentage cumulative frequency at $u_0$ which is the probability of a value below $u_0$, that is:

$$p(\text{value} < u_0) = P_0$$

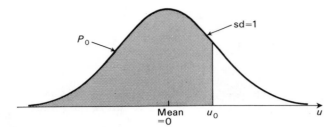

**Fig. 9.20.** Probabilities and the standardized normal distribution curve.

The probability of a value at or above $u_0$ is:

$$p\,(\text{value} > u_0) = 1 - P_0$$

and the probability of a value between $u_0$ and $u_1$ is;

$$p\,(u_0 < \text{value} < u_1) = P_1 - P_0$$

where $P_1$ is the area under the curve below $u_1$.

The variable $u$ is effectively the nunber of sds a value is from the mean. For variables with a different mean and variance, equivalent probabilities are deduced by calculating how many sds each value is from its mean and treating these as values of $u$.

For example, suppose systolic blood pressure in adult males is normally distributed with mean 130 and sd 15. To calculate the probability of an individual value less than 160 mm Hg note that this is 30 mm Hg, i.e. two sds above the mean. This implies that:

$$p\,(\text{value} < 160) = p\,(u < 2)$$

and since from tables:

$$p\,(u < 2) = 0.977$$

it can be deduced that

$$p\,(\text{value} < 160) = 0.977$$

and the required probability is 97.7 per cent.

With knowledge of the population distribution these techniques allow the probabilities of individual sample values to be deduced.

However, the problem is really in the opposite direction. The need is to deduce the population characteristics from the sample values. A method is required to assess how close sample values such as the mean are to the unknown population equivalents.

This is done by considering how the values of a sample estimate might vary if further samples were taken from the same population. Each sample will differ and estimates from them will vary.

### Estimation and sampling distributions

It is simplest to start by considering how the sample mean varies in a sequence of samples all taken the same way from the same population. The result can be generalized to any estimate, for example, a regression coefficient, a difference between means, etc. calculated from a sample. Suppose a sequence of samples of four values ($n = 4$) is taken from the systolic blood pressure distribution and the mean calculated

for each. These sample means will themselves have a distribution which, because it can only arise as a result of repeated sampling, is known as a *sampling distribution*. In this distribution of means samples with all values at one extreme of the population distribution will be rare. As a result the sample means will be more tightly clustered about the population mean than the individual observations. In addition, as long as the sampling was properly random the mean of the sampling distribution will be the same as the population mean. Because of this the sample mean is said to be an unbiased estimate of the population mean. It can be shown in fact that if the sampling is repeated indefinitely the sampling distribution of the mean will tend to a smooth curve with the same mean as the population of individual values, but a smaller standard deviation. In fact, it can be shown mathematically that this standard deviation of the mean is:

$$\text{sd (mean SBP)} = \text{sd (SBP)}/\sqrt{\text{sample size } n}$$

So for samples of size 4 and sd = 15:

$$\text{sd (mean SBP)} = 15/\sqrt{4} = 15/2 = 7.5$$

half the spread of the population.

Remember the complete sampling distribution only exists in theory. In practice there is only a single sample mean which is one observation from the distribution.

The narrower the spread of this distribution the nearer the single value available is likely to be to the truth. This spread represented by the standard deviation of the sampling distribution indicates how precise a single sample mean is as an estimate. It indicates the likely error in the estimate. Largely because of this the standard deviations of sampling distributions are almost universally referred to as standard errors:

$$\text{se (mean)} = \text{sd (mean)} = \text{sd (original variable)}/\sqrt{n}$$

Thus the standard error of a mean (or of any other estimate) indicates its precision as an estimate. For samples of 100 values ($n = 100$) the sample means would have had a standard deviation of 15/10 or 1.5, a very small spread. The estimate can be made as precise as required by increasing the sample size.

So the standard error of a sample mean is:

$$\begin{aligned} \text{se (mean)} &= \text{sd (original variable)}/\sqrt{(\text{sample size})} \\ &= \text{sd}/\sqrt{n} \end{aligned} \tag{9.1}$$

which can be deduced mathematically by the application of some fairly general rules. The same techniques can be used to deduce the standard errors of regression coefficients, differences between means and so on. In fact for any value calculated from a sample appropriate standard errors can be obtained.

### Confidence intervals

Although the estimate is chosen as the 'best guess' at the population value it will not usually be exactly right. In practice the standard error and the estimate are used to obtain a range of values defining an interval on the original variable scale which will contain the unknown population value with some chosen probability.

Fortunately for reasonably large samples ($n > 30$) and some fairly mild assumptions the sampling distributions of many common estimates are close to normal. This means, for example, that the sample value will only fall outside the range:

True value $- 1.96$ ses   to   true value $+ 1.96$ ses

for 5 per cent of such samples. With some algebra it follows that the interval:

estimate $- 1.96$ ses   to   estimate $+ 1.96$ ses

will include the true population value in 95 per cent of such samples. This means that one can be 95 per cent confident that an interval calculated in this way will include the true population value. Other confidence intervals such as 99 per cent are obtained by taking, instead of 1.96, the appropriate centile of the standard normal distribution.

These calculations need the population standard deviation of the original variable. Since this is rarely known it is necessary to use the sample value as an estimate. This does not matter very much for large samples, but if the sample size falls below about $n = 30$ it may. As a result for small samples the standard normal distribution cannot be used. It is necessary to use what is known as the '$t$' distribution. The centiles of the normal distribution, such as $|u_{0.975}| = 1.96$, have to be replaced by the equivalent centiles of the '$t$' distribution appropriate to the sample size. None the less the appropriate 97.5 centiles are all close to 2. These centiles are commonly denoted by $t_{f, 0.975}$ where $f$ is known as the degrees of freedom and represents the amount of information available to estimate the population sd used in the calculation of the standard error. The degrees of freedom are invariably the total sample size less the number of values estimated from the sample. From tables (Lindley and Miller 1964) it can be seen that:

$$t_{20, 0.975} = 2.09$$
$$t_{30, 0.975} = 2.04$$
$$t_{40, 0.975} = 2.02$$
$$t_{60, 0.975} = 2.00$$
and $\qquad t_{240, 0.975} = 1.96 = u_{0.975}$

so as the degrees of freedom increases beyond 240, the '$t$' distribution becomes the same as the normal distribution.

## Sample sizes for estimation

The sample size for an estimation is determined by the precision required. The usual approach to defining precision is to stipulate that there should be a high probability (often 95 per cent) that the estimate is close to the true value. Close is usually defined as within some small percentage such as 5 per cent of the correct value. Clearly this means that the approximate size of the value being estimated must be known.

Consider the problem of estimating a population mean from a sample. Ninety five per cent of means from unbiased samples will be within 1.96 standard errors of the true value. This implies that if $1.96 \times$ se is less than 5 per cent of the true value the precision will be as specified.

If $M$ represents the value to be estimated then the sample will be large enough if:

$$1.96 \times \text{sd}/\sqrt{n} \leqslant 0.05 \times M$$

i.e. if:

$$n \geqslant (1.96)^2 \times \text{sd}^2/(0.05 \times M)^2 \qquad (9.2)$$

With this sample size one can be 95 per cent confident that the estimate will be within 5 per cent of the truth.

### Example

To estimate the mean systolic blood pressure for men between 30 and 60 years old to within 5 per cent with 95 per cent confidence. From previous work it is known that the true value ($M$) is about 150 mm Hg and that the standard deviation is about 15.

Using eqn. 9.2 this means that the sample size needs to be:

$$n \geqslant (1.96 \times 15)^2/(0.05 \times 150)^2 = 16$$

This is very small so 5 per cent in this context is not a very stringent requirement. Requiring a higher degree of precision, for example, that the estimate must be accurate to 1 per cent implies a sample size of:

$$n \geqslant (1.96 \times 15)^2/(0.01 \times M)^2 = 400$$

### Significance tests

The probability of a sample 95 per cent confidence interval not containing the true population value is less than or equal to 5 per cent. This means that for any hypothetical population value it is possible to judge whether the sample estimate is surprisingly far from it by seeing whether it falls outside the 95 per cent confidence interval. If a value hypothesized for the population falls outside the interval then the probability of the sample giving this interval and hence the estimate – assuming the population value correct – is less than 5 per cent so:

$$p \text{ (estimate} \quad \text{population value)} \leqslant 0.05$$

or as it is frequently written ($p < 0.05$).

A significance test is a procedure which can be applied, assuming that the hypothesis to be tested is true, to the calculation of the probability ($p$) of sample values as far or further from those expected. Some value, called a test statistic which has a known sampling distribution is calculated from the sample. This is frequently the number of standard errors an estimate is from the population value expected from the hypothesis. The $p$ value can then be obtained from the sampling distribution of the test statistic. If the $p$ value is less than 5 per cent then the sample value is taken as evidence significant at the 5 per cent level that the hypothesis is untrue.

In 5 per cent of tests using a 5 per cent significance level, surprising values of the test statistic will occur even though the hypothesis is correct. This error, of concluding that an hypothesis is not true when it is, is known as a type I error. Therefore, if a test uses a 5 per cent level of significance there will be a 5 per cent risk in the test of a type I error. Notice that the risk may be set as required in a test by altering the level of significance to be used. Finally there is a risk that even when the hypothesis is false, samples may be obtained which produce unsurprising values of the test statistic. This leads to the error of accepting as true a hypothesis which is actually false. This is a type II error. The size of sample needed to give a reliable test of some hypothesis must take both types of error into account. Sample size calculations for significance testing are discussed in a later section.

There is a close relationship between confidence interval calculations and significance tests. Any hypothesis that predicts a population value can be tested by inspecting whether the value falls inside the appropriate confidence interval. Using the 99 per cent confidence interval this is equivalent to $p < 0.01$.

Suppose a study is estimating the population mean systolic blood pressure for adult males. For a large sample ($n > 30$) with mean 120 mm Hg and standard error 2.0 the 95 per cent confidence interval is:

$$120 \pm 1.96 \times 2.0 \text{ or } 116.1 \text{ to } 123.9.$$

The probability of results as extreme as 120 if the true value is 130 is less than 5 per cent since 130 is well outside the interval. The estimate 120 mm Hg is significantly different from 130 mm Hg at the 5 per cent level, it is surprisingly far from the population value of 130 ($p < 0.05$). It is reasonably clear that the sample is from a population with a lower mean value than 130 mm Hg. However, it must be remembered that by definition 5 per cent of the confidence intervals will exclude the true value. This is the type I error above. If this system is used to take decisions they will be wrong 5 per cent of the time.

Although the use of confidence intervals is quite sufficient it is common to calculate the $p$ values directly. As implied above this is most frequently done by calculating, as a test statistic, how many standard errors separate the estimate and the hypothetical value

$$\frac{\text{estimate} - \text{hypothetical value}}{\text{se of the estimate}}$$

What centile this is of the '$t$' or standard normal distribution is then determined from tables which for a given value of the variable give the probability of values below it say $P$.

The probability of values equal to or above that obtained is then $1 - P$ which is the probability of surprisingly high values. Surprisingly low values will also be possible so the probability of values as surprising as that observed will be twice $1 - P$ or:

$$p = 2(1 - P).$$

These are the basic concepts of statistics. It is now necessary to consider how these techniques are used to answer practical questions from real data.

## TYPES OF ANALYSES

### Measured outcomes

#### Simple regression

Figure 9.21 shows some data on chromosome abnormalities and blood lead levels from female workers in a battery factory.

The research question was: 'Does lead exposure damage chromosomes?'.

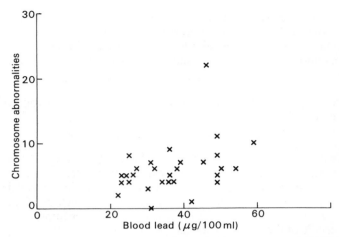

**Fig. 9.21.** Chromosome abnormalities per 100 cells and blood lead levels. (Source: Forni *et al.* (1975).)

If it is assumed that current lead levels in the blood reflect overall exposure then the question can be expressed as: 'In the population of all such subjects as these is the number of chromosome abnormalities higher, on average, in those with high blood lead levels than it is in those with low levels?'.

This is the same as asking: 'Is the trend in these points sufficiently non-horizontal to indicate a real trend in the population?'.

To answer the question it is necessary to fit the least squares regression line and test whether the sample regression coefficient is consistent with a true value of zero. Alternatively it is simply necessary to show that a non-zero trend model fits the data significantly better than a horizontal line model to demonstrate that the apparent trend is unlikely to be due to chance.

To demonstrate how a regression line is fitted a number of algebraic definitions are needed. The variance of a set of values has already been introduced as:

Sum for all values (value − mean value)$^2$/(no. of values − 1)

which for values of a variable $y$ becomes:

$$\text{Sum } (y - \bar{y})^2/(n - 1) \tag{9.3}$$

where $\bar{y}$ (pronounced $y$ bar) is the conventional abbreviation for the mean of a sample of $y$ values. The sum of squared deviations construction is so common in statistical calculations that it is convenient to have a special notation. This text will use:

$$Syy = \text{Sum } (y - \bar{y})^2 \tag{9.4}$$

and for an $x$ variable:

$$Sxx = \text{Sum } (x - \bar{x})^2 \tag{9.5}$$

and finally:

$$Sxy = \text{Sum } (y - \bar{y})(x - \bar{x}). \tag{9.6}$$

The sum of squared deviations minimized when we fit a regression line is essentially $Sdd$ but it is more often called the residual sum of squares ($RSS$) or $Sr$.

In general:

$$Sr = \text{Sum } (y - \text{value predicted by the model})^2$$

which for a simple regression line becomes:

$$Sr = \text{Sum } (y - \text{height of line})^2.$$

Now to fit the regression line of the form:

$$y = a + bx$$

to describe the trend in chromosome abnormalities as blood lead increases means choosing the most appropriate values for $a$ and $b$. The principle of least squares means that $a$ and $b$ are required to make the sum of the squared deviations $Sr$ a minimum. For this line the residual sum of squares is:

$$Sr = \text{Sum } (y - a - bx)^2. \tag{9.7}$$

It can be shown mathematically that this is a minimum when the slope:

$$b = Sxy/Sxx \tag{9.8}$$

and the intercept:

$$a = \bar{y} - b\bar{x}. \tag{9.9}$$

The minimum value of $Sr$ when $a$ and $b$ take these values is:

$$Sr = Syy - Sxy^2/Sxx. \tag{9.10}$$

The residual sum of squares is the basic measure of how well a model, in this case $y = a + bx$, fits the data. If points are scattered about the line, $Sr$ will be large indicating a bad fit. If the points fall more or less on a straight line $Sr$ will be small indicating that a straight line model fits the data well.

The variance of the deviations about the line is called the residual variance and denoted by:

$$s^2 = Sr/(n - 2) \tag{9.11}$$

where $n - 2$ is known as the degrees of freedom and is the amount of information available to estimate the residual variance. This is the number of observations (or points on the plot) less the number of parameters in the model that need to be estimated. Here it was necessary to estimate two parameters, the intercept and the slope.

The residual variance can be used to calculate the standard error of $b$ which is:

$$se(b) = \sqrt{(s^2/Sxx)} \tag{9.12}$$

For the Italian data on women battery factory workers, with $y = $ chromosome abnormalities (ABS)/100 cells and $x = $ blood lead levels (BL) in $\mu g/100$ ml, the values required in the analysis to fit a simple regression line are:

$$n = 30 \qquad \bar{y} = 5.97 \qquad \bar{x} = 36.37$$

with:

$$Syy = 432.97 \qquad Sxx = 3302.96 \qquad Sxy = 460.37$$

The estimates of $a$ and $b$ are therefore:

$$b = Sxy/Sxx = 460.37/3302.96 = 0.14$$
$$a = \bar{y} - b\bar{x} = 5.97 - 0.14 \times 36.37 = 0.90$$

from eqn. 9.10:

$$Sr = 432.97 - 460.37^2/3302.96 = 368.80$$

so:

$$s^2 = Sr/(n - 2) = 368.80/28 = 13.17$$

and:

$$se(b) = \sqrt{(s^2/Sxx)} = 0.06$$

The line representing the apparent trend 'best' in the least squares sense is therefore:

$$\text{ABS} = 0.90 + 0.14 \times \text{BL}$$

where ABS stands for chromosome abnormalities and BL for blood lead levels. Assuming that the sampling distribution of $b$ is near enough normal, the 95 per cent confidence interval for the 'true' value of the slope is:

$$0.14 - 1.96 \, (0.06) \text{ to } 0.14 + 1.96 \, (0.06)$$

or $\qquad\qquad 0.02 \qquad$ to $\qquad 0.16$

since this does not include zero it is a reasonably strong indication that the population trend is not zero. That is, the observed trend is significantly different from a population value of zero at the 5 per cent level. A sample regression slope could not easily occur this far from zero by chance ($p < 0.05$).

The significance test of the zero slope hypothesis is performed by calculating how many standard errors the slope 0.14 is from the expected zero, that is:

$$\frac{\text{observed slope} - \text{expected slope}}{se \, (\text{slope})} = \frac{0.14 - 0}{0.06} = 2.33$$

which is, as the confidence interval also showed, well above 1.96. There is therefore strong evidence of a trend in the population represented by this sample. Higher numbers of chromosome abnormalities will be found in individuals such as these with the higher blood lead levels.

There was one 'outlying' individual on the plot with 22 abnormalities. If the results had been less conclusive it might have been wise to repeat the analysis excluding this individual. Her effect on the analysis could then be assessed and the interpretation modified appropriately. Note that for samples this size the $t$ distribution should be used. The $t$ distribution centile equivalent to the standard normal 1.96 for 28 df is 2.05 (about 5 per cent higher), but the conclusions are exactly the same.

Whether these results really mean that lead in the blood damages chromosomes is still not clear. Partly for this reason it is customary to describe significant trends as indicating a real association between the variables to make it clear that the existence of a trend in the population in no way proves a 'causal relationship'. This one fact must be added to the whole body of knowledge on the subject before conclusions can be carried that far.

Apart from tests of the assumptions that the population line is straight and not a curve, that there is a similar residual variance at all $x$ values and that the underlying distribution is normal, this analysis is complete.

In fact since any trend is indicative of the relationship, in this case between lead exposure and chromosome abnormalities, whether or not it is straight hardly matters. Whether the residuals have a normal distribution is more crucial since inferences from confidence intervals and significance tests all assume that they do. How to test these assumptions will be discussed later. Meanwhile it is useful to consider how this analysis can be approached in a more general way applicable to most common problems. In some circumstances the question cannot be phrased so it becomes a test of a single parameter. In those cases the question has to be expressed as a comparison of different models.

In the lead data example the equivalent model comparison is between a model of the form:

$$y = a + bx$$

which is a sloping straight line and the model:

$$y = a$$

which represents a horizontal line.

If there is a significant trend the second model will fit the data significantly worse than the first. How well a model describes data is measured by the residual sum of squares – the smaller $Sr$ is the better the fit. Comparisons of the fit of two models are made by comparing their residual sums of squares.

As should be clear from this example the more parameters in a model the smaller the residual sum of squares $Sr$ can be made. Choosing the intercept and the slope, two parameters for a sloping line makes it possible to fit the model closer to the data points than when the fitting process is restricted to choosing one parameter, the intercept, for a horizontal line. From the model:

$$y = a + bx$$

the residual sum of squares is:

$$Sr = 368.75$$

and the residual variance is:

$$s^2 = 13.17.$$

From the horizontal line model when the intercept (height of the line) is simply the mean of $y$, the residual sum of squares is:

$$Sr = 433.0$$

that is, an increase of 64.25.

The increase has associated with it one degree of freedom since one parameter has been dropped from the more complicated model. On the hypothesis that the trend is a chance event in this particular sample 64.25 is a further estimate of the residual variance. This means that if the hypothesis is true $64.25/s^2$ should be about one since it is the ratio of two estimates of the same variance: the value in this example is $64.25/13.17$ or 4.88.

The numerator which is the increase in $Sr$ resulting from simplifying the model has one degree of freedom. The denominator which is the residual variance from the most complicated model has $n - 2$ which is 28 degrees of freedom. If the 'no-trend' hypothesis is true this variance ratio can be

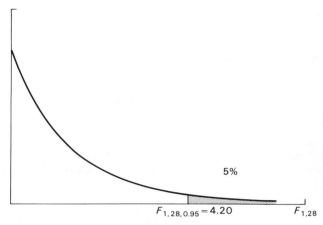

Fig. 9.22. $F$ distribution with one and 28 degrees of freedom.

shown to have a sampling distribution with a particular mathematical form called the $F$ distribution with in this case 1 and 28 degrees of freedom. This can be used to assess how surprising an observed variance ratio is to give what is known as an $F$ test.

The $F$ distribution for 1 df and 28 df is illustrated in Fig. 9.22. The 95th centile of the $F$ distribution is 4.20 and less than 5 per cent of $F$ values calculated in this way from a sample should occur this far above one. This implies that the value 4.88 is surprisingly large ($p < 0.05$) if the population has no trend. It suggests that the horizontal – line model ·is incorrect. Surprisingly low values can occur, but they have little meaning. If anything they imply that the model fits the data surprisingly well given the amount of variation present. They are generally treated as insignificant.

The interpretation of this analysis is that it is either necessary to assume a freak sample or that the non-zero trend model was necessary to describe this data. In practice it would be taken as reasonably strong evidence that there was a trend in the population. The estimated regression coefficient with a confidence interval should then be obtained to demonstrate the magnitude of the effect.

This model comparison approach to the analysis is best presented in tabular form giving what is known as an 'analysis of variance' but is actually an analysis of residual sums of squares. Denoting the residual sum of squares from Model 1 as $S_1$ and the sum of squares divided by the degrees of freedom for a model as the mean square ($MS$) the analysis is given in Table 9.5.

**Table 9.5.** *Analysis of variance to test for a linear trend in chromosome abnormalities by blood lead (BL) levels*

| Model | SS | df | MS | F |
|---|---|---|---|---|
| 1. Intercept and trend on BL – sloping line | $S_1 = 368.75$ | 28 | $s^2 = 13.17$ | |
| 2. Intercept, but no trend – horizontal line | $S_2 = 433.00$ | 29 | | |
| (2 – 1) Due to trend | 64.25 | 1 | 64.25 | $F_{1,28} = 64.25/13.17 = 4.88$ |

To construct such analysis of variance tables it is only necessary to obtain the residual sum of squares for the two models. A test of the parameters omitted when model 1 is changed to the simpler model 2 is then immediately available as:

$$F_{1,28} = (S_2 - S_1/s^2). \qquad (9.13)$$

Since, all that is needed for this approach is the residual sum of squares for each model, it is not even necessary to fit them. In practice they are fitted because it is necessary to know the likely magnitudes of the effects not just whether they exist or not.

### Non-linear regression

In a given analysis a straight line trend may well be inadequate, a curved trend line might fit the data better. To test this a model representing a curved trend is fitted and the fit is compared with that of a straight-line model. The simplest model for a curved trend is known as a quadratic and takes the form:

$$y = a + bx + cx^2$$

In the lead data example this is equivalent to:

$$ABS = Intercept + b.BL + c.BL^2$$

with ABS and BL standing for chromosome abnormalities and blood lead levels respectively. The model is fitted exactly as before with $a$, $b$, and $c$ chosen so that the residual sum of squares is minimized.

The formulae are rather more complicated than for the straight line model so although this model can be fitted by hand it is tedious. With a professionally produced package program on a computer it is very easy and it is not necessary to know the formulae in detail.

The hypothesis that there is no curvature in the population can be tested very easily by calculating

$$t = \frac{c - \text{expected } c}{se(c)} = \frac{c - 0}{se(c)}$$

and since we have fitted three parameters this has $n - 3$ degrees of freedom where $n$ is the number of data points. The fitted model for the lead data gives:

Intercept $a = 2.77$
Linear coefficient $b = 0.03$
Quadratic coefficient $c = 0.0014$ with $se(c) = 0.0066$

so for the '$t$' test of curvature:

$$t = \frac{0.0014 - 0}{0.0066} = 0.2 \qquad \text{with 27 df}$$

This is very far from the value needed for significance which is a little above 2.0 ($t_{0.975} = 2.05$ on 27 df). Obviously there is little evidence that the population trend is not a straight line.

### Comparing two groups

The above analysis of the lead study data looked at the association between chromosome abnormalities and blood lead levels. However, current blood lead may not reflect long-term exposure. Figure 9.23 compares the individuals from lead free

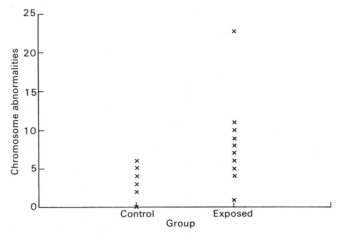

**Fig. 9.23.** Chromosome abnormalities and exposure group.

areas in the factory with those exposed to lead in their work. The values for the exposed individuals appear to be slightly higher with a wider spread. To investigate this more precisely it is necessary to calculate the mean and standard deviations for the two groups (Table 9.6).

**Table 9.6.** *Chromosome abnormalities (ABS) in female battery factory workers by exposure group. (Findings when one woman with ABS=22, was excluded are shown in parentheses)*

|        | Not exposed | Exposed | All |
|--------|-------------|---------|-----|
| Number | 12 (12) | 18 (17) | 30 (29) |
| Mean | 4.00 (4.00) | 7.28 (6.41) | 5.97 (5.41) |
| sd | 1.71 (1.71) | 4.36 (2.43) | 3.87 (2.44) |

The question becomes: 'Are the means surprisingly different?' This is tested by fitting a model of the form:

$$\text{mean ABS} = \text{reference value} + \text{group effect}$$

Taking the 'reference value' as the mean for the first group (not exposed), the group effect is zero for that group and equal to the difference between the two means for the second group. Fitting this model by least squares is exactly the same as allowing each group to have its own mean. The model is:

$$\text{mean ABS} = 4.00 + 0 \qquad \text{for group 1}$$
$$\text{mean ABS} = 4.00 + (7.28 - 4.00) \qquad \text{for group 2}$$

Each mean minimizes the sum of squared deviations within its own group $Syy_1$ and $Syy_2$ (say) so the total residual sum of squares $Sr = Syy_1 + Syy_2$ is a minimum.

The variances for the groups separately are calculated as $Syy_1/(n_1 - 1)$ for group 1 and $Syy_2/(n_2 - 1)$ for group 2. To compare the group means it is necessary to assume one underlying residual variance. On this assumption both samples contain information on the residual variance and the information is pooled as the overall residual sum of squares $Sr$ to estimate it. The 'pooled' estimate of variance is therefore $Sr$ divided by its degrees of freedom.

For the above model the number of degrees of freedom is

$n_1 + n_2 - 2$ because there are $n_1 + n_2$ values in total and two parameters, the two means, have been estimated. Now:

$$Syy_1 = 32.00 \text{ and } Syy_2 = 323.61$$

So:

$$Sr = Syy_1 + Syy_2 = 355.6$$

and since $n_1 = 12$ and $n_2 = 18$

$$s^2 = Sr/(n_1 + n_2 - 2) = 355.6/28 = 12.7 \qquad (9.14)$$

The difference between the means, which is the group 2 effect, since the reference value is the group 1 mean, is:

$$\text{Difference} = 7.28 - 4.00 = 3.28$$

this has the standard error:

$$se \, (\text{Difference}) = \sqrt{(s^2(1/n_1 + 1/n_2))} \qquad (9.15)$$
$$= \sqrt{(12.7(1/12 + 1/18))} = 1.33$$

A significance tests of the hypothesis that the population difference is zero is obtained as:

$$t = \frac{\text{Difference} - \text{Hypothesized Difference}}{se \, (\text{difference})} = \frac{3.28 - 0}{1.33} = 2.47$$

and the probability of values as far from zero as 2.47 occurring by chance, obtained from tables of the $t$ distribution with 28 degrees of freedom is about 0.02 so $p < 0.05$. The difference is significant at the 5 per cent level ($p < 0.05$) on the assumption that the two samples came from populations with identical variances.

However, the two groups actually have very different variances (Table 9.6) and the assumption should be tested. This is done using a form of the $F$ test. If the population variances are the same the variances from the two groups are estimating the same thing. Their ratio in that case will be an observation from an $F$ distribution and should have a value close to one. If the hypothesis of equal population variances is false, the variance ratio will deviate from one. Whether this gives large or small values depends on which way the variance ratio is calculated: large/small or small/large. Since this is arbitrary, surprisingly small values are just as interesting, in this context, as surprisingly large values.

It is usual to calculate the ratio with the larger variance as the numerator. The probability of $F$ values as high as that is then obtained from tables and doubled to give $p$, the probability of variances as different as observed occurring by chance. This means that the probability of values as high as the ratio calculated must be less than 0.025 for the probability of obtaining variances this different by chance to be less than 0.05.

The standard deviations of the two groups were 1.71 and 4.36 so the variance ratio (large/small) is:

$$F = (4.36/1.71)^2 = 6.50$$

with $18 - 1 = 17$ and $12 - 1 = 11$ degrees of freedom. The tables show that only 2.5 per cent of values from the $F_{17, 11}$ distribution should occur above 3.33. This implies that our variances are significantly different at the 5 per cent level ($p < 0.05$). The assumption of equal variances is clearly unsafe and some corrective action is required.

In these data the difference in the variances is largely due to one very high value of ABS (22) in the exposed group. If she is removed (Table 9.6), then, although the standard deviations are still different the $F$ value:

$$F_{16, 11} = (2.43/1.71)^2 = 2.02$$

is less than the 95th centile of $F_{16, 11}$ which is 2.37. Thus the probability of variances this different by chance is at least $2 \times 0.05$ or 0.10. There is now no real evidence of unequal variances and no reason not to perform the standard analysis.

The residual sum of squares reduces to 126.12 with 27 degrees of freedom so the residual variance becomes 4.67. The difference between the means is $6.41 - 4.00 = 2.41$ and the standard error of this difference is now:

$$se \, (\text{difference}) = \sqrt{(4.67(1/12 + 1/17))} = 0.81$$

The $t$ test becomes, $t = 2.41/0.81 = 2.98$, which is in fact even more significant than before because removing the extreme point has reduced the standard error more than it has the difference.

The above analysis fitting a single model is possible and sufficient because the question of interest can be reduced to a test of a single parameter. However, when several groups have to be compared this is not really possible and the model comparison approach is required.

In a model comparison analysis of these data there are two models. The first is the one assuming the population means to be different

1.   mean ABS = reference value + group effect
where the reference value is the group 1 mean. As before the residual sum of squares for this model is $Syy$ for group 1 plus $Syy$ for group 2 and calling this $S_1$:

$$S_1 = 126.12$$

(omitting the individual with ABS = 22). The residual variance from this model is $s^2 = 4.67$.

The second model, assuming no difference, is:

2.   mean ABS = reference value
where the reference value is the overall mean of the two groups estimating the supposedly constant population mean. The residual sum of squares for this model is the value of $Syy$ calculated from both groups combined into one sample. Calling this $S_2$:

$$S_2 = 167.03$$

and the analysis of variance table is as given in Table 9.7. Since $|F_{1, 27, 0.99}| = 7.68$ this gives a probability of a difference of this magnitude, given the hypothesis of no difference between

**Table 9.7.** *Analysis of variance for comparing the mean number of chromosome abnormalities in two groups*

| Model | RSS | df | MS | Variance ratio |
|---|---|---|---|---|
| 1. Groups different | 126.12 | 27 | 4.67 | |
| 2. Groups same | 167.03 | 28 | | |
| (2 − 1) Due to difference | 40.91 | 1 | 40.91 | $F_{1,27} = 40.91/4.67 = 8.76$ |

the populations, of $p < 0.01$. This is the same $p$ value as for $t = 2.98$ obtained using the alternative $t$ test of the relevant parameter in a single fitted model. They are the same test in two different forms.

### Comparing three or more groups

Consider data from an Italian study designed to assess the effects of well-publicized hypertension clinics on blood pressure levels in the community. There is some evidence that systolic blood pressure increases with age in a non-linear way. For this reason the analyses were performed using age groups rather than exact ages. At the beginning of the study the mean systolic blood pressure (SBP) for males in the control district that had no clinic was as shown in Table 9.8.

**Table 9.8.** *Mean systolic blood pressure by age in males from a study of the effect of hypertension clinics*

|  | Age group (years) | | | | | |
|  | 20–29.9 | 30–39.9 | 40–49.9 | 50–59.9 | 60+ | All |
|---|---|---|---|---|---|---|
| Number | 340 | 303 | 302 | 207 | 288 | 1440 |
| Mean | 141.9 | 146.0 | 150.1 | 149.2 | 156.9 | 148.5 |
| sd | 20.4 | 19.9 | 22.7 | 21.4 | 24.7 | 22.4 |

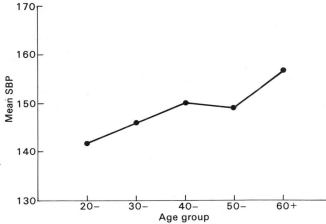

**Fig. 9.24.** Mean systolic blood pressure by age in males from a study of hypertension clinics.

There is a tendency for the mean value to increase with age (Fig. 9.24). The sds are all about the same so an assumption of equal variances is reasonable. The appropriate model is:

1.   mean SBP = reference value + group effect

and because it simplifies the interpretation of the fitted parameters the group 1 mean (men aged 20–29 years) is taken as the 'reference value'. The 'group effects' are then the differences between the mean of that particular group and the group 1 mean, that is, the reference value. The model then has five parameters:

the reference value (the mean for group 1)
the group 2 effect $G_2$ (the group 2 mean – reference value)
the group 3 effect $G_3$ (mean for group 3 – reference value)

the group 4 effect $G_4$ (mean for group 4 – reference value) and group 5 effect $G_5$ (mean for group 5 – reference value).

To fit the model, estimates for these five parameters must be obtained as the means and differences implied above with the residual sum of squares ($Sr$) and hence the ses of the parameter estimates. Since the model essentially allows each group to have its own mean, $Sr$ is the sum of the $Syy$s obtained separately from each of the groups. Calling this $S_1$ and its degrees of freedom $f_1$ where:

$$f_1 = \text{(total number of values – the no. of parameters)}$$

gives:

$$S_1 = 685\,211 \text{ with } f_1 = (1440 - 5) = 1435$$

The residual variance is thus:

$$s^2 = 685\,211 / 1435 = 477.5$$

The simpler model where differences are assumed to be chance is simply one overall mean:

2.   mean SBP = reference value

with the overall mean as the reference value which represents a single horizontal line. How well this fits the data is measured by the residual sum of squares about the overall mean. This is simply $Syy$ from all 1440 individuals treated as one sample which is $S_2 = 723\,110$. The analysis of variance is given in Table 9.9.

**Table 9.9.** *Analysis of variance comparing mean systolic blood pressures in five age groups*

| Model | SS | df | MS | F |
|---|---|---|---|---|
| 1. Groups different | $S_1 = 685\,211$ | 1435 | $s^2 = 477.5$ | |
| 2. One overall mean | $S_2 = 723\,110$ | 1439 | | |
| (2 – 1) Due to group differences | $S_2 - S_1 = 37\,899$ | 4 | 9475 | 19.8 |

$F$ values of 19.8 with 4 and 1435 df are extremely unlikely to occur by chance ($p \ll 0.01$). The sample sizes are so large that the small but consistent changes in SBP are highly significant. A linear trend model:

3.   mean SBP = intercept + $b$ age

taking individuals in the same age group as having the same age gives a test of whether the population trend is in any way curved.

Treating the data as one large sample and fitting a simple regression line the residual sum of squares from eqn 9.10 is:

$$S_3 = Syy - Sxy^2/Sxx$$

and for these data:

$$S_3 = 688\,123$$

Since two parameters have been fitted this has

$$1440 - 2 = 1438 \text{ df}$$

**Table 9.10.** *Analysis of variance testing whether mean systolic blood pressure follows a linear trend over five age groups*

| Model | SS | df | MS | F |
|---|---|---|---|---|
| 1. Groups different (any trend) | 685 211 | 1435 | $s^2 = 477.5$ | |
| 3. Linear trend | 688 123 | 1438 | | |
| (3 − 1) Due to non-linearity | 2912 | 3 | 970.7 | 2.03 |

The analysis of variance is given in Table 9.10. Since *F* with 3 and 1435 df needs to exceed 2.60 for significance at the 5 per cent level there is little evidence that a linear trend is not adequate. The estimated slope is:

$$b = Sxy/Sxx = 0.68 \text{ mm Hg/year}$$

and from eqn 9.11:

$$se(b) = 0.08$$

The analysis shows that the means differ significantly and that the way they differ is adequately represented by a linear trend. This implies that the slope of the linear trend is significantly non-zero and the direct test is:

$$t = 0.68/0.08 = 8.5 \ (p < 0.01)$$

### Comparing groups allowing for trends

Consider the problem of comparing lung function, in particular FEV, between smokers and non-smokers. The underlying question is: 'Does smoking affect lung function?' It appears that the study simply requires samples of smokers and non-smokers to test whether their respective populations differ.

However, for an efficient analysis, the samples need to be as similar as possible in other respects so that, for example, a preponderance of males in the smokers will not bias the comparison. It is possible to avoid this bias by restricting the study to one sex. Unfortunately this approach cannot be used to avoid bias due to such things as height. Some height differences will inevitably occur. It is possible to ensure that the groups have the same range of heights which avoids the problem of systematic bias. Nonetheless the variation in lung function is increased as a result of height differences. This decreases the sensitivity with which group differences can be detected.

Quantitative variables interfering with group comparisons in this way are known as covariates and analyses involving them are known as analyses of covariance. The analysis of covariance uses regression techniques to deduce from the data in this example: (i) whether FEV changes with height in the same way for both groups; and if it does (ii) what FEV differences would be seen between smokers and non-smokers if they all had the same height. Four main circumstances can arise illustrated in Fig. 9.25.

The biases illustrated in Fig. 9.25 can be avoided by designing the study to keep the height distributions of the groups similar. In practice it is more important to remove the variation due to covariate differences to increase the sensitivity with which the analysis estimates and tests the group differences.

If the trend lines in two groups are parallel the groups differ by the same amount at all heights. As long as both groups have the same range of height it is possible to predict how they will differ without specifying a height. To investigate this it is necessary to compare the fit of parallel and non-parallel models. Assuming straight line trends, an assumption that would need testing in practice, the models are:

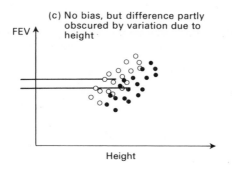

(a) A real difference obscured by height differences

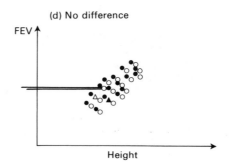

(b) An apparent difference created by height differences

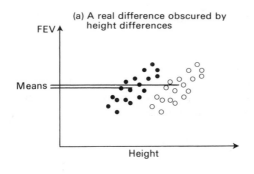

(c) No bias, but difference partly obscured by variation due to height

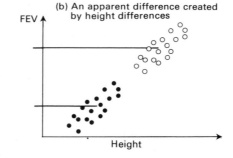

(d) No difference

**Fig. 9.25.** Two group scatter diagrams to illustrate the ways in which a covariate may influence a group comparison.

1. *Non-parallel*
   Mean FEV=Group intercept+Group slope×Height
   That is each group has its own slope and intercept.
2. *Parallel*
   Mean FEV=Group intercept+Common slope×Height
   That is each group has its own intercept, but the same slope.

If there are $n = n_1 + n_2$ points in total the residual sum of squares for model 1 is:

$$S_1 = \text{Sum for both groups } (Syy - Sxy^2/Sxx)$$

with $n - 4$ df because four parameters have been fitted, two slopes and two intercepts. The residual variance about this model is $s^2 = S_1/(n - 4)$.

The residual sum of squares from model 2 is $S_2 = \text{Sum } Syy - (\text{Sum } Sxy)^2/\text{Sum } Sxx$ where 'Sum' implies that the $Syy$, $Sxx$, and $Sxy$ are calculated for each group separately and then summed. $S_2$ has $n - 3$ df since in this model only three parameters are required, two intercepts and one slope. The test of parallelism, from eqn 9.13, is:

$$F_{1, n-4} = (S_2 - S_1)/s^2$$

which is compared with the appropriate $F$ distribution centile.

If it seems reasonable to accept that the population trends are parallel, then the estimated slope is from eqn 9.8:

$$b = \text{Sum } Sxy/\text{Sum } Sxx$$

and from eqn 9.12:

$$se(b) = \sqrt{(s^2/\text{Sum } Sxx)}$$

The group difference allowing for height is then constant for all heights and most easily calculated as the difference between the intercepts. This is:

Mean FEV difference − slope × Mean height difference.

Although the algebra is beyond the scope of this text it can be shown that the variance of this is:

$$var(diff) = s^2(1/n_1 + 1/n_2 + (\text{mean height difference})^2/\text{Sum } Sxx)$$

from which we can obtain:

$$se(diff) = \sqrt{(var\,(diff))}$$

which gives us a $t$ test of the group differences allowing for height.

For more complex situations with several groups and possibly more than one covariate the group differences are more easily tested by model comparison. Considering the single covariate case to avoid excessive complications a third model is fitted assuming that all intercepts and slopes are the same in the population. This means that only one intercept and one slope need to be estimated. To fit them the groups are ignored and all the data combined as one. The model is:

3. *Coincident trend lines*
   Mean FEV = Intercept + Slope × Height.

The residual sum of squares from this model is:

$$S_3 = Syy \text{ all data} - (Sxy \text{ all data})^2/Sxx \text{ all data}$$

with $n - 2$ df. The test for group differences is again an $F$ test performed by obtaining the difference between the $Sr$ for the two models and dividing by the residual variance obtained from the most complex model, in this case model 1 as in eqn 9.13:

$$F_{1, n-4} = (S_3 - S_2)/s^2.$$

Expressed as an analysis of variance (Table 9.11) it is easier to see how this approach may be generalized to more than two groups.

**Table 9.11.** *Analysis of covariance table construction for comparing groups allowing for the interfering effect of a covariate*

| Model | SS | df | MS | F |
|---|---|---|---|---|
| 1. Non-parallel | $S_1$ | $n - 4$ | $s^2 = S_1/(n - 4)$ | |
| 2. Parallel | $S_2$ | $n - 3$ | | |
| (2 − 1) Due to non-parallelism | $S_2 - S_1$ | 1 | $S_2 - S_1$ | $F_{1,n-4} = (S_2 - S_1)/s^2$ |
| 3. Same intercept and slope | $S_3$ | $n - 2$ | | |
| (3 − 2) Due to group differences | $S_3 - S_2$ | 1 | $S_3 - S_2$ | $F_{1,n-4} = (S_3 - S_2)/s^2$ |

Example

Mean FEV values were obtained for 50 males of whom five were regular smokers (Table 9.12). The smokers have slightly lower FEV values than the non-smokers, but the comparison makes no allowance for differences in height. The mean heights are in fact different, the smokers being slightly shorter on average. The analysis is given in Table 9.13.

**Table 9.12.** *Mean FEV values for 50 males by smoking behaviour together with mean height in inches*

| | Non-smokers | Smokers |
|---|---|---|
| Number | 45 | 5 |
| Mean | 3.34 | 3.23 |
| sd | 2.33 | 2.83 |
| Mean height | 70.6 | 69.0 |

**Table 9.13.** *Analysis of covariance comparing FEV in cigarette smokers and non-smokers allowing for height differences*

| Model | SS | df | MS | F |
|---|---|---|---|---|
| 1. Non-parallel trends with height | 12.91 | 46 | $s^2 = 0.28$ | |
| 2. Parallel trends | 12.99 | 47 | | |
| (2 − 1) Due to non-parallelism | 0.08 | 1 | 0.08 | $F \ll 1$ |
| 3. Same intercept | 13.03 | 48 | | |
| (3 − 2) Due to group difference | 0.04 | 1 | 0.04 | $F \ll 1$ |

Since $F$ values will exceed one for surprising values and both these $F$ values are less than one there is no evidence that the trends have different slopes or the smokers and non-smokers in general differ on the FEV scale.

### Groups in a cross classification

The effects of intervention in an Italian hypertension study were assessed at the end of a five-year period. Samples of males and females were obtained from the control and intervention areas. The mean systolic blood pressure values for those aged 60 years and above are given in Table 9.14. This is a $2 \times 2$ classification because the table has two rows and two columns. The groups are defined by the categorical variables sex in one direction and treatment in the other. For historical reasons variables used to classify individuals are known as factors and their values, the actual categories, are known as levels.

**Table 9.14.** *Mean systolic blood pressures by sex and intervention group of subjects in a hypertension study*

|        |        | Area |              |
|--------|--------|---------|--------------|
|        |        | Control | Intervention |
|        | Number | 200     | 223          |
| Male   | Mean   | 158.5   | 150.1        |
|        | sd     | 24.2    | 21.0         |
|        | Number | 191     | 283          |
| Female | Mean   | 167.4   | 154.7        |
|        | sd     | 27.5    | 21.5         |

To assess the effects of intervention it is necessary to investigate whether the difference between the intervention and control areas is the same in both sexes. If it is, an overall estimate of the effect using data from both sexes is required. This must then be tested against zero to assess whether the hypothetical population of such individuals treated in this way would show a non-zero effect. If the effects are different for the two sexes they have to be estimated and tested for each sex separately.

Figure 9.26 shows that the intervention means are well below those of the equivalent control groups. The females

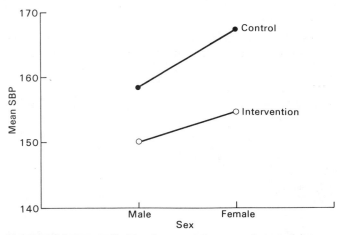

**Fig. 9.26.** Mean systolic blood pressure by sex and treatment group from a study of hypertension.

have consistently higher values than the males and there is a slight suggestion that the intervention/control difference is greater in the females. This makes the lines joining the sample means non-parallel.

To test this non-parallelism or interaction between the effects of treatment and sex two models must be fitted. These are a non-parallel model where each group has its own mean and a model where the population means are constrained to fall on parallel lines.

The parameter representing the deviation from parallelism is the difference, on Fig. 9.26, between the control/intervention interval for the females and that for the males. Consequently if $T$ is the treatment effect in the males (that is, the control mean – the intervention group mean) and $T+I$ is the equivalent effect in the females then $I$ is the deviation from parallelism. Because it represents an influence of the factor sex on the treatment effect (cf. synergy and antagonism in pharmacology) it is often referred to as an interaction. The sex effect ($S$ say) is taken as the difference between the sexes in the intervention group. The model is:

1. Mean  SBP = Reference  value + Sex  effect + Treatment effect + Sex × Treatment interaction.

which represents four equations for the four sex/treatment combinations

$$\text{male intervention } \text{mean} = rv$$
$$\text{male control } \text{mean} = rv + T$$
$$\text{female intervention } \text{mean} = rv + S$$
$$\text{female control } \text{mean} = rv + S + T + I$$

The estimate of the interaction may be calculated from

$I$ = (Control mean – Intervention mean) females –
      (Control mean – Intervention mean) males

which from these data gives:

$$(167.4 - 154.7) - (158.5 - 150.1) = 12.7 - 8.4 = 4.3.$$

The $Sr$ from this model is:

$$S_1 = \text{Sum of } Syy \text{ from the four groups} = 488\,486.2$$

with $n - 4$ df, where $n$ is the total number of subjects in all four groups and four is subtracted because four parameters need to be estimated. The residual variance is therefore:

$$s^2 = S_1/(n-4) = 488\,486.2/893 = 547.0$$

which can be used to obtain a standard error for $I$ which is:

$$\text{se}(d) = \sqrt{(s^2(1/n_1 + 1/n_2 + 1/n_3 + 1/n_4))} = 3.16$$

So a test of the hypothesis that the true deviation from parallelism is zero is:

$$t = (d-0)/se(d) = 4.3/3.16 = 1.36.$$

Since there are 893 df the '$t$' distribution is the same as the standard normal distribution (see pp. 154–5). This means the value would have to exceed 1.96 for significance at the 5 per cent level. Since it does not there is little evidence of an interaction. The effect of intervention if any is the same for both sexes.

The parallel line model is:

2. Mean SBP = Reference value + Sex effect + Treatment effect.

Unfortunately there is no simple formula for $Sr$ from this model and the analysis cannot easily be done without a statistical package on a computer. When there are only two treatment groups a technique due to Yates (described very thoroughly by Snedecor and Cochran 1967) using averages of the mean differences weighted according to the group sizes can be used. It is however laborious and not very general. The $Sr$ from this model $S_2$ (say) will have $n-3$ df. The three fitted parameters will be the reference mean, the average difference between the sexes, and one treatment effect averaged over both sexes. The effects can be tested using:

$$t = \text{estimate}/se(\text{estimate})$$

or, for the generality required for comparing several groups, by fitting models without them. To test the treatment effect it is necessary to fit:

3. Mean SBP $= rv +$ Sex effect

with $Sr = S_3$ and $n-2$ df.

The $F$ test for the treatment effect is then:

$$F_{1, n-4} = (S_3 - S_2)/s^2$$

Exactly the same procedure can be used to test the sex effect. The full analysis of variance is given in Table 9.15.

**Table 9.15.** *Analysis of variance comparing means in a two-way classification*

| Model | SS | df | MS | F |
|---|---|---|---|---|
| 1. With interaction | $S_1$ | $n-4$ | $s^2 = S_1/(n-4)$ | |
| 2. No interaction | $S_2$ | $n-3$ | | |
| (2−1) Due to interaction | $S_2 - S_1$ | 1 | $S_2 - S_1$ | $F_{1,n-4} = (S_2 - S_1)/s^2$ |
| 3. No treatment effect | $S_3$ | $n-2$ | | |
| (3−2) Due to treatment | $S_3 - S_2$ | 1 | $S_3 - S_2$ | $F_{1,n-4} = (S_3 - S_2)/s^2$ |
| 4. No sex effect | $S_4$ | $n-2$ | | |
| (4−2) Due to sex | $S_4 - S_2$ | 1 | $S_4 - S_2$ | $F_{1,n-4} = (S_4 - S_2)/s^2$ |

### Example

The actual analysis for the Italian SBP data is given in Table 9.16. Since the 95th centile $F_{1,893}$ is 3.84, there is no evidence of interaction. The other two $F$ values are highly significant indicating that both the differences between the treatment groups and between the sexes are highly significant ($p < 0.001$).

The treatment effect is estimated using Model 2 and was found to be:

$$10.6 \text{ with se } 1.58$$

which means that, all else being equal, individuals receiving the second treatment, the intervention, will be on average, 10.6 mm Hg below the control group. The approximate 95 per cent confidence interval for the 'true' effect of intervention is:

$$\text{estimate} \pm 2 \text{ ses which gives } -7.44 \text{ to } -13.76.$$

**Table 9.16.** *Analysis of variance comparing mean systolic blood pressure in groups classified by sex and treatment*

| Model | SS | df | MS | F |
|---|---|---|---|---|
| 1. With interaction | 488 486.2 | 893 | $s^2 = 547.0$ | |
| 2. No interaction | 489 499.2 | 894 | | |
| (2−1) Due to interaction | 1013.0 | 1 | 1013.0 | $F_{1,893} = 1.85$ |
| 3. No treatment | 514 316.2 | 895 | | |
| (3−2) Due to treatment | 24 817.0 | 1 | 24 817.0 | $F_{1,893} = 45.4$ |
| 4. No sex | 498 866.2 | 895 | | |
| (4−2) Due to sex | 9367.0 | 1 | 9367.0 | $F_{1,893} = 17.1$ |

The 'true' difference between the sexes is estimated in a similar way showing females to be higher on average by 6.5 mm Hg with an approximate 95 per cent confidence interval of $6.5 \pm 1.57$ mm Hg.

The general principles of the above analyses apply to much more complicated situations. A study design may lead to cross classifications with many more than two factors. Any of the factors may have more than two levels. As well as a cross-classification there may be one or more covariates to allow for in the analysis. Even so the pattern of the analysis is more or less the same. With a computer the appropriate residual sums of squares can be obtained together with estimated parameters representing the group differences of interest and their standard errors.

### Repeated or paired measurements

Repeated observations are made on the same subjects when changes over time are of interest. In addition subjects may be matched in pairs or larger groups to increase the precision of an investigation.

An important reason for performing analyses using covariates or interfering factors is to explain and remove some of the variation observed in the response variable and thus increase the precision of the analysis. In comparisons of a treatment with a control the main source of variation is between the individuals within the groups. There may be a clear difference between the means of the control and treatment groups, but the degree of overlap among individual values may well mean that the observed difference cannot be distinguished from possible chance effects.

In certain circumstances it is possible to use each individual as his or her own control. Or, as in studies of twins there may be a very well defined pairing. This means that the part of the response unique to the individual (or the pair) appears in both the control and the treatment measurement and cancels out when the difference is calculated. As Fig. 9.27 shows, the consistent way in which the lines joining paired points slope upwards gives a much stronger impression of a genuine treatment effect than the points alone.

The questions dictating which models need to be fitted and compared are: (i) Is the effect of treatment the same for all subjects? That is, are the population lines parallel? (ii)

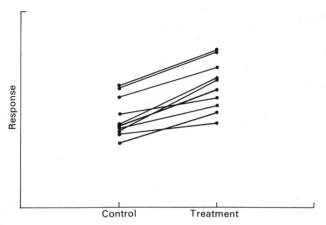

**Fig. 9.27.** Paired observations plotted against treatment category.

Assuming the effect is the same for all is it non-zero? That is, are the population lines non-horizontal?

The first question cannot be answered if, as is usual, there is only one measurement for each subject within a group. In a non-parallel line model every pair of points has its own line which fits them exactly and there are no deviations. This means there is no information about the underlying variation and inferences cannot therefore be made about the population. To address this particular question it is necessary to replicate some of the measurements.

To answer the second question it is necessary to fit a set of parallel lines to the pairs of points. The model is:

1.  Mean $Y = rv +$ Subject effect + Treatment effect

where the 'treatment effect' is actually the mean of the treatment/control differences. The subject effects represent the height of the lines in Fig. 9.27. It is not necessary to estimate these effects they are included in the model to keep them out of the residual sum of squares and hence reduce the residual variance. There are $2n$ points from $n$ subjects, the model requires $n$ parameters for the subjects and 1 for the treatment group difference. Thus the residual sum of squares $S_1$, has $2n - (n + 1) = n - 1$ df.

The model appropriate to the hypothesis that the treatment has no effect is:

2.  Mean $Y = rv +$ Subject effect

which is simply a set of horizontal lines. The model requires one parameter for each subject so the residual sum of squares $S_2$ has $2n - n = n$ df. The analysis of variance is given in Table 9.17.

This is a very simple example. In practice there may well be subpopulations such as sex represented in the sample and it will be necessary to check that effects are the same in each. There will frequently be more than two treatment groups.

The model comparison approach can be extended quite simply to handle both situations. It does, however, need quite sophisticated computing facilities.

In this simplest of cases, the test of the treatment effect can be expressed as what is known as the paired $t$-test. Denoting the treatment/control difference for each subject by $d$, then:

$$\text{Treatment effect} = \text{Mean } d$$

and the test of the estimate against zero is

$$t = \text{Mean } d / \sqrt{(s_d^2 / n)}$$

where $s_d$ is the standard deviation of the $n$ differences.

### Example

In an investigation of the accuracy of blood pressure measurements, two measurements of systolic blood pressure were taken about five minutes apart. These replicated readings ought to differ in a purely random way unless the process of measurement affects the value. The comparison here is not between two treatments but between the first and second reading. The mean values are given in Table 9.18. If these are treated as two independent groups the apparent decrease is far from significant.

**Table 9.18.** *Means of paired blood pressure readings*

|        | 1st reading | 2nd reading |
|--------|-------------|-------------|
| Number | 10          | 10          |
| Mean   | 157.6       | 152.1       |
| sd     | 17.0        | 17.0        |

Table 9.19 gives the analysis of variance obtained by fitting the models with subject parameters to take account of the pairing. The 95 centile of this $F$ distribution is, $F_{1,\,9,\,0.95} = 5.12$, the 90 centile is 3.35 and hence, $0.05 < p \leqslant 0.10$. The model with a reading effect fits better, but not startlingly so. The evidence is ambiguous. It is probably necessary to repeat the investigation with a larger sample before coming to a conclusion on the existence or otherwise of a reading effect.

**Table 9.19.** *Analysis of variance to test for a change over time in duplicate systolic blood pressure readings*

| Model | SS | df | MS | F |
|-------|-----|-----|-------|-----|
| 1. Reading effect | 299.3 | 9 | 33.25 | |
| 2. No reading effect | 450.5 | 10 | | |
| (2 – 1) Due to reading effect | 151.2 | 1 | 151.2 | $F_{1,9} = 4.55$ |

Treating the analysis as a straight paired $t$ test the mean difference is:

$$d = -5.55 \quad (1\text{st} - 2\text{nd reading})$$

**Table 9.17.** *Analysis of variance for paired measurements*

| Model | SS | df | MS | F |
|-------|-----|-------|-------|-----|
| 1. Parallel lines | $S_1$ | $n-1$ | $s^2$ | |
| 2. Horizontal lines | $S_2$ | $n$ | | |
| (2 – 1) Due to slope of lines | $S_2 - S_1$ | 1 | $S_2 - S_1$ | $F_{1,n-1} = (S_2 - S_1)/s^2$ |

with the residual sum of squares of the differences about their mean of:

$$Sdd = 598.6 \text{ with 9df}$$

the variance of the differences therefore is:

$$s_d^2 = 598.6/9 = 66.5$$

and:

$$t = d/\text{se}(d) = 5.5/\sqrt{(66.5/10)} = 2.13.$$

This must be compared with the 97.5 centile of the $t$ distribution with 9df which is 2.26. Thus, as for the $F$ test $p$ obtained in this way is greater than 0.05. In fact this $t$ value is the square root of the above $F$ value ($2.26^2 = 5.12$) illustrating that $F$ and $t$ here are effectively the same test and will always produce the same answer.

### Sample size calculations for comparing means

Sample sizes for significance tests of means are calculated in much the same way as they are for estimation (see p. 155) with one extra complication. The probability of accepting an incorrect hypothesis, that is a type II error, must be taken into account. Since the standard error of the test statistic is a function of the sample size $n$ and the residual variance, which must be known or estimated, the calculation amounts to solving, for $n$:

$$\frac{\text{smallest interesting value of the test statistic} - \text{value expected if hypothesis true}}{\text{standard error of test statistic}} \geqslant Za + Zb.$$

The values $Za$ and $Zb$ are centiles of the standard normal distribution which are determined by the size of the type I and II errors considered acceptable. The $t$ distribution might be more appropriate. However, since the $t$ distribution centiles can only be determined if the degrees of freedom and hence the sample size is known, the argument becomes circular. It is simpler to use the normal distribution and remember that the calculated sample sizes may be slightly smaller than is necessary.

$Za$ will usually be 1.96 for a type I error of 5 per cent. Demanding an 80 per cent chance of detecting when the hypothesis is false, which implies a type II error of 20 per cent, means that $Zb$ must be taken as 0.84, the 80th centile of the standard normal distribution.

For a paired $t$ test, as above, the expected difference, given the usual hypothesis of no effect, is zero. If the smallest interesting difference is $D$, a 5 per cent significance level is to be used ($Za = 1.96$), and an 80 per cent chance of detecting a real difference as large as $D$ is required ($Zb = 0.84$) then the sample size $n$ (the number of pairs) must satisfy:

$$(D - 0)/(s_d^2/\sqrt{n}) \geqslant 1.96 + 0.84.$$

Note that $D$ is assumed positive which makes no difference and simplifies the calculations. This requires that:

$$n \geqslant (1.96 + 0.84)^2 \times 2s_d^2 / D^2.$$

### Example

Suppose it is of importance to detect a difference of 5 mm Hg between paired blood pressure measurements. With type I and II errors of 5 and 20 per cent, this requires a sample size of:

$$n \geqslant (1.96 + 0.84)^2 \times 2 \times 66.5/25 = 41.7.$$

Thus at least 42 pairs of measurements are required.

If two independent groups are to be compared (see pp. 159–61), the calculations are similar except that the form of the standard error becomes that given in eqn 9.14. Using $D$ as the smallest interesting difference, the sample size is obtained by solving:

$$(D - 0)/\sqrt{[s^2(1/n_1 + 1/n_2)]} \geqslant Za + Zb$$

for $n_1$ and $n_2$.

Since analyses are most efficient if the sample sizes are equal, assuming them both equal to $n$ the number in each group must satisfy:

$$n \geqslant (Za + Zb)^2 \, 2s^2/D^2.$$

### Example

In a study to assess the effect of jogging on systolic blood pressure, two independent groups, one of joggers and one of non-joggers would be compared. The appropriate test statistic would be the difference between the means. This is known as a two group $t$ test. If $D$ is set at 5 mm Hg, the two error levels I and II taken as 5 and 20 per cent and the residual variance taken from previous studies as 225, then the number in each group must be:

$$n \geqslant (1.96 + 0.84)^2 \times 2 \times 225/25 = 141.1.$$

That is, 142 subjects are required in each group.

The analyses in the preceding sections cover most of the situations that arise in practice when responses are measured.

## Qualitative responses – two category outcomes

### Maximum likelihood estimation

Exactly the same questions arise for qualitative as for quantitative responses, and the same general approach is used as covered above. There are, however, a few essential differences which must be discussed.

Typically two category outcomes arise when the effects of some treatment or experience are judged according to whether an individual responds or not, has a symptom or not, and so on. The outcome variables are responses with the values yes or no. It is conventional to represent such variables numerically as 0 and 1. Obviously they cannot have normal distributions and the principle of least squares cannot be used, but apart from this the conceptual approach to the analysis is identical to that for measured outcome variables.

In fact the underlying distribution is binomial and instead of mean values it is the proportion of individuals in each category that are of interest. In the population these proportions are the probabilities or 'risks' of individuals picked at random belonging to the specified category. An algebraic model is needed to describe how the 'risk' of an individual being in category 1 (responding, having a symptom, etc.)

changes from one group to another or according to values of some measured $x$ variable or covariate.

To fit these models (that is, estimate the parameters) the 'maximum likelihood principle' is used instead of least squares. Essentially this means assuming not only that the sample obtained is not peculiar, but also that it is the most likely sample to occur. Once the form of the conditional distributions is determined – in this case binomial – the probability of the sample can be calculated for any algebraic model describing the pattern in the population 'risks', for example:

population risk = some function of $(a + bx)$

The values of the parameters $a$ and $b$ are then chosen to maximize this probability or likelihood. Apart from this difference the process follows much the same lines as the 'least squares' approach.

To illustrate the analysis of this type of data, consider several groups of similar men exposed to differing levels of pollution classified according to whether they have persistent cough or not. If there is a positive relationship, the proportion with cough will start close to some minimum (it cannot go below zero) for low pollution levels, start to rise at some point and then level off as it approaches some upper limit (it cannot exceed 1.0) for high levels of pollution. This produces an 'S' or sigmoid-shaped curve which is characteristic of data where the response variable is constrained between two limits – in this case 0 and 1. From a sample it may appear that there is some sort of relationship even when there is none. The curve may be a chance deviation from a horizontal line. A test is needed to assess whether there really is an effect of exposure on the risk of response. This is obtained by using an algebraic model to describe the curve. The parameters representing how increasing the dose affects response can then be estimated and tested.

If subpopulations are represented in the sample, it will be necessary to compare two or more such dose–response curves. For example, the effect of pollution on respiratory symptoms might have to be assessed using a sample containing smokers and non-smokers. Smokers might well have a consistently higher risk. It is necessary to allow for this when assessing the apparent dose–response relationship. There will be two 'sigmoid' curves representing how risk changes with pollution, one for each of the smoking groups. This pair of curves will have to be described with algebraic models in order to allow for the smoking effect while assessing the effect of pollution. At the tails of such curves the risks are very close to zero or one. Small changes in these may be, proportionally, very important. It is necessary to take into account that a change in risk from 0.01 to 0.02 (1 to 2 per cent) is in fact a doubling of the risk while the same absolute change in the middle of the curve, say 0.50 to 0.51 (50 to 51 per cent), is a relatively trivial proportional change in risk.

In practice this is allowed for by converting the values to the 'logistic scale'. Using the variable $y$ to represent values on this scale, the $y$ values for the proportion with cough, i.e. $p(\text{cough})$, are calculated as:

$$y = \log[p(\text{cough})/(1 - p(\text{cough}))]$$

where the function log() is the 'natural' logarithm to the base '$e$' and the function $p/(1 - p)$ is known as the odds. So:

if $p(\text{cough}) = 0.01$ then $y = \log(0.01/0.99) = -4.6$
if $p(\text{cough}) = 0.50$ then $y = \log(0.5/0.5) = 0.0$

and

if $p(\text{cough}) = 0.99$ then $y = \log(0.99/0.01) = +4.6$.

This pulls the lower tail of the curve down and pushes the upper tail up with an overall effect of straightening the sigmoid curves.

The order of points on the curve is unchanged by moving from the $p$ to the $y$ scale. An increase on the logistic scale automatically implies an increase on the risk scale.

Transforming proportions to the logistic scale:

$$y = \log(p/(1 - p))$$

turns a sigmoid curve into a straight line. The reverse transformation which is:

$$p = 1/(1 - \exp(-y))$$

turns a straight line to a sigmoid curve. The exponential function exp() is the 'anti-log' for logarithms to the base '$e$'. This means that trends in proportions can be assessed and compared by fitting straight line models:

$$y = a + bx$$

on the logistic scale and using the reverse transformation specific risks can be estimated or compared.

All the analyses of the section on measured outcomes can be applied to proportions using this approach. Any proportion can be considered as a point on a sigmoid curve and the same approach can be used for comparing two or more groups, possibly in some cross classification, at the same time as allowing for the effects of covariates.

Because maximum likelihood is used to fit the models and not least squares, the residual sum of squares cannot be used to indicate how well a model fits the data. It is necessary to use what Nelder and Wedderburn (1972) have called the 'deviance' defined as:

$$\text{Deviance} = -2 \times \log(\text{likelihood})$$

where the 'likelihood' is the probability of the sample for the given model.

The analysis of variance to compare two models produces a ratio which is an observation from an $F$ distribution if the two models fit the data equally well. In the analysis of deviance for qualitative response variables the difference between two deviances is, near enough, an observation from a distribution known as the chi-squared distribution. This is a widely used distribution so tables (Lindley and Miller 1964) are available from which centiles and $p$ values can be obtained.

Unfortunately, most practical problems involving proportions can only be handled with the aid of a computer and a good statistical package. Only if the problem is greatly simplified can the analysis be performed by hand. The following sections will cover the general approaches first and then indicate how simpler analyses can be performed at the cost of a few assumptions.

*Comparing two groups allowing for a covariate*

Table 9.20 gives some simulated data on the prevalence of cough in children exposed to different levels of pollution. The proportions increase steadily with increasing pollution and they might well arise from the tails of 'sigmoid' curves.

**Table 9.20.** *Prevalence of respiratory symptoms (cough) in children by pollution level and smoking in the home (simulated data). Proportion with the symptom (number at risk)*

| | | SO$_2$ pollution level | | |
|---|---|---|---|---|
| | | Low (100 $\mu g/m^3$) | Medium (200 $\mu g/m^3$) | High (300 $\mu g/m^3$) |
| Smoking in the home | No | 0.05 (37) | 0.20 (25) | 0.33 (12) |
| | Yes | 0.09 (32) | 0.29 (28) | 0.53 (17) |

The questions are:
(i) Is the effect of pollution the same in both groups? That is, on the logistic scale are the equivalent population lines parallel?
If parallelism can be assumed:
(ii) Is there an effect of pollution? That is, are the equivalent population lines non-horizontal?
and
(iii) Is there an effect of exposure to smoking? That is, are the equivalent population lines separated vertically?
For this analysis it is necessary to fit the models
(1) *Non-parallel* – a different pollution effect in each smoking group

$$y = rv + \text{smoking effect} + \text{smoking group pollution effect}$$

$rv$ is the reference value which is the predicted proportion for the low pollution/no smoking reference group transformed to a value on the logistic scale.
(2) *Parallel*

$$y = rv + \text{smoking effect} + \text{pollution effect}$$

(3) *Horizontal* – no pollution effect

$$y = rv + \text{smoking effect}$$

and
(4) *Coincident lines* – no smoking effect

$$y = rv + \text{pollution effect}.$$

The analysis was performed using a computer and the statistical package GLIM (Baker and Nelder 1978). Other packages such as BMD-P (Dixon 1981) can be used to perform the same analyses, but not so easily. GLIM requires as input the numbers at risk and the numbers responding (that is those with symptoms) for each cell of the two way table (Table 9.20) to fit the models and obtain their deviances. From these the analysis of deviance in Table 9.21 can be constructed.

From line (2–1), there is no evidence of non-parallelism. The difference between the two deviances gives a chi-squared value of 0.04 which is trivial compared to the 95th centile of the chi-squared distribution with one degree of freedom which is

**Table 9.21.** *Analysis of deviance for comparing prevalences of respiratory symptoms in children classified by exposure to air pollution and cigarette smoking*

| Model | Deviance | df | Approximate chi-squared |
|---|---|---|---|
| 1. Different pollution effects non-parallel | 0.40 | 2 | |
| 2. Identical effects parallel | 0.44 | 3 | |
| (2 – 1) Due to different effects | 0.04 | 1 | 0.04  (cf. Chi $S_{1,\,0.95} = 3.84$) |
| 3. No pollution effect horizontal | 17.64 | 4 | |
| (3 – 2) Due to pollution effect | 17.20 | 1 | 17.20  ($p < 0.01$) |
| 4. No smoking effect coincident lines | 2.38 | 4 | |
| (4 – 2) Due to smoking effects | 1.94 | 1 | 1.94  not significant |

3.84. Whatever the association it is the same whether or not the child is exposed to cigarette smoking in the home.

From line (3–2) omitting the pollution effect from the parallel line model gives a much worse fitting model. Values as large as the chi-squared value testing the slope of the pollution trend against zero, that is 17.6, should occur, by chance, in less than 0.1 per cent of such investigations. The 99.9 centile of the chi-squared distribution on 1 df is only 10.83. This simulated data very strongly indicate that at these levels there is an association between increasing pollution levels and increasing risk of having a symptom.

The effect of smoking in the home is not so clear. The smoking effect, that is, the separation of the two lines, appears to be no more than could easily occur by chance. The chi-squared value of 1.94 on 1 df is well below the 3.84 required for significance.

The parallel line model (2) is adequate to describe the data and it provides estimates of the effects. The model is, on the logistic scale,

$$y = a + smk + b \times \text{pollution}$$

where $a$ is the intercept for the no smoking group; $smk$ the smoking effect, is the vertical separation of the lines; and $b$ is the slope or regression coefficient of the pollution trends.

The computed analysis gives estimates with approximate standard errors as:

$$a = -3.87 \qquad \text{with } se(a) = 0.69$$
$$smk = 0.61 \qquad\qquad se(smk) = 0.44$$
$$b = 0.0113 \qquad\qquad se(b) = 0.0029$$

The pollution effect can be tested by comparing $b$ with 0 using the standardized normal distribution ($u$):

$$u = 0.0113/0.0029 = 3.90 \qquad (\text{cf.} 1.96).$$

This gives an equally significant result to that of the chi-squared test. They are essentially two ways of doing the same thing.

The test of the smoking effect, $0.61/0.44 = 1.39$, is

consistent with this chi-squared result, well below 1.96. The confidence interval which therefore includes zero is

$$0.61 \pm 1.96 \times 0.44$$
or                      $-0.25$ to $1.47$.

However, the data are consistent with quite large values, up to 1.47. It is wise to investigate what these effects on the logistic scale mean in terms of estimated risks.

Taking pollution at $100 \ \mu g/m^3$, the low category on the logistic scale, the model predicts that for the no smoking (ns) group:

$$y_{ns} = -3.87 + 0.0113 \times 100 = -2.74$$

and for the smoking (s) group:

$$y_s = -3.87 + 0.61 + 0.0113 \times 100 = -2.13$$

If $y = \log(p/(1-p))$ then the value of $p$ is:

$$p = 1/(1 + \exp(-y))$$

so:

$$p_{ns} = 1/(1 + \exp(+2.74)) = 0.061$$

and

$$p_s = 1/(1 + \exp(+2.13)) = 0.106.$$

This means that the estimated risks of having the symptom 'cough' are 6.1 and 10.6 per cent respectively. And although it does not reach significance in this data set the effect of exposure to smoking is estimated as an increase in risk of 4.5 per cent. The risk of 6.1 per cent has nearly doubled going from children not exposed to smoking to those who are. If this represents a real effect it is obviously important.

The ratio of the two risks is known as the relative risk – that is the risk of the exposed relative to that of those not exposed. This is calculated as:

$$\text{relative risk} = 0.106/0.061 = 1.74$$

which is nearly 2 indicating that the risk is nearly doubled.

An approximation of the relative risk is provided by the odds ratio which, for the smoking factor, is:

$$(p_s/(1-p_s))/(p_{ns}/(1-p_{ns})).$$

Because the analysis uses the logistic scale this is in fact:

$$\exp(smk) = \exp(0.61) = 1.84$$

which is rather larger than the relative risk. None the less for small risks (about 5 per cent or less) the odds ratio is a good approximation to the relative risk.

There are a number of tests specifically designed for comparing such estimates of relative risk with the value expected if the true risks are identical – that is 1. (For further discussion see Chapter 8 on case-control studies.) Apart from slightly differing assumptions they are effectively the same test as that derived from the model comparison in the analysis of deviance. In addition, fitting and comparing models has allowed the use of all the data from several pollution groups. The model comparison approach is much more general. It can be extended to cover very complicated data sets and it allows estimates of all the various effects to be obtained in a relatively straightforward way.

From the parallel line model, approximate confidence intervals for the estimates of risk and relative risk can be obtained. However, this can only be done indirectly by first calculating the confidence limits on the logistic scale as:

$$\text{estimate} + 1.96 \ se(\text{estimate})$$

and then converting the limits of the confidence interval back to the risk scale. The predicted $y$ value for the no smoking group is:

$$y = a + b \times 100.$$

The standard error of $y$, $se(y)$, which is the square root of the sampling variance of $y$, is a function of the sampling variances of $a$ and $b$ with what is known as their covariance. The interdependence of estimates has not been discussed, but they must be taken into account when standard errors of functions of estimates are required. For a full discussion see Armitage (1971). All that is needed are the covariances of the estimates and these are readily obtained during computer analysis. For $y = a + bx$ the variance of $y$ ($\text{var}(y)$) is then calculated by:

$$\text{Var}(y) = \text{var}(a) + 2x \times \text{covariance}(a, b) + x^2 \times \text{var}(b).$$

For this analysis, the computer produced the values:

$$\text{var}(a) = 0.48$$
$$\text{var}(b) = 8.3 \times 10^{-6}$$
$$\text{cov}(a, b) = -0.0017$$

So   $\text{var}(y) = 0.48 + 200(-0.0017) + 100^2 \times 10^{-6} \times 8.30$
$$= 0.22$$
and   $se(y) = \sqrt{(\text{var}(y))} = 0.47.$

The 95 per cent confidence interval for $y$ in the no smoking group is therefore:

$$-2.74 \pm 1.96 \times 0.47$$
or
$$-3.66 \text{ to } -1.82$$

Converting back to the risk scale, the equivalent confidence interval for the risk in this group is 0.025 to 0.139. In the group exposed to smoking the equivalent figures are 10.6 per cent for the best estimate of risk with a confidence interval of 5.0 to 21.3 per cent. This gives an estimated relative risk of 10.6/6.1 = 1.75.

It is not simple to obtain a confidence interval for the true relative risk, but it is quite straightforward for the odds ratio. On the logistic scale, the effect of smoking is 0.61 with a confidence interval of $0.61 \pm 1.96 \times 0.44$ or $-0.25$ to $1.47$. The odds ratio is estimated as $\exp(0.61)$ and $\exp(-0.25)$ to $\exp(1.47)$, that is 0.77 to 4.35, are approximate confidence limits.

The data are reasonably consistent with a true odds ratio as low as 0.77, that is, the no smoking group running less risk than the smoking group, or as high as 4.35, that is, the group exposed to smoking running more than four times the risk of those not exposed. This means that the odds ratio is not significantly different from 1.

The conclusions from these simulated data are first that there is strong evidence of a pollution effect – going from low to medium to high pollution in these individuals at least doubles then trebles the risk in both the smoking and non-smoking groups. Secondly there is some suggestion that a larger study might identify an important effect of exposure to smoking since these results are not inconsistent with a four-fold increase in risk of cough in those exposed to smoking compared with those not so exposed.

### Comparing two proportions

If data were only available for the high pollution group as in Table 9.22, the problem reduces to comparing two proportions. The prevalence of cough is 4/12 or 33.3 per cent in the non-smoking homes and 9/17 or 52.9 per cent in the smoking homes. The question is: 'Are these two proportions more different than could easily occur by chance?'

**Table 9.22.** *Numbers of children with cough according to whether they were exposed to smoking in the home and, in parentheses, the numbers expected if there was no association between exposure and risk of cough*

|        |       | Smoking in the home |         |       |
|--------|-------|------------|---------|-------|
|        |       | No         | Yes     | Total |
| Cough  | Yes   | 4 (5.4)    | 9 (7.6) | 13    |
|        | No    | 8 (6.6)    | 8 (9.4) | 16    |
|        | Total | 12         | 17      | 29    |

The hypothesis to test is that there is a single 'true' risk which is the same for both groups and that the differences arose by chance. This single risk, assuming the hypothesis true, is best estimated by using all the data, i.e. by $13/29 = 44.8$ per cent.

This means that on average in studies like this 44.8 per cent of each group would be expected to fall in the cough category. On this basis the expected numbers can be calculated for each cell of the table: 5.4 is 44.8 per cent of 12, 7.6 is 44.8 per cent of 17 and so on. The problem becomes one of assessing whether the cell frequencies are surprisingly far from those expected. For each cell the measure of how far apart the observed and expected frequencies are is taken as:

$$\frac{(\text{observed frequency} - \text{expected frequency})^2}{\text{expected frequency}}$$

or more simply:

$$(O - E)^2/E.$$

This summed over all the cells of the table gives a measure of how the table as a whole deviates from what should be expected if the hypothesis were true, that is:

$$\text{Sum for all cells of } (O - E)^2/E$$

which can be shown to have a chi-squared distribution on one degree of freedom. This is because the analysis is essentially comparing a model with two different proportions or parameters, with a model with one proportion or parameter. Measures of the difference between these two models have one degree of freedom. In this case:

$$\text{chi-squared} = (4 - 5.4)^2/5.4 + (9 - 7.6)^2/7.6$$
$$+ (8 - 6.6)^2/6.6 + (8 - 9.4)^2/9.4 = 1.09$$

which is a long way from significance at the 5 per cent level (cf. 3.84).

Practical problems rarely reduce to the comparison of two proportions without gross simplification. None the less, a number of alternatives to this test have been developed over the years. There is also a lot of discussion as to which is right. Fortunately it rarely matters. Yates (1934) pointed out that Sum $(O - E)^2/E$ was more nearly a chi-squared variable if the test was slightly modified by subtracting 0.5 from the frequencies on the diagonal with the largest product, in this case the 8,9 diagonal. This is probably the most sensible test to use in this context. If a computer is available and it still seems appropriate to treat the analysis as nothing more than the comparison of two proportions then a test known as Fisher's exact test is more precise.

Fisher's test calculates the exact probability of this or more surprising tables occurring given the marginal totals and the hypothesis. It therefore gives $p$ values directly. Those requiring the algebraic details should consult Armitage (1971).

### Sample sizes for comparing proportions

The exact solution to this problem leads to a very complicated formula which can be found in a paper by Casagrande *et al.* (1978). For most practical purposes it will be sufficient to use a calculation analogous to that for comparing means. The sample sizes obtained will be slightly smaller than optimum, but this can be regarded as an increase in the risk of a type II error. If this matters the risk can be set higher and the calculations repeated. The calculations are based on expressing the chi-squared test above in the form:

$$\frac{\text{estimate} - \text{expected value}}{se \text{ (estimate)}}$$

where the estimate is the difference between two proportions and usually the expected value is zero. The test statistic is:

$$(r_1/n_1 - r_2/n_2)/\sqrt{[p(1 - p)(1/n_1 + 1/n_2)]}$$

where $p$ is $(r_1 + r_2)/(n_1 + n_2)$. For quite small proportions and values of $n_1$ and $n_2$ this has a sampling distribution close to normal. This means that the statistic may be tested against 1.96 for a 5 per cent significance level. As for comparing means, it is efficient to keep the groups the same size. The number in each group must then satisfy:

$$D/\sqrt{[p(1 - p)2/n]} \geqslant Za + Zb$$

where $Za$ and $Zb$ are centiles of the standard normal distribution determined by the choice of what risks of type I and II errors are acceptable. In this calculation $p$ is taken as the average of the two proportions expected if the hypothesis is false. The number must satisfy:

$$n \geqslant (Za + Zb)^2 \times 2p(1 - p)/D^2.$$

### Example

What sample size is needed to detect a difference in the prevalence of respiratory symptoms between children in two towns with differing air pollution levels? If the prevalence is about 20 per cent and the smallest interesting difference is 5 per cent than $p = 0.20 + 0.05/2 = 0.225$. If the acceptable risks of type I and II errors are 5 per cent and 20 per cent, then the number in each group must satisfy:

$$n \geqslant (1.96 + 0.84)^2 \times 2 \times 0.225(1 - 0.225)/(0.05)^2$$

which gives $n \geqslant 1093.7$. Thus 1094 subjects are needed in each group and 2188 in total.

This and the section on sample size for comparing means (p. 167) give a simplified guide to sample size calculations. Lachin (1981) gives a very comprehensive guide.

### Repeated observations

An individual may be classified as having a symptom or not several times during a course of treatment. This produces an analysis problem analogous to that of repeated measurements. Using a subject parameter in the model allows it to be analysed in much the same way using an analysis of deviance instead of the analysis of variance. Odds ratio estimates for risks before and after some treatment or exposure may then be obtained as the square root of the equivalent estimate in the section above on comparing two groups allowing for a covariate (pp. 169–71). In practice, a modified form of model fitting is used for this type of data which also arises in matched case-control studies discussed in the next section and a separate chapter. A comprehensive discussion of the model fitting approach in this context is given by Breslow and Day (1980), and the method of analysis with the computer package GLIM is fully described by Adena (1982).

In the simplest case analogous to the paired $t$ test problem a simple technique known as McNemar's test may be used.

### Example using McNemar's test

Geriatric patients in the community often have complex drug regimens to follow. Table 9.23 gives some data from a study to assess whether a specially designed, patient held, treatment record affects the error rate when the patients are questioned on their regimen.

**Table 9.23.** *Distribution of subjects according to errors made on their regimen before and after provision of a patient-held treatment record*

| | | After record | |
| --- | --- | --- | --- |
| | | Errors | No errors |
| Before record | Errors | 4 | 4 |
| | No errors | 0 | 2 |

It is possible to analyse these data using a model fitting approach, but in this simple case it is not necessary. On the hypothesis that the subjects are equally likely to make errors before and after as many should improve as get worse. This means that those who changed should be equally divided between the two types of change possible.

In these data four changed – they all became better at identifying their drug dosages. The probability of a result as surprising as this if there was only a 50 per cent chance of getting better is required. This is exactly the same as the probability of getting heads in all four tosses of a coin which is $0.5 \times 0.5 \times 0.5 \times 0.5 = 0.0625$ and the probability of a result this surprising is $p = 0.0625$ which is at least interesting although not less than 0.05.

If the effect was genuinely of this magnitude a larger sample might well have shown it to be significant.

### Comparing proportions from separate samples —case-control or retrospective studies

If cases with a particular disease or condition and controls are not matched to have the same values of potentially interfering factors such as age and sex, the data from case-control studies are analysed in exactly the same way, using the model fitting approach, as any other set of proportions taking cases/(cases +controls) as the proportions. Odds ratios, assessing the effects on risk of factors in the model, are obtained from the fitted model as described earlier (p. 170).

If the cases and controls have been matched in some way according to factors which might be related to the risk of becoming a case then the correct analysis is more complicated. Further discussion may be found in Chapter 8, Breslow and Day (1980), and Adena (1982).

### More than two categories of outcome

Categorical outcomes arise when individuals can respond to treatment or experience in several ways not easily measured. For example a treatment for Hodgkin's disease may be assessed according to whether the patients 'died', 'got worse', 'stayed the same' or 'showed signs of remission'. The clinicians overall classification is preferred in this case to a single measure of well-being such as white cell count.

It is always possible to combine some of the categories so there are only two, for example, 'no remission' and 'remission'. This permits the response to be treated as a proportion and allows the use of the methods in the previous section. In practice this is often the most sensible thing to do although it does waste information. Alternatively, some way must be found for describing responses in many categories by models.

Consider data from a trial comparing two treatments, A and B, for Hodgkin's disease. The outcomes, assessed after a fixed period of treatment, were 'no response or died', 'partial remission' and 'complete remission'. The results are given in Table 9.24.

It is necessary to compare how the two groups are distributed among the response categories. This is best done

**Table 9.24.** *Distribution of Hodgkin's disease patients by treatment and remission category (treatment group percentages in parentheses)*

| | Remission category | | | |
| --- | --- | --- | --- | --- |
| Treatment | 1. None/died | 2. Partial remission | 3. Complete remission | Total |
| A | 16 (40) | 9 (23) | 15 (37) | 40 (100) |
| B | 11 (24) | 4 ( 9) | 31 (67) | 46 (100) |

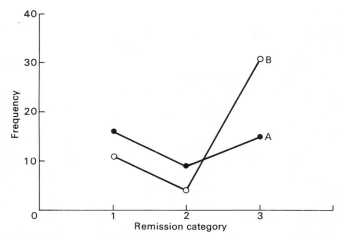

**Fig. 9.28.** Frequency of Hodgkin's disease patients against remission category by treatment group. (Source: British National Lymphoma Investigation (1975).)

by plotting the frequencies against the remission category for each of the treatment groups. Joining the points within each treatment group makes the diagram easier to interpret (Fig. 9.28).

The true responses are represented on the horizontal axis. However, if the frequencies on the $y$ axis are considered as the response variable then the pattern to be described by an algebraic model has exactly the same form as discussed in previous sections for means and proportions. The $y$ variable in this context is a 'count' or frequency.

For proportions obtained from counts in two categories of response it was necessary to use the logistic scale to fit the models. For frequencies it is necessary to use another scale and the most useful and appropriate is the logarithmic scale. This is logical because changes in frequencies seen when moving to groups at higher risk are likely to be proportional. On the frequency scale distances representing the same proportional difference will change with the frequency. On the log (frequency) scale these distances will stay constant which means that constant proportional effects will give parallel line models. For this reason this analysis has come to be known as 'log linear modelling'.

Notice that if there had been many more subjects in treatment group A the frequencies would all be larger. The A line would have been much higher than the B line, even if the treatments were equally effective. Because of this it is the parallelism of the lines that is the main interest not their separation.

To test whether there are significant differences in the shapes of the distribution it is necessary to compare models with and without interaction parameters. Because the height of the lines does not matter it is not necessary to treat it as a random variable and waste information estimating some 'true' height. This is avoided by forcing the model fitting process to choose estimates for the 'height' parameters so the model fits or predicts the observed total frequencies exactly.

Apart from the use of the log scale, the constraints on the models and the interactions being the model parameters of prime interest, the analysis is much the same as for

proportions. Maximum likelihood and the analysis of deviance are used to produce approximate chi-squared tests of the interaction parameters quantifying the hypothesis of interest.

*Comparing two groups with three outcomes*

In the above example the models to be compared are

(1) *Non-parallel lines*
$$y = rv + \text{treatment effect} + \text{remission category effect} + \text{treatment} \times \text{remission category interaction}$$

and

(2) *Parallel lines*
$$y = rv + \text{treatment effect} + \text{remission category effect}.$$

Model 1 requires six parameters. Since there are only six points it will fit the data exactly and there are no degrees of freedom and no deviance.

A computer analysis gave the deviance from the parallel line model as 8.17 on 2df so the analysis of deviance is as in Table 9.25.

**Table 9.25.** *Analysis of deviance comparing the frequency distribution of Hodgkin's disease patients among three remission categories for two treatment groups*

| Model | Deviance | df | Chi-squared |
|---|---|---|---|
| 1. Non-parallel | 0 | 0 | |
| 2. Parallel | 8.17 | 2 | |
| (2 − 1) Due to non-parallelism | 8.17 | 2 | 8.17 |

Since the 95th centile of the chi-squared distribution with 2 df is 5.99, the outcome distributions of the two treatment groups are significantly different ($p < 0.05$). It only remains to make quantitative statements about how the 'relative risk' of ending up in the various remission categories varies according to treatment using the estimated frequencies from the non-parallel model and the treatment group totals, which give, in this simple case, estimates of risk equal to the percentages in Table 9.24.

This approach easily extends to more complex problems, for example, if initial severity subgroups had to be taken into account.

*Comparing frequencies in a two-way classification*

If the data are as simple as in the above example, the frequencies can be compared directly with a chi-squared test

**Table 9.26.** *Distribution of Hodgkin's disease patients by treatments and remission category with, in parentheses, frequencies expected assuming equally effective treatments*

| | Response | | | |
|---|---|---|---|---|
| | 1 | 2 | 3 | Total |
| A | 16 (12.6) | 9 (6.0) | 15 (21.4) | 40 |
| B | 11 (14.4) | 4 (7.0) | 31 (24.6) | 46 |
| Total | 27 | 13 | 46 | 86 |
| % | 31.4 | 15.1 | 53.5 | 100 |

using expected frequencies calculated assuming the hypothesis to be tested as true (Table 9.26).

On the hypothesis that the treatments are equally effective, 31.4 per cent, 15.1 per cent, and 53.5 per cent of individuals would be expected to fall into the three response categories whatever the treatment (Table 9.26). This means that 31.4 per cent of the 40 receiving treatment A are expected to fall into response category 1:

$$\frac{31.4}{100} \times 40 = \frac{27}{86} \times 40 = 12.6$$

in category 2, 15.1 per cent of 13 = 6, and so on.

As when comparing two proportions (pp. 171–2), the test of whether the frequencies are surprisingly far from those expected on the hypothesis of equally effective treatments is:

$$\text{chi-squared} = \text{Sum } (O - E)^2 / E = 8.03.$$

This is not quite the same as the analysis of deviance chi-squared value, because the analyses make slightly different assumptions. However, the conclusion is much the same and unless 5 per cent is inappropriately regarded as a 'magic' cut-off point these two approaches will usually lead to the same conclusions.

### Survival or event data

These data arise when individuals observed over time are at risk of some event. The event may be death, menarche, coronary heart attack, and so on. After death or menarche the individual is no longer at risk. The event cannot occur again. A coronary heart attack could in fact be the first of many, but if observation of the subject is discontinued after the event it can be treated as terminal and standard analyses used.

If these data consist of numbers dying in a fixed period then the analysis is simply a comparison of proportions. The techniques of the section on qualitative two category responses (pp. 167–72) will usually suffice. Annual mortality rates from different geographical areas can be analysed in this way, treating them as proportions, but there may be complications as discussed by Pocock *et al.* (1981). None the less, the analysis of mortality data of this sort by a model-fitting approach avoids the use of standardizing techniques whereby mortality figures were traditionally adjusted for age and sex effects before group comparisons were made notably using standardized mortality ratios (SMRs). Such adjustments make possibly unwarranted and certainly untested assumptions about the effects of age and sex being the same in all the groups to be compared and for that reason must be used with care.

When the individuals are at risk of the event for varying periods of time the problem cannot easily be considered as an analysis of proportions. There are two main types of problem. In the first it is assumed that within the groups to be compared the risk is constant over time. In the second case the risk changes with time. The remaining discussion will be restricted to these two types of survival data.

*Constant risks*

From the number experiencing the event in a group of individuals observed for varying lengths of time the risk per unit time for an individual in the group can be estimated by dividing the number of deaths by the accumulated time at risk. The modelling approach to analysing such data requires that the number of deaths in each group is taken as the response variable and the accumulated time at risk used as a covariate.

In the occupational health study data in Table 9.27 the deaths were classified according to factory and age at the start of the observation period. The table also gives the total man years at risk (MYR) within each group. Since the response variable is a count, the appropriate analysis requires fitting the models on the log scale using $y = \log (\text{deaths})$ as the response variable.

**Table 9.27.** *Number of deaths by age group and factory from a study of occupational mortality with man years at risk in parentheses*

| Age at start of study (years) | Factory | |
|---|---|---|
| | 1 | 2 |
| 50–59.9 | 7 (4045) | 7 (3701) |
| 60–69.9 | 27 (3571) | 37 (3702) |
| 70–79.9 | 30 (1777) | 35 (1818) |
| 80–89.9 | 8 ( 381) | 9 ( 350) |

The questions to be answered are: 'Is the effect of age the same in both factories?' If it is: 'Are the risks, allowing for age, different in the two factories?' The models to answer these are:

(1) *Non-parallel age trends*
　　$y = \log (\text{MYR}) + rv + \text{factory effect}$
　　　　　　　　　　　　$+ \text{factory specific slope} \times \text{age}$
assuming straight line age trends.

(2) *Parallel age trends*
　　$y = \log (\text{MYR}) + rv + \text{factory effect}$
　　　　　　　　　　　　$+ \text{slope} \times \text{age}$

(3) *No factory effect*
　　$y = \log (\text{MYR}) + rv + \text{slope} \times \text{age}$
and for completeness

(4) *No age effect*
　　$y = \log (\text{MYR}) + rv + \text{factory effect}.$

When these models are fitted the analysis of deviance in Table 9.28 is obtained.

The 95th centile of the chi-squared distribution with one degree of freedom is 3.84 and values less than this could well occur by chance. Obviously the age effect producing a chi-squared value of 89.19 is very marked and real. The factory effect gives a chi-squared of 1.73 which does not appear to indicate much. However, the initial deviance of 12.70 on four degrees of freedom indicates that the first model is a long way from the data points. The linear age trends do not fit the data well so the subsequent analysis must be treated with caution. In fact fitting an age-squared term to allow for curvature

**Table 9.28.** *Analysis of deviance comparing mortality in two factories allowing for different age structures*

| Model | Deviance | df | Chi-squared |
|---|---|---|---|
| 1. Non-parallel linear age trends | 12.70 | 4 | |
| 2. Parallel trends | 12.71 | 5 | |
| (2 − 1) Due to non-parallelism | 0.01 | 1 | 0.01 |
| 3. No factory effect | 14.44 | 6 | |
| (3 − 2) Due to factory effect | 1.73 | 1 | 1.73 |
| 4. No age effect | 101.90 | 6 | |
| (4 − 2) Due to age effects | 89.19 | 1 | 89.19 |

gives a much smaller deviance and the model with such a term, but assuming a zero difference between the two factories:

(5) $y = \log (MYR) + rv + b \times age + c \times age^2$

fits the data well with a deviance of 2.09 on five degrees of freedom. There is therefore very little evidence of a factory effect.

### Observed and expected deaths

In simple cases a hypothesis may be used to deduce the number of deaths expected and these used to calculate $(O - E)^2/E$ for appropriate groups. This can then be used to obtain a simple chi-squared test.

In the above example the hypothesis to be tested was that the risks were equal in the two factories. The risk for each age group per man year is calculated as:

sum of deaths/sum of MYRs.

The expected deaths in each factory are obtained from this multiplied by the appropriate MYR. For the 50-year-olds in factory 1 this gives:

$$\text{expected deaths} = 4045 \times \frac{(7 + 7)}{(4045 + 3701)} = 4045 \times 0.0018 = 7.3$$

Similarly for factory 2:

$$\text{expected deaths} = 3701 \times 0.0018 = 6.7$$

and so on for all age groups.

The overall chi-squared to test the hypothesis of no factory effect on risk is the sum of the eight $(O - E)^2/E$ values which is:

$$(7 - 7.3)^2/7.3 + (7 - 6.7)^2/6.7$$
$$+ (27 - 31.4)^2/31.4 + (37 - 32.6)^2/32.6$$
$$+ (30 - 32.1)^2/32.1 + (35 - 32.9)^2/32.9$$
$$+ (8 - 8.9)^2/8.9 + (9 - 8.1)^2/8.1$$
$$= 1.70.$$

This has four degrees of freedom because there were eight observations and to calculate the chi-squared value it was necessary to estimate four parameters (the risks for the four age groups). The conclusions are the same, but this approach is impossibly tedious if there are many more than two groups

to compare. The modelling approach is almost inevitable for a thorough analysis which estimates the magnitude of the various effects.

### Changing risks – survival curves

For each individual, data of this type will consist of the length of time observed and reason lost to observation. The period of observation may start at birth, diagnosis, start of treatment, or some other appropriate point in time. An individual who dies is then lost to observation. When a study is concluded observation stops on the survivors and some may drop out during the course of the study.

To investigate survival in a group of individuals observed for differing periods of time life-table survival curves are used. The survival curve is a plot against time elapsed from diagnosis, or other appropriate points, of the percentage of individuals surviving. The life-table calculations to obtain these percentages from individuals observed for varying lengths of time are moderately simple, but not obvious.

Consider a number of subjects entering and leaving a trial at different times as in Fig. 9.29. Using time since entry as the horizontal scale gives a modified plot (Fig. 9.30) from which the number of subjects at risk and dying in each week since entry

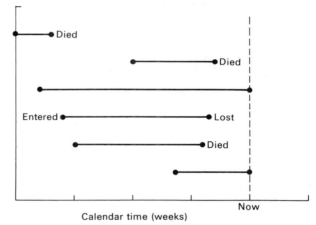

**Fig. 9.29.** Observation periods of subjects in a trial.

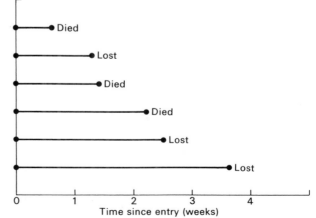

**Fig. 9.30.** Observation periods of subjects in a trial from time of entry.

can be seen. In the first week after entry six were at risk and one had died. This gives an estimated death rate of 0.17 and hence a survival rate of 0.83. In week two there were four at risk all the time, one for half a week and one died giving a death rate of 1/4.5 = 0.22 and a survival rate for individuals getting that far of 0.78.

The chance of an individual surviving the second week which requires he or she survives both the first and the second is 0.83 × 0.78 = 0.65. This is the estimated cumulative survival rate. Plotting it against time from treatment gives the survival curve. Conventionally individuals lost in any interval are treated as having been at risk for half the interval.

The life-table for cancer of the prostate patients in the radiotherapy group of a trial comparing radiotherapy and hormone treatments is given in Table 9.29. The adjusted number at risk is the number entering the interval minus half the number lost to observation during it. Plotting the percentage surviving (S) against the upper end of the time intervals gives the survival curve shown in Fig. 9.31. It is not appropriate to draw a smooth curve through the points since such curves give a spurious impression of accuracy.

**Table 9.29.** *Life table for cancer of the prostate patients in the radiotherapy group of a clinical trial*

| Time since entry (years) | No. died | No. at risk | No. lost | Adj. no. at risk | Estimated probability of Death | Estimated probability of Survival | Estimated proportion of survivors at end of interval |
|---|---|---|---|---|---|---|---|
| 0–1 | 3 | 44 | 3 | 42.5 | 0.071 | 0.929 | 0.929 |
| 1–2 | 2 | 38 | 10 | 33.0 | 0.061 | 0.939 | 0.873 |
| 2–3 | 1 | 26 | 3 | 24.5 | 0.041 | 0.959 | 0.837 |
| 3–4 | 3 | 22 | 3 | 20.5 | 0.146 | 0.854 | 0.715 |
| 4–5 | 2 | 16 | 4 | 14.0 | 0.143 | 0.857 | 0.613 |
| 5–6 | 1 | 10 | 1 | 9.5 | 0.105 | 0.895 | 0.548 |
| 6–7 | 1 | 8 | 1 | 7.5 | 0.133 | 0.867 | 0.475 |
| 7–8 | 0 | 6 | 3 | 4.5 | 0.000 | 1.000 | 0.475 |
| 8–9 | 1 | 3 | 1 | 2.5 | 0.400 | 0.600 | 0.285 |
| 9–10 | 1 | 1 | 0 | 1.0 | 1.000 | 0.000 | 0.000 |

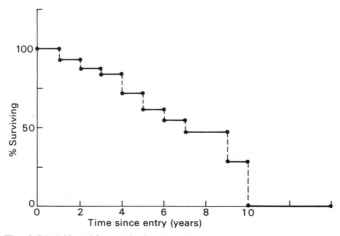

**Fig. 9.31.** Life-table survival curve for the radiotherapy group in a trial of treatments for cancer of the prostate.

Comparisons of a small number of survival curves can be made by hand using what is known as the 'log rank' test. On the hypothesis of no difference between two curves the number of deaths expected in each group can be calculated. By calculating $(O - E)^2/E$ for each group a chi-squared test on one degree of freedom comparing the curves can be obtained. The method can be used to compare survival curves within a cross-classification of treatment or other groups but it is not simple. The method is described in detail by Peto *et al.* (1976).

At the cost of a few testable and often reasonable assumptions a full modelling approach can be used analogous to those discussed in earlier sections. This approach was introduced by Cox (1972) and is discussed by Anderson *et al.* (1980) and Kalbfleisch and Prentice (1980). Although these texts are rather mathematical, computer programs are now available that make it possible to fit sequences of models to survival data with relative ease. This approach provides quantitative estimates with standard errors thus aiding considerably the interpretation and presentation aspects of the analysis.

## CONCLUSION

Obviously special problems require special techniques which cannot be discussed here. None the less, the range of problems discussed and the appropriate analytical approaches cover the major part of statistical activity in public health research and epidemiology. With reasonable computing facilities most practical problems you meet can be tackled using these methods.

## REFERENCES

Adena, M.A. and Wilson, S.R. (1982). *Generalised linear models in epidemiological research: case-control studies.* The Instat Foundation, Sydney, Australia.

Anderson, S., Auquier, A., Hauck, W.W., Oakes, D., Vandaele, W., and Weisberg, H.I. (1980). *Statistical methods for comparative studies.* Wiley, New York.

Armitage, P. (1960). *Sequential medical trials.* Blackwell Scientific Publications, Oxford.

Armitage, P. (1971). *Statistical methods in medical research.* Blackwell Scientific Publications, Oxford.

Baker, R.J. and Nelder, J.A. (1978). *The GLIM system manual for release 3.* Numerical Algorithms Group, Oxford.

Breslow, N.E. and Day, N.E. (1980). *Statistical methods in cancer research,* Vol. 1. *The analysis of case-control studies.* IARC Scientific Publications No. 32. International Agency for Research on Cancer, Lyon.

British National Lymphoma Investigation (1975). Value of prednisone in combination chemotherapy of stage IV Hodgkin's disease *Br. Med. J.* **iii**, 413.

Casagrande, J.T., Pike, M.C., and Smith, P.G. (1978). An improved approximate formula for calculating sample sizes for comparing two binomial distributions. *Biometrics* **34**, 483.

Cox, D.R. (1972). Regression models and life tables (with discussion) *J. R. Statist. Soc. B.* **34**, 187.

Dixon, W.J. (ed.) (1981). *BMDP statistical software.* University of California Press, Berkeley.

Forni, A. and Sciame, A. (1975). Chromosome and biochemical

studies in women occupationally exposed to lead. *Arch. Environ. Health* **35**, 139.

Kalbfleisch, J. and Prentice, R.L. (1980). *The statistical analysis of failure time data.* Wiley, New York.

Lachin, J.M. (1981). Introduction to sample size determination and power analysis for clinical trials. *Clin. Trials* **1**, 93.

Lindley, D.V. and Miller, J.C.P. (1964). *Cambridge elementary statistical tables.* Cambridge University Press.

Nelder, J.A. and Wedderburn, R.W.M. (1972). Generalised linear models. *J. R. Statist. Soc. A.* **135**, 370.

Peto, R., Pike, M.C., Armitage, P., *et al.* (1977). Design and analysis of randomised clinical trials requiring prolonged observation of each patient: II Analysis and examples. *Br. J. Cancer* **35**, 1.

Pocock, S.J. (1984). *Clinical trials: a practical approach.* Wiley, New York.

Pocock, S.J., Shaper, A.G., Cook, D.G., *et al.* (1980). British Regional Heart Study – geographical variations in cardio-vascular mortality and the role of water quality. *Br. Med. J.* **280**, 1243.

Pocock, S.J., Cook, D.G., and Beresford, S.A.A. (1981). Regression of area mortality rates on explanatory variables: what weighting is appropriate? *Appl. Statist.* **30**, 286.

Ryan, T.A., Joiner, B.L., and Ryan, B.F. (1981). *Minitab reference manual.* Minitab Project, Pennsylvania.

Snedecor, G.W. and Cochran, W.G. (1967). *Statistical methods,* 6th edn. Iowa State Press, Ames.

Yates, F. (1934). Contingency tables involving small numbers and the chi-squared test. *J. R. Statist. Soc. Suppl.* **1**, 217.

# Social science techniques

# 10 Economic studies

M. F. Drummond

## INTRODUCTION

'Is this procedure cost-effective?' is a comment more often overheard in debates concerning the provision of health services these days. This increased interest in the economic aspects of health services has been mirrored by a rapid growth in recent years in the publication of economic studies of health care alternatives. In a search of the literature for the period 1966–78, Warner and Hutton (1980) found more than 500 relevant references, growing from half a dozen per year at the beginning of the period, to close to 100 in each of the most recent two years. They also found that the growth had been more rapid in medical than non-medical journals.

This chapter reviews studies which assess the relative merits and demerits of health care programmes or treatments from an economic perspective. This general approach to the analysis of alternative strategies is known as the *cost-benefit approach* or *economic appraisal* and embodies specific analytical forms such as *cost-benefit analysis* and *cost-effectiveness analysis*. First, the reasons for wishing to apply this approach to health care choices will be discussed. Second, the methodological principles underlying both the general approach and its specific forms will be outlined, illustrated by reference to published studies. Finally, the contribution of this approach to health service decision making will be considered and the problems and prospects for its use in the future discussed.

## THE BACKGROUND TO THE USE OF ECONOMIC APPRAISAL IN HEALTH CARE

The main reason for wishing to apply economic appraisal to choices in health care is that resources are *scarce*. That is, there are not, and never will be, enough resources to satisfy human wants completely. This means that choice between alternative programmes both within and outside the health care system is inescapable, since more resources devoted to one beneficial activity automatically means that benefits which would arise from the use of those same resources in another activity are foregone. Within the health care field scarcity often manifests itself in terms of budget restrictions or shortages of money, but it is important to recognize that the economist's notion of cost goes deeper than money expenditures. To an economist, the cost of an activity is the benefits that the resources consumed by the activity would generate in their best alternative use. It just happens that money expenditures are often a convenient measuring rod for costs since market exchanges will, under

certain conditions, reflect the value of resources and, in developed economies, generate money prices. However, to emphasize the conceptual difference between cost and money expenditure, economists often use the terms 'opportunity cost' or 'resource cost'.

If one accepts the notion of scarcity, it is clear that it is no longer sufficient to compare options in health care solely on the basis of the benefits they generate; comparisons should be made on the basis of benefits *and costs*, since costs merely reflect lost benefits elsewhere. It is not difficult to find practical examples of this; the undisciplined use of high-technology diagnostic aids may mean that there are fewer resources to devote to the development of community services for the elderly or mentally handicapped. However, at least one commentator (Williams 1974) has argued that decisions in the health care field are too often made on the basis of one option being more beneficial than another – irrespective of cost – or of being cheaper and disregarding relative benefits. Doctors are more prone to the first error, accountants and health ministries to the second. Nevertheless, even if one accepts that health care alternatives should be compared on the basis of relative costs and benefits, there are numerous problems in converting this undeniable logic into analyses whose results can be trusted and used. Economic appraisal takes on a wide brief in attempting to assess all the costs and benefits of treatment or planning options, not only to the health sector but also to patients, families, other public sector agencies, and the community at large. There are obvious problems both in assessing the impact on health of treatment alternatives and in attempting to bring all costs and benefits into a common unit for comparison. Whereas health service costs and savings may be readily converted into money terms, patient and family items such as the time taken to obtain treatment or nurse sick relatives and the benefits of reducing pain and suffering are much more difficult to evaluate, as will be seen from the examples given later.

## THE METHODOLOGY OF ECONOMIC APPRAISAL IN HEALTH CARE

In principle the methodology of economic appraisal is quite simple; namely, to select two or more alternatives for appraisal, to assess the costs and benefits of the alternatives, and to make a comparison based on relative costs and benefits. However, a number of important methodological issues need to be resolved at each stage. These are discussed below, by reference to studies of increasing degrees of complexity.

## Cost analysis

One of the simplest situations for the application of economic appraisal is that where the choice between alternatives is dependent largely on relative costs, rather than relative benefits. Consider, for example, a recent study of alternative methods of providing long-term domiciliary oxygen therapy (Lowson *et al.* 1981). Medical research has shown that patients with chronic bronchitis can benefit from long-term oxygen treatment in the home (up to 15 hours a day). Yet there are three quite distinct methods of service delivery; cylinder oxygen, liquid oxygen, and the oxygen concentrator, a machine which extracts oxygen from air. There is no reason to suppose that the relative medical effectiveness of the treatment methods differs, since under all three the patient receives a steady supply of oxygen *via* a face mask. However, it is likely that the costs differ between methods, because cylinders and liquid oxygen represent a steady resource commitment through time, whereas concentrators require a large capital outlay in terms of equipment and workshop facilities but may have lower running costs in the long term. In addition, since the service facilities required for the concentrator option are shared by all the patients on the therapy in a given location, the unit cost per patient per annum is likely to fall as more patients are given the therapy. The results of the cost analysis undertaken by Lowson *et al.* are given in Fig. 10.1. For all but small numbers of patients, the concentrator option is to be preferred on cost grounds. Therefore, it can be seen that in some situations merely revealing the costs of options can provide useful information for decision making purposes.

However, even in this simple costing example a number of methodological issues arise; three in particular are worth exploring. First, *whose* costs should be considered? It is clear that health sector costs are relevant to the choice of treatment made, but what about the costs borne by the patients, such as electricity consumption in the concentrator option? The view taken by Lowson *et al.* was that all resources consumed, no

matter on whose budget they fall, are relevant to the choice. That is, the appraisal was being performed from the viewpoint of society at large. This is the correct standpoint for economic appraisal, although it is possible to find in the literature more restricted forms of analysis, performed from the point of view of the hospital, the health sector or the government. While legitimate exercises in their own right, such studies are not economic appraisals. Above all, it is important that analyses state the viewpoint from which they are undertaken (Stoddart 1982). This is particularly important when analysing institutional versus domiciliary care options for patient groups such as the elderly, where one of the options is much more intensive than the other in its use of family resources (say) in informal nursing care and in other community support services, including voluntary help.

Second, how are cost flows compared through time? The concentrator option requires a large outlay at the beginning of the therapy, whereas the other options require a steady annual resource outlay. It is usually argued that, as individuals or as a society, we prefer to postpone costs (or conversely, bring benefits forward). That is, even in the absence of inflation we would prefer to receive $100 this year rather than $100 next year; in economists' language we are said to have a *positive (marginal) rate of time preference*. The normal method of incorporating this notion into economic appraisals is to *discount* costs and benefits in the future *to present values*. In effect this implies treating costs and benefits in the future as though they have slightly less weight than those in the present. (Those requiring more explanation of discounting and the method of calculating present values should consult Drummond (1980).) In the example described above a discount rate of 7 per cent was used to convert the initial capital outlays to an annual charge to reflect not only the actual sums involved, but also the fact that they occur sooner rather than later. This approach gives the same result as discounting all the recurring annual outlays to present values and is more convenient in this case since the initial capital outlays for the concentrator option are the only costs which do not occur each and every year. There is a large literature on the choice of discount rate in economic appraisals and the debate is too complex to reproduce here. (See Fleming (1977) for a recent review.) However, most studies in the health care field have used rates between 4 and 10 per cent and it is often worthwhile investigating whether the study result is sensitive to the choice of rate. In this particular case the study result was not very sensitive to choice of rate, but other choices in health care, such as those between a curative option and a preventive one aimed at the same disease, may well be. The reason is that a preventive option requires large resource outlays *now* in return for potential benefits (in reduction of disease) *in the future*.

Finally, the cost estimates derived in the study by Lowson *et al.* incorporate a number of key assumptions. First, the costs depend on the existing facilities available, especially for the concentrator option. Therefore, in the study two assumptions were made about the availability of technician time and workshop space. (The different assumptions generated the two curves labelled A and B in Fig. 10.1.) Second, it is implicitly assumed that this treatment will be given; the issue of whether it is worthwhile providing oxygen therapy to chronic bronchitics

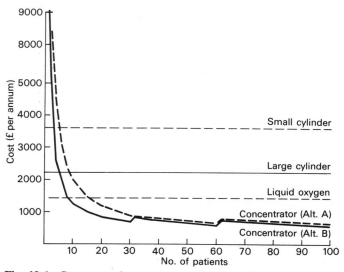

**Fig. 10.1.** Cost per patient per annum for all methods of providing oxygen. (Source: Lowson *et al.* (1981).)

at all, given other treatment priorities, is not addressed. Usually such issues are not presented as 'all or nothing' questions, but those of *how much* one should pursue particular activities. A good example of how simple costing studies can inform this kind of debate is given by Neuhauser and Lewicki (1975). They examined the costs of pursuing a protocol of six sequential tests for detecting asymptomatic colonic cancer. Each test can detect about 92 per cent of the cancers being looked for in the screened population, so that the second test detects about 92 per cent of the 8 per cent not detected by the first test and so on. The costs include the screening itself and barium enemas for all positive cases. After six sequential tests the mean cost (that is, total costs divided by total cases detected by all six tests) was estimated at less than $2500. But the *marginal* cost (that is, the extra cost per case detected by the sixth test and the figure relevant to deciding whether to perform six tests or five) was over $47 million. The difference between marginal costs and average costs is an important one to note. In the case of provision of concentrators, for example, the marginal cost of adding an extra patient to the therapy is lower than the average cost owing to the fact that the initial investment in service facilities can be shared by more than one patient.

Therefore it can be seen that even simple costing exercises require a number of methodological issues to be resolved, such as defining the *range* of costs to be considered, making allowances for differential *timing* of resource outlays and matching the costs to the decision being considered (i.e. identifying the marginal costs). However, at the same time the examples cited show that costing studies can, in certain situations, generate useful information.

### Cost-effectiveness analysis

A slightly more complex situation is one where again it is implicitly assumed that a given treatment or health care planning objective will be pursued, but that no prior assumptions can be made about relative effectiveness of the alternative treatments or programmes. Here a cost-effectiveness study is usually carried out. There are a number of good examples of such studies from the field of elective surgery, where economic appraisals have been undertaken in conjunction with randomized controlled clinical trials. Consider, for example, the study by Russell *et al.* (1977) on day case surgery for hernias and haemorrhoids. The results of the medical evaluation were that there was no significant difference in outcome (as assessed by number of complications) between day-case hernia patients (eight-hour stay) and those treated by traditional in-patient methods (see Table 10.1). Given equivalence in medical outcome, it was possible to estimate the relative resource use in the two alternatives so as to advise on relative cost-effectiveness. It was found that although the day-case patients consumed more community services, in GP consultations and district nurse visits, these extra costs were far outweighed by the savings in hospital care. This particular study also employed an innovative approach to estimating the *marginal* savings in hospital resources from day-case surgery. (Clearly shortening stays will not save the equivalent of *average* hospital cost per day as merely the 'hotel' element of cost is

**Table 10.1.** *Results of a comparison of day-case and long-stay surgery for patients with hernia and haemorrhoids*

| | Planned length of stay | | |
|---|---|---|---|
| | Day-case patients | Long-stay (trial patients) | Long-stay (excluded patients) |
| No. of patients | 55 | 56 | 54 |
| Complications (however slight) | | | |
| Hernia | 12 out of 32 | 11 out of 35 | 17 out of 44 |
| Haemorrhoids† | 13 out of 23 | 6 out of 21 | 4 out of 11 |
| Length of convalescence | | | |
| < 4 weeks | 8 | 11 | 7 |
| 4–8 weeks | 22 | 21 | 12 |
| > 8 weeks | 14 | 12 | 12 |
| Special arrangements made for return home | 30 | 30 | 32 |
| Average additional expenditure | £4.67 | £5.12 | £4.33 |
| Preferred length of stay | | | |
| Shorter than occurred | 2 | 11 | 1 |
| Same as occurred | 27 | 41 | 41 |
| Longer than occurred | 26‡ | 4 | 12 |
| Average no. of GP consultations | | | |
| Home | 0.87 | 0.55 | 0.60 |
| Surgery | 1.49 | 1.31 | 1.39 |
| Average no. of district nurse visits | 5.96 | 1.79 | 2.07 |

†Differences almost significant at 5 per cent level.
‡Including 17 who would have preferred 24 hours.
Source: Russell *et al.* (1977).

being escaped.) Rather than basing their estimate of savings on average costs, Russell *et al.* argued that a movement towards the treatment of more day cases would either (i) enable a five-bed ward to be closed or (ii) enable construction of a new five-bed ward to be avoided. It was estimated that the net saving from day-case surgery would be between £19 and £24 per case (1973 prices), depending upon which of these two outcomes resulted from the change in surgical policy.

There are other interesting examples of cost-effectiveness analysis undertaken when two medical procedures produce equivalent medical outcomes. Waller *et al.* (1978) considered in addition patients' views on shortened hospital stays for hernia, haemorrhoids, and varicose veins surgery and found that when patients' costs were considered, the overall cost advantage of short-stay surgery (48 hours postoperative stay) was only slight. It can be seen that in certain situations it can be highly advantageous to link economic appraisal to clinical trials (Drummond and Stoddart 1982). It should also be noted that cost-effectiveness analyses, and the other forms of economic appraisal to be discussed below, are dependent on having good evidence on the effectiveness of medical interventions. In that respect economic appraisal is a complement to, and not a substitute for, some of the other approaches to evaluation described in this volume.

But what if the alternatives being considered have different relative effectiveness. One of the pioneering cost-effectiveness studies by Klarman *et al.* (1968) addressed this issue. The study concerned the choice between different mixes of transplantation, centre dialysis, and home dialysis for patients with chronic renal failure. For the patients surveyed, transplantation gave a longer survival time (17 years on average compared with nine on dialysis) although it had a higher initial cost. The authors

**Table 10.2.** *Cost-effectiveness of treatments for chronic renal failure*

|  | Cost per year of life gained |
| --- | --- |
| Transplantation | $ 2600 |
| Centre dialysis | $11 600 |
| Home dialysis | $ 4200 |

Source: Klarman *et al.* (1968).

argued that since the main objective of treatment for chronic renal failure was to extend life, a legitimate comparison would be in terms of cost per year of life gained. On this basis transplantation appears to be a good buy (see Table 10.2). The logic is that, given a fixed budget, the number of years of life gained would be maximized by selection of the maximum transplantation route.

Such an approach is useful in those situations where there is a clear objective of medical intervention, such as to extend life. For example, Gravelle *et al.* (1982) have recently compared different tests in breast cancer screening in terms of cost per woman-year of life saved. However, there are many health care investment decisions for which the *quality* of life gained may differ between medical procedures for the same condition, or between conditions. The treatments for chronic renal failure are a case in point; most people would argue that the quality of life gained by transplants is higher than that gained by dialysis. In the early work, Klarman *et al.* (1968) made a fairly arbitrary judgement, that a year gained by transplant is equivalent to 1.25 years gained by dialysis, but later researchers, such as Torrance *et al.* (1973) and Bush *et al.* (1973) have attempted to estimate these relative valuations empirically by asking physicians or patients. One approach might be to pose the question 'how many years on dialysis would you exchange for one by transplant; another might be to obtain a linear ranking of health states by presenting the individual with a choice between a certainty of being in one health state and a 'gamble' of either being worse off or better off. The relative valuations of states are obtained by varying the probabilities assigned to the gamble until the respondent is indifferent between the gamble and the certainty. Such approaches are known as 'health status' or 'utility' measurement and are reported more fully by Berg (1973) and Culyer (1978).

An example of a more recent study which uses this approach to benefit measurement is that by Stason and Weinstein (1977). Their purpose was to apply cost-effectiveness analysis to the management of essential hypertension, both to determine how resources can be used most efficiently within a programme to treat hypertension and to provide a yardstick for comparison with alternative health-related uses of these resources. The central benefit measurement issue concerns the fact that although blood pressure screening and control may extend life, the medication also has certain unpleasant side-effects. Also, extension of life is not the only potential benefit of lowered blood pressure, since non-fatal (but disabling) strokes and myocardial infarctions may also be averted. Therefore, a utility analysis was performed and the results expressed in terms of cost per quality-adjusted life year (see Fig. 10.2). As in the study by Klarman *et al.* (1968), the adjustment chosen was

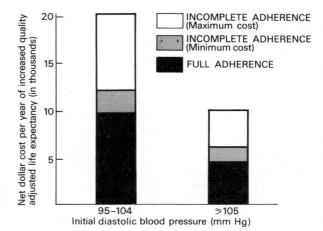

**Fig. 10.2.** Cost per quality-adjusted life year by management of hypertension (40-year-old subjects; discount rate of 5 per cent assumed). (Source: Stason and Weinstein (1977).)

not based on thorough empirical analysis, but at least the authors did explore the sensitivity of their results to the assumption made. In fact, sensitivity analysis was a central feature of this particular study, given the uncertainties about patient compliance with therapy, medical treatment costs, and valuation of adverse subjective medication side-effects. Variations in a number of these factors were found to have a substantial impact on the cost-effectiveness ratio. Nevertheless the study was able to generate useful insights into the efficiency of different ways of managing hypertension. One of the main findings was that an intervention to improve patient compliance with anti-hypertensive therapy may be a better use of limited resources than maximum efforts to detect hypertension by extending screening programmes. The question of whether treatment of hypertension represents an efficient use of health resources was answered only indirectly by the analysis. The cost per quality-adjusted life year (assuming difficulties with patient compliance) was found to be $10 500 for patients with diastolic blood pressures above 105 mm Hg and $20 400 for those with diastolic blood pressures between 95 and 104 mm Hg. Whether or not this is a reasonable price to pay depends on the subjective valuation one places on life and the returns from other life-saving investments.

## Cost-benefit analysis

Discussion of those cost-effectiveness studies which employ benefit measurement in terms of 'utilities' raises the wider issue of valuation of health benefits. The broadest kind of comparison between programmes would be one in which all the costs and benefits were valued in the same unit (e.g. money terms). In theory one should then be able to assess whether particular investments in health treatments or programmes are worth undertaking when compared to other uses for the same scarce resources.

Very few studies succeed in tackling this wide brief, but one which comes close is the study by Weisbrod *et al.* (1980) on alternatives in the treatment of psychiatric illness. This study compared conventional hospital-based treatment with a community-based alternative called 'Training in Community Living', and was linked to a controlled prospective evaluation. A wide range of costs and benefits were quantified in money terms. These included the direct costs of the alternative programmes, the costs imposed on other public sector agencies (such as social service agencies and sheltered workshops), law enforcement costs resulting from offences committed by patients, patient maintenance costs, and costs imposed on the family. The money benefits included earnings resulting from return to employment. Of course some items could not be valued in money terms, although many were quantified in physical units; these included the number of arrests, suicides, days in employment, indicators of 'improved consumer decision making' and patient mental health (e.g. presence of clinical symptoms and patient satisfaction). (See Table 10.3).

Therefore, this study investigates fairly fully the relevant changes in a comparison of the economic efficiency of treatments (see Fig. 10.3). The main finding was that although the community-based programme cost about $800 more per annum per patient, the monetary benefits were around $1200 per patient per annum. A number of the forms of benefits and costs that were measured in quantitative but non-monetary terms showed additional advantages of the community-based experimental programme. At the same time the authors are careful to point out that the generalizability of a single experiment is limited, that the analysis can be viewed from different perspectives (e.g. society, the government budget, and the patient), and that those costs and benefits for which it was impossible to provide monetary values should not be ignored.

Discussion of cost-benefit analysis raises two key issues (i) is it possible to obtain reliable money estimates for all the benefits of health services and (ii) *whose values* are the appropriate ones to use? With regard to the first issue, it has often been argued that it is impossible to place a value on the 'intangible' elements of the benefits of health services, such as the reduction of pain and suffering or the extension of life itself. However, it should be noted that, implicitly at least, a valuation *is* being placed on these items every time a health care investment decision is

**Table 10.3.** *Costs and benefits per patient (12 months after admission) for alternative mental illness programmes. (After Weisbrod et al. 1980)*

| Category | Conventional hospital-oriented programme | Community-based programme |
|---|---|---|
| **Money costs (C)** | | |
| Direct treatment costs | $3138 | $4798 |
| Indirect treatment costs (Falling on other agencies) | $2142 | $1838 |
| Law enforcement costs | $ 409 | $ 350 |
| Patient maintenance costs | $1487 | $1035 |
| Lost family earnings | $ 120 | $ 72 |
| **Money benefits (B)** | | |
| Patient earnings | $1168 | $2364 |
| **Net money cost** | | |
| (C – B) | $6128 | $5729 |
| | | |
| **Non-money costs** | | |
| No. of arrests | 1.2 | 1.0 |
| Suicide | 1.5 | 1.5 |
| **Non-money benefits** | | |
| Days in employment | 87 | 216 |
| Patient satisfaction | Significantly higher with community programme | |
| Clinical symptomatology | Significantly better with community programme (on seven of 13 measures) | |

made. Returning to the example of screening for cancer of the colon cited earlier, a decision to endorse a protocol of six sequential tests rather than five is implicitly valuing the extra lives saved in excess of $47 million. Conversely, Cochrane and Holland (1971) calculated that the cost of saving the life of a patient with porphyria variegata, by population screening, was around £250 000, yet community screening for the disease had never been tried in the USA or UK. They pointed out that this 'suggests a conscious or unconscious recognition of the financial factor'. It is apparent that, although valuations are *implicitly* being placed on health service outputs every day, there are likely to be many inconsistencies. This has led some economists to undertake studies which reveal these implicit valuations so that decision makers can give them more active

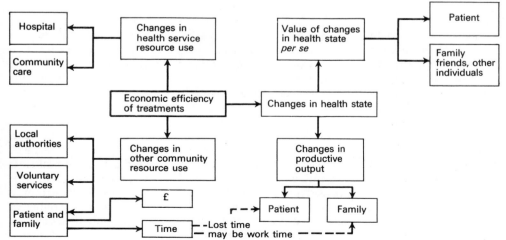

**Fig. 10.3.** The relevant changes in a comparison of the economic efficiency of treatments. (Source: Drummond (1980).)

consideration. For example, Buxton and West (1975) calculated the implicit social value of a year of life on renal dialysis; that is, the amount which, as a community, we are currently paying to keep patients alive under this particular regimen. It was found to be £2600 and £4720 per annum respectively for home and hospital dialysis in the UK. Buxton and West point out that these figures should then be compared with those implied by other life-saving health treatments. It is interesting to note that whilst the UK had restrictions on the growth of dialysis, the cost per life implied by building safety measures following the collapse of an apartment block in London was around £20 million (Mooney 1977).

From time to time economists have attempted to place a money value on life directly. The most popular approach in the early literature was to take discounted future earnings (either gross or net of the individual's consumption) as an estimate of the loss to the community from premature death of an individual. (The logic was the 'value' of the lost life years averted related to the productive output of the individual during that time.) This approach has always been recognized as, at best, partial and at worst, misleading (Mishan 1971). (See Drummond (1981a) for more discussion of this point.) Certainly the approach can give answers which may mislead decision makers. For example, in a study of the size and distribution of benefits from US medical research into cancer and heart disease, Holtmann (1973) found that if cancer were eliminated the average White male would gain about $561 and the average Black male about $316 (present values using 5 per cent discount rate). The corresponding figures for cardiovascular disease were $1034 and $508. However, Holtmann states that 'we should note that the higher returns for White males should not be taken as a justification for investing more in treatment of Whites at the expense of Blacks', presumably because if Blacks had equal opportunities in the labour market the figures may be different.

An alternaive approach is to elicit from individuals values for their own lives, either by inference from their actions (e.g. attitudes towards personal safety) or by asking them directly. (See, for example, the work of Jones-Lee (1976).) Progress is being made in overcoming the considerable measurement problems inherent in such approaches, but for the time being the main contribution of economists is more likely to be in making previously hidden values explicit.

This leads on to the other major issue raised by cost-benefit analysis; that of *whose* values should be used? Economists typically start from the premise that the consumer is the best judge of the utility that he or she obtains from a particular good or service. In fact cost-benefit analysis is firmly based in the theoretical traditions of Paretian welfare economics. Here the purpose of cost-benefit analysis is *to identify potential Pareto improvements*; that is, situations where the maximum total sum of money that the gainers from a project would be prepared to pay to ensure that the project were undertaken exceeds the minimum total sum of money that the losers from it would accept as compensation to allow it to be undertaken. Therefore, this perspective requires that benefits from health services be valued in terms of consumers' willingness-to-pay. Not all economists would totally adhere to these principles

when judging health service investments, but most would argue that consumers' values are too often neglected by policy makers (at the planning and clinical levels) who merely replace them with their own. All economists would prefer values to be *made explicit*, no matter whose values are used. (See Drummond (1981a) for more discussion of this point.) One advantage of the cost-effectiveness approach using utilities (as described above) is that the technical and value judgements implicit in measuring health service benefits are clearly identified and can be discussed in the constructive arena of multidisciplinary activity.

Finally, and most fundamentally, economic appraisal in health care is an *aid* to decision making and not a substitute for it. Resource allocation decisions in health care are likely to depend on a number of considerations and the main contribution of economic appraisal is to provide an assessment of the consequences, *in terms of economic efficiency,* of various choices. The other major consideration is *equity,* and on occasions economists have explored the equity-efficiency trade-off skillfully. A good example is in the study by Rich *et al.* (1976) of alternative screening procedures for asymptomatic bacteriuria in schoolgirls. The most cost-effective method, an unsupervised test, has a lower detection rate in children from low-income groups. The authors present this information to the decision maker in a way which highlights the key issues involved in choice of test.

## THE CONTRIBUTION OF ECONOMIC APPRAISAL TO HEALTH SERVICE DECISION MAKING

### Judging the quality of the literature

It is clear from the discussion above that undertaking an economic appraisal in health care requires numerous methodological judgements on the part of the analyst, many of which can be debated. Recent reviews of the literature (Drummond 1980, 1981b; Warner and Hutton 1980) have shown published studies to be of a variable quality. How, therefore, can the non-economist critically appraise the quality of this growing body of literature? A simple checklist of questions to ask of any published study has been offered by Drummond and Mooney (1981) and is elaborated upon here.

(i) *Is it clear what question the study is designed to answer?* In particular, it is important to be clear on whether the study takes as given that a particular treatment objective is to be met to a given extent, or whether it attempts to question the objective. This determines whether or not the study should employ the broader cost-benefit methodology. (It should be noted that *study title* is a notoriously bad guide to methodological content!)

(ii) *Is the study placed in any particular planning or clinical context?* It has already been pointed out that clear statement of the *viewpoint* from which the study is being undertaken is helpful, as this determines which costs and benefits should be considered. Also it is helpful if the study gives clues as to how its results should be interpreted in the context of planning or clinical decisions. For example, does a result that day-case surgery is more cost-effective than in-patient surgery mean that every patient (suffering with the given condition) should be treated as a day-case? Probably not, but it may mean that planners should provide facilities for the expansion of day-case surgery and that clinicians should scrutinize patients to ascertain which ones would be suitable for the new treatment. In general, to what extent do the authors of the study recognize the dangers in generalizations of study results to other settings?

(iii) *What is the quality of the underlying technical (medical) evidence on which the study is based?* It was mentioned above that it is often advantageous to link economic appraisals to controlled clinical trials. If this is not the case, how does the study cope with the uncertainties in the medical evidence on which it is based.

(iv) *What range of costs and benefits is considered?* Are those costs and benefits which are difficult to measure or value 'lost' when the results of the study are discussed? Are capital as well as recurrent costs considered? Are costs and benefits falling outside the agency undertaking the appraisal considered, if a social viewpoint is being adopted? Is the issue of differential timing of costs and benefits alluded to, and what adjustments are made?

(v) *Does the study make explicit the value judgements being made and identify the sources of values?* It was mentioned above that there may often be no unambiguously 'right' way of measuring and valuing some costs and benefits. Does the study encourage readers to question some of the judgements made, or are they presented with *the* result?

(vi) *Is a sensitivity analysis performed?* It is unlikely that any study is carried out from the position of perfect information. Therefore, how does the study cope with uncertainties in medical evidence, in expected health sector costs or in future technological change? A common approach is to undertake a sensitivity analysis of the way study results change with variations in key parameters. It may be possible to demonstrate that although some factors are unknown, they may not affect study conclusions very much. Conversely, the discovery that the economic results are highly sensitive to particular factors might be a strong argument for investing more effort in obtaining better estimates of their likely range of values.

## Problems and prospects of applying economic appraisal in health service decision making

There is now a substantial body of literature relating to issues in the economic burden of disease, prevention, diagnosis, treatment, and rehabilitation. However, despite the increasing popularity of economic appraisal among health service and medical researchers, there is very little evidence of its being used in planning or clinical decisions. Warner and Luce (1982) cite the work of Eddy (1980), as a good example of economic analysis being presented in a form and quality which enabled decision makers to appreciate its relevance. It contributed to decisions by Blue Cross–Blue Shield and the American Cancer Society to alter their recommendations on screening practices. However, Warner and Luce point out that both in terms of its technical competence and its policy impact, Eddy's work remains a distinct deviation from the norm. Whilst also recognizing the variable quality of the existing literature (a point discussed above), Drummond (1983) cites additional

evidence from Europe, such as the decision by the Department of Health and Social Security in the UK to place on trial a new approach (rather like economic appraisal) to the appraisal of planning options where one of these is a large capital scheme, such as building or extending a hospital (DHSS 1981). Perhaps, given the methodological comments made above, a promising approach may be to build an economic element into medical research design where this appears to be relevant. Requests for research monies from one of the Ministry of Health's committees in Ontario (Canada) are evaluated not only in terms of their methodological soundness, but also in terms of whether 'the proposal is likely to have an important economic impact in reducing the costs or increasing the efficiency of health services' and the grant application has to provide, where appropriate, 'an adequate cost-effectiveness, cost-benefit, or cost-utility analysis' (Ontario Ministry of Health 1982).

The main focus of this chapter has been on outlining the methodology of economic appraisal and on giving examples of studies undertaken to date. It is clear that refinements in methodology can be, and are being, made. However, the major challenge, if economic appraisal is to make a lasting contribution to health service decision making, will be in finding better ways of disseminating the 'way of thinking' implicit in economic studies and in making the studies themselves more relevant to decisions taken at the planning and clinical levels.

## REFERENCES

Berg, R.L. (ed.) (1973). *Health status indexes*. Hospital Research and Educational Trust, Chicago.

Bush, J.W., Chen, M.M., and Patrick, D.L. (1973). Cost effectiveness of a PKU program. In *Health status indexes* (ed. R.L. Berg) p. 172. Hospital Research and Educational Trust, Chicago.

Buxton, M.J. and West, R.R. (1975). Cost-benefit analysis of long-term haemodialysis for chronic renal failure. *Br. Med. J.* **ii**, 376.

Cochrane, A.L. and Holland, W.W. (1971). Validation of screening procedures. *Br. Med. Bull.* **27**, 3.

Culyer, A.J. (1978). *Measuring health: lessons for Ontario.* Toronto University Press for Ontario Economic Council.

Department of Health and Social Security (1981). *Health services management: health building procedures.* HN(81)30. DHSS, London.

Drummond, M.F. (1980). *Principles of economic appraisal in health care.* Oxford University Press.

Drummond, M.F. (1981a). Welfare economics and cost-benefit analysis in health care. *Scottish J. Political Economy* **28**, 125.

Drummond, M.F. (1981b). *Studies in economic appraisal in health care.* Oxford University Press.

Drummond, M.F. (1983). Economic appraisal and health service decision making. *Effective Health Care* **1**, 25.

Drummond, M.F. and Mooney, G.H. (1981). Economic appraisal in health care. 1. A guide to the methodology of economic appraisal. *Hosp. Health Serv. Rev.* **77**(9), 277.

Drummond, M.F. and Stoddart, G.L. (1982). *Economic analysis and clinical trials.* QSEP Report No. 34. McMaster University, Faculty of Social Sciences, Hamilton, Ontario.

Eddy, D. (1980). *Screening for cancer: theory, analysis and design.* Prentice-Hall, Englewood Cliffs, NJ.

Fleming, J.S. (1977). What discount rate for public expenditure? In *Public expenditure: allocation between competing ends* (ed. M. Posner) p. 45. Cambridge University Press.

Gravelle, H.S.E., Simpson, P.R., and Chamberlain, J. (1982).

Breast cancer screening and health service costs. *J. Health Econ.* **1**, 185.

Holtmann, A.G. (1973). The size and distribution of benefits from U.S. medical research: the case of eliminating cancer and heart disease. *Public Finance* **28**, 354.

Jones-Lee, M.W. (1976). *The value of life: an economic analysis.* Martin Robertson, London.

Klarman, H.E., Francis, J.O'S., and Rosenthal, G.D. (1968). Cost effectiveness analysis applied to the chronic renal disease. *Med. Care* **6**, 48.

Lowson, K.V., Drummond, M.F., and Bishop, J.M. (1981). Costing new services: long-term domiciliary oxygen therapy. *Lancet* **ii**, 1146.

Mishan, E.J. (1971). Evaluation of life and limb: a theoretical approach. *J. Political Economy* **79**, 687.

Mooney, G.H. (1977). *The valuation of human life.* Macmillan, London.

Neuhauser, D. and Lewicki, A.M. (1975). What do we gain from the sixth stool guaiac? *N. Engl. J. Med.* **293**, 226.

Ontario Ministry of Health (1982). *Health care systems research grant review committee: criteria for assessment of applications.* Toronto, Canada.

Rich, G., Glass, N.J., and Selkon, J.B. (1976). Cost effectiveness of two methods of screening for asymptomatic bacteriuria. *Br. J. Prev. Soc. Med.* **30**, 54.

Russell, I.T., Devlin, H.B., Fell, M., Glass, N.J., and Newell, D.J. (1977). Day case surgery for hernias and haemorrhoids: a clinical, social and economic evaluation. *Lancet* **i**, 844.

Stason, W.B. and Weinstein, M.C. (1977). Allocation of resources to manage hypertension. *N. Engl. J. Med.* **296**, 732.

Stoddart, G.L. (1982). Economic evaluation methods and health policy. *Evaluation and the Health Professions* **5**, 393.

Torrance, G.W., Sackett, D.L., and Thomas, W.H. (1973). Utility maximisation model for program evaluation: a demonstration application. In *Health status indexes* (ed. R.L. Berg) p. 156. Hospital Research and Education Trust, Chicago.

Waller, J., Adler, M., Creese, A., and Thorne, S. (1978). *Early discharge from hospital for patients with hernia or varicose veins.* HMSO, London.

Warner, K.E. and Hutton, R.C. (1980). Cost benefit and cost effectiveness analysis in health care: growth and composition of the literature. *Med. Care* **18**, 1069.

Warner, K.E. and Luce, B.R. (1982). *Cost benefit and cost effectiveness analysis in health care: principles, practice and potential.* Health Administration Press, Ann Arbor.

Weisbrod, B.A., Test, M.A., and Stein, L.I. (1980). Alternative to mental hospital treatment. II Economic benefit-cost analysis. *Arch Gen. Psychiat.* **37**, 400.

Williams, A.H. (1974). The cost benefit approach. *Br. Med. Bull.* **30**, 252.

# 11 Sociological investigations

Donald L. Patrick

## THE LEGACY OF CONCERNS

Sociological investigations in public health are concerned with how and why people are healthy, that is, the scientific, social, economic, political, and ethical issues involved in the promotion, processing, distribution, use, and effectiveness of public health activities to prevent illness and to promote health. This encyclopaedic list of issues is not the exclusive province of trained and practising *sociologists,* or even of concern only to the broader group of *social scientists,* including anthropologists, economists, psychologists, and social administrators, most of whom are represented in this textbook. Sociological concerns are present whenever and wherever health and illness are related to the social, economic, and political world in which we live. Thus, sociology plays an important role in the history of public health while public health concerns appear in the history of sociology.

### Sociology in public health

The relationship between social factors and health became a consideration as soon as human societies responded to the need to protect the health of the community. Every civilization has had diseases peculiar to it, and adaptation to these diseases has varied within the changing social climate of different cultures and of different social groups within a particular culture. The magicians hired to deal with disease in the early civilizations along the Nile, the Aesculapean temples which performed functions of hospitals around 700 B.C., the medical officers of health appointed in the wake of the Industrial Revolution in Great Britain, and the World Health Organization, whose efforts extend from distribution of the 'magic bullets' to the 'promotion of health for all by the year 2000', have all organized their activities, implicitly or explicitly, around observations that illness is differently distributed in society. This fact has influenced both the public health and sociological traditions.

One of the greatest sociological investigations ever conducted in public health was the survey carried out by Sir Edwin Chadwick and published in 1842 as *Report on the sanitary condition of the labouring population of Great Britain.* The *Report* was compiled on the evidence of the union medical officers who were urged by Chadwick, then Secretary to the Poor Law Commission, to send in an account of the medical conditions to be found in their areas (Brockington 1966). Chadwick, analysing the comparative chances of life in different classes of the community, wrote: 'Whatever influence occupation and other circumstances may have upon mortality, no one can inspect the registers without being struck by the deteriorated value of life in inferior localities, even where the inhabitants were the same in condition with those who lived in better conditions' (Chadwick 1842). The *Report's* ultimate outcome was the Public Health Act of 1848 in which the British government, for the first time, charged itself with a measure of responsibility for safeguarding the health of the population. Chadwick's investigations addressed questions not only about mortality but also about housing, occupation, education, the prevention of epidemics, and the prevention of robberies and murder (Richardson 1887). His objective was unity of action for the prevention of evil, and his survey evidence was important in mobilizing such action. Similarly, in the US, Lemuel Shattuck, in his *Report of the Sanitary Commission of Massachusetts*, 1850 (reprinted by Harvard University Press 1948), used extensive social survey data which was to play a major role in the establishment of official public health agencies.

### Public health in sociology

Public health concerns have played a less direct role in the sociological tradition; none the less, the relationship between social factors and health has influenced the thinking of some of sociology's greatest figures. Karl Marx, exhausted by a variety of illnesses, some of which stemmed from his miserable living conditions, observed conditions of work and their consequences for workers in terms of mortality and morbidity. Marx and Engels developed crucial insights into the conflicts and inbuilt contradictions of capitalist society (Engels 1845; Wilson 1940). Emile Durkheim (1851), the first French academic sociologist, demonstrated that the rate of suicide varies universally with the degree of social integration or cohesion, that is the extent to which different groups in society, such as religious groups, have a hold on their individual members and integrate them fully within their boundaries. Those members of society who are well integrated into a group are less likely to commit suicide in the face of tragedy or frustration. Durkheim explained the rate of suicides cross-nationally by relating suicide levels to religion, season of the year, time of day, sex, education, and marital status. He concluded (1951:373) '. . . it is because society, weak and disturbed, lets too many persons escape too completely from its influence. Thus, the only remedy for the ill is to restore enough consistency to social groups for them to obtain a firmer grip on the individual, and for him to feel himself bound to them'. These observations, originally published in 1897, have spawned a long tradition of aetiological studies of suicide by both sociological and public health practitioners (Maris and Lazerwitz 1981; Sainsbury *et al.* 1983).

## SOCIOLOGY WITHIN THE PUBLIC HEALTH PERSPECTIVE

Sociology was important in the early writings of social epidemiologists such as Sir John Snow's *On the mode of communication of cholera* (1855), in which he traced London's horrific cholera epidemic to users of a public pump with contaminated water. However, sociologists themselves are relatively late arrivals in medicine and public health. McIntyre (1894) presented a formal definition of 'medical sociology' as a science investigating both the environmental and social aspects of disease causation and the progress society makes in affecting disease. Not until the mid-1950s, however, did sociologists begin to establish themselves in academic institutions (Elling and Sokolowska 1978), with the greatest growth in the US and Canada (Pflanz 1974; Olesen 1975). Even then, the predominant concerns, as described by Robert Straus (1957), were the sociologies *of* and *in* medicine. Sociology of medicine (1957:203) is '. . . concerned with studying such factors as the organizational structure, role relationships, value systems, rituals and functions of medicine' while sociology in medicine is the introduction and use of sociological concepts, principles, and research in medicine, including the teaching of medical students, studies of health behaviour, and social epidemiology. This basic dichotomy, elaborated by Kendall and Reader (1979) and sometimes updated to the sociologies of and in *health*, describes the major activities of medical sociologists as reflected in textbooks on medical sociology (Wilson 1970; Susser and Watson 1971; Tuckett 1976; Cockerham 1978; Denton 1978; Mechanic 1978; Freeman *et al.* 1979; Wolinsky 1980; Patrick and Scambler 1982).

Sociology became more important within the public health perspective when the major killers of the day – once the communicable diseases of smallpox, diphtheria, tuberculosis, and malaria – changed into the currently important health problems of heart disease, cancer, and mental illness which represent chronic, degenerative processes, insidious in their beginnings, long-term in their treatment, and largely irreversible in their progress (Suchman 1967*a*). The shift in prevalence of chronic, degenerative disease blurs the distinction between prevention and treatment, places greater emphasis on the social environment, brings problems such as alcoholism and drug addiction into the scope of public health programmes, and focuses health concerns on social problems. Another major influence on public health sociology was the Second World War. War activity exposed many social conditions associated with illness as well as the disabling conditions of many draftees and recruits. Suchman (1963), in a comprehensive description and analysis of sociology and public health, notes that social problems have tended to replace or at least equal medical problems as the objectives for public health activity, and this is why sociology entered the field of public health.

Sociology contributes content, methodology, skills, and perspective to public health as it does to law, family, religion, education, and the other institutions of society. Surveys of the field are numerous and informative (Freeman and Reeder 1957; Jaco 1958; Roemer and Elling 1963; Mechanic 1966; Suchman 1967*a*; Susser 1974*a*; 1974*b*; Mechanic and Levine 1977; Clausen 1980; Elinson 1980; Illsley 1980), and the research literature continues to expand both in new journals and articles within established journals. (The major sources are listed in an appendix at the end of this chapter.) While special interest areas abound, the uses and contributions of sociology can be identified within four major aspects of public health described briefly below.

### Social epidemiology

Sociology has been concerned first and foremost with the social and economic influences and forces in the prevention of death, disease, illness, and disablement. Sociological investigations, at first concerned mainly with the aetiology of mental illness, focus on important factors such as age, sex, social class, ethnicity, occupation, urban–rural residence, and social support in the aetiology and course of disease. Sociological studies have proved valuable in generating and testing hypotheses, not only about the distribution and aetiology of disease, but also about the behaviour of people with a health problem, and about the structure and functioning of the activities organized to meet the problem. A variety of methods described later in this chapter have been used, although retrospective social surveys are employed most often to investigate causal relationships between social factors and health status. Social epidemiological surveys have been conducted in relation to heart disease (Jenkins 1976), cancer (Shapiro 1983), mental illness (Hollingshead and Redlich 1958; Srole *et al.* 1962; Leighton *et al.* 1963), accidents (Spence *et al.* 1954), alcoholism (Cahalan *et al.* 1969), disablement (Nagi 1976), and drug addiction (Kellam *et al.* 1983). In addition, social variables are included in almost all epidemiological survey work (Graham and Reeder 1979). While most of these surveys are concerned with social and psychological factors in the aetiology of disease, an increasing number of social and behavioural scientists are studying the factors which influence the course of disease and disablement (Kasl 1983).

Social factors may create or encourage a predisposition for a disease; may themselves cause disease directly; may transmit the causes of diseases; and may influence the course of disease (Grotjahn 1915). While social factors have been used most often in conjunction with biological risk factors employing a biomedical perspective on disease causation, social scientists, particularly those interested in mental illness, are concentrating more and more on the social context in which illness is defined and in which disease and illness varies (Mishler *et al.* 1981). In either perspective, efforts are more often directed toward the identification and subsequent modification of psychosocial factors rather than on screening and early detection (Cassel 1976).

## Health beliefs and health behaviour

Social patterns of health beliefs and health behaviour are another principal area of sociological concern in public health. The social processes which affect the values and beliefs of whole societies as well as the behaviour of individuals are important in all areas of public health. Past and present beliefs affect both consumers and providers in the recognition of illness, the seeking of care and treatment, and the evaluation of outcome. Much social science theory has been formulated and manipulated to account for the way individuals perceive and act on illness, for example, the concepts of *labelling* (Schur 1971; Scheff 1974), *role* (Parsons 1951, 1975), *deviance* (Lemert 1951), and *stigma* (Goffman 1963).

Health, illness, and sick role behaviour (Kasl and Cobb 1966), symptom experience (Zborowski 1952), illness behaviour (Mechanic 1960), and patient career (Parsons 1951) have been employed to study social processes and behaviour patterns underlying illness recurrence and service use, often with a social anthropological eye on the cultural meaning of illness or a psychological emphasis on perception and learning. The development of health promotion techniques such as health hazard or health risk appraisal (Wagner *et al.* 1982) has been based on studies of preventive health beliefs and on behaviours such as smoking, alcohol intake, family history, exercise, frequency of health examinations, and self-examination, and their possible relationship to health status.

The seeking and using of public health services have been major topics of sociological investigation. Mechanic (1976*a*, 1978, 1983) has used a sociopsychological approach to the study of illness behaviour, and the decisions that are made by persons in the social process of becoming ill. Suchmann (1965*a*, *b*, 1967*b*) has attempted to capture structural factors, sociocognitive factors, and group interaction factors, as well as actual behaviours associated with illness. Individuals engage in health-related activities for three major reasons (Kasl and Cobb 1966): (i) to prevent illness or to detect it at an asymptomatic stage (health behaviour); (ii) in the presence of symptoms, to obtain diagnosis, and to discover suitable treatment (illness behaviour); and (iii) in the presence of defined illness, to undertake/receive treatment aimed at restoration of health or at halting disease progression (sick-role behaviour). Models of health-related behaviour are numerous and complex (Becker and Maiman 1983). The modelling of health services utilization has been approached with painstaking research in the US by a wide variety of investigators (Andersen 1968; Aday and Andersen 1975; Wolinsky 1976, 1978; Andersen and Anderson 1979). Much of this research is directed toward individual, private health services rather than the traditional public health services of immunization, water treatment, sanitation services, or screening programmes. A notable exception is the work surrounding the health belief model (Becker 1974) which was developed to explain preventive health behaviour and the failure of the public to accept disease screening for tuberculosis, hypertension, or asymptomatic disease, and disease preventive measures such as polio or flu vaccination. The health belief model is based on the social psychological field theory of Kurt Lewin (1951). It takes into account the perceived susceptibility and seriousness of disease, perceived benefits and barriers to taking action, cues motivating action, and sociocultural background of individuals in predicting the likelihood that they will take a recommended preventive action (Becker *et al.* 1977; Becker 1979). Although there are weaknesses in the health belief model, including the lack of evidence that attitudes and beliefs influence behaviour (Wolinsky 1980), this tradition of public health research has continued and expanded to take into account other competing theories (Becker and Maiman 1983).

## Organization and evaluation of public health activities

A third area of sociological investigation concerns the structure and function of public health activities, including the evaluation of services, assessments of the self-perceived needs of clients, and studies of occupational structure and practice. The organizational dynamics of public health services have not received as much attention from social scientists as hospitals or educational and industrial organizations, nor have studies been conducted on public health practitioners such as those mounted on medical students, nurses, and intermediate health workers. The complex network of community health, welfare, and social service organizations and agencies, including many public health activities, have been studied from many points of view. Sociologists in the 1950s and 1960s examined the problems of co-ordination, co-operation, and conflict among different organizations (Kimball 1955; Levine *et al.* 1963; Mott 1970). More recent investigations have concerned the representation of the community, the design, implementation and evaluation of specific services, and the growing number of self-help groups who have joined the more traditional voluntary organizations in consumer-initiated activities involving health promotion and mutual support (Levin *et al.* 1976; Robinson 1977). Investigations clearly must now account for 'many new actions and organizations and a scenario for health as an increasingly populist and pluralistic phenomenon' (White *et al.* 1979).

A major field of activity for social scientists in the health field, including sociologists, is evaluative research (Suchman 1967*b*; Shortell and Richardson 1978; Rossi and Freeman 1982). The size and complexity of modern health services, the growth in expenditure, the vast expansion of technology and applied medical science, increased public accountability, and development of evaluation research methodology have all contributed to the political process of determining the worth of health activity (Patrick 1982). While hospital and primary care services and programmes have received the most attention from social scientists, public health activities such as screening programmes, community health education, and emergency services have also been major subjects of evaluation. Methods of evaluative research have been developed and tested by social scientists working outside the health field

(Campbell and Stanley 1966; Riecken and Boruch 1974; Cook and Campbell 1979; Patton 1980; Cronbach 1982). The evaluation of public health interventions presents unique theoretical and methodological problems which require evidence from complicated and necessarily ingenious research designs (Webb *et al.* 1966; Cook and Campbell 1979).

### Public health policy

Perhaps the most intractable issue for sociologists in public health is the relationship between the health of a population and what society does about it (Elinson 1980; Levine *et al.* 1983). The development of public health policy, investigation of its successes and failures, the decision-making process, and the process of policy implementation have all been the subject of sociological investigation, primarily at the local level. Through lack of confidence or lack of encouragement, there have been few opportunities for sociologists to contribute to or to evaluate national health policy (Elinson 1980; Ilsley 1980). The establishment of national or regional commissions on health problems has brought the involvement of some social scientists but primarily from economics, political science, and public administration. The sociological analysis of policy tends to be based on official statistics and the trends, variations, and outcomes of policy. The relationship between the economy and health policy in modern society has been receiving considerable attention (Brenner 1977, 1979; Eyer 1977). Economic change, unemployment, and illness, particularly mental illness, have been studied extensively since the Great Depression of the 1930s (Komora and Clark 1935; Faris and Dunham 1939; Pierce 1967). The health consequences of unemployment are being investigated with growing frequency, again with a legacy from the 1930s (Komarovsky 1940; Kasl *et al.* 1975; Gore 1978). This issue will clearly continue to consume greater sociological research activity in the future.

## SOCIAL CLASS AND SOCIAL INEQUALITY: A CENTRAL THEME

Many different sociological concepts of health and illness have been used in the wide array of investigations around the four main areas of concern briefly reviewed above. The underlying sociological theories are mainly 'theories of the middle-range' (Merton 1968), which are testable relationships between sociological concepts such as stressful life events, social support, or social class, and health outcomes such as psychiatric disorder, death, disablement, or dissatisfaction. These middle-range theories have stimulated long traditions of productive research with a predominantly analytical perspective of social epidemiology or the study of health status across various social groups. The lack of a general or integrative theory of health and illness has been noted by Pflanz (1974, 1975), Frankenberg (1974), Johnson (1975), and Freidson (1978). This lack of theoretical development and integration has meant that sociological investigations are loosely connected and less likely to contribute to a cumulative scientific tradition in which pieces of a puzzle fit together to form a bigger picture. In most cases theory has been invoked in order to explain data, and the

adequacy of theory has been judged for individual pieces of research. The exceptions are long-term investigations into a single area such as the social origins of depression (Brown and Harris 1978). Organizational and financial support for such cumulative research traditions around one or several investigators are, however, rarely available.

While no global theory has emerged in relation to public health and sociology, a central sociological *theme* in the prevention of illness and promotion of health is socioeconomic status, or social class, which is a major aspect of the social structure of societies. Societies are distinguished by the age, sex, ethnic, educational, religious, geographical, and class status of groups, and by the major institutions which govern social relationships – the state, the family, the economy, the religious, educational, medical, and cultural systems. These social factors are, not surprisingly, the basic variables in social epidemiological investigations of the patterns of health and disease. Sociological investigations have concentrated above all on socio-economic status or the relationship between different groups in society to ownership and means of production and exchange.

Social class, among all the divisions of social structure, has been viewed as containing the culture of the society – the social relations, norms, values, obligations, and sanctions which each generation transmits to the next. Since the nineteenth century, investigations into the nature of the link between social class and health have preoccupied both sociologists and epidemiologists alike. A single chapter on the main areas and techniques of sociological investigations in public health cannot begin to address in depth the complex issues involved in this relationship. This single theme will be used, however, throughout the remainder of this chapter to illustrate sociological methods and their use in efforts to prevent disease and to promote health.

## SOCIOLOGICAL METHODS: GENERAL CONCERNS

### Quantity and quality

The major contribution of sociology to measurement and methodology is the variety of approaches that have been used in the 'real world'. On the one hand, methods, sometimes referred to as positivist, are used to gather observations and assign numerical quantities to them. On the other hand, observations on the motives, meanings, emotions, and subjective aspects of individuals are represented in the notational system of everyday language. As noted by Illsley (1980:140): 'Sociologists have responded to problems of epistemology and data validity by developing a range of approaches, from the expert manipulations of demographic facts and social survey methods through symbolic interactionism (taking the role of the other) to phenomenology and the attempt to approach the phenomena of the social world without importing the analyst's own preoccupations, assumptions, and values'.

Investigations into social class and health have used every available measure in a wide variety of research designs and methodological approaches (Kosa and Zola 1976). Antonovsky (1967) has conducted an extensive review of the literature on socio-economic status and life expectancy, and all available measures led him to conclude that higher socio-economic status was a major causal factor in staying alive longer. But just what does this clear social class gradient mean? First the meaning of socio-economic status or social class must be explored, and secondly the meaning of the causal relationship requires explanation.

## Social class

Measures of social class, a highly complex construct or set of concepts, are likely never to reflect the deepest meaning of social class within the broader society or to the occupants of social class positions whether it be high, medium, or low. In the broadest historical picture most societies have been structured in some way, for example, feudal society in the Middle Ages or the ancient caste civilization in Hindu Culture. Weber (1947) delineated three main dimensions of this stratification: social class, social status or honour, and the political power of organized groups. Class, status, and power are generally inter-related – an unskilled factory worker, for example, usually although not inevitably has low status and relatively minor political power – and the three analytical dimensions are distinct and can vary independently (Bendix and Lipset 1967). Sociologists differ in their theories of social class, and consequently the precise definition also varies.

For many analysts, modern industrial society is divided into stereotyped groups such as the 'working class', 'blue- or white-collar', 'professional' or 'middle class'. These divisions, generally based on occupation, reflect occupational prestige and an associated general life-style such as home ownership, income, living conditions, working conditions, and educational level. Social class can also be characterized by a group's relationship to the modes of production of society's wealth (Giddens 1973). Derived from the work of Marx, the population can be divided into a relatively small capitalist class who own and control land, industries and financial institutions and a working class who engage in wage labour. These alternative divisions form hierarchies of prestige, regardless of their theoretical content, and this prestige can come from many aspects of life, including family history, ethnic origin, military training, religious affiliation, or from membership in particular groups (Miliband 1977). The intergenerational transmission of class and other origins of social mobility affect these hierarchies and their description, an example being the recent discussion in the US of an emerging 'underclass' (Auletta 1982). Detailed descriptions of the lives of people in the under-class or in different disadvantaged (or sometimes advantaged) positions such as those by Coles (1977) are examples of attempts to plumb the meaning of social class for the people themselves. They are rewarding to read alongside statistical tables of social class data as reminders of the complex and varied processes which envelop the often used factor or variable of social class.

Research investigations into social class require an index of social position, occupation, education, income, housing tenure, or some combination of these indicators. By far the most widely used index is occupation, a good example being the Registrar General's classification of the population in Britain into five social classes (one of which is subdivided into manual and non-manual) according to the general social standing of different groups of occupations. Married women are assigned according to their husband's occupation/class, children to that of their father, and the retired and unemployed to that of their last significant period of employment. In the US, social scientists have worked with numerous combinations of the education–income–occupation complex in an attempt to build a satisfactory classification for women and men. Other attempts have been made to refine the measurement of social class to get away from the dependency on classification of occupations (Goldthorpe and Hope 1974). In studies of health and disease, all these indices have been applied, and apart from a few discrepant results, consistent differences are found between the classes in morbidity and mortality.

## Cause and effect

The consistently demonstrated relationship between social class and health status raises the question of the cause and effect meaning of the data. The significant correlation between low social class, low life expectancy, and high morbidity is sometimes attributed to differential access to or use of health services, suggesting that equality of access will level off the differences. Comparisons before and after the National Health Service (NHS) and welfare state were instituted in Britain show, however, that traditional differences in death rates by social class continue, albeit at lower absolute levels of mortality (Morris 1979). The professions do well, while unskilled workers and their families do particularly badly. Indeed, the Working Group on Inequalities in Health (Townsend and Davidson 1982) noted the striking lack of improvement, in some cases even deterioration, in the health experience of occupational classes IV and V relative to occupational class I, as judged by mortality indicators. Mortality statistics and data from the National Health Interview Survey in the US indicate that the Great Society reforms promulgated by the Johnson Administration during the 1960s improved but did not close the gap between the poor and non-poor, while at the same time, use of doctors and hospitals by the poor increased (Lerner and Stutz 1977; Wilson and White 1977). Thus, alternative explanation of the social class gradient must be entertained in relation to the characteristics and processes which affect disease and distribution by class.

Disease-specific studies testing alternative theories have been conducted on a number of clinical conditions, although coronary heart disease and mental illness have received major attention (Susser and Watson 1971; Susser et al. 1983). In relation to coronary heart disease, diet (Feinleib et al. 1977; Shekelle et al. 1981), body weight (Stunkard et al. 1972), exercise (Morris et al. 1973), blood pressure (Cassell et al. 1971), smoking (Cartwright et al. 1959), and emotional strain (Jenkins 1976) have all been examined as ways of life which vary with social class. Susser et al. (1983) conclude that the immediate reasons for the social class distribution of coronary heart disease should be related to the broader socio-economic context in which these risk factors operate, suggesting that occupational and specific group and life-style studies are necessary to unravel the association.

The association between social status and psychological disorder has been well studied (Dohrenwend and Dohrenwend 1969; Brown and Harris 1978; Wheaton 1978). Two causal interpretations of the social class gradient in health status compete: 'social class determines health' and 'health determines social class'. The former explanation, presented by Antonovsky (1967) for life expectancy in general, links social class with preventive health behaviour, sanitation, and access to medical care. In relation to mental illness, the material conditions of poverty (Dohrenwend 1983), job loss (Cobb and Kasl 1977), stressful life experience (Dohrenwend and Dohrenwend 1974, 1981), divorce (Goode 1956), and bad childhood experiences (Rutter and Madge 1976) have been implicated. Brown and Harris (1978) have shown that working class women exhibit greater psychological vulnerability and experience a combination of life stresses without as much environmental support as middle-class women, and consequently suffer a higher incidence and prevalence of clinical depression.

Evidence of the concentration of schizophrenic disorders in the lowest social class (Faris and Dunham 1939; Dohrenwend and Dohrenwend 1969) has been used to support the drift or 'health determines class' hypothesis (Lawrence 1958) that those who have the disorder drift downward in socio-economic status during their lifetime because of difficulty getting or maintaining jobs and secure living conditions. Studies have shown that drift does occur (Goldberg and Morrison 1963; Harkey et al. 1976) and that diagnoses and treatments drift and change across the careers of schizophrenic patients (Sheehan 1982). But this explanation alone does not suffice to account for the strength of the observed relationship between social class and health. It is likely that many factors are implicated in the onset and course of schizophrenia, including genetic susceptibility, stressful life experiences, the lack of social resources, and inability to cope resulting from disturbed family socialization experience (Kohn 1972; Dohrenwend 1983).

The difficulties in assessing the causal direction of relationships between social class and health are similar to the problems encountered in testing causal hypotheses about the relationships between public health interventions directed toward providing equality of opportunity and their effects on outcomes. For such interventions – for example, increasing child benefits, positive discrimination in health services for the poor, individual educational programmes for children and adults, community health education campaigns, the self-care movement, school milk – determination of the validity of any relationship requires data from many experiments and quasi-experiments performed in numerous settings.

## Research design

True experimental designs with random assignment to treatment or control groups are rare in sociological investigations precisely because the real world does not often lend itself to the controlled conditions of an experiment. Randomization is not always considered ethical, feasible, or desirable in social treatment. The high cost of labour-intensive research teams in collecting data from large population groups is often prohibitive and the lack of stability and certainty in research careers, funding agencies, and client support all work against the implementation of social experiments. For example, randomizing access to health care for disadvantaged groups in a single population clearly would be unethical given that barriers to care would constitute the control. Social experiments in which treatment was withheld have occurred in the past (DHEW 1973) to the discredit of public health researchers in the US. While randomized, experimental designs have been used in evaluating social action programmes, these have been conducted when conditions have been optimal for achieving control in the field setting (Gilbert et al. 1975). The Rand Health Insurance Study in the US, a controlled experiment concerning cost sharing in health insurance policies, is a national social experiment involving some 8000 individuals in six US communities (Newhouse 1974). Early findings indicate that cost sharing, that is, family out-of-pocket expenditure for medical bills, clearly reduces medical care expenditures. The effect of variations in cost sharing on participants' health status is not yet known (Newhouse et al. 1982). This study is an example both of a true experiment with a controlled intervention and of the high cost and complexity of large-scale social experimentation.

The lack of opportunity for experimentation does not detract from the usefulness of sociological investigations in public health, as Patrick and Elinson (1979:443) note: 'Although experimentation is properly revered, too often the form is honored more than the substance. A carefully controlled experiment on a trivial manipulable variable contributes far less than a careful inferential analysis of the association of non-manipulable but non-trivial variables. For instance, one does not abandon research on the association between smoking and cancer because randomization and the classic experimental design are not possible.'

A large number of quasi-experimental research designs not requiring random assignment are available (Cook and Campbell 1979). Two major principles are involved in using this type of research design (Patrick 1981). The first is that the logic for establishing causality requires that all plausible alternative explanations of the relationship between cause and effect or treatment and outcome be specified, and evidence to counter these rival explanations considered or demonstrated. Most important, the rival hypotheses or threats to internal validity must be ruled out – for example, screening programmes for hypertension may attract predominantly health conscious, white, or otherwise low-risk clients, and the failure to show any effect of the programme may be the result of selection artifacts or of the low-risk group screened.

Knowledge of the precise theoretical meaning of the constructs used in research is necessary in order to link a particular study to others based on the same ideas. Thus, differences among investigations using an occupational index of social class reflecting social standing of occupation and their consequences for life-style are easier to interpret than differences from studies using other measures unless the hypothesized relationship between measures – such as occupation and housing tenure – are specified.

The second major principle governing the use of quasi-experimental designs is that of assessing the consistency of findings from studies across times and across research settings, methods, and populations. These issues of external validity are crucial to interpreting results. Studies of stressful life events have been plagued by a host of measurement and theoretical conflicts, including the nature of the events which should be studied, weighting or non-weighting of events, and the timing of observations (Dohrenwend and Dohrenwend 1981). Despite these difficulties, evidence from different cultures, investigations, and times shows that lower social class persons experience more events as well as more distress than higher social class persons (Langner and Michael 1963; Dohrenwend and Dohrenwend 1969; Brown *et al.* 1975; Brown and Harris 1978; Kessler 1979; Kessler and Cleary 1980). These consistent findings give high external validity to the association.

Quasi-experimental research designs are most useful when the opportunity exists for collecting additional data on the potential threats to internal validity, when standardized measures of cause and effect are used for comparability, when different populations are studied, and when different intervention strategies or hypotheses are compared. The Stanford Community Studies (Farquhar 1978, 1980) illustrate such a strategy for experimentation under conditions that do not satisfy the more rigorous but more restrictive criteria for controlled experiments. This study involved three communities, two of which were exposed to mass-media campaigns directed at cigarette smoking, blood cholesterol levels, and high blood pressure while the third had no special campaign. One of the 'experimental' communities also had personal counselling for a sample of high-risk individuals. The mass media and counselling interventions were successful in achieving immediate reductions in the risk of cardiovascular disease.

## METHODOLOGICAL APPROACHES

The choice of research methods is never atheoretical or neutral. Training and familiarity with one methodological tradition can blind researchers to evidence from research endeavours which use unfamiliar, new, or newly-revised methods. Different disciplines and research practitioners in different eras, cultures, and applied settings tend to lay claim to a method or set of methods in convincing others that their approach is the most appropriate and that their evidence represents the 'truth'. This parochialism in method – stemming from diferences in the philosophy of science, in the need for disciplinary identity, and in socio-political beliefs – is the best argument for training in a wide variety of research methods, which should lead to greater methodological awareness and flexibility in investigations and research critiques.

Sociological investigators have been exceedingly creative in their use of methods, perhaps because the real world setting for most studies demands this. Five main approaches have been used with a broad range of variation within each

approach: historical research, demography and administrative statistics, social survey methods, qualitative or observational/participation methods, and policy analysis. These are not exclusively sociological or social science methods, since a number of natural scientists and health professionals have developed and used them as well. Each approach will be described briefly and illustrated using, to whatever extent possible, sociological investigations concerning social class and health, including health promotion and disease prevention programmes as well as social epidemiological investigations.

### Historical methods

Personal documents such as diaries, autobiographies, letters, essays, speeches, and historical records such as registration documents, minutes of meetings, newspaper clippings, agency records, and other documents found in libraries and collections, both public and private, are rich sources of data for both generating and testing hypotheses. All written material, whether or not presented in the scientific literature, is history, and scientists read, interpret, conclude, and report using written materials, so in this sense all scientists are historians (Barzun 1977). The studies noted previously of working class populations in England and the US in the eighteenth and nineteenth centuries provide a brilliant historical record of the observed relationship between poor housing, sanitation, water, income, and working conditions, and poor health, death, or life expectancy. In another example, Edward Jarvis (1855) noted that there were 64 times as many cases of insanity in the lower (pauper) class in proportion to its numbers in comparison to the independent class. These historical writings help us to deal with the problems of the present and future by playing a part in the creation of 'ideology' or 'utopia' (Dewey 1938). The past is reconstructed in terms of the present using projective interpretations.

Waitzkin (1981), in an interesting historical review of the social origins of illness, used the collected works of Rudolf Virchow, Salvador Allende, and Fredrich Engels to compare and contrast these thinkers' views of social aetiology, multifactorial causation, social epidemiology, strategies of sociomedical change, and other aspects of the disease-generating conditions of the workplace and environment. Virchow emphasized the inequalities in the distribution and consumption of social resources and their effects on 'crowd diseases' such as typhus, scurvy, tuberculosis, and cholera. Allende linked underdevelopment and the international economic order, including extraction of wealth from the developing world, to ill health. Engels concentrated on industrialism, economic production, and the miseries of working-class life. The biographies and historical periods of these men are as divergent as their theoretical stances, but taken together their writings anticipated many concerns of people currently examining the social causation of disease. This historical analysis is important in providing continuities in the link between social structure and disease as well as in reminding us that reconstructed models of aetiology may be necessary for meaningful solutions.

The burgeoning world literature and technological innovation in systematic library research such as the MEDLINE system of the US National Library of Medicine or the citation indexes in social science and science contribute greatly to the power of the individual researcher in seeking evidence. The mere manipulation of all this evidence, including notes and bibliographical references, can be awesome. Mills (1959) has recommended using files as a research journal in which the grandest and littlest bits of ideas and records can be stored, re-sorted, sifted, and used in writing, generating research proposals, and interpreting other types of evidence. Meta-analysis, a set of techniques for reviewing research in which data from different studies are statistically combined, is emerging as a useful means of reviewing the evidence for conclusions drawn from a series of related studies (Glass et al. 1981).

### Demography and administrative statistics

A considerable amount of statistical data is available on the members of most modern, industrial societies. These data are accumulated primarily for purposes of administration and historical record, although field researchers can use them to good effect. Perhaps the most stunning example in sociology of the flexible and truly productive use of available statistics is Durkheim's work on suicide (1951). Starting with his theories of group cohesiveness and suicide rates, he examined available international records and modified and refined his theory in the light of this evidence.

Statistical data on social class and health are available from population surveys and censuses in many industrial nations. Some countries, such as Britain, are fortunate in having administrative reviews over time of mortality related to occupation and the classification of occupations into socio-economic groups – OPCS, *Decennial Supplements, Occupational Mortality (passim)*. The analysis and interpretation of statistical returns on mortality, however, poses theoretical and methodological problems (Alderson 1972; Leete and Fox 1977; OPCS 1978). Table 11.1 illustrates data produced in the Registrar General's Decennial Supplements in England and Wales between 1931 and 1971 on trends in inequality in male mortality, as measured by the relative changes in the mortality of different social or occupational classes (Towns-

end and Davidson 1982). In general, these standardized mortality ratios show a regular upward trend with downward social class. The mortality of the different occupational classes is shown relative to the national rate for England and Wales. At first glance, from the unadjusted data it would appear that inequality in mortality between occupational classes widened sharply between 1949 and 1953 and 1959 and 1963. Changes were introduced in 1960 in the classification of occupations, however, and these account for most of the change in the relative mortality experience of classes I and II over the period 1959–63 and 1970–72. In 1961, about 26 per cent of the occupations were allocated to a class different from that to which they would have been allocated in the 1950 classification. In certain professional groups such as doctors, lawyers, teachers, and clergy, however, the improvements in social classes I and II cannot be accounted for by differences in classification. Further adjustments confirm the social class gap, but it is still difficult to attribute excess mortality to occupation, primarily since other factors contribute to premature illness and death. These measures of occupation are also cross-sectional and do not take into account mobility between occupations during life, changes in the composition of the labour force, or possible selection effects such that poor health produced a smaller class of unskilled workers. The evidence on disease-specific mortality ratios would also indicate that where death rates are falling, class differentials increase, and where they are rising, the reverse is true. A cultural lag in the diffusion of medical evidence across the social classes is one often-mentioned hypothesis for this latter trend (Blaxter 1981). These statistical data also do not reflect what it is about occupational conditions that affects health status. Job type, conditions, security, and benefits may all affect occupational risk, and further research is required to illuminate these administrative statistics. Nevertheless, such statistics remain the best evidence of structured inequality in health chances and pose important policy questions about conditions of poverty and possible course of action because they illustrate the point made so forcibly by Townsend (1979:31): 'Poverty can be defined objectively and applied consistently only in terms of the concept of relative deprivation'.

Interpretation of administrative data involves a complex interweaving of theory and methodological technique.

**Table 11.1.** *Mortality of men aged 15–64 years by occupational class – England and Wales 1931–71*

| Occupational class | Standardized mortality ratios | | | | | |
| --- | --- | --- | --- | --- | --- | --- |
| | 1930–32 | 1949–53* | 1959–63 unadjusted | adjusted † | 1970–72 unadjusted | adjusted † |
| I    Professional | 90 | 86 | 76 | 75 | 77 | 75 |
| II   Managerial | 94 | 92 | 81 | – | 81 | – |
| III  Skilled manual and non-manual | 97 | 101 | 100 | – | 104 | – |
| IV   Partly skilled | 102 | 104 | 103 | – | 114 | – |
| V    Unskilled | 111 | 118 | 143 | 127 | 137 | 121 |

*Corrected figures as published in *Registrar General's Decennial Supplement, England and Wales, 1961: Occupational Mortality Tables*. HMSO, London (1971), p. 22.

†Occupation in 1952–63 and 1970–72 have been reclassified according to the 1950 classification.

Source: Townsend and Davidson (1982).

Statistical analysis of trend data on unemployment and mortality using time series techniques has been used by both Brenner (1977) and Eyer (1977) to reach different conclusions about economic cycles and health. Brenner (1977, 1979) has argued that the variation in annual overall mortality rates in the US, England and Wales, and Sweden can be explained in terms of changes in the annual level of employment, given that a time lag of five years is allowed for unemployment to have an effect on health. Eyer (1977) has challenged the use of a five-year time lag on the grounds that the health consequences of unemployment generally occur within a much shorter time. Instead, Eyer argues that death rates increase at the time when employment rates are high through worker migration and stressful work conditions and their consequences in alcohol and tobacco consumption. No amount of technique can answer the competing theoretical questions. Evidence on the health effects of unemployment must be obtained from different countries, investigators, data sets, and analytical techniques in order to reach conclusions about economy and health which should guide policy decisions and social action.

## Social survey methods

Surveys, both cross-sectional and longitudinal, based on self-administered questionnaires or conducted by interview, are the most commonly used designs in sociological investigations. The assumption behind the use of structured interview schedules or questionnaires is that respondents share a common vocabulary and understanding of the research process so that the questions elicit ranges of responses which are similar for each person interviewed. This assumption often breaks down, exactly because respondents do *not* share common meanings, histories, moods, or even cultures. A good example of this is the seemingly simple question posed in many surveys: 'Who is the head of this household?' To the middle class, white, native English-speaking household group, the response to this question may be straightforward, or the interviewer may have probes or decision rules to arbitrate and decide. Even so, room-mates or unrelated members of co-operative households may not identify a head. English-speaking, Puerto Rican immigrants in the US often assume 'head' to mean landlord (Smith 1975). Thus, a simple question can evoke different ranges of response in deceptive ways. While techniques of interviewer training, questionnaire piloting and even *post hoc* assessment of interviewer effects can go a long way toward standardizing the interview process, no amount of methodological sophistication can force homogeneity in memory, or understanding and willingness to reveal information. Respondents are seldom from the same social class as investigators, a fact which can influence how much shared meaning there is for questions and responses. In some situations, a less standardized or structured approach to questionnaire or interview design that gives respondents more responsibility and freedom of expression is appropriate.

Semi-structured, in-depth interviewing is only one variant of the many survey research methods which generate data on samples of populations or large enough numbers of respondents to subdivide the data by sex, occupation, age, ethnic group, or area of residence. An example of this approach is provided by George Brown and his colleagues who have designed contextual measures of life events for use in psychiatric epidemiological studies (Brown 1974; Brown and Harris 1978; Brown 1981). This work starts from the premise that conceptual and methodological shortcomings detract from the dictionary approach to assigning meaning to life events which is used by many researchers following the now classic paper by Holmes and Rahe (1967). The contextual approach, the origins of which arise out of the phenomenological work of Alfred Shutz (1954, 1972), moves the locus of measurement from the respondent, who replies to a checklist of events in the usual survey, to the interviewers, who in as informal a way as possible ask a lengthy list of questions about events with a particular kind of meaning decided by the researchers before the field work begins. The interviewer in this approach is the measuring instrument, and the job of interviewing is to ask questions until enough information is obtained to rate the qualities of life events. The ratings are made by people not involved in the interview, and the reports of inter-rater reliability are encouraging. The question of validity is more difficult to assess and it rests on the demonstration of construct validity as Brown (1981:196) admits: 'The issue of validity is more complicated and ultimately, we believe, depends on the persuasiveness of theory stemming from research using the measures'. The main conclusion of this line of inquiry to date is that social stresses, mainly important losses and disappointments, are important in the onset of psychiatric disorder. The generalization of this finding across different investigations and research settings, using the tape-recorded interview and researcher-rating technique developed by these investigations, will address the question of validity. Using the characteristics of ordinary conversation in the survey research process has great potential, provided the intensive training of interviewers can be accomplished, and researchers, independent raters, and time are available in the investigation.

Others who have worked on the standardized questionnaire have defined the interview as a conversation with a purpose (Cannel and Kahn 1968). Great advances have been made in the construction of questions which are open-ended – for example, unrestricted in response – and close-ended – for example, forced-choice (Schuman and Presser 1981; Sudman and Bradburn 1982). This research is crucial to the rapidly expanding use in the US of health interviews by telephone (Groves and Kahn 1979), and to the surveys conducted in response to the demands of funding agencies for large amounts of quantifiable data collected over a short period of time at relatively low cost. Advances have also been made in the use of informants (Sirken 1981) and health diaries (Verbrugge 1980; Sudman and Lannom 1980). Most importantly, extensive research is being done on the effects of interviewers themselves on the respondents to surveys and the contributions to survey error made by interviewer variability (Andersen *et al.* 1979). Such studies are crucial to all survey research whether it be standardized or non-standardized.

A large number of textbooks on survey research methods are available (Babbie 1973; Moser and Kalton 1975; Backstrom and Hursh-Cesar 1981). In addition, published reports of national conferences on health survey research methods held in the US summarize the most important advances in standardized, structured surveys in the health field (NCHSR, *passim*). A great deal can also be learned about the application of survey methods to a variety of health problems from reading systematically the works of Ann Cartwright and her colleagues in London (Cartwright 1967, 1970, 1976, 1983; Cartwright and Anderson 1981).

Survey research is sometimes considered synonymous with sociological or social science methodology. This is not only because of the methodological parochialism mentioned earlier or the availability of computer-assisted statistical tools for analysing structured survey data. Survey data tend to take on the quality of fact. Medical and natural scientists are often most comfortable with the so-called 'hard' data of structured social surveys and administrative statistics. Social surveys have the advantage of a long tradition in data generation and analysis, but the meaning and interpretation of these data are no less a problem than research based on the other methods reviewed here. Surveys are one route to knowledge, no more and no less.

### Qualitative methods

Efforts to decide and explain the reality of health-related interactions or service settings have evolved multiple methodological strategies which can be classified as qualitative or observational. Anthropologists have long engaged in ethnographic studies of different cultures and societies. Sociologists – building on the early work of G.H. Mead, John Cooley, and Herbert Blumer, and later work by Anselm Strauss, Howard Becker, and Erving Goffman – have used these techniques in intensive studies of small samples to learn the actor's point of view and to develop what Weber called *verstehen*, both an empathetic appreciation and causal explanation of social processes (Weber 1964). These methods, reviewed by Schwartz and Jacobs (1979), include participant observation and interviewing, biographies and life histories, audio-visual techniques, unobtrusive observation, still-picture photography, and various combinations of these techniques which illustrate unlimited ingenuity. Qualitative studies of health-related interactions and service settings have contributed to an understanding of the viewpoints of both patients and providers in every day medical practice (Robinson 1971; Wadsworth and Robinson 1976; Davis and Horobin 1977) and the 'illness' careers of patients and non-patients with polio (Davis 1963), tuberculosis (Roth 1963), epilepsy (West 1976; Scambler and Hopkins 1980), mental illness (Estroff 1981; Sheehan 1982), drug problems (Becker 1963), and other health problems. Other studies have examined intensively health providers and delivery settings (Goffman 1963; Sudnow 1967; Roth 1972). In a two-year participant observation study, Millman (1977) explored the closely related topics of physician mistakes and patient trust. She showed the lines of defence that physicians employ in coping with error and how patients' assertions and questions reflected patient anxiety and distrust. Taken together, these studies demonstrate how the context of the interaction between patients and providers and the rituals and routines of health settings influence attitudes, service use, health status, and health knowledge. Observational studies in socio-economic status and health have been conducted concerning the illness behaviour which arises out of the culture of poverty, a phrase first introduced in 1959 by Oscar Lewis in his studies of Mexican and Puerto Rican families (1959, 1961, 1964, 1965) and then adopted by Michael Harrington in his book *The other America* (1962) which played a seminal role in sparking the national anti-poverty programme in the US. The culture, or more accurately the subculture of poverty, can be characterized as a way of life passed down from generation to generation along family lines as an adaptation and a reaction of the poor to their marginal position in a class-stratified society. It is not only a matter of economic deprivation; in fact, there are positive aspects and rewards which develop as survival tactics. The historical contexts and conditions for a developing culture of poverty have been described by Lewis (1965). The recent participant observation work by Auletta (1982) on the 'underclass' shows that the subculture changes both in membership and survival tactics, although the conditions of deprivation may have transcended rural–urban differences, time, and national differences.

Rainwater (1968) and Strauss (1969) applied the culture of poverty ideas to observational studies in health. They both focused on the cultural gap between low-status users and professional medical practitioners in the US to explain the lower use of health services by those whose feelings of powerlessness and low self-esteem arose from the culture of poverty. Rainwater described this distinctive culture in relation to the public health clinics where the poor sought treatment which was curt, cursory, and enveloped by a culture of its own in which the standards of scientific medicine prevailed. The result was the refusal of or delay in consultation and acceptance of poor health (Rainwater 1968:263): 'Just as lower class people become more resigned to a conception of themselves as persons who do not function very well socially or psychologically, they become resigned if necessary to bodies that do not function very well physically'. Strauss (1969) studied a small sample of more stable working class people and their attitudes toward official medical services. He found that these people put a low emphasis on health as a life-goal, had a low level knowledge about illness and services, found access to professional care difficult, and disliked the stigma of 'charity' which they experienced in the bureaucracy and attitudes of the professional staff.

These studies inevitably suggest changes in the organization and delivery of services and health education programmes to fit the perceptions and expressed needs of poor people. Such efforts are rewarding and worthwhile in humanizing health care (Howard and Strauss 1975), but the very nature of the culture of poverty and its roots in the larger economic and social order of society makes it unlikely that services directed toward individual preventive and illness behaviour will have lasting impact on the health effects of the cycle of disadvantage.

Qualitative studies have been maligned for the opposite reasons that quantitative methods have been revered: they are 'subjective' rather than 'objective', they do not permit easy replication, they are based on samples that are too small, and they cannot be generalized. These criticisms reflect a misunderstanding or distrust of the worth of finding out how health providers and prospective or actual patients take in what is going on around them and act on their perceptions. The motives, meanings, emotions, and other subjective aspects of the lives of individuals and groups are powerful influences on action, and on the understanding of success and failure in purposive action (Patton 1980). Qualitative studies on health and health care will continue to enlighten our thinking and provide explanations of how and why social inequalities persist.

## Policy analysis

Policy analysis is the study of the nature, causes, and effects of alternative public policies, and such analysis of policies directed toward the prevention of illness and the promotion of health is ever-increasing (Carter and Peel 1976; Knowles 1977; Mechanic 1979; Hunter 1980). While the field of public policy analysis is being pursued vigorously, particularly by economists, the methods used in applying social science methodology to policy are evolving into a subspeciality (Zeckhauser and Stokey 1978; MacRae 1979). The methods themselves are no different from those used in other social science fields, but the question of choosing the best policy among a set of alternatives, sometimes deductively or before the policies are adopted, raises distinctive methodological problems (Burt 1974).

The first task of policy analysis is choosing the policy problem itself, and this aspect dominates the formal methodology which follows. Although there is no 'method' for choosing the right problem, the experience and talent of the investigator in a specific field is often an advantage in formulating a problem on which information is available and action is possible. Consequently, most policy analysis is retrospective, but the investigator may have had long experience with the policy problem. Foltz (1982), for example, has analysed the early periodic screening, detection, and treatment programme for children implemented in the US during the 1960s, and her analysis developed out of her knowledge of and experience with other public health policy alternatives for children.

Developing clear 'valuative' criteria for the comparison of policy results is the next stage, and highly developed techniques from operations research and economics are available to help with this methodological task. 'Objective function' or maximization techniques, cost-benefit and cost-effectiveness analysis, and value analysis methods from applied welfare economics described in the previous chapter provide systematic tools. The availability of these tools does not solve the problem of whether or not the right measures have been used in the first place. For example, mortality, morbidity, disability, dissatisfaction, happiness, or some other subjective health indicators can be used in assessing the results of public assisted health care. When policies are to be judged in terms of their effects on people, then the thorny questions of how human life and health are to be valued become inevitable (Fuchs 1974; Mooney 1977). Social science investigators in the health field have developed valuational

techniques for health states which do not depend on monetary terms (Kaplan et al. 1976; Torrance 1976; Patrick 1979), and the values have been used in maximization models of alternative programmes (Chen and Bush 1976).

In policy analysis, the expected consequences of possible alternative policies are compared after being predicted by models of causation, and complex methods of simulation and gaming have been developed to predict programme results. Estimating the consequences of policies involving services may depend on the results of sociological studies of provider and consumer behaviour, both qualitative and quantitative. One frequently used economic model in the US is that of the free, competitive market, including departures from this model and the means of coping with them. Application of this model to health care financing in the US has produced fierce policy debate about competition and regulations (Enthoven 1980; McClure 1980) illustrating the fine line between policy analysis and policy advocacy. Sociological studies of consumer attitudes and behaviour contribute to the prediction of policy effects, particularly unanticipated consequences (Klein 1979). Many models of public provision exist, and the prediction of their consequences in health care ranges from evaluating specific services and large decision-making procedures to the analysis of conflicts and competing interests of the different groups concerned with health care.

The final stage in analysing policy implementation involves estimating the political feasibility for enacting a chosen policy, and such estimation cannot be easily systematized. How policy determines politics and vice versa is likely to be specific to particular political situations, personalities, and events, and generalized methods will be elusive.

The War on Poverty and the Great Society programmes, created or expanded in the US during the administration of President Lyndon B. Johnson, have provoked a great deal of retrospective policy analysis, partly because of their expense but also because they represent a recent attempt to renew the American 'dream' of equal opportunity. The overall objective of these programmes was improved access to services and health improvements for the disadvantaged, an equally important problem for countries with national health systems such as Britain. Davis and Schoen (1978) have summarized the basic health and poverty issues and the public programmes of the Great Society from 1965 to 1975 that attempted to break the link between low income and poor health: Medicaid, Medicare, the maternal and child health programmes, and the neighbourhood health centres. Using administrative statistics such as those described earlier in this chapter, these authors showed that all the programmes have made improvements in increasing the availability of health care to the poor and disadvantaged, while Medicare and Medicaid have protected many elderly and poor people from the financial burden of large medical bills. The neighbourhood health centres, in addition to delivering better services to extremely poor communities, provided many poor with employment and enabled them to upgrade their educational and job skills. The benefits of these programmes were unevenly distributed, however, and did not reach all the groups of people for which they were intended. Inefficiency in national and local administration of the programmes and spiralling health care cost were unwelcome consequences of these major policy initiatives. The effects of separate programmes for the poor were also deleterious (Davis and Schoen 1978:215): 'Covering the poor and the disadvantaged separately from the rest of the population leads the public programs to absorb rapid increases in expenditures and undermines their ability to deliver care to all'. The authors recommended that all the programmes be combined into a national health insurance scheme that would service the poor and non-poor alike and would promote the reallocation of resources from overserved to underserved geographical areas. This recommendation spawns an entirely new set of alternative policies for national health insurance, some of which are currently being debated under conditions of rising or continuing unemployment or uncertain and unstable economic conditions.

Policy analysts use almost any available source document that defines and impinges on public policy alternatives. Legislative and other official documents form one important source, while public speeches and televised interviews provide another, almost instantaneous data source in which the shape of health policy can be discerned. To the student of public health, much of policy analysis looks like an insider's knowledge of programme options and of the personalities involved in the decision-making process. Ironically it is often the outsider, such as De Tocqueville's appraisal of democracy in America, who can best see the outline of alternative policy options and their possible consequences, sometimes even predicting the next option successfully. Perhaps this is because the outsider can return home safely without facing the inevitable muddle of part-success and part-failure which accompanies most policy change and which, in turn, prompts the next round of decision-making.

## USE OF SOCIOLOGICAL EVIDENCE

This chapter has briefly described the concerns, concepts, and methods of sociological investigations in public health using, wherever possible, examples from studies on social class and health status and health care. Not all the methods and examples bear directly on the prevention of disease and the promotion of health. Most sociological investigations on social class are concerned either with documenting the fact that socially patterned differences in health status exist, or with attempting to explain why they do in order to shed light on the causal mechanisms. The latter investigations also often suggest feasible interventions or policies that will close the gap in physical, social, and mental well-being between the poor and non-poor, but this is not always the case.

The theme of social class and social inequality will certainly continue to dominate sociological method and theory in health just as it has since the nineteenth century. As General William Booth, founder of the Salvation Army, wrote in 1890 (p. 15): 'If this were the first time that this wail of hopeless misery had sounded on our ears the matter would have been less serious. It is because we have heard it so often that the case is so desperate. The exceeding bitter cry of the disheartened has come to be as familiar in the ears of men as

the dull roar of the streets or as the moaning of the wind through the trees . . . Only now and then, on rare occasions, when some clear voice is heard giving more articulate utterance to the miseries of the miserable men, do we pause in the regular routine of our daily duties, and shudder as we realize for one brief moment what life means to the inmates of the slums.' The convergence of evidence periodically reviewed and re-reviewed shows the same gap even though mortality rates have declined significantly and access or opportunity for health care has in many places improved. In order to make explicit the consequences for disease prevention and health promotion, future sociological investigations in public health will have to be designed so that the best use of sociological evidence will be made.

Improved data sources, methodology, techniques of analysis, and dissemination of scientific evidence will put demands on investigators to design and produce studies which answer basic aetiological questions. Such expectations spill over from the natural sciences where careful development and the right combination of laboratories, tissue cultures, bioassay techniques, electron microscopy, and other technological tools have produced great scientific advances, with the consequent accolades, prestige, and opportunity for further research. Scientific revolutions and Nobel Prizes do not await the investigator who shows that the personality characteristics, social networks, religion, and housing of some poor people raise their risk for developing hypertension or coronary heart disease. The immediate utility of the finding would not be obvious to the decision-maker since personalities, social networks, religion, and housing are notoriously hard to change or affect. Rather, another piece of the class–psychosocial factor–disease link might fall into place, and a long tradition of replications and partial replication studies might follow, particularly if a methodological advance has been made along the way.

Aetiological studies of all the critical variables involved in the social causation of disease and illness are difficult to mount and accomplish. More fruitful is the painstaking examination of a single idea or set of ideas by a group of investigators over a long period of time with regular state-of-the-field assessments. The work on life events and mental illness, one example of a cumulative social epidemiological subspecialty, illustrates how much personal dedication, public and private investment, and time are necessary to unravel the causal process. Golden and Dohrenwend (1981) suggest path-analysis for testing six alternative hypotheses concerning the life stress process. This provides another step, specific choice of methodology aside, for furthering the research tradition to include social support, personality factors, and the qualities of life events themselves in multifactorial studies of psychiatric disorder. George Brown (1981) makes the case for contextual studies of life events which combine the survey approach with the qualitative, phenomenological orientation to sociological knowledge. These suggestions are not responses to the disappointment felt by some that over two decades of empirical studies leave the causal significance of stressful life events for psychiatric illness at best ambiguous. Rather, they show that investigations into the aetiology and onset of psychiatric, or any other chronic illness, will require long periods of time to determine new critical variables, create data sets, and analyse relationships.

While there are many gaps in the explanation of how social class determines lifelong health choices, research directions have been suggested. Blaxter (1981:221) notes in her extensive review on *The health of children*: 'We do have considerable evidence about the correlates of ill health in early childhood, and about the extent of inequality. For these reasons, a good case can be made, in light of current knowledge, for focusing attention upon children and particularly the under-fives.' The literature on social inequality and perinatal mortality, morbidity, and early childhood illness would suggest a trend in this direction (Townsend and Davidson 1982). Antenatal care, childhood accidents, child morbidity patterns, the adolescent and early adulthood experience of handicapped children, and the cycle of transmitted deprivation are important topics for research. Piece-by-piece opportunities, collaborations among social and medical scientists, and effective production of research results are necessary to meet this agenda.

The identification of psychosocial factors in disease and illness causation is only the precursor to eliminating or modifying those factors which facilitate the occurrence of disease. For instance, changing the amount and quality of family support, though difficult, is certainly possible. Psychiatrists have mobilized whole families in support of a psychiatrically disturbed member, and family members themselves have brought about support changes as, for example, the change depicted in the documentary film, *Best boy*. In this film, a middle-aged, mentally handicapped man was gradually exposed to new friends and independent living in a sheltered environment in advance of the death of his one surviving parent.

Controlled studies of innovations in social support systems, 'access' studies, and investigations into bureaucratic arrangements for service delivery, practitioner supply, and service effectiveness can be turned into social experiments. To do this implies that the investigator will have some control over implementing the programme or randomizing participants into experimental and control conditions in order to eliminate contaminating influences on the outcome of the intervention (Campbell 1969; Riecken and Boruch 1974; Rossi and Freeman 1982). The interventions studied are not usually radical innovations, but instead are modest efforts to increase efficiency or control cost (Freeman and Solomon 1979). It is clear that evaluation studies share with psychosocial epidemiological studies the same incremental, one-step-at-a-time cumulative knowledge process.

True and quasi-experimentation on policy-based questions, particularly those concerned with socio-economic status and health, are the major challenges for sociological investigators in the decades ahead. This social experimentation is different from the evaluation of health programmes which seek to find better ways to control or lessen harmful, individual or family practices such as alcoholism, drug addiction, and smoking. It is also different from studies of the efforts to promote health practices such as exercise, weight control, health screening, and other detection, diagnosis, prevention, and treatment programmes (Freeman and Rossi 1981; Breslow 1983). Social

experiments on health policy challenge fundamental norms in health care and in the socio-economic order to change existing public policy. Medicaid represents one of the boldest social innovations for providing health care to the poor ever attempted in the US, and the evaluation of its successes and failures still has an impact on planning for the future (Davis and Schoen 1978). Current efforts to improve health care delivery are likely to be more modest and less innovative than those in the 1930s or 1960s (Aday *et al.* 1980; Aiken *et al.* 1980). Nevertheless, social experiments are necessary to determine the different effects of service arrangements and financing on lower- and higher-income families – to evaluate combined housing, health, and social service care for the elderly and disabled poor; to assess the effects of child care support programmes for single-parent mothers or fathers receiving public assistance who wish to work; to eliminate work hazards and poor working conditions such as those experienced by some migrant workers; and to determine the effects of providing preventive and primary health care services to poor children, workers, and the elderly. These are the 'bold' social experiments which will accompany the more modest programme evaluations which are important for their frequent immediate effects on the lives of individuals.

Social experiments, and other types of sociological investigations, do not address the questions of standards or the basic values of a society. The choice and definition of the values to be served – for example, equality of distribution of resources or reverse discrimination for disadvantaged groups in gaining access to opportunities – are not technical matters of research. While research can uncover the basis for social objectives, investigations do not set the objectives. The challenge for all public health investigations, particularly those likely to influence decisions, is to find the best link between the standards or objectives and the research assessment. For example, the evaluation of the effectiveness of health services is best conducted when the objectives of the service are set by funding agents, decision-makers, administrators, sponsors of the service, and the participants themselves.

The recognition of the mix of social and health objectives is resulting in an important role for sociological investigations in efforts to increase opportunities for health within our society. Understanding persistent patterns of disadvantage in health will require all types of investigation. Historical studies of the general nature, conditions, and styles of living which have evolved in different societies at different times are necessary. Quantitative exploratory and explanatory surveys will be needed to discover the complex multicausal chain between the social and economic order and health status. Qualitative studies of the values and beliefs but, most of all, the coping strategies of people living in poverty will be valuable for understanding how people find their own solutions to seemingly intractable problems and suggesting how to provide that opportunity or power to others. Policy studies on the inequality of opportunity, particularly those that spawn social experiments in the health care field, are crucial to developing continuity in health chances. Many of these investigations will be long-term, particularly the social epidemiological and social policy evaluations. As competition for research resources gets keener because funds are not being made available, methodological and interdisciplinary struggles may ensue on how best to conduct research into health inequalities. To capitalize on the advances already made in reducing the health gap between the social classes and to broaden the research mosaic to encompass health in its most global socio-economic terms, the full range of sociological investigations and investigators will be necessary. Only with the combination of method, theory, meaning, and action are we likely to find and implement solutions with lasting impact on health for all.

## APPENDIX

### Major sources of research literature in sociology and public health

*American Journal of Epidemiology*
*American Journal of Public Health*
*American Sociological Review*
*Epidemiology and Community Health*
*Health and Society*
*Health Education Quarterly*
*Health Services Research*
*International Journal of Health Services*
*Journal of Health and Social Behavior*
*Journal of Human Stress*
*Medical Care*
*New England Journal of Medicine*
*Sociology of Health and Illness*
*Social Science and Medicine*

## REFERENCES

Aday, L. and Andersen, R. (1975). *Development of indices of access to medical care.* Health Administration Press, Ann Arbor, Michigan.

Aday, L.A., Andersen, R., and Fleming, G.V. (1980). *Health care in the US: equitable for whom?* Sage Publications, Beverly Hills, CA.

Aiken, L.H., Blendon, R.C., Freeman, H.E., and Rogers, D.E. (1980). Evaluating a private foundation's health program. *Evaluation Progr. Planning* 3 (2), 119.

Alderson, M.R. (1972). Some sources of error in British occupational mortality data. *Br. J. Ind. Med.* **29**, 245.

Andersen, R. (1968). *A behavioral model of families' use of health services.* Center for Health Administration Studies, University of Chicago.

Andersen, R. and Anderson, O. (1979). Trends in the use of health services. In *Handbook of medical sociology*, 3rd edn (ed. H. Freeman, S. Levine, and L. Reeder) p. 371. Prentice-Hall, Englewood Cliffs, NJ.

Andersen, R., Kasper, J., and Frankel, M. (1979). *Total survey error.* Jossey-Bass, San Francisco, CA.

Antonovsky, A. (1967). Social class and the major cardiovascular diseases. *J. Chronic Dis.* **21**, 65.

Auletta, K. (1982). *The underclass.* Random House, New York.

Babbie, E. (1973). *Survey research methods.* Wadsworth, Belmont, CA.

Backstrom, C. and Hursh-Cesar, G. (1981). *Survey research.* 2nd edn. Wiley, New York.

Barzun, J. (1977). *The modern researcher,* 3rd edn. Harcourt, Brace, and Jovanovich, New York.

Becker, H.S. (1963). *Outsiders: studies in the sociology of deviance.* Free Press, New York.

Becker, M. (ed.) (1974). The health belief model and personal health behavior. *Health Educ. Monogr.* **2**, 326.

Becker, M. (1979). Psychosocial aspects of health-related behavior. In *Handbook of medical sociology*, 3rd edn (ed. H. Freeman, S. Levine, and L. Reeder) p. 253. Prentice-Hall, Englewood Cliffs, NJ.

Becker, M. and Maiman, L. (1983). Models of health-related behavior. In *Handbook of health, health care and the health professions* (ed. D. Mechanic) p. 539. Free Press, New York.

Becker, M., Maiman, L., Kirscht, J., Haefner, D., and Drachman, R. (1977). The health belief model and prediction of dietary compliance: a field experiment. *J. Health Soc. Behav.* **18**, 348.

Bendix, R. and Lipset, E. (eds.) (1967). *Class, status, and power: a reader in social stratification,* 2nd edn. Routledge, London.

Blaxter, M. (1981). *The health of the children: a review of research on the place of health in cycles of disadvantage.* Heinemann Educational, London.

Booth, General W. (1890). *In darkest England and the way out.* Funk and Wagnalls, London.

Brenner, M. (1977). Health costs and benefits of economic policy. *Int. J. Health Serv.* **7**, 581.

Brenner, M. (1979). Mortality and the national economy. *Lancet* **ii**, 568.

Breslow, L. (1983). The potential of health promotion. In *Handbook of health, health care, and the health professions* (ed. D. Mechanic) p. 50. Free Press, New York.

Brockington, F. (1966). *A short history of public health.* Churchill, London.

Brown, G.W. (1974). Meaning, measurement and stress of life events. In *Stressful life events: their nature and effects* (ed. B.S. Dohrenwend and B.P. Dohrenwend) p. 217. Wiley, New York.

Brown, G.W. (1981). Contextual measures of life events. In *Stressful life events and their contexts* (ed. B.S. Dohrenwend and B.P. Dohrenwend) p. 187. Prodist, New York.

Brown, G. and Harris, T. (1978). *Social origins of depression.* Tavistock, London.

Brown, G.N., Ni Bhrolchain, M., and Harris, T. (1975). Social class and psychiatric disturbance among women in an urban population. *Sociology* **9**, 225.

Burt, M.R. (1974). *Policy analysis: introduction and applications to health programs.* Information Resource Press, Washington, DC.

Cahalan, D., Cisin, I., and Crossley, H. (1969). *American drinking practices: a national study of drinking behavior and attitudes.* Rutgers Center for Alcohol Studies, New Brunswick, NJ.

Campbell, D. (1969). Reforms as experiments. *Am. Psychol.* **24**, 409.

Campbell, D. and Stanley, J. (1966). *Experimental and quasi-experimental designs for research.* Rand McNally, Chicago.

Cannell, C. and Kahn, R. (1968). Interviewing. In *Handbook of social psychology, Vol. II* (ed. G. Lindzey and E. Aronson). p. 526. Addison-Wesley, Reading, MA.

Carter, C.O. and Peel, J. (eds.) (1976). *Equalities and inequalities in health: proceedings of the 12th Annual Symposium of the Eugenics Society.* Academic Press, London.

Cartwright, A. (1967). *Patients and their doctors: a study of general practice.* Routledge and Keagan Paul, London.

Cartwright, A. (1970). *Parents and family planning services.* Routledge and Keagan Paul, London.

Cartwright, A. (1976). *How many children?* Routledge and Keagan Paul, London.

Cartwright, A. (1983). *Health surveys in practice and in potential.* Kings Fund, London.

Cartwright, A. and Anderson, R. (1981). *General practice revisited.*

Tavistock, London.

Cartwright, A., Martin, E.M., and Thomson, J.G. (1959). Distribution and development of smoking habits. *Lancet* **ii**, 725.

Cassel, J. (1976). The contribution of the social environment to host resistance. *Am. J. Epidemiol.* **104**, 107.

Cassel, J., Heyden, S., Bartez, A.G., *et al.* (1971). Incidence of coronary heart disease by ethnic group, social class and sex. *Arch. Intern. Med.* **128**, 901.

Chadwick, E. (1842). *Report on the sanitary conditions of the labouring population of Great Britain.* (New Edition 1965 ed. M. Flinn.) Edinburgh University Press.

Chen, M. and Bush, J. (1976). Maximizing health system output with political and administrative constraints using mathematical programming. *Inquiry* **13** (3), 215.

Clausen, J. (1980). Some current issues in medical sociology. In *Sociological theory and research* (ed. H. Blalock Jr) p. 361. Free Press, New York.

Cobb, S. and Kasl, S. (1977). *Termination: the consequences of job loss.* OHEW (NIOSH) Publication No. 77–224, Cincinnati, OH.

Cockerham, W. (1978). *Medical sociology.* Prentice Hall, Englewood Cliffs, NJ.

Coles, R. (1977). *Children of crisis.* Little Brown, Boston, MA.

Cook, T. and Campbell, D. (1979). Quasi-experimentation: design and analysis issues in field settings. Rand McNally, Chicago.

Cronbach, L. (1982). *Designing evaluation of educational and social programs.* Jossey-Bass, San Francisco.

Davis, A. and Horobin, G. (eds.) (1977). *Medical encounters.* Croom Helm, London.

Davis, K. and Schoen, C. (1978). *Health and the war on poverty: a ten-year appraisal.* The Brookings Institution, Washington, DC.

Davis, F. (1963). *Passage through time: polio victims and their families.* Bobbs-Merrill, New York.

Denton, K. (1978). *Medical sociology.* Houghton Mifflin, Boston.

Department of Health, Education and Welfare (1973). *Final report of the Tuskegee Syphillis Study Ad Hoc Advisory Panel.* Department of Health, Education and Welfare, Washington, DC.

Dewey, J. (1938). *Logic, the theory of inquiry.* Holt, New York.

Dohrenwend, B.P. (1983). The epidemiology of mental disorder. In *Handbook of health, health care, and the health professions* (ed. D. Mechanic) p. 157. Free Press, New York.

Dohrenwend, B.P. and Dohrenwend, B.S. (1969). *Social status and psychological disorder.* Wiley-Interscience, New York.

Dohrenwend, B.S. and Dohrenwend, B.P. (eds) (1974). *Stressful life events: their nature and effects.* Wiley, New York.

Dohrenwend, B.S. and Dohrenwend, B.P. (eds.) (1981). *Stressful life events and their contexts.* Prodist, New York.

Durkheim, E. (1951). *Suicide: a study in sociology.* Free Press, New York.

Elinson, J. (1980). Medical sociology: theoretical underdevelopment and some opportunities. In *Social theory and research* (ed. H. Blalock Jr) p. 373. Free Press, New York.

Elling, R. and Sokolowska, M. (eds.) (1978). *Medical sociologists at work.* Transaction Books, New Brunswick, NJ.

Engels, F. (1845). *The condition of the working class in England in 1844.* (trans. and ed. W. Henderson and W. Chaloner, 1968). Stanford University Press.

Enthoven, A.C. (1980). *Health plan: the only practical solution to the soaring cost of medical care.* Addison-Wesley, Reading, MA.

Estroff, S. (1981). *Making it crazy: an ethnography of psychiatric clients in an American community.* University of California Press, Berkeley, CA.

Eyer, J. (1977). Does unemployment cause the death rate peak in each business cycle? A multifactorial model of death rate change. *Int. J. Health Serv.* **7**, 625.

Fabrega, H. (1974). *Disease and social behavior: an interdisciplinary perspective.* MIT Press, Cambridge, MA.

Faris, R. and Dunham, H. (1939). *Mental disorders in urban areas.* University of Chicago Press.

Farquhar, J.W. (1978). The community-based model of life style intervention trials. *Am. J. Epidemiol.* **108**, 103.

Farquhar, J.W. (1980). Changing cardiovascular risk factors in entire communities: The Stanford Three-Community Project. In *Childhood prevention of atherosclerosis and hypertension* (ed. R.M. Lower and R.B. Shekelle) p. 435. Raven Press, New York.

Feinleib, M., Garrison, R.J., Fabsitz, R., *et al.* (1977). The NHLBI twin study of cardiovascular disease risk factors: methodology and summary of results. *Am. J. Epidemiol.* **106**(4), 284.

Foltz, A. (1982). *Ounce of prevention.* MIT Press, Cambridge, MA.

Fox, J. (1977). *Occupational mortality 1970–72. Population trends No. 9.* HMSO, London.

Frankenberg, R. (1974). Functionalism and after? Theory and developments in social science applied to the health field. *Int. J. Health Serv.* **3**, 411.

Freeman, H. and Reeder, L. (1957). Medical sociology: a review of the literature. *Am. Sociol. Rev.* **22**, 73.

Freeman, H.E. and Rossi, P.H. (1981). Social experiments. *Milbank Mem. Fund. Qt.* **59**, 340.

Freeman, H.E. and Solomon, M.A. (1979). The next decade in evaluation research. *Eval. Progr. Plan.* **2**, 225.

Freeman, H., Levine, S., and Reeder, L. (eds.) (1979). *Handbook of medical sociology,* 3rd edn. Prentice Hall, Englewood Cliffs, NJ.

Freidson, E. (1970). *Profession of medicine.* Dodd Mead, New York.

Freidson, E. (1978). The development of design by accident. In *Medical sociologists at work* (ed. R. Elling and M. Sokolowska) p. 115. Transaction Books, New Brunswick, NJ.

Fuchs, V.R. (1974). *Who shall live? Health economics and social choice.* Basic Books, New York.

Giddens, A. (1973). *The class structure of the advanced societies.* Barnes and Noble Books, New York.

Gilbert, J.P., Light, R.J., and Mosteller, F. (1975). Assessing social innovations: an empirical base for policy. In *Evaluation and experiment* (ed. C.A. Bennett and A.A. Lumsdaine) p. 39, Academic Press, New York.

Glass, G.V., McGaw, B., and Smith, M.L. (1981). *Meta-analysis in social research.* Sage Publications, Beverly Hills, CA.

Goffman, E. (1963). *Stigma: notes on the management of spoiled identity.* Prentice-Hall, New York.

Goldberg, E. and Morrison, S. (1963). Schizophrenia and social class. *Br. J. Psychiatr.* **109**, 785.

Golden, R.R. and Dohrenwend, B.S. (1981). A path analytic method for testing causal hypotheses about the life stress process. In *Stressful life events and their contexts* (ed. B.S. Dohrenwend and B.P. Dohrenwend) p. 258. Prodist, New York.

Goldthorpe, J. and Hope, K. (1974). *The social grading of occupations.* Clarendon Press, Oxford.

Goode, W. (1956). *Women in divorce.* Free Press, New York.

Gore, S. (1978). The effect of social support in moderating the health consequences of unemployment. *J. Health Soc. Behav.* **19**, 157.

Graham, S. and Reeder, L. (1979). Social epidemiology of chronic diseases. In *Handbook of medical sociology,* 3rd edn (ed. H. Freeman, S. Levine, and L. Reeder) p. 71. Prentice-Hall, Englewood Cliffs, NJ.

Grotjahn, A. (1915). *Soziale pathologie,* 2nd edn. August Hinschwald Verlag, Berlin.

Groves, R.M. and Kahn, R.L. (1979). *Surveys by telephone: a national comparison with personal interviews.* Academic Press, New York.

Harkey, J., Miles, D., and Rushing, W. (1976). The relation

between social class and functional status: a new look at the drift hypothesis. *J. Health Soc. Behav.* **17**, 194.

Harrington, M. (1962). *The other America: poverty in the United States.* Macmillan, New York.

Hollingshead, A. and Redlich, F. (1958). *Social class and mental illness.* Wiley, New York.

Holmes, T.H. and Rahe, R.H. (1976). The social readjustment rating scale. *J. Psychosom. Res.* **11**, 213.

Howard, J. and Strauss, A. (eds.) (1975). *Humanizing health care.* Wiley, New York.

Hunter, D. (1980). *Coping with uncertainty: policy and politics in the national health service.* Research Studies Press, New York.

Illsley, R. (1980). *Professional or public health?* Nuffield Provincial Hospital Trust, London.

Jaco, E. (1958). Areas for research in medical sociology. *Sociol. Soc. Res.* **42**, 441.

Jarvis, E. (1855). *Insanity and idiocy in Massachusetts: report of the Commission on Lunacy, 1855.* (Reprinted 1971.) Harvard University Press, Cambridge, MA.

Jenkins, C. (1976). Recent evidence supporting psychologic and social risk factors for coronary disease. *N. Engl. J. Med.* **295**, 987; 1033.

Johnson, M. (1975). Medical sociology and sociological theory. *Soc. Sci. Med.* **9**, 227.

Kaplan, R.M., Bush, J.W., and Berry, C.L. (1976). Health status: types of validity and the Index of Well-being. *Health Serv. Res.* **11**(4), 478.

Kasl, S. (1983). Social and psychological factors affecting the course of disease: an epidemiological perspective. In *Handbook of health, health care, and the health professions* (ed. D. Mechanic) p. 683. Free Press, New York.

Kasl, S. and Cobb, S., (1966). Health behavior, illness behavior, and sick role behavior. *Arch. Environ. Health* **12**, 246.

Kasl, S., Gore, S., and Cobb, S. (1975). The experience of losing a job: reported changes in health, symptoms, and illness behavior. *Psychosom. Med.* **37**, 106.

Kellam, S., Simon, M., and Ensminger, M. (1983). Antecedents of teenage drug use and psychological well-being: a ten-year community wide perspective study. In *Origins of psychopathology: research and public health* (ed. D. Ricks and B.S. Dohrenwend) p. 17. Cambridge University Press, New York.

Kendall, P. and Reader, G. (1979). Contributions of sociology to medicine. In *Handbook of medical sociology,* 3rd edn (ed. H. Freeman, S. Levine, and L. Reeder) p. 1. Prentice-Hall, Englewood Cliffs, NJ.

Kessler, R.C. (1979). Stress, social status and psychological distress. *J. Health Soc. Behav.* **20**, 100.

Kessler, R.C. and Cleary, P.D. (1980). Social class and psychological distress. *Am. Sociol. Rev.* **45**, 463.

Kimball, S. (1955). An Alabama town surveys its health needs. In *Health, culture and community* (ed. B. Paul) p. 269. Russell Sage Foundation, New York.

Klein, R. (1979). Control, participation, and the British National Health Service. *Health Soc.* **57**(1), 70.

Knowles, J.H. (ed.) (1977). *Doing better and feeling worse: health in the United States.* Horton, New York.

Kohn, M. (1972). Class, family and schizophrenia: a reformulation. *Soc. Forces* **50**, 295.

Komarovsky, M. (1940). *The unemployed man and his family.* Dryden Press, New York.

Komora, P. and Clark, M. (1935). Mental disease in the crisis. *Ment. Hyg.* **19**, 289.

Kosa, J. and Zola, I. (eds.) (1976). *Poverty and health: a sociological analysis,* 2nd edn. Harvard University Press, Cambridge, MA.

Langner, T.S. and Michael, S.T. (1963). *Life stress and mental health.* Free Press, New York.

Lawrence, P. (1958). Chronic illness and socioeconomic status. In *Patients, physicians and illness* (ed. E. Jaco) p. 37. Free Press, New York.

Leete, R. and Fox, J. (1977). *Registrar General's social classes: origins and uses. Population trends No. 8.* HMSO, London.

Leighton, D.C., Harding, J.S., Macklin, D.B., MacMillan, A.M., and Leighton, A.H. (1963). *The character of danger.* Basic Books, New York.

Lemert, E. (1951). *Social pathology.* McGraw-Hill, New York.

Lerner, M. and Stutz, R.N. (1977). Have we narrowed the gaps between the poor and the nonpoor? Part II. Narrowing the gaps, 1959–61 to 1969–71: mortality. *Med. Care* **15**, 620.

Levin, L., Katz, A., and Holst, E. (1976). *Self-care: lay initiatives in health.* Prodist, New York.

Levine, S., Feldman, J., and Elinson, J. (1983). Does medical care do any good? In *Handbook of health, health care, and the health professions* (ed. D. Mechanic) p. 394. Free Press, New York.

Levine, S., Paul, B., and White, P. (1963). Community interorganizational problems in providing medical care and social services. *Am. J. Public Health* **53**, 1183.

Lewin, K. (1951). *Field theory in social science.* Harper and Row, New York.

Lewis, O. (1959). *Five families: Mexican case studies in the culture of poverty.* Basic Books, New York.

Lewis, O. (1961). *The children of Sanchez.* Random House, New York.

Lewis, O. (1964). *Pedro Martinez.* Random House, New York.

Lewis, O. (1965). *La Vida: a Puerto Rican family in the culture of poverty.* Random House, San Juan and New York.

McClure, W. (1980). *Comprehensive and regulatory strategies for medical care.* InterStudy, Excelsior, Minn.

McIntyre, C. (1894). The importance of the study of medical sociology. *Bull. Am. Acad. Med.* **1**, 425.

MacRae, D. (1979). Concepts and methods of policy analysis. *Society* **16**(6), 17.

Maris, R. and Lazerwitz, B. (1981). *Pathways to suicide.* Johns Hopkins University Press, Baltimore, MD.

Mechanic, D. (1960). The concept of illness behavior. *J. Chronic Dis.* **15**, 189.

Mechanic, D. (1966). The sociology of medicine: viewpoints and perspectives. *J. Health Hum. Behav.* **7**, 237.

Mechanic, D. (1976). Stress, illness and illness behavior. *J. hum. Stress* **2**, 2.

Mechanic, D. (1978). *Medical sociology: a comprehensive text,* 2nd edn. Free Press, New York.

Mechanic, D. (1979). *Future issues in health care: social policy and the rationing of medical services.* Free Press, New York.

Mechanic, D. (1983). The experience and expression of distress: the study of illness behavior and medical obligation. In *Handbook of health, health care and the health professions* (ed. D. Mechanic) p. 591. Free Press, New York.

Mechanic, D. and Levine, S. (eds.) (1977). Issues in promoting health: committee reports of the medical sociology section of the American Sociology Association. *Med. Care* **15** (Suppl.), 1.

Merton, R. (1968). *Social theory and social structure,* enlarged edn. Free Press, New York.

Miliband, R. (1977). *Marxism and politics.* Oxford University Press, New York.

Millman, M. (1977). *The unkindest cut: life in the backrooms of medicine.* Morrow, New York.

Mills, C.W. (1959). *The sociological imagination.* Oxford University Press, New York.

Mishler, E., AmaraSingham, L., Hauser, S., Liem, R., Osherson, S. and Waxler, N. (1981). *Social contexts of health, illness, and patient care*. Cambridge University Press.

Mooney, G. (1977). *The valuation of human life*. Macmillan, Basingstoke.

Morris, J.N. (1979). Social inequalities undiminshed. *Lancet* i, 87.

Morris, J.N., Adam, C. Chave, S.P.W., Sirey, C., Epstein, L., and Sheehan, D.J. (1973). Vigorous exercise in leisure time and the incidence of coronary heart disease. *Lancet* i, 333.

Moser, C.A. and Kalton, G. (1975). *Survey methods in social investigations*, 2nd edn. Heinemann, London.

Mott, B. (1970). Coordination and inter-organizational relations in health. In *Inter-organizational research in health: conference proceedings* (ed. P. White and G. Vlasak). p. 55. National Center for Health Services Research, Washington, DC.

Nagi, S. (1976). An epidemiology of disability among adults in the US. *Health Soc.* 54(4), 439.

National Center for Health Services Research (passim). *Health survey research methods. Reports of biennial conferences*. US Department of Health and Human Services, Hyattsville, MD.

Newhouse, J.P. (1974). A design for a health insurance experiment. *Inquiry* 11, 5.

Newhouse, J.P., Manning, W.G., Morris, C., *et al.* (1982). *Some interim results from a controlled trial of cost sharing in health insurance*. Rand Corporation Report-2847-HHS, Santa Monica, CA.

Office of Population Censuses and Surveys (passim). *Occupational mortality: decennial supplements*. HMSO, London.

Office of Population Censuses and Surveys (1978). *Occupational mortality: decennial supplement 1970–72*. HMSO, London.

Olesen, V. (1975). Convergences and divergences: anthropology and sociology in health care. *Soc. Sci. Med.* 9, 7.

Parson, T. (1951). *The social system*. Free Press, New York.

Parsons, T. (1975). The sick role and the role of the physician reconsidered. *Milbank Mem. Fund Q.* 53, 257.

Patrick, D. (1979). Constructing social metrics for health status indexes. In *Socio-medical health indicators* (ed. J. Elinson and A.E. Siegmann) p. 75. Baywood, New York.

Patrick, D. (1981). Quasi-experimental evaluation of public health interventions (Methodes d'evaluation ne component pas de randomisation). *Rev. Epidemiol. Sante Publique* 29, 245.

Patrick, D. (1982). Evaluation of health care. In *Sociology as applied to medicine*. (ed. D. Patrick and G. Scambler) p. 238. Ballière-Tindall, London.

Patrick, D.L. and Elinson, J. (1979). Methods of sociomedical research. In *Handbook of medical sociology*, 3rd edn (ed. H.E. Freeman, S. Levine, and L.G. Reeder) p. 437. Prentice-Hall, Englewood Cliffs, NJ.

Patrick, D. and Scambler, G. (eds) (1982). *Sociology as applied to medicine*. Ballière-Tindall, London.

Patton, M. (1980). *Qualitative evaluation methods*. Sage, Beverly Hills, CA.

Pflanz, M. (1974). A critique of Anglo-American sociology. *Int. J. Health Serv.* 4, 565.

Pflanz, M. (1975). Relations between social scientists, physicians, and medical organizations in health research. *Soc. Sci. Med.* 9, 7.

Pierce, A. (1967). The economic cycle and the social suicide rate. *Am. Sociol. Rev.* 32, 457.

Rainwater, L. (1968). The lower class: health, illness and medical institutions In *Among the people* (ed. I. Deutscher and E. Thompson) p. 259. Basic Books, New York.

Richardson, B. (1887). *The health of nations: a review of the works of Edwin Chadwick*. Longmans Green, London.

Riecken, H.W. and Boruch, R.F. (eds.) (1974). *Social experimentation: a method for planning and evaluating social intervention*. Academic Press, New York.

Robinson, D. (1971). *The process of becoming ill*. Routledge and Keagan Paul, London.

Robinson, D. (1977). *Self-help and health*. Martin Robertson, London.

Roemer, M. and Elling, R. (1963). Sociological research on medical care. *J. Health Hum. Behav.* 4, 49.

Rossi, P. and Freeman, H. (1982). *Evaluation: a systematic approach*. 2nd edn. Sage, Beverly Hills, CA.

Roth, J. (1963). *Time-tables*. Bobbs-Merrill, Indianapolis, Ind.

Roth, J. (1972). Some contingencies of the moral evaluation and control of clientele: The case of the hospital emergency service. *Am. J. Sociol.* 77, 839.

Rutter, M. and Madge, N. (1976). *Cycles of disadvantage*. Heinemann, London.

Sainsbury, P., Jenkins, J., and Baert, A. (1983). *Suicide trends in Europe: a study of the decline in suicide in England and Wales and the increase elsewhere*. European Office, World Health Organization, Copenhagen.

Scambler, G. and Hopkins, A. (1980). Social class, epileptic activity, and disadvantage at work. *Epidemiol. Community Health* 34, 129.

Scheff, T. (1974). The labeling theory of mental illness. *Am. Sociol. Rev.* 39, 444.

Schuman, H. and Presser, S. (1981). *Questions and answers: experiments on question form, wording and context*. Academic Press, New York.

Schur, E. (1971). *Labeling deviant behavior*. Harper and Rowe, New York.

Schutz, A. (1954). Concept and theory formation in the social sciences. *J. Philosophy* 51, 257.

Schutz, A. (1967). *The phenomenology of the social world* (trans. G. Walsh and F. Lehnert). Northwestern University Press, Evanston, ILL.

Schwartz, H. and Jacobs, J. (1979). *Qualitative sociology*. Free Press, New York.

Shapiro, S. (1983). Epidemiology of ischemic heart disease and cancer. In *Handbook of health, health care and the health professions* (ed. D. Mechanic) p. 120. Free Press, New York.

Shattuck, L. (1948). *Report of the Sanitary Commission of Massachusetts, 1850*. Harvard University Press, Cambridge, MA.

Sheehan, S. (1982). *Is there no place on earth for me?* Houghton-Mifflin, Boston.

Shekelle, R.B., Shyrock, A.M., Paul, O., *et al.* (1981). Diet, serum cholesterol and deaths from coronary heart disease. The Western Electric Study. *N. Engl. J. Med.* 304, 65.

Shortell, S. and Richardson, W. (1978). *Health program evaluation*. Mosby, St. Louis.

Sirken, M. (1981). Network sampling in health surveys. In *Health survey research methods. Third biennial conference* (ed. S. Sudman) p. 136. National Center for Health Services Research, DHSS Pub. No. (PHS) 81-3268, Hyattsville, MD.

Smith, H.W. (1975). *Strategies of social research: the methodological imagination*. Prentice-Hall, New Jersey.

Snow, J. (1855). *On the mode of communication of cholera*, 2nd edn. Churchill, London.

Spence, J., Walton, W., Miller, F., and Court, S. (1954). *A thousand families in Newcastle-Upon-Tyne: an approach to the study of health and illness in children*. Oxford University Press, London.

Srole, L., Langner, T., Michael, S., Opler, M., and Rennie, T. (1962). *Mental health in the metropolis*, Vol. 1. McGraw-Hill, New York.

Straus, R. (1957). The nature and status of medical sociology. *Am. Sociol Rev.* 22, 200.

Strauss, A.L. (1969). Medical organization, medical care and lower income groups. *Soc. Sci. Med.* 3, 143.

Stunkard, S., D'Aquili, E., Fox, S., and Filion, R. (1972).

Influence of social class on obesity and thinness in children. *J. Am. Med. Assoc.* **221**, 578.

Suchmann, E. (1963). *Sociology and the field of public health.* Russell Sage Foundation, New York.

Suchmann, E. (1965a). Stages of illness and medical care. *J. Health Hum. Behav.* **6**, 114.

Suchmann, E. (1965b). Social patterns of illness and medical care. *J. Health Hum. Behav.* **6**, 2.

Suchmann, E. (1967a). Preventive health behavior: a model for research on community health campaigns. *J. Health Hum. Behav.* **8**, 197.

Suchmann, E. (1967b). *Evaluative research.* Russell Sage, New York.

Sudman, S. and Bradburn, N. (1982). *Asking questions: a practical guide to questionnaire design.* Jossey-Bass, San Francisco.

Sudman, S. and Lannom, L. (1980). *Health care surveys using diaries.* DHHS Publication No. (PHS) 80-3279. National Center for Health Services Research, Hyattsville, MD.

Sudnow, D. (1969). *Passing on: the social organization of dying.* Prentice-Hall, New Jersey.

Susser, M. (1974a). Introduction to the theme: a critical review of sociology in health. *Int. J. Health Serv.* **4**, 407.

Susser, M. (1974b). A critical review of sociology in health. *Int. J. Health Serv.* **4**, 403.

Susser, M. and Watson, W. (1971). *Sociology in medicine,* 2nd edn. Oxford University Press, London.

Susser, M., Hopper, K., and Richman, J. (1983). Society, culture and health. In *Handbook of health, health care and the professions* (ed. D. Mechanic) p. 23. Free Press, New York.

Torrance, G. (1976). Social preferences for health states. An empirical evaluation of three measurement techniques. *Socio-Economic Plan. Sci.* **10**, 129.

Townsend, P. (1979). *Poverty in the United Kingdom.* Penguin Books, Harmondsworth.

Townsend, P. and Davidson, N. (eds.) (1982). *Inequalities in health: The Black Report.* Penguin, Harmondsworth.

Tuckett, D. (ed.) (1976). *Introduction to medical sociology.* Tavistock, London.

Verbrugge, L.M. (1980). Health diaries. *Med. Care* **18** (1), 73.

Wadsworth, M. and Robinson, D. (1976). *Studies in everyday medical life.* Martin Robertson, London.

Wagner, E., Beery, W., Schoenbach, V., and Graham, R. (1982). An assessment of health hazard/health risk appraisal. *Am. J. Public Health* **72**, 347.

Waitzkin, H. (1981). The social origins of illness: a neglected history. *Int. J. Health Sci.* **11**, 77.

Webb, E., Campbell, D., Schwartz, R., and Sechrest, L. (1966). *Unobtrusive measures: nonreactive research in the social sciences.* Rand McNally, Chicago.

Weber, M. (1947). *The theory of social and economic organization* (trans. A.M. Henderson and T. Parsons). Oxford University Press, New York.

West, P. (1976). The physician and the management of childhood epilepsy. In *Studies in everyday medical life* (ed. M. Wadsworth and C.D. Robinson). Martin Robertson, London.

Wheaton, B. (1978). The sociogenesis of psychological disorder: reexamining the causal issues with longitudinal data. *Am. Sociol Rev.* **43**, 383.

White, P., Levin, L., and Levine, S. (1979). Community health organizations and resources. In *Handbook of medical sociology* (ed. H. Freeman, S. Levine, and L. Reeder) p. 347. Prentice-Hall, Englewood Cliffs, NJ.

Williamson, D. and Danaher, K. (1978). *Self-care in health.* Croom Helm, London.

Wilson, E. (1940). *To the Finland station.* Harcourt Brace Jovanovich, New York.

Wilson, R.N. (1970). *The sociology of health: an introduction.* Random House, New York.

Wilson, R.W. and White, E.L. (1977). Changes in morbidity, disability and utilization differentials between the poor and nonpoor: Data from the Health Interview Survey: 1964 and 1973. *Med. Care* **15**, 636.

Wolinsky, F. (1976). Health services utilization and attitudes toward health maintenance organizations: a theoretical and methodological discussion. *J. Health Soc. Behav.* **17**, 221.

Wolinsky, F. (1978). Assessing the effects of predisposing, enabling, and illness-morbidity characteristics on health service utilization. *J. Health Soc. Behav.* **19**, 384.

Wolinsky, F. (1980). *The sociology of health: principles, professions and issues.* Little Brown, Boston.

Zborowski, M. (1952). Cultural components in responses to pain. *J. Soc. Issues* **8**, 16.

Zechhauser, R. and Stokey, E. (1978). *Methods: a primer for policy analysis.* Norton, Boston.

# 12 Education and communication studies

John W. Farquhar, Nathan Maccoby, and Peter D. Wood

## INTRODUCTION

Much of the premature death and disability experienced throughout the world has a social and behavioural basis. These problems therefore require applications of social science theory, data, and methods to achieve change on a scale sufficient to affect the public's health. Our research group at Stanford has been investigating such applications within communities directed toward cardiovascular disease for many years. Examples discussed here are drawn largely from this experience. This chapter describes methods of education and communication that can help to achieve changes in attitude, knowledge, and behaviour. This will allow assessment of potential causal links between social, environmental, or behavioural factors, and the dependent variables of disease outcomes, such as stroke or heart attack, or the physiological states, such as elevated blood pressure, that underlie these disease states. A comparison of these methods will be made with those employed in analogous studies throughout the world. The considerable gap in our knowledge and experience in these methods will be described and the research needed to close some of these gaps will be suggested.

A broad definition of education and communication will be used, encompassing the recruiting, persuading, and organizing needed to achieve lasting change within the complex system that a community or region represents. Although the methods are directly applicable to planned experiments, in principle they would apply to non-experimental disease control interventions directed toward various social, political, or geographical units. These units could be smaller than or larger than the moderate-sized communities that have been the site of the Stanford studies. The methods, although derived from experience in the field of cardiovascular disease, will certainly be applicable to other public health issues.

## THEORETICAL FOUNDATIONS

Success in community-based studies, which are inherently complex, is more likely if the investigators seek theoretical guidelines. Many theories of learning, are available (McGuire 1981) and a variety of theoretical bases for community change also exist (Rogers 1983). Given the need to reach individuals and to collaborate with (and change) community institutions, the community study requires insights from both sources. We therefore present here a theoretical framework to assist the designer of community-based communication and education studies. The Stanford group has termed the practical application of theoretical foundations for community organizational change as 'community organization for health'. We term our derivative of theoretical foundations for how to reach and how to teach individuals as 'health communication – behaviour change'. In the sections that follow we will make it clear that the investigator must link these two derivatives of theory to forge their successful application in community studies. Such hybrids, especially those providing recently developed and effective behaviour change methods, are rather rare in the research literature. Therefore, past theoretical formulations should be seen only as imperfect blueprints for the investigator, who must be ultimately guided by the incomplete evidence currently available and by the apparent rationale for methods such as we present here.

### Community organization for health

We have relied most heavily on diffusion theory (Rogers and Kincaid 1981; Rogers 1983) and the community self-development field (Kahn 1969; Litwak and Rothman 1970; Spergel 1977; Warren 1978; Rothman 1979; Green *et al.* 1980) as guides. These literatures are too extensive to review completely but each contains some major principles most germaine to the novel but needed research on the application of community organization to public health described in this chapter.

The central theme of diffusion theory applicable to community organization for health is that communication leading to persuasion and learning flows through natural social networks and that opinion leaders within the system are needed as collaborating allies to achieve adequate adoption of the health innovations being advocated. The central theme of the community self-development field is that community residents and organizations must collaborate with the agencies advocating change in order to achieve successful maintenance of change.

Some practical generalizations flow from these themes. For example, data from diffusion research (Rogers 1983) would lead us to choose change agents (the health professionals that represent the investigators' programme) who are perceived by community residents as having credibility for the safety and the prudence of the changes being advocated. This important goal may be achieved by employing and training one or more existing community health professionals as key initiators of change. A new change-agent acquires the research agency's novel health technology but retains a prior trust as a member of that community. This trust must exist for a change agent among the community's opinion leaders in order to achieve the diffusion and adoption goals implied in diffusion theory's central theme. The rejection of water boiling in a Peruvian village, described by Rogers (1983), is an example of a failure due to lack of attention to this principle. In this now classic example, a village extension worker failed to win support of key village opinion leaders whose influence led to rejection of the innovation (Rogers 1983).

Another lesson from diffusion research is that the generation of interpersonal communication should be an explicit goal of much of one's educational programme. As examples one can cite use of schoolchildren to bring notices of health education events to their families, such as scheduled television programmes. Or one can add an admonition to 'tell a smoker friend' to a newspaper advertisement about a new smoking cessation learning opportunity.

A practical generalization that is derived from the community self-development literature is that territorial conflict among various health organizations can inhibit collaborative adoption of novel health programmes of the delivery agency (the experimenters). An example of a solution is that the external agency, through recognition of the organizations' power structures and linkages, helps to create a consortium of leaders from each health agency such that new and valued resources entering the system are allocated by consensus. Another generalization from community self-development is that incentives should be provided to community organizations to enhance the likelihood of collaboration. Among many possible examples are provision of training, materials, funds, or status to key individuals within such organizations.

### Health communication – behaviour change

Despite the wide variety of seemingly polarized and inconsistent views of human nature (McGuire, in press), the past few decades of new research in the field of attitude and behaviour change have given the social science experimenter a guide to reasonably effective methods of achieving cost-effective change in knowledge, attitude, and behaviour (Paisley 1981).

The health communication – behaviour change formulation offers a perspective on how individuals and groups change knowledge, attitudes, and behaviour. Our picture of this process draws heavily on the prior work of others: the excellent unified theory of human behaviour provided by Bandura's expanded social learning theory (Bandura 1977, 1978); the hierarchy of learning model of Ray and colleagues (1973); the extensively documented communication-persuasion model of McGuire (1969, in press) and the attitude change model of Ajzen and Fishbein (1980). The health communication – behaviour change formulation presented here emphasizes the features that are relevant to community-based education and health communication. There are several underlying assumptions implicit in these portrayals of the change process:

(a) A need and the potential for change exist.
(b) Initial and final states are measurable.
(c) Educating forces have adequate social legitimacy.
(d) Adequate time exists within the design for the change to occur.

Health education programmes often will encompass multiple objectives in a population whose members vary greatly in their awareness, knowledge, and behaviours relative to each objective. Education programme planning therefore requires dividing the audience into smaller units that share relevant characteristics. Rational education decisions (message content, choice of media channel) can then be made and educational activities presented in a logical sequence. Messages can be designed to address the needs of various parts of the total audience at various stages in a matrix, by topic area. When used in this way, the health communication – behaviour change formulation is a helpful organizing scheme for audience segmentation, message design, and sequencing of instructional events.

This approach proposes a series of steps that people go through as they gradually adopt the advocated attitudes and/or behaviour. These are described below, but note that the concept of behaviour change as an orderly sequence of steps is admittedly an idealized version of real life. The sequence of steps may vary, or one or two steps will be much more important than others. Also, one message may perform more than one function. This approach, in its linear portrayal, deviates from the one in which reciprocal sharing between elements in communication systems occurs as described in the community organization section and, as such, it is incomplete. However, it does help us to develop a clearer picture of how to devise a course of action. As we proceed in a research study, we can also use it as an evaluation framework to observe the shift of population groups over time in the direction of the intended project goals.

Table 12.1 outlines the essential components of the health communication – behaviour change formulation. The steps or behaviour change objectives are listed in the right-hand column. The middle column lists the corresponding communication function required to meet those objectives. The

**Table 12.1.** *The health communication – behaviour change formulation*

| Communication inputs | Communication functions (for the sender) | Behaviour objectives (for the receiver) |
|---|---|---|
| Messages Media Community Events | 1. Determine receiver's needs | 1. Become aware |
| | 2. Gain attention (set the agenda) | 2. Increase knowledge |
| | 3. Provide information | 3. Increase motivation and interest |
| | 4. Provide incentives | 4. Learn and practise skills |
| | 5. Provide training | 5. Take action, assess outcomes |
| | 6. Provide cues to action | 6. Maintain action, practise self-management skills |
| | 7. Provide support, self-management | 7. Become an opinion leader (exert peer group influence) |
| | | 8. Give feedback to sender |

column on the left notes that instructional products and events must be designed, produced, and distributed, in sequence, to perform the functions listed.

*Determination of receiver's needs.* The experimenter (the sender) must determine the interests and knowledge and skill needs of the audience before a health communication programme can begin.

*Agenda-setting.* The agenda-setting function is to gain the public's attention and focus it on certain specific issues and problems. The existence of the problem must be established in the public's mind, and an awareness must be created of potential solutions being promoted. Generally, in developed societies the mass media play an important agenda-setting role. As political scientist Bernard Cohen (1963) puts it:

The press may not be successful in telling people what to think, but it is stunningly successful in telling its readers what to think about.

When attention is brought to the issue either by mass media or through interpersonal means, and people begin thinking about it, then the first step in the behaviour change process is underway.

*Information.* Once a particular topic or subject matter is on the public agenda, an educational programme must present information, in layman's terms, that makes the issue interesting and understandable. Messages need to be designed that make the issue personally meaningful and that set the stage for action. The messages must be retained in a way that predisposes the person to act in a different way in the future.

*Incentives.* Change is more likely when individuals perceive clearly the personal and social benefits of change, which can be enhanced by appropriate communications.

*Skills.* Where changes in complex habits of long standing are involved, it may be necessary to provide skills training in how to start making changes, both by providing modelling, and step-by-step instruction, and by promoting the availability of guided practice, self-help, and professional resources (Bandura 1977).

*Action.* Ideally, this phase of an overall strategy would provide educational messages that act as cues to trigger specific actions. Messages would indicate clear action paths to stimulate the trial adoption of new behaviours (Cartwright 1949).

*Maintenance.* At this stage, teaching is required to provide a sense of social support and approval, and as a reminder of both the short-term and long-term personal and social benefits of the changes undertaken. Both gaining self-efficacy (Bandura 1978) and learning self-management methods (Farquhar 1978) are important aspects of the maintenance phase. Some recent work suggests that this type of maintenance training is better begun early in the learning process. For example, Killen *et al.* (in press) found that early training in relapse prevention helps forestall relapses in smoking cessation. Specific training in counter-arguing skills has been found to aid the achievement of stable change (Roberts and Maccoby 1974; Telch *et al.* 1982).

In health education programmes with multiple objectives, everything cannot be done at once, for everyone. Planners need to have a rational basis for making selections from among competing choices and for sequencing actions over

time. The health communication – behaviour change framework can be a general guide. It suggests how to break the large community health education task down into manageable pieces, and helps to pinpoint where to start, and with what messages.

*Applications.* Table 12.2 shows the behavioural objectives of a cardiovascular disease prevention programme on the top, and the steps in the individual's desired behaviour change process down the left side.

**Table 12.2.** *Framework of education*

| Behavioural steps | Smoking control | Diet | Weight | Exercise | Stress control | Blood pressure |
|---|---|---|---|---|---|---|
| Awareness | | | | | | |
| Knowledge | | | | | | |
| Motivation | | | | | | |
| Skills | | | | | | |
| Action | | | | | | |
| Maintenance | | | | | | |

This table shows an example of planning organized around specific objectives. In this case, the objectives are changes in risk factor status (smoking, weight, etc.). This divides the general audience into risk-factor categories. Communication needs are assessed by noting how the population is distributed along the behaviour change states within each risk-factor area. Additional sub-divisions would be needed along other dimensions (for example, English or Spanish-speaking, male or female).

An example from one of Stanford's community-based projects serves to show how this table helps in distinguishing between needed behavioural processes when designing an education programme. First, formative questionnaire data revealed widespread lack of awareness of the distinction between low-level and aerobic exercise. Messages conveying this information were therefore created and used. Second, data revealed a widespread belief that beneficial exercise was often painful and associated with muscle building. Messages counteracting this belief were therefore created and distributed. Lastly, data revealed considerable readiness to start exercise but showed a strong desire for geographical convenience and social support. Accordingly, a neighbourhood exercise programme and its associated media support were created. Thus, this project demonstrates how some of the different behavioural stages listed in Table 12.2 are selected for emphasis in planning a project, dependent upon the outcomes of baseline data and upon the theoretical formulations underlying health communication and behaviour change.

### A hybrid of organizational and educational principles

The novel and highly important aspect of our recommended research strategy is that the need for provision of curricula, training of instructors, and provision of skills training for the general public loom large as a dimension not covered by the theory and practice of the social reform literature and the diffusion/adoption literature cited. Thus we propose a new terminology within a framework that identifies the temporal sequence of events. In this terminology organizing, as a process, leads to development of local forces and to educational programmes as products. The development, since it entails change within community agencies, is termed 'endogenous'. The organizing, originating from an agency seeking change, is termed 'exogenous'. Education products are either collaborative, endogenous, or exogenous, depending on their origin. Figure 12.1 displays this conceptual blend of organizational process and educational products that we consider.

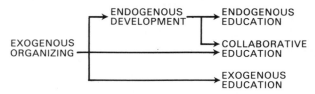

**Fig. 12.1.** Sequence and products of community organizing in comprehensive community health education.

An example of exogenous organizing leading to endogenous development, which in turn leads to collaborative education, is the joint establishment with a local health department of smoking classes in a community. The external experimenters help with training, curriculum development, evaluation, and curriculum revision, but the classes are staffed and clients are recruited by the local agency. An example of exogenous organizing leading to exogenous education would be found in a programme of supplying health columns to newspapers. Exogenous organizing is needed to recruit the newspapers and to remain sensitive to their wishes regarding frequency of columns, but the responsibility is almost entirely the experimenter's for continuation.

The temporal sequence for the activities and products is generally one in which an initial surge of activity by the originating agency is replaced over time by increasing collaboration and is finally replaced by new educational activities that originate within newly transformed community institutions. These relationships are depicted in Fig. 12.2. The research stages in which exogenous, collaborative, and lastly endogenous education predominate are termed *initiation, collaboration,* and *transformation,* respectively. The duration of each stage will vary greatly with circumstances of the topic,

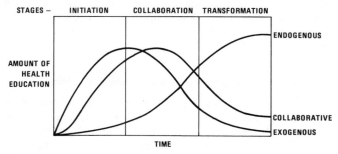

**Fig. 12.2.** Research stages in community studies.

locale, and resources. For many experimental conditions we would predict that from two to five years will be needed for each stage. Research design and evaluation challenges will vary considerably as a function of research stage.

## METHODS FOR ACHIEVING CHANGE IN COMMUNITY-BASED STUDIES

This section lists the operational steps needed to design and carry out community-based health education studies. Evaluation methods and design issues are described elsewhere (Farquhar 1978; Williams *et al.* 1981) and will not be covered here save for a description of formative evaluation, a method needed for successful development of educational methods and products. These steps are derived from our 13 years of experience in carrying out one completed study, the Stanford Three Community Study (Farquhar *et al.* 1977; Maccoby *et al.* 1977) and in the design and implementation of an ongoing eight-year study, the Stanford Five City Project (Farquhar 1978; Maccoby and Solomon 1981; Farquhar *et al.* 1983). Although the methods will be derived from studies on cardiovascular disease prevention, they are relevant to any study in which life-style change within a sizeable proportion of the population is the goal.

The methods will be described in the sequence in which such activities usually occur, including information on activities before and following the receipt of funding by the research group. The model being described is that of a field demonstration project with a strong evaluation component, the 'experimental paradigm' of Flay and Cook (1981). In such a project, a considerable proportion – usually in excess of 50 per cent – of the total costs are assigned to measurement and evaluation.

### Planning

*Initial planning phase (prior to financial support)*

The project begins as an idea held by one or more members of the research team. This idea can grow to involve a nucleus of potential principal investigators. This *Planning Group* or *Steering Committee* must meet for at least six months and is responsible for the following sequence of tasks:

1. Clarification of overall research goals, including scientific rationale, ethical acceptability, and assessment of community need and interest. The group must identify the many disciplines in medicine and the social sciences needed to carry out such work, and they must decide if their institution has the ability and interest needed to enter this challenging field. The group must obtain early co-operation with the community or other experimental group or locale and accept that this partnership will limit the freedom for unilateral action ordinarily treasured by research scientists. With diligence, this group could proceed within six months through the stage of proposal preparation and submission to a supporting agency. The proposal must contain assurance of community support, which necessitates tentative community selection and the first stages of recruitment of key community opinion leaders and gatekeepers (Rogers 1983). The ideal sequence is that funds

for a year-long planning period be obtained that would allow a final research project proposal to be prepared with greater assurance.

2. Research project proposal writing and submission.

3. Maintaining contact with recruited community leaders. Expect an awkward interim period while community opinion leaders may begin to wonder if they have been forgotten. The recruiting process itself may in fact trigger certain community groups to launch programmes of the type planned. This can occur in either treatment or control communities, of course.

4. Research project proposal evaluation: convincing the proposal's evaluation group that the study is worthwhile.

### Final project planning (following award of funding)

The Planning or Steering Committee is advised to form a larger group of investigators for a minimum of four to six months of final planning before formal field operations begin. Two steps are needed here.

The first step is to complete the community recruiting phase. Within control communities this step is one solely of re-affirmation of intent to obtain archival information or survey data. It is advisable to label the control communities as reference communities to avoid unnecessary provocation of feelings of deprivation. The programme of surveying and measurement of risk-factor status should be identified as a screening service that will uncover some heretofore unrecognized risk for the individuals within the sample surveyed. The opinion leaders of the reference communities should of course be informed of the forthcoming contribution to science. Since the research institution cannot provide supplementary educational services to the entire world, the reference communities can readily accede to the logistical arguments and be willing to accept the screening activities and epidemiological data as benefits that warrant their co-operation.

Within treatment communities the recruitment tasks are more complex. The first task is to identify through opinion leader surveys (Rogers 1983) an individual community resident who has opinion leader status and the skills of a community organizer and health educator. This individual, the 'change agent' identified in the theory section, should be hired at an early stage in order to create a foundation for the true community/research agency partnership. This change agent or community co-ordinator should be part of this next stage in which the level of interest and degree of co-operation of local health agencies, schools, and media outlets will be determined. The co-ordinator is now starting the endogenous development stage of the community organization process described in the theoretical section.

The second step is the establishment of expert groups to complete pre-field planning. These planning tasks are as follows:

1. A survey design and data management group must refine the statistical power calculations, define the survey and evaluation instruments, and hire and train survey and evaluation staff. This process will take 6–12 months depending on the complexity of the survey.

2. An education group should establish task forces for identifiable parts of the education programme to produce a set of planning guides that specify the broad education goals

on the basis of current knowledge in various fields. In a cardiovascular disease prevention study, these task forces would include smoking, weight control, nutrition, hypertension, stress, youth education, and community organization.

3. The final planning stage begins by setting specific goals and objectives. For a comprehensive cardiovascular disease control project, this means setting goals for changes in each of the risk factors (for example, a 7 per cent decline in systolic blood pressure) and then creating a list of objectives that can be expected to achieve the goals (such as, reduce salt intake by 50 per cent). The researcher should list health behaviour objectives that could reasonably be expected to achieve the goals. These objectives should include knowledge, attitude, and behaviour changes desired. These risk-factor goals and objectives now constitute the planning guides for the project.

4. The Steering Committee assembles the planning guides to determine if any additional pre-field studies are needed.

5. The pre-field studies are assigned to either the survey/measurements group or to the education group. The two most likely pre-field activities will be testing survey instruments and educational methods. The former are usually readily completed within a few months as a needed predecessor of the surveys. The latter often require many months for completion and can begin on the expectation that a field education process of some years' duration can accept results from pre-field studies even if they post-date the beginning of field operations. Also, at least one baseline survey must be completed before the education programme begins, allowing additional time for these studies.

Following the planning stage, and as pre-field studies begin to reach completion, the education programme will come to consist of a number of (interrelated) projects. Each project needs to have a list of distinct objectives of its own. This enables the programme directors to compare projects and set priorities. Each project and the overall objectives are periodically re-evaluated to ensure adequate progress. For example, one objective might be to make people aware that exercise is good for the heart as a way to motivate them to begin exercising. A baseline population survey might, however, reveal that this attitude is common, but that even people with this attitude still do not begin to exercise. This would require a change in the objective and the content of the education programme. Thus planning becomes a data-based management system with continuous feedback from formative evaluation. This evaluation-planning process is best conducted as a six-month time scale. Thus long-term plans for each year are converted into an overall six-month timeline. Each education group professional should translate the master timeline into a personal six-month one, allowing the researchers to evaluate the practicality of each six-month plan. Priorities can then be established and re-evaluated every six months. The general method we recommend for ongoing planning is that separate weekly meetings should be held by staff involved in education/organization and survey/evaluation. A small executive committee should oversee both meetings and should meet separately, including heads of the two major divisions, to formulate policy and allocate resources.

## Formative evaluation methods

Formative, as distinct from summative, evaluation provides data for designing educational programmes and materials to meet specific objectives and for monitoring the progress of the educational programme. A general criticism in the literature of health communication campaigns (Atkin 1979) is that they usually lack formative evaluation. Therefore the materials and programmes produced are often not able to meet the campaign objectives.

There are at least seven specific topics where formative evaluation assists the design, development, production, and distribution of the education programme. Each topic is briefly described below.

1. *Audience needs analysis.* Understanding of the audience's attitudes, beliefs, self-efficacy ratings, and knowledge is invaluable in developing effective programmes and mass communication media.

2. *Audience segmentation.* This research is aimed at identifying sub-sections of the community with factors in common such as needs, risk, demographic characteristics, and media use. This allows programmes and materials to be developed which are best for each sub-audience. For example, teenage smoking cessation programmes must differ greatly from those for adult men or pregnant women.

3. *Programme design.* Here one gathers information needed to design programmes, such as weight control classes or neighbourhood exercise groups, to best fit the needs of any sub-group. This research typically addresses questions such as the proper name, location, and time for the programme, and appropriate educational methods and materials.

4. *Programme testing.* This research tests an early version of a programme with relevant audiences such as existing community groups. Such testing helps determine both whether and why a programme was a success or a failure, and predicts future effectiveness.

5. *Message design and pre-testing.* Formative research for message design and pre-testing is conducted to improve the effectiveness of mass media messages. Researchers begin with objectives for a particular message and attempt to answer questions raised in the communication research literature dealing with source, message, channel, and receiver factors (for example: McGuire 1969, in press; Schramm 1972; Zimbardo *et al.* 1977). These would typically involve questions about the content and method of delivery of the message. Prototypes of a message are next developed and pretested by a variety of methods ranging from focus group discussions (that is, small group discussions focused on a predetermined set of critical issues which are led by trained leaders) to paper and pencil tests of target audience samples. The pre-test data are used to revise the message prior to its use.

6. *Community event analysis.* Community events include such things as health fairs, classes, and lectures. One should ask which factors motivated participants to attend, how did they learn about the event, what did they think about it, how will this experience influence their future participation, and how did the event influence their desire and skills to change their behaviour? The methods used to evaluate community events include questionnaires, face-to-face interviews, focus group discussions, and follow-up telephone surveys as well as unobtrusive measures.

7. *Media event analysis.* A similar follow-up as for community events should be conducted for each major media event, such as a televised 'how to stop smoking' programme. This has much to teach the experimenter on how to best reach, motivate, and teach individuals to change.

## Pre-field studies

The need for pre-tests of survey instruments and for development of education methods was stated above. In this section we describe examples from Stanford's community studies of educational method development to demonstrate the utility of such studies in translation of behavioural science theory into action.

The first example is derived from the Stanford Three-Community Study, which was in the field from 1972 through to 1975. The design of this study required a comparison of the efficacy of face-to-face instruction under an umbrella of mass media (print, television, and radio) with that of mass media alone in achieving change in knowledge, attitude, and behaviour. Our prior assumption was that the advantages inherent in face-to-face instruction would achieve considerably greater change than the inherently cheaper mass media alone, thus giving us a standard for a comparison of considerable health relevance. In order to apply the face-to-face methods in the community setting to be used in 1972, we first tested the methods in a worksite setting near Stanford University. The methods, termed *intensive instruction,* were patterned after Bandura's social learning theory (1977) and furnished specific information to each individual on his or her risk status and provided extensive modelling, guided practice in new behaviours, and group and spouse support. The pretest was successful in achieving change (Meyer and Henderson 1972). It succeeded not only in training our instructors and giving us protocols and manuals, but also showed us that Bandura's methods could be applied to cardiovascular disease in a setting reasonably close to the one we would experience in our field experiment. The linkage of the laboratory to field is of course a major goal of community studies, and the pre-field study is sometimes a necesary intermediate stage. One principle demonstrated by this study is that a pre-field test of methods is needed if they have not been adequately developed. A research group can develop its own index of confidence largely by determining the stage that research and development has reached on the topic in question. A safe generalization is that the field trial in public health has not had an adequate use, leading to public policy devisions or adoption of attempts at producing innovations without field trials (Farquhar 1978). Therefore, the courage to do more field trials is more needed than is concern over whether trial methods are sufficiently advanced to warrant their use.

The second example is derived from Stanford's current, larger, and more ambitious community study, the Five City Project (Farquhar 1978, in press; Maccoby and Solomon 1981; (Farquhar *et al.* 1983). In this study, as part of a broad community-wide education programme, we planned to create an ambitious school-wide curricular change to promote adoption of healthy habits regarding smoking, nutrition, and exercise. An inadequate number of established methods applicable to young people were found. Accordingly, a programme for smoking prevention aimed at seventh grade students was successfully developed in a school near Stanford University (McAlister *et al.* 1979; Telch *et al.* 1982). This study contributed a body of methods directly relevant to the community study and again successfully demonstrated the transferability of basic behavioural science research, in this case in methods of counter-argument (Roberts and Maccoby 1974), into field studies. This study introduced an additional but perhaps critical technological wrinkle. Students were taught to invent counter-arguments and to use them when they were needed. Thus, the study further demonstrated that specific behavioural science technology may be an important ingredient in success.

A major principle of pre-field studies is their utility in sharpening the researcher's skills, thereby enhancing the probability of success. Once the field operations begin, formative research continues to perform this function. However, researchers are advised to continue their own laboratory development and to borrow from experiences of other investigators. The natural human tendency toward insularity and excessive pride is an important potential barrier to success. The admonition is therefore to adopt, adapt, and advance; an admonition applicable both to the researcher and to the community residents.

## Field studies

It is indeed a difficult challenge to carry out a successful experiment on the effects of an integrated multifaceted education and communication project in a community or set of communities. It is difficult to achieve either an adequate evaluation component in both reference and treatment communities or an adequate amount of education and organization. Guidance on methods and a judgement of what kind and what amount of education and organization will suffice is therefore important.

To achieve the goals set during the pre-field planning phase, the investigators must continue the previously described planning process and must develop an adaptive response to early results. Continuation of formative research insures the plan will change in accord with results of early effort and unforeseen developments.

### How much education and organization is needed?

An over-riding question is how the education/organization group can decide when an adequate amount of education or organization has been provided to give assurance that the goals of the study will be achieved. Considerable uncertainty should be anticipated given the complexity and uncertainties of community studies. However, the experimenters are advised to address this question in their planning and they must create a reasonable model from their past experience, from pre-field studies, and from their evaluation of work done by other investigators.

An example of a dose-response relationship can be derived from the two-year results of education delivered in the Stanford Three-Community Study (Farquhar *et al.* 1977;

Maccoby *et al.* 1977). The design of the study was that two communities were the recipients of various printed and radio and television-based health education. This media education was the product of close collaboration with local media groups. In one community a small sample of high-risk individuals received supplementary face-to-face instruction in a setting in which an analogue of community organization was provided. Two major pieces of printed material, booklets of about 50 pages each, were distributed to the cohorts of adults aged 35–59 years who were the subjects of repeated surveys. These booklets were a general cardiovascular disease risk factor booklet *The Heart of the Matter*, and a very well received loose-leaf recipe book, the *Cook's Book*. Generally distributed printed material included a weekly newspaper *Doctor's column* and a weekly *Dietitian's column*, bus cards that appeared over a three-month period, and one billboard in each of the two treatment towns that was present for about six months. Electronic media included 50 different television spots (public service announcements) which appeared repeatedly at a rate of about 20 per week, three hours of television programming time, and 100 radio spots and several hours of radio programme time. A sub-set of the surveyed cohort who were at high risk for cardiovascular disease were given a three-month programme of about 25 hours of face-to-face instruction with special attention to skills training and generation of social support.

The results of the education programme over a two-year period demonstrated a surprisingly large decrease in a composite risk score for cardiovascular disease. This was of about 25 per cent for those exposed to only the mass-media campaign and about 30 per cent for those who also received intensive instruction. The risk reduction in the community provided with mass media education was comprised almost equally of contributions from blood pressure reduction, blood cholesterol reduction and decreased cigarette use. Among the individuals who received additional intensive instruction, a larger proportion of change was due to decreased cigarette use. Changes were reasonably well maintained during a third year of decreased education, especially for the intensively instructed group (Meyer *et al.* 1980; Williams *et al.* 1981).

Therefore, it appears that the amount of education provided, as described, was sufficient to produce impressively large decreases in predicted future risk of cardiovascular disease in a free-living adult population. The change when relying only on media education was especially surprising, given the generally poor results of prior media-based health campaigns (Griffiths and Knutson 1960; Robertson *et al.* 1974). Although no fixed standard of comparison is available, due to a combination of the difficulty in quantifying the amount of education and a general lack of well-evaluated health education studies, it does appear that in areas of generally high public interest a reasonably small amount of well designed printed, television and radio-based health education combined with a small amount of community organization and personal influence can produce substantial changes in knowledge, behaviour, and physiological states that confer risk (Farquhar *et al.* 1977; Maccoby *et al.* 1977). Confidence in the generalizability of this conclusion is weakened by the obvious question of whether this particular set of media was unusually effective, or whether the population was unusually susceptible. Another, and more plausible, explanation for enhanced effect that requires consideration as a factor that was causally related to the changes observed is the role of inter-personal influence exerted by repeated surveying, although the reference community's surveyed sample was also so exposed.

Nevertheless, an interaction between a small amount of sensitization produced by the experience of an hour of contact with a survey centre environment and the subsequent exposure to mass media could be important. We explored this factor in the Three Community Study by inclusion of a small after-only sample at the end of one year of surveying. From this analysis we estimated the benefits of sensitization to be in the order of a 33 per cent improvement in results, assuming the trend would continue beyond one year of educational exposure. Thus a media-only package of the sort we described without survey contact might achieve a two year decrease in risk of perhaps 18 per cent. For research purposes one might be satisfied with changes that are much less than this but which would yet be statistically significant. In this Stanford Study, however, the overall change was at least double that considered adequate to show a change in cardiovascular events within six years (Farquhar 1978). It would thus appear that an adequate total effect was created by the education provided. The estimation of relative efficacy of print versus electronic media, for example, or of other parts of the fine structure of multi-media education, is even more difficult and inexact than estimating effects of an entire programme. Attempts to relate effects to specific educational programmes must involve an assessment of the role of diffusion and of the resultant secondary gain in effect within a communicating system.

As indicated in our remarks on community organization theory, we assume that diffusion of effect from the initial primary exogenous education will result in the creation of secondary change agents and opinion leaders within the system. Indeed, we suggest that the cost-savings that ensue from reaching the stage of community transformation represent the ultimate utility of a community setting in contrast to a medical model applied to a high-risk minority of the population. The Three-Community Study offers evidence for this diffusion effect, as studied by network analysis (Meyer *et al.* 1977). Although up to half of the short-term effect of exogenous education in a community may be due to secondary factors, we are much more persuaded that long-term continuation is dependent upon the change in social norms that occurs when social support for an innovation becomes widespread. A community setting provides this opportunity for social support generation in a manner difficult to achieve in other settings, even in worksites or in the family, where some social support opportunities exist.

In summary, a modest amount of mediated education supplied to a population exposed to a rather small amount of personal contact will diffuse its effects into this population and be well maintained. If reasonably large amounts of face-to-face personal attention (nine or ten lessons during three months) is added, this effect should be enhanced. The probably optimum effect will come from a judicious com-

bination of community organization to supply an impetus to diffusion and adoption, combined with adaptive exogenous education. Considerable research will be needed to clarify the optimum mix of effort. Clearly one can anticipate differences related to the social change being sought and to the country and population in which the experiment is carried out. Nevertheless, considerable confidence can be generated in the research capabilities for education and communication programmes applied at the community level.

### Process evaluation

Evaluation usually is either summative or formative. Formative evaluation has been discussed above. Summative evaluation is the measure of outcomes – the impact of the total programme. We previously described many of the evaluative procedures used in the Three Community Study, including both standard statistical methods (Farquhar *et al.* 1977; Maccoby *et al.* 1977; Meyer *et al.* 1980) and ancillary evaluation measures which strengthened the internal validity of the study (Farquhar 1978; Williams *et al.* 1981). Most of these methods deal only with the first main question in evaluation: 'Did the programme work?'. Clearly, a highly important question for the policy maker and a principal challenge to community research of a quasi-experimental nature is to increase the sensitivity and breadth of the evaluation instruments used in answering this question.

Therefore, a second question – 'Why did it work or fail?' – is also important and is most often ignored in risk reduction evaluations. This kind of evaluation is often called process evaluation and it may include both qualitative studies such as case studies and ethnography as well as quantitative methods (Reichardt and Cook 1979). If process evaluation is omitted, the benefits from the programme are lessened since it loses its value as a model for the design of future studies. Because of this concern, it is essential to identify a number of steps in the process of change and measure each of these steps. For example, while the ultimate outcome variable may be change in morbidity and mortality due to heart disease and stroke, it is also important to measure intermediate stages such as success in community organization, knowledge, attitude change, skills learning, and performance and maintenance of these skills. One needs to know who changed and in response to what influences. It is also important to evaluate the success of achieving stable and meaningful change in community practices and institutions as a measure of success in leaving behind a programme that runs partly or totally on its own energies. While one cannot guarantee a totally clear explanation of success or failure, there will be at least some important clues to provide guidance for future research.

### Principles of field operations

In this section we attempt descriptions of important principles of methods of field operations, drawing from experiences of our research group. We present these in lieu of a manual of operations, which would not be generalizable, and they are designed to clarify aspects of these methods that are not always obvious from theory, although many are derived from extensive empirical evidence, at times only in retrospect. The principles are not listed in order of importance, nor do they have any temporal or structural sequence.

*Establish credibility—The experimenter has a double burden.* The community requires high scientific or source credibility, and a university-based research group can achieve this goal. Public opinion polls in the US place physicians and scientists at the top of the credibility ladder, thus the health content of the type of experiments we are describing allows these individuals to be placed in key roles. In the research of our group, physician members have played important roles to considerable advantage in credibility formation and as participants in exogenous and collaborative media. However the 'safety' credibility of individuals or groups radically different in customs or social status may be low (Rogers 1973). The solution is achieved through using as change agents local citizens who establish the new information and technology as legitimate, safe, and locally relevant. The experimenters provide scientific credibility but are not inherently linked to community needs and interests. On the practical side these goals are achieved through frequent joint appearances and media linkages between the researchers and the community co-ordinators. Rogers (1973, 1983) extensively reviews credibility issues.

*Produce mediated education collaboratively—It's not 'mine' but 'ours'.* Too often, researchers choose media before the goals of the programme are specifically defined, and before adequate co-operative arrangements are made with local media sources. This mistake spawns a large number of ineffective programmes and fails to lead toward the desired maintenance.

*Expect the unexpected—Jeanne D'Arc may be right around the corner.* The essence of an adaptive community organization method is that potential key opinion leaders or gatekeepers may turn up suddenly and the researchers must be ready to alter their plans. Which organizations, such as worksites, hospitals, media outlets, or voluntary health associations will want to adopt a new prevention-oriented agenda? The organizers cast their bread upon the waters and the loaves come back on unexpected waves. Other empty waves come back to drown your hopes, thus the Education group's six- and 12-month plans must be flexible. A few examples derived from Stanford's Five City Project will be described in order to demonstrate the types of unexpected events that one might encounter.

1. A local health department received funds from the federal government to create a smoking cessation programme, allowing us to create effective adult smoking cessation classes earlier than expected. Resources were allocated to accelerate development of our smoking cessation methods, training protocols, and manuals.

2. A local community college surprised us with their readiness for adoption of a novel weight control correspondence course.

3. A single Spanish language series on smoking cessation generated about 600 letters to the originating radio station, a factor of 10 greater than expected. This response redirected our future efforts.

4. A local newspaper refused an offer of material suitable for a weekly health column, necessitating alternative media methods and outlets. Unexpected events are not always pleasant.

*How do you decide on the general content of education campaigns—Use the GRAS principle (GRAS—generally recognized as safe).* In education and communication research programmes directed at communities one cannot obtain the informed consent of each citizen. Therefore the ethical experimenter must restrict the investigation to tests of policy changes, organizational changes, or individual behaviour changes that are generally accepted by society as being safe. The community study is therefore primarily useful in determining generalizable and cost-effective means of achieving lasting change. Only secondarily can such research be used to test hypotheses of putative benefit to an individual of an advocated change. They can be used as ancillary support for such benefits but more commonly they primarily test whether individual changes can in the aggregate produce detectable benefits in the system as a whole. Tests on fluoridation, automobile driving habits, seat-belt use, or programmes directed toward alcohol abuse should be contemplated only after an adequate consensus has been reached on their general advisability. In experiments on life-style change to decrease the probability of development of chronic disease, such as cardiovascular disease or certain types of adult-onset cancers, the topics should also be generally accepted as having benefit, or at least that the recommended change does not cause harm. Examples of positions taken by the Stanford group in community research on cardiovascular disease are as follows: (a) maintenance of some form of exercise, common to younger people, is beneficial as one grows older; (b) non-smoking is natural and healthful; (c) weight gained after age 20 years is ordinarily harmful; and (d) a prudent reduction in salt, sugar, saturated fat, and total fat, and an increase in dietary fibre and complex carbohydrate intake is likely to be beneficial.

The research group may develop an adequate consensus on education content only by close scrutiny of the relevant scientific evidence and established policies of governmental health groups, scientific groups, and voluntary health agencies. An example of an excellent analysis of the health policy implications of the scientific data on cardiovascular disease risk factors may be found in a recent piece by Blackburn (1979).

*How do you decide the specific content of education campaigns?—Seek the critical mass.* If a community is not ready for an innovation, however beneficial it might be, don't squander resources on a futile endeavour. If a respected leader is a smoker, try something else. Don't try to teach Bedouins how to ice skate. Seek to create adoption of innovations that have begun and which have affected a sufficient proportion of the population to give a chance to observe a change in a community system within a four-year period. The sufficient proportion or critical mass for predicting the successful subsequent wide diffusion of a health innovation is probably on the order of 15 per cent of the population having already adopted the innovation (Rogers 1983). Baseline survey data and subsequent formative evaluation can contribute to these decisions.

*Have a passionate belief in the virtues of your educational goals—'Health professional heal thyself'.* A scientist must of course measure his data with accuracy and objectivity. If, however, an educator wishes to teach a person to change, it cannot be done without advocacy. Nor can the teacher teach, in an abstract manner, the principles of life-style change that require the learner to be exposed to modelling and to undergo guided practice in a new behaviour (Bandura 1977). Acquisition of motor skills is enhanced by active learning. We ask our airline pilots and our surgeons to become trained before we put ourselves in their care, similarly the life-style health educator/communicator needs to practice in order to become effective. In the Stanford studies we have therefore advocated a 'health professional heal thyself' stance as an appropriate precursor to major community education. This admonition applies initially to research staff and later to community health professionals. A more general admonition is 'prospective change agent, change thyself'.

*Provide education in surges of external effort devoted to a single theme—Overloaded circuits burn adoption fuses.* Although a general background of education covering many topics can be provided, successful focusing of the education's effort and optimum learning requires phased cycles emphasizing a single topic. The Stanford projects have generally used three-month cycles of emphasis covering topics such as hypertension, exercise, nutrition, weight control, or smoking control that recur each year.

*Adopt the natural rhythm of the system.* Forces external to the community or innate structural or climatic characteristics of the community may determine choice of campaigns. In the US, beginning in 1979, the month of May has been designated as 'high blood pressure month'; accordingly our hypertension cycle begins in May. Our exercise cycle begins in the spring when the winter rainy season has ended; and programmes in schools are determined by the school year and by pre-established patterns of instruction.

*Look for structural obstacles—Is the environment against you?* The experimenter must look for non-communication obstacles to change. For example, one may find that healthy alternative foods (for example, non-fat yoghurt) are not available in a community, in which case no amount of education will produce this change in behaviour. If community organization cannot solve this problem by encouraging grocers to select such products, then a campaign to encourage customers to ask their grocers for these foods might be launched, or a combined strategy might be planned. Or, in another example, installation of bicycle paths might be sought through an analogous strategy.

*Don't be frightened by vested interests.* Appropriate community organization can determine what will meet with appropriate community reception even if a small minority will be opposed. It is important to know the nature and strength of any opposition. It is common, in our group's experience, for scientists falsely to assume that the position of opposition created by a national industry spells inevitable doom for any life-style change (such as smoking cessation) that will affect the profits of that industry. If the conditions of appropriate ethical standards, scientific consensus, and public acceptance are met, then the experimenter can be optimistic about the success of inclusion of a topic that runs counter to the wishes of a nationally-based pressure group. It is also evident that innoculation against persuasion applies in a manner similar to that in infectious disease. If the opposition's arguments are mentioned and refuted, their attempts at counter persuasion can often be blunted (Roberts and Maccoby 1974; McGuire in press).

*Use a marketing perspective—Will anyone pay attention?* Education research has shown that people learn as well from drab texts as from attractive ones provided they can be motivated to read them (Maccoby 1950). The less motivated citizen, however, will respond differentially to factors such as the size, colour, print size, and convenience of media material. The Stanford group uses social marketing methods (Kotler 1975; Solomon 1981) to define the characteristics optimum for acceptance of media materials and of programmes. Social marketing principles also lead the experimenter to provide tangible incentives to organizations to collaborate. An example from our studies is that a local television station was given incentives for continued collaboration by our provision of space for commercial announcements within an hour-long television programme that we supplied. On another occasion the eagerness of a local television station to collaborate in production of an anti-smoking series was enhanced by our inclusion of their newscaster as narrator.

*Encourage endogenous modification of exogenous programmes—'Reinvention' is a desirable ideal.* When a local group modifies or embellishes a product or programme that began with the researcher, the collaborative goal has been reached. The process of modification in fact usually results in an improved product for that community.

*Promote synergistic interaction among elements.* As indicated in the Introduction, the community locale has inherent advantages, in that the community's networks of communication are natural diffusion-adoption pathways. As an example, we have found that our smoking cessation effort grew synergistically through a conscious effort to cross-publicize. A television segment of smoking publicized both smoking cessation classes and printed material on smoking cessation. The latter publicized the classes, and participants in the classes publicized the television segment, the classes, and the printed material through their own personal networks.

*Don't raise expectations unduly—'Can we have the programme tomorrow?'* Our group found that an initial recruiting foray often led to a disappointed gatekeeper who was more eager to receive our 'exogenous materials or curricula' than we were ready to deliver. The solution to this problem comes from cautious promotion, aggressive preparation, and readiness to meet unexpected interest with rapid development.

*Develop a cost-benefit perspective—How much does it cost, and was it worth it?* Successful community transformation implies decreased continued external costs, assuming that local institutions such as schools, hospitals, and health departments will transform activities to better ends with the same personnel, facilities, and local financial support. A strict interpretation of costs would not count transformation of this sort as a decreased cost, since equivalent human energy and capital is being expended. This decreased cost is thus contingent upon the experimenter demonstrating a change that either does or can be predicted to decrease direct or indirect costs of the health problem being addressed. The means of answering the question of costs is implicit in achieving the research goals of the experiment, as well as a system of counting costs of exogenous organizing and education.

*Do not exclude commercial resources as a component of community transformation—'Let a thousand flowers bloom'.* In various cultures a population will find, to a varying degree, that convenience or preference or necessity will lead to efficient delivery of health education via profit-making organizations. The usual research team will not often be open to this option and may therefore miss the opportunity it provides. A restaurant that offers healthier menu selections, a retail food outlet, a sporting goods store or local media outlets are part of the life-style 'delivery system'. If they are provided with workable ideas, these organizations can be an important part of a health maintaining social system of a community. A campaign to increase use of helmets by bicycle riders would be useless without a provider. Other commercial resources, such as health clubs and weight-reduction salons should be considered in the array of profit-making organizations that deliver health education. The research group should consider these as secondary providers whose role may complement that provided by the extensive array of free or low-cost community supported organizations, such as schools and community colleges, that exist in comunities of the US.

## REVIEW OF COMPREHENSIVE COMMUNITY-BASED HEALTH EDUCATION AND COMMUNITY ORGANIZATION RESEARCH PROGRAMMES FOR CARDIOVASCULAR DISEASE PREVENTION

Two projects, the Stanford Three Community Study (Farquhar *et al.* 1977; Maccoby *et al.* 1977) and the Finnish North Karelia Project (Puska *et al.* 1978, 1981), began in 1972 and were in operation for three and five years, respectively. A group of eight comparable multifactor studies with an emphasis on comprehensive educational methods, including mass media, have since begun in Australia, South Africa, Switzerland, the Federal Republic of Germany, and the US. Many other studies are in the planning phase or are underway in Europe (WHO 1977). Although some of these will surely be comparable with previous studies, others will either not have reference communities or will stress methods of detection and clinical management of high-risk individuals rather than comprehensive public health education and community organization as the means of changing cardiovascular disease risk. Three of the four current US studies are now funded by the National Heart, Lung and Blood Institute and are loosely bound in a confederation for sharing evaluation methods. These three are: (i) the Stanford Five-City Project, start date 1978 (Farquhar 1978); (ii) the Minnesota Heart Health Study, under the aegis of Dr Henry Blackburn, start date 1980; and (iii) the Pawtucket Heart Health Study, under the aegis of Dr Richard Carleton of Providence, Rhode Island, start date 1980. A fourth US study, now partly funded through the State of Pennsylvania Health Department, is under the aegis of Drs Paul Stolley and Albert Stunkard of the University of Pennsylvania.

Table 12.3 lists these ten projects and identifies the years of education, country of origin, numbers of communities, and numbers of residents. It is noteworthy that in only one of the ten studies, that in Switzerland, was random assignment used (Gutzwiller 1979). In this instance the random assignment was within two pairs of French or German-speaking villages, chosen for demographic similarity within each language group.

Of these projects only the Stanford Three-Community

**Table 12.3.** *Description of ten community-based multifactor health education studies* *

| Description | Country | Years of education | Reference |
|---|---|---|---|
| 1. Stanford Three Community Study: three towns, two treatment, one reference, $n = 45\,000$. | USA (California) | 1972–75 | Farquhar *et al.* (1977) |
| 2. North Karelia Project: two counties, one treatment, one reference, $n = 433\,000$. | Finland | 1972–82 | Puska *et al.* (1981) |
| 3. North Coast Project: three towns, two treatment, one reference, $n = 70\,000$. | Australia | 1977–80 | Egger *et al.* (1983) |
| 4. Swiss National Research programme: four towns, two treatment, two reference, $n = 40\,000$. | Switzerland | 1978–80 | Gutzwiller *et al.* (1979) |
| 5. Community Health Improvement Project: two counties, one treatment, one reference, $n = 224\,000$. | USA (Pennsylvania) | 1979– | Stunkard *et al.* (In press) |
| 6. Heidelberg Study: three towns, two treatment, one reference, $n = 30\,000$. | Federal Republic of Germany | 1980– | Nussel (1981) † |
| 7. South African Study: three towns, two treatment, one reference, $n = 16\,000$. | South Africa | 1980–83 | Rossouw (1981) |
| 8. Stanford Five City Project: five cities, two treatment, three reference, $n = 350\,000$. | USA (California) | 1980–86 | Farquhar (1978) |
| 9. Minnesota Heart Health Study: two towns, two cities, two suburbs, paired treatment and reference, $n = 356\,000$. | USA (Minnesota) | 1982–89 | Blackburn (In press) |
| 10. Pawtucket Heart Health Study: two cities, one treatment, one reference, $n = 173\,000$. | USA (Rhode Island and Massachusetts) | 1982–86 | Carleton (In press) |

*This list is necessarily incomplete and represents projects personally known to the authors of studies based on communities, including at least one reference area, and involving use of comprehensive public health education and community organization methods.
†Personal communication.

Of these projects only the Stanford Three-Community Study and the first five years of the North Karelia study are fully reported (Farquhar *et al.* 1977; Puska *et al.* 1981). Changes in cardiovascular risk factors were comparable in these two studies. The next few years, however, will undoubtedly provide many new insights and new challenges as these and other projects unfold. For example, the Finnish study has reported preliminary findings from a second five years of education which reveal favourable changes in cardiovascular disease endpoints (Puska *et al.* in press). The Australian project, now completed, was successful in achieving change in smoking rates (Davidson, personal communication, 1982). An ambitious multi-city project is in the final stages of planning in the Federal Republic of Germany (Kreuter, personal communication, 1983) and other comprehensive programmes are underway in Portugal, Italy, the German Democratic Republic, Yugoslavia, Cuba, and the Peoples Republic of China (Puska, personal communication, 1983).

## REVIEW OF COMPREHENSIVE HEALTH EDUCATION AND COMMUNITY ORGANIZATION RESEARCH PROJECTS IN NON-CARDIOVASCULAR DISEASE PUBLIC HEALTH ISSUES

Despite the importance of issues such as alcohol abuse, family planning, automobile seat belt use, nutrition, accident prevention, immunization, or fluoridation, it is surprising and disappointing to find very few comprehensive, well supported, conceptually sophisticated, and adequately evaluated research studies. Too often the story is one of an inadequate conception of the public's needs or receptivity, and an inadequate amount and quality of mediated education. Equally often one finds an inadequate stimulation of inter-personal influence, and a grossly inadequate evaluation coupled with a premature spread of a method to a national level prior to adequate field testing.

The field of family planning, of all public health topics mentioned, has the most complete array of experiments covering single or multimedia education or community organization methods within countries of varying levels of development (Rogers 1973). These have been recently reviewed by Taplin (1981). She concludes that the field of family planning is now moving away from clinic-centred approaches toward a comprehensive combined multimedia and community organization method similar to that which has evolved for the field of cardiovascular disease prevention. Within the definition of community-centred and well-evaluated studies in family planning she cites the Esfahan campaign of 1970 in Iran as an example of a multimedia campaign whose success rested on successful pre-testing and successful integration of the mediated education into the community (Taplin 1981). At the other extreme, the example of the successful acceptance of family planning in a small Korean village, the 'miracle of Oryu Li', has been cited (Rogers and Kincaid 1981) as an example of success based on generation of inter-personal influence through community organizing and a virtual absence of external media. In this study, it is important to note that extensive national publicity and frequent visitors to the village may well have reinforced the villager's early changes. Taplin

concludes that even in the relatively well-studied issue of family planning that ' . . . there is no systematic evaluation and analysis that compares the different models with one specific set of developed criteria: the evaluation tools, content, and criteria are not uniform throughout the various projects'. She goes on to suggest that despite the uncertainty and clear need for greater research, that the trend toward community centred approaches and use of media and marketing techniques and attention to the social structure of the receivers is likely to be correct (Taplin 1981).

A growing interest in nutrition education experiments at the community level in developing countries has appeared in the last decade, and a transition similar to that within family planning has occurred. Again, the number of comprehensive well evaluated studies is low but one can make a comment similar to the one made about family planning regarding appropriate content for successful education and communication (Rasmuson 1977).

The theme that emerges from the community-based health communication research of the past 30 years is that a judicious combination of well-formulated mass media and of an appropriate type of community organization is most cost- and effort-effective in achieving measurable differences in experimental and control conditions within a reasonable period of time. These conclusions stem from observations of failures as well as successes in all three categories of: (i) a reasonably pure exogenous mass media-only programme (devoid of planned community organization); (ii) a mix of planned exogenous media and planned community organization; and (iii) a reasonably pure community organization-only programme. The failures usually stem from neglect of the appropriate theory or strategy as embodied in the examples and principles described in this chapter. The failure of many community fluoridation programmes in the US (Crain and Rosenthal 1966) can now be understood as due in part to näivete in regard to the need to identify and persuade minority community groups that hold negative opinions but may have considerable influence. Other failures are due to an inadequate dose of education and organization. In many instances the evaluation was adequate only to say that the programme succeeded or failed but, due to absence of process evaluation, there is no way to determine why this happened. It is also clear that prior expectations may colour the conclusions. For example, the Salk polio vaccination campaign of the 1950s in the US was judged to be failing 18 months after its initiation because half of the target population had not been vaccinated. The effect of the campaign accelerated over time and led to the virtual disappearance of poliomyelitis in the US within a few years. Was this a failure? Of additional interest is that the acceleration of adoption of vaccination during the late phases of the campaign was attributed to those who had received vaccination becoming effective protagonists (Glasser 1958). This is an example of diffusion and adoption via newly generated opinion leaders (Rogers 1983). It appears that successful media-only programmes such as the Salk vaccination and of various family planning studies are associated with the generation of a considerable amount of validating and persuasive inter-personal contact (Meyer *et al.* 1977). Such findings bear out the findings and predictions of

Cartwright (1949), a pioneer in the social psychology of communication.

Past experiences, however they are seen in research project outcomes, lead us toward a consideration of the future challenges for research.

## CONCLUSIONS AND FUTURE CHALLENGES

The conclusion is inescapable that, compared to earlier decades, more effective methods in education and communication in public health are now available. A compelling corollary is that research in this area now can be increased in scope and complexity. This is the natural path of science: to open new avenues of research when the vehicles to allow that path to be taken are available.

Given this new capacity and new confidence, we suggest that effective community-based education and communication programmes may be assured if the investigators take the following six steps: (i) become proficient in the use of effective mediated and face-to-face teaching methods; (ii) establish a sound and ethical content of instruction; (iii) collaborate with local forces in programme development; (iv) use communication pathways natural to the system; (v) activate opinion leadership and accelerate diffusion and adoption of the desired health innovations; and (vi) assist in community transformation. These steps are but one way to summarize the more detailed methods and principles described in earlier sections of this chapter.

As in other branches of developing scientific disciplines the new capacity for research greatly expands the scope of questions to be answered. For example, policy makers in health have a great unmet need for more generalizable data (Farquhar 1978). There is also a need for a societal counterforce to the new potency of commercially generated pressures. Over 50 billion dollars is spent annually in the US by commercial advertisers (McGuire, in press). The average American adult watches four hours of television daily (Neuman 1982), and a considerable proportion of the total health knowledge and attitudes of Americans is derived from television and radio (Chaffee 1982). This pre-occupation with electronic media is not restricted to citizens of the US. A recent tricultural study of determinants of learning among children in Taiwan, Japan, and the US revealed more television viewing by mothers and their children in the Japanese sample than in the sample from the US (Stevenson, personal communication, 1982). As McGuire (in press) points out, large parts of the modern world are now engulfed in the latest and most pervasive and most flourishing of the 'four great eras of persuasion'. He describes our seeming plight as a boon compared to the alternative of dampening human spirits and creativity as communications are stilled. Given this century's burgeoning growth of electronic media and information technology, including the ubiquitous computer, Graubard and others (1982) have called this 'information revolution' the major challenge and 'central fact' of this century, deserving attention by scholars in all disciplines. Thus, the wise recourse is that public health research workers learn to cope with this communication technology and information overload and to turn it to our benefit, where this

is possible. Research in education and communication can give us these coping skills and can teach us how to preserve a nation's health by harnessing the new information technologies to better serve man.

Beyond a need for a counterforce to unwanted persuasion and a need for increased awareness of the potential role of health communication lies a set of specific unmet research questions that the new technologies of health communication can address. Some of these issues and questions are: (i) study of how the emerging new information systems, such as home computers, home-learning centres, and cable television will influence the ways that people acquire good and bad health habits; (ii) how can social isolates and educationally deprived minorities within communities be provided with equitable distribution of health improvement services? (A different definition of this problem is that ways of preventing 'communication effects gaps' must be sought (Rogers 1983).); (iii) how can a community-wide programme avoid tyrannizing a minority? (The experimenter and social planner must seek new ways of studying this issue.); (iv) more research is needed to measure costs and benefits of community-based research; (v) an extensive increase in qualitative evaluation such as ethnographic methods will be needed to gain insights into the process of change; (vi) research expansion into the community control of self-destructive behaviours is greatly needed; (vii) a special challenge exists for research in the means of prevention of the acquisition of harmful health habits by young people; (viii) an expansion of research is needed in ways to improve the effectiveness, at reasonable cost, of providing mass skills training through the media; (ix) the determinants of maintenance of change, including methods of achieving lasting community transformation, need a considerable amount of study; (x) differentiation of methods appropriate to nations at different stages of development is greatly needed; and lastly, (xi) the means of transfer of research knowledge into public policy needs thorough investigation.

We cannot answer all these questions in a single way nor as rapidly as we would like. The challenges are clear, and given newly available skills, the opportunities are many. However, we believe that the public health advances we all seek will be attainable only by direction of research resources into community-based education and communication. Given the evident world-wide impact of social problems on the public's health, it is urgent that social science techniques of this sort become an important and familiar part of the public health armamentarium.

*Acknowledgement*

This work is supported by grant HL21906 from the National Heart, Lung and Blood Institute, National Institutes of Health, USA.

## REFERENCES

Ajzen, I. and Fishbein, M. (1980). *Understanding attitudes and predicting social behavior.* Prentice Hall, Englewood Cliffs, NJ.
Atkin, C. (1979). Research evidence on mass mediated health com-

munication campaigns. In *Communication yearbook III* (ed. D. Nimmo). Transaction Books, New Brunswick, NJ.

Bandura, A. (1977). *Social learning theory*. Prentice Hall, Englewood Cliffs, NJ.

Bandura, A. (1978). The self system in reciprocal determinism. *Am. Psychol.* **33**, 344.

Blackburn, H. (1979). Diet and mass hyperlipidemia: a public health view. In *Nutrition, lipids, and coronary heart disease* (ed. R. Levy, B. Rifkind, B. Dennis, and N. Ernst) p. 309. Raven Press, New York.

Blackburn, H. The Minnesota Heart Health Program: a research and demonstration project in cardiovascular disease prevention. In *Behavioral health: A handbook of health enhancement and disease prevention* (ed. J.D. Matarazzo, N.E. Miller, S.M. Weiss, J.A. Herd, and S.M. Weiss). John Wiley, Silver Spring, MD. [In press.]

Carleton, R. Lay volunteer delivery of a community-based cardiovascular risk factor change program: the Pawtucket experiment. In *Behavioral health: A handbook of health enhancement and disease prevention* (ed. J.D. Matarazzo, N.E. Miller, S.M. Weiss, J.A. Herd, and S.M. Weiss). John Wiley, Silver Spring, MD. [In press.]

Cartwright, D. (1949). Some principles of mass persuasion. *Hum. Relations* **2**, 253.

Chaffee, S.H. (1982). Television's health promoting possibilities. In *Television and behavior: ten years of scientific progress and implications for the eighties*, Vol. I summary report, p. 9. DHHS publication 82-1195. Washington, DC.

Cohen, B.C. (1963). *The press, the public, and foreign policy*. Princeton University Press, NJ.

Crain, R.L. and Rosenthal, D.B. (1966). Structure and values in local political systems: the case of fluoridation decision. *J. Politics* **28**, 169.

Egger, G., Fitzgerald, W., Frape, G. *et al.* (1983). Results of a large scale media antismoking campaign: North Coast "Quit For Life" Programme. *Br. Med. J.* **286**, 1125.

Farquhar, J.W. (1978). The community-based model of life-style intervention trials. *Am. J. Epidemiol.* **108**, 103.

Farquhar, J.W., Fortmann, S.P., Wood, P.D., and Haskell, W.L. (1983). Community studies of cardiovascular disease prevention. In *Prevention of coronary heart disease* (ed. N.M. Kaplan and J. Stamler) p. 170. Saunders, Philadelphia.

Farquhar, J.W., Maccoby, N., and Solomon, D.S. (in press). Community applications of behavioural medicine. In *Handbook of behavioural medicine* (ed. W.D. Gentry). Guilford Press, New York.

Farquhar, J.W., Maccoby, N., Wood, P.D., *et al.* (1977). Community education for cardiovascular health. *Lancet* **i**, 1192.

Flay, B.R. and Cook, T.D. (1981). Evaluation of mass media prevention campaigns. In *Public communication campaigns* (ed. R.E. Rice and W.J. Paisley), p. 239. Sage Publications, Beverley Hills, CA.

Glasser, M.A. (1958). A study of the public's acceptance of the Salk vaccine programs. *Am. J. Public Health* **48**, 141.

Graubard, S.R. (1982). Preface to the issue: print culture and video culture *Daedalus* Fall issue, V.

Green, L.W., Kreuter, M.W., Deeds, S.G., and Partridge, K.B. (1980). *Health education planning: a diagnostic approach*. Mayfield Publishing, Palo Alto, CA.

Griffiths, W. and Knutson, A.L. (1960). The role of mass media in public health. *Am. J. Public Health* **50**, 515.

Gutzwiller, F., Junod, B., and Schweizer, W. (1979). Prevention des malades cardio-vasculaires. *Les cahiers medico-sociaux* **23** eine annee, No. 2. Geneve, Suisse.

Kahn, A.J. (1969). *Theory and practice of social planning*. Russell Sage Foundation, New York.

Killen, J.D., Maccoby, N., and Taylor, C.B. (in press). Nicotine chewing gum and self-regulation training in smoking relapse prevention. *Behav. Therapy*.

Kotler, P. (1975). *Marketing for nonprofit organizations*. Prentice Hall, Englewood Cliffs, NJ.

Litwak, E. and Rothman, J. (1970). Toward the theory and practice of coordination between formal organizations. In *Organizations and clients* (ed. W.R. Rosengren and M. Lefton) p. 137. Merrill Publishing, Columbus, Ohio.

McAlister, A.L., Perry, C., and Maccoby, N. (1979). Adolescent smoking: onset and prevention. *Pediatrics* **63**, 650.

Maccoby, N. (1950). Comparing 'finished' versus working copy versions of a persuasive message. (Unpublished Report.) Communication Research Center, School of Public Communication, Boston University, Mass.

Maccoby, N. and Solomon, D.S. (1981). Heart disease prevention: community studies. In *Public communication campaigns* (ed. R.E. Rice and W.J. Paisley). Sage Publications, Beverly Hills, CA.

Maccoby, N., Farquhar, J.W., Wood, P.D., and Alexander, J.K. (1977). Reducing the risk of cardiovascular disease: effects of a community-based campaign on knowledge and behavior. *J. Community Health* **3**, 100.

McGuire, W.J. (1969). The nature of attitude change. In *The handbook of social psychology* (ed. G. Lindzey and E. Aronson) p. 136. Addison Wesley, Reading, Mass.

McGuire, W.J. (1981). Theoretical foundations of campaigns. In *Public comunication campaigns* (ed. R.E. Rice and W.J. Paisley) p. 41. Sage Publications, Beverly Hills, CA.

McGuire, W.J. (in press). The nature of attitudes and attitude change. In *The handbook of social psychology*, 3rd edn (ed. G. Lindzey and E. Aronson). Addison Wesley, Reading, Mass.

Meyer, A.J. and Henderson, J.B. (1974). Multiple risk factor reduction in the prevention of cardiovascular disease. *Prev. Med.* **3**, 225.

Meyer, A.J., Maccoby, M., and Farquhar, J.W. (1977). The role of opinion leadership and the diffusion of innovations in a cardiovascular health education campaign. In *Communication yearbook I* (ed. D. Nimmo) p. 579. Transaction Books, New Brunswick, NJ.

Meyer, A.J., Nash, J.D., McAlister, A.L., Maccoby, N., and Farquhar, J.W. (1980). Skills training in a cardiovascular health education campaign. *J. Consult. Clin. Psychol.* **48**, 129.

Neuman, W.R. (1982). Television and American culture: the mass medium and the pluralist audience. *Public Opinion Q.* **46**, 471.

Paisley, W.J. (1981). Public communication campaigns: the American experience. In *Public communication campaigns* (ed. R.E. Rice and W.J. Paisley) p. 15. Sage Publications, Beverly Hills, CA.

Puska, P., Tuomilehto, J., Salonen, J., and Nissinon, A. Ten years of the North Karelia Project: results with community-based prevention of coronary heart disease in Finland. *Scand. J. Soc. Med.* [In press.]

Puska, P., Virtamo, J., Tuomilehto, J., Maki, M., and Neittaanmaki, L. (1978). Cardiovascular risk factor changes in three year follow-up of a cohort in connection with a community programme (the North Karelia Project). *Acta Med. Scand.* **204**, 381.

Puska, P., Tuomilehto, J., Salonen, J. *et al.* (1981). *The North Karelia Project: evaluation of a comprehensive community programme for control of cardiovascular diseases in 1972–1977 in North Karelia, Finland*. Public Health in Europe. WHO/ERO Monograph Series, Copenhagen.

Rasmuson, M. (1977). *Current practice and future directions of nutrition education in developing countries: a research and policy assessment*. Academy for Educational Development, Washington, DC.

Ray, M.L., Sawyer, A.G., Rothschild, M.L., Heeler, R.M., Strong, E.C., and Redd, J.B. (1973). marketing communication and the hierarchy of effects. In *New Models for mass communication research* (ed. P. Clarke) p. 147. Sage, Beverly Hills, CA.

Reichardt, C.S. and Cook, T.D. (1979). Beyond qualitative *versus* quantitative methods. In *Qualitative and quantitative methods in evaluation research* (ed. T.D. Cook and C.S. Reichardt) p. 7. Sage Publications, Beverly Hills, CA.

Roberts, D. and Maccoby, N. (1974). Information processing persuasion: counterarguing and behavior. In *New models for communication research* (ed. P. Clarke) p. 269. Sage Publications, Beverly Hills, CA.

Robertson, L.S., Kelley, A.B., O'Neill, B., Wixom, C.W., Eisworth, R.S., and Haddon, W. Jr (1974). A controlled study of the effect of television messages on safety belt use. *Am. J. Public Health* **64**, 1071.

Rogers, E.M. (1973). *Communication strategies for family planning.* Free Press, New York.

Rogers, E.M. (1983). *Diffusion of innovations,* 3rd edn. Free Press, New York.

Rogers, E.M. and Kincaid, D.L. (1981). *Communication networks: toward a new paradigm for research.* Free Press, New York.

Rossouw, J.E., Jooste, P.L., Kotze, J.P., and Jordaan, P.C.J. (1981). The control of hypertension in two communities: an interim evaluation. *S. Afr. Med. J.* **60**, 208.

Rothman, J. (1979). Three models of community organization practice, their mixing and phasing. In *Strategies of community organization* (ed. F.M. Cox, J.L. Erlich, J. Rothman, and J.E. Tropman) p. 25. Peacock Publishers, Illinois.

Schramm, W. (ed.) (1972). *What the research says about quality in instructional television.* University Press of Hawaii, Honolulu.

Solomon, D.S. (1981). A social marketing perspective on campaigns. In *Public communication campaigns* (ed. R.E. Rice and W.J. Paisley) p. 281. Sage Publications, Beverly Hills, CA.

Spergel, I.A. (1977). Social planning and community organization: community development. In *Encyclopedia of social work* (ed. J.B. Turner) p. 1425. National Association of Social Workers, Washington, DC.

Stunkard, A.J.., Felix, M.R.J. and Cohen, R.Y. Mobilizing a community to promote health: The Pennsylvania County health Improvement Program (CHIP). In: *Prevention in health psychology.* (ed.) J.C. Rosen and L.J. Slomon. University Press on New England, Hanover, VT: [In press]

Taplin, S. (1981). Family planning communication campaigns. In *Public communication campaigns* (ed. R.E. Rice and W.I. Paisley) p. 127. Sage Publications, Beverly Hills, CA.

Telch, M.J., Killen, J.D., McAlister, A.L., Perry, C.L., and Maccoby, N. (1982). Long-term follow-up of a pilot project on smoking prevention with adolescents. *J. Behav. Med.* **5**, 1.

US Public Health Service (1979). *Smoking and health: a report of the Surgeon General.* DHEW publication No. (PRS) 79-50066. Washington, DC.

Warren, R. (1978). *The community in America,* 3rd edn. Rand McNally, Chicago, Ill.

Williams, P.T., Fortmann, S.P., Farquhar, J.W., Varady, A., and Mellen, S. (1981). A comparison of statistical methods for evaluating risk factor changes in community-based studies: an example from the Stanford Three Community Study. *J. Chronic Dis.* **34**, 565.

World Health Organization (1977). *Comprehensive cardiovascular community control programmes. Meeting in Koli, Finland, August, 1975* (ICP/CVD 019). WHO, Geneva.

Zimbardo, P., Ebbeson, E., and Maslach, C. (1977). *Influencing attitudes and changing behavior.* Addison Wesley, Reading, Mass.

# 13 Operational and system studies

Shan Cretin

## INTRODUCTION

Operational research was first recognized as a distinct discipline during the Second World War. Scientists, long engaged in the design of weapons, began to apply scientific methods of anaylsis to the deployment of weapons and to overall military operations, with the goal of providing military commanders with a quantitative basis for decisions (Morse and Kimball 1951). A decision problem (for example, how to search for U-boats in the North Atlantic or what size to make a convoy) was recast into a mathematical model. The key variables in the problem, including the appropriate measure of the effectiveness of the operation, were quantified, and the relationships among the variables were described using mathematical expressions. These formulae comprised a mathematical model of the real decision problem and could be manipulated to predict the impact of a given decision on the measure of effectiveness. The success of operational research in the Second World War demonstrated that many apparently complex problems could be usefully analysed using simple models to approximate the critical variables and relationships.

After the Second World War operational research was extended to non-military problems. Hospitals and health care systems were quickly identified as fruitful areas for analysis, with the first published reports of health applications appearing in the early fifties. Bailey (1951, 1952) used the mathematical theory of queues to explore various out-patient appointment systems and to analyse the use of single versus multiple occupancy rooms in hospitals. Other studies applied operational research techniques to models of epidemics (Abbey 1952; Taylor 1958), emergency admissions (Newell 1954) and inventory control in general (Flagle 1960), and in blood banks (Rockwell et al. 1962; Elston and Pickrel 1963).

Most uses of these early applications of operational research used mathematical models based on probability or statistical theory. Today, operational research studies use a variety of mathematical tools, some adapted from traditional mathematical fields and some newly developed. The techniques most commonly employed are: (i) probability models, which use queueing theory, Monte Carlo simulations, and statistics; (ii) optimization models, which use mathematical programming, dynamic programming, graph and network theory; (iii) differential equation methods and dynamic systems simulation; (iv) decision analyses, which use models based on Bayesian and statistical decision theory, game theory, and utility theory.

The remainder of this chapter will be divided into three parts. The first section will review the most frequently used operational research techniques, with references to sources of more detailed information about each. The second part will review the types of public health problems that have been addressed using operational research methods, with references to some typical studies. The third section will discuss the potential and the problems surrounding applications of operational research methods in public health.

## REVIEW OF OPERATIONAL RESEARCH TECHNIQUES

There are several excellent textbooks surveying the methods of operational research. Duckworth and colleagues (1977) and Ackoff and Rivett (1962) provide overviews of methods and applications aimed at managers. Hillier and Lieberman (1974) and Wagner (1975) are good references for basic methods. Larson and Odoni (1981) focus on techniques useful in the analysis of urban problems. Warner and Holloway (1978) stress methods and applications in health administration. In addition, there are scores of books and hundreds of articles devoted to specific techniques, models, and problems. In the brief review of techniques which follows, reference is made to a few of these more advanced texts.

### Probability models

Uncertainty is a feature of life. Many important administrative and policy decisions in health care are complicated by chance elements beyond the control of the decision-maker. Recent work by psychologists (Tversky and Kahneman 1974) has demonstrated biases and inconsistencies in our intuition about probabilities. This failure of intuition may explain why operational research models employing probability theory to analyse chance events have resulted in some of the most substantial improvements in operating systems.

#### Stochastic processes

Stochastic, or probabilistic, processes evolve over time in a way that is not completely predictable. Some simple probabilistic processes have proved to be useful models of real events. These models have been carefully described and well analysed over the years, so that once the model is known to apply, many results can be inferred. The Bernoulli process, the

Poisson process, and the Markov process are three models that have been used extensively in health applications.

In the simplest probability models, successive events are assumed to be independent of each other. The classic example is coin flipping, modelled by a Bernoulli process: the outcome (heads or tails) on one toss does not alter the probability of heads or tails on the next toss.

In a Bernoulli process, the outcome is a result of some discrete event. When tossing coins, for example, 'heads' or 'tails' cannot occur at any instant, but only as a result of the action of 'flipping the coin'. For this reason, the Bernoulli process cannot be used to model events which can occur at any moment in time, such as a request for emergency medical service. The Poisson process extends the notion of independent events to continuous time by assuming that the number of events in one time period is independent of the number of events in any other non-overlapping time period. Poisson arrivals (sometimes called 'random arrivals') have been used to model the arrival of women in spontaneous labour at an obstetrics service, as well as requests for ambulance or other emergency medical care.

The Poisson and Bernoulli processes are called memoryless. While such memoryless processes may be adequate for many situations, there are times when probabilities of future events will depend on past outcomes. The Markov model is a simple probability model with 'memory'. A Markovian world is assumed to consist of a set of discrete, non-overlapping states. At any time the world is described as being in exactly one of these states. For example, a Markovian model of a person's state of health might consist of four states: disease-free, pre-symptomatic, symptomatic, dead. Starting in one of the states, the system undergoes changes of state (or state transitions) according to a set of probability rules. The Markov process is allowed to have a limited memory – that is, the probability of transition to a particular state is allowed to depend on which state the system is in just before the transition. Some Markovian systems undergo transitions only at discrete times (similar to the Bernoulli process), while others may undergo transitions at any time.

Drake (1967) and Feller (1968) provide introductions to applied theory. Other useful references on stochastic processes are Parzen (1962), Bailey (1964), Cox and Miller (1965), Howard (1960, 1971), and Ross (1970).

## Queuing systems

The application of stochastic models to the analysis of queues for service has been quite fruitful and queuing theory has become a distinct and expanding field of inquiry. A. K. Erlang did much of the early work in this field in conjunction with his studies of the Copenhagen telephone system (Brockmeyer et al. 1948).

The simplest queuing system has one server who handles requests for service sequentially. To simplify the analysis, both arrivals and service are assumed to be 'memoryless'. The arrival of customers is modelled by a Poisson process. Service times for each customer are assumed to drawn independently from a negative exponential distribution, a distribution with the property that no matter how long service has been in progress, the expected remaining time in service is the same. Given the average arrival rate of customers and the mean service time, one can then calculate the distribution of the length of the queue, the distribution of customer waiting times, as well as characteristics of the server's busy and quiet periods.

More complex queuing systems have been analysed which allow multiple servers, more general arrival and service time distributions, batch arrivals of customers, balking or reneging by customers who wait too long in the queue, and even hierarchical queuing networks. For these more complex systems, less complete mathematical results are available, but many approximate results have been obtained. Many complex queuing networks are now analysed using computer simulation methods and this will be discussed in the section on Monte Carlo simulations.

Cox and Smith (1961) provide a concise introduction to queuing theory, while Cooper and Kleinrock (1975) give fuller treatment to the subject. Newell (1971) emphasizes approximate solution methods.

A special class of queuing models of particular relevance to the analyses of ambulance systems is the spatially distributed queue. In this case, chance is involved not only in the timing of the requests, but also in the location from which the requests originate. The geography of the region is important in describing the location of calls for service and in determining the distribution of response times. Servers are no longer indistinguishable, although they provide the same service, since each potential server may be at a different distance from an incoming call. Models of spatially distributed queues have been developed to analyse the effects of call volume, number, and location of servers and dispatching strategies on the efficiency and equity of service. Larson and Odoni (1981) give a description of models and methods. The Rand Fire Project report (Walker et al. 1979) describes the use of these and similar models in analysing fire services.

## Monte Carlo simulations

The behaviour of systems involving chance elements can often be analysed by simulating the operation of the system. Simulation is also used to analyse complex deterministic systems, as in dynamic systems simulation, discussed below. Coin flipping could be simulated using digits from a table of random numbers, by labelling odd digits as 'heads' and even digits as 'tails'. Alternatively, a computer could be programmed to simulate coin flipping in a similar way using internally generated random numbers.

Simulation is usually an analysis of last resort, used when a system is too complex for the simpler mathematical models with closed form solutions. Complex queueing networks are frequently simulated. In theory a simulation can be carried out 'by hand', but in practice simulations are usually computer operations, using one of several simulations languages (GPSS, SIMSCRIPT, GASP). Simulations in these languages are 'event paced'. First, the logical structure of the system is described and the beginning state of the system is specified. The simulation then focuses on events that change the state of the system (for example, arrival of a new customer or completion of service on a current customer). Various statistics describing the operating characteristics of the system are compiled during the simulation and reported when a predetermined span of simulation time has elapsed.

In effect, running a simulation is like collecting experimental data on an operating system. As in any experiment, the interpretation of the result depends on the design of the experiment and the sample size. Interpretation of simulation results may also depend on how the data used in constructing the simulation were obtained. With a little care, a simulation can give a reliable picture of how the model behaves. As with all operational research, the crucial question is also the most difficult to answer: how well does the model represent the real system?

Emshoff and Sisson (1970) or Hammersley and Handscomb (1964) provide a general introduction to simulation methods. Manuals for specific simulation languages are also useful guides – for example, Kiviat *et al.* (1969) on SIMSCRIPT II or Pritsker (1973) on GASP.

### Competing risk and other life-table models

Historically, life-tables have been used by demographers and biostatisticians to calculate life expectancies and survival curves. With some modifications, the basic life-table models can incorporate the notion of competing causes of death (Chiang 1968; Manton *et al.* 1976). The age-specific mortality from any particular cause of death may further be described as a function of various risk factors (such as blood pressure or smoking habits). Several operational research studies have incorporated competing risk/life-table methods in larger models designed to estimate the costs and benefits of risk factor intervention programmes (Weinstein and Stason 1977; Berwick *et al.* 1980; Eddy 1980).

### Inventory theory

Inventory theory, like queueing theory, is organized around an area of application rather than a method. Inventory models include both deterministic models (which assume that the demand for a good is completely predictable) and probability models (which allow demand and various time lags to be stochastic). The basic components of most inventory models include ordering costs, storage costs for items on hand, shortage costs, outdating costs (for perishable goods, such as whole blood) and the cost of capital (the discount rate). The models are analysed to determine the least-cost inventory policy, including the size and timing of orders.

Inventory models have been developed to analyse one-time ordering decisions, multiple cycle ordering decisions, single and multiple product systems. When an inventory problem is too complex to fit any of the existing models, then computer simulation can provide a means of analysis. Buffa (1968) reviews inventory theory and practice, and Vienott (1966) reviews theory.

### Optimization models

Many of the probability models just discussed are descriptive rather than prescriptive. A queueing model, for example, would be useful in describing the trade-off between customer waiting time and server idle time, but would not indicate the 'optimal' number of servers for a given workload. The value of the model is in predicting the effects of uncertain events so that a few known alternatives can be evaluated. In some

decisions, uncertainty about the outcome of a strategy is not the major difficulty. The outcome for any given alternative is easy to calculate, but the decision-maker is cursed with too many choices. In this kind of problem, mathematical modelling can provide an efficient way to find the optimal alternative from a large (perhaps infinite) number of possibilities. Optimality is defined in terms of a mathematical expression (an 'objective function') which is to be made as large (or as small) as possible.

### Mathematical programming

Mathematical programming includes a variety of techniques used to determine the optimal allocation of resources. The form of these models is always the same: maximize or minimize an objective function subject to a series of constraints. The specific techniques (linear programming, quadratic programming, integer programming, or non-linear programming) rest on different assumptions about the mathematical form of the objective function and constraints, and therefore involve different solution methods. Linear programming models are usually the simplest to solve and are often used to approximate more complex integer or non-linear problems.

A classic linear programming problem is the 'product mix' decision. Suppose, for example, that a potter has 80 pounds of clay and 10 hours available to prepare pottery for a craft show. She can make vases (each uses a pound of clay and takes five minutes) or bowls (each takes a pound and a half of clay and 15 minutes). If bowls sell for 20 dollars and vases for 10, how many of each should she make to maximize her revenue?

In this example, the decision variables are the number of vases to be made ($V$) and the number of bowls ($B$). The objective is to maximize revenue, a linear function of the two decision variables ($20B + 10V$). There are two constraints, time and material, which may be expressed as linear inequalities:

$$\text{Time: } \tfrac{1}{12}V + \tfrac{1}{4}B \le 10$$
$$\text{Clay: } \quad V + \tfrac{3}{2}B \le 80.$$

If this problem is solved using linear programming techniques, the optimal values for the decision variables will take on fractional values. When it is important to restrict the solution to integral values, the same formulation of the objective function and constraints could be solved using integer programming methods.

In the simple example just given, the decision problem is not very difficult. Once the problem is formulated mathematically, it can be solved by hand using algebraic or graphical techniques. However, many applications of linear programming involve hundreds of decision variables and constraints. The solution of problems of this magnitude only became feasible with the development of the simplex algorithm (Dantzig 1963), an extremely efficient solution method when used on high-speed computers.

Although linear programming provides a powerful tool for analysing questions of resource allocation, many practical problems violate the assumptions of the model. A common problem is the need to restrict the solution to integer values. This is demonstrated in the example above, and is even more pronounced when the variable represents the number of surgical suites. In other cases, the constraints are not linear. For example, the potter may find that each additional bowl takes a little less time than the preceding bowl, because of a learning effect. While solution methods for non-linear and integer programming problems do exist, except for some rather special cases, these algorithms are far less efficient than linear programming techniques.

Luenberger (1973) provides a valuable introduction to both linear and non-linear programming. Garfinkel and Nemhauser (1972) have produced a good text on integer programming.

### Graphs and networks

A graph is a set of nodes or points with lines or branches connecting certain pairs of points. A network is a graph with some type of flow along its branches. A highway system is an example of a network, with roads as branches, intersections as nodes, and traffic flowing along the roads. Network theory provides an excellent means of analysing many problems related to transportation, such as finding the shortest route from one point to another or finding the shortest tour through a network ( a path that visits every node). Network theory is also the basis for a technique widely used in coordinating and scheduling interrelated activities. This method has been popularized as PERT (program evaluation and review technique) or CPM (critical path method).

PERT systems begin by representing a project as a network. Each node represents an event – for example, the beginning of the project, the end of the project, or the completion of some intermediate activity. Each activity or task is represented by a directed branch (a line with an arrow) starting from the node marking completion of all necessary predecessor tasks and ending at a task completion node. If the duration of each sub-task is known, network theory can be used to calculate the earliest possible completion time for the whole project, the earliest and latest starting time for each sub-task, and the critical path. Activities on the critical path have no slack time, meaning that if the starting time on one of these activities is delayed, the completion of the entire project is delayed.

Although the critical path is found as a result of an optimization technique, the major use of PERT systems is as an aid to scheduling, not as an optimization tool. Sometimes a range of times for each sub-task is the basis for 'best case' and 'worst case' analyses. Alternatively, the cost of speeding up certain sub-tasks can be balanced against the effect on project completion time.

Network analyses have also been applied to assignment problems (assigning personnel to tasks) and to facility location problems (finding the best location for fire stations in a region). Assignment problems and certain transportation problems can be solved using adaptations of linear programming algorithms. Ford and Fulkerson (1962) cover network theory in general. CPM/PERT is reviewed by Moder and Phillips (1970) and Pocock (1962). Larson and Odoni (1981) provide a good review of routing problems and facility location problems in an urban context.

### Dynamic programming

Dynamic programming is a technique for maximizing the overall effectiveness of a series of interrelated decisions. In a dynamic programming problem the decisions take place in stages. The choices available and the results of a decision at each stage depend on the current state of the system. After the decision has been made, the state of the system changes (either deterministically or according to a set of known probabilities). The complexity of the problem is not the result of uncertainty but of the number of possible decision sequences which must be evaluated. If there are only four stages with four possible decisions at each stage, there are 256 distinct sequences.

Finding the optimal solution to a dynamic programming problem is not a simple matter of applying a standard algorithm as was the case for linear programming. Although there is a general approach, it must be tailored to each individual problem. The solution procedure starts by finding the best decisions for each possible state at the last decision stage and works backward. The best decision set at the $n$th stage is found by building on the best decisions found for stage $n + 1$.

An extension of dynamic programming to allow an infinite number of recurring decision stages is found in Markovian decision models. Some decisions with continuous outcomes can also be modelled using continuous state dynamic programming. Howard (1960, 1971) discusses both dynamic programming and Markovian decision theory.

### Differential equations and difference equations

Differential equations and difference equations have been used in modelling electrical, mechanical, and fluid systems for many years. Differential equations are useful in describing systems in which key variables change continuously over time, and in which the rate of change of a variable may depend on the level of that variable and on the level and rates of other variables. Difference equations are simply approximations to differential equations in which time is only allowed to change in discrete units.

A simple example of a system well modelled by differential equations is a world populated by caterpillars and birds. If some external force suddenly depletes the bird population, the caterpillars will thrive. This, in turn, will allow the small remaining bird population to grow. Such a system may oscillate for some time before reaching a stable equilibrium. The size of the oscillations and the length of time taken for the system to stabilize will depend on the size of the external force and on the exact relationship between bird and caterpillar populations.

In the late 1950s, Forrester (1961) began using difference equations to model the responses of industrial firms to management policies. Since that time, the applications have been extended to many other settings, including health care. The models of such systems are too complex to be solved mathematically, and analysis is usually done using simulation. The computer language DYNAMO was developed especially for this purpose.

### Decision analysis

Decision analysis is a general approach to the problem of decision-making when there is uncertainty. Imbedded in this widely accepted approach to structuring the problem are several thorny and highly controversial topics. How does one estimate the degree of uncertainty in the absence of data? What criteria should be applied in finding the 'best decision'? How does one value outcomes, especially when there are multiple dimensions – for example, mortality, money, impaired function?

Decision analysts structure a problem by first separating decisions, chance events, and outcomes. Decisions and chance events are then displayed using a sequential 'tree'. Branches representing alternatives and chance occurrences radiate from appropriately sequenced 'decision' and 'chance' nodes respectively. Each end point of the tree is labelled with the appropriate outcome. Each chance branch is labelled with its probability of occurring. Decision branches are unlabelled initially. At the end of the analysis the 'best' alternative is identified at each decision node.

When the outcome is a single dimension (profit in a business decision or winnings in a gamble), the best decision is often defined as that which maximizes the expected value of the outcome. A common extension of decision analysis uses the decision-maker's 'utility' for the outcome, rather than the outcome itself. In this case the best decision is the one which maximizes expected utility.

The concept of utility makes it easier to apply decision analysis to problems with inherently qualitative outcomes and to incorporate multi-dimensional outcomes. However, the problem of eliciting a decision-maker's utilities for complex outcomes is itself quite difficult. Psychologists have challenged the ability of utility theory to model the preferences people express in real decision situations (Tversky and Kahneman 1981).

Another controversial area in the practice of decision analysis is the problem of estimating probabilities in the absence of data. It is common practice to include subjective or intuitive estimates of probabilities when no other means of estimation are possible. However, the method of eliciting these subjective probabilities may bias the estimates (Tversky and Kahneman 1974) and hence the analysis. For this reason, many applications of decision analysis include extensive sensitivity analysis to test the stability of the optimal policy. An excellent introduction to decision analysis is given by Raiffa (1968).

### Game theory

Game theory involves the analysis of decisions against opponents or competitors. Decisions by one party will interact with decisions by the other party to produce the outcomes. In two person zero-sum games, the winnings of one party must equal the loss of the opponent. Other games include co-operative games, non-zero sum games, and games involving more than two players. In game theory (as in decision analysis) the analysis specifies the decision strategy which maximizes one player's gain in the face of the opponents' best strategies. One promising application of game theory is in predicting behaviour of an industry to changes in regulations or reimbursement methods. Luce and Raiffa (1957) offer an extensive treatment of game theory and decision-making.

## REVIEW OF PUBLIC HEALTH APPLICATIONS

Over the last three decades there have been many reviews of health applications of operational research. Some reviewers focused on a particular technique or problem, such as statistics (Bailey 1956), queuing theory (Bailey 1954), mathematical programming (Boldy 1976), decision analysis (Krischer 1980), or facility location (ReVelle et al. 1977). Others have conducted more general surveys levened with varying degrees of philosophical comment (Flagle 1962, 1967; Horvath 1965, 1967; Denison et al. 1969; McLaughlin 1970; Shuman et al. 1975; Fries 1976, 1979, 1981; Boldy 1981; Boldy and O'Kane 1982). Several reviews have looked primarily at applications in hospitals (Nuffield Provincial Hospitals Trust 1955, 1962, 1965; Bailey 1957a; Luck et al. 1971; Stimson and Stimson 1972). Several critical reviews – notably, Stimson and Stimson (1972); Shuman et al. (1975); Boldy (1981) – have been motivated by the apparent discrepancy between the large number of published studies and the considerably smaller number of successful implementations.

Since there are so many existing reviews (including several recent efforts), I will not attempt to be comprehensive in this chapter. Rather, for each application area, I will highlight some representative studies.

### Health facilities management

Many early operational research studies, especially in the United States, addressed problems that arise in the management of hospitals and clinics. This emphasis may be explained in part by the importance of the hospital and clinic in medical care systems. It is also true that problems in hospitals and clinics (scheduling, inventory control) often have parallels in business and industry. Many hospital applications represented efforts to transfer models and solutions from business to health settings.

### Outpatient appointment systems

The design of efficient appointment systems has engaged analysts for three decades. Queueing and simulation studies abound (Bailey 1952; Welch and Bailey 1952; Blanco White and Pike 1964; Welch 1964; Fetter and Thompson 1965, 1966; Rockart and Hoffman 1969; Walter 1973; Fries 1981), and a considerable amount of data on the performance of operating systems has been collected (Nuffield Provincial Hospitals Trust 1965; United Hospital Fund of New York 1967; Johnson and Rosenfeld 1968). Recently, Fries and Marathe (1981) used a dynamic programming approach to compare the performance of block appointment systems. Most studies have elaborated (without fundamentally altering) Bailey's original queueing formulation. Given the demand for services and the distribution of service times, the model describes the relationship between patient waiting time and provider idle time under various appointment systems. A wide array of other variables may be added to the basic model: patient and provider punctuality, the fraction of patients who arrive without appointments, the fraction of patients who fail to keep appointments, service times dependent on patient characteristics.

Regardless of the model used or the site of the study, analysts have come to the same general conclusions:(i) patients are quite punctual, physicians are not; (ii) minor changes in clinic procedures will usually eliminate excessive patient delays without significantly increasing the idle time of providers.

Despite the agreement among the analysts, long delays persist in many clinics, including some of those studied. Operational research analysts have been quick to assume that the staff and administration of the clinic are interested in reducing patient waiting time and in increasing their own productivity. This may not be the case. Under a system of prepaid health care (the National Health Service in Great Britain or health maintenance organizations in the United States), increasing the number of patient visits will only increase workload, not income. Staff may consciously or unconsciously use long patient waiting time to hold down demand for services. Recommended changes, however minor, must be carried out by the staff. If the staff are not interested, the implementation is likely to falter.

When clinic staff recognize a problem in the appointment system, an operational analysis can aid in identifying and evaluating possible solutions (Henderson 1976). In one successful project, staff involvement led to a model which focused on the patient's delay in getting an appointment, rather than on waiting time in the clinic. The mark of a good operational research analysis is that it solves the problem of interest to the manager, rather than one of interest to the analyst.

### In-patient admission/discharge scheduling

Interest in the efficient scheduling of in-patients arises in over-crowded facilities and also in underutilized facilities. In hospitals with high occupancy rates (90 per cent or more), efficient scheduling may be viewed as an alternative to capital investment in new facilities. Hospitals with low average occupancy face a different problem: wide fluctuations in the size of patient populations are likely to occur, making staffing difficult. In this case, scheduling of patients can result in a more stable operation.

Many different models have been used in the analysis of in-patient scheduling: queueing (Young 1965), simulation (Smith and Solomon 1966; Webb et al. 1977), Markov probability (Kolesar 1970; Shonick and Jackson 1973; Esogbue and Singh 1976). Some models also employ statistical or time-series forecasting methods in predicting future demand as part of the scheduling problem (Shonick and Jackson 1973; Kao and Pokladnik 1978).

Despite the variety of models, there is common ground. Most analysts consider at least two classes of admission separately – elective and emergency. A further division into medical versus surgical admissions is frequently used. Future demand in each category is forecast from past experience. Future census is forecast from future emergency demand, future scheduled demand, and length of stay estimates. Measures of the effectiveness of the scheduling system include resulting in-patient census, rate of turnaway for emergencies, and length of waiting time for electives.

The simplest systems generate fixed rules about the maximum number of elective patients who can be scheduled on a given day. The most elaborate systems consider each potential admission separately, using individual patient data to project length of stay and then scheduling the patient so that the probability of facility overflow never exceeds a preset value (Rubenstein 1976).

The fixed rule systems are most commonly used. The more complex systems are necessarily limited to hospitals with on-line computerized admission and pre-admission systems. Implementation studies done at two hospitals suggest that systems with heavy day-to-day data requirements in underutilized hospitals are not as likely to be successful as simpler systems implemented in overcrowded facilities (Griffith et al. 1975).

### Facility sizing

Most of the scheduling and appointment models discussed assume that the size of the facility is fixed. While efficient scheduling can increase the apparent capacity of a facility, there are times when a hospital or clinic can only meet a growing demand by expanding. Many of the models used in evaluating appointment systems or admissions scheduling systems can be adapted to the problem of establishing an appropriate facility size (Fetter and Thompson 1966; Shonick and Jackson 1973; Esogbue and Singh 1976). These models are limited, however, because they focus on a single facility. A more efficient health system is achieved by fixing individual facility size as part of a regional plan, as discussed in the section on regional health planning.

Several studies have tried to establish appropriate sizes for various units within a hospital. Operating suites have been analysed using queueing theory (Whitson 1965), dynamic programming (Esogbue 1969), and simulation (Goldman and Knappenberger 1968). Maternity services have been analysed using queueing models (Thompson et al. 1960) to determine the number of labour, delivery, and postpartum beds required. Markov and semi-Markov probability models have been used to predict the resources needed for coronary patients (Kao 1972). As an example of what might be done using a linear programming model, Dowling (1971) determined the numbers of appendectomies, cholecystectomies, and tonsillectomies that could be performed subject to constraints in the numbers of operating suites, recovery beds, and hospital beds.

Most 'size' analyses assume that the pattern of demand for services is fixed. However, reducing the fluctuations in demand through better scheduling may increase the effective capacity of a facility without increasing its size. Simulation studies have been used to evaluate facility size under various scheduling policies (surgical suites: Kwak et al. 1976; radiology: O'Kane 1981). Such comprehensive models are more realistic and therefore more appealing. However, they may be less likely to be used than simpler models. Because complex models take longer to develop and require more extensive data collection, they cannot be used when quick answers are needed.

### Staffing

Staffing is a major concern in most health facilities. Nurse staffing, in particular, has been the subject of many operational research analyses – see, for example, Hershey et al. (1981). Warner and Holloway (1978) use a three-level classification of staffing decisions: (i) long-range planning of the numbers and types of nursing personnel needed on each unit; (ii) deriving work schedules for each individual nurse; (iii) allocation of nurses to units at the start of each shift. In addition, modelling has been applied to a fourth area: (iv) predicting the supply of personnel.

A quantitative approach to long-range staffing requires quantification of the nursing tasks needed on a unit. The simplest formulations relate nursing needs to the number of patients. More sophisticated approaches attempt to determine the nursing needs of each patient or class of patients. Simulation or statistical concepts can be used to incorporate the inevitable fluctuation in demand for nursing services (Smallwood et al. 1971; Hershey et al. 1974).

The scheduling problem consumes considerable time and effort in most hospitals. A common solution is to have each employee rotate through a fixed set of weekly schedules. Various heuristic and mathematical programming techniques have been used to help in formulating sets of schedules that meet staffing needs (Maier-Rothe and Wolfe 1973; James et al. 1974). This approach is fair in that each employee cycles through the same set of schedules; it does not, however, exploit differences in personal preferences. Warner (1976) has developed and implemented a system to assign schedules based on individual preferences for long weekends, night shifts, and other characteristics. Nurses are asked to assign numerical weights to reflect their preferences, and a mathematical programming algorithm is then used to maximize the sum of these weights while meeting minimal coverage requirements.

The need to allocate nurses on a shift by shift basis arises because the number and type of patient assigned to each ward or floor can be expected to fluctuate. In addition, some nurses may be absent from an assigned shift. Many hospitals cope with this problem by having a pool of 'floaters', nurses who are not assigned to a particular unit until the start of the shift. Trivedi and Warner (1976) use an integer programming model to assign floaters based on the quantified needs of each unit.

Staffing also must be determined for other areas of the hospital. Queueing and simulation studies have been used in staffing operating rooms (Whitston 1965), messenger services (Gupta et al. 1971), and out-patient clinics (Keller and Laughhunn 1973).

The issue of physician staffing has not received much attention. In the United States, most physicians have a voluntary rather than salaried or contractual relationship with hospitals. Fetter and Thompson (1966) did look at physician staffing in the out-patient clinics of a teaching hospital.

Statistical and probability models have been used to forecast the supply of physicians and other health professionals. The report of the Graduate Medical Education National Advisory Committee (GMENAC) modelled both the expected supply of physicians and the anticipated demand (Tarlov 1980a, b) in order to make national policy recommendations on the need for physicians and other personnel. Kane and colleagues (1980) made similar projections for geriatric manpower.

## Patient flow models

Patient flow models do not, in themselves, address operational questions. However, estimates derived from such models may be useful (in conjunction with other models and data) in planning and staffing facilities. Analyses of such operational decisions often hinge on having an explicit model of how patients flow through the facility. Markov and semi-Markov models are frequently proposed as good methods of analysing patient flow. Fetter and Thompson (1965) proposed simulating a Markovian model of patient transition through a facility organized around Progressive Patient Care (a patient classification system based on the nursing needs of the patient). More recently, Weiss et al. (1982) used a semi-Markov model to predict patient flow through a hospital.

When used to focus on particular patient subgroups, patient flow models blur the distinction between clinical and operational models. Kao (1972), for example, analysed the flow and recovery of coronary patients. Kastner and Schachtman (1982) looked at the flow of patients with hospital-acquired infections.

## Ancillary and support services

Ancillary departments of hospitals present special cases of the general problems of sizing, scheduling, staffing, and inventory control. Simulation has been a popular tool for studying the size and operation of radiology departments (Jeans et al. 1972), laboratories (Fetter and Thompson 1965; Rath et al. 1970), blood banks (Jennings 1973), and pharmacies (Myers et al. 1972). A complex hierarchical queueing model was used to study the operation of telemedicine systems (Willemain 1974).

Inventory theory has proved useful in evaluating hospital support services such as oxygen supplies (Kilpatrick and Freund 1976). The costs of ordering, storage, and shortage are considered in determining the best supply policy. Smith et al. (1975) used inventory theory to develop a stock control system for hospitals which was widely implemented in Britain.

## Regional health planning

In the United States regional health planning has fallen in and out of favour several times in the last three decades. Despite these ups and downs, the interest in quantitative models in health planning has grown steadily. Early efforts in modelling health care systems were primarily academic exercises (Navarro 1969). As a result, Shuman et al. (1975) found that few operations research models had resulted in useful aids for planners. More recent reports paint a brighter picture. Boldy and Clayden (1979) noted that in Great Britain, where regional health planning has long been accepted, the number of operational research projects devoted to 'strategic studies' in health care has increased, while the number of 'hospital-based, tactical studies' has declined. In planning ambulance services, Raitt (1981) reports several implementations of a queueing model developed for the National Health Service.

Because the hospital is often the building block in regional planning, there is some interest in determining which populations are apt to be served by which hospital, especially in multi-hospital regions. Simple statistical models have been used in defining hospital service areas (Meade 1974; Griffith 1978). In the US, particularly in regions with an excess number of hospital beds, hospitals have developed 'marketing strategies' to compete for patients (and physicians) based in part on service area statistics.

In both the UK and the US, as in other industrialized countries, the emphasis in regional health planning has been on assessing the health needs of a population and then allocating resources to meet those needs most effectively. Operational research models have been used both in the needs assessment and in the resources allocation phases of this process. The analysis of ambulance systems has engendered such an extensive literature that I treat it as a separate planning area. There are few examples of operational research models applicable to the planning needs of developing countries, except in the area of epidemic control, discussed below.

### Population-based needs assessment

Most planning projects start with an estimate of future needs. Because the determination of health needs has proved to be exceptionally difficult, planners have used past utilization (or demand) for health services as a surrogate for needs. Many economists believe that demand, not need, is the most appropriate yardstick for measuring and allocating medical care. Williams (1974), however, finds the classical economic concept of demand inadequate and concludes that some of the issues raised by 'needologists' have merit. Multivariate statistical and econometric methods have been widely used to project future demand for health care from past usage and a few population characteristics such as age, sex, and socio-economic status (Rosenthal 1964; Wirick 1966; Dove and Ritchie 1972).

Several studies have used probability models, usually Markov models, to predict the need or demand for particular medical services (Navarro 1969; Liebman and Logan 1976). Smallwood et al. (1971) proposed a semi-Markov model of 'disease dynamics' which could be used to project need for nursing or medical care. The full implementation of this model would require data on the dynamics of scores of disease groupings, however, and this limits its practicability.

Another approach to assessing needs has been the use of hybrid models, combining traditional epidemiological methods and data with probability models linking the incidence or prevalence of disease with the need for health services. The IIASA Health Care Systems Modelling Team used this approach (Shigan et al. 1979). Roberts and Cretin (1980) use life-table methods to predict the need for paediatric cardiac surgery, combining epidemiolocal data on the incidence of congenital heart disease, clinical reports on survival after surgical intervention, and subjective estimates of the fraction of patients operated on at each age. Similar models were presented in a series of reports on the use of health outcomes (usually obtained from vital statistics) as a basis for planning (Harris et al. 1977). These techniques have been used in US Health Systems Agencies (for example, Los Angeles County 1978).

### Facility location

A wide variety of operational research models have been applied to the facility location problem. Many variants of mathematical programming and network theory have been used to specify sets of hospital locations which would minimize travel time (Calvo and Marks 1973; Elshafei 1977) or maximize consumer preferences (Parker and Srinivasan 1976). Abernathy and Hershey (1972) compare the locations resulting from four different criteria for placement.

Unfortunately, the facility location problem addressed by most existing operational research models is not the problem faced by the planner. The health planner interested in where to locate facilities faces a complex problem subject to many constraints. Most facilities are not easily moved, so the question really only applies to new or replacement facilities. Even so, in most urban settings, the number of locations actually available for expansion is limited. An additional problem has been the failure to incorporate realistic models of patient and physician behaviour in choosing facilities.

Health maintenance organizations have spurred interest in the facility location question, not only for hospitals but for out-patient facilities, as well (Shuman et al. 1973). Dokmeci (1977) used a non-linear mathematical programming model to determine the number, size, and location of medical centres, hospitals, and health clinics. This model chose an allocation which minimized the sum of facility and transportation costs. Buchanan (1980) developed a series of algorithms for both the timing and location of expansions for HMO facilities.

### Ambulance system design and operation

Ambulance services present a number of design and operational problems. How many vehicles are needed in a region? Where should the vehicles be stationed? How should they be dispatched? In the last 15 years, all of these problems have been adressed with the help of quantitative models, usually simulation, queueing models, or network models (Savas 1969; Toregas et al. 1971; Fitzsimmons 1973; Swoveland et al. 1973; Larson 1975; Groom 1977). In addition, statistical models have been used to predict demand for emergency medical care (Kamenetzky, et al. 1982).

Analysts of ambulance systems benefited greatly from the work done in modelling other urban emergency services, mainly fire and police patrol services. Models originally developed for one service were easily adapted to another because the key elements of the systems are the same: vehicles must make their way to emergency calls which may occur at any time and from any location in the region. Although the ultimate goals of the systems are different (to reduce crime, to limit fire damage, to save lives), the operators of these systems tend to think in terms of the same intermediate objective: minimize response time. The success of operational research models in ambulance systems springs in large part from the fact that emergency medical systems administrators had an agreed upon, easily quantifiable objective which could be incorporated into a mathematical model.

In the case of ambulance systems, the good fit between the mathematical model and the real concerns of the decision-makers has borne fruit. In both the US and the UK, the recommendations resulting from ambulance system modelling have been successfully implemented (Brandeau and Larson 1978; Jarvis *et al*. 1975; Raitt 1981).

### Epidemic control

Epidemiologists and biomathematicians have used mathematical models in investigating the behaviour of epidemics since the nineteenth century (Valinsky 1975). By the late 1950s, both deterministic and probabilistic models of the spread of epidemics had been developed and refined (Abbey 1952; Bailey 1957*b*). The models were so complex that they could not be solved for realistic situations. However, computer simulations of the models were feasible (Taylor 1958; Garg *et al*. 1967; Revelle *et al*. 1969; Cvjetanovic *et al*. 1972; Coffey 1973; Elveback *et al*. 1976).

The more recent work on modelling epidemic control programmes has included an economic component, evaluating the costs of various control strategies as well as the cost of the epidemic (Chorba and Sanders 1971; Horowitz and Montgomery 1974; Frerichs and Prawda 1975). Simulations of epidemics are closer to dynamic system simulations than to the usual Monte Carlo simulation based on a queueing model. Differential equations or difference equations are often incorporated to model disease incubation periods and lags in the effectiveness of control programmes.

### Clinical decision-making

The study of medical decision-making has blossomed in the last decade. Applications of operational research methods, especially decision analysis, to the diagnosis and treatment of disease are described in several texts (Lusted 1968; Barnoon and Wolfe 1972; Weinstein *et al*. 1980). The use of statistically-based algorithms and computer-aided diagnosis are widely reported in the medical literature (for example, Walmsley *et al*. 1977; Pozen *et al*. 1980; Christiansen-Szalanski *et al*. 1982). In addition, simulation studies, Fourier analysis, and other mathematical techniques are used in the interpretation of data from electrocardiograms (Wolf *et al*. 1977), X-rays (Chan and Doi 1981; Kalender 1981; Kulkarni 1981) and CAT scans (Willis *et al*. 1981).

The early applications of decision analysis to problems of medical management had a distinctly academic air. While physicians try to decide each case on its individual characteristics, the decision analyst seemed to approach clinical decision-making on an aggregate basis, as if there was only one 'best answer' which applied over the whole population. Recently, the emphasis has shifted to the development of interactive tools to assist the physician decision-maker (Pauker and Kassirer 1981). There is some indication that these tools are most useful to physicians-in-training (Walmsley *et al*. 1977; Goldman *et al*. 1981). Clinical decision-making methods have also been extended to quality of care assessment (Greenfield *et al*. 1982). With the growing availability of computer systems in hospitals, the place of computer-based decision aids in medical training and medical practice seems assured.

### Programme evaluation and policy analysis

The most important public health decisions are those involving the future directions for national health policy. The way in which health care is financed, for example, has consequences for the health and finances of a nation. Decisions regarding national policy on screening or treatment for a specific disease or decisions on which types of biomedical research to fund may also have major impact on the public's health. These policy decisions are, almost by definition, complex. Decision-makers at this level often confront conflicting objectives, competing interest groups, and divergent views of justice, equity, and human behaviour.

What role, if any, can operational research play in the resolution of policy debates? Few analysts (and fewer decision-makers) believe that a mathematical model can generate optimal (or even acceptable) solutions to such complex decisions. However, many analysts (and a few decision-makers) now believe that mathematical models can be useful in organizing the problem, analysing relevant data, and evaluating the readily quantified consequences of an action.

Most examples of operational research models used in policy analysis involve interdisciplinary projects. Economic and political theories are usually incorporated, as are epidemiological and statistical models. In some of these analyses, operational research plays a relatively minor role; in others, the operational research component is the means for organizing contributions from other fields. In a few examples, the entire analysis revolves around a particular mathematical approach, such as Markov models, dynamic system simulations or integer programming. Many economic analyses of health care financing and health insurance use simulation (for example, Drabek *et al*. 1974; Feldman and Dowd 1982).

Whether simple or complex, the models are rarely intended to be used as decision-making machines. Rather they are designed for use in an iterative or interactive mode as an aid to effective decision-making. While this caveat applies to every application of operational research, it is especially pertinent when reviewing policy models.

The allocation of research grants in biomedical and health services research was an early area of interest. Utility theory, economic theory, and other scaling techniques were suggested as means to develop funding priorities (Stimson 1969; Keeler 1970; Cutler *et al*. 1973). Shachtman (1980) reports a decision analysis which helped secure funding for a national survey on nosocomial infection. In the United States, the continuing study of the peer review process (Carter 1974) and the use of consensus panels at the National Institutes of Health bear the stamp of this earlier work.

Early programme evaluation studies tended to use 'pure' operational research models. Markov models were proposed as a general approach to programme evaluation (Navarro 1969; Ortiz and Parker 1971). Markov models were also poposed to evaluate mental health programmes (Trinkl 1974), tuberculosis control programmes (Bush *et al*. 1972), geriatric programmes (Meredith 1971; Burton *et al*. 1975), and as a method for generating a measure of benefit for health programmes in general (Chen *et al*. 1975). Dynamic system simulation was used to model narcotics addiction and control

(Levin *et al.* 1972), conversion to a health maintenance organization (Hirsch and Miller 1974), and the delivery of dental care (Hirsch and Killingsworth 1975). Mathematical programming models have been used to analyse a voucher system for financing medical care (Whipple 1975). Chen and Bush (1976) used 0–1 integer programming to specify which groups should be screened for phenylketonuria or tuberculosis.

Some of these early simple models have been the foundation for more complex, interdisciplinary models. Burton's Markov model of geriatric care has subsequently evolved into a complex methodology for planning geriatric care (Burton and Dellinger 1981). Boldy and colleagues (1981) describe the 'balance of care' model used to assist the UK in allocating resources among various health and social services. Although this is not an optimization model, it grew out of a traditional mathematical programming approach to resource allocation (McDonald *et al.* 1974). Both the geriatric care model and the balance of care model have been used by decision-making agencies.

Nursing homes and long-term care have attracted considerable interest in the US. Willemain (1980) has used modelling to predict the effects of two different reimbursement strategies in nursing homes. Keeler and colleagues (1981) used simple models to explore the mix of long-stay patients in nursing homes.

Case mix in hospitals has been the subject of a series of studies by a group at Yale University (Fetter *et al.* 1980). This work resulted in a set of diagnosis-related groups which form the basis for an experimental hospital reimbursement scheme now being tested in New Jersey. Klastorin (1982) proposes a very different approach to grouping hospitals for reimbursement or cost-containment purposes. Cluster analysis is used to group hospitals on the basis of price-related variables (prices of inputs, degree of union involvement, urban versus rural setting).

Several studies have used probability and statistical models to organize a large body of inconclusive scientific data bearing on a policy issue. Cretin (1974, 1977) reviewed the clinical literature on the effectiveness of prehospital cardiac care and hospital coronary care units, and then used a hypothetical life table to evaluate the effectiveness of prehospital versus in-hospital care in terms of life-years saved. Weinstein and Stason (1976) used a similar approach in comparing strategies for the screening and treatment of hypertension. They incorporate techniques from decision analysis to arrive at 'quality adjusted life years'. Berwick *et al.* (1980) reviewed the literature linking cholesterol and heart disease, and analysed alternative policies for screening and treating hypercholesterolaemic children. Eddy (1980) developed a generic Markov model for analysing cancer screening programmes. Using data from the clinical literature to estimate the parameters for specific cancers, he then estimated optimal screening strategies for several major cancers.

Policy models that incorporate extensive reviews of the clinical and epidemiological data can serve two purposes. First, the models can help the policy-maker distill the scientific data. This is especially useful when there is an extensive and apparently contradictory body of work. Second, the models can help in identifying the strengths and weaknesses of the scientific evidence, suggesting directions for future studies. Such work has already highlighted one important fact – unanswered questions which are critical to the development of sound public policy in an area are not necessarily the questions of most interest to scientists or clinicians.

This review of health applications of operational research has been of necessity incomplete. The bibliographies mentioned at the beginning of this section are good sources of additional information. In addition, the following journals often include articles using operational research methods: *Health Services Research, Medical Care, Journal of Medical Decision Making, Methods of Information in Medicine*. Operational research journals may also contain reports of health applications, especially *Management Science, Operations Research, Journal of Operational Research,* and *Operational Research Quarterly*. Unfortunately, selection of reports for publication is often based on the originality of the modelling approach rather than on utility of the model to the decision-maker. Many good accounts of implementations of operational research receive limited distribution as technical reports.

## PROBLEMS AND PROSPECTS

Applications of operational research to public health problems have enjoyed mixed success. Operational research analysts and public health practitioners have worried over the discrepancy between the many published accounts of health applications and the few successful implementations. The problem is a reflection of the gap between academic operational research (theory) and applied operational research (practice) which exists in all areas of application. However, the usual difficulties take a special form in health care systems.

One problem, partly semantic and partly practical, is the notion of 'optimization' inherent in many mathematical models. Models that optimize are necessarily limited to a single measure of effectiveness. The concepts of 'maximize' and 'minimize' run into difficulty when more than one variable is involved. It is easy to identify the tallest person in a room (the one of maximum height) or the heaviest person (the one of maximum weight). If, however, we define 'bigness' as a two part concept involving weight and height, we may not be able to identify the 'biggest' person (unless the tallest is also the heaviest).

The world of public health seems inherently multidimensional. The outcomes of disease inevitably encompass mortality, morbidity, and costs. The goals of health agencies are most often in terms of balancing several outcomes, not in terms of maximizing or minimizing a single variable. We strive for complete physical, psychological, and social well-being, or for the best possible medical care at the least possible cost. Operational researchers have been quick to point out the logical impossibility of such goals and to recast the goal into logically acceptable form – minimize the cost of care subject to certain constraints. While such a formulation may, in fact, be adequate for the problem at hand, there is a fundamental difference between the concepts of optimization and balancing which the operational researcher needs to acknowledge.

The analyst also needs to acknowledge that solutions which are optimal in the model are not necessarily optimal in the world. The model is an imperfect representation of the real problem, and it is crucial to test the sensitivity of an 'optimal' solution to assumptions and parameters in the model which may well be wrong. For this reason, the best use of operational research models, including optimization models, may be in an interactive mode or, as Boldy (1981) terms it, a 'what-if' mode. This may help humble the analyst who claims to have an optimal solution and raise healthy scepticism in the decision-maker anxious to believe the claim.

A second difficulty arises because different observers have different opinions about whether health services are inputs to or outputs from the medical care system. Epidemiologists, for example, tend to treat medical services as inputs (or costs) which will eventually produce improved health status as an output (or benefit). Health administrators are more likely to take personnel and facilities as inputs which produce health services as outputs. Operational research studies have tended to follow the latter perspective. Both points of view are valid. However, when differences in perspective are not explicitly recognized, conflict and poor communication may result.

A third result is the difficulty in quantifying many important parameters. While some analysts think the main difficulty has been too little quantification – that is, reluctance of health practitioners to clear up fuzzy thinking and put a number on some factor – I believe that there has also been too much misleading quantification.

It is relatively easy to quantify concrete things by counting, weighing, or measuring. However, some of the concepts involved in health and the delivery of health services are quite abstract: patient satisfaction, quality of care, and health status, for example. The simplicity of the labels belie the richness of the underlying concepts. It is tempting to believe that any concept described by a single word or phrase can automatically be captured by a single number. Unfortunately, this is not the case.

When a concept, such as quality of care, can only be realistically represented by an elaborate measurement scheme, it is appropriate to look for simpler, approximate representations. The problem is that approximation of complex concepts has not always been carried out responsibly. This is not solely a problem of operational research and Gould (1981) gives a thorough analysis of the misuse of measures of intelligence.

A good approximation should retain the essential while cutting away the non-essential. This requires that the essential part of a concept be identified with the application in mind. The most critical component of the quality of medical care is different in an emergency department and a nursing home. Approximations are often chosen with little consideration of their appropriateness, but rather because the data were readily available. The problem of using less than adequate approximations is compounded when the analysts fail to distinguish clearly between the underlying concept and the approximate measure. The danger is that the analyst and the decision-maker may come to believe that this measure is the concept.

The fourth problem arises in all applications of operational research. Operational research is supposed to be a service to a decision-maker. Models are meant to solve the problems perceived by the manager of the system. There is a tendency,

especially among academic operational researchers, to solve problems of interest to the analyst. This problem was exacerbated in health applications of operational research in the United States by the manner in which much of the early work was funded. Individual hospitals, by and large, did not see the possibilities for quantitative analysis. Major funding was through research grants to the analysts. The hope was that these research projects would demonstrate the value of operational research in health, and lead operating institutions to fund their own operational research units. This has happened, but very slowly. Many of the projects were never implemented or only implemented with half-hearted support from key decision-makers in the organization studied.

Despite these problems, operational research has now become an accepted part of public health, particularly health administration. The maturation and expansion of health operational research has undoubtedly benefited from the expanding role of computers in hospitals. The presence of computers in hospitals encourages the development of more ambitious models which can only be implemented with the help of computers. In addition, the use of the computer to collect and store information in hospitals gives the analyst access to data which was previously unavailable or at least difficult to extract. The ready access to clinical information has contributed to the rapid growth of clinical decision models and computer-aided diagnosis.

Clinicians and administrators have gradually learned the value and the limitations of operational research. Operational researchers have come to respect the uniqueness and complexity of the health field. This atmosphere of mutual respect and realistic expectations bodes well for the effectiveness of future collaborations.

## REFERENCES

Abbey, H. (1952). An examination of the Reed–Frost theory of epidemics. *Hum. Biol.* **24**, 20.

Abernathy, W. and Hershey, J. (1972). A spatial-allocation model for regional health services planning. *Operations Res.* **20**, 629.

Ackoff, R. L. and Rivett, P. (1962). *A manager's guide to operations research.* Wiley, New York.

Bailey, N.T.J. (1951). On assessing the efficiency of single-room provision of hospital wards. *J. Hygiene* **49**, 452.

Bailey, N.T.J. (1952). A study of queues and appointment systems in outpatient departments, with special reference to waiting times. *J. R. Stat. Soc.* (B) **14**, 185.

Bailey, N.T.J. (1954). Queueing for medical care. *Appl. Stat.* **3**, 137.

Bailey, N.T.J. (1956). Statistics in hospital planning and design. *Appl. Stat.* **5**, 146.

Bailey, N.T.J. (1957*a*). Operational Research in hospital planning and design. *Operational Res. Q.* **8**, 149.

Bailey, N.T.J. (1957*b*). *The mathematical theory of epidemics.* Griffin, London.

Bailey, N.T.J. (1964). *The elements of stochastic processes with applications to the natural sciences.* Wiley, New York.

Barnoon, S. and Wolfe, H. (1972). *Measuring the effectiveness of medical decisions: an operations research approach.* Thomas, Springfield, Illinois.

Berwick, D.M., Cretin, S., and Keeler, E.B. (1980). *Cholesterol, children and heart disease: an analysis of alternatives.* Oxford University Press, New York.

Bianco White, M.F. and Pike, M.C. (1964). Appointment systems in outpatient clinics and the effect of patients' unpunctuality. *Med. Care* **2**, 133.

Boldy, D. (1976). A review of application of mathematical programming to tactical and strategic health and social service problems. *Operational Res.* **27**, 439.

Boldy, D.P. (1981). *Operational research applied to health services.* St. Martin's Press, New York.

Boldy, D., Canvin, R., Russell, J., and Royston, G. (1981). Planning the balance of care. In Operational research applied to health services (ed. D. Boldy) p. 84. St. Martin's Press, New York.

Boldy, D. and Clayden, D. (1979). Operational research projects in health and welfare services in the United Kingdom and Ireland. *J. Operational Res. Soc.* **30**, 505.

Boldy, D.P. and O'Kane, P.C. (1982). Health operational research – a selective overview. *Eur. J. Operational Res.* **10**, 1.

Brandeau, M. and Larson, R.C. (1978). *Implementing the hypercube queueing model to plan ambulance districts in Boston.* Report PPR 7804. Public Systems Evaluation, Inc., Cambridge, Mass.

Brockmeyer, E., Halstrom, H.L., and Jensen, A. (1948). *The life and works of A.K. Erlang.* Trans. Danish Acad. Tech Sci. No. 2. Copenhagen.

Buchanan, J. (1980). Planning inpatient capacity expansion in health maintenance organisations. Unpublished dissertation. Graduate School of Management, University of California, Los Angeles.

Buffa, E.S. (1968). *Production-inventory systems: planning and control.* Irwin, Homewood, Illinois.

Burton, R.M., Damon, W.W., and Dellinger, D.C. (1975). Patient states and the technology matrix. *Interfaces* **5**, 43.

Burton, R.M. and Dellinger, D.C. (1981). Planning the care of the elderly. In *Operational research applied to health services* (ed. D. Boldy) p. 129. St. Martin's Press, New York.

Bush, J. W., Fanshel, S., and Chen, M.M. (1972). Analysis of a tuberculin testing program using a health status index. *Socio-Economic Planning Sci.* **7**, 49.

Calvo, A. and Marks, D.H. (1973). Location of health care facilities: an analytic approach. *Socio-Econ. Planning Sci.* **7**, 407.

Carter, G. M. (1974). *Peer review, citations and biomedical research policy: N.I.H. grants to medical school faculty.* R-1583-HEW. Rand Corporation, Santa Monica, California.

Chan, H.P. and Doi, K. (1981). Monte Carlo simulation studies of backscatter factors in mammography. *Radiol.* **139**, 195.

Chen, M.M. and Bush, J.W. (1976). A mathematical programming approach for selecting an optimal health program case mix. *Inquiry* **13**, 215.

Chen, M.M., Bush, J.W., and Patrick, D.L. (1975). Social indicators for health planning and policy analysis. *Pol. Sci.* **6**, 71.

Chiang, C.L. (1968). *Introduction to stochastic processes in biostatistics.* Wiley, New York.

Chorba, R.W. and Sanders, J.L. (1971). Planning models for tuberculosis control programs. *Health Serv. Res.* **6**, 144.

Christensen-Szalanski, J.J., Diehr, P.H., Wood, R.W., and Tomkins, R.K. (1982). Phased trial of a proven algorithm at a new primary care clinic. *Am. J. Public Health* **72**, 16.

Coffey, R.J. (1973). Model of communicable diseases spread in a rural population. In *Health care delivery planning* (ed. A. Reisman and M. Kiley) p. 287. Gordon and Breach Science Publishers, New York.

Cooper, R.N. (1972). *Introduction to queueing theory.* Macmillan, New York.

Cox, D.R. and Miller, H.D. (1965). *Theory of stochastic processes.* Wiley, New York.

Cox, D.R. and Smith, W.L. (1961). *Queues.* Chapman and Hall, London.

Cretin, S. (1974). *A model of the risk of death from myocardial infarction.* Innovative Resource Planning Project Technical Report No. TR-09-74. MIT Operations Research Center, Cambridge, Massachusetts.

Cretin, S. (1977). Cost/benefit analysis of treatment and prevention of myocardial infarction. *Health Serv. Res.* **12**, 174.

Cutler, R.S., Martino, V.A., and Webb, A.M. (1973). Biomedical research relevance assessment. In *Health care delivery planning* (ed. A. Reisman and M. Kiley) p. 89. Gordon and Breach Science Publishers, New York.

Cvietanovic, B., Grab, B., Uemura, K., and Butchenko, B. (1972). Epidemiological model of tetanus and its use in the planning of immunization programmes. *Int. J. Epidemiol.* **1**, 125.

Dantzig, G.B. (1963). *Linear programming and extensions.* Princeton University Press, Princeton, New Jersey.

Denison, R.A., Wild, R., and Martin, M.J.C. (1969). *A bibliography of operational research in hospitals and the health services.* University of Bradford Management Centre, Bradford, England.

Dokmeci, V.F. (1977). A quantitative model to plan regional health facility systems. *Management Sci.* **24**, 411.

Dove, H.G. and Richie, C.G. (1972). Predicting hospital admission by state. *Inquiry* **9**, 51.

Dowling, W.L. (1971). The application of linear programming to decision-making in hospitals. *Hosp. Admin.* **16**, 66.

Drabek, L., Intriligator, M.D., and Kimbell, L.J. (1974). *A forecasting and policy simulation model of the health care sector.* Lexington Books, Lexington, Massachusetts.

Drake, A.W. (1967). *Fundamentals of applied probability theory.* McGraw-Hill, New York.

Duckworth, W.E., Gear, A.E., and Lockett, A.G. (1977). *A guide to operational research,* 3rd edn, Chapman and Hall, London.

Eddy, D.M. (1980). *screening for cancer: theory analysis and design.* Prentice Hall, Englewood Cliffs, New Jersey.

Elshafei, A.N. (1977). Hospital layout as a quadratic assignment problem. *Operational Res. Q.* **28**, 167.

Elston, R.C. and Pickrel, J.C. (1963). A statistical approach to ordering and usage policies for a hospital blood bank. *Transfusion* **3**, 41.

Elveback, L.R., Fox, J.P., Ackerman, E., langworthy, A., Boyd, M., and Gatewood, L. (1976). An influenza simulation model for immunization studies. *Am. J. Epidemiol.* **103**, 152.

Emshoff, J.R. and Sisson, R.L. (1970). *Design and use of computer simulation models.* MacMillan, New York.

Esogbue, A. (1969). Dynamic programming and optimal control of variable multichannel stochiastic service systems with applications. *Mathematical Biosci.* **5** 133.

Esogbue, A. and Singh, A.J. (1976). A stochiastic model for an optimal priority bed distribution problem in a hospital ward. *Operations Res.* **24**, 884.

Feldman, R.D. and Dowd, B.E. (1982). Simulation of a health insurance market with adverse selection. *Operations Res.* **30**, 1027.

Feller, W. (1968). *An introduction to probability theory and its applications.* Vol. 1, 3rd edn. Wiley, New York.

Fetter, R. B. and Thompson, J.D. (1965). The simulation of hospital systems. *Operations Res.* **13**, 689.

Fetter, R.B. and Thompson, J.D. (1966). Patients' waiting time and doctors' idle time in the outpatient setting. *Health Serv. Res.* **1**, 66.

Fetter, R., Shin, Y., Freeman, J., Averill, R., and Thompson, J. (1980). Case mix definition by diagnosis related groups. *Med. Care* **18**, 2 suppl., 1.

Fitzsimmons, J. (1973). A methodology for emergency ambulance deployment. *Management Sci.* **19**, 627.

Flagle, C.D. (1960). The problem of organization for inpatient care. In *Management science: models and techniques* (ed. C.W. Churchman and M. Verhulst) Vol. 2. Pergamon Press, New York.

Flagle, C.D. (1962). Operations research in the health services. *Operations Res.* **10**, 591.

Flagle, C.D. (1967). A decade of operations research in health. In *New methods of thought and procedure* (ed. F. Zwicky and A.G. Wilson) p. 33. Springer, New York.

Ford, L.R. Jr and Fulkerson, D.R. (1962). *Flows in networks.* Princeton University Press, Princeton, New Jersey.

Forrester, J. (1961). *Industrial dynamics.* MIT Press, Cambridge, Mass.

Frerichs, R. and Prawda, J. (1975). A computer simulation model for the control of rabies in an urban area of Colombia. *Management Sci.* **22**, 411.

Fries, B.E. (1976). Bibliography of operations research in health care systems. *Operations Res.* **24**, 801.

Fries, B.E. (1979). Bibliography of operations research in health care systems: an update. *Operations Res.* **27**, 408.

Fries, B.E. (1981). *Applications of operations research to health care delivery systems.* Springer, Berlin.

Fries, B.E. and Marathe, V.P. (1981). Determination of optimal variable-sized multiple-block appointment systems. *Operations Res.* **29**, 324.

Garfinkel, R.S. and Nemhauser, G.L. (1972). *Integer programming.* Wiley, New York.

Garg, M.L., Thompson, D.J., and Gezon, H.M. (1967). Assessing the influence of treatment on the spread of staphylococci in newborn infants by simulation *Am. J. Epidemiol.* **85**, 220.

Goldman, J. and Knappenberger, H.A. (1968). How to determine the optimum number of operating rooms. *Modern Hosp.* **111**, 114.

Goldman, L., Waternaux, C., Garfield, F. *et al.* (1981). Impact of a cardiology data bank on physicians' prognostic estimates — evidence that cardiology fellows change their estimates to become as accurate as the faculty. *Arch. Intern. Med.* **141**, 1631.

Gould, S.J. (1981). *The mismeasure of man.* Norton, New York.

Greenfield, S.G., Cretin, S., Worthman, L., and Dorey, F. (1982). The use of an ROC curve to express quality of care results. *Med. Decision Making* **2**, 13.

Griffiths, J.R. (1978). *Measuring hospital performance.* An Inquiry Book, Blue Cross Association, Chicago.

Griffith, J.R., Munson, F.C., and Hancock, W.M. (1975). *Cost control in hospitals.* Health Administration Press, Ann Arbor, Michigan.

Groom, K.N. (1977). Planning emergency ambulance services. *Operational Res. Q.* **28**, 641.

Gupta, I., Zareda, J., and Kramer, N. (1971). Hospital manpower planning by use of queuing theory. *Health Serv. Res.* **6**, 76.

Hammerslev, J.M. and Handscomb, D.C. (1964). *Monte Carlo methods.* Methuen, London.

Harris, L.J., Keeler, E.B., Kisch, A.E., Michnich, M.E., de Sola, S.F., and Drew, D.E. (1977). *Algorithms for planners: an overview.* R-2215/1. Rand Corporation, Santa Monica, California.

Henderson, K.M. (1976). Some aspects of clinic management. In *Selected papers on operational research in the health services* (ed. B. Barber) p. 161. Operational Research Society, Birmingham.

Hershey, J.C., Abernathy, W.A., and Baloff, N. (1974). Comparison of nurse allocation policies — a Monte Carlo model. *Decision Sci.* **5**, 58.

Hershey, J., Pierskalla, W., and Wandel, S. (1981). Nurse staffing management. In *Operational research applied to health services* (ed. D. Boldy) p. 189. St. Martin's Press, New York.

Hillier, F.S. and Lieberman, G.J. (1974). *Operations research,* 2nd edn. Holden-Day, San Francisco.

Hirsch, G.B. and Killingsworth, W.R. (1975). A new framework for projecting dental manpower requirements. *Inquiry* **12**, 126.

Hirsch, G.B. and Miller, S. (1974). Evaluating HMO policies with a computer simulation model. *Med. Care* **12**, 668.

Horowitz, J.S. and Montgomery, D.C. (1974). A computer simulation model of a rubella epidemic. *Comput. Biomed. Res.* **4**, 188.

Horvath, W.J. (1965). British experience with operations research in the health services. In *Medical care research* (ed. K.L. White) p. 55. Pergamon press, New York.

Horvath, W.J. (1967). Operations research in medical and hospital practice. In *Operations research for public systems* (ed. P.M. Morse) p. 127. MIT Press, Cambridge, Mass.

Howard, R. (1960). *Dynamic programming and Markov processes.* MIT Press, Cambridge, Mass.

Howard, R. (1971). *Dynamic probabilistic systems.* Vols I and II. Wiley, New York.

James, S., Outten, W., Davis, P.J., and Wands, J. (1974). House staff scheduling: a computer-aided method. *Ann. Intern. Med.* **80**, 70.

Jarvis, J.P., Stevenson, K.A., and Willemain, T.R. (1975). *A simple procedure for the allocation of ambulances in semi-rural areas.* Technical report TR-13-75. MIT Operations Research Center, Cambridge, Mass.

Jeans, W.D., Berger, S.R., and Gill, R. (1972). Computer simulation model of an x-ray department. *Br. Med. J.* **i**, 674.

Jennings, J.B. (1973). Blood bank inventory control. *Management Sci.* **19**, 637.

Johnson, W.L. and Rosenfeld, L.S. (1968). Factors affecting waiting time in ambulatory care services. *Health Serv. Res.* **3**, 286.

Kalender, W. (1981). Monte Carlo calculations of x-ray scatter data for diagnostic radiology. *Phys. Med. Biol.* **26**, 835.

Kamenetzky, R.D., Shuman, L.J., and Wolfe, H. (1982). Estimating need and demand for prehospital care. *Operations Res.* **30**, 1148.

Kane, R., Solomon, D., Beck, J., Keeler, E., and Kane, R. (1980). The future need for geriatric manpower in the United States. *New Engl. J. Med.* **302**. 1327.

Kao, E.P.C. (1972). A semi-Markov model to predict recovery progress of coronary patients. *Health Serv. Res.* **7**, 191.

Kao, E.P.C. and Pokladnik, F.M. (1978). Incorporating exogenous factors in adaptive forecasting of hospital census. *Management Sci.* **24**, 1677.

Kastner, G.T. and Shachtman, R.H. (1982). A stochastic model to measure patient effects stemming from hospital acquired infections. *Operations Res.* **30**, 1105.

Keeler, E. (1970). *Models of disease costs and their use in medical research resource allocation.* Rand Corporation, Santa Monica, California.

Keeler, E.B., Kane, R.L., and Solomon, D.H. (1981). Short- and long-term residents of nursing homes. *Med. Care* **19**, 363.

Keeney, R.L. (1982). Decision analysis: an overview. *Operations Res.* **30**, 803.

Keller, T.F. and Laughhunn, D.J. (1973). An application of queuing theory to a congestion problem in an out-patient clinic. *Decision Sci.* **4**, 379.

Kilpatrick, K.E. and Freund, L.E. (1967). A simulation of oxygen tank inventory at a community general hospital. *Health Serv. Res.* **2**, 298.

Kiviat, P.J., Villaneauva, R., and Markowitz, H. (1969). *The SIMSCRIPT II programming language.* Prentice-Hall, Englewood Cliffs, New Jersey.

Klastorin, T.D. (1982). An alternative method for hospital partition determination using hierarchical cluster analysis. *Operations Res.* **30**, 1134.

Kleinrock, L. (1975). *Queueing systems.* Wiley, New York.

Kolesar, P. (1970). A Markovian model for hospital admission scheduling. *Management Sci.* **18**, B374.

Krischer, J.P. (1980). An annotated bibliography of decision analytic applications to health care. *Operations Res.* **28**, 97.

Kulkarni, R.N. (1981). Monte Carlo calculation of the dose distribution across a plane bone-marrow interface during diagnostic x-ray examinations. *Br. J. Radiol.* **54**, 875.

Kwak, N.K., Kuzdrall, P.J., and Schmitz, H.H. (1976). A GPSS simulation of scheduling policies for surgical patients. *Management Sci.* **22**, 982.

Larson, R. (1975). Approximating the performance of urban emergency service systems. *Operations Res.* **22**, 845.

Larson, R.C. and Odoni, A.R. (1981). *Urban operations research.* Prentice-Hall, Englewood Cliffs, New Jersey.

Levin, G., Hirsch, G., and Roberts, E. (1972). Narcotics and the community: a system simulation. *Am. J. Public Health* **62**, 861.

Liebman, J.S. and Logan, E. (1976). Analyzing the start-up effects of new patients on an ambulatory care program. *Med. Care* **14**, 839.

Los Angeles County (1978). *Health systems plan component, cardiovascular surgery and cardiac cathetarization services.* Health Systems Agency, Los Angeles.

Luce, R.D. and Raiffa, H. (1957). *Games and decisions.* Wiley, New York.

Luck, G.M., Luckman, J., Smith, B.W., and Stringer, J. (1971). *Patients, hospitals and operational research.* Tavistock publications, London.

Luenberger, D.G. (1973). *Introduction to linear and nonlinear programming.* Addison-Wesley, Reading, Mass.

Lusted, L.B. (1968). *Introduction to medical decision making.* Thomas, Springfield, Illinois.

McLaughlin, C.p. (1970). Health operations research and systems analysis literature. In *Systems and medical care* (ed. A. Sheldon, F. Baker, and C.P. McLaughlin) p. 27. MIT Press, Cambridge, Mass.

Maier-Rothe, C. and Wolfe, H.B. (1973). Cyclical scheduling and allocation of nursing staffing. *Socio-Econ. Planning Sci.* **7**, 471.

Manton, K.G., Tolley, H.D., and Poss, S.S. (1976) Life table techniques for multiple cause mortality. *Demography* **13**, 541.

Meade, J. (1974). A mathematical model for deriving hospital service areas. *Int. J. Health Serv.* **4**, 353.

McDonald, A.G., Cuddeford, G.C., and Beale, E.M.L. (1974). Balance of care: some mathematical models of the National Health Service. *Br. Med. Bull.* **30**, 262.

Meredith, J. (1971). A Markovian analysis of a geriatric ward. *Management Sci.* **19**, 604.

Moder, J.J. and Phillips, C.R. (1970). *Project management with CPM and PERT,* 2nd edn. Van Nostrand, New York.

Morse, P.M. and Kimball, G.E. (1951). *Methods of operations research,* 1st edn, revised. MIT Press, Cambridge, Mass.

Myers, J.E., Johnson, R.E., and Egan, D.M. (1972). A computer simulation of outpatient pharmacy operations. *Inquiry* **9**, 40.

Navarro, V. (1969). Planning personal health services: a Markovian model. *Med. Care* **7**, 242.

Newell, D.J. (1954). Provision of emergency beds in hospitals. *Br. J. Prev. Soc. Med.* **8**, 77.

Newell, G.F. (1971). *Applications of queueing theory.* Chapman and Hall, London.

Nuffield Provincial Hospitals Trust (1955). *Studies in the functions and design of hospitals.* Oxford University Press, London.

Nuffield Provincial Hospitals Trust (1962). *Towards a clearer view: the organization of diagnostic x-ray departments.* Oxford University Press, London.

Nuffield Provincial Hospitals Trust (1965). *Waiting in out-patient departments.* Oxford University Press, London.

O'Kane, P.C. (1981). Hospital studies. In *Operational research applied to health services* (ed. D. Boldy) p. 159. St. Martin's Press, New York.

Ortiz, J. and Parker, R. (1971). A birth-life-death model for planning and evaluating of health service programs. *Health Serv. Res.* **6**, 120.

Parker, B.R. and Srinivasan, V. (1976). A consumer preference approach to the planning of rural primary health-care facilities. *Operations Res.* **24**, 991.

Parzen, E. (1960). *Modern probability theory and its application.* Wiley, New York.

Pauker, S.G. and Kassirer, J.P. (1981). Clinical decision analysis by personal computer. *Arch. Intern. Med.* **141**, 1831.

Pocock, J.W. (1962). PERT as an analytical aid for program planning – its payoff and problems. *Operations res.* **10**, 893.

Pozen, M.W., D'Agostino, R.B., Mitchell, J.B. *et al.* (1980). The usefulness of a predictive instrument to reduce inappropriate admissions to the coronary care unit. *Ann. Intern. Med.* **92**, 238.

Pritsker, A.A.B. (1973). *The GASP IV user's manual.* Pritsker and Associates, West Lafayette, Indiana.

Raiffa, H. (1968). *Decision analysis.* Addison-Wesley, Reading, Mass.

Raitt, R. (1981). Ambulance service planning. In *Operational research applied to health services* (ed. D. Boldy) p. 239. St. Martin's Press, New York.

Rath, G.L., Balbas, J.M.A., Ikeda, T., and Kennedy, G.O. (1970). Simulation of a hematology department. *Health Serv. Res.* **5**, 25.

ReVelle, C.S., Feldmann, F., and Lynn, W. (1969). An optimization model of tuberculosis epidemiology. *Management Sci.* **16**, B190.

ReVelle, C.S., Bigman, D., Schilling, D., Cohon, J., and Church, R: (1977). Facility location: a review of context free and EMS models. *Health Serv. Res.* **12**, 129.

Roberts, N. and Cretin, S. (1980). The changing face of congenital heart disease. *Med. Care* **18**, 930.

Rockart, J.F. and Hoffman, P.B. (1969). Physician and patient behavior under different scheduling systems in a hospital outpatient department. *Med. Care* **7**, 463.

Rockwell, T.H., Barnum, R.A., and Giffin, W.C. (1962). Inventory analysis applied to hospital whole blood supply and demand. *J. Ind. Engineering* **13**, 109.

Rosenthal, G.D. (1964). *The demand for general hospital facilities.* Hospital Monograph Series No. 14. American Hospital Association, Chicago.

Ross, S. (1970). *Applied probability models with optimization applications.* Holden-Day, San Francisco.

Ross, S. (1972). *Introduction to probability models.* Academic Press, New York.

Rubenstein, L.S. (1976). *Compurerized hospital inpatient admissions scheduling system—a model.* No. 76-9010. University Microfilms International, Ann Arbor, Michigan.

Savas, E.S. (1969). Simulation and cost-effectiveness analysis of New York's emergency ambulance service. *Management Sci.* **15**, B608

Shachtman, R.H. (1980). Decision analysis assessment of a national medical study. *Operations Res.* **28**, 44.

Shigan, E.N., Hughes, D.J., and Kitsul, P.J. (1979). *Health care systems modeling at IIASA: a status report.* SR-79-4. International Institute for Applied systems Analysis, Laxenburg, Austria.

Shonick, W. and Jackson, J.R. (1973). An improved stochastic model for occupancy-related random variables in general-acute hospitals. *Operations Res.* **21**, 952.

Shuman, L.J., Hardwick, P., and Huber, G.A. (1973). Location of ambulatory care centres in a metropolitan area. *Health Serv. Res.* **8**, 121.

Shuman, L.J., Speas, R.D., and Young, J.P. (1975). *Operations research in health care: a critical analysis.* Johns Hopkins University Press, Baltimore, Md.

Smallwood, R.D., Sondik, E.J., and Offensend, F.L. (1971). Towards an integrated methodology for the analysis of health-care systems. *Operations Res.* **19**, 1300

Smith, A.G., Gregory, K., and Maguire, J.D. (1975). Operational research for the hospital supply service. *Operational Res.* **2**, 375.

Smith, W.G. and Solomon, M.B. Jr (1966). A simulation of hospital admission policy. *Communications A.C.M.* **9**, 362.

Stimson, D.H. (1969). Utility measurement in public health decision making. *Management Sci.* **16**, B17.

Stimson, D.H. and Stimson, R.H. (1972). *Operations research in hospitals: diagnosis and prognosis.* Hospital Research and Educational Trust, Chicago.

Swoveland, C., Uyeno, D., Vertinsky, I., and Vickson, R. (1973). Ambulance location: a probabilistic enumeration approach. *Management Sci.* **20**, 686.

Tarlov, A.R., (Chairman) (1980a). *Summary report,* Vol. 1. Graduate Medical Government Printing Office, Washington, DC.

Tarlov, A.R. (Chairman) (1980b). *Modeling, research and data technical panel,* Vol. 2. Graduate Medical Education National Advisory Committee. US Government Printing Office, Washington, DC.

Taylor, W.F. (1958). SOme Monte Carlo methods applied to an epidemic of acute respiratory disease. *Hum. Biol.* **30**, 185.

Thompson, J.D., Fetter, R.B., McIntosh, C.S., and Pelletier, R.J. (1963). Use of computer simulation techniques in predicting requirements for maternity facilities. *Hospitals* **37**, 132.

Toregas, C., Swain, R., ReVelle, C., and Bergman, L. (1971). The location of emergency service facilities. *Operations Res.* **19**, 1363.

Trinkl, F.H. (1974). A stochastic analysis of programs for the mentally retarded. *Operations Res.* **22**, 1175.

Trivedi, V.M. and Warner, D.M. (1976). A branch and bound algorithm for optimal allocation of float nurses. *Management Sci.* **22**, 972.

Tversky, A. and Kahneman, D. (1974). Judgement under uncertainty: heuristics and biases. *Science* **185**, 1124.

Tversky, A. and Kahneman, D. (1981). The framing of decisions and the psychology of choice. *Science* **211**, 453.

United Hospital Fund of New York (1976). *Systems analysis and the design of outpatient department appointment and information systems.* The Fund, Training Research and Special Studies Division, New York.

Valinsky, D. (1975). Simulation. In *Operations research in health care: a critical analysis* (ed. L. Shuman, R. Speas, and J. Young) p. 114. Johns Hopkins University Press, Baltimore, Md.

Veinott, A.F. Jr (1966). The status of mathematical inventory theory. *Management Sci.* **12**, 745.

Walker, W.E., Chaikan, J.M., and Ignall, E.J. (1979). *Fire department deployment analysis.* North Holland, New York.

Walmsley, G.L., Wilson, D.H., Gunn, A.A., Jenkins, D., Horrocks, J.C., and De Dombal, F.T. (1977). Computer aided diagnosis of lower abdominal pain in women. *Br. J. Surg.* **64**, 538.

Wagner, H.M. (1975). *Principles of operations research,* 2nd edn. Prentice-Hall, Englewood Cliffs, New Jersey.

Walter, S.D. (1973). A comparison of appointment schedules in a hospital radiology department. *Br. J. Prev. Soc. Med.* **27**, 160.

Warner, D.M. (1976). Scheduling nursing personnel according to nursing preference: a mathematical programming approach. *Operations Res.* **24**, 842.

Warner, D.M. and Holloway, D.C. (1978). *Decision making and control for health administration.* Health Administration Press, Ann Arbor, Michigan.

Webb, M., Stevens, G., and Bramson, C. (1977). An approach to the control of bed occupancy in a general hospital. *Operational Res.* **28**, 391.

Weinstein, M.C. and Stason, W.B. (1976). *Hypertension: a policy perspective.* Harvard University Press, Cambridge, Mass.

Weinstein, M.C., Fineberg, H.V., Elstein, A.S. *et al.* (1980). *Clinical decision analysis.* Saunders, Philadelphia.

Weiss, E.N., Cohen, M.A., and Hershey, J.C. (1982). An iterative estimation and validation procedure for specification of semi-Markov models with applications to hospital patient flow. *Operations Res.* **30**, 1082.

Welch, J.D. (1964). Appointment systems in hospital outpatient department. *Operational Res.* **15**, 224.

Welch, J.D. and Bailey, N.T.J. (1952). Appointment systems in hospital outpatient departments. *Lancet* **i**, 1105.

Whipple, D. (1973). A voucher plan for financing health care deliver. *Socio-Econ. Planning Sci.* **7**, 681.

Whitston, C.W. (1965). An analysis of the problems of scheduling surgery. *Hosp. Management* **99**, 58.

Willemain, T.R. (1974). Approximate analysis of a hierarchical queueing network. *Operations Res.* **22**, 522.

Willemain, T.R. (1980). A comparison of patient-centered and case-mix reimbursement for nursing home care. *Health Serv.* **15**, 365.

Willemain, T.R. and Larson, R.C. (eds.) (2977). *Emergency medical systems analysis.* Lexington Books, Lexington, Mass.

Williams, A. (1974). 'Need' as a demand concept (with special reference to health). In *Economic policies and social goals* (ed. A. Culyer) p. 60. Martin Robertson and Company, London.

Willis, K., du Boulay, G.H., and Teather, D. (1981). Initial findings in the computer-aided diagnosis of cerebral tumours using CT scan results. *Br. J. Radiol.* **54**, 948.

Wirick, G.C. (1966). A multiple equation model of demand for health care. *Health Serv.* **1**, 301.

Wolf, H.K., Gregor, R.D., and Chandler, B.M. (1977). Use of computers in clinical electrocardiography: an evaluation. *Can. Med. Assoc. J.* **117**, 877.

Young, J.P. (1965). Stabilization of inpatient bed occupancy through control of admission. *Hospitals* **39**, 41.

# 14 Management science and planning studies

Paul R. Torrens and Robert J. Maxwell

## HISTORY AND BACKGROUND

Until relatively recently in the history of public health, management and planning have not been formally recognized as being important to the successful control of common health problems. For generations, great attention was paid to scientific developments which put new and effective tools for the control of communicable diseases into the hands of public health workers. In more recent generations, the focus of attention has shifted to the social policy issue of assuring equal access for all the public to the benefits of these scientific discoveries.

By contrast, comparatively little attention has been paid to the techniques which would allow these scientific discoveries to be provided in a more effective or more efficient fashion. Until recently, very little formal training was provided to public health workers in the newly emergent field of management and planning, and in many cases there was a strong feeling that these new disciplines were appropriate only to large corporations and commercial enterprises, not to a human service endeavour such as public health.

This is not to say that public health workers were not actually managing or planning, or that they were not in fact using the equivalent of these techniques in their work. In retrospect, it seems clear that these processes and techniques have always been an important part of public health work but have not been recognized and valued as such. Their use has probably suffered by the lack of direct recognition of their existence and importance, but they have been utilized none the less.

In recent years, there has been a surge of interest in management and planning as legitimate aspects of public health in their own right. A special commission on higher education for public health of the Milbank Memorial Fund reported in 1976 that there seemed to be three basic knowledge areas that were central to the purposes of public health: (i) the measurement and analytical sciences of epidemiology and biostatistics; (ii) social policy and the history and philosophy of public health; (iii) principles and practice of management and organization for public health (Milbank Memorial Fund Commission 1976).

Similar surveys or studies of various aspects of public health programmes and personnel around the world, sponsored variously by the Kellogg Foundation in the US, the King's Fund in England, and the WHO in Europe, have all stressed the great importance of improved management practices throughout all areas of health care (Commission on Education for Health Administration 1975; King's Fund 1977; WHO 1976). John Evans of the World Bank, writing in 1981 in a special report for the Rockefeller Foundation, on *Measurement and Management in Medicine and Health Services,* suggests that organized health programmes around the world will not reach their fullest potential until they have the benefit of better trained and more effective managers.

In the US, since the passage of the Medicare national health insurance programme for the elderly in 1965, interest in management and planning has been very evident. Training programmes in schools of public health have greatly expanded their course offerings in management and administration, and many have encouraged their students to take additional course work in graduate schools of management (even though the latter's occasional designation as schools of 'business administration' have sometimes made this course of action seem less appropriate than it really is). Several of the major graduate schools of public health in the US (UCLA and Columbia among them) have developed joint MPH/MBA (Master of Public Health/Master of Business Administration) degree programmes that allow students to obtain graduate training and academic degrees in both public health and management. Some prominent graduate schools of management in the US, such as the Wharton School of Finance at the University of Pennsylvania, have developed programmes of management education that focus on public health and curative medicine as their primary area of interest.

This vigorous development of academic programmes has been accompanied, as one might expect, by the publication of a number of textbooks on management of health programmes. These texts range from the more general texts dealing with management principles (Levey and Loomba 1973; McCool and Brown 1977; Rakich *et al.* 1977; Kovner and Neuhauser 1978; Levey and McCarthy 1980; Longest 1980; Kaluzny *et al.* 1982), to textbooks dealing with such specialized topics as strategic planning (Flexner 1981; Fournet 1982), marketing (Cooper 1979; MacStravic 1977, 1980), quantitative methods for planning (Griffith 1972), management of human resources (Rubin *et al.* 1978), decision making and managerial control (Warner and Holloway 1978) and organizational development (Wieland 1981).

The field of public health practice has changed in a manner that parallels the changes in academic training. In the US for some years, the qualifications for major positions in local, state, or national public health agencies have not been the traditional ones of biostatistics, epidemiology, environmental engineering, and maternal and child health. Now instead, potential employers of public health practitioners look for skills in organizing budgetary projections and controlling finances, experience in long-range planning and strategy, and competence in organizational development and the leadership of people. The ability to recognize and appreciate the traditional purposes and objectives of public health are still important, but increasingly it is the ability to manage and plan for large-scale public health enterprises that is more highly valued.

Since these changes in attitude and approach to much of the practice of public health have taken place, it is important to identify and strengthen those management and planning disciplines that have become so central to effective functioning in the 'new' public health. What are these disciplines and areas of expertise in management and planning that are important to the modern public health practitioner? In particular, for the purposes of this chapter, what are those techniques of management and planning that need to be brought more firmly and directly into the centre of public health practice?

Here, we will explore those management techniques and practices which should be part of the equipment of every public health practitioner. The approach used will be first to consider those areas of knowledge, skill, or procedure that have already been identified as being important in the broader non-public health management world. Examples of their application to public health programmes will be cited wherever this has taken place, and in those cases in which little or no formal transfer has taken place, discussion will be focused on what should take place in the future. In all the discussion, attempts will be made to show the logic and general applicability of standard management principles and practice to public health, while at the same time commenting on the unique environment (public health programmes) to which they will be applied.

In the material that follows, the discussion will focus first on the nature of managerial work, particularly within the public health organization. Then the discussion will turn to the nature of organizations, particularly health care organizations. Finally, blending together what is known and what has been discussed about managers and organizations, the third section will discuss future needs in the management science and planning area as it applies to public health.

## THE NATURE OF MANAGERIAL WORK

Writing in 1980, Longest suggests that there are three ways of looking at managerial work, whether in health care programmes or in other settings, and that the appraisal of a particular manager or managerial piece of work must include all three in some form or another. The three areas of study are: (i) the *roles* a manager plays in the course of managerial work; (ii) the *functions* that a manager actually carries out in completing that work; and (iii) the *skills* that a manager must employ in completing these functions.

In the sections that follow, we will review each of these three aspects of managerial work, and then show how a knowledge of these three areas can be used to construct a means of evaluating managers and their work; to develop improved programmes for training and educating prospective managers;

and to form the basis for the improved design of managerial positions in public health organizations. Although the discussion may seem somewhat academic in places, it is important for the reader to understand each of the three areas, in order to understand and utilize the synthesis being proposed at the end of the section.

### Managerial roles

As suggested both by Longest and by Kaluzny *et al.* (1980, 1982), it is possible to learn a great deal about the nature of managerial work by understanding the various roles that a manager must assume in the course of that work. They point out that, just as an actor plays a role, a manager must adopt certain patterns of behaviour when a particular managerial position is assumed, those patterns of behaviour often arising out of the necessities of the job to be done.

The classic work in this area has been done by Mintzberg, who reviewed the various roles of managers in general and then developed a very useful typology by which to analyse the manager's work. Through intensive case studies of a set of executives in different organizational settings, he identified ten different managerial roles and then proceeded to group them into logical clusters, as summarized in Table 14.1 (Mintzberg 1973).

**Table 14.1.** *Managerial roles*

| |
|---|
| **Interpersonal roles** |
| Figurehead |
| Liaison |
| Leader |
| **Informational roles** |
| Monitor |
| Disseminator |
| Spokesperson |
| **Decisional roles** |
| Entrepreneur |
| Disturbance handler |
| Resource allocator |
| Negotiator |

Mintzberg argues that all managers have authority, either formal or informal, over the units they manage and that this authority forces them into certain *interpersonal* roles that are necessary for the successful completion of the managerial task. The first of these interpersonal roles is that of *figurehead* and refers to the manager's role as the symbolic head of the organization. In this role, the manager is obligated to perform a number of routine functions of a ceremonial, legal, or social nature, to represent the organization or unit to the outside environment whenever some official representation is required.

The second interpersonal role is that of *liaison* and refers to the need for the manager to interact with peers and with other people outside the organization to exchange information and maintain contact. This is different from the figurehead role in the sense that liaison is an active, participatory, communicative role, while the role as a figurehead is more passive and ceremonial.

The third interpersonal role identified by Mintzberg is that of *leader* and refers to the manager's role primarily within the base organization itself. In this role, the manager is seen as the primary administrative figure in the organization, the person responsible for the direction of the organization's total activities. This is different again from the figurehead role, since it is active, essential, and internal.

The second set of roles have been designated by Mintzberg as *informational,* and relate to the manager's ability to gather information, disseminate it, monitor its flow and use within the organization, and establish new sources of information as appropriate or needed.

The first informational role for the manager is that of *monitor* and refers to the manager's ability to seek and receive current information about the organization and its function; the manager thereby has a thorough understanding of the entire organization, hopefully more complete than anyone else within that organization.

The second informational role for the manager is that of *disseminator* and refers to the manager's ability to transmit factual and interpretational information to members of the organization. By the careful selection and dissemination of appropriate information, the manager can guide members of the organization to areas that are felt to be most productive, keep them away from areas of less interest, and encourage a greater involvement in the organization as a whole.

The third of this category of roles is that of *spokesperson,* and refers to the transmission of information to outsiders about the organization's work plans and operating status. This is obviously somewhat similar to the liaison role but is in fact different enough to warrant a separate role designation. It is entirely possible to serve as the liaison with another organization or group, while not passing along formal information about the base group's work plans or operating status. The liaison role can be essentially neutral with regards to the communication of information, thereby making it necessary to emphasize the spokesperson role as that of the formal communicator of detailed information outside the organization or unit.

These two key roles are really preliminary to Mintzberg's third set, which are the *decisional* roles. These are connected with the manager's ability to make and implement decisions within an organizations and to exercise real authority within that organization.

The first of these decisional roles is that of *entrepreneur* and refers to the manager's ability to initiate change within the organization, to develop new programmes or procedures, and to move the organization or unit into new activities or endeavours that should eventually benefit the organization and enhance its objectives.

The second decisional role is that of *disturbance handler* and refers to the manager's ability (and indeed, responsibility) to take corrective action when the organization faces unanticipated problems, either externally or internally. One of the manager's key roles is to identify disruptive patterns of activity or behaviour and, more appropriately, to prevent these disruptive patterns from damaging the fabric and functioning of the organization.

The third decisional role, according to Mintzberg, is that of

*resource allocator,* and refers to the manager's ability to direct the organization's resources of money, personnel, space, and equipment towards those purposes and people that are deemed most important to the organization's objectives. This is generally considered to be the source of a manager's real internal power, although many others, such as the control of information, are felt by some to be equally important.

The fourth and final decisional role is that of *negotiator,* which refers to the manager's responsibility for representing the organization at major negotiations with other organizations or groups. Again, this is a different role from that of liaison, since this is a more active posture of putting forward the organization's needs and desires, and seeking to obtain the best deal possible for that organization. It is also a different role from that of spokesperson, which is more of a passive, information-handling posture and not necessarily one of actively engaging in the bargaining and manoeuvring which characterize the negotiator role. The negotiator role seeks to obtain the best arrangement possible for the organization; it is a role that expects that a trophy or an achievement of some sort will be brought home to the organization.

Research has shown that not every managerial position includes the same set of roles to the same degree. Each managerial position requires a different 'mix' of managerial roles, and the same position may require different combinations of roles at different times. Kaluzny (1982) refers to a paper by Forrest and Johnson in which they reviewed the different activities of managers in several different kinds of health organizations and found that there were significant differences in the roles that the managers played and in the work they actually conducted. These findings were similar to those of Kuhl, also referred to by Kaluzny (1982), who reviewed the work of managers in different types of health care organizations and who also found some significantly different sets of roles and functions depending upon the nature of the organization itself. At the same time, both studies reported that there were general similarities in the types of roles required by similar organizations or agencies, so that although managers of individual hospitals might vary significantly from one another, managers of hospitals in general shared many similar clusters of roles.

Although a great deal of research has not been carried out thus far into the various roles of the manager in health care, the approach has significant merit for gaining better understanding of managerial activities in the future. For example, if the actual role content of the various types of managerial positions in health care were better understood and more clearly described, candidates could perhaps be better selected and better prepared to assume those positions. Kurtz (1980) and Slater (1980) have separately studied the personal characteristics of two populations of physician managers and have shown that it is possible to categorize them according to certain management-related styles and attitudes. Their work suggests that it may be possible to make a better match of physician managers (and perhaps all managers) in the future, by identifying individual manager's strengths and weaknesses and then projecting them into the various roles that they must assume in various managerial positions.

Recent studies in the UK by Stewart *et al.* (1980) and Schulz and Harrison (1983) demonstrate how differently individual chief officers in the health care field perceive and discharge their roles. Stewart, in particular, emphasizes the substantial scope for personal choice in how managers use their time and in the styles that they adopt. Often these choices go by default. Presumably managers should take account of the needs of their organization at the time; their own personal characteristics, and the characteristics of their immediate colleagues; and should make conscious choices about the roles that they will fill.

## Managerial functions

A second means of understanding and improving managerial work in public health is the analysis of the manager's *functions*. This analysis looks not so much at the roles or postures that a manager must assume while managing, but rather at what the manager actually does while filling those roles. It focuses more directly on the *practice* of management than does the study of roles; it deals with those actions and activities of the manager that are generally recognized as making up the manager's daily work. As with all such classifications, it suggests a tidier and more rigid situation than exists in life. The analysis is nevertheless helpful for the range of facets of management that it describes.

The classic description of managerial functions has been developed by Koontz and O'Donnell (1955) who suggested that the main functions of a manager are planning, organizing, staffing, directing, and controlling. Although this description has since been broadened and elaborated, it still forms one of the fundamental, traditional ways of viewing a manager's actions and of understanding those actions better. In recent years, however, a great range of additional functions has been identified and the complexity of management functions has been frequently commented upon.

In general, these managerial functions (see Table 14.2) seem to fall into two categories: (i) future-oriented, planning, projective types of activities; (ii) present-oriented, maintenance, daily operational types of activities. Just as was the case in the review of managerial roles, a better understanding of these individual managerial functions and of the clusters of managerial functions that make up a particular management job will allow us better to understand and improve managerial performance.

The *future-oriented* management functions are those functions focused more on where the organization is going (or

### Table 14.2. *Managerial functions*

**Future-oriented management functions**
Planning and organizational goal-setting
Organizational design and development
Leadership and motivation
Management of change

**Present-oriented management function**
Organizing
Decision-making
Directing
Controlling
Conflict resolution

at least, should go in the future) than on maintaining its present status. These functions are: planning and organizational goal-setting; organizational design and development; leadership and motivation; and management of change.

The most important of these future-oriented functions and the one around which all others must revolve is *planning and organizational goal-setting*. This function involves considering where the organization should be going and how it should get there. It requires a thorough review of present and future resources and how they might best be organized to continue the advance of the organization. It includes the development of a strategy for moving in that direction and the role each part of the organization is to play in doing so. It also certainly includes the development of long-range financial forecasts and is usually linked together with the budgeting process by which financial resources are allocated within the organization.

Internationally the most extensive and coherent example of health service planning is in the USSR and the other communist countries of eastern Europe. Theirs is, on the whole, a model of 'top-down', national planning with objectives set in terms of provision (for example, medical manpower or beds per 10 000 population). It is a model that can be operationally strong, in that it can lead to action, and conceptually weak, because there is seldom any sound basis for the norms of provision that are adopted. Sweden also has a long-established interest in health planning; it has been influenced by the setting of normative targets of provision, yet has been more decentralized and collaborative in its approach (Navarro 1974). Other countries have recently taken a growing interest in health planning, starting (typically) from the planning of hospital building, through medical manpower planning to service planning. The WHO has supported this trend, by documenting the approaches taken by different countries and by expounding what it considers good practice (see for example WHO 1972, 1980).

Although there has been great interest in health planning in the US, this has generally been area-wide rather than institutional or organizational planning. In recent years, more attention has been directed towards institutional strategic planning, both within industry in general (Steiner 1979) and within health organizations in particular (Goldsmith 1981; Flexner *et al.* 1981; Fournet 1982).

In the UK, on the other hand, planning, based on a national analytical model, was seen as a logical accompaniment to the integration of health services in the 1974 reorganization of the National Health Service (NHS) (DHSS 1976). More recently there has been criticism of the shortcomings of the NHS planning system on the grounds of rigidity, cumbersomeness, and unreality (Lee and Mills 1982). Some of the criticisms concern the way in which planning has been implemented, and the timing: the official British model was much better suited to an era of slow, incremental growth, than to nil growth or service reduction. The criticisms also raise deeper, more fundamental questions. New approaches to health planning are needed in concepts as well as in practice, less concerned with setting a long-term direction and sticking to it, and more concerned with planning for flexibility and learning in uncertain times.

The second future-oriented management function is

*organizational design and development.* This function naturally follows the development of plans for the organization's future and involves the creation of an organizational structure and identification of its shortcomings, together with the initiation of steps to create change in all or part of the present structure. Although a number of prominent researchers have studied organizational behaviour and design in other types of settings (March and Simon 1958; Etzioni 1961, 1964; Katz and Kahn 1966; Lawrence and Lorsch 1969; Schein 1970; Minzberg 1979), relatively little has been done in health care organizations until recently. The Health Services Research Unit at Brunel University, has done pioneering work in this field (Rowbottom *et al.* 1973).

The development of new units or programmes within hospitals (such as intensive care units, hospice programmes or community mental health centres) represents one form of organizational design effort by managers; the merger or affiliation of several hospitals into one multi-unit organization or chain represents another. A number of health care workers have begun to write about various aspects of this process (Mount 1976; Tichy 1977; Starkweather 1981), and the literature on the subject is beginning to grow.

The third future-oriented management function is that of *leadership and motivation of personnel* within an organization, although this function might also be described as a more present-oriented, maintenance function. In this aspect of the manager's activities, efforts are directed towards inspiring and motivating people to give their best efforts in the future, to commit themselves fully to the goals and the purposes of the organization, and to co-operate with the plans and objectives that have been laid down for the future. Rubin *et al.* (1972, 1974, 1978) has written extensively about this aspect of management as has Beckhard (1972, 1974) and Weiss *et al.* (1974).

The fourth and final future-oriented management function is that of the *management of change.* In many ways, this function is clearly part of organizational design and of leadership and motivation, but it has become such an important function that it is worth singling out as separate. One of the major characteristics of health care and public health at the present time is the continuous stream of major changes that are taking place: new technology is being developed; new methods of financing or new regulatory restraints are being put into place; new pressures from the public are building up for different types of services. The manager plays a key role in preparing the organization and the workers within it for change, so that they are both encouraged and enthused by its prospect. Bennis *et al.* (1966, 1976) have provided the classic discussion of change in general, as have Rubin *et al.* (1974, 1978) with regard to health systems in particular.

The *present-oriented management* functions are those that focus more on the maintenance of the organization's ability to function in the short run and less on the direction in which the organization should be heading over the longer term. In many ways, it is the more mundane, less exciting part of management but an absolutely critical part none the less.

The *organizing function* of the manager depends upon the fact that the organization's goals and directions have already been set; now it is up to the manager to bring together the personnel and the resources in such a way as to accomplish the objectives laid out by the organization's plan. Within the organizing function, the manager takes on two separate tasks: first, deciding what type of organizational structure is best to get the work done; second, gathering the people and resources together into that organizational format and assigning the specific tasks, delegating the specific responsibility and authority to the individual workers or to specific work groups – all these are included in the manager's organizing function.

The *decision-making function* of the manager is obviously both a long-range, future-directed function, and a short-term, present-oriented function (Warner and Holloway 1978). On a daily basis, there are a myriad of individual details that require decisions. For a manager these include the establishment of a system for determining which decisions should be brought forward for the manager's attention and which should be handled by subordinates; it also includes the actual process of decision-making by the manager.

The *directing function* of the manager, another of the traditional functions outlined by Koontz, involves the conveying of instructions to members of the organization concerning how work is to be carried out, how things are to be done. In this function, the manager must express his or her will about the style and substance of the work being carried out, making it clear what the instructions are and what is expected of those doing the work. Directing is making explicit how the manager wishes the job to be done; it is the communication of details about the work, together with a statement of authority of the manager's position.

The *controlling function* involves the review of what is being done within the organization and making the appropriate changes (Anthony and Herzlinger 1975). It involves the reception of information on a regular basis about the organization's operation, the evaluation of that information in comparison to pre-set goals and objectives, and the issuance of corrective directions wherever appropriate. In the area of finance, for example, it involves the continuous review of financial reports, the comparison of these reports with pre-set objectives or indicators, and the initiation of corrective actions with regard to expenditures, prices, inventories, and the like. Controlling is perhaps the area of expression of a manager's authority that most directly impacts on people within organizations; for that reason, it is also very closely tied up with the manager's personality and the overall personnel atmosphere within an organization.

Perhaps one of the most important functions of the manager is that of *conflict resolution*; between individuals, between sub-units of the organization, or between the manager's organization and other similar organizations in the environment. Although it is usually felt that the planning, organizing, and controlling functions of a manager are most important on a long-term basis, it is usually the conflict resolution function that is the most visible in the short term; it is often the function that requires the most time and that drains the most energy from the manager. In this function, the manager is called upon to bring together opposing parties, to reconcile opposing viewpoints, and to develop consensus between opposing values. It is the most 'people'-connected function of the manager and is the one that most usually takes the manager out of the office and into the lives of the workers in the organization (Robbins 1974).

## Managerial skills

The third method suggested by Longest for looking at managerial work is to appraise managerial skills. He suggests a typology created by Katz (1974) that identifies three types of skills an effective manager must use.

*Technical skills* are the abilities to use the methods, processes, and techniques of a particular field in managerial work; in the case of public health work, for example, these might include the traditional areas of biostatistics, epidemiology, environmental health, maternal and child health, and the like. It might also include some of the technical areas related to management, such as financial management and accounting, certain quantitative methods for planning or decision-making, or perhaps certain specialized systems for conflict resolution.

Katz's second area of managerial skills is described as the *human skills*. These involve the ability to get along with other people, to understand them, and to motivate them towards the organizational objective (or at least the organizational objective as the manager sees it). This collection of skills is utilized by the manager not so much in the abstract aspects of management that involve technical or conceptual abilities, but in translating these aspects into terms and conditions and attitudes that the people in the organization will understand and respond to.

The third area of managerial skills described by Katz is the *conceptual skills*. This is the mental ability to visualize the complex interrelationships that exist in the work place – that is, among people, among departments or units of an organization, and even between a single organization and the environment in which it exists. Conceptual skills permit the manager to understand how the various factors in a particular situation fit together and impact on each other; it also allows the manager to know what to do about them.

Just as with the managerial roles and functions, there is an appropriate but differing 'mix' of managerial skills that is necessary for each administrative position in public health. For example, in one community at one time, the medical officer of health or the local health commissioner may be faced with a problem that is really more *technical* in nature than anything else: what type of polio vaccine to use in a programme for infants and pre-school children; what type of tuberculosis screening mechanism; what type of family planning materials or programmes. The main thrust of the managerial challenge may be a technical one, with the public health administrator functioning more as a technical expert than anything else.

In another instance, the managerial challenge may be the need to provide fluoridation for the local water supply in order to reduce the incidence of dental caries. In this case, the local public health officer may not need technical skills at all; the technical, scientific work in this area has already been done and is well discussed in the literature. In this jurisdiction at this time, the need may be more for *human skills,* skills that will bring together the divergent opinions and groups in the community, and that will allow a major public health benefit to be successfully implemented in that community.

Finally, in another circumstance the medical officer of health or the local public health commissioner may be called upon to use *conceptual skills* that are quite different from either of the other two types of skills. For example, the health officer may understand that the community needs to develop a comprehensive programme of cancer prevention, early diagnosis, early treatment, and (if necessary) comprehensive care up to and including hospice care. There will be a number of complex interrelationships that will need to be worked out, an overall system designed, and perhaps an organizational structure created either to oversee the effort or actually to carry it out. Here the manager will need to use *conceptual skills* in identifying the problem, understanding what needs to be done, and organizing a system that will accomplish the necessary objective.

## Summary

More effective management of health care programmes and institutions depends upon more effective health care managers. A better understanding of managerial roles, functions and skills is a first step towards improvement of the work of health care managers, as it makes possible better evaluation of managers and their work, better programmes for training and educating prospective managers, and improved design of managerial positions in public health organizations.

For example, if one better understands the various roles, functions, and skills that make up a particular management job, one can design a form of managerial evaluation that is much more specific and pertinent to the task. If it is known that the particular position calls for a manager whose main roles are mainly that of liaison and to act as figurehead and spokesperson for the organization, the incumbent can be evaluated on how those roles are carried out. If that same position is translated into the managerial functions of planning and organizational goal-setting, as well as leadership and motivation, the evaluation can focus on these future-oriented functions and not concentrate so much on present-oriented ones. If the managerial skills that are necessary for this same position are felt to be more technical and conceptual in nature and are not felt to be so human or people-oriented, the evaluation can be shaped accordingly.

In the same fashion, if a training programme for a particular type of position is being established, it will be important to know the mix of managerial roles, functions, and skills that are necessary for maximum success in that particular position. Once these are known, an educational curriculum or training programme can be developed to cover these more important areas; an education or training framework can be created that will alert the prospective manager to the specific challenges of the position and will prepare him or her for those challenges in a more focused manner. Rather than a wide array of different educational and training experiences which may have little or nothing to do with the eventual managerial practice, a more pertinent and specifically-directed training can be offered and, it is to be hoped, a better prepared manager will be the result.

Finally, a better understanding of managerial roles, functions, and skill will allow for the improved design of managerial positions in public health organizations. Positions can be created in which a more specific set of expectations can be drawn up and a more specifically-trained set of individuals recruited to fill those positions. A better knowledge of the contents of management work might force organizations to analyse their management needs much more carefully and draw up their management tables much more precisely; it might allow for more specific assignment of responsibility and authority, as well as the clearer definition of each individual manager's part in the organization *vis à vis* all others. A better understanding of managerial work might force public health organizations to look at their entire structure, particularly in light of some of the considerations to be discussed in the next section below.

## THE NATURE OF ORGANIZATIONS

A second method of understanding the administration and planning of health service programmes is to look not so much at the manager, but the organization and the environment in which management takes place. In this approach, interest is focused more on organizational issues than managerial issues, and a rather different set of research and analytical skills and approaches are called into play.

Until relatively recently, little work was done on health service organizations *as organizations,* compared to other types of industrial or political organizations. Hospitals have attracted some attention because of their unusual and intriguing organizational complexity (Georgopoulos and Man 1962; Georgopoulos 1972, 1975; Rowbottom *et al.* 1973; Shortell and Brown 1976). But there has been comparatively little organizational research into health agencies other than hospitals, and particularly, into public health institutions.

This is actually more apparent than real, when one reviews the literature on patient care in organizations. Literature that deals with specific attempts to understand or improve some aspect of patient care is usually considered under the rubric of 'patient care', 'medical care', or 'public health' research; in fact, it contains a great deal of organizational analysis, generally of an applied nature. That is, the research was not carried out primarily to understand the organization better, but was specifically done to improve a particular service process. It is almost as if the first and more basic step of building up a significant body of fundamental knowledge has been by-passed, and the research methodology has moved almost immediately into a study of applications of basic knowledge. If the applied research has sometimes turned out to be faulty or not as valuable as it might have been, the explanation may lie in the lack of a well-understood and well-described basic set of facts regarding health service organizations to begin with.

## Basic organization theory

Towards the end of the last century and into the beginnning of this one, workers in various parts of the world began to develop a body of general knowledge of organization theory that has served as the foundation for most modern approaches to organizations. In recent years, the more classical ideas of the early years have been challenged and modified considerably, so that present organization theory is a mixture of the older, more classical ideas that have now been tempered and adapted in light of newer findings. The major developer of classic organization theory was Max Weber, a German sociologist. Weber developed the idea of the bureaucratic model of organizations, as the ideal one for his time, since it presented a method for the rational organization of collective energies and activities. ('Bureaucratic' here being used in the general sense and not necessarily limited to governmental bureaucracies, as the term has come to be utilized in more recent years.)

In Weber's ideal model of organizations, several principles predominated: (i) *specialization and division of labour* (that is, tasks are broken down into specific pieces of work and the various specific jobs are assigned clearly and definitely to individual workers or work groups); (ii) *hierarchical organization and chain of command* (organizations are structured in a hierarchy, with each succeeding higher level having authority and control of the units beneath it on the table of organization); (iii) *consistent set of organizational rules* (the organization has a set of explicit statements that govern conduct of life within the organization and without which the organization could not function effectively); (iv) *managerial impersonality* (the manager should assume a somewhat impersonal attitude towards those working under his or her direction, so that personal attributes of either the manager or the managed do not interfere with the task-orientation of the organization); (v) *assumption of authority on the basis of competence* (that is, managerial authority and the management positions in which that authority resides should be assigned on the basis of competence in the work; in the same fashion, tenure in a position should be dependent upon effectiveness in meeting the objectives of the organization).

Inherent in this bureaucratic, traditional model of organizations were certain principles or ideas that have become widely accepted and applied throughout organizations all over the world. The division of labour and the increasing specialization of tasks is one that is universally accepted, as is the need for co-ordinating control to bring together all these various specialized tasks. The principle of unity of command is also generally accepted. The principle operates on the basis that each worker in the organization has one person administratively responsible for him or her and it is clear to each worker just who that controlling person is. The distinction between 'line' and 'staff positions' (that is, the distinction between those who have the responsibility for keeping the organization operating and those who are technical experts or consultants to the operating line staff) has been open to widespread discussion and challenge in recent years, but continues to be a fundamental assumption in most organizations. Limitations on the span of control exercised by an individual manager is another principle that is inherent in many of the classical interpretations of the bureaucratic model of organizations. Finally, the delegation of management decisions and actions downward to the lowest appropriate organizational level is an additional principle that has become accepted in all organizational thinking.

## Objections to classical organization theory

Almost from the beginning, there have been objections to classical organization theory, generally on the grounds that it was too mechanistic in its approach, too impersonal in its application. Various workers have pointed out that organizations are not simply physical constructions that deal only in physical, tangible activities; these workers have stressed that organizations are really collections of people and it is the personal aspects of work, the individual and group interactions, attitudes and values, that more accurately describe and define an organization. Latterly, behavioural scientists and others have played a major part in re-assessing the classical bureaucratic model and in developing alternative models of organizational analysis and behaviour (Homans 1950; Maslow 1954; McGregor 1960; Likert 1961, 1967; Perow 1970; Peters and Waterman 1982).

One of the major objections of behavioural scientists to the classic theory of organization is that it ignores what is now known as the informal organization, in favour of studying only the formal organization (Blau and Scott 1962). The formal organization is the structure as it is supposed to be, in theory or on paper or in the mind of some distant manager or authority figure. The informal organization is that spontaneous interaction of people and situations that more accurately resembles how work is accomplished, how authority is really exercised and received, and how an organization actually 'lives'. The general feeling among more modern organizational thinkers is that a complete view of any organization must include both the formal structure (as outlined in the organization chart, job descriptions, formal work rules, operating policies, and the like) and the informal structure (the actual interrelationships of people, authority, and work activities).

Certainly one of the most important contributions in recent years to organizational thinking has been the application of general systems theory to organizations, since it has provided a much more useful and relevant view of organizations and a method of analysing their behaviour (Johnson *et al.* 1967; Churchman 1968; Kast and Rosenzweig 1974). In general, systems theory suggests that organizations are systems or sets of interrelated and inter-dependent parts that, taken together, form the complex whole. Each part of the system (that is, sub-system) has a life and momentum and set of relationships of its own, while at the same time, it is affected by, and in turn affects, all other parts of the complex. It suggests that systems such as organizations are living, changing, interactive complexes, and also suggests that the nature of that interaction can be delineated and often quantified. At the same time, it allows for formal and informal aspects of an organization to be combined, doing

away with the necessity of an artificial distinction between these two important components of organizational life.

The importance of the open systems model of organization is apparent from a number of viewpoints. First, it more accurately displays organizations as complex interactions of many component parts and many forces and influences. Second, it allows these interactions to be more accurately described and permits a more realistic portrait of the organization to be presented. Third, it permits a more total perspective of the organization to be developed for both planning and management purposes, so that the implications of any one action in one part of the system can be traced into other, related parts of the system. Fourth, it allows workers and managers in one part of the system better to understand how their actions affect the total organization and vice versa. Finally, it allows for organizational design that is more pertinent to the operating needs and realities of the organization than is possible in the usually conventional two-dimensional models.

## The characteristics of health care organizations

It is virtually impossible to develop a list of characteristics of health care organizations that will apply equally well to all such organizations, since the diversity among health care organizations in general and public health organizations in particular, is very great. There are, however, a number of characteristics that have been identified as being somewhat common among all health care organizations and a further set of characteristics that are common among public health agencies and organizations.

It is important for those interested in the management and planning of public health organizations to be aware of and to understand their characteristics, since they are symptomatic of forces and influences that shape these agencies and determine their existence. The characteristics themselves are perhaps not so important as what has brought them about. Knowing these characteristics allows us to understand the dynamic shaping forces better; knowing these forces better allows us to develop more appropriate and effective public health organizations in the future.

*In general, public health organizations are altruistic in nature and not profit- or productivity-motivated.* This means that they are seen differently from other organizations, both by those within them and those without, including researchers. Workers within these organizations frequently refuse to believe that many of the principles that apply to other organizations are relevant for them, since the purposes of their organizations are so different. In general, workers within public health organizations are intent on the delivery of a service to a public or a population that needs it, and matters such as organizational efficiency or resource constraints are not seen as legitimate reasons for altering organizational behaviour. There is a moral imperative to health work that is seen as preempting many of the principles that govern the operation of other types of organizations.

However, although public health organizations themselves are altruistic in purpose, they are often forced to utilize harsh methods to reach their altruistic aims. Sometimes these methods and approaches are directly contradictory to their normal operating mode and cause serious organizational confusion of attitude and purpose.

For example, every *governmentally-sponsored* public health organization occasionally carries out a police-like function to enforce certain ordinances and laws; in this role, it must assume a somewhat formidable police-like posture. At the same time, the same organization may be trying to convince mothers to bring in their babies voluntarily for well-child examinations or trying to convince people to stop smoking. On the one hand, the organization is ordering people to behave in a certain way under threat of legal action, while on the other hand, it is trying to convince people to behave voluntarily in certain ways that will benefit them. The organizational confusion that can arise from this contradiction should be obvious.

*Second, most public health organizations are governmentally-sponsored, or they are at least very closely connected with some social or political set of values.* That is, the operations of these agencies are very much influenced and directed by a broader set of social and/or political decisions that provide the framework within which the public health agency functions. The public health agency is not free to embark on whatever course of action or whatever direction it wishes, strictly by the will of the people within the organization. The framework or the environment for its work is set outside the organization and then passed along to it.

A further sub-set of these social purposes is the reality that the public health agency or organization usually focuses its attention more forcibly and aggressively on certain sub-sets of the population being served, with the result that the agency sometimes becomes identified with the individual sub-sets of the population and not with the population as a whole. In the US, for example, although public health organizations work very assiduously to improve the health of the public as a whole, they work most energetically to improve the health of the poorer and disadvantaged portions of the public. As a result, public health work in the US is not seen as an activity that has equal relevance to all parts of the population; it is seen more as a 'poor people's programme', or one that focuses on tuberculosis or venereal disease, or some other similar sub-set. This means that the organization may then be able to call upon the active emotional support and involvement of a comparatively limited part of the population at large, because only a limited part of the population feels that its activities are relevant to them.

*Another characteristic of public health organizations is that their operations are technically- or scientifically-determined.* That is, the whole purpose of the organization is influenced by the technology or the scientific discoveries that have been deemed to be important for a particular population to receive. The development of a polio vaccine in a laboratory somewhere in the world will immediately mean that public health agencies all over the world must begin to consider the addition of polio vaccination efforts to their array of products and services.

This scientific determinism has two important impacts on public health organizations. First, it may well determine the operating structure of the organization by forcing the creation of one type of programme or unit, either where none has existed before or where something rather different has been in operation. The arrival of a new birth control method or the development of some new vaccine will frequently call forth a new organizational unit to administer that new service, occasionally drawing off staff and resources from other already-existing units in the organization. A second aspect of this technical determinism relates to the social and professional distance between those who develop the new technology or science and those who must apply it. For example, the development of the polio vaccine was the result of the efforts of a large number of scientific researchers and technical experts; the implementation of a polio vaccination effort by a public health agency depends upon the work of a large number of non-technical personnel, or at least lower-level technical personnel than those who originated the product to be delivered. The translation of very sophisticated technical ideas and products into terms and procedures that are genuinely understood by lower-level workers is a major feature of public health agencies and organizations throughout the world.

*Another characteristic of public health organizations is the difficulty in evaluating or appraising their work, given the long-term nature of the results.* It is perhaps easy to measure the effectiveness of a public health organization in finding and removing a contamination of the drinking water supply in a particular town. It is harder to measure the impact of a public education campaign aimed at reducing the amount of cigarette smoking in a particular population, since the effect may be stretched out over so long a period of time. It is often easy to measure the effort expended (for example, the number of educational sessions on cigarette smoking), but it may not be possible to measure the results of that effort (which is obviously the more important aspect of the educational work).

*A final organizational characteristic of public health organizations is their often archaic structure* and their retention of organizational units that perhaps no longer have any relevance. In the US, a review of the organizational structure of many public health organizations will reveal units that have existed for 50 years next to ones that have been created only recently; it may reveal units that were initially organized to tackle one particular disease pattern (for example, infectious disease) still in existence long after other health problems (for example, alcoholism or chronic disease) have assumed a more important position. Structures would be found that are composed of professional personnel of one kind (for example, public health nursing) immediately next to another unit that operates a programme of services (for example, maternal and child health). The structure of public health organizations seems to evolve by indirection rather than by direction; it seems to be more an incidental happening than a deliberate attempt to develop the more pertinent organizational form to meet the particular organizational purpose.

In the next section, we will discuss a means for analysing or reviewing public health organizations from the point of view of their organizational structure, with the hope that more pertinent and appropriate structures can be developed.

## FRAMEWORK FOR ANALYSING ORGANIZATIONS

For the future, it will be important for managers and others interested in health service organizations to be able to conduct a systematic review of organizations and their operations (Litterer 1965). To assist managers in their analysis, and to point out to researchers important aspects of health care organizations that are worth study, it will be useful to have a framework for analysis of health care organizational structures.

In general, there are four parts of the analysis of any organization, health services organization or otherwise. The first three deal with the organization's history, its environment, and its formal organizational structure. The fourth and much more comprehensive portion of the organization analysis involves an orderly review of the organization's ten major operational or functional systems. All elements of this analytical frame are given in Table 14.3.

**Table 14.3.** *Framework for appraisal of public health organizations*

| | |
|---|---|
| **A** | Developmental history of the organization |
| **B** | Environmental factors affecting the organization |
| **C** | Formal organizational structure |
| **D** | Organizational systems |
| | 1. Task completion process |
| | 2. Distribution of power |
| | 3. Planning and decision-making pattern |
| | 4. Resource distribution and resource allocation method |
| | 5. Internal management structure |
| | 6. Communications network |
| | 7. Interpersonal/intergroup/interorganizational relationships |
| | 8. Evaluation and control systems |
| | 9. Conflict resolutions systems |
| | 10. Organizational redesign and new products system |

### Developmental history of organizations

One of the first items to be studied in any review or analysis of an organization is its developmental history. Any organization will have gone through a series of developmental steps to bring it to its present situation. None of these steps would have been purely accidental and all of them would reflect important changes in the organization itself or the environment in which it functions.

A careful historical review will tell a great deal about an organization's past, but more important, about its present as well. A review of its organizational changes over the years, the growth of the services or products it has offered, a description of the personnel involved in its leadership – all of these will provide important clues to an organization's present situation and its future opportunities.

### Environmental factors affecting the organization

The next area to review in investigating any organization is the environment in which it exists and the forces that presently impinge upon it. In general, the key environmental factors are social, economic, political, and physical, but any aspect of the general environment in which an organization exists should be reviewed, if felt to be important.

A good place to start is to consider the economy upon which the organization is dependent. Is the economy strong and growing, or is it weak and unstable? Does it hold prospects for providing increasing financial support in the future, or will the organization be lucky to continue to obtain its present funding? Are there prospects that the organization can assist in the economic development of the area, or will it always be a drain on economic growth?

In the same fashion, a review should be made of political, social, and other factors affecting the organization. Is it an agency of government and, if so, is the governmental structure stable and supportive? What are the political imperatives for the present government and how do they impact on the public health organization? Does the organization fit in well with the social and cultural values that are currently important in the community to be served, and does it have a means of determining whether its programmes are congruent with these social and cultural values?

With regard to the physical environment, does the public health organization have an appropriate physical setting in which adequately to conduct its work? Is the physical geography and topography a factor to be considered in its work, or is it a relatively neutral feature? If the organization is not appropriately located, would it take major changes to bring it into a setting in which it would work better? Are there other major physical environmental considerations that affect its operations, such as availability of fuel, supplies, shelter, and the like? If so, what are the implications for its structure and mode of working?

### Formal organizational structure

Although the formal organization is only half the picture (the informal organization being the other half), it is important clearly to identify what the formal organizational structure is supposed to be. An attempt should therefore be made to obtain such items as organization charts, job descriptions, procedure manuals, and other written and documentary material that describe the organization.

With these in hand, it should be determined how closely the present structure actually approximates to what appears in the written materials. Does the structure truly resemble the organization chart? Are the personnel listed in that chart actually still in place, or have they changed positions? How often is the organization chart brought up to date and how much attention does anyone pay to it? Is there any attempt to review and reorganize these charts, procedure manuals, job descriptions, and other formal procedures on a regular basis? What major discrepancies are there between the formal structure and the way that things are actually done?

### Organizational systems

Once these three basic background areas of development history, environmental forces, and formal organizational structure have been reviewed one can look at the internal systems of the public health organization itself. These are the functioning networks, the formal or informal coming together of people and problems that *in toto* really comprise the organization.

### Task process

The first organizational system to examine is the process (or processes) by which the organization's primary tasks are performed. It may seem strange to underline this need to review how an organization carries out its primary work, but in many ways the pendulum has swung so far the other way (for example, the study of personal interactions) that less attention is paid to a searching review of how the work gets done. Too many managers and researchers work in organizations without carefully examining the steps by which their organizations function on a daily basis.

### Distribution of power

One of the most important features of organizations is the distribution of power, both formal and informal (Khan and Boulding 1964). Every organization will have a formal arrangement for distributing power that is generally related to supervisory authority, ability to expend resources, power to hire or fire, power to approve or disapprove new projects, and the like. As much as possible, these arrangements must be clearly understood.

In addition to the formal distribution of power, what can be learned about informal power and influence? Is there a particular person who has significant ability to speed up or impede organizational functioning? Are there structural aspects of the organization that have allowed power or influence to concentrate in one unit or person more by default than by intent? Are there forces, psychological or political, that affect the ways in which power is actually applied?

### Planning and decision-making pattern

A third important area to review is how the organization's long range intentions are developed and implemented. Are they the results of a formal process or does a long-range direction seem to emerge by some kind of informal concensus? Is planning primarily a budgetary function, or is it separate? If it is separate, at what point are the two processes joined?

How are decisions made within the organization and by whom? What types of decisions are made on which levels? Do individuals within the organization know accurately what power they have to make decisions or must they guess what is expected of them, each time risking some significant over-expression of their authority? Are decisions in the organization really made by default, by delay, or by being unwilling to make active, positive decisions?

### Resource distribution and resource allocation methods

A fourth area to analyse is the distribution of resources and the method by which resources are allocated. Although the formal organization chart will portray the supposed relation of one organizational unit to another, it does nothing to describe the allocation of resources among all the units. It is therefore useful to obtain the financial reports and personnel rosters for the organization under study, and to attempt to recreate the pattern of resource distribution throughout the organization. If it is possible to break down these reports by service programme or product line (for example, health education efforts or vaccine efforts), it is also helpful since it shows whether or not an organization's priority statements are reflected in the way its resources are allocated.

In parallel with the mapping of planning and decision-making, it is also of value to learn how resources of various kinds are actually allocated through the organization. Is there a formal budgetary process by which funds, personnel, and equipment are assigned, or is the process more informal? Does it take place once a year or throughout the year? Is there a single person involved in these decisions or many people? Are financial resources handled one way, personnel another, and space/equipment/supplies a third? What policies appear to govern current decisions: for example, do resource allocations suggest some major changes in policy or a continuation of the status quo? Do people in the organization know how resources are allocated, and do they think the process is fair and equitable?

### Internal management structure

It is useful to know what the basic management structure of the organization really is: which people are part of central management and which part of local management. How far down into the organization does top management feel that the 'management' system extends? Do the employees involved agree that they are part of management, or do they see themselves as mainly involved in professional or technical work within their particular unit? Do managers in one portion of the organization know who are the managers in a distant part of the organization and do they have a chance to exchange experiences? Is there a clear pattern of upward management mobility, or is it unclear how one moves through the management structure?

### Communication networks

Some organization theorists think that an organization can be well pictured by mapping its communications and the actions stemming from them. Are there clear patterns of communication from the top of the organization to the bottom? From the bottom to the top? From one organizational sub-unit to another sub-unit organization? Are there formal methods of communication from the organization outward to the environment and to the public that the organization wishes to serve? Are there easy methods of communication back to the organization from that public? Is communication felt to be important or something that simply happens on an *ad hoc* basis? Is the philosophy of the organization to keep people comprehensively informed or just tell them about those matters in which they have direct involvement? Does anyone regularly review communications systems and networks to see if some change needs to be made?

### Interpersonal/intergroup/interorganizational relationships

A complete analysis of any organization should include a review of the interpersonal relations within it (Davis 1967). Do people see themselves in the midst of colleagues and supporters, or beset by adversaries on all sides? Is there an atmosphere of mutual respect and co-operation, of common purpose and objectives, or is it one of isolation and alone-ness!

At the same time as one is looking at individual inter-actions, it is also important to look at the interactions of groups (for example, interactions of professional workers with non-professionals) and of one profession with another (nurses with doctors, for example). Does the organizational structure encourage the creation of separate groups of personnel and how does this affect its functioning? Does the existence of sub-groups create a sense of close support for the individual, or does it serve to pigeon-hole and isolate people even more?

Are workers within a governmentally-sponsored public health organization discouraged from having contacts (whether task-related or professional) with people in other governmental or private organizations? What is done to encourage co-operative efforts between workers in the public health organization and in other organizations?

### Evaluation and control systems

In every effective modern organization, there should be some organized effort to measure the outcome of the organization's work, to determine whether its objectives are being met, either in total or in part. There should also be some method of feeding back this evaluative information into the management and planning structure so that appropriate changes and corrections can be made.

A thorough review should attempt to identify the major evaluative systems that may be in place within the organization, to learn how they function, what information is developed, and how that information is utilized. This review should include a determination of whether the organization is interested in evaluating its activities for internal, self-protective reasons or whether it genuinely conducts its evaluations to determine whether it is meeting the needs of the public that it serves. The timeliness, appropriateness, and completeness of the evaluation system needs to be determined, together with the effectiveness of whatever corrective actions the evaluation calls into play.

### Conflict resolutions

One of the natural outcomes of organizational life is conflict – between individuals, between groups of individuals, and between organizational units. Sometimes the conflict is based on personal differences and variations in style of work, while at other times it is based on different beliefs as to how the work should be done, where the organization should be going, or how it is going to get there.

In every organization, there will exist some formal or informal mechanisms for handling conflict and, it is to be hoped, for resolving it (Robbins 1974). A thorough review should attempt to document these conflict resolution systems, whether formal or informal, and to evaluate their effective-ness. Are there appropriate systems in place for identifying potential sources of conflict early, and for correcting or ameliorating them? Are there ways of containing conflict so that its existence does not do major damage to the broader aspects of the organization? Are there systems in place by which each episode of conflict leads to a better understanding of the organization by its managers; by which each episode leads to action to prevent future conflict?

### Organization re-design and new products

Finally, every effective organization must continually seek to renew itself, to realign its resources and organizational structure, to introduce new services, programmes, or products. No organization can afford to remain static and unchanged for long, and certainly public health organiza-tions, with their rapidly changing environments and challenges, are not exceptions.

A careful review or investigation of any public health organization must then ask itself: how is this organization systematically preparing itself for the future? What informa-tion does an organization continuously seek with regard to its future directions, and what steps does it take once it has this information? Is there an organized, continuous effort to consider the long-term plans of the organization and to shape its structure accordingly? How do new ideas and new approaches get circulated for discussion and consideration, and how does a decision get made to try some new approach? Are innovation and new product development seen as a benefit to the organization or a bother? Is everyone involved in preparing for the future, or is it felt to be the responsibility of a special separate planning or research/demonstration unit?

Obviously a great deal more could be said about organizations in general and public health organizations in particular. The important message to take away from this discussion is not merely that there is a body of technical or professional knowledge about organizations, but that the way in which public health agencies are organized is important. The organization is the vehicle by which public health work gets done. The more effective and streamlined the vehicle, the more powerful the outcome.

Public health workers cannot afford to be passive about the organization in which they work. They should spend as much time studying, understanding, and trying to improve it as they spend on their professional work. These two aspects, the work itself and the organization through which it is accomplished, go hand in hand and are interdependent.

## MANAGEMENT ISSUES FOR THE FUTURE IN PUBLIC HEALTH

Looking forward into the future, there are a number of com-paratively new areas that will be increasingly important to the management and administration of public health programmes around the world. If public health programmes improve in the future, if public health managers become more effective in their work, it will mostly be as a result of their efforts in these newer areas of management. The areas that will require special attention are: (i) population monitoring, priority setting and strategic choice, and resource allocation; (ii) cost-benefit/cost-effectiveness analysis and programme evaluation; (iii) responsiveness to public opinion at both the individual and collective levels, communications skills, and political sensitivity.

## Population-monitoring, priority setting, strategic choice, and resource allocation

As societies and countries become wealthier, they move out of the era in which infectious diseases (particularly among the young) are the most important health problems and move into one in which the chronic, long-term diseases such as cancer, heart disease, stroke, and renal disease take precedence. Unfortunately, most public health systems throughout the world, in developed as well as developing countries, do a much better job of measuring their acute infectious problems than they do of monitoring their chronic long-term disabling ones.

For the future, effective public health organizations will have to develop and maintain much more appropriate and relevant data systems about the real health problems of their particular society. In societies for which hypertension, depression, alcoholism, and motor vehicle accidents are much more important than typhoid and measles, it will be necessary to develop information systems that concentrate on these newer problems, not on those which were prevalent in the past. This will challenge the epidemiologists to develop new kinds of data systems regarding the new threats to health in the modern world and to present this information in a fashion that is more useful to health planners, managers, and governments in the future. The 1971 conference sponsored by the International Epidemiological Association on 'The Uses of Epidemiology in the Planning of Health Services' is an example of a good beginning in this area, as are the writings of Knox and White (IEA 1972; White and Henderson 1976; Knox 1979).

Not only must different types of epidemiological data be gathered, they must be used as a basis for making sensible choices about priorities and strategies; they must be tied into a system that allocates resources to various parts of a country or to various programmes of service on the basis of real need, as documented by epidemiological as well as economic data. It is, for example, scandalous that in most relatively poor countries the lion's share of the few resources available goes to mimicking the hospital services of wealthier countries, rather than tackling problems of water supply and child health (Bryant 1969). Although it may seem an unlikely grouping, the public health priorities of the future should be the joint efforts of the epidemiologists, the economists, the administrators, and the politicians (Cooper and Rice 1976; Hartunian et al. 1981). At the present time, there is virtually no country of the world that utilizes such a system well, but perhaps the Research Allocation Working Party (RAWP) methodology in the UK approaches this ideal of epidemiology with resource allocation better than most (DHSS 1976a; Brotherston 1978). Once adopted such a method should be reviewed regularly and its effects monitored. It must not be allowed to go unquestioned.

### Cost-benefit/cost-effectiveness analysis and programme evaluation

In the same vein of improved priority setting and resource allocation, there will have to be much greater interest in, and usage of, the techniques of cost-accounting and cost-benefit/cost-effectiveness analysis.

In the past, decisions concerning individual programmes were generally made only on the basis of an initial assessment of that programme itself, or at least seemingly so. There were relatively few attempts to review later whether the returns from the investment of time, money, and personnel had been worth the effort. Similarly there was little interest in comparing the returns or results from one potential programme with another, to see which yielded a better return on society's investment of its capital. There was often no real understanding in public health circles that, by choosing to perform one service or programme, one was simultaneously choosing not to perform another. There was little attempt to weigh the merits of programmes against one another (or even against not doing anything at all) in establishing priorities for the public health organization to attack during the next budget year.

In future, this type of narrow, incremental thinking will have to be put aside, as it becomes increasingly apparent that the resources for health are simply not adequate to do everything. It will now be incumbent on a society to appraise the comparative benefits of the various things that it can do, before it sets its mind to do anything. The society may still choose to do something that is less 'productive' because it is committed to helping one area of the country or one part of the population, but at least now it should be able to make these choices knowingly. In order to function in this new era, public health managers will have to have a much greater knowledge of cost-accounting and other quantitative techniques for management and planning. They must be much better able to document the real costs of health programmes and to project much more accurately the real benefits of such efforts (Dunlop 1975; Warner and Luce 1982). Fortunately, in recent years well-organized, rigorous studies have begun to appear in the area of cost-benefit/cost-effectiveness analysis of public health programmes that might well serve as good example for the future (Hornbrook et al. 1982; Kottke et al. 1982; Smith et al. 1982).

Although there have been various public health leaders interested in evaluation in the past, the subject has not been given the degree of attention it deserves. George James, the Commissioner of Public Health in New York City in the 1960s, was a strong advocate of programme evaluation in public health and together with Suchman (1967) was responsible for a surge of interest in the subject. Until recently, however, it has not been a standard part of the typical public health practitioner's equipment. Now with the generally tightening budgets and with the need to expend resources more carefully by means of programmes that are more accurately designed and more vigorously appraised, programme evaluation is coming back into its own (Fink and Kosecoff 1978; Shortell and Richardson 1978).

For the future, it seems clear that every public health practitioner will have to know how to design and carry out programme evaluation, and indeed that every new programme will have built into it from the beginning the means by which it can be evaluated. It is probable that in the near future, anyone proposing a new programme of service or care will not only have to show what it can do, but also show how it will be determined whether it has done it or not. More and more, public health programmes will probably be created on a somewhat temporary basis, their long-term future being assured only after evaluation reports are in, proving that the continuation of the programme is worth the expense. For the public health practitioner of the future, working in this type of setting, a knowledge of programme evaluation and its implementation will be essential.

### Responsiveness, communication, and political sensitivity

Although the term 'consumer marketing' conjures up images of salesmen, of advertising, or of vigorous public relations campaigns by business concerns to sell a product, in fact the term has a different meaning and an important role in the future of public health practice. Indeed, much of the success of public health programmes in the years to come may depend upon public health practitioners being able to 'market' them better.

Basically, marketing consists of several aspects. On the one hand, it involves a careful appraisal of what people want and need, and also what they are capable and potentially willing to buy or use. On the other hand, it means a careful appraisal of what the organization has to offer, and what new programmes or services it can develop to meet the needs of that public. It means the development of a strategy for presenting the new programme or service in such a way that people want to utilize it, and a careful continuing assessment of what the public thinks of it in practice.

Most of the interest or awareness about marketing in the past has centred around the third of these four elements, the creation of a campaign to convince people to buy or utilize a product. For those not directly connected with marketing, the other elements are forgotten. So much interest has focused on the actual selling of the product that the more important aspects of need assessment, product development, and consumer reaction have been forgotten. It has recently become more and more apparent that there is an important role for marketing the human services sector, particularly those programmes that depend at least partially on the compliance or co-operation of individuals (Kotler 1975; Peters and Waterman 1982). In the health area, a number of writers have suggested that the diagnostic part of the marketing effort for health programmes – for.example, surveys to determine the role of cigarette smoking in people's lives – are just as important as the attempts to develop new products to meet that need – such as, the development of new programmes to help people to stop smoking (MacStravic 1977, 1980; Cooper 1977). The actual 'selling' of the programme may be the easiest part of the entire marketing effort, but will be pointless without a broader awareness of the marketing context.

For the public health practitioner of the future, it will be fundamental to search out what is wanted and needed in the community now, rather than what has always been standard in the past. If some of the major problems of modern society are related to life-style then it becomes a major public health concern to identify what can be done to help people live more healthily. This means that new programmes of exercise, diet, stress reduction, and other forms of life-style modification

may be required to meet the newly identified need of the public. If the problem for a substantial minority is unemployment and lack of a valued role, then we must rethink employment and occupation.

At the same time, it will be necessary for the public health practitioner to know better how to make contact with the public in a fashion that attracts people to the product that the public health practitioner has to sell. If the aim is to reduce excessive drinking, the practitioner then must learn how to develop programmes that are attractive enough to interest the public and the government. Public programmes must be offered in a fashion that is in keeping with the ability of the public to understand, to accept, and to participate in them. Constantly those involved in public health must listen to public reactions and learn from them (Schon 1971).

Finally, public health practitioners must never forget that they are public servants, who must by definition work in a political setting. They will therefore do well to study political commentaries and case studies. Fortunately there are some excellent ones by politicians (Crossman 1971; Powell 1976; Castle 1980), and political scientists and policy analysts (Allison 1971; Neustadt and Fineberg 1978; Allen 1979; Ham 1981; Silverstein 1981; Klein 1983). It is far too easy to assume that if a public health proposal or programme fails, it is because of the irrationality of the politicians and the public. To the contrary, it may well be that the public health professionals have been blind to the broader public context and are politically inept.

### SUMMARY

In the last 50 years there have been major advances in the management and administration of organizations, but mostly in commerce and industry. It is only in recent years that much of this management advance has been evident in the health sector, and then primarily in the area of diagnostic and therapeutic services, particularly those offered by hospitals; thus far, very little impact has been made on public health organizations and practitioners in their work. For the future, public health practitioners around the world will have to become more conversant with the newer management practices that have been developing in recent years, and more adept at translating them into the particular setting of public health, so that their programmes will have maximum impact.

### REFERENCES

Allen, D. (1979). *Hospital planning*. Pitman Medical, London.

Allison, G.T. (1971). *Essence of decision*. Little, Brown, Boston.

Anthony, R. and Herzlinger, R. (1975). *Management control in non-profit organizations*. Richard Irwin Publishers, Homewood, Ill.

Beckhard, R. (1972). Organizational issues in the team delivery of comprehensive health care. *Milbank Mem. Fund Q.* **1**(3), 297.

Beckhard, R. (1975). Strategies for large-system change. *Sloan Management Rev.* **16**(2). 118.

Bennis, W. (1966). *Changing organizations*. McGraw-Hill, New York.

Bennis, W., Benne, K., Chin, R., and Corey, K. (1976). *The planning of change,* 3rd edn. Holt, Rinehart, and Winston, New York.

Blau, R. and Scott, W. (1962). *Formal organizationa.* Chandler Publishing Company, San Francisco.

Brotherston, J. (ed.) (1978). *Morbidity and its relationship to resource allocation. (Papers and proceeding of a workshop.)* The Welsh Office, Cardiff.

Bryant, J.H. (1969). *Health and the developing world.* Cornell University Press, New York.

Castle, B. (1980). *The Castle diaries 1974–76.* Weidenfeld and Nicolson, London.

Churchman, C. (1968). *The systems approach.* Delacorte Press, New York.

Commission on Education for Health Administration (1975). *The report of the Commission on Education for Health Administration,* Vol. I–II. Health Administration Press, Ann Arbor.

Cooper, D. and Rice, D. (1976). The economic cost of illness revisited. *Soc. Security Bull.* **39,** 21.

Cooper, P. (1979). *Health care marketing.* Aspen Systems Corporation, Germantown, Md.

Crossman, R. (1977). *The diaries of a Cabinet Minister,* Vol. 3. Hamish Hamilton and Jonathan Cape, London.

Davis, K. (1967). *Human relations at work: the dynamics of organizational behavior,* 3rd edn. McGraw-Hill, New York.

Department of Health and Social Security (1976a). *Sharing resources for health in England. Report of the Resource Allocation Working Party.* HMSO, London.

Department of Health and Social Security (1976b). *The NHS planning system.* DHSS, London.

Dunlop, D. (1975). Benefit-cost analysis: a review of its applicability in policy analysis for delivering health services. *Soc. Sci. Med.* **9,** 133.

Etzioni, A. (1961). *Comparative analysis of complex organizations.* Free Press, Glencoe.

Etzioni, A. (1964). *Modern organizations.* Prentice-Hall, Englewood Cliffs, NJ.

Evans, J.R. (1981). *Measurement and management in medicine and health services.* The Rockefeller Foundation, New York.

Fink, A. and Kosecoff, J. (1978). *An evaluation primer.* Capitol Publications, Washington, DC.

Flexner, W., Berkowitz, E., and Brown, M. (eds.) (1981). *Strategic planning in health care management.* Aspen Systems Corp., Rockville, Md.

Fournet, B. (1982). *Strategic planning in health services management.* Aspen Systems Corp., Rockville, Md.

Georgopoulos, B. and Mann, F. (1962). *The community general hospital.* Macmillian, New York.

Georgopoulos, B. (1972). *Organization research on health institutions.* Institute for Social Research, University of Michigan, Ann Arbor.

Georgopoulos, B. (1975). *Hospital organization research: review and source book.* Saunders, Philadelphia.

Goldsmith, S. (1981). *Health care management: a contemporary perspective.* Aspen Systems Corp., Rockville, Md.

Griffith, J. (1972). *Quantitative techniques for hospital planning and control.* Lexington Books, D.C. Heath and Co., Lexington, Mass.

Ham, C. (1981). *Policy making in the National Health Service.* Macmillan, London.

Hartunian, N., Smart, C., and Thompson, M. (1981). *The incidence and economic costs of major health impairments: a comparative analysis of cancer, motor vehicle injuries, coronary heart disease, and stroke.* Lexington Books, D.C. Heath and Co., Lexington, Mass.

Homans, G. (1950). *The human group.* Harcourt Brace Jovanovich, New York.

Hornbrook, M., Dodd, R., Jacobs, P., Friedman, L., and Sherman, K. (1982). Reducing the incidence of non-A, non-B post-transfusion hepatitis by testing donor blood for alanine aminotransferase. *N. Engl. J. Med.* **307,** 1315.

International Epidemiological Association (1972). *Uses of epidemiology in planning health services,* Vol. I–II, Edition *Savremena Administracija.* The Publishing House, Belegrade.

Johnson, R., Kast, F., and Rosenzweig, J. (1967). *The theory and management of systems,* 2nd edn. McGraw-Hill, New York.

Kahn, R. and Boulding, E. (1964). *Power and conflict in organizations.* Basic Books, New York.

Kaluzny, A. and Veney, J. (1980). *Health service organizations: a guide to research and assessment.* McCutchan Publishing Corp., Berkeley.

Kaluzny, A., Warner, D., Warren, D., and Zelman, W. (1982). *Management of health services.* Prentice-Hall, Englewood Cliffs, NJ.

Kast, F. and Rosenzweig, J. (1974). *Organization and management: a systems approach,* 2nd edn. McGraw-Hill, New York.

Katz, R. (1974). Skills of an effective administrator. *Harvard Business Review,* September–October.

Katz, D. and Kahn, R. (1978). *The social psychology of organizations,* 2nd edn. Wiley, New York.

King's Fund Working Party (1977). *The education and training of senior managers in the National Health Service, report of a Working Party.* King Edward's Hospital Fund for London.

Klein, R. (1983). *The politics of the National Health Service.* Longman, London.

Knox, E.G. (1979). *Epidemiology in health care planning.* Oxford University Press.

Koontz, H. and O'Donnell, C. (1955). *Principles of management: an analysis of managerial functions,* 1st edn (many subsequent editions). McGraw-Hill, New York.

Kotler, P. (1975). *Marketing for non-profit organizations.* Prentice-Hall, Englewood Cliffs, NJ.

Kottke, T., Puska, P., Feldman, R., Salonen, J., and Tuomilehto, J. (1982). A decline in earning losses associated with a community-based cardiovascular disease prevention project. *Med. Care* **20,** 663.

Kovner, A. and Neuhauser, D. (1978). *Health services management: readings and commentary.* Health Administration Press, Ann Arbor.

Kurtz, M. (1980). A behaviorial profile of physicians in management roles. In *The physician in management* (ed. R.S. Schenke) American Academy of Medical Directors, Falls Church, Va.

Lawrence, P. and Lorsch, M.J. (1969). *Organization and environment: managing differentiation and integration.* Richard Irwin Publishers, Homewood, Ill.

Lawrence, P. and Lorsch, M.J. (1969). *Developing organizations: diagnosis and action.* Addison-Wesley, Reading, Mass.

Lee, K. and Mills, A. (1982). *policy making and planning in the health sector,* Croom Helm, London.

Levey, S. and Loomba, N. (1973). *Health care administration: a managerial perspective.* Lippincott, Philadelphia.

Levey, S. and McCarthy, T. (1980). *Health management for tomorrow.* Lippincott, Philadelphia.

Likert, R. (1961). *New patterns of management.* McGraw-Hill, New York.

Likert, R. (1967). *The human organization.* McGraw-Hill, New York.

Litterer, J. (1965). *The analysis of organizations.* Wiley, New York.

Longest, B. (1980). *Management practices for the health professional.* Reston Publishing Co., Reston, Va.

McCool, B. and Brown, M. (1977). *The management response: conceptual, technical, and human skills of health administration.*

Saunders, Philadelphia.

McGregor, D. (1960). *The human side of enterprise.* McGraw-Hill, New York.

MacStravic, R. (1977). *Marketing health care.* Aspen Systems Corp., Germantown.

MacStravic, R. (1980). *Marketing by objectives for hospitals.* Aspen Systems Corp., Germantown.

March, J. and Simon, H. (1958). *Organizations.* Wiley, New York.

Maslow, A. (1954). *Motivation and personality.* Harper and Row, New York.

Milbank Memorial Fund Commission on Higher Education for Public Health (1976). *Report.* Milbank Memorial Fund, New York.

Mintzberg, H. (1973). *The nature of managerial work.* Harper and Row, New York.

Mintzberg, H. (1979). *The structuring of organizations: a synthesis of research.* Prentice-Hall, Englewood Cliffs, NJ.

Mount, B. (1976). The problem of caring for the dying in a general hospital; the palliative care unit as a possible solution. *Can. Med. Assoc. J.* **115,** 119.

Navarro, V. (1974). *National and regional health planning in Sweden.* DHEW, Washington.

Neustadt, R.E. and Fineberg, H.V. (1978). *The swine flu affair.* DHEW, Washington.

Perow, C. (1970). *Organizational analysis: a sociological view.* Wadsworth Publishing Co., Belmont. Ca.

Peters, T.J. and Waterman, R.H. (1982). *In search of excellence.* Harper and Row, New York.

Powell, T. E. (1976). *Medicine and politics: 1975 and after.* Pitman Medical, London.

Rakich, J., Longest, B., and O'Donovan, T. (1977). *Managing health care organizations.* Saunders, Philadelphia.

Robbins, S. (1974). *Managing organizational conflict.* Prentice-Hall, Englewood Cliffs, NJ.

Rowbottom, R., Balle, J., Cang, S. *et al.* (1973). *Hospital organization.* Heinemann, London.

Rubin, I. and Beckhard, R. (1972). Factors influencing the effectiveness of health teams. *Milbank Mem. Fund Q.* **1**(3), 251.

Rubin, I., Plovnick, M., and Fry, R. (1974). Initiating planned change in health care systems. *J. Appl. Behav. Sci.* **10,** 107.

Rubin, I., Fry, R., and Plovnick, M. (1978). *Managing human resources in health care organizations: an applied approach.* Reston Publishing Co., Reston, Va.

Schein, E. (1970). *Organizational psychology.* Prentice-Hall, Englewood Cliffs, NJ.

Schon, D.A. (1971). *Beyond the stable state.* Temple Smith, London.

Schultz, R. and Harrison, S. (1983). *Teams and top managers in the National Health Service.* Project Paper No. 41. King's Fund, London.

Shortell, S. and Brown, M. (1976). *Organizational research in hospitals.* Blue Cross Association, Chicago.

Shortell, S. and Richardson, W. (1978). *Health program evaluation.* Mosby, St. Louis, Mo.

Silverstein, A.M. (1981). *Pure politics and impure science.* John Hopkins University Press, Baltimore.

Slater, C. (1980). The physician manager's role: results of a survey. In *The physician in management* (ed. R.S. Schenke). American Academy of Medical Directors, Falls Church, Va.

Smith, P., Keyes, N., and Forman, E. (1982). Socioeconomic evaluation of a state-funded comprehensive hemophilia-care program. *N. Engl. J. Med.* **306,** 575.

Starkweather, D. (1981). *Hospital mergers.* Health Administration Press, Ann Arbor.

Steiner, G. (1979). *Strategic planning: what every manager must know.* Free Press, New York.

Stewart, R., Smith, P., Blake, J., and Wingate, P. (1980). *The district administrator in the National Health Service.* King's Fund, London.

Suchman, E.A. (1967). *Evaluation research: principles and practice in public service social action programs.* Russell Sage Foundation, New York.

Tichy, N. (1977). *Organizational design for public health care: the case of the Martin Luther King Health Center.* Praeger, New York.

Warner, D. and Holloway, D. (1978). *Decision making and control for health administration.* Health Administration Press, Ann Arbor.

Warner, K. and Luce, B. (1982). *Cost-benefit and cost-effectiveness analysis in health care: principles, practice, and potential.* Health Administration Press, Ann Arbor.

Weiss, H., Beckhard, R., Rubin, I., and Kyte, A. (1974). *Making health teams work.* Ballinger, Cambridge, Mass.

White, K. and Henderson, M. (1976). *Epidemiology as a fundamental science.* Oxford University Press, New York.

Wieland, G. (ed.) (1981). *Improving health care management: organization development and organization change.* Health Administration Press, Ann Arbor.

World Health Organization (1972). *Approaches to national health planning.* Public Health Papers No. 46. WHO, Geneva.

World Health Organization (1976). *The education and training of public health medical officers, report of a working party.* ICP/HMD.037, WHO Regional Office for Europe, Copenhagen.

World Health Organization (1980). *The planning of health services: studies in 8 European countries.* WHO Regional Office for Europe, Copenhagen.

# Field investigations of physical, chemical, and biological hazards

# 15 Viral diseases of public health importance

George E. Kenny and Marion K. Cooney

## INTRODUCTION

The control and prevention of viral diseases is simultaneously a very old and a very new field. Although the first useful vaccine was produced by Jenner for smallpox, the majority of the known viruses have been discovered in the last 30 years. Additional agents are still being discovered. Rational control is only possible by an understanding of the epidemiology of the infections, pathogenesis of the agents, and their biochemical nature: determinations which require the ability to isolate (or detect) the agent, to propagate the virus in quantity, and to conduct suitable field studies to assess the impact of the agent.

From the time of Pasteur to the mid-1940s, viruses could be propagated only to a limited extent in embryonated eggs and experimental animals. The heroic efforts applied to poliomyelitis, using non-human primates as host systems for virus studies, provided a base of information which enabled virologists to take immediate advantage of cell culture systems when these became available in the late 1940s. Modern virology dates from the application of cell culture techniques. A great variety of viruses were isolated throughout the 1950s and 1960s spurred by the success of the poliovirus vaccines produced in monkey kidney cell cultures. Many viruses such as Coxsackie A viruses, all of the Coxsackie B viruses, influenza and para-influenza viruses, and mumps virus could readily be isolated in monkey kidney cells.

The advent of the HeLa cell was most important because this cell line was immortal and capable of indefinite propagation (other immortal cell lines have subsequently been found to be of great importance). This provided both research laboratories and diagnostic laboratories with an invaluable tool for isolation and propagation of a variety of agents. In the early 1960s, Hayflick and Moorhead established techniques for propagating cells in limited passage, which retained their diploid chromosome number, and were therefore very similar to primary cell cultures in susceptibility to virus infections, but could be preserved in liquid nitrogen, revived, and continued in their passage history. The most used of these diploid cell lines is WI-38 (WI stands for Wistar Institute). Diploid fibroblasts were not only more sensitive for detection of certain viruses (herpes viruses, most ECHO viruses, and certain adeno-viruses) than HeLa cells or primary monkey kidney cells, but were required for demonstration of the rhinoviruses.

Individual lines and strains of the available cell culture types vary in their susceptibility to 'wild' viruses. Thus, the well-equipped diagnostic laboratory maintains several cell lines – a

primary culture, a diploid cell line, and a HeLa cell culture – to accommodate the variety of agents likely to be circulating in the community. The main advantage of cell culture technology is that it is much less expensive and usually more sensitive than animal inoculation. However, animal inoculation is still employed for certain viruses such as rabies and arboviruses.

Agents also exist which cannot be detected in any known cell culture system. Morphological methods based on light micro-scopy have been used for a long time to detect pathognomic inclusion bodies in cells (methods presently replaced to a large extent by the fluorescent antibody technique). Electron micro-scopy has added another tool particularly when used in combination with specific antibody ('immune electron micro-scopy'). The antibody causes aggregation of scarce virus particles so that the clumps can be detected and identified in the electron microscope. A most important advance (mostly in the 1970s) was the development of direct antigen-detection methods. This methodology received great impetus from studies with hepatitis B viruses which cannot be cultivated in cell cultures but sufficient viral proteins are synthesized in the host which can be detected by highly sensitive immunological methods. Both the radioimmunoassay and enzyme-linked immunosorbent assay (ELISA) have been most important in developing direct detection methods.

Future advances in detection of viruses will continue to focus on the development of new and more sensitive cell culture systems. However, much greater emphasis will be placed on direct detection of viruses using monoclonal antibodies in sensitive immunological methods. These developments will lead to much greater availability of inexpensive diagnostic methods which will do much to aid our understanding of viral infections; a development which in turn will lead to more effective prevention.

### Serodiagnosis

Detection of viral antibodies is a useful device for assessing individual infections and, more importantly, the prevalence of past infections in populations. For the individual case, the detection of a significant antibody increase between acute and convalescent sera is a major means of establishing an association between a recent illness and a given viral agent. Such serodiagnoses are particularly useful in detecting infections in which the agent cannot be isolated or where appropriate specimens have not been collected. Detection of presence or absence of antibody is important in diseases such as rubella because if it is known that antibody is present before pregnancy it can be assumed that there has been no damage to the fetus by rubella because reinfection with this virus is unknown. For population studies, detection of antibodies provides an excellent picture of the prevalence of a given agent over the past history of a population. Collection of sequential sera permits the detection of antibody increases over time and hence assessment of the incidence of recent infections with specific agents.

There is a major caveat concerning the use of significant antibody rises between acute and convalescent sera. Since certain bacteria and viruses are polyclonal B cell activators, it is possible that significant antibody rises generated to a given agent may be the result of polyclonal activation and not of a recent infection with the agent showing the rise. A different agent may have caused the primary problem. The total significance of such 'false-positive' serological antibody increases is not presently known; however, it appears that the problem may be most marked with antigens containing carbohydrate determinants. Testing of antisera with a variety of antigens may help to distinguish false-positives from real antibody increases.

The major problem in devising control methods for virus infections lies in the fact that our understanding of the prevalence and persistence of various viruses in the community is still very limited particularly for more recently identified agents. Few comprehensive studies have been conducted to determine the full range of agents detectable in a given disease syndrome. Most studies have focused on a very limited range of agents because of cost and technical difficulty of managing large studies. Such studies can be conducted provided that sufficient funds are available and below we will show examples of comprehensive studies of respiratory viruses.

## Infection versus disease

The hallmark of most viral infections is that many individuals are infected but few become ill. One of the more exaggerated cases is that of poliovirus, where most infections are subclinical and only a few persons develop poliomyelitis. In contrast, in diseases such as measles, chickenpox, and rubella, infection usually results in clinical symptoms and disease. For viruses causing repeated infections such as parainfluenza and respiratory syncytial virus, the incidence of clinical disease may be much lower on reinfections in adults. On the other hand, presence of antibody (either maternal or induced by immunization) in young infants has been hypothesized to be a prerequisite for severe disease.

## RESPIRATORY AGENTS

In this chapter, respiratory viruses are defined as those agents which have a method of spread which is primarily respiratory (Table 15.1) even though the ultimate disease is not respiratory (for example, smallpox). Further, some of the agents such as adenoviruses may have a primary route of spread by the oral-faecal route but the agents may cause respiratory infections.

## The common cold

Although the common cold is generally considered to be a mild disease, it is the largest health problem of an infectious nature faced by western society today. The economic cost of

**Table 15.1.** *Viral respiratory agents and diseases*

| Agent | Disease | Prime age group | Virus detection* |
|---|---|---|---|
| Influenza viruses | Influenza | All | Cell culture (embryonated egg) |
| Rhinoviruses | Common cold | All | Cell culture |
| Parainfluenza viruses | Croup, pneumonia<br>Mild URI | Children<br>Adults | Cell culture |
| Mumps virus | Mumps, URI<br>Aseptic meningitis | Children | Cell culture (embryonated egg) |
| Measles virus | Measles | Children | Cell culture (low efficiency) |
| Rubella virus | German measles | Children, adults | Cell culture |
| Respiratory syncytial virus | Pneumonia | Children | Cell culture (low efficiency) |
| Coronaviruses | Cold-like syndromes | Children<br>Adults | Rare cell culture isolates |
| Adenoviruses | Pneumonia †<br>Eye infections | Children, adults | Cell culture |
| Herpes virus Type I ‡ | Herpes | All ages | Cell culture |
| Cytomegalovirus | Cytomegalic inclusion disease<br>Opportunistic infections | Fetal<br>Immunocompromized persons | Cell culture |
| Epstein–Barr virus | Mononucleosis | Young adults | Serology |
| Variola virus | Smallpox | All ages | Cell culture |
| Varicella/zoster virus | Chicken pox<br>Shingles | Children<br>Adults | Cell culture (low efficiency) |

*Detection of agent by culture in laboratory.

† Although symptoms are respiratory, agent appears to be an enteric agent.

‡ Type II herpesviruses are genital agents primarily. Type I viruses may also have genital spread.

rhinovirus infections (days lost from work or school, and purchase of cold remedies) is enormous. An insidious consequence, which cannot be evaluated is the impairment in efficiency and judgement in persons who try to carry out their normal responsibilities when affected by this 'trivial' disease. The major cause of the common cold is the rhinovirus group which includes more than 100 serotypes. Effective control by vaccines has been thought to be impossible because of: (i) the large number of serotypes; (ii) the multiplicity of serotypes circulating concurrently in a community; and (iii) the lack of medical consultation for symptoms of the common cold. However, the rhinovirus serotypes show extensive grouping by serological cross-reactions; thus, it might be possible to prepare a vaccine to a number of crucial types and obtain significant prevention. Further, some types are more common than others. The common cold shows peak incidence with the onset of cold seasons, a fact without apparent explanation.

Although the mechanism of spread had been assumed to be by aerosol from sneezing, it now appears that self-inoculation (nose-picking among other possibilities) from hand to hand contact or contact with contaminated fomites is important. This concept is supported by evidence that during high incidence of rhinovirus infections many serotypes, each limited to a few households, circulate in the community. Cate has suggested that 'self-control' of rhinovirus infections might be accomplished through strict attention to personal hygiene such as frequent handwashing.

A variety of other agents also cause common cold-like syndromes. The most important of these may be the parainfluenza viruses. Although description of diseases caused by coronaviruses has been difficult because the agents have not been isolated, serological surveys have shown that these agents also may cause a substantial amount of cold-like disease.

## Influenza

Influenza remains the most dramatic of viral respiratory diseases occurring in major epidemics as shifts in the virus occur. Major influenza A epidemics occur at two to three yearly intervals. In between epidemic peaks, small outbreaks occur in specific localities. Influenza A viruses are unique in that they show both antigenic drift (small antigenic changes on haemagglutinin and neuraminidase antigens) and antigenic shift (large changes in antigenic structure on either or both antigens). Pandemics usually follow a major shift, particularly a 'double shift', that is, changes in both antigens. Four different haemagglutinins are known: $H_0$, $H_1$, $H_2$, $H_3$. There is less variation in neuraminidase and only two, $N_1$ and $N_2$, are known. Four different influenza viruses are known to have infected man – they are $H_0N_1$ (1933), $H_1N_1$ (1947), $H_2N_2$ (1957 – Asian flu), and $H_3N_2$ (1968 – Hong Kong flu). A fifth variant is known if we include $H_{sw}N_1$ thought to have been responsible for the 1918 pandemic. It has been postulated that the number of antigenic variants may be limited and that a cycle of influenza viruses may occur. Thus, when $H_{sw}N_1$ appeared in 1976 it was feared that a major pandemic similar to the 1918 pandemic might occur. A vaccine was prepared and used (primarily in the US), but the virus did not spread and instead a virus similar to the 1947 $H_1N_1$ appeared and

spread two years later. Although the various haemagglutinins are quite distinct antigenically, the antigens appear to contain enough common determinants that the prime immune response in man to haemagglutinin is focused on the first infecting A virus. Thus each successive infection with another A virus generates a major recall of antibodies to the initial infecting strain for that individual (original antigenic sin). Influenza B viruses do not show antigenic shift but are subject to antigenic drift and epidemics occur at three to five yearly intervals.

## Severe respiratory disease

In the 1940s, the term primary atypical pneumonia was defined to include those pneumonias which did not resemble classic pneumococcal pneumonia. Over the past 40 years, a number of agents have been identified which cause portions of the syndrome, atypical pneumonia. In young children the most important agents of pneumonia are viruses with parainfluenza viruses and respiratory syncytial viruses playing the major role. Reinfection with these agents in later life results in mild cold-like infections. In young adults (particularly military recruits), adenoviruses may play an important role. A non-viral agent, *Mycoplasma pneumoniae*, is the most important cause of atypical pneumonia in this age group.

## Prospects for control of respiratory infections

It is reasonable to assume that agents which are able to reinfect and cause disease will be difficult to control by vaccine. Thus, the success of vaccines for rubella and rubeola may have resulted from the fact that neither of these agents is able to reinfect. In contrast, vaccines for influenza have had low efficacy rates (protection rates over 50 per cent are considered good) depending upon the match of the vaccine with the potential infecting influenza virus. Since most of the respiratory agents with the exception of influenza are relatively difficult to cultivate on a large scale, efforts at producing vaccines have been concentrated on live attenuated vaccines.

## ENTERIC VIRUSES

The viral agents which are transmitted by the faecal-oral route differ from those which cause respiratory infections in that they must survive the acid conditions in the stomach. Thus the enterovirus group of the picornaviruses are acid-stable in contrast to the acid lability of the rhinoviruses. As for the respiratory agents, the enteric agents are difficult to classify since some agents (for example, certain ECHO viruses) may cause respiratory infections. We have classified the viruses by primary site of infection recognizing that other routes of infection may occur (Table 15.2). These agents can be differentiated into several classes.

1. Agents which multiply in the gut and are shed in the faeces but are not associated with diarrhoeal disease (for example, adenoviruses and enteroviruses). Both of these classes of agents can be isolated from the throat as well early

**Table 15.2.** *Viral enteric agents and diseases*

| Agent | Disease | Prime age group | Virus detection* |
|---|---|---|---|
| Polioviruses | Poliomyelitis | Children, adults † | Cell culture |
| Enteric cytopathic human orphan viruses (ECHO) | Aseptic meningitis, respiratory infections | Children, adults | Cell culture |
| Coxsackie virus | Pleurodynia, aseptic meningitis, common-cold like | Children, adults | Cell culture (suckling mice) |
| Hepatitis A | Hepatitis | Children, adults | Antigen detection only |
| Rotaviruses | Diarrhoea | Children, adults | Antigen detection only |
| Norwalk agent | Diarrhoea | Children, adults | Antigen detection only |
| Reoviruses | Respiratory (?) | Children, adults | Cell culture |

*Detection of agent by culture in laboratory.

†Prime age groups infected depend upon amount of virus circulating in community. The less the sanitation, the younger the age group infected and paradoxically the less clinical disease.

in infection. In addition, adenoviruses are often associated with conjunctivitis or pharyngo-conjunctival fever and may be recovered from the conjunctiva as well.

2. Certain viruses, such as, rotaviruses, and the non-cultivatable adenoviruses are associated with diarrhoea. They cannot be readily isolated in cell culture but can be detected by electron microscopy and/or enzyme-linked immuno-sorbent assay.

## Hepatitis

Three major forms of viral hepatitis are known: hepatitis A (infectious hepatitis), hepatitis B (serum hepatitis), and non-A, non-B hepatitis. Hepatitis A virus is now classified as an enterovirus. The disease is a typical enteric infection with the hepatitis resulting from antigen–antibody complexes. Although the acute disease may be severe, complications are relatively rare. In contrast, hepatitis B is a life-threatening disease with potentially severe complications extended over a long time period. Three outcomes can result from hepatitis B infection: (i) no symptoms and development of immunity; (ii) hepatitis with eventual development of immunity after a period of hepatitis antigen carriage; and (iii) life-long carriage of hepatitis B surface antigen. Chronic carriers of surface antigen are at risk not only to progressive hepatitis but also to hepatoma (hepatocellular carcinoma) incidence of which is greatly increased in those who carry hepatitis B antigen. Much less is known about non-A, non-B hepatitis. The agent appears to be a DNA-containing virus similar to hepatitis B. A recently recognized disease is caused by the 'Delta' agent. From what is presently known this agent can only replicate in persons who carry hepatitis B surface antigen. Thus, the agent appears to be defective in that it requires hepatitis B virus as a helper. Infection with Delta agent can result in clinical hepatitis. The relationship of Delta agent to hepatoma and severe hepatitis is presently unknown.

Hepatitis A virus appears to spread as a typical enterovirus (faecal–oral route of transmission), while the other agents (hepatitis B; non-A, non-B; and Delta agent) are spread by serum products. However, other modes of infection are also important. A major mode of transmission of hepatitis B in the Orient is from an antigen positive mother to her infant. In that setting, the infant has a high probability of becoming a chronic antigen carrier with no symptomatology. It may be 40 or 50 years later that hepatoma is observed (primarily in male offspring). Apparently antigen carrying females continue the cycle by infecting some of their offspring. The high incidence of hepatitis B antigen carriage in active male homosexuals also suggests alternative methods of transmission other than blood products.

Clearly, hepatitis B virus poses a major public health problem which will become more acute in western societies if the basic epidemiology of the agent changes to one more like that observed in the Orient.

### Diagnosis of hepatitis infections

The knowledge we have of hepatitis B infections has been primarily gained by the use of advanced methods of sero-diagnosis. Through radio-immunoassay and enzyme-linked immunosorbent assay, it has been possible to detect antigens (core antigen, surface antigen, early (e) antigen) and their corresponding antibodies. This has been a major triumph since the agent has yet to be propagated in the laboratory. However, from a public health point of view, the present tests are expensive and not widely available. Preparation of antigen by recombinant DNA methods is proceeding rapidly and should lead to improved availability of diagnostic reagents.

### Prevention of hepatitis

Prevention of hepatitis A might be accomplished using killed vaccines in a manner similar to that used for polioviruses since the virus can be grown in cell culture. Prevention of hepatitis B by vaccine is much more complex because of the difficulties in cultivating the virus. Two lines of approach are being used: preparation of vaccine from human blood plasma from hepatitis B surface antigen carriers, and production of the viral proteins by recombinant DNA technology. Understanding of the immune response will be most important since the clinical outcome of persons who persistently carry hepatitis B surface antigen is much more serious than in those persons who develop sufficient immunity to eliminate antigen carriage. Treatment of infants, who are at risk of becoming permanent carriers of surface antigen, with immune globulin appears to reduce the chance of the infant becoming an antigen carrier. Fortunately, a natural animal model for hepatitis B infections exists in the eastern woodchuck where a similar agent is detectable, with antigen carriage and eventual development of hepatoma. This model system may permit the elucidation of the association of hepatoma with hepatitis B type viruses. One important question is: does the virus itself provide the transforming event or does chronic infection set up conditions for eventual hepatoma? In the human system, determination of the role of antigenic variation in the viruses will be most important in devising strategies of prevention. Efforts at preventing non-A, non-B hepatitis, and Delta agent infections await further developments in the assessment of their role in human disease.

## NEW EMERGING DISEASES

### Acquired immunodeficiency syndrome (AIDS)

In 1980, a new and distinct clinical syndrome was recognized in the US and Europe which is characterized by a profound immunosuppression. Patients with the disease characteristically present with opportunistic infections including *Pneumocystis carinii* and *Candida*. Another major finding is a high incidence of Kaposi's sarcoma, in a severe and progressive form. Ordinarily, Kaposi's sarcoma is a relatively mild skin tumour occasionally found in middle-aged males. The disease has been observed in active male homosexuals, persons who receive frequent blood transfusions, and in some Haitian males. The immune dysfunction(s) involves a relative decrease in the number of T helper cells as well as changes in T cell responsiveness to T-cell independent immunogens. The spread of the disease from area to area is strongly suggestive of an infective agent or agents. Further, the clinical syndrome is so distinctive that it is likely that the disease is new at least in western society.

The search for possible agents has been intense. Data have been accumulated which show that a retrovirus is a possible candidate. First, some 30 per cent of patients with AIDS showed antibody to a human retrovirus (human T-cell leukaemia virus) whereas only one of the controls showed antibody. Secondly, retroviruses have been isolated from several patients, and finally retrovirus genomic material has been found in cells from several patients. Although retroviruses are an attractive candidate as an agent for AIDS, because of the similarities of the immunosuppression to that seen in cats infected with feline leukaemia virus, a similar human agent found in Japan does not appear to be associated with AIDS. It is possible that the retroviruses are detected because of the immunosuppression which might be caused by another agent. However this may turn out, it is likely that the agent is new or a variant of some previously known agent.

Clearly, any efforts at preventing AIDS must focus on determining the responsible agent(s) and the mode of spread. The high mortality and apparently rapid spread of the agent in target populations suggest that this is a most important public health problem.

### Viruses and cancer

The findings that hepatitis B is associated with hepatoma and that some infectious agent may ·be associated with AIDS provide the first evidence of an infectious nature for some human tumours. Although Epstein–Barr (EB) virus is known to infect humans and cause infectious mononucleosis, its association with two other cancers suspected to have infectious origins, nasopharyngeal carcinoma and Burkitt lymphoma, is much less clear. Similarly, the association of herpes simplex type II with cervical carcinoma provides only limited evidence for a role of that virus in cancer. Although certain human adenoviruses are known to cause tumours in hamsters, extensive studies have shown no evidence for adenovirus DNA in human tumours.

The difficulty in associating human tumours with viruses lies in the lack of appropriate models for study. However, in animals an extensive association of tumours with viruses has been established. For example, an avian herpesvirus (Marek disease virus) causes neoplastic transformation of T cells accompanied by a severe immunodepression (which may facilitate the disease and might relate to AIDS, discussed above). Retroviruses are also tumour agents of animals (mice, cats, birds, etc.). The development of animal models will certainly provide important leads to the assessment of the role of viruses in cancer. An important new concept is that the transformation of a cell to an invasive tumour is a multistep process. A further critical concept which links virology with environmental carcinogenesis theories is that mutagens and viruses are not necessarily independent agents in the aetiology of cancer. Viral infection is required before a carcinogen can induce transformation of certain cells in culture. In some of these cases, neither the carcinogen nor the virus alone could cause a tumour.

Since viruses can clearly provide a critical event in the development of tumours in animals and some association of viruses can be found with human tumours, intensive studies will be required to assign a role for viruses in some human tumours. Only after such studies have been provided will it be possible to intervene in the process of causation of cancers.

### Slow viral infections

Subacute sclerosing panencephalitis follows measles infection by several years. Measles antigens are detectable from the brain and an agent apparently closely related to measles virus has been recovered by co-cultivation. A more unusual agent is associated with Creutzfeld–Jakob disease, a fatal presenile dementia in mid-life. The agent is apparently not a conventional virus but appears to be an agent composed of protein. The agent is highly resistant to disinfectants such as formaldehyde, alcohols, and detergents, and a variety of other agents. The agent is susceptible to oxidizing agents such as hypochlorite and to autoclaving. Creutzfeld–Jakob disease is rare but has been spread by corneal transplants and by instruments used in neurosurgery. Similar agents are involved in the slow virus disease of sheep (scrapie).

## VIRUS DISEASES OF ANIMALS FOR WHICH MAN IS AN ACCIDENTAL HOST

The natural hosts for rabies appear to be bats and a number of other species of wild animals. Humans are infected by bite.

**Table 15.3.** *Virus isolation from family studies of influenza and rhinovirus infections*

| Year | Total isolates | RV | HSV | Flu | Para | Adeno | Cox | Echo | Other |
|------|------|------|------|------|------|------|------|------|------|
| 1975 (Sept–Dec) | 47 | 18 | 8 | 0 | 17 | 0 | 2 | 1 | 1 |
| 1976 (Jan–Dec) | 479 | 234 | 53 | 60 | 47 | 25 | 21 | 26 | 13 |
| 1977 (Jan–Dec) | 457 | 308 | 55 | 13 | 2 | 32 | 20 | 18 | 9 |
| 1978 (Jan–Dec) | 322 | 202 | 53 | 33 | 3 | 16 | 2 | 7 | 6 |
| 1979 (Jan–Apr) | 105 | 27 | 9 | 66 | 0 | 1 | 0 | 0 | 2 |
| Total | 1410* | 789 | 178 | 172 | 69 | 74 | 45 | 52 | 31 |

RV – Rhinovirus; HSV – Herpes simplex; Flu – Influenza A and B; Para – Parainfluenza 1, 2, 3; Adeno – Adenovirus; Cox – Coxsackie; Echo – Echo viruses; Other – includes poliovirus, rubeola, respiratory syncytial virus, and cytomegalovirus.
*Isolation from 17 823 respiratory specimens from ill persons and their family contacts: 8 per cent isolation rate.

Although it is not known whether subclinical infections occur, humans who develop symptoms nearly always die (though recently a few patients have survived with intensive support of vital functions). Prevention is difficult in areas where rabies is enzootic in a variety of animals. Vaccination of pets is most important. Treatment of humans bitten by suspect animals is more complex because laboratory diagnosis is not useful from patient specimens except retrospectively from deceased patients. If the animal can be captured, detection of rabies virus will indicate possible infection. If the animal cannot be found, the decision to treat is independent of laboratory data, and dependent upon observational data. Treatment with rabies vaccine is required if the animal is positive or circumstances strongly indicate infection. The incubation period is ordinarily sufficiently long to permit formation of antibodies and prevention of disease.

The arthropod-borne viruses (arboviruses – see chapter 16 for a detailed description) are a most important group because they can multiply both in vertebrates and arthropods. The viruses of yellow fever, the various equine encephalitis viruses, and dengue are important agents in this group. Man is usually an accidental and terminal host for these agents. Yellow fever is an exception since a human infected from monkeys in a jungle can serve as a focus for further mosquito-borne spread from man to man (urban yellow fever). Diagnosis can be accomplished by isolation of the virus or demonstration of an antibody increase. Arenaviruses (the haemorrhagic fever agents) cause severe and frequently fatal disease. Arenaviruses primarily cause chronic disease in rodents, and man is an accidental host. Infection is spread to humans through urine and other excretions of rodents. Although man is an accidental host, Lassa virus can spread from man to man. All of the agents discussed in this paragraph are highly hazardous to handle in the laboratory and only a few regional laboratories are suitably equipped.

## PUBLIC HEALTH RESPONSIBILITIES IN VIRAL SURVEILLANCE

If an overall goal of public health laboratory science is the prevention of disease, then surveillance is required to determine which diseases are prevalent. This role is carried out by regional and national laboratories to the extent that such laboratories serve as reference centres for local laboratories. However, regional laboratories are rarely in a position to sample more than the most spectacular diseases and epidemics. What is required is a surveillance system in defined populations to assess the incidence and prevalence of diseases due to various agents. Such undertakings are invariably expensive not only in terms of laboratory resources but also in terms of specimen collection. The Seattle family studies is an example of such a surveillance system. Mild respiratory diseases were found to be caused by a great variety of agents (Table 15.3). If prevention of mild disease were a public health goal, one would clearly focus on rhinoviruses which appear to be the major agents.

## PROSPECTS FOR PREVENTION OF VIRAL DISEASES

The elimination of smallpox was a major public health triumph, and was possible for a number of reasons: (i) an effective attenuated vaccine was available; (ii) prolonged asymptomatic excretion of the viruses from carriers did not occur; (iii) the virus had no reservoir in nature; and (iv) a concentrated effort was directed at eliminating the disease. A similar but less total success has been achieved with poliovirus infections. Although the choice of live or attenuated vaccines has been contentious, both vaccines proved to be effective in greatly reducing paralytic disease but were not effective in eliminating the wild virulent viruses. A further example of a less effective but useful vaccine is that against rabies. Rabies vaccine evolved from the attenuated vaccine of Pasteur (which had the drawback of causing severe immune neurological reactions), through the attenuated vaccine propagated in duck embryo, to the present relatively safe and effective human diploid cell vaccine.

Future vaccine developments will focus on the use of recombinant DNA technology to produce abundant supplies of specific viral proteins. The advantage of this technology is that it is not necessary to propagate the agent to clone the genetic information required. Hepatitis B genomes have been cloned already. Another important development is the use of synthetic polypeptides for immunization. Such polypeptides can be synthesized either from information obtained from direct protein sequences of important viral peptide antigens, or deduced from the structure of the nucleic acid.

However, vaccines are not practical for agents which cause chronic infections or reinfect with disease. More detailed knowledge of the immune response to specific viruses and viral components will be required before such vaccines can be developed if they prove to be possible at all.

## FURTHER READING

Davis, B.D., Dulbecco, R., Eisen, H.N., and Ginsberg, H.S. (1980). *Microbiology,* 3rd edn. Harper and Row, Hagerstown, Md.

Evans, A.S. (ed.) (1982). *Viral infections of humans: epidemiology and control.* Plenum, New York.

Fenner, F. and White, D.O. (1976). *Medical virology,* 2nd edn. Academic Press, New York.

Fox, J.P. and Hall, C.E. (1980). *Viruses in families.* PSG Publishing Company, Littleton, Mass.

Fox, J.P., Hall, C.E., Cooney, M.K., and Foy, H.M. (1982). Influenza virus infections in Seattle families, 1975–1979. *Am. J. Epidemiol.* **116**, 212.

Koprowski, C. and Koprowski, H. (eds.) (1975). *Viruses and immunity.* Academic Press, New York.

Knight, V. (ed.) (1973). *Viral and mycoplasmal infections of the respiratory tract.* Lea and Febiger, Philadelphia.

Lennette, D.A., Specter, S., and Thompson, K.D. (eds.) (1979). *Diagnosis of viral infections. The role of the clinical laboratory.* University Park Press, Baltimore, Md.

Lennette, E.H., Balows, A., Hauseler, W.J. Jr, and Truant, J.P. (eds.) (1980). *Manual of clinical microbiology,* 3rd edn. American Society for Microbiology, Washington, DC.

Lennette, E.H., Balows, A., Hausler, W.J. Jr, and Truant, J.P. *cedures for viral rickettsial and chlamydial infections,* 5th edn. American Public Health Association. Washington, DC.

McLean, D.M. (1980). *Virology in health care.* Williams and Wilkins, Baltimore, Md.

Mims, C.A. (1982). *Pathogenesis of infectious disease.* Academic Press, New York.

# 16 Arboviruses

## M.G.R. Varma and H.E. Webb

### DEFINITION

Arboviruses are defined as animal viruses transmitted biologically by blood-sucking arthropods; hence the name *Ar-* (arthropod) *bo-* (borne) viruses. They are world-wide in distribution and include the causative agents of some of the most devastating and important epidemic and enzootic diseases. They form a biological rather than a natural taxonomic group and include members of different families such as Togaviridae, Bunyaviridae, Rhabdoviridae, and Reoviridae, some members of which may not be associated with arthropods at all.

The American Committee on Arthropod-borne Viruses lists 446 viruses. Most of these are not true arboviruses and do not comply with the guide lines for confirmation of an agent as an arbovirus. Some are listed as arboviruses (e.g. Entebbe bat and Rio Bravo viruses) because of their relationship with known arboviruses, although they are not associated with blood-sucking arthropods. Others appear to be listed simply because they were isolated in laboratories or by virologists primarily interested in arboviruses (for example, Lassa, Ebola, Lagos bat, and Mount Elgon bat viruses).

The following are guide lines for determining whether a virus is an arbovirus:

1. Isolation from naturally infected arthropods.

2. Demonstration of virus multiplication in salivary glands or body of experimentally infected arthropods and transmission of the virus to susceptible vertebrates during feeding by infected arthropods.

3. Demonstration of stage-to-stage (trans-stadial, horizontal) and/or transovarial (hereditary, vertical) transmission of the agent in infected arthropods.

4. Demonstration of biological arthropod transmission by wild-caught naturally infected arthropods feeding on a susceptible vertebrate host.

5. Demonstration of viraemia in vertebrate hosts compatible with blood-sucking habits of arthropods.

6. Antigenic relationship to a proven arbovirus.

7. Strong epidemiological association such as increase in numbers of arthropods and arthropod-vertebrate contact compatible with arthropod transmission.

Arboviruses may not satisfy all the above criteria, but proven biological transmission in the laboratory, i.e. infection by feeding on a viraemic host and transmission after a varying period of time, during feeding on a susceptible host is taken as evidence for arbovirus status of an agent. This will confirm the presumptive and circumstantial evidence provided by the other criteria.

Analysis of all the evidence for the 446 viruses shows that 26 (6 per cent) are not, or probably not, arboviruses and only 109 (24 per cent) are proven arboviruses. Seventy-three (16 per cent) are probable arboviruses and a further 238 (53 per cent), possible arboviruses. Additional data are required for a more precise rating of these agents.

### HISTORICAL REVIEW

The first arbovirus to be isolated was bluetongue virus which causes disease in livestock, and the first arbovirus causing human disease to be isolated was yellow fever (YF) virus. Devastating epidemics of yellow fever or 'yellow jack' occurred in the new world following its introduction from Africa with the slave traffic. This aroused a great deal of concern and interest about the nature of the aetiological agent and the method of its transmission. Discovery of the role of mosquitoes in the transmission of yellow fever was the starting point in our knowledge of arbovirus infections in animals. Despite the interest in arboviruses, only 16 had been isolated up to the end of the Second World War (Table 16.1), most of them of veterinary importance, although some such as Japanese encephalitis (JE) and Russian Sring–Summer encephalitis (RSSE) viruses, both causes of human disease, were isolated during this period. With the development of 17D vaccine against yellow fever by the Nobel Prize winner, Dr Max Theiler at the Rockfeller Foundation Virus Laboratories in New York, and the subsequent control of the disease in humans, the Rockfeller Foundation turned its attention to other tropical arboviruses. Since 1950 the Foundation has established several regional virus laboratories in tropical America, Africa, India, and Asia. Our considerable knowledge about arboviruses is almost entirely due to the work of these laboratories and of the distinguished scientists who worked there. The majority of

**Table 16.1.** *Isolation of viruses by decade*

| Decade | Number |
| --- | --- |
| 1900–09 | 1 |
| 1910–19 | 2 |
| 1920–29 | 3 |
| 1930–39 | 10 |
| 1940–49 | 19 |
| 1950–59 | 109 |
| 1960–69 | 206 |
| 1970–79 | 96 |
| Total | 446 |

arbovirus isolations, 315 out of 446 were made during the two decades 1950–69. Although some of the isolates are associated with human and/or animal diseases, there are many which are not and are viruses 'looking for a disease'. During 1970–79, there was more emphasis on ultrastructural, biochemical, and physicochemical investigations of known arboviruses.

With the emergence of dengue haemorrhagic fever as a major paediatric problem in many parts of the world over the last 20 years, there has been a resurgence of interest in the ecology of arboviruses and of the diseases they cause.

## Properties and classification of arboviruses

The term 'arbovirus' is an ecological label and arboviruses form a biological rather than a taxonomic group. They may contain RNA or DNA which may be single- or double-stranded. They may be small (20–100 nm) or large (150 nm or more) and, although usually spherical, some are bullet-shaped. The virions may be naked or enveloped.

The arboviruses in general are thermolabile and are destroyed very quickly outside the body of the vertebrate or invertebrate hosts. A majority are inactivated by lipid solvents such as ether or sodium deoxycholate, indicating the presence of a lipid containing coat or envelope associated with infectivity. However, some proven arboviruses do not have this property.

Almost all arboviruses are lethal for infant mice (1–2 day old) by the intracerebral route, although the degree of pathogenicity may vary with different viruses or strains of the same virus. Fresh isolates of some strains of dengue viruses may not produce a recognizable disease in infant mice, but may do so after a period of adaptation by repeated passage. This makes isolation of these viruses in mice difficult or at best unreliable. Most arboviruses will produce a cytopathic effect in one or more of the several vertebrate cell lines of mammalian or avian origin such as Vero cells (African green monkey kidney), LLC-MK2 cells (Rhesus monkey kidney), PS cells (pig kidney), BHK-21 cells (baby hamster kidney) or primary CEC (chick embryo fibroblast cells).

## CLASSIFICATION

The classification of arboviruses is based on cross-reactions in one or other of three serological tests – haemagglutination inhibition (HI), complement fixation (CF), and neutralization (N). Casals and Brown (1954), divided the then known arboviruses into groups on the basis of serological relationships. The first three were given letter designations, A, B and C, and subsequent groups were known by their type viruses – for example, Bunyamwera group. Viruses which did not react with any known arbovirus were classified as 'ungrouped'. One of the drawbacks of a classification based on serological relationships is that viruses such as Rio Bravo or Entebbe bat are classified as arboviruses, when all other evidence suggests that they are not.

With more advanced techniques in biochemistry and the application of electron microscopy, a more rational classification based on structure and physicochemical properties has been proposed which on the whole agrees with the serological classification. The viruses have been given a family, a genus, and an antigenic group based on serological cross-reactivity (Table 16.2). Most of the arboviruses come under the family Togaviridae. This includes the group A (genus Alphavirus) and the group B (genus Flavivirus) of Casals and Brown. In addition the family includes the newly designated genera Rubivirus (rubella virus) and Pestivirus (bovine diarrhoea, hog cholera, and border disease viruses) which are not arboviruses. The togaviruses are spherical, enveloped, and consist of an isometric core 30–40 nm in diameter to which is applied a lipid bilayer from which glycoprotein spikes project. The enveloped virions have a diameter of 60–80 nm. The genome is a single molecule of single-stranded RNA. The alphaviruses and flaviviruses include many of the major human arboviral pathogens.

The family Bunyaviridae is the largest taxonomic grouping and includes the Bunyamwera and C groups of Casals and Brown as well as several other minor groups. There are at least 150 members all of which are arboviruses. They are spherical, about 100 nm in diameter and consist of a dense core and a ragged closely adherent envelope with projections. The single-stranded RNA is probably in three circular segments. They are sensitive to lipid solvents. The genera Bunyavirus, Nairovirus, and Phlebovirus contain many of the viruses causing disease in humans and animals, such as California encephalitis, Congo–Crimean haemorrhagic fever, sandfly fever, Rift Valley fever, and Nairobi sheep disease.

The third family containing arboviruses is the Reoviridae. They possess a double-stranded rather than single-stranded RNA genome with several segments. They are resistant to lipid solvents. The genus Orbivirus contains the arboviruses in the family. The best known members of the genus are the viruses of blue tongue and African horse sickness, both associated with *Culicoides* midges and of considerable veterinary importance. Colorado tick fever virus, another member of the genus, is transmitted by Dermacentor ticks and causes disease in man.

Members of the family Rhabdoviridae are enveloped, rod-shaped virions. They are about 200–400 nm long and 70–100 nm wide, and resemble bullets. The genome of single-stranded RNA is unsegmented. The viruses are sensitive to lipid solvents. The genus Vesiculovirus contains the arthropod-borne animal viruses and include vesicular stomatitis virus affecting livestock and Chandipura virus causing disease in humans. The genus also contains several antigenically related viruses such as Kern Canyon and Mount Elgon bat viruses and several fish viruses none of which are arthropod-borne.

The family Arenaviridae is often listed under arboviruses. Although some members have been isolated from arthropods, there is no evidence to date that arthropods are involved in the transmission cycle. Members are spherical or pleomorphic and have single-stranded RNA with one to four segments. One property which they share with most arboviruses is sensitivity to lipid solvents. Rodents are the natural hosts and transmission is usually contaminative, through urine. The viruses causing lymphocytic choriomeningitis, which although not arthropod-borne can replicate in ticks and tick cells (Reiss-Gutfreund *et al.* 1962; Rehcek 1965) and the two South American haemorrhagic fevers of man, Junin and Machupo, are arenaviruses. Perhaps the best known arenavirus is Lassa fever virus.

**Table 16.2.** *Abbreviations and taxonomic status of the more important arboviruses associated with disease in man*

| Name | Abbreviation | Family | Taxonomic status | |
|------|-------------|--------|-------|-------|
| | | | Genus | Antigenic group |
| Bunyamwera | BUN | Bunyaviridae | *Bunyavirus* | Bunyamwera |
| Bwamba | BWA | Bunyaviridae | *Bunyavirus* | Bwamba |
| California encephalitis | CE | Bunyaviridae | *Bunyavirus* | California |
| Chandipura | CHP | Rhabdoviridae | *Vesiculovirus* | Ves. Stomati |
| Chikungunya | CHIK | Togaviridae | *Alphavirus* | A |
| Colorado tick fever | CTF | Reoviridae | *Orbivirus* | CTF |
| Crimean–Congo haemorrhagic fever | CCHF | Bunyaviridae | *Nairovirus* | CCHF |
| Dengue 1, 2, 3, 4 | DEN – 1, 2, 3, 4 · | Togaviridae | *Flavivirus* | B |
| Eastern equine encephalitis | EEE | Togaviridae | *Alphavirus* | A |
| Hazara | HAZ | Bunyaviridae | *Nairovirus* | CCHF |
| Japanese encephalitis | JE | Togaviridae | *Flavivirus* | B |
| Kyasanur Forest disease | KFD | Togaviridae | *Flavivirus* | B |
| La Crosse | LAC | Bunyaviridae | *Bunyavirus* | California |
| Louping ill | LI | Togaviridae | *Flavivirus* | · B |
| Mayaro | MAY | Togaviridae | *Alphavirus* | A |
| Murray Valley encephalitis | MVE | Togaviridae | *Flavivirus* | B |
| Omsk haemorrhagic fever | OMSK | Togaviridae | *Flavivirus* | B |
| O' nyong nyong | ONN | Togaviridae | *Alphavirus* | A |
| Oropouche | ORO | Bunyaviridae | *Bunyavirus* | Simbu |
| Rift Valley fever | RVF | Bunyaviridae | *Phlebovirus* | PHL |
| Rocio | ROC | Togaviridae | *Flavivirus* | B |
| Ross River | RR | Togaviridae | *Alphavirus* | A |
| Russian Spring–Summer encephalitis | RSSE | Togaviridae | *Flavivirus* | B |
| Sandfly fever (Naples) | SFN | Bunyaviridae | *Phlebovirus* | PHL |
| Sandfly fever (Sicilian) | SFS | Bunyaviridae | *Phlebovirus* | PHL |
| St. Louis encephalitis | SLE | Togaviridae | *Flavivirus* | B |
| Spondweni | SPO | Togaviridae | *Flavivirus* | A |
| Venezuelan equine encephalitis | VEE | Togaviridae | *Alphavirus* | A |
| Western equine encephalitis | WEE | Togaviridae | *Alphavirus* | A |
| West Nile | WN | Togaviridae | *Flavivirus* | B |
| Yellow Fever | YF | Togaviridae | *Flavivirus* | B |

## ARBOVIRUSES AND HUMAN DISEASE

Arboviral diseases are zoonotic infections, that is, they are primarily animal diseases transmissible to man by haematophagous arthropods. The only exception is dengue which until recently was known as a disease affecting man only. However, dengue-2 virus has been isolated from forest monkeys in Malaysia and it appears that dengue might have a 'wild' maintenance cycle involving forest-breeding *Aedes* mosquitoes and forest monkeys (Halstead 1981).

Because of the zoonotic nature of many arbovirus infections, it is of the utmost importance that there should be close co-operation and communication between veterinary and public health workers. Many arbovirus diseases of man may not be diagnosed at all as being of viral origin. Others may be misdiagnosed if the clinician and/or pathologist does not suspect a particular disease. For example, yellow fever has been misdiagnosed in Trinidad as typhoid with jaundice, malaria with jaundice, and acute yellow atrophy. Detailed case histories with background information will alert an inquisitive clinician, but many do not realize the relevance or importance of such information in correct diagnosis. The Rift Valley fever (RVF) outbreak in humans in Egypt in 1977 was not recognized earlier because veterinary authorities and public health officials failed to connect extensive abortion in sheep and cattle and death of some animals with acute liver necrosis, with febrile illness in humans (Shope *et al.* 1982). It is easier to identify such connections when the illness occurs in particular groups of people such as animal handlers, butchers, and veterinarians.

Any arbovirus is capable of infecting man, although the number actually responsible for natural cases is only a fraction of the total. The Subcommittee on Arbovirus Laboratory Safety, reporting in 1980, listed 54 arboviruses which have caused a staggering total of 753 human cases with 16 deaths as a result of laboratory accidents. The major arboviruses involved are listed in Table 16.3. These represent only the reported cases – actual numbers are probably much higher. Venezuelan equine encephalitis (VEE) with 150 cases and one death and

**Table 16.3.** *Major causes of human infection and deaths following laboratory accidents with arboviruses. (After Sub-Committee on Arbovirus Laboratory Safety)*

| Virus | Total infections (deaths) to 1980 | Source | |
|-------|-----------------------------------|---------|------|
| | | Aerosol | Other/ unknown |
| Ven. equine encephalitis | 150 (1) | 57 | 93 |
| Chikungunya | 39 | 7 | 32 |
| Dengue | 11 | 1 | 10 |
| Japanese encephalitis | 22 | 0 | 22 |
| West Nile | 18 | 1 | 17 |
| Yellow fever | 38 (8) | 0 | 38 |
| Tick-borne encephalitis | 37 (2) | 1 | 36 |
| Kyasanur Forest disease | 133 | 23 | 110 |
| Louping ill | 22 | 0 | 22 |
| Rift Valley fever | 47 (1) | 0 | 47 |
| Colorado tick fever | 16 | 0 | 16 |
| Piry | 13 | 3 | 10 |
| Vesicular stomatitis | 46 | 2 | 44 |
| Orungo | 13 | 0 | 13 |

Kyasanur Forest disease (KFD) with 133 cases accounted for over a third of the laboratory acquired human infections. Aerosol constituted a major source of infection in the laboratory, and direct entry into the bloodstream by arthropod bite or needle prick is not necessary for successful infection. The arboviruses associated with human disease acquired naturally are given in Table 16.2. The majority are caused by viruses in the family Togaviridae.

Many human infections with arboviruses may be symptomless and are diagnosed retrospectively on seropositivity. Clinical aspects may range from febrile illness with or without rash (O'nyong nyong fever, Chikungunya fever, dengue), encephalitis (Japanese encephalitis, tick-borne encephalitis) to haemorrhagic fevers (yellow fever, Omsk haemorrhagic fever). In the case of the encephalitic phenomenon these are always part of a second phase of the illness after the viraemia has finished and immunity has developed. It gives a biphasic picture with sometimes as much as a two-week gap between the first febrile illness and the onset of the neurological complications. In the haemorrhagic infections many different factors may play a part, for example, leukopenia with thrombocytopenia in a population already anaemic and malnourished. Thus infections will affect different communities in different ways. For example, Kyasanur Forest disease had a haemorrhagic component occurring naturally in Indians who had low haemoglobins and were undernourished. There was also the biphasic component with florid central nervous system involvement as seen with other viruses of the tick-borne encephalitis complex. In many of the laboratory cases of infection with this virus a haemorrhagic diathesis was not a feature, probably related to their better initial state of health. Different strains of a single virus or even the same strain may produce a variety of symptoms in man. In the case of diseases classed as arboviral encephalitides, the encephalitic syndrome represents the extreme disease condition with inapparent or mild systemic infections outnumbering those with central nervous system involvement in a ratio of 25–400 to 1 (Chamberlain 1968).

## RECENT EPIDEMICS CAUSED BY ARBOVIRUSES

The last 10–15 years have seen some spectacular achievements in the field of human viral diseases, such as the eradication of smallpox. However, there have also been several outbreaks of arboviral diseases which have caused concern and bewilderment, particularly as some of the outbreaks occurred in areas where the viruses were unknown before. Among the contributing factors must be the development of resistance to insecticides by mosquitoes which are one of the major groups of arbovirus vectors. There are now 121 resistant strains of insects important to public health and the number of resistant culicine mosquitoes (which includes the vectors of many arboviruses) has gone up from 19 species in 1968 to 41 in 1975 (Agarwal 1979). Unfortunately vector control is still the major and, in some cases, the only means of controlling arboviral diseases in animals. Human beings, if educated, can protect themselves successfully against the bites of arthropods. There is still no known reliable and acceptable drug therapy for arboviruses and effective vaccines have been developed and are available for large scale use only against a few. In any case,

immunization without total eradication leads to lowering of herd immunity with the subsequent danger of explosive outbreaks in the event of reintroduction of the virus into a susceptible population.

### Dengue and dengue haemorrhagic fever (DHF)

Dengue is endemic throughout the tropics, particularly Asia, the Caribbean, and the Pacific. In its classical form, it is a mild disease, usually affecting adults and older children. In 1953, an epidemic of an apparently new and severe disease syndrome characterized by fever, shock, acute haemorrhage, and high mortality and affecting young children, occurred in Manila in the Philippines. A second outbreak occurred in 1956 during which dengue viruses were isolated from patients' sera and from *Aedes aegypti* mosquitoes. The disease came to be known as dengue haemorrhagic fever (DHF) and during the next 20 years appeared in many of the urban centres of South-East Asia. It is one of the leading causes for admission to hospital and death in children in tropical Asia (Halstead 1982). Dengue haemorrhagic fever was reported from urban Bangkok in 1958, and between 1977 and 1980, in Thailand, some 100 000 children were admitted to hospital with the condition, of whom more than 1500 died. Between 1960 and 1973, the disease appeared in Singapore, Penang, Indonesia, urban Rangoon, Kuala Lumpur, and the West Pacific. The outbreak of a severe haemorrhagic disease which occurred in Calcutta in 1963–64 is believed to have been due to dengue. It is now one of the major paediatric problems in South-East Asia and West Pacific with over 600 000 admissions to hospital and 20 000 deaths in 12 countries in the two regions (Halstead 1982). The recent outbreak in Cuba in 1981 with over 340 000 cases and 156 deaths mostly in children under 15 years, is the first record of this form of the disease in the Caribbean (WHO 1981a), although the classical mild form is endemic in that region.

In 1977–78 there was a large outbreak of dengue in the Caribbean which by 1980 had reached Mexican communities on the US border. What caused concern was that the serotype involved was type 1, unknown in that region before and believed to have been introduced to Jamaica from Nigeria by participants returning from an international arts festival. In early 1981 infection due to dengue 4, another serotype new to the Caribbean was diagnosed in two US travellers to the French Caribbean island of St. Barthelemy (CDC 1981). Dengue 4 is common in South-East Asia, South Pacific and Africa, and was most probably introduced into St. Barthelemy from French Polynesia. By late 1981 to early 1982, dengue 4 was the predominant virus in outbreaks in the Caribbean (CARED 1982). Since dengue haemorrhagic fever may result from sequential infection with two serotypes, the introduction of dengue 1 and dengue 4 into a dengue 2 area like the Caribbean, is potentially dangerous.

### Japanese encephalitis (JE)

The disease is endemic in Japan and many South-East Asian countries. There has been serological evidence of Japanese encephalitis virus activity in southern India since 1955. Recent epidemics in India since 1973 have been characterized by high mortality and involved several states (some in the north) and were particularly severe in two states in north India and east India with over 5000 cases and nearly 1300 deaths in 1978 alone (Sankaran 1978). The 1979 outbreaks were less severe with 995 cases and 242 deaths (WHO 1980a).

### Yellow Fever (YF)

Although urban yellow fever has been controlled by immunization, spectacular outbreaks such as the one in Ethiopia in 1960–62 with 15 000 deaths (Serie et al. 1964) still occur and yellow fever is still enzootic in parts of Africa and tropical America with human cases occurring every year. A review of cases from 1965 to 1979 has shown that little progress has been made in reducing the risk of yellow fever (WHO 1980b). In Ghana alone in 1979 there were 494 human cases with 120 deaths. The same year a total of 711 cases with 281 deaths were reported from West Africa and South America (WHO 1981b). The actual numbers may be higher. Monath et al. (1980), estimated that the yellow fever outbreak in Gambia in 1978–79 probably involved 8400 cases and 1600 deaths. The vector of urban yellow fever and dengue, Ae. aegypti, is reinvading countries from where it had been eradicated. In Colombia for instance, the threat of urban yellow fever is very real, since for the first time in 50 years, jungle yellow fever appeared practically on the shores of the Caribbean, near cities which Ae. aegypti had reinvaded (Groot 1980).

### Rift Valley fever (RVF)

Rift Valley fever caused by another mosquito-borne arbovirus, is primarily a disease of sheep and other domestic livestock. In man it was until recently, believed to be a relatively benign disease. It is enzootic in many parts of Africa as far north as the Sudan and spectacular epizootics have occurred in domestic livestock from time to time. In 1977 an outbreak was reported in Egypt for the first time causing enormous losses in sheep and cattle, but also thousands of human cases with nearly 600 reported deaths. (Shope et al. 1982). A second smaller outbreak followed in 1978 (WHO 1981c).

### Epidemic polyarthritis

This is caused by a mosquito-borne virus, Ross River (RR) virus and is endemic in Australia. In Fiji in 1979, a large outbreak of the disease occurred involving 30 000 people. The disease was also reported in New Zealanders returning from Fiji. This was the first time that Ross River virus had been recorded from outside Australia.

### Saint Louis encephalitis (SLE)

The disease is endemic in the USA where an extensive outbreak occurred in 1975 with an estimated total of 2131 cases and 171 deaths. The disease spread northwards to Canada for the first time involving 68 laboratory confirmed cases and five deaths in Ontario.

### Oropouche fever (ORO)

Oropouche virus was first isolated from the blood of a febrile human in Trinidad. Between 1961 and 1978 there were seven outbreaks of the disease in Para State, Brazil and serological evidence indicated that approximately 370 000 persons became infected in six of the outbreaks (Pinheiro et al. 1981). Although no fatalities occurred, some patients were severely ill.

### Rocio encephalitis (ROC)

Beginning in 1975, several epidemics of human encephalitis occurred in the coastal areas of Sao Paolo State, Brazil. The agent which was isolated from a patient who died, was named Rocio virus and is considered to be a recent introduction to the area. One epidemic alone involved a total of 825 cases and 95 deaths (Lopez et al. 1981).

### Tick-borne arbovirus diseases

Tick-borne encephalitis (TBE) in Europe has received a great deal of publicity recently. Reports in the press suggest that the disease is spreading westwards in Europe. While there is little evidence for spread, it is true that the disease is being diagnosed more frequently and in new areas and has become a considerable public health problem.

Kyasanur Forest disease (KFD) erupted as a new unrecognized illness in man and monkeys in a forested area of South India in 1957. Expansion of the infected area has continued and in the first half of 1978, 600 cases were recorded with 14 deaths.

In the appendix (p. 272) can be found a short account of each important human arboviral illness. This includes a short description of the virus, its world distribution, the known mosquito vectors, animal reservoirs, and public health significance.

What are the reasons for the spread of known arboviral diseases into new areas and for the emergence of 'new' ones? The proximity of Virus Research Centres and their interest in unusual outbreaks is one reason (Smith 1978). The outbreaks of the 'new' diseases, Marburg, Lassa, and Ebola have made trained medical personnel in developing and developed countries aware of the existence of unrecognized viral disease entities previously classified as fevers of unknown origin. A disease new to an area may be revealed because a major disease has been removed uncovering a residuum of different but clinically similar illnesses (Smith 1972). There are improved and rapid methods of diagnosis which were unavailable previously.

The development of insecticide resistance in arbovirus vectors is another contributory factor. There is an increasing interest in the human ecosystem and in the impact of ecological and behavioural changes on the natural history of human disease.

## CHANGES IN ECOSYSTEM

It has been estimated that in the next 20 years the present world population of 4.2 billion will increase to 6.2 billion of which

4.85 billion will be in developing countries (Pearson 1969). Food production, despite the Green Revolution, has not kept pace with the burgeoning population. The need to increase the amount and quality of food and for economic growth by industrialization, have called for large scale expansion of agricultural and engineering resources to provide more and better food and power (mainly hydroelectric) for industrial purposes. Storage of vast quantities of water in reservoirs (man-made lakes) and the use of this water for agricultural irrigation of the surrounding areas, while encouraging human settlement and crop cultivation, are also creating ideal conditions for increase in the population of aquatic invertebrates such as the mosquito vectors of arboviruses. Many of the irrigation schemes are associated with rice cultivation. The recent epidemics of Japanese encephalitis in India are believed to be due to an increase in the mosquito vector population breeding in flooded areas. An increase in the mosquito vectors of arboviruses and infection in the human population with rice field development has been observed in America (Hardin *et al.* 1967), in Czechoslovakia (Trpis 1960), and France (Hannoun *et al.* 1964). The dramatic change in mosquito populations biting man after a dry area has been irrigated was shown by Surtees (1970*a*), in Kisumu, Kenya. The population of *Anopheles gambiae*, the vector of O'nyong nyong fever, a mosquito-borne arboviral disease, increased in many newly irrigated areas.

The outbreak of the tick-borne Kyasanur Forest disease in south India is believed by Boshell (1969) to have been due to an increase in human population in the area and the consequent alteration of the ecosystem providing conditions suitable for the overt expression of a hidden enzootic process.

The opening up of vast new areas by the construction of highways, for example, across the Amazon basin, is not only altering the natural environment, but also bridging natural barriers to the spread of diseases. Dixon *et al.* (1981), point out that along the Transamazon Highway in Brazil, the original clearing of the land, future expansion of cleared areas and hunting are the activities most likely to involve contact with the forest and most likely to result in arbovirus infection.

Climatic conditions can also play a part in the spread of arbovirus disease into new areas as in the case of the Saint Louis encephalitis outbreak in Ontario, Canada in 1975. The summer in 1975 was unusually early and weatherwise this was the equivalent of displacing South-West Ontario several hundred miles southwards into the regions of the USA where the disease is prevalent (Bristow 1979).

### Increased travel and population movements

The post-war years have witnessed considerable increase in human mobility, either voluntarily through international and national travel for business, pleasure or as migrant labour, or forced, as a result of civil wars, insurrections or the expulsion of large numbers of people from their native lands for ethnic, religious or political reasons. In the past, travel and population movements were of necessity slow and the travel period itself was a 'quarantine' of sorts. Persons who became ill during the journey either recovered or died before they reached their destination and there was little risk of introducing a disease into new areas. Present day jet travel has made it possible for man and animals to be transported over extremely long distance in 24 hours while incubating a disease and remaining symptomless, thus introducing an infection into a new area. When a susceptible vector is present in the receptive area, the risk of an outbreak is very real. The outbreaks of dengue 1 and dengue 4 in the Caribbean, where they were unknown previously, is believed to have been due to the introduction of these serotypes into the region from Nigeria and French Polynesia respectively by returning air passengers and the presence of large numbers of the vector mosquito, *Ae. aegypti*. Between 1976 and 1979 there were 26 imported cases of dengue in Canada, mostly from Jamaica (WHO 1980*c*). The potential for the spread of arboviruses into new areas and for their subsequent persistence has been recently reviewed by Johnson and Chanas (1981). Since many arboviruses are zoonotic infections, spread may also occur through movements of animals, naturally as in the case of intercontinental migration of birds which are hosts to a variety of arboviruses and arbovirus vectors such as ticks, or by the movement of infected livestock. Hoogstraal *et al.* (1979), have suggested that the Rift Valley fever outbreak in Egypt in 1977 originated from infected camels trekking northwards into Egypt.

### Increased urbanization

Better health and an expanding economy and industrialization in many developing tropical countries have led to large rural populations moving into urban or periurban areas and creating slums. In India, for example, about a third of the population of Bombay and over half that of Calcutta are migrants (Chandrasekhar 1971). Increasing urbanization and the attendant socio-economic changes have resulted in an increase in the *Ae. aegypti* mosquito populations which would explain the recent extensive outbreaks of dengue and dengue haemorrhagic fever. The high density of human population in urban centres provides an abundance of blood meal sources for the man-biting *Ae. aegypti* which has a short flight range. Many new towns in the tropics have piped water supplies, but water for domestic use is still collected from street hydrants and stored in water containers in and around houses providing mosquito breeding places. With rising standards of living, tinned food has become a feature of life and discarded tins provide additional prolific breeding sites for the mosquitoes (Surtees 1970*b*). Increase in motor transport in developing countries, particularly in towns, has produced large tyre depots, another favourite breeding site for *Ae. aegypti*, as well as a means for dispersal of mosquito eggs to new areas. There is also evidence that with increasing urbanization, the more competitive, domestic, man-biting *Ae. aegypti* (which is also a more efficient vector of dengue and is invariably associated with dengue haemorrhagic fever), has replaced *Ae. albopictus* in many towns of South-East Asia (Gilotra *et al.* 1967; Bunnag 1978).

### Changes in human behaviour

Tick-borne arboviruses are usually maintained as cryptic foci in forests. In the past, the people at risk were pastoralists and hunters who intruded into these areas and were bitten by infected ticks.

Changes in human behaviour as well as ecological changes have had a profound impact on the incidence of tick-borne arboviruses. This is well illustrated in the case of tick-borne encephalitis in Europe. An affluent society with more time for leisure activities such as tourism, walking in the forests, and camping, and increased motor and bus travel, have resulted in much clinical tick-borne encephalitis being diagnosed in picnickers and campers from urban centres. New foci of tick-borne encephalitis are being recognized in Europe, most probably due to increased tourism and other leisure activities which bring man into contact with foci of infection in forests and with infected ticks. Recreational parks with considerable populations of rodent hosts of arboviruses and their tick vectors may have foci of tick-borne arboviruses. Not only are such amenities being created, but they are also being increasingly used. Cases of Colorado tick fever caused by a tick-borne arbovirus have been confirmed in employees of the Rocky Mountain National Park in the USA and in tourists (McLean et al. 1981). There are numerous camping grounds in the Park and with increasing outdoor recreational activities, the three million people who visit the Park annually are at risk.

## ECOLOGY OF ARBOVIRUSES

The ecological aspects of arboviruses have been summarized by Smith (1959) and Chamberlain (1958). All arboviruses with the probable exception of dengue, are zoonotic infections and have complex infection cycles involving one or more wild vertebrate and invertebrate hosts. In nature, the viruses are maintained by alternating cycles in vertebrate hosts and haematophagous arthropod hosts. Survival of the virus depends on the stability of the vertebrate–arthropod–virus community or biocenose in particularly favourable environments or biotopes. In the natural maintenance cycle, the maintenance hosts (vertebrate and arthropod) are not adversely affected and are reservoirs of infection; for example, monkey-mosquito reservoir of yellow fever, bird–mosquito of Eastern equine encephalitis, rodents–ticks of Russian Spring–Summer encephalitis. Arthropods themselves may function as reservoirs of infection by transmitting the viruses transovarially from generation to generation. This has been well documented for the tick-borne arboviruses (Burgdorfer and Varma 1967). There is increasing evidence that some mosquito-borne viruses are also transmitted transovarially.

Incidental hosts are tangentially infected from a maintenance cycle without being directly involved in it. With most arboviruses, man is an incidental host, in a sporadic infection. In an epidemic, man is the vertebrate element in an incidental biocenose, for example, urban yellow fever. Some arthropods may also be incidental hosts, acquiring the virus with a bloodmeal, without actually being able to maintain and transmit it.

Both vertebrate and arthropod hosts may also be long-range hosts and serve to introduce an arbovirus into new areas, for example, migrant birds and tick ectoparasites carried by them.

Link hosts are involved when an arbovirus maintained in one biocenose gains access to another biocenose. For example, yellow fever in Uganda is maintained in the forst canopy by a monkey–*Aedes africanus* cycle. *Aedes simpsoni* acts as a link host, biting both man and forest monkeys, raiding banana plantations on the forest fringe. Infected man then initiates a rural cycle (incidental biocenose) of yellow fever involving the domestic *A. aegypti*.

Amplifier hosts, usually vertebrates, increase the amount of virus circulating in a biocenose so that the infection overflows into neighbouring populations of incidental hosts. In Japan, epidemics of Japanese encephalitis are usually preceded by intense transmission among heron nestlings. Domestic animals such as pigs also serve both as link and amplifier hosts of Japanese encephalitis in Japan (Konna et al. 1966). Some incidental hosts of the virus may also function as amplifier hosts by increasing the vector population. Cattle, for example, are only incidental hosts of Kyasanur Forest disease virus, but they are the major host for the adult stages of the vector tick.

The maintenance cycles of any one arbovirus may involve several wild vertebrate hosts and several arthropod species. These complex cycles make it very difficult to control or eradicate arboviral diseases.

### Vertebrate hosts

Wild birds and rodents are the vertebrate hosts of a large number of arboviruses (Table 16.4). Birds are particularly involved in a large number of mosquito-borne viruses and rodents in tick-borne viruses. The importance of wild vertebrate hosts in the maintenance of arboviruses depends on their population, their reproduction rate and levels of viraemia in the infected individuals. For successful long-term maintenance, a sufficient population of non-immune hosts should be available. Vertebrates infected with arboviruses either die of the infection or become immune and in either case they are no longer involved in the maintenance cycle. A high birth rate as in rodents and birds ensures a steady supply of non-immune juveniles. For successful infection of blood-sucking arthropods, virus must be present in the circulation. The higher and longer the viraemia, the better the chances of infecting large numbers of arthropods.

**Table 16.4.** *Viruses isolated from naturally infected vertebrates*

| | |
|---|---|
| Man | 98 |
| Other primates | 13 |
| Rodents | 90 |
| Birds | 70 |
| Bats | 32 |
| Marsupials | 21 |
| Liverstock | 36 |
| Others | 35 |
| Total | 395 |

### Arthropod hosts

Mosquitoes and ticks are the two major groups of arbovirus vectors, followed by phlebotomine sandflies and *Culicoides* midges (Table 16.5). The feeding habits of the arthropods are closely related to their importance as arbovirus vectors. They must, for example, feed preferentially on the known

**Table 16.5.** *Viruses isolated from wild caught arthropods*

| | |
|---|---|
| Mosquitoes | 216 |
| Ticks | 98 |
| Phlebotomine sandflies | 31 |
| *Culicoides* midges | 24 |
| Others | 15 |
| Total | 384 |

vertebrate hosts of the viruses. Different species may act as vectors of the same virus in different areas. The ability of any arthropod to transmit an arbovirus in the laboratory only suggests its potential – it may not be a vector in nature.

When an arthropod feeds on a viraemic vertebrate, virus is taken into the alimentary canal of the arthropod with the blood meal. The higher the viraemia, the more the chances of infecting the arthropod. The amount of virus needed to infect an arthropod is called the 'infection threshold'; this varies from species to species. The lower the infection threshold, the more efficient the vector. On the basis of viraemia levels and infection thresholds, it is possible to grade the vertebrate hosts and arthropod hosts in order of importance. A combination of high viraemia in the vertebrate, a low infection threshold for the arthropod vector, and a preference for the arthropod to feed on the particular vertebrate species, is the ideal situation for maintenance and spread of an arbovirus.

Following a blood meal on a viraemic host the virus has to pass through various barriers in the body of the arthropod before it reaches the salivary glands. Transmission is through the injection of infective salivary secretions during feeding. The gut of the arthropod is the first barrier which the virus encounters. Once it passes this barrier, the salivary glands may be another barrier to successful infection. If the virus is able to gain entry into the salivary glands and multiply there, the arthropod is able to transmit by bite. The ganglionic mass ('brain') of vector arthropods often contains large concentrations of virus. The reason for this neurotropic behaviour of viruses in arthropods is not clear. Since ganglionic mass infection is always accompanied by salivary gland infection, examination of head squashes of mosquitoes by immunofluorescence can be taken as presumptive evidence of salivary gland infection and ability to transmit.

The period elapsing between an infecting blood meal and the time when virus has reached the salivary glands and transmission is possible by bite, is called the extrinsic incubation period. This varies with the virus and in general depends on the temperature; the higher the temperature, the shorter the extrinsic incubation period.

In the case of mosquitoes, sandflies, and midges, only the blood-feeding adult females are able to acquire the infection and transmit it by bite. All stages of ticks, immature as well as adult males and females, feed on blood. Any stage can acquire the infection and pass it on to the next stage (transstadial transmission) which then transmits it to a vertebrate during feeding.

The reasons for the susceptibility of some arthropods and not others to arboviruses are not clearly understood. One may be that the virus in the vertebrate host and the vector arthropod are ecologically isolated in space and/or time (Varma 1972). This isolation operates directly by reducing or eliminating 'effective contact' between virus and arthropod. Intrinsic factors in the virus and in the arthropod vector may also increase or reduce effective contact and are thus important in the transmission cycle.

## INVESTIGATIONAL METHODS IN ARBOVIRUS EPIDEMIOLOGY

Arbovirus investigations are a team effort involving clinicians, epidemiologists, and entomologists/zoologists. Heightened awareness and a high index of suspicion are prerequisites on the part of clinicians and public health workers. The first priority for early recognition of potentially dangerous epidemics is to educate health and administrative personnel, particularly in the developing world, of the need for surveillance and reporting of any acute febrile disease. This can easily be done by policemen, teachers or villagers given simple but clear instructions (Smith 1978). There must be a trained person to report to who can then marshall a small but well-trained team able to respond at short notice at national, state or provincial level.

The occurrence of cases at a time when there are high populations of blood-sucking insects, and a history of arthropod bites prior to onset of symptoms will suggest the arthropod-borne nature of the infection. Diseases such as malaria or relapsing fever could be excluded by blood smear examination. If an arboviral aetiology is suspected, attempts should be made to isolate the agent, usually from blood.

### Isolation

By the time a patient presents at a hospital or clinic with symptoms, the viraemic phase of the infection may be over and it may not be possible to isolate virus from the blood. A blood sample is nevertheless taken for isolation and/or serology. In the absence of a positive virus isolation, seroconversion or a rise in titre between paired acute and convalescent sera will provide evidence of infection. For isolation, blood or serum is inoculated with the least possible delay into 1–2-day-old suckling mice by the intracerebral route, and into vertebrate and arthropod cell cultures. If there is delay, the specimens (blood or autopsy material such as brain tissue) are stored at −70°C until they can be processed. The shorter the period between obtaining the specimen and inoculation, the better the chances of isolating virus. Race *et al.* (1979), isolated dengue 1 virus by direct inoculation of AP-61 mosquito cell cultures with whole blood obtained by finger prick from a patient attending a Health Centre in Trinidad.

Exposure of sentinel animals (mice, hamsters, monkeys) in areas where they are likely to be bitten by infected arthropods, is another way of isolating an arbovirus or of obtaining evidence of viral activity by seroconversion.

Recently, arthropod cell cultures grown at 28°C have been increasingly used for the isolation of arboviruses such as dengue which are difficult to isolate in mice or vertebrate cell cultures. Mosquito cell cultures have been shown to be also a more sensitive isolation system for other arboviruses, such as, yellow fever (Varma *et al.* 1976), and Japanese encephalitis viruses (Hsu *et al.* 1978). One of the disadvantages of arthropod cell culture systems is that although viruses will replicate in the cells often to high titres, only a few will produce a visible cytopathic effect. However, inoculation of mosquito cells with human sera and mosquito suspensions and examination by immunofluorescence has been used for rapid isolation and identification of dengue viruses (Hebert *et al.* 1980). Several mosquito and tick cell lines are now available and all known arboviruses will replicate in one or other of these lines. This in itself will provide strong circumstantial evidence for the arbovirus status of an isolate.

A fourth system for the isolation of mosquito-borne viruses is the inoculation of non-biting mosquitoes such as *Toxorhynchites* spp and examination of their head squashes by the immunofluorescence test after a suitable interval. The method is complicated but highly sensitive and a positive result will indicate the mosquito-borne status of an isolate. Monoclonal antibodies to arboviruses are becoming increasingly available and have been successfully used for identifying the dengue serotypes by immunofluorescence tests on mosquito head squashes and mosquito cell cultures.

Some arboviruses may have temperature sensitive (ts) mutants or variants occurring in nature. Igarashi *et al.* (1981) found that mosquito cell cultures at 28°C were more efficient than mice in isolating such mutants or variants of Japanese encephalitis virus from wild caught mosquitoes.

## Identification

When an agent is isolated, tests on filter passing ability, and sensitivity to lipid solvents and to heat will indicate whether it is an arbovirus or not. Serological tests such as haemagglutination-inhibition (HI), complement fixation (CF) or neutralization (N) will help to place the agent in one of the groups of arboviruses and show if it is a known arbovirus, related to a known arbovirus but distinct or whether it is a new virus, unrelated to any known arbovirus. Monoclonal antibodies are making identification easier and have been used in combination with immunofluorescence for identifying the different serotypes of dengue.

As part of the epidemiological studies, attempts should be made in parallel to isolate the aetiological agent from likely species of vertebrates (domestic and wild) and from arthropods. Sometimes direct evidence of the involvement of particular species of vertebrates is suggested by illness and death among the animals, for example, monkeys and yellow fever in South America, monkeys and Kyasanur Forest disease in India. However, animals may often be symptomless. Arthropods to study in depth would be those biting man. Serological relationships of the virus will indicate if it is mosquito-borne, tick-borne or transmitted by sandflies. Efforts could then be concentrated on the particular group of arthropods.

If and when viruses have been isolated from man, other vertebrates and arthropods, the next step is to demonstrate that they are identical. This would provide additional evidence for an arboviral aetiology of the human infection.

## Vertebrate investigations

Information on population and species composition of vertebrates can usually be obtained by trapping (rodents) or netting/shooting (birds). The animals are examined for ectoparasites. Blood is taken for virus isolation/serology and brain and spleen removed for virus isolation. Procedures for collecting vertebrates and processing them are given by Sudia *et al.* (1970). While it may not always be possible to isolate virus from vertebrates, evidence for infection can be obtained by serological tests.

## Arthropod investigations

Epidemics during the rainy season will suggest the involvement of mosquitoes and during the dry season, that of ticks. Arthropods are collected using various trapping devices, or bait animals. Analysis of the collections will provide information on population fluctuations, species composition, biting preferences of various species, time of biting activity and so on. Fed specimens are usually discarded or allowed to digest their blood meal before being processed, since an isolate from fed specimens could come from the blood meal and not from the tissues. Isolation of a virus from non blood-sucking males of mosquitoes and sandflies would suggest that the virus was passed transovarially from the previous generation. Methods for collecting and processing arthropods are given by Sudia and Chamberlain (1967).

## Seroepidemiology

Serological tests have a dual function – identifying isolates and obtaining evidence of recent or past infection. In the absence of a positive isolation from a patient, seroconversion of a rise in titre of specific antibody in paired acute and convalescent sera, may be the only definitive evidence of infection with an arbovirus. During epidemics and interepidemic periods, serological surveys help to determine antibody rates and by inference attack rates in the population. This is particularly important when the infection is inapparent or mild, not requiring a visit to the clinic or hospital.

The three main serological tests used are the haemagglutination-inhibition (HI), complement fixation (CF), and neutralization (N) tests. The other tests, the ELISA test (Enzyme Linked ImmunoSorbent Assay) and IFAT (Indirect Fluorescent Antibody Test) are being increasingly used. These last two are highly sensitive and could be developed for use in the field.

### Haemagglutination–inhibition test

Several viruses, including most arboviruses, agglutinate red cells and this property can be utilized for quantitation of specific antibody, the so-called haemagglutination–inhibition antibody. Arboviral haemagglutinins are prepared usually from infected mouse brain. The sera to be tested may contain nonspecific inhibitors which should be removed before testing. The HI test is invaluable as a screening procedure for sera and as a means of classifying and identifying arboviruses.

### Complement fixation test

This is sometimes used for the rapid identification of newly isolated viruses using infected mouse brain suspension as a crude antigen. Complement fixation antibody has a short duration and its presence therefore indicates a recent infection with the virus.

## Neutralization test

Apart from the HI test, this is the one most used in viral identification and seroepidemiology. It is not an *in vitro* test, except when cell cultures are used. Neutralizing antibody is highly specific and is accepted as the antibody responsible for the protective action of immune serum. Suitably prepared serum–virus mixtures are inoculated into a host system, usually mice, which will serve as an indicator of presence or absence of active virus in the mixture, i.e. whether neutralization of infectivity has or has not been achieved in the mixtures. Cell cultures are also used in neutralization tests. Neutralization is indicated by a reduction in the number of plaques produced by the serum–virus mixture in cell monolayers. This is the plaque reduction neutralization test (PRNT). Neutralizing antibody may persist for many years. It usually provides the only means of measuring the extent to which a population has been exposed to a virus.

### Behavioural investigations

In depth investigations of arbovirus epidemiology should include socio-cultural and behavioural studies of the human population. Arthropods often bite at particular times of the day. Infection is most likely if man is exposed by behavioural activities in the habitat during peak biting times of the arthropods. If a mosquito bites only out of doors at a time when people are inside their homes, infection is less likely. In certain societies, women work in the fields and are more likely to be bitten by outdoor day-biting mosquitoes. Behaviour and certain occupations may bring man into contact with infected arthropods, for example woodcutters in forests and yellow fever in South America. In many South-east Asian countries boys and men sleep out of doors in the hot season, increasing exposure to night-biting mosquitoes. Domestic pigs, hosts of Japanese encephalitis, are kept by certain communities and not others and may be a factor in epidemics of the disease. Apart from behavioural factors, there may be ethnic factors in epidemiology of arbovirus disease, which should also be investigated.

## SOME RECENT TRENDS IN ARBOVIRUS RESEARCH

The recent serious epidemics of dengue haemorrhagic fever and of other arboviral diseases, including the 'emergence' of new ones have generated renewed interest in the epidemiology and pathology of this group of viruses.

The discovery that dengue haemorrhagic fever occurs in individuals infected for a second time by one of the four serotypes of dengue, or in infants with maternally acquired antibody, has created considerable interest in the role of immune complexes in viral pathogenesis. According to Halstead (1982), passively or actively acquired non-neutralizing antibody forms immune complexes with dengue viruses. These have an affinity for reticuloendothelial cells, the dengue target cells, and result in acute vascular permeability. Thus infection-enhancing antibody acts to increase the severity of dengue disease. The paradoxical increase in viral replication when viruses are complexed with sub-neutralizing levels of antibody, antibody-dependent enhancement (ADE), has been observed in vitro with other flaviviruses, alphaviruses, and bunyaviruses (Peiris *et al.* 1981). Thus, ADE may be involved in the pathogenesis of viral disease and the implications of vaccination with live attenuated strains in populations with low levels of viral antibody should be considered.

Monoclonal antibodies to viruses are becoming increasingly available. Arboviral monoclonal reagents will provide a resource of exquisitely specific reagents which can be used to clearly define antigenic variations in arbovirus types derived from various geographical areas, from different types of host or from epidemic and endemic situations. They will also help to locate particular viral epitopes and identify the regions responsible for virulence, immunogenecity, etc.

Man is a host to a variety of microbial pathogens and parasites and the efect of these on the course of arboviral infections has not received the attention it deserves. The role of ecological changes in the natural history of arboviral diseases is being increasingly recognized and studied.

Two of the more important developments in the arthropod aspects of arboviral research have been the study of vector competence and of transovarial transmission.

Most of the original work on transmission of arboviruses by vectors has been with laboratory colonized arthropods and mouse-adapted strains of viruses. The effects of selection pressure by colonization or adaptation were either not recognized or not investigated. $F_1$ adults and unadapted or low passage strains of viruses are used now in vector studies. Clearly defined differences in the ability of geographical strains of the same mosquito species to transmit arboviruses have been demonstrated (Gubler and Rosen 1976; Tesh *et al.* 1976; Aitken *et al.* 1977; Grimstad *et al.* 1977). Kramer and Scherer (1976) used vector competence as a marker for distinguishing Central American and Mexican epizootic and enzootic strains of Venezuelan equine encephalitis.

Although there have been occasional reports of the transovarial transmission of arboviruses in mosquitoes, it is only during the last decade that a considerable amount of positive evidence has accumulated (Leake 1983). Yellow fever, Japanese encephalities, dengue 2, Murray Valley encephalitis, and St. Louis encephalitis have been transovarially transmitted in mosquitoes in the laboratory, while extensive field and laboratory studies with the California encephalitis group of viruses have shown that transovarial transmission occurs in nature. Transovarial transmission in mosquitoes may play a role in the overwintering of arboviruses in temperate regions and also act as a maintenance mechanism in nature. The reasons for the successful demonstration of transovarial transmission recently may well be due to the more sensitive low-temperature assay systems such as mosquito cell cultures and the mosquito inoculation techniques.

Many arboviruses reach high concentrations in the nerve mass or 'brain' of their arthropod hosts. The effect this may have on altering the behaviour of the arthropods has not been adequately studied. Increased probing behaviour of mosquitoes infected with La Crosse virus was shown by Grimstad *et al.* (1980). The increased probing results in multiple transmissions, but may also reduce the mosquito population gradually since infected mosquitoes are unable to engorge fully. Such studies are of fundamental importance in the epidemiology of arboviruses. Indeed arboviruses are known to persist in the central nervous systems of many vertebrates after the infection is over. More use should be made of this fact if virus isolation is required. Modern central nervous system cell culture techniques which get rid of accompanying antibody will sometimes enable virus to be isolated when normal fragmentation techniques done in the presence of antibody fail.

Host antigen is present in various enveloped viruses. The effect of host-associated factors on infectivity of mosquito-transmitted viruses has been little studied. Feinsod *et al.* (1975), found that Sindbis virus propagated in *Ae. aegypti* mosquitoes was neutralized by serum made against whole-body extracts and saliva of the mosquito. When propagated in Vero cells, the virus was not neutralized by such sera. Ashcroft (1979) notes that Indian indentured labour arriving in the West Indian colonies in the nineteenth century was little affected by outbreaks of yellow fever which was rampant among European arrivals. Dengue antibodies may be responsible for this protection. However, prolonged exposure of the Indians to the bites of the vector *Ae. aegypti* in India is another possible explanation. Clearly more studies are needed to understand this phenomenon.

## CONTROL

### Vaccines

Apart from urban epidemics where man is at least temporarily the maintenance host (for example, yellow fever), vaccination of man has no effect on the ecosystems responsible for maintenance of the virus. Although the 17D vaccine against yellow fever is safe and effective, the disease has not been eradicated. But it is possible to prevent large scale urban epidemics of the disease. A carefully chosen combination of live and inactivated vaccines may give a fairly broad protection within a group. Development of vaccines has also been helped by military requirements where a large number of susceptible persons may have to be moved quickly into an endemic or enzootic area. A live vaccine against dengue is being developed, but the part which immunological phenomena play in the pathogenesis of arbovirus diseases (notably dengue haemorrhagic fever) suggests that this is a risk to be considered very seriously. Some vaccines are available for limited use for the protection of laboratory personnel. A Japanese encephalitis vaccine and tick-borne encephalitis vaccine are available commercially. However, one of the major problems in providing vaccines is the relative poverty of many of the populations in which the infections are most common. Because of the risk of allergic encephalomyelitis, cell culture vaccines are being developed to replace the earlier brain tissue vaccines.

Since it is impossible to eradicate arboviral diseases with their wild maintenance cycles, vaccination should be used to protect particular groups of people at risk, e.g. tourists, campers, etc. in the case of tick-borne encephalitis, or to prevent urban epidemics, for example, yellow fever or dengue. A vaccine could also be used for immunizing domestic hosts of an arboviral disease, for example, pigs against Japanese encephalitis.

### Vector control

In spite of the development of insecticide resistance in many vectors, this remains the only method of controlling many arboviral diseases. The dengue epidemics in the Caribbean were very effectively controlled by the use of malathion against the adult mosquitoes and by treatment of breeding places. A recent development in vector control is the use of *Bacillus thuringiensis israelensis* as a mosquito larval insecticide. Alternative methods such as biological control using larvivorous fish are also being explored.

Tick vectors are more difficult to control, particularly when they are found in forests and do not parasitize domestic animals. Spraying of forests with DDT has been used by Russian scientists for reducing vector tick populations. Against ticks, the most effective method for humans would appear to be personal protection, using repellents such as DEET which are available commercially. This of course also applies to humans for protection against mosquito and midge bites as well.

## APPENDIX – CLINICAL ARBOVIRUS ILLNESSES

### California group viral infections (California encephalitis and La Crosse viruses)

This group of viruses comprises 12 serotypes within the virus family Bunyaviridae (Porterfield *et al.* 1976).

#### Distribution

US, Canada, Trinidad, Europe, Africa, and Finland (Hammon and Reeves 1952; Thompson and Inhorn 1967; Berge 1975).

#### Incubation period

Uncertain.

#### Clinical illness

It presents with headache, fever, and general symptomatology of a meningo-encephalitis, with upper motor neurone signs and occasionally chorea. Abnormal neurological signs may persist after recovery.

#### Mosquito vectors

*Aedes triseriatus* is likely to be the most important vector in California but other *Aedes* spp may be involved (Thompson *et al.* 1972).

#### Reservoir

Chipmunks and squirrels are most commonly involved.

#### Public health significance

This is a severe enough illness to require admission to hospital. As it involves children more severely they must be protected against mosquito bites. Mosquitoes are most active in forested areas, but have a limited flight range. Local areas can be treated by insecticides to reduce the oviposition sites. These are usually in water contained in tree holes or paraphernalia, such as tins, tyres, broken glass and plastic containers, discarded from tourist activities. These latter types of breeding sites can be removed. It is a reportable disease.

## Chikungunya

This virus is classified in the genus Alphavirus in the family Togaviridae.

### Distribution

South-east Asia, Vietnam (Deller and Russell 1967), Thailand (Halstead *et al.* 1969), Africa including Tanzania, Zimbabwe, Transvaal (McIntosh *et al.* 1963), Zambia, and Congo, India, Calcutta, Vellore, Madras, Pondischerry (Thiruvengadam *et al.* 1965; Jadhav *et al.* 1965; Sarkar *et al.* 1965), and also in Sri Lanka (Ceylon).

### Incubation period

3–12 days.

### Clinical illness

*1st phase:* Symptoms include fever, severe joint, limb, and spine pains which can completely immobilize the patient. This phase may last six to ten days.

*2nd phase:* This quite often occurs after an afebrile period of two to three days, and in the majority is associated with an irritating maculopapular rash over the body particularly on the extensor surface of the limbs. Joint pains may persist occasionally without fever for up to four months. On rare occasions, probably related to the general health of the patients involved, myocarditis and peripheral circulatory failure has been seen (Thiruvengadam *et al.* 1965; Ramachandra Rao *et al.* 1965). Occasionally encephalitis and haemorrhagic manifestations are seen during the second phase (Halstead *et al.* 1965; Sarkar *et al.* 1965). The death rate has been estimated at 0.4 per cent but in patients under one year it may be as high as 2.8 per cent and similarly over the age of 50 years the mortality may increase.

### Mosquito vectors

In Asia the vectors in urban epidemics are *Ae. aegypti* and various Culex spp. In Africa, the vector in forest areas is *Ae. africanus* and in the Sudan *Ae. leuteocephalus*.

### Reservoir

This includes baboons, monkeys, rodents, bats, and reptiles.

### Public health aspects

Epidemics of this disease can involve thousands of people and thus cause both economic loss and pressure on medical services. To date it is not a notifiable disease but in areas where there is a potential for infection medical services should keep alert. If reports are submitted to WHO they will be published in the *Weekly epidemiological record*. The Centers for Disease Control, Atlanta, Georgia 3033 also like to be informed of new epidemics, new vectors or unusual cases.

## Colorado tick fever

This virus is classified in the genus Orbivirus in the family Reoviridae.

### Distribution

In mountainous or high land regions (approximately 4000 to over 10 000 feet) in at least 11 western states of the USA and in the provinces of Alberta and British Columbia in Canada (Topping *et al.* 1940; Florio and Miller 1948; Florio *et al.* 1950).

### Incubation period

3–6 days after tick bite.

### Clinical illness

Onset is sudden with high fever, severe headache, photophobia, ocular pain, myalgia, arthralgia, and mild conjunctivitis. The disease is often biphasic with a 2–3 day febrile period followed by a 1–2 day gap and then a further fever with worse symptoms. In this second phase particularly in children there may be a typical meningo-encephalitic illness. Occasionally there is a maculopapular rash, splenic enlargement and haemorrhagic manifestations (Spruance and Bailey 1973; Goodpasture *et al.* 1978).

### Tick vector

This is usually by adult *Dermacentor andersoni* ticks (Eklund *et al.* 1955).

### Reservoir

Small mammals including squirrels and chipmunks, porcupines, rabbits, and deer can be infected (Burgdorfer and Eklund 1960).

### Public health significance

There are no very significant community or economic effects from this disease. Nevertheless it remains an important medical problem and in areas where there is a high incidence it could inhibit development because of occupational groups put at risk.

## Dengue

This virus is classified in the genus Flavivirus of the family Togaviridae.

### Distribution

Throughout the world except Antarctica. Recently epidemics have occurred in Asia, the Caribbean, and Pacific Islands. The haemorrhagic dengue is now endemic in many parts of tropical Asia, particularly Thailand (Siler *et al.* 1926; Halstead 1965; 1981).

### Incubation period

2–7 days.

### Clinical illness

It is characterized by a biphasic fever, headache, generalized myalgia and/or arthralgia and a maculopapular rash which disappears over five days and sometimes associated with desquamation of the epithelium. Occasionally there is epistaxis, petechial, and purpuric lesions in the ordinary disease. A very much more severe and lethal form is known as haemorrhagic dengue. This starts in a mild form like any other mild virus pyrexia of unknown origin. Two to five days later a rapid deterioration occurs with physical collapse. The features of shock are present with cold extremities, flushed face with a bleeding diathesis into skin and mucous membranes. The blood pressure falls and the pulse becomes weak and rapid. After 24–36 hours recovery may occur but depending on the medical facilities available up to 40 per cent of children may die. This severe aspect of dengue is thought to have a basic immunopathogenic mechanism (Rush 1789; Cohen and Halstead 1966; Halstead *et al.* 1969).

### Mosquito vectors

*Aedes aegypti* and *Ae. albopictus* are the principal vectors during the day. Other *Aedes* spp have been implicated (Halstead 1966).

### Reservoir

In the jungle, monkeys are liable to be important. In urban areas humans have adequate viraemia to infect mosquitoes.

### Public health significance

Ordinary dengue is of no great significance but the cases of the 'shock' syndrome with its high incidence of morbidity in areas poorly served with hospitals requires active steps to be taken. The WHO have asked for these cases to be reported and three news letters are currently published. Attempts to eradicate *Ae. aegypti* to prevent dengue in 1972 cost $436 million whereas the damage to tourism and medical care of patients due to this disease was $450 million in the Americas.

## Eastern equine encephalitis

This virus is classified in the genus Alphavirus of the family Togaviridae.

### Distribution

Canada, throughout the USA, particularly the Atlantic seaboard (Giltner and Shahan 1936), Trinidad, Guyana, Mexico, Panama, Brazil, Peru, Columbia, and Argentina (Hayes, 1981).

### Incubation period

Uncertain.

### Clinical illness

In the severe cases onset is abrupt with high fever followed by all the features of meningitis including coma, convulsions, and neurological damage. In those in which a recognizable disease develops the mortality rate approaches 80 per cent. Mental retardation, convulsions, and paralysis are common sequelae particularly of younger children. In the older groups, infections have less sequelae.

### Mosquito vectors

*Culiseta melanura* and certain species of *Aedes* and *Culex* may be involved.

### Reservoir

There is a definite association with salt marshes and the spread depends on infected birds. In winter, virus is present in small rodents, reptiles, and amphibia. It is only when the endemic spread becomes explosive that man and horses are likely to be involved. The disease is commonest in the late summer.

### Public health significance

This is an unpleasant form of encephalitis. Vaccines have been produced to prevent horses becoming infected and for laboratory workers, but they are not in general use. It is a reportable, communicable disease in most of the states in the USA. News media in the presence of proven cases tend to cause alarm amongst the public and severe economic consequences among such industries as the hotel business. In the vector population, bird infection rates including those in pheasant flocks and levels of antibodies in these reservoirs may help to indicate the incidence of infection.

## Epidemic polyarthritis

Ross River (RR) virus, the cause of this disease, is classified in the genus Alphavirus in the family Togaviridae.

### Distribution

Australia, Fiji, Samoa, Cook Islands, Tonga, Melanesian Islands, New Zealand (Doherty 1981).

### Incubation period

Uncertain.

### Clinical illness

A mild illness with slight fever, sore throat, and pain and swelling particularly of the small joints of the hand. Sometimes a maculopapular rash or occasionally a vesicular rash appears. Parasthesiae and pain in the palms and soles of the feet may be present suggesting a possible very mild neuropathy. The patients are usually better after 10–14 days. Although chronic joint disease has not been reported, relapsing joint disease over the first year does occur. It is probable that many people have a febrile illness with this virus without other specific exanthemata. It seems likely that the joint pains are immunologically determined manifestations as they are more common in adults than in young children (Edwards 1928; Anderson *et al.* 1957; Thomson *et al.* 1979).

### Mosquito vectors

Probably *Aedes* and *Culex* spp, for example, *Ae. vigilax* and *Cx. annulirostris* (Doherty *et al.* 1963; Gard *et al.* 1973).

### Reservoirs

These are still uncertain but rodents and mammals are generally likely to be involved (Doherty *et al.* 1966).

### Public health significance

Although not a serious disease it is perhaps the most common arboviral disease in Australia. The fact that it has spread rapidly through the Pacific into places which have non-immune populations causing large epidemics indicates how alarmingly easily these things can happen. One of the early epidemics occurred in the immediate vicinity of the large international airport at Nandi in Fiji. This creates the real possibility of spreading the disease by air travel. The spraying of the insides of planes to eradicate mosquitoes is important.

## Japanese encephalitis

This virus is classified in the genus Flavivirus of the family Togaviridae.

### Distribution

The virus is found in Japan, Far East, Guam, USSR, Malaysia, India, and Western Pacific Island areas (Pond *et al.* 1954; Hammon *et al.* 1958; Green *et al.* 1963).

### Incubation period

4–14 days.

### Clinical illness

Characteristically, onset is sudden, with fever, headache, and other signs of meningeal irritation. Convulsions occur in children. Upper motor neurone involvement with extra pyramidal disturbances are a feature of the central nervous system disturbance. Mortality rate of those with meningo-encephalitis is around 20 per cent in children and up to 50 per cent in the age groups over 50 years. Sequelae are common and include both motor and psychological disturbances (Weaver *et al.* 1958).

### Mosquito vectors

*Culex tritaeniorhynchus* and *Cx. vishnui* group of mosquitoes are the most important vectors (Gressler *et al.* 1958). Other species of *Culex, Aedes, Anopheles,* and *Mansonia* have been found to be infected and are probably involved.

### Reservoir

Pigs and many birds including herons and egrets may be the chief source of virus. Other domestic animals can become infected and humans themselves may play a part in epidemics. In certain Far Eastern areas, human antibodies to this virus will be present in 90 per cent of the human population.

### Public health significance

Vaccines are being developed but have not been tried adequately as yet. Up to 50 per cent of litters of swine may die during active seasons of this virus. Protection against mosquito bites is essential particularly in immigrant and tourist populations where natural immunity has not developed.

## Murray Valley encephalitis

This virus is classified in the genus Flavivirus of the family Togaviridae. It is closely related to Japanese and St. Louis encephalitis and West Nile virus (Pond *et al.* 1955).

### Distribution

Australia, Papua New Guinea (French 1952; French *et al.* 1957).

### Incubation period

Uncertain.

### Clinical illness

Onset is sudden with headaches, fever, and symptoms of a meningo-encephalitis. Paresis of both upper and lower motor neurones may occur and breathing and swallowing may become impaired. In early epidemics fatalities were as high as 60 per cent, but with modern intensive care the mortality rate is less than 20 per cent. However, as a result of increased survivors, the number of people with both upper and lower motor neurone and psychiatric sequalae have increased.

### Mosquito vectors

*Culex annulirostris* is the major vector but *Ae. normanensis* may also be involved (Doherty *et al.* 1963).

### Reservoir

Birds, particularly herons, cormorants, and other water birds are the reservoir of this virus (Marshall and Woodroofe 1975; Gard *et al.* 1976).

### Public health significance

In epidemic proportions it can be a severe enough problem to affect the tourist trade and gaining workers for agricultural work. Control must come from stopping mosquitoes feeding in the shallow pools in urban and rural areas. It is notifiable in all mainland Australian states.

## Oropouche fever (Febu de Mojui)

This virus is classified in the genus Bunyavirus of the family Bunyaviridae (Pinheiro 1981).

### Distribution

Trinidad, Northern Brazil, and Colombia.

### Incubation period

Uncertain.

### Clinical illness

There is an abrupt onset of fever, headache, myalgia, arthralgia, and photophobia. The illness lasts 2–7 days and to date is not thought to cause fatalities.

### Vectors

Mosquitoes and possibly *Culicoides* midges are thought to be involved and *Cx. paraensis* may be the main vector.

### Reservoir

Monkey, sloths, and birds are probably the main reservoir, but other animals may be involved.

### Public health significance

In Brazil the epidemics have been severe and many people have required admission to hospital. This has affected the local manpower availability.

## O'nyong-nyong

This virus is classified in the genus Alphavirus of the family Togaviridae.

### Distribution

Uganda, Kenya, Tanzania, and Malawi (Haddow *et al.* 1960).

### Incubation period

Similar to Chikungunya virus.

### Clinical illness

The clinical expression is similar to Chikungunya, but also includes lymphadenitis. Joint pains, epistaxis, and a rash are frequently a feature of this disease.

### Mosquito vectors

The vectors are *An. gambiae* and *An. funestus*.

## Orungo

This virus is classified in the genus Orbivirus of the family Reoviridae.

### Distribution

Nigeria, Guinea, and Uganda.

### Incubation period

Uncertain.

### Clinical illness

This is characterized by fever, headache, nausea, vomiting, and myalgia. There is frequently a fine papular rash involving the face, chest, and abdomen which appears about the third day of the illness. Conjunctivitis and skin hyperaesthesia may be present. The fever may last up to one week (Fabiyi 1981).

### Mosquito vectors

*Aedes dentatus* and *Anopheles* spp are involved.

### Reservoir

Probably human beings and animals (monkeys and sheep particularly) are part of the transmission cycles of the virus.

### Public health significance

Unpleasant epidemics of disease occur, particularly in rural workers.

## Rift Valley fever

This virus until recently was classified in the ungrouped arthropod-borne viruses. Now it seems likely that it is similar to viruses in the family Bunyaviridae (Murphy *et al.* 1973).

### Distribution

Throughout Africa including Nigeria, Egypt, and the Sudan. The first detailed account of the disease was described in sheep in the Rift Valley in Kenya, 1930 (Daubney *et al.* 1931).

### Incubation period

2–7 days.

### Clinical illness

*1st phase:* fever, back and joint paints, and headache which lasts approximately one week.

*2nd phase:* after 1–2 days remission, similar symptoms for 1–2 days with nausea, occasionally an haemorrhagic diathesis with evidence of liver and renal damage. Sometimes vision is disturbed with evidence of a retinitis and cotton wool exudates in the region of the macula. Meningo-encephalitis sometimes occurs with focal motor signs and hallucinations (Van Velden *et al.* 1977; Laughlin *et al.* 1979; Siam and Meegan 1980).

### Mosquito vectors

Over 20 species of mosquitoes have been implicated as possible vectors of this disease. *Culex pipiens, Cx. theileri, Ae. caballus* and other mosquitoes of the *Culex* and *Aedes* group may be involved. Biting flies have been suspected of transmitting the virus from animal to animal during epidemics (Peters and Meegan 1981).

### Reservoir

This is chiefly a disease of sheep, cattle, and goats, although camels and antelopes can become infected.

### Public health significance

There is severe loss of life in cattle and sheep with considerable risk to personnel involved with these animals at farms, in the veterinary profession, or in abattoirs. Some laboratory infections have occurred. Infection occurs mostly by contact with infected organs and aerosols. The virus has been isolated from milk but there is no positive evidence to date that the disease is transmitted in this way. A live virus vaccine is available for sheep and goats, but may result in fetal destruction in pregnant animals. An attenuated vaccine is available for cattle and pregnant animals. Recently a human vaccine has been tried in South Africa but its efficiency has not as yet been determined. The spread north of Rift Valley fever from the Sub-Saharan areas of Africa is a cause for concern and there is a need for vigilance in the mediterranean countries and other parts of the world.

## Rocio encephalitis

This virus is classified in the genus Flavivirus of the family Togaviridae.

### Distribution

Brazil (Sao Paulo area particularly).

### Incubation period

7–14 days.

### Clinical illness

Frequently infections may be sub-clinical, but death from an encephalitis may occur. The illness usually starts abruptly with fever, headache, nausea, vomiting, and, if the central nervous system is involved, a stiff neck. Coma and death may ensue. In those who have had an encephalitic illness there may be considerable impairment of cerebral function (Lopes *et al.* 1981).

### Vectors

These are uncertain, but a haematophagus insect, probably a mosquito, is thought to be involved.

### Reservoir

Wild birds have antibodies to this virus but more investigation of this disease needs to be done.

### Public health significance

The attack rate has been high and has severely affected local communities. Morbidity and mortality is much higher when adequate medical treatment is not available. The epidemics have occurred in tourist areas and have affected this source of finance considerably.

## St. Louis encephalitis

This virus is classified in the genus Flavivirus of the family Togaviridae.

### Distribution

USA, Mexico, Panama, South America, Canada, and West Indies. It is one of the most important mosquito-borne human encephalitides in the US (Muckenfuss *et al.* 1938; Bond 1969; Monath 1980).

### Incubation period

Uncertain.

### Clinical illness

This virus usually causes a mild illness with fever and headache lasting for several days. Meningo-encephalitis can develop and may cause deaths. There are no particular symptoms or signs which might differentiate this encephalitis from other meningo-encephalitides (Brinker and Monath 1980).

### Mosquito vectors

*Culex tarsalis* and, in the urban areas, *Cx. pipiens* and *Cx. quinquefasciatus* (sometimes *Cx. nigripalpus*) are involved. Virus has been isolated from other mosquito species (Kemp 1981).

### Reservoir

The virus occurs in terns, house sparrows, and other nesting birds (Bowen and Francy 1980).

### Public health significance

It is a notifiable disease in the USA and up to 1000 cases are reported each year. It is therefore a significant human disease problem. Protection against mosquitoes and destroying their breeding sites is important in control.

## Spondweni virus

This virus is classified in the genus Flavivirus of the family Togaviridae.

### Distribution

Southern and Western Africa.

### Incubation period

Uncertain.

### Clinical illness

Symptoms include fever, headache, nausea, dizziness, myalgia, photophobia, and pain behind the eyes. In a recent case in an American there was a rash over the trunk and face but more marked in the legs. The pharynx had a greyish mucoid lining which bled easily if touched (Wolfe *et al.* 1982).

### Vector

Virus has been isolated from *Mansonia uniformis, M. africana, Ae. circumluteolus,* and other *Aedes spp.*

### Reservoirs

These are uncertain but domestic livestock do have antibodies.

### Public health significance

This is uncertain as yet, but it is likely to be diagnosed more frequently and non-immune populations coming to work in infected areas will be at risk.

## Tick-borne encephalitis complex

The viruses of this group are classified in the genus Flavivirus of the family Togaviridae.

### Distribution

Far East, Asia and Europe, England and Scandinavia (Zilber and Soloviev 1946; Svedmyr *et al.* 1958).

### Incubation period

7–14 days.

### Clinical illness

The disease of the Far East variety, Russian Spring–Summer, is more severe than that seen in Central Europe. Both have a biphasic illness.

*1st Phase:* severe headache, fever, nausea, vomiting, weakness, hyperaesthesia, and photophobia.

*2nd Phase:* when it occurs some days later is typical of meningo-encephalitis which may include both lower and upper neurone lesions. Epileptic attacks may be part of the neurological illness. These may persist in the long term as may cervical segment lower motor neurone paralysis particularly, and upper motor neurone damage in the form of hemiplegias.

Many cases only have the first phase. Some present clinically in the second phase.

### Vectors

Ixodid ticks are the main vectors – *I. persulcatus* in the East and *I. ricinus* in the West. However, species of *Dermacentor* and *Haemaphysalis* are also involved.

### Reservoirs

Ticks and wild vertebrate hosts particularly rodents are involved. Overwintering of the virus can occur in hedgehogs and dormice. Birds, bats and domesticated animals can all become involved.

### Public health significance

In Central Europe the disease is often transmitted in goats' milk (Pogodina 1961), so pasteurization is very important. Protection against ticks for country workers is necessarily combined with reduction in the high tick population by insecticides if this is feasible. The tick-borne encephalitis complex consists of seven types all associated with human disease: Powassan – Canada (Casals 1960), Louping ill – Central and Far Eastern encephalitis, Omsk haemorrhagic fever (Chumakov 1958), Negishi – Japan, Kyasanur Forest disease – Mysore, India (Work and Trapido 1957). In Omsk haemorrhagic fever and Kyasanur Forest fever the disease has haemorrhagic manifestations. Both these diseases, particularly Kyasanur Forest disease, have central nervous system complications in a significant number of cases (Webb *et al.* 1961). In the USSR and European countries, tick-borne encephalitis is a reportable disease. Human vaccines are available now and are expected to be helpful.

## Venezuelan equine encephalitis

This virus is classified as a species in the Venezuelan equine encephalitis complex of the alphavirus group of the family Togaviridae. Subtype I is Venezuelan equine encephalitis, Subtype II is often known as the Florida strain, and Subtype III is usually called Mucambo virus (Kubes and Rios 1939).

### Distribution

It is endemic in Central and South America, and parts of North America, and has occurred particularly in Venezuela, Colombia, Equador, Panama, Brazil, Mexico, Florida, Texas and Trinidad.

### Incubation period

1–4 days.

### Clinical illness

It presents with fever, severe headache, myalgia, and respiratory symptoms. Meningo-encephalitis can occur particularly in children but is much less common in adults. The mortality is usually very low but in undernourished populations and with little medical care deaths can occur (Sanmartin 1972).

### Mosquito vectors

*Culex melanoconion* and *Deinocereites* spp are probably the main vectors in rodent-to-rodent transmission. Horse-to-horse transmission can occur as can transplacental transmission of virus. Horses are a major reservoir of infection. Both domestic and wild dogs and pigs develop high blood virus titres. Over 150 different animal species have been found to be infected in the field. Birds have low viraemias but could infect mosquitoes. These may spread the disease and cause the new epidemics (McConnell and Spertzel 1981).

### Public health significance

Some 60 000 human cases were recorded in Columbia, Venezuela, and Equador between 1962 and 1970. In Mexico in 1969–70, 16 922 human cases were reported. There were around 500 deaths and 42 deaths respectively in these epidemics. Many smaller epidemics have occurred elsewhere. Over the period 1967–71 figures approaching 200 000 horses may have died. It can be seen that the combination of these two figures related to work, management, veterinary and medical care is a very significant problem. It is now a reportable disease in the USA. The disease can be controlled by the intelligent use of vaccines in horses. This has prevented spread of the disease. This is a costly programme but if properly applied would appear to far outweigh the cost of epidemics affecting horses, humans, and other animals.

## Vesicular stomatitis virus

This virus is classified in the Rhabdoviridae family which includes Piry virus. This latter virus has caused non-lethal laboratory infections and antibodies have been demonstrated in humans in the Amazon basin of Brazil.

### Distribution

North and South America, and Asia (Hanson 1975).

### Incubation period

As little as 30 hours.

### Clinical illness

Fever, headache, eye and chest pain, and vomiting are the chief symptoms. In a minority of cases vesicles may be present on the tongue and the mucosa of the mouth and pharynx. The illness is frequently biphasic but the whole course of the disease only lasts approximately six days (Hanson *et al.* 1950; Yuill 1981).

### Vectors

Although as yet unproven, phlebotomine sand flies almost certainly play a part both as a vector and a reservoir of the virus. The virus has been isolated from *Culex* mosquitoes. Direct contact cases occur amongst animals (Meyer *et al.* 1960).

### Public health significance

It may occur amongst cattle, horses, and handlers and laboratory workers. Disease amongst farm animals, sheep, and pigs can result in destruction of stock and thus be very expensive to the economy. Milk production can be significantly decreased. Vaccines are available and have some beneficial effect.

## Wesselsbron fever

This virus is classified in the group Flavivirus of the family Togaviridae.

### Distribution

Chiefly central and South Africa including Madagascar but is also present in Thailand (Weiss *et al.* 1956; Smithburn *et al.* 1957).

### Incubation period

2–4 days or slightly longer.

### Clinical illness

It presents with fever, headache, and pain in joints, muscles, and eyes. Sometimes a maculopapular rash develops and patients have complained of increased sensitivity of the skin. There is occasionally a second phase with a meningo-encephalitic illness and the liver may become involved.

### Mosquito vectors

*Aedes* spp.

### Reservoir

Sheep, in which the disease causes a severely debilitating illness, are the main reservoir. Cattle are involved as is the gerbil, wild ducks, and coots. Humans circulate high titres of virus and may be involved in mosquito infections.

### Public health significance

It causes a disease of sheep and a vaccine has been developed for use in adults, sheep, and lambs. It is not recommended for use in gestating sheep as it causes meningo-encephalitis of the fetus and abortion.

## Western equine encephalitis

This virus is classified in the genus Alphavirus of the family Togaviridae.

### Distribution

Canada – particularly Manitoba, Saskatchewan, Alberta, and British Columbia; US; Central and South America to Argentina (Hayes 1981).

### Incubation period

Uncertain.

### Clinical illness

It is characterized by sudden onset of fever, headache, and general symptoms of meningo-encephalitis. Tremors and convulsions may occur especially in babies. Neurological and psychological sequelae occur particularly in babies. The incidence may be up to 55 per cent. In adults sequelae may be found in approximately 5 per cent.

### Mosquito vectors

These include *Cx. tarsalis, Culiseta melanura,* and other mosquitoes of these two genera. *Aedes* and *Anopheles* species may be slightly involved.

### Reservoir

Wild birds, domestic fowl, and nestling house sparrows act as a reservoir for this virus.

### Public health significance

Horses can be protected by vaccines and vaccines have been used to protect laboratory workers. Control of mosquito vectors is the best method of reducing the risk to humans. Epidemics can be large and frightening. During 1952 in California 348 human cases were confirmed (Kokernot *et al.* 1953). In 1975–76 approximately $70 million was spent on mosquito control in USA and Canada (Directory of Mosquito Control Agencies 1977). Control is expensive.

## West Nile virus

This virus is classified in the genus Flavivirus. It is closely related to Japanese and St. Louis encephalitis viruses.

### Distribution

Africa, Europe, and Asia (Smithburn *et al.* 1940).

### Incubation period

3–6 days, sometimes biphasic.

### Clinical illness

It presents with sudden onset of fever, headaches, retrobulbar and muscular pain, sore throat, nausea, and vomiting. A maculopapular rash may then develop on the trunk and extend to face and limbs. Arthralgia sometimes occurs. The disease is usually mild in the young but in older age groups a second phase with mild meningo-encephalitis can develop but sequaelae have not been seen.

### Mosquito vectors

Vectors include *Culex* spp and other ornithophilic mosquitoes (Taylor *et al.* 1956).

### Reservoir

Birds including domestic poultry are a reservoir of the virus (Taylor *et al.* 1956).

### Public health significance

Large human epidemics are rare. Mosquitoes should be controlled and care should be taken by people handling poultry carcasses and involved in research. Areas where abnormally high rains may occur and those newly opened to irrigation may cause a risk for West Nile infections provided that the appropriate ornithophilic mosquitoes and reservoir host are present.

## Yellow fever

This virus is classified in the genus Flavivirus of the family Togaviridae.

## Distribution

East, Central, and West Africa south of the Sahara, Caribbean, Mexico, Central America, Panama, Atlantic and Pacific coasts of South America, Columbia, Brazil, and Paraguay. There are two types – urban and sylvan (Strode 1951).

## Incubation period

3–6 days but can be as long as 10–13 days.

## Clinical illness

It is usually mild presenting with headache, fever, backache, nausea, and sometiems epistaxis. There may be a second phase associated with severe jaundice and a haemorrhagic tendancy including vomiting blood. Death may occur within nine days. It is a notifiable disease.

## Mosquito vectors

In urban areas *Ae. aegypti* is the chief vector (Reed 1901). In sylvan areas of Africa, forest canopy mosquitoes are the vector and *Ae. africanus* in the Western areas. *Haemogogus* spp and to a lesser extent *Ae. luteocephalus* and *Sabethes chloropterus* are also involved (Bauer 1928; Robin and Beran 1981) and other African vectors are *Ae. simpsoni* and *Ae. taylori*.

## Reservoir

In urban epidemics man and mosquitoes form a reservoir while in sylvan epidemics this is supplemented by non-human primates.

## Public health significance

It is a notifiable disease. Excellent vaccines are available and are compulsory for those travelling through an endemic area and for those born in endemic areas. Control of *Ae. aegypti* breeding sites in urban areas is very helpful.

## REFERENCES

Agarwal, A. (1979). Pesticide resistance on the increase, says UNEP. *Nature* **279**, 280.

Aitken, T.G.H., Downs, W.G., and Shope, R.E. (1977). *Aedes aegypti* strain fitness for yellow fever virus transmission. *Am. J. Trop. Med. Hyg.* **26**, 985.

Anderson, S.G. and French, E.L. (1957). An epidemic exanthem associated with polyarthritis in Murray Valley, 1956. *Med. J. Aust.* **2**, 113.

Ashcroft, M.T. (1979). Historical evidence of resistance to yellow fever acquired by residence in India. *Trans. R. Soc. Trop. Med. Hyg.* **73**, 247.

Bauer, J.H. (1928). Transmission of yellow fever by mosquitoes other than *Aedes aegypti. Am. J. Trop. Med.* **8**, 261.

Berge, T.O. (ed.) (1975). *International catalogue of arboviruses including certain viruses of vertebrates* (2nd edn, Pub. No. (CDC) 75-8301) Public Health Service, US Department of Health, Education and Welfare, Atlanta.

Bond, J.O. (1969). St. Louis encephalitis and dengue fever in the Caribbean area: evidence of possible cross-protection. *WHO Bull.* **40**, 160.

Boshell, J.M. (1969). Kyasanur Forest disease: ecological considerations. *Am. J. Trop. Med. Hyg.* **18**, 67.

Bowen, G.S. and Francy, D.B. (1980). Surveillance. In *St. Louis encephalitis* (ed. T.P. Monath) p. 473. American Public Health Association, Washington, DC.

Brinker, K.R. and Monath, T.P. (1980). The human disease: acute central nervous system infection. In *St. Louis encephalitis* (ed. T.P. Monath) p. 503. American Public Health Association, Washington, DC.

Bristow, G.E. (1979). Climatological conditions in south western Ontario in 1975. Their possible impact on the outbreak of St. Louis encephalitis. In *Arboviral encephalitis in Ontario with special reference to St. Louis encephalitis* (ed. M.S. Mahdy, L. Spence, and J.M. Joshua) p. 70. Ministry of Health, Ontario.

Bunnag, T. (1978). Disease ecology and control. A nidal base approach to arthropod-borne virus infection. *J. Med. Assoc. Thailand* **61**, 555.

Burgdorfer, W. and Eklund, C.M. (1959). Studies on the ecology of Colorado tick fever virus in Western Montana. *Am. J. Hyg.* **69**, 127.

Burgdorfer, W. and Varma, M.G.R. (1967). Trans-stadial and transovarial development of disease agents in arthropods. *Ann. Rev. Entomol.* **12**, 347.

CAREC (1982). Dengue. *Surveillance Report* **8**, 5.

CDC (1981). Dengue type 4 infections in US travellers to the Caribbean. *Morbidity and Mortality Report* **30**, 249.

Casals, J. (1960). Antigenic relationship between Powassan and Russian Spring–Summer encephalitis viruses. *Can. Med. Assoc. J.* **82**, 355.

Casals, J. and Brown, L.V. (1954). Haemagglutination with arthropod-borne viruses. *J. Exp. Med.* **99**, 249.

Chamberlain, R.W. (1968). Arboviruses, the arthropod-borne animal viruses. *Curr. Topics Microbiol. Immunol.* **42**, 38.

Chandrasekhar, A. (1971). Some aspects of urbanisation of population in India. In *The International Population Conference, London 1969*. Volume 4, Section 10.2. International Union for Scientific Study of Populations, Leige.

Chumakov, M.P. (1958). Tick-borne haemorrhagic diseases in the U.S.S.R. *Rep. 6th Int. Congr. trop. Med. Malar.*

Cohen, S.N. and Halstead, S.B. (1966). Shock associated with dengue infection. I. The clinical and physiologic manifestations of dengue haemorrhagic fever in Thailand, 1964. *J. Pediatr.* **68**, 448.

Daubney, R., Hudson, J.R., and Garnham, P.C. (1931). Enzootic hepatitis or Rift Valley fever. An undescribed virus disease of sheep, cattle and man from East Africa. *J. Pathol. Bacteriol.* **34**, 545.

Deller, J.J. Jr and Russell, P.K. (1967). Fevers of unknown origin in American soldiers in Vietnam. *Ann. Intern. Med.* **66**, 1129.

Directory of Mosquito Control Agencies in the US and Canada (1977). *American Mosquito Control Association Newsletter* (ed. T.D. Mulhern) **July 1977**, 2.

Dixon, K.E., Llewellyn, C.H., Travassos Da Rosa, A.P.A., and Travassos Da Rosa, J.F. (1981). A multidisciplinary program of infectious disease surveillance along the Transamazon highway in Brazil: epidemiology of arbovirus infections. *PAHO Bull.* **15**, 11.

Doherty, R.L. (1981). Epidemic polyarthritis. Arboviral zoonoses in Australia. *CRC Handbook series in zoonoses: viral zoonoses* (ed. J.H. Steele and G.W. Beran) p. 473. CRC Press, Boca Raton, FL.

Doherty, R.L., Gorman, B.M., Whitehead, R.H., and Carley, J.G. (1966). Studies of arthropod-borne virus infections in Queensland. V. Survey of antibodies of group A arboviruses isolated from mosquitoes in man and animals. *Aust. J. Exp. Biol. Med. Sci.* **44**, 365.

Doherty, R.L., Carley, J.G., Mackerras, M.J., Trevethan, P., and Marks, E.N. (1963). Studies of arthropod-borne viruses in

Queensland. III. Isolation and characterization of virus strains from wild-caught mosquitoes in north Queensland. *Aust. J. Exp. Biol. Med. Sci.* **41**, 17.

Edwards, A.M. (1928). An unusual epidemic. *Med. J. Aust.* **1**, 664.

Ekland, C.M., Kohls, G.M., and Brennan, J.M. (1955). Distribution of Colorado tick fever and virus-carrying ticks. *JAMA* **157**, 335.

Fabiyi, A. (1981). Other arboviral zoonoses in Africa. *CRC handbook series in zoonoses: viral zoonoses* (ed. J.H. Steele and G.W. Beran) p. 259. CRC Press, Boca Raton, FL.

Feinsod, F.M., Spielman, A., and Swaner, J.L. (1975). Neutralisation of Sindbis virus by antisera to antigens of vector mosquitoes. *Am. J. Trop. Med. Hyg.* **24**, 533.

Florio, L. and Miller, M.S. (1948). Epidemiology of Colorado tick fever. *Am. J. Public Health* **38**, 211.

Florio, L., Miller, M.S., and Mugrage, E.R. (1950). Colorado tick fever. Isolation of the virus from *Dermacentor andersoni* in nature and a laboratory study of the transmission of the virus in the tick. *J. Immunol.* **64**, 257.

French, E.L. (1952). Murray Valley encephalitis: isolation and characterization of the aetiological agent. *Med. J. Aust.* **1**, 100.

French, E.L., Anderson, S.G., Price, A.V.G., and Rhodes, F.A. (1957). Murray Valley encephalitis in New Guinea. I. Isolation of Murray Valley encephalitis virus from the brain of a fatal case of encephalitis occurring in a Papuan native. *Am. J. Trop. Med. Hyg.* **6**, 827.

Gard, G., Marshall, I.D., and Woodroofe, G.M. (1973). Annually recurrent epidemic polyarthritis and Ross River virus activity in a coastal area of New South Wales. II. Mosquitoes, viruses and wildlife. *Am. J. Trop. Med. Hyg.* **22**, 551.

Gard, G.P., Giles, J.R., Dwyer-Gray, R.J., and Woodroofe, G.M. (1976). Serological evidence of interepidemic infection of feral pigs in New South Wales with Murray Valley encephalitis virus. *Aust. J. Exp. Biol. Med. Sci.* **54**, 297.

Gilotra, S.K., Rozeboom, L.E., and Bhattacharya, N.C. (1967). Observations on possible competitive displacment between populations of *Aedes aegypti linnaeus* and *Aedes albopictus* Skuse in Calcutta. *WHO Bull.* **37**, 437.

Giltner, L.T. and Shahan, M.S. (1936). The present status of infectious equine encephalomyelitis in the United States. *J. Am. Vet. Med. Assoc.* **41**, 363.

Goodpasture, H.C., Poland, J.D., Francy, D.B., Bowen, G.S., and Horn, K.A. (1978). Colorado tick fever: clinical, epidemioligic, and laboratory aspects of 228 cases in Colorado in 1973–1974. *Ann. Intern. Med.* **88**, 303.

Green, J.J., Wang, S.P., Yen, C.H., and Hung, S.C. (1963). The epidemiology of Japanese encephalitis virus in Taiwan in 1961. *Am. J. Trop. Med. Hyg.* **12**, 668.

Gressler, I., Hardy, J.L., Hu, S.M.K., and Scherer, W.F. (1958). Factors influencing transmission of Japanese B encephalitis virus by a colonized strain of *Culex tritaeniorhynchus* Giles, from infected pigs and chicks to susceptible pigs and birds. *Am. J. Trop. Med. Hyg.* **7**, 365.

Grimstad, P.R., Ross, Q.E., and Craig, G.B. (1980). *Aedes triseriatus* (Diptera: Culicidae) and La Crosse virus. II Modification of mosquito feeding behaviour by virus infection. *J. Med. Entomol.* **17**, 1.

Grimstad, P.R., Craig, G.B., Ross, Q.E., and Yuill, T.M. (1977). *Aedes triseriatus* and La Crosse virus: geographic variation in vector susceptibility and ability to transmit. *Am. J. Trop. Med. Hyg.* **26**, 990.

Groot, H. (1980). The reinvasion of Colombia by *Aedes aegypti*: aspects to remember. *Am. J. Trop. Med. Hyg.* **29**, 330.

Gubler, D.J. and Rosen, L. (1976). Variation among geographic strains of *Aedes albopictus* in susceptibility to infection with dengue virus. *Am. J. Trop. Med. Hyg.* **25**, 318.

Haddow, A.J., Davies, C.W., and Walker, A.J. (1960). O'nyong-nyong fever: epidemic virus disease in East Africa: I. Introduction. *Trans. R. Soc. Trop. Med. Hyg.* **54**, 517.

Halstead, S.B. (1965). Dengue and haemorrhagic fevers in Southeast Asia. *Yale J. Biol. Med.* **37**, 434.

Halstead, S.B. (1966). Mosquito-borne haemorrhagic fevers of South and Southeast Asia. *WHO Bull.* **35**, 3.

Halstead, S.B. (1981). Dengue and dengue haemorrhagic fever. In *CRC handbook series in zoonoses. Section B: Viral zoonoses*, Vol. 1 (ed. J.H. Steele and G.W. Beran) p. 421. CRC Press, Boca Raton, FL.

Halstead, S.B. (1982). WHO fights dengue haemorrhagic fever. *WHO Chron.* **36**, 65.

Halstead, S.B., Nimmannitya, S., and Margiotta, M.R. (1969). Dengue and chikungunya virus infection in man in Thailand 1962–1964. Observations on disease in out-patients. *Am. J. Trop. Med. Hyg.* **18**, 972.

Halstead, S.B., Scanlon, J.E., Umpaivit, P., and Udomsakdi, S. (1969). Dengue and chikungunya virus infection in man in Thailand, 1962–1964. IV. Epidemiologic studies in the Bangkok metropolitan area. *Am. J. Trop. Med. Hyg.* **18**, 997.

Hannoun, C., Panther, R., Mouchet, J., and Eazan, J.P. (1964). Isoliment en France au virus West Nile a partir de malades et du vecteur *Culex modistus ficalbi*. *C.R. Acad. Sci.* **259**, 4170.

Hammon, W. McD. and Reeves, W.C. (1952). California encephalitis virus; a newly described agent. *California Med.* **77**, 303.

Hammon, W.M., Tigertt, W.D., and Sather, G.E. (1958). Epidemiologic studies of concurrent virgin epidemics of Japanese B encephalitis and of mumps on Guam, 1947–1948, with subsequent observations including dengue, through 1957. *Am. J. Trop. Med. Hyg.* **7**, 441.

Hanson, R.P., Rasmussen, A.F., Brandly, C.A., and Brown, J.W. (1950). Human infection with the virus of vesicular stomatitis. *J. Lab. Clin. Med.* **36**, 754.

Hanson, R.P. (1975). Vesicular stomatitis. In *Diseases of swine* (ed. H.W. Dunne and A.D. Leman) p. 308. Iowa State University Press, Ames, Iowa.

Hardin, F.W., Hepburn, H.R., and Etheridge, B.J. (1967). A history of mosquitoes and mosquito-borne diseases in Mississippi 1699–1965. *Mosquito News* **27**, 60.

Hayes, R.O. (1981). Eastern and Western encephalitis. *CRC handbook series in zoonoses: viral zoonoses* (ed. J.H. Steele and G.W. Beran) p. 29. CRC Press, Boca Raton, FL.

Hebert, S.A., Bowman, K.A., Rudnick, A., and Burton, J.J.S. (1980). A rapid method for the isolation and identification of dengue viruses employing a single system. *Malaysian J. Pathol.* **3**, 67.

Hoogstraal, H., Meegan, J.M., Khalil, G.M., and Adham, F.K. (1979). The Rift Valley fever epizootic in Egypt 1977–78. 2. Ecological and entomological studies. *Trans. R. Soc. Trop. Med. Hyg.* **6**, 624.

Hsu, S.H., Huang, W.C., and Cross, J.H. (1978). The isolation of Japanese encephalitis virus from Taiwan mosquitoes by mosquito cell cultures and mouse inoculation. *J. Med. Entomol.* **14**, 698.

Igarashi, A., Sasao, F., Fukai, K., Buei, K., Ueba, N., and Yoshida, M. (1981). Mutants of Getah and Japanese encephalitis viruses isolated from field-caught *Culex tritaeniorhynchus* using *Aedes albopictus* clone C6/36 cells. *Ann. Virol.* **132E**, 235.

Jadhav, M., Namboodriapd, M., Carman, R.H., Carey, D.E., and Myers, R.M. (1965). Chikungunya disease in infants and children in Vellore: a report on clinical and haematological features of virologically proved cases. *Indian J. Med. Res.* **53**, 764.

Johnson, B.K. and Chanas, A.C. (1981). *Abstracts on Hygiene and*

*Communicable Diseases* **56**, 165.

Kemp, G.E. (1981). Saint Louis encephalitis (SLE). *CRC handbook series in zoonoses: Section B: viral zoonoses* (ed. J.H. Steele and B.W. Beran) p. 71. CRC Press, Boca Raton, FL.

Kokernot, R.H., Shinefield, H.R., and Longshore, W.A. Jr (1953). The 1952 outbreak of encephalitis in California. Differential diagnosis. *Calif. Med.* **79**, 73.

Konno, J., Endo, K., Agatsuma, H., and Ishida, N. (1966). Cyclic outbreaks of Japanese encephalitis among pigs and humans. *Am. J. Epidemiol.* **84**, 292.

Kramer, L.D. and Scherer, W.F. (1976). Vector competence of mosquitoes as a marker to distinguish Central American and Mexican epizootic from enzootic strains of Venezuelan encephalitis virus. *Am. J. Trop. Med. Hyg.* **25**, 336.

Kubes, V. and Rios, F.A. (1939). The causative agent of infectious equine encephalomyelitis in Venezuela. *Science* **90**, 20.

Laughlin, L.W., Meegan, J.M., Strausbaugh, L.J., Morens, D.M., and Watten, R.H. (1979). Epidemic Rift Valley fever in Egypt; observations of the spectrum of human illness. *Trans. R. Soc. Trop. Med. Hyg.* **73**, 630.

Leake, C.J. (1983). *Virus vectors*. Academic Press, London.

Lopes, O.S. (1981). Rocio viral encephalitis. Arboviral zoonoses in South America. *CRC handbook series in zoonoses: Section B Viral zoonoses* (ed. J.H. Steele and G.W. Beran) p. 171. CRC Press, Boca Raton, FL.

Lopes, O.S., Sacchetta, L.A., Francy, D.B., Jakob, W.L., and Calisher, C.H. (1981). Emergence of a new arbovirus disease in Brazil. III. Isolation of Rocio virus from *Psorophora ferox* (Humboldt, 1819). *Am. J. Epidemiol.* **113**, 122.

McConnell, S. and Spertzel, R.O. (1981). Venezuelan equine encephalomyelitis (VEE). CRC handbook series in zoonoses: Section B: Viral zoonoses (ed. J.H. Steele and G.W. Beran) p. 59. CRC Press, Boca Raton, FL.

McIntosh, B.M., Paterson, H.E., Donaldson, J.M., and De Sousa, J. (1963). Chikungunya virus: viral susceptibility and transmission studies with some vertebrates and mosquitoes. *S. Afr. J. Med. Sci.* **28**, 45.

McLean, R.G., Francy, D.B., Bowen, G.S., Bailey, R.E., Calisher, C.H., and Barnes, A.M. (1981). The ecology of Colorado tick fever in Rocky Mountain National Park in 1974. Objectives, study design, and summary of principal findings. *Am. J. Trop. Med. Hyg.* **30**, 483.

Marshall, I.D. and Woodroofe, G.M. (1975). Epidemiology of arboviruses. *Rep. John Curtin Sch. Med. Res. Aust. Nat. Univ.* 92.

Meyer, N.L., Moulton, W.M., Jenney, E.W., and Rodgers, R.J. (1960). Outbreaks of vesicular stomatitis in Oklahoma and Texas. In *Proc. U.S. Livestock Sanit. Assoc.* **64**, 324.

Monath, T.P. (1980). *Epidemiology*. In *St. Louis encephalitis*, (ed. T.P. Monath) p. 239. American Public Health Association, Washington, DC.

Muckenfuss, R.S., Smadel, J.E., and Moore, E. (1938). The neutralization of encephalitis virus (St. Louis, 1933) by serum. *J. Clin. Invest.* **17**, 53.

Murphy, F.A., Harrison, A.K., and Whitfield, S.B. (1973). Bunyaviridae: morphologic and morphogenetic similarities of Bunyamwera serologic supergroup viruses and several other arthropod-borne viruses. *Intervirology* **1**, 297.

Peiris, J.S.M., Gordon, S., Inkeless, J.E., and Porterfield, J.S. (1981). Monoclonal anti-Fc receptor IgG blocks antibody enhancement of viral replication in macrophages. *Nature* **289**, 189.

Pearson, L.B. (1969). *Report of the Commission on International Development*. Pall Mall Press, London.

Peters, C.J. and Meegan, J.M. (1981). Rift Valley fever. *CRC handbook series in zoonoses: Section B: Viral zoonoses,* (ed. J.H. Steele and G.W. Beran) p. 403. CRC Press, Boca Raton, FL.

Pinheiro, F.P., Travassos Da Rosa, A.P.A., and Travassos Da Rosa, J.F.S. (1981). Oropouche virus. I. A review of clinical, epidemiological and ecological findings. *Am. J. Trop. Med. Hyg.* **30**, 149.

Pinheiro, F.B. (1981). Oropouche fever. Arboviral Zoonoses in South America. *CRC handbook series in zoonoses: Viral zoonoses* (ed. J.H. Steele and G.W. Beran) p. 177. CRC Press, Boca Raton, FL.

Pogodina, V.V. (1961). Epidemiology and prevention of alimentary infections of tick-borne encephalitis, *J. Hyg. Epidemiol. Microbiol. Immunol.* **5**, 75.

Pond, W.L., Russ, S.B., Rogers, N.G., and Smadel, J.E. (1955). Murray Valley encephalitis virus: its serological relationship to the Japanese–West Nile-St. Louis encephalitis group of viruses, *J. Immunol.* **75**, 78.

Pond, W.L., Russ, S.B., Lancaster, W.E., Audy, J.R., and Amadel, J.E. (1954). Japanese encephalitis in Malaya. II. Distribution of neutralizing antibody in man and domestic animals. *Am. J. Hyg.* **59**, 17.

Porterfield, J.S., Casals, J., Chumakov, M.R. *et al.* (1976). Bunyaviruses and Bunyaviridae. *Intervirology* **6**, 13.

Race, M.W., Williams, M.C., and Agostini, C.F.M. (1979). Dengue in the Caribbean: virus isolation in a mosquito (*Aedes pseudoscutellaris*) cell line. *Trans. R. Soc. Trop. Med. Hyg.* **73**, 18.

Rao, T.R., Devi, P.S., and Singh, K.R.P. (1968). Experimental studies on the mechanical transmission of chikungunya virus by *Aedes aegypti*. *Mosquito News* **28**, 406.

Reed, W. (1901). Propagation of yellow fever virus; observations based on recent researches. *Med. Rec.* **60**, 201.

Rehcek, J. (1965). Cultivation of different viruses in tick tissue cultures. *Acta Virol.* **9**, 332.

Reiss-Gutfreund, R.J., Andral, L., and Serie, C., (1962). Etude d'un virus presentant les caracteristiques de la choriomeningite lymphocytaire (C.M.L.) isole en Ethiopie. *Ann. Inst. Pasteur, Paris* **102**, 36.

Robin, Y. and Beran, G.W. (1981). Yellow fever. *CRC handbook series in zoonoses: Viral zoonoses* (ed. J.H. Steele and G.W. Beran) p. 85. CRC Press, Boca Raton, FL.

Ross, R.W. (1956). The Newala epidemic. III. The virus: isolation, pathogenic properties and relationship to the epidemic. *J. Hyg.* **54**, 177.

Rush, B. (1789). An account of the bilious remitting fever, as it appeared in Philadelphia in the summer and autumn of the year 1780. *Medical Inquiries and Observations, Philadelphia*, **102**.

Sankaran, B. (1978). Follow-up on Japanese B encephalitis – India. *Morbidity and Mortality Weekly Report* **27**, 64.

Sanmartin, C. (1972). Diseases hosts: man. In *Venezuelan encephalitis*, p. 231. Pan American Health Organization, Washington, DC.

Sarkar, J.K., Chatterjee, S.N., Chakravarti, S.K., and Mitra, A.C. (1965). Chikungunya virus infection with haemorrhagic manifestations. *Indian J. Med. Res.* **53**, 921.

Serie, C., Andral, L., Lindrec, A., and Neri, P. (1964). Epidemie de fièvre jaune en Ethiopie (1960–1962). Observations preliminaires. *WHO Bull.* **30**, 299.

Shope, R.E., Peters, C.J., and Davies, F.G. (1982). The spread of Rift Valley fever and approaches to its control. *WHO Bull.* **60**, 299.

Siam, A.L. and Meegan, J.M. (1980). Rift Valley fever virus infection causes ocular manifestations. *Trans. R. Soc. Trop. Med. Hyg.* **74**, 540.

Siler, J.F., Hall, M.W., and Hitchens, A.P. (1926). Dengue: its history, epidemiology, mechanisms of transmission, etiology, clinical manifestations, immunity, and prevention. *Philipp. J. Sci.* **29**, 1.

Smith, C.E.G. (1959). Arthropod-borne viruses. *Br. Med. Bull.* **15**, 235.

Smith, C.E.G. (1972). Changing patterns of disease in the tropics. *Br. Med. Bull.* **28**, 3.

Smith, C.E.G. (1978). 'New' viral zoonoses: past, present and future. In *Microbial ecology* (ed. M.W. Loutid and J.A.R. Miles) p. 170. Springer, Berlin.

Smithburn, K.C., Hughes, T.P., Burke, A.W., and Paul, J.H. (1940). A neutropic virus isolated from the blood of a native of Uganda. *Am. J. Trop. Med. Hyg.* **20**, 471.

Smithburn, K.C., Kokernot, R.H., Weinbren, M.P., and de Meillon, B. (1957). Studies on arthropod-borne viruses of Tongaland. IX. Isolation of Wesselsbron virus from a naturally infected human being and from *Aedes* (B) *circumluteolus*. *S. Afr. J. Med. Sci.* **22**, 113.

Souza Lopes, O. (1981). Rocio viral encephalitis. Arboviral zoonoses in South America. *CRC handbook series in zoonoses: Viral zoonoses.* (ed. J.H. Steele and G.W. Beran) p. 171. CRC Press, Boca Raton, FL.

Spruance, S.L. and Bailey, A. (1973). Colorado tick fever. A review of 115 laboratory confirmed cases. *Arch. Intern. Med.* **131**, 288.

Strode, G.K. (1951). *Yellow fever.* McGraw-Hill, New York.

Sub-Committee on Arbovirus Laboratory Safety (1980). Laboratory safety for arboviruses and certain other viruses of vertebrates. *Am. J. Trop. Med. Hyg.* **29**, 1359.

Sudia, W.D. and Chamberlain, R.W. (1967). *Collection and processing of medically important arthropods for arbovirus isolation.* US Public Health Service, Atlanta, Georgia.

Sudia, W.D., Lord, R.D., and Hayes, R.O. (1970). *Collection and processing of vertebrate specimens for arbovirus studies.* US Public Health Service, Atlanta, Georgia.

Surtees, G. (1970a). Large scale irrigation and arbovirus epidemiology, Kano Plain, Kenya. I. Description of the area and preliminary studies on the mosquitoes. *J. Med. Entomol.* **7**, 509.

Surtees, G. (1970b). Mosquito breeding in the Kuching area, Sarawak, with special reference to the epidemiology of dengue fever. *J. Med. Entomol.* **7**, 273.

Svedmyr, A., von Zeipel, G., Holmgren, B., and Lindahl, J. (1958). Tick-borne meningoencephalomyelitis in Sweden. *Arch. Gesamte Virusforsch.* **8**, 565.

Taufflieb, R., Cornet, M., Le Gonidec, G., and Robin, Y. (1973). Un foyer selvatique de fièvre jaune au Senegal oriental. *Cah. ORSTOM, Ser. Entomol. Med. Parasitol.* **11**, 211.

Taylor, R.M., Work, T.H., Hurlbut, A.S., and Rizk, F. (1956). A study of the ecology of West Nile virus in Egypt. *Am. J. Trop. Med. Hyg.* **5**, 579.

Tesh, R.B., Gubler, D.J., and Rosen, L. (1976). Variation among geographic strains of *Aedes albopictus* in susceptibility to infection with Chikungunya virus. *Am. J. Trop. Med. Hyg.* **25**, 985.

Thiruvengadam, K.V., Kalyanasundaram, V., and Rajgopal, J. (1965). Clinical and pathological studies on chikungunya fever in Madras City. *Indian J. Med. Res.* **53**, 720.

Thompson, W.H. and Inhorn, S.L. (1967). Arthropod-borne California group viral encephalitis in Wisconsin, *Wis. Med. J.* **66**, 250.

Thompson, W.H., Anslow, R.O., Hanson, R.P., and DeFoliart, G.R. (1972). La Crosse Virus isolations from mosquitoes in Wisconsin, 1964-68. *Am. J. Trop. Med. Hyg.* **21**, 90.

Thomson, K.B., Austin, F.J., Maguire, T., and Miles, J.A.R. (1979). Epidemic polyarthritis in Fiji and New Zealand. *N.Z. Med. J.* **90**, 30.

Topping, N.H., Cullyford, J.S., and Davis, G.E. (1940). Colorado tick fever. *Public Health Rep.* **55**, 2224.

Trpis, M. (1960). Bitting mosquitoes of the rice fields and possible means of their control. (An ecological study.) *Biol. Proc.* **6**, 4.

Van Velden, D.J.J., Meyer, J.D., Olivier, J., Gear, J.H.S., and McIntosh, B. (1977). Rift Valley fever affecting humans in South Africa: a clinicopathological study. *S. Afr. Med. J.* **51**, 867.

Varma, M.G.R. (1972). Invertebrate host specificity in arthropod-borne animal viruses. *Monogr. Virol.* **6**, 49.

Varma, M.G.R., Pudney, M., Leake, C.J., and Peralta, P.H. (1976). Isolations in a mosquito (*Aedes pseudoscutellaris*) cell line (Mos. 61) of yellow fever virus strains from original field material. *Intervirology* **6**, 50.

Weaver, O.M., Haymaker, W., Pieper, S., and Kurland, R. (1958). Sequelae of the arthropod-borne encephalitides. V. Japanese encephalitis. *Neurology* **8**, 887.

Webb, H.E. and Lakshmana Rao, R. (1961). Kyasanur Forest disease: a general clinical study in which some cases with neurological complications were observed. *Trans. R. Soc. Trop. Med. Hyg.* **55**, 284.

Weiss, K.E., Haig, D.A., and Alexander, R.A. (1956). Wesselsbron virus – a virus not previously described associated with abortion in domestic animals. *Onderstepoort J.* **27**, 183.

Wolfe, M.S., Calisher, C.H., and McGuire, K. (1982). Spondweni virus infection in a foreign resident of Upper Volta. *Lancet* **ii**, 1306.

Work, T.H. and Trapido, H. (1957). Kyasanur Forest disease: a new infection of man and monkeys in tropical India by a virus of the Russian Spring–Summer complex. *Public Health Med. Sci.* **17**, 80.

WHO (1980a). Surveillance of Japanese encephalitis. *WHO Weekly Epidemiol. Record* **53**, 48.

WHO (1980b). Yellow fever in 1979. *WHO Weekly Epidemiol. Record* **55**, 355.

WHO (1980c). Human arbovirus surveillance. *WHO Weekly Epidemiol. Record* **55**, 76.

WHO (1981a). Dengue fever surveillance in the American region. *WHO Weekly Epidemiol. Record* **56**, 298.

WHO (1981b). Yellow fever in 1980. *WHO Weekly Epidemiol. Record* **56**, 259.

WHO (1981c). Rift Valley fever surveillance. *WHO Weekly Epidemiol. Record* **56**, 214.

Yuill, T.M. (1981). Vesicular stomatitis. *CRC handbook series in zoonoses: Viral zoonoses* (ed. J.H. Steele and G.W. Beran) p. 125. CRC Press, Boca Raton, FL.

Zilber, L.A. and Soloviev, V.D. (1946). Far Eastern tick-borne spring–summer (spring) encephalitis. *Am. Rev. Sov. Med.* Special Suppl. **5**, 1.

# 17 The principles of an epidemic field investigation

Michael B. Gregg

## INTRODUCTION

This chapter contains a simple, practical, and, essentially, a non-technical discussion of how to prepare for and perform an epidemic field investigation. To emphasize certain major issues, attention will be focused on a presumed point-source (common-source) epidemic of a bacterial disease, recognized and reported by local health authorities to a regional (district, provincial, or state) health department with a concomitant request for epidemiological assistance. The purpose of establishing such a setting stems from the fact that this frequent and typical scenario highlights some key operational and public health issues health officials should recognize and address as integral aspects of any field investigation – besides the obvious epidemiological considerations. Therefore, not only is the discussion directed towards the description of a logical progression of tasks the epidemiologist should perform, but considerable attention is also directed towards important operational and public health policy concerns. Although this chapter centres about the occurrence of an acute bacterial disease epidemic in a community, the epidemiological and public health principles apply equally well to other infectious or non-infectious disease epidemics and to occurrences of disease extending over much longer periods of time.

## BACKGROUND CONSIDERATIONS

### Overall purposes and methodology

As mentioned in earlier chapters, the purposes of epidemiology are to determine the causative agent of a disease, its source, its mode of transmission, who is at risk of developing disease, and what exposures predispose to disease. With answers to these questions, the epidemiologist hopes to control and prevent disease. Clearly, these purposes also apply to field investigations of, for example, bacterial disease epidemics. Fortunately, in most bacterial disease outbreaks, the clinical syndromes are easily identifiable, the bacterial agents can be readily isolated and characterized, and the source, mode of transmission, and risk factors of the disease are usually well known and understood. Therefore, epidemiologists are often quite well prepared for their field investiga-

tions by having the proper information, tools, and techniques to define the circumstances surrounding any given outbreak. However, when the clinical diagnosis and/or laboratory findings are unclear, the epidemiologist's task becomes much more difficult, often requiring careful consideration of the clinical presentation of disease in order to obtain key information regarding the source, mode of spread, and population(s) at risk of disease. For example, bacterial contamination of food or water is usually manifested by signs and symptoms referable to the gastrointestinal tract. Pathogenic bacteria transmitted in air often affect the respiratory tract and sometimes the skin, eyes, or mucous membranes. Skin abrasions or lesions may suggest animal or insect transmission. So the clinical manifestations of disease may serve as critical leads for epidemiologists who may at times have no other information to guide them regarding the circumstances surrounding the epidemic. Regardless of how secure the clinical diagnosis may be, however, the epidemiologist's thought process must include clinical, laboratory, and epidemiological considerations – almost always applied on an ongoing basis during the entire investigation – each providing leads and pathways to take or reject, so that ultimately the natural history of the epidemic will be understood.

Although epidemiologists perform several separate operations (which are listed below), in broad strokes they do two things. First, they collect information that describes the setting of the outbreak, namely, over what time period people became sick, where they acquired disease, and what the characteristics of the ill people were. These are the descriptive aspects of the investigation. Very often, simply by knowing these facts (and the diagnosis), the epidemiologist can determine the source and mode of spread of the agent, and can identify those primarily at risk of developing disease. Common sense will often give these answers, and relatively little, if any, further analysis is required.

However, on occasion, it will not be readily apparent where the agent resided, how it was transmitted, who was at risk of disease, and what the risk factors were. Under these circumstances, a second operation, analytical epidemiology, must be used. As has been described in other chapters and volumes of this series, epidemiological analyses require comparisons of ill and well persons, exposed and not exposed. In an epidemic, the epidemiologist usually compares ill and well people – both believed at risk of disease – to determine what exposures ill people had that well people did not have. These comparisons are made using appropriate statistical techniques, and if the differences between ill and well are greater than one would expect by chance, the epidemiologist can draw certain inferences regarding the transmission and exposure of the disease.

### The pace and commitment of a field investigation

An underlying theme woven through the entire chapter emphasizes the need to act quickly, to establish clear operational priorities, and to perform the investigation responsibly. This should not imply the haphazard collection and inappropriate analysis of data, but rather the use of simple and workable case definitions, case-finding methods, and analyses. If at all possible, collection, analyses, and recommendations should be performed in the field as part of the investigation. There is often a strong tendency to collect what is believed to be the essential information in the field and then retreat to 'home base' for analysis – particularly with the availability of sophisticated computers. However, the local constituency may view such action as lack of interest or concern, or even possessiveness. Equally important, the investigator's premature departure makes any further collection of data or direct contact with study populations and local health officials difficult, if not impossible. Once home, the epidemiology team has lost the urgency and momentum to perform, the sense of relevancy of the epidemic, and, most of all, the totally committed time for the investigation. Every field investigation should be completed not only to the satisfaction of the epidemiologist, but particularly to the satisfaction of the local health officers as well. Every field investigator should contemplate what the local health department must face if the investigative team leaves without providing reasonably final results and firmly based recommendations.

### RECOGNITION AND RESPONSE TO A REQUEST FOR ASSISTANCE

#### The report

The regional health officer may learn of an epidemic from a variety of sources such as the local health department, a private physician, a hospital administrator, a concerned citizen, or perhaps even the news media. Generally, the most direct and reliable source of information is a local health official, who will often have a 'working' diagnosis, an estimate of the number of cases, the background expected number of cases, and the affected population. Reports of a possible or real epidemic from others such as private physicians, hospitals, and the like may reveal only a segment of the overall picture of the epidemic or may, indeed, not reflect the existence of an epidemic at all. Therefore, when reports such as these are received at the regional level, the regional official should contact the pertinent local health officials as soon as possible and inform them of the reports and requests. Thereupon, local officials will usually attempt

to verify such reports and, if they find them to be true, will investigate the epidemic themselves. Even if no epidemic is ultimately recognized or no request for assistance results as a consequence of the contact between regional and local health departments, the regional health official has clearly discharged an important responsibility by reporting back to those with the primary charge for investigation, control, and prevention.

#### The request

However, if the local health official requests assistance in investigating a presumed outbreak, the regional epidemiologist, before making any decision, should try to acquire as much information as possible regarding the diagnosis, the normal occurrence of disease, and the primarily affected population. Laboratory tests used to suggest or confirm the diagnosis and some knowledge of the working hypothesis as to the source of the causative agent and its mode of spread may also be extremely useful. Quite frequently local health departments will have performed a preliminary and sometimes relatively extensive investigation before calling for assistance and will be able to provide a considerable amount of valuable information – to be used in planning for the appropriate allocation of professional personnel, supplies, and the probable time needed for an investigation.

It is particularly important at this juncture to find out exactly why the request for assistance is forthcoming. Does the local health department simply need an extra pair of hands to perform or complete the investigation or has it been unable to uncover the nature or source of infection or the mode of spread, thereby limiting adequate control or prevention? Perhaps the health department wants to share the responsibility of the investigation with a more seasoned and knowledgeable health authority so as to be relieved of local political or scientific pressure. Occasionally, legal or ethical issues may have become prominent in the early investigation, and those responding to requests for help must be aware of these possibilities. Rarely, an epidemic may even be declared or announced by local authorities or citizens and assistance sought in order to publicize perceived adverse health conditions, to awaken provincial or national health leaders, or even to secure funds. Regardless of the motivation behind a call for assistance, there must be an established official basis for such a request and official local permission for an epidemiological investigation. Many a field study has been aborted simply because either those requesting assistance had no authority to do so or state, regional, or national teams were investigating without local permission.

#### The response and the responsibilities

The relationships between regional and local health departments vary not only from region to region within countries but also from country to country. In general, the larger health districts help serve the smaller ones in time of need; yet the sensitivities between these two authorities are frequently delicate, particularly as they relate to perceived competence, local jurisdiction, and ultimate authority. In discussions of potential collaborative investigations, the regional health officer must decide, on the basis of prevailing local-provincial amenities and agreements and his best judgment, the most appropriate response. Without undue detail, however, there are several important reasons why requests for a field investigation should be answered, if not encouraged.

(a) To control and prevent further disease.

(b) To provide agreed upon or statutorily mandated services.

(c) To derive more information about interactions among the human host, the infectious agent, and the environment.

(d) To assess the quality of communicable disease epidemiological surveillance at the local level.

(e) To maintain or improve such epidemiological surveillance by personal and direct contact.

(f) To establish a new system of epidemiological surveillance.

(g) To provide training opportunities, under proper supervision in practical field epidemiology.

If the regional health officer decides to provide field assistance, both he or she and the local health official should discuss and hopefully agree upon: (i) what resources (including personnel) will be available locally; (ii) what resources will be provided by the regional team; (iii) who will direct the day-to-day investigation; (iv) who will provide overall supervision and ultimately be responsible for the investigation; (v) how the data will be shared and who will be responsible for their analysis; (vi) whether a report of the findings will be written, who will write it, and to whom will it go; and (vii) who will be the senior author of a scientific paper, should one be written. These are extremely critical issues, some of which cannot be totally resolved before the investigative team arrives on the scene; however, they must be addressed, discussed openly, and agreed upon as soon as possible.

## Preparation for the field investigation

No attempt is made here to describe in detail what personnel or equipment should be deployed for the field investigation. These decisions will clearly depend upon the presumed cause, magnitude, geographical extent of the epidemic, and the local and regional resources available. Rather, the emphasis focuses upon the necessary collaborative relationships between health professionals at the regional office and key instructions to the investigating team before they depart.

### Collaboration and consultation

Virtually all bacterial disease outbreaks require the support of a competent laboratory. Even if local laboratories are believed capable of processing and identifying specimens collected during the investigation, it is strongly advised that the regional epidemiological team, upon being informed of the proposed investigation, should immediately contact their counterparts within the regional laboratories. These bacteriologists or microbiologists should be requested to provide any needed guidance and laboratory assistance. It is preferable to obtain assurance of co-operation and commitment at this time rather than in the midst of the field investigation or near the end when specimens have already been collected and await testing. Not only must the bacteriologists schedule the processing of specimens, but also recommend what kinds of specimens are needed and how they should be collected and processed for maximum usefulness to the investigation. There may be also substantive basic or applied research questions that could be appropriately addressed and answered during the field investigation. These issues should be discussed in detail with the bacteriologists, and every effort made to enlist and support their interest.

Advice on statistical methods may be also sought at this time, particularly if questionnaires will be created or if large populations will be sampled. The same philosophy applies also to contacting other health professionals, such as veterinarians, mammalogists, or entomologists, whose expertise can be crucial to a successful field investigation. Moreover, serious consideration should be given to including such professionals on the investigative team if needed and if comparable local personnel are not available. It is particularly important to determine whether such scientists should be part of the initial team so that appropriate information and particularly specimens can be collected concomitantly with other relevant epidemiological information.

Other persons who can be extremely important in the overall management of a field investigation are information or news media specialists. Particularly when large outbreaks of disease are to be investigated that will likely attract even moderate local or regional attention in the news media, the presence of an experienced and knowledgeable information officer who can respond to public inquiries and meet with the news media on a regular basis can be invaluable.

Parenthetically, some consideration should always be given to including secretarial and/or administrative personnel on the investigating team—not only in order to utilize their services in the field but to expose them to a real-life investigation. By such experience they will almost invariably return home with a better understanding of field work and an increased ability to support technical personnel in the regional offices.

### Basic administrative instructions

Once the field team has been designated, certain key instructions concerning the investigation should be emphasized.

1. Identify the team leader and the person to whom he or she should report regularly at the regional level.

2. Specify when and how communications should be established with the regional home base for information and guidance. Do not permit the investigating team to notify, as it is convenient, the regional supervisors of the progress of the investigation. Establish within reason fixed times and places for regular communication regardless of whether new facts or findings have been uncovered. There may be just as important reasons for the home base to communicate with the field team as the reverse.

3. Emphasize the need for the team to meet with appropriate local health officials immediately upon arriving in the field. If the local official has not already been identified, instruct the team leader to determine as soon as possible who at the local level will be in charge and who has the authority to give the epidemiologists the clinical, laboratory, and epidemiological information needed for the investigation. Encourage the team to identify and meet with all persons they

may need co-operation from in the investigation. Such persons include: local health department directors and/or chiefs of epidemiology, laboratory services, vital statistics, nursing, and maternal and child health. Other important persons would often include the mayor, the local medical society, or hospital administrators and staff. It is highly preferable to take the day or so needed to meet these persons initially – so that key doors will be opened – than to spend valuable time later in the investigation mending bridges.

4. Have the team leader identify the appropriate local person to speak for the entire investigative team when necessary. In general, the regional team should try to avoid direct contact with the news media and should always defer to local health officials. The investigative team is usually working at the request and under the aegis of the local health authorities, and, therefore, it is the local officials who not only know and appreciate the local aspects of the epidemic but are the appropriate persons to comment on the findings of the investigation. In the most practical sense, the less the news media make contact with the investigative team, the more can be done at the pace and discretion of that team.

5. Before leaving to conduct an investigation, the team leader or preferably his or her immediate supervisor should write a memorandum summarizing how and when the region was contacted, what information was provided by the local health department, what the proposed response by the region is, what the agreed upon commitments of both local and regional health authorities are, who is on the field team, and when the latter are expected to arrive in the field. This memorandum should be distributed to key supervisors in both regional and local health offices and to others who may have a need to know.

## THE FIELD INVESTIGATION

Before the actual field activities are discussed, it should be borne in mind that the order of the tasks should not be considered fixed or binding but rather logical in terms of field operations and epidemiological thinking. The epidemiologist may perform several of these functions simultaneously or in different order during the investigation and may even institute control and prevention measures soon after beginning the investigation on the basis of intuitive reasoning and/or common sense. No two epidemiologists will take the same pathway of investigation. Yet, in general, the data they collect, the analyses they apply, and the control and prevention they recommend will likely be similar.

Since, by definition, the epidemic in question has resulted from a point source and may be continuing or nearly over before the field team arrives, the field investigation will be retrospective in nature. This should alert the epidemiologist to some fundamental aspects of any investigation that occurs 'after the fact'. First of all, because many illnesses and critical events have already occurred, virtually all information acquired and related to the epidemic will be based upon the memory of health officers, physicians, and patients, each of whom may have different recollections, views or perceptions of what transpired, what caused the disease, and even who or what was responsible for the epidemic. In practical terms, epidemic-related information may conflict, may not be accurate, and certainly cannot be expected to reflect the precise recounting of past events. Yet, just as the clinician may ask patients what they think is making them sick, the epidemiologist will do well to ask members of the affected community what they think caused the epidemic.

For the young, inexperienced medical epidemiologist steeped in the tradition of molecule and millimole determinations, the 'more-or-less' measurements of the field epidemiologist can initially be major hurdles to the successful field investigation. However lacking in accuracy these data may be, they are the only data available, and must be collected, analysed, and interpreted with care, imagination, and caution.

## Determine the existence of an epidemic

In most instances, local health officials will know whether more cases of disease are occurring than would normally be expected. Since most local health departments have ongoing records of the occurrence of communicable disease, comparisons by week, month, and year can be made to determine whether the observed numbers exceed the normally expected level. Although strict laboratory confirmation may be lacking at this time, an increase in the number of cases of a disease reasonably accurately reported by local physicians should stimulate further inquiry. It should be borne in mind, however, that the terms 'epidemic' and 'outbreak' are quite subjective, not only depending upon how local health officials view the normal rises and falls in disease incidence, but upon whether such changes are deemed worthy of investigation. One must be acutely aware of artefactual causes of increases or decreases in numbers of reported cases, such as changes in local reporting practices, increased interest in certain diseases because of local or national awareness, or changes in methods of diagnosis. Even the presence of a new physician or clinic in the community may lead to a substantial increase in numbers of cases of a particular disease reported, yet not represent a true increase above normal in the number of cases that actually occur.

In certain situations, however, it may be difficult to document rapidly the existence of an epidemic. The epidemiologist may need to acquire information from such sources as school or factory absentee records, out-patient clinic visits, hospitalizations, laboratory records, or death certificates. Sometimes a simple survey of practising physicians will strongly support the existence of an epidemic, as would a similar rapid survey of houses or households in the community. Frequently, such quick assessments entail asking for information about signs and symptoms rather than about specific diagnoses. For example, such inquiry might involve asking physicians or clinics if they are treating more people than usual with sore throats, gastroenteritis, fever with rash, etc., in order to obtain an index of disease incidence. Although not specific for any given bacterial disease, such surveys can often document the occurrence of an epidemic. Sometimes it is extremely difficult to establish satisfactorily the existence of an epidemic. Yet because of local pressures, epidemiologists may be obliged to continue the investigation even if they believe that no significant health problem exists.

### Confirm the diagnosis

Every effort possible should be made to confirm the clinical diagnosis by standard laboratory techniques such as serology and/or isolation and characterization of the bacterium. Newly introduced, experimental, or otherwise not broadly recognized confirmatory tests should not be used for this purpose – at least not at this stage in the investigation. If at all possible, the field epidemiologist should visit the laboratory and verify the laboratory findings. Not every reported case has to be confirmed. If most patients have the expected or similar clinical signs and symptoms and, perhaps, 15–20 per cent of the cases are laboratory confirmed, there is no pressing need at this time in the investigation to require more confirmation; this should be ample confirmatory evidence. The medical epidemiologist should also attempt to examine several representative cases of the disease as well. Clinical assumptions should not be made; the diagnosis should be verified by the investigator or a qualified physician with the epidemiologist. Nothing convinces epidemiologists and responsible health officers more than an eyewitness confirmation of clinical disease by the investigating team.

### Determine the number of cases

Now the epidemiologist must create a workable case definition, decide how to find cases, and inquire about and count cases. The simplest and most objective criteria for a case definition are usually the best (for example, fever, X-ray evidence of pneumonia, white cells in the spinal fluid, number of bowel movements per day, blood in the stool, skin rash). However, the epidemiologist should be guided by the accepted, usual presentation of the disease, with or without standard laboratory confirmation, in the case definition. Where time may be a critical factor in a rapidly unfolding field investigation, a simple, easily applicable definition should be used – recognizing that some cases will be missed and some false cases included. The following factors can help to determine the levels of sensitivity and specificity of the case definition:

(a) What is the usual apparent-to-inapparent clinical case ratio?

(b) What are the important and obvious pathognomonic or strongly clinically suggestive signs and symptoms of the disease?

(c) What bacterial isolations, identification, and serological techniques are easy, practicable, and reliable?

(d) How accessible are the patients or those at risk; can they be recontacted after the initial investigation for follow-up questions, examination, or serology?

(e) In the event that the investigation requires long-term follow-up, can the case definitions be applied easily and consistently by individuals other than the current investigating team?

(f) Is it absolutely necessary that all patients be identified during the initial investigation or would only those seen by physicians or hospitalized suffice?

These considerations and others will likely play an important role in how cases will be defined and how intensive case investigation will be. However, no matter what criteria are used, the case definition must be applied equally and without bias to all persons under investigation.

Methods for finding cases will vary considerably according to the disease in question and the community setting. In many field investigations the techniques for identifying cases will be relatively self-evident. Most outbreaks involve certain clearly identifiable groups at risk, and it is simply a matter of intensifying reporting from physicians, hospitals, laboratories, or school and industrial contacts, or perhaps using some form of public announcement to identify most of the remaining, unreported cases. However, there may be times when more intensive efforts – such as physician, telephone, door-to-door, culture, or serological surveys – may be necessary to find cases. Regardless of the method, some system(s) of case identification should be established for the duration of the investigation and perhaps for some time afterwards.

In the vast majority of instances, simply determining the number of cases does not provide adequate information. Since control and preventive measures depend upon knowing the source and mode of spread of an agent as well as the characteristics of ill patients, the process of case finding should include the acquisition of pertinent information likely to provide clues or leads to the natural history of the epidemic and, particularly, relevant characteristics of those affected. First, basic information regarding each patient's age, sex, residence, occupation, date of onset, etc., should always be secured to define the simple and basic descriptive aspects of the epidemic. However, if the disease under investigation is usually water- or food-borne, questions should be asked about exposure to various water and food sources. Or if the disease is most frequently transmitted by person-to-person contact, questions should be devised that will help the investigators determine the frequency, duration, and nature of personal contacts and thus perhaps explain why certain persons became ill. If the nature of the disease is not known or cannot be comfortably presumed, a variety of questions covering all possible aspects of bacterial disease transmission and risk must be asked.

### Orient the data in terms of time, place, and person

Having determined reasonably accurately the number of cases of disease there are and an attack rate, the field epidemiologist should now record the descriptive aspects of the investigation, namely, characterize the epidemic in terms of when patients became ill, where patients resided or became ill, and what characteristics the patients possess. There may be a tendency to wait until the epidemic is over or until all likely cases have been reported before performing such an analysis. This tendency should be strongly avoided for a variety of reasons but mainly because further inclusion of a proportionately small number of cases will usually not affect the analysis or recommendations.

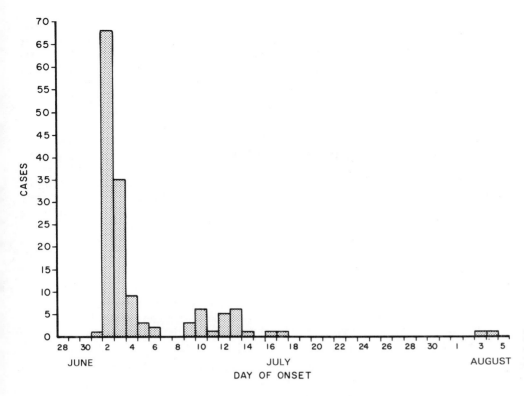

**Fig. 17.1.** Cases of pontiac fever, by day of onset, Oakland County (Michigan) Health Department, 28 June–5 August 1968.

*Time*

In most instances it will be very valuable to describe the cases in terms of onset by constructing a graph that depicts the occurrence of cases over an appropriate time interval (Fig. 17.1). This 'epidemic curve', as it is frequently called, may provide a considerably deeper appreciation for the magnitude of the outbreak, its possible mode of spread, and the possible duration of the epidemic than would a simple listing of cases. A remarkable amount of information can be inferred from such a pictorial representation of times of onset of disease. If the incubation period of the disease is known, relatively firm inferences can be made regarding the likelihood of a point-source exposure, person-to-person spread, or a mixture of the two. Also, if the epidemic is in progress, the epidemiologist may be able to predict, using the epidemic curve, how many more cases are likely to occur. Finally, a pictorial representation of cases over time serves as an excellent means of ready communication to non-epidemiologists, administrators, and the like who need to grasp in some fashion the nature and magnitude of the epidemic. The epidemic curve in Fig. 17.1 portrays cases of Pontiac fever (subsequently confirmed Legionnaires' disease) that occurred in Pontiac, Michigan, July and August 1968, by day of onset (Glick *et al.* 1978). As can be seen, the epidemic was explosive in onset suggesting (i) a virtually simultaneous common-source exposure of many persons; (ii) a disease with a short incubation period; and (iii) a continuing exposure spanning several weeks.

*Place*

Not infrequently, cases of disease develop in unique locations in the community, which, if properly depicted and analysed, may provide major clues or evidence regarding the source of the agent and/or the nature of exposure. Water supplies, milk distribution routes, sewage disposal outflows, prevailing wind currents, air-flow patterns in buildings, and ecological habitats of animals may play important roles in disseminating bacterial pathogens and determining who is at risk of acquiring disease. If cases are plotted geographically, a pattern of distribution may emerge that approximates these known sources and routes of potential exposure that may help identify the vehicle or mode of transmission.

Figure 17.2 illustrates the usefulness of a 'spot map' early in the investigation of an outbreak of shigellosis in Dubuque, Iowa, in 1974 (Rosenberg *et al.* 1972). Initially the investigation revealed that cases were not clustered by area of residence or age or sex. A history of drinking water gave no useful clue as to a possible source and mode of transmission. However, it was later learned that many cases had been exposed to water by recent swimming in a camping park located on the Mississippi River. As can be seen on Fig. 17.2, the river sites where 22 culture positive cases swam within three days of onset of illness strongly suggested a common source of exposure. Ultimately the epidemiologists incriminated the Mississippi River water by documenting gross contamination by the city's sewage treatment plant five miles upstream and by isolating *Shigella sonnei* from a sample of river water taken from the camping park beach area.

*Person*

Lastly, the epidemiologist should examine the character of the patients themselves in terms of a variety of attributes, such as age, sex, race, occupation, or virtually any other

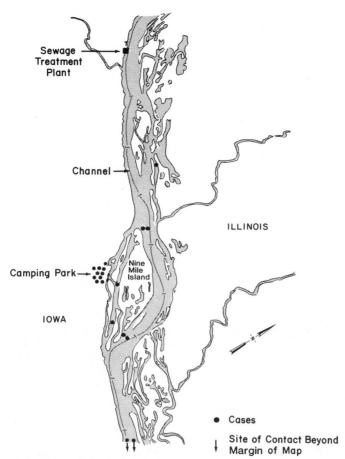

**Fig. 17.2.** Mississippi River sites where 22 culture-positive cases swam within three days of onset of illness.

characteristic that may be useful in portraying the uniqueness of the case population. Some diseases primarily affect certain age groups or races; frequently, occupation is a key characteristic of people with certain bacterial diseases. Unfortunately, the list of human characteristics is nearly endless. However, the more epidemiologists know about the bacterial disease in question – that is, the reservoir, mode(s) of spread, persons usually at greatest risk – the more specific and pertinent information they can seek from the cases to determine whether any of these characteristics predisposes to illness.

### Determine who is at risk of becoming ill

It is at this juncture in the investigation that epidemiologists may begin to apply analytical techniques. They now know the number of people ill, when and where they were when they became ill, what their general characteristics are, and usually they have a firm diagnosis or a good 'working' diagnosis. These data frequently provide the investigators with enough information to feel relatively sure how and why the epidemic started. For example, often this information will strongly suggest that only people in a particular community supplied by a specific water system were at risk of getting sick, or that only certain students in a school or workers in a single factory

became ill. Perhaps it was only a group of people who attended a local restaurant who reported illness. In other words, the simple descriptive aspects of the epidemic frequently identify those most likely to be at risk of disease. However, no matter how obvious it might appear that only a single group of persons were at risk, the epidemiologist should apply analytical methods to support this conclusion.

For example, if fever, abdominal cramps, and diarrhoea occur among 35 residents of a housing subdivision 'A' (presumably caused by water contaminated with *Shigella*) and no similar illness was reported from subdivision 'B' over the same time period, the initial conclusion would logically be that only subdivision 'A' residents were at risk of developing disease. However, only after a proper survey is applied to the residents of subdivision 'B' or even elsewhere in the community, looking for the same illness and comparing illness rates for such groups, can one legitimately infer that the at-risk population were all residents of subdivision 'A'.

### Develop a hypothesis that explains the specific exposure that caused the disease and test this hypothesis by appropriate statistical methods

The next analytical step is often the most difficult one to perform. By now epidemiologists should have an excellent grasp of the epidemic and an overall feel for the most likely source and mode of transmission. However, they must still determine the most likely exposure that caused disease. A classic example of what is meant here would be an investigation of an outbreak of nausea, vomiting, and diarrhoea among people who had attended a church supper presumedly caused by staphylococcal contamination of food(s) eaten at the supper. Since the disease was most likely acquired by eating or drinking something (because of the signs and symptoms) and because no other cluster of similar disease had occurred elsewhere in the community, the investigator focused attention only on those who attended the supper. He hypothesized that the exposure necessary to develop the observed symptoms was consumption of some food(s) contaminated with staphylococcal enterotoxin. Therefore, he asked the ill people what they had eaten or drunk at the church supper (that is, what they had been exposed to) and compared their food histories with those people who had not become ill but had also attended the church supper. Comparisons of food histories (eating rates) between the ill and the well participants were made and statistically analysed. The food histories were found to be very different (and unlikley to be different simply by chance alone). Thus, the inference was drawn that a particular food or drink was the exposure that caused the illness.

Several other examples of epidemiological investigations of bacterial diseases may serve to emphasize the importance of developing hypotheses and testing them.

In August 1980, a community hospital in the State of Michigan recognized seven cases of group A streptococcal post-operative wound infections which had occurred over the previous four months (Berkelman *et al.* 1982). This represented more cases then usual, and an investigation was started. Using a standard case definition the epidemiologists ultimately identified 10 cases that had occurred over this time period, all of whom were patients on several surgical wards. This geographical clustering plus the fact that the infections developed within one and two days following surgery suggested a common source of exposure, presumably in the operating rooms. Although streptococcal disease can rarely be transmitted by inanimate objects, within the hospital setting, the most frequent source of streptococci is man and the most common mode of spread is person-to-person. Therefore, the epidemiologists hypothesized that the probable risk factor unique to these patients was contact with or exposure to an infected or colonized member of the hospital's professional staff sometime during surgery. After selecting appropriate non-streptococcal-infected post-surgical patients as controls, the investigators compared both ill and well in regard to what exposure they had had with a total of 38 surgeons, anaesthesiologists, and nursing staff during surgery for the epidemic period. Exposure rates were not statistically different between cases and controls except for one nurse. This nurse was cultured and found to be an anal and vaginal carrier of a strain of beta haemolytic streptococci identical to the epidemic strain. Following appropriate treatment this strain of streptococci could no longer be cultured from her. She returned to work and six months later two more cases of post-operative beta haemolytic streptococcal infection occurred, caused, however, by a different serotype. The nurse was cultured again and found to be a vaginal and anal carrier of this different strain.

The recent investigation of an epidemic of *Listeria monocytogenes* is a classic example of how the epidemiological method, simple inferences, and persistent re-examination of data can point to a hitherto unknown source and mode of spread of disease. Thirty-four cases of perinatal listeriosis and seven cases of adult disease occurred between 1 March and 1 September 1981, in several maritime provinces of Canada (Schlech *et al.* 1983). These cases represented a several-fold increase over the number of cases diagnosed in previous years suggesting some common exposure. Although *L. monocytogenes* is a common cause of abortion and nervous system diseases in cattle, sheep, and goats, the source of human infection has been obscure. The epidemiologists, therefore, undertook an investigation to determine if cases had had contact with one another or whether there had been a common environmental source which would explain their disease. Cases could not be linked together by person-to-person contact, they shared no common water source, and food exposures, as determined from a general food history, were not different between cases and controls. However, a second, more detailed food history and subsequent intensive interrogation of cases and controls revealed that there was a statistically significant difference between cases and controls regarding exposure to cole slaw. Even though this food had never been previously incriminated as a source of *Listeria*, it was the only food item statistically incriminated and essentially the only lead the investigators had at the time. Armed with this association, the epidemiologists subsequently found a specimen of cole slaw in the refrigerator of one of the patients which grew out the same serotype of *Listeria* found in the epidemic cases. No other food items in the refrigerator

were positive for *Listeria*. The cole slaw had been prepared by a regional manufacturer who had obtained cabbages and carrots from several wholesale dealers and many local farmers. Although environmental cultures from the cole slaw plant failed to reveal *Listeria* organisms, two unopened packages of cole slaw from the plant subsequently grew *L. monocytogenes* of the same epidemic serotype. A review of the sources of the vegetable ingredients was made, and a single farmer was identified who had grown cabbages and also maintained a flock of sheep. Two of his sheep had previously died of listeriosis in 1979 and 1981; also, he was in the habit of using sheep manure to fertilize his cabbage.

Although it cannot definitely be proven that this particular farm was the source of the *Listeria* organisms that caused the epidemic, the hypothesis that cole slaw was the source and the statistical test which supported this hypothesis provided the necessary impetus to continue an investigation that ultimately uncovered a single highly suggestive source of the bacterium, and strongly supported listeriosis as a zoonotic infection transmitted from infected animals via contaminated vegetables to man.

Lastly, a similar logic in a much more difficult situation was applied to an outbreak of Legionnaires' disease among conventioneers attending meetings in Philadelphia, Pennsylvania, in July 1976 (Fraser *et al.* 1977). From the very beginning to the end of the field investigation, neither the clinical presentation nor laboratory results provided the epidemiologist with a diagnosis. However, initially it appeared and was epidemiologically established that disease was not transmitted from person to person; yet being a conventioneer who stayed at or visited the Bellevue Stratford Hotel in Philadelphia conferred an increased risk of disease. But this conclusion did not provide enough information about the source or mode of spread of the agent to be particularly useful. To put it another way, just a person's presence in the Bellevue Stratford did not help explain what the specific exposure was or how the disease was acquired. A Legionnaire could easily have eaten a meal, consumed water from the hotel, or simply breathed in the hotel – all possible exposures to the agent that could place a person in the high-risk category of becoming ill. Therefore, a series of hypotheses was proposed to determine whether eating meals, drinking water, or simply being in the hotel conferred increased risk of developing illness among the Legionnaires. When the final analysis was done, there was no significant difference between ill and well Legionnaires in terms of eating or drinking at the hotel. However, spending at least one hour in the hotel lobby conferred a much greater risk of disease than would have been expected by chance alone. Therefore, the investigators inferred that being in the lobby of the hotel was the necessary exposure for acquiring disease. This, coupled with the clinical features of the disease (pneumonia), implied that the agent was airborne and was transmitted through the air-conditioning system. Although the bacterium responsible for Legionnaires' disease was not isolated from the Bellevue Stratford Hotel air-conditioning system at that time, it was later recovered from lung tissue of several diseased Legionnaires. Moreover, subsequent investigations of similar epidemics of Legionnaires' disease elsewhere have not only confirmed the epidemiological pattern of this disease, but *Legionella* bacteria have been isolated from similar air-conditioning systems.

Again, this phase of the investigation clearly poses the greatest challenge to epidemiologists. They must review their findings carefully, weigh the clinical, laboratory, and epidemiological features of the disease, and hypothesize possible exposures that could plausibly cause disease. In other words, they must seek, from the patients' histories, exposures that could conceivably predispose to illness. If exposure histories for ill and well are not significantly different, the epidemiologist must develop new hypotheses. This may require imagination, perseverance, and sometimes resurveying those at risk to obtain more pertinent information.

## Compare the hypothesis with the established facts

Having determined by epidemiological and statistical inference the probable exposure responsible for disease, the epidemiologist must now 'square' the hypothesis with the clinical, laboratory, and other epidemiological facts of the investigation. In other words, do the proposed exposure, mode of spread, and population affected fit well with the known facts of the disease? For example, if in the gastroenteritis outbreak, referred to above, the analysis incriminated an uncooked food left at room temperature for 18–24 hours and previously known to promote growth of staphylococci, the hypothesis fits well with our understanding of staphylococcal food poisoning. However, if the analysis incriminated coffee or water – highly unlikely sources of staphylococcal enterotoxin – the epidemiologists must then reassess the findings, perhaps secure more information, reconsider the clinical diagnosis, and certainly pose and test new hypotheses.

In the rare field investigation, when the disease is unknown, the epidemiologist will clearly find it more difficult to fit the hypothesis to the natural history of the disease in question. All that can be hoped is that the clinical, laboratory, and epidemiological findings portray a coherent, plausible, and physiologically sound series of findings and events that make sense.

## Plan a more systematic study

The actual field investigation and analyses may be completed by now, requiring only a written report (see below). However, because there may be a need to find more patients, to define better the extent of the epidemic, or because a new laboratory method or case-finding technique may need to be evaluated, the epidemiologists may want to perform more detailed and carefully executed studies. With the pressure of the investigation somewhat relieved, the field team may now consider surveying the population at risk in a variety of ways to help improve the quality of data and answer particular questions. Perhaps the most important reasons to perform such studies are to improve the sensitivity and specificity of the case definition and establish more accurately the true number of persons at risk, i.e. to improve the quality of numerators and denominators. For example, serosurveys coupled with a more complete clinical history can often sharpen the accuracy of

the case count and define more clearly those truly at risk of developing disease. Moreover, repeat interviews of patients with confirmed disease may allow for rough quantitation of degrees of exposure or dose responses – useful information in understanding the pathogenesis of certain diseases.

## Preparation of a written report

Frequently, the final responsibility of the investigative team is to prepare a written report to document the series of events associated with the epidemic and its management. It is beyond the scope of this chapter to provide a detailed set of guidelines on scientific report writing. However, in most instances there are several important reasons a report should be written as soon as possible.

### Administrative/operational purposes

#### A document for action

Not infrequently, control and preventive efforts will only be taken by the responsible health authorities when a report of all relevant findings has been written and submitted for consideration. This can and should place a heavy but necessary burden on the epidemiologists to complete their work with dispatch. Even if all possible cases have not yet been found or some laboratory results are still pending, reasonable written assumptions and recommendations can usually be made without fear of retraction or subsequent major change.

#### A record of performance

In this day of input and output measurements, programme planning, programme justifications, and performance evaluations, there is often no better record of accomplishment than a well-written report of a completed field investigation. The number of investigations performed and the time and resources expended not only document the magnitude of health problems, changes in disease trends, and the results of control and prevention efforts, but serve as concrete evidence of programme justification and needs.

#### A document for potential medical/legal issues

Presumably, epidemiologists investigate epidemics with objective, unbiased, and scientific purposes and similarly prepare written reports of their findings and conclusions objectively, honestly, and fairly. Such information may prove absolutely invaluable to consumers, practising physicians, or local and regional health department officials in any legal action regarding health responsibilities and jurisdictions. In the long run, the health of the public is best served by simple, careful, honest documentation of events and findings made generally available for interpretation and comment.

### Scientific/epidemiological purposes

#### Enhancement of the quality of the investigation

Although not fully explained and rarely referred to, the actual process of writing and viewing data in written form often generates new and different thought processes and associations in the mind of the epidemiologist. The discipline of commiting to paper the clinical, laboratory, and epidemiological findings of an epidemic investigation almost always will bring to light not only a better understanding of the natural unfolding of events, but their importance in terms of the natural history and development of the epidemic. The actual process of creating scientific prose, summarizing data, and creating tables and figures representing the known established facts forces the epidemiologist to view the entire series of events in a balanced, rational, and explainable way – considerably more so than an oral report given to the local health department the day of departure from the field. Occasionally, previously unrecognized associations will emerge from a careful and step-by-step written analysis that may be critical in the final interpretation and recommendations. The exercise of writing what was done and what was found will sometimes uncover facts and events that were more or less assumed to be true but not specifically sought for during the investigation. This in turn may stimulate further inquiry and fact finding in order to verify these assumptions.

### An instrument for teaching epidemiology

There would hardly be disagreement among epidemiologists that the exercise of writing the results of an investigation constitutes an essential building block in learning epidemiology. Much the way a lawyer prepares a brief, the epidemiologist should know how to organize and present in logical sequence the important and pertinent findings of an investigation, their quality and validity, and the scientific inferences that can be made by their written presentation. The simple, direct, and orderly array of facts and inferences will not only reflect on the quality of the investigation itself but on the writer's basic understanding and knowledge of the epidemiological method.

### Execute control and preventive measures

It is not the purpose of this chapter to elaborate on this aspect of the investigation. Nevertheless, the underlying purposes of all epidemic investigations are to control and/or prevent further disease.

## CONCLUSION

In summary then, the process of performing a thorough and successful epidemic field investigation has two major components. The first is the operational aspect that includes knowing why the investigation should be performed, who are the principal health officers involved, and who will assume the primary responsibility for data collection, interpretation, and implementation of control and preventive measures. The epidemiologist must also identify other health professionals who will provide the necessary laboratory and field support early in the planning stage.

Secondly, the field investigation is a direct application of the epidemiological method very often with an implied relatively circumscribed timetable. This forces the investigation team (i) to establish workable case-finding techniques; (ii) to collect data rapidly but carefully, and (iii) to describe these cases in a general sense regarding the time and place of occurrence and those primarily affected. Usually, the bacterial agent is known

and its sources and modes of transmission are well established, allowing the epidemiologist to identify the source and mode of spread rapidly. However, when the clinical disease is obscure and/or the origin of the bacteria ill-defined, the epidemiologist may be hard-pressed to create a hypothesis that will not only identify the critical exposure and show statistical significance, but will logically explain the occurrence of the epidemic. Although scientific proof of causation in the strictest sense will not be established by such retrospective investigations, in most instances the careful development of epidemiological inferences coupled with persuasive clinical and laboratory evidence will almost always provide convincing evidence of the source and mode of spread of disease.

## APPENDIX I. IMPORTANT BACTERIAL DISEASES

The following pages describe 11 bacterial diseases or conditions that could be considered the most important to the industrialized world in regard to frequency of occurrence, duration of morbidity, and general impact upon the health economy. No attempt has been made to quantitate their importance in any formal way; however, they represent the author's best assessment following discussions with experts in the field of bacterial diseases.* Although there may be differences of opinion regarding the importance of some of the bacterial diseases discussed herein, an attempt was made to direct the attention of the reader to bacterial pathogens that appear to be emerging as important problems for the next several decades. In particular, *Campylobacter* infections have, within the recent past, become recognized as important agents of gastrointestinal disease in the industrialized world. Likewise, the sexually transmitted chlamydial infections of the genitourinary tract are of increasing importance occurring substantially more frequently than even gonorrhoea in the US and parts of Europe.

The diseases are listed in alphabetical order and not by any implied order of importance. The description of these conditions is short and in outline form because it is not the purpose of this chapter nor the text to which it belongs to describe such diseases in any clinical, laboratory, or epidemiological detail. There are a variety of excellent texts that can provide the reader with extensive, detailed descriptions of these diseases, and for those who want more information, they are listed at the end of this chapter.

It should also be added that one category of diseases discussed in the following pages concerns nosocomial bacterial infections. This is clearly the only group of diseases not caused by a single or closely related group of bacterial agents. The purpose for including nosocomial bacterial infections is that they represent an important continuing and probably slowly expanding disease problem, particularly for hospitals in the developed world that care for the elderly, the chronically ill, and those with altered or diminished immune mechanisms.

*Exact incidence of some of these diseases is not really known for the US. However, the Centers for Disease Control in Atlanta, Georgia, USA, has attempted to make estimates of certain bacterial disease occurrence using a variety of sources and techniques for its own programme and planning purposes. Some of these estimates have been used in the discussions that follow.

As long as these kinds of patients constitute an ever increasing portion of medical responsibility within the hospital setting, and as long as medical science continues to prolong life, we can expect to see increasing problems associated with nosocomial infections.

## Bacterial nosocomial infections

### Clinical picture

A variety of clinical presentations occur as a result of bacterial nosocomial infections, but the great majority relate to urinary tract infection (UTI), surgical wounds, and lower respiratory tract infections. Primary bacteraemia, although considerably less common, is a very serious manifestation of nosocomial infections as well. Urinary tract infections, that comprise approximately 42 per cent of known bacterial infections, are generally mild, often asymptomatic, and resolve spontaneously. However, some develop ascending infection, resulting in pyelonephritis or secondary bacteraemia. Surgical wound infections, comprising 24 per cent of bacterial nosocomial infections, vary according to surgical procedure and location of surgery. However, presentation is relatively characteristic with low-grade fever, redness, swelling, and pain at the surgical operative sight. Lower respiratory infections, usually characterized by pneumonia, lung abscesses, empyema, or bronchitis, equal about 10 per cent of bacterial nosocomial infections. Clinical presentation will vary considerably and is often obscure or difficult to diagnose because of underlying medical and/or surgical conditions. Primary bacteraemia (5 per cent of all bacterial infections) is a very serious complication within the hospital and often appears as spiking fever, shaking chills, and even profond hypotension.

### Agent

Among the Gram-negative bacteria *Escherichia coli, Pseudomonas aeruginosa,* and species of *Enterobacter, Proteus,* and *Providencia,* are the most frequently isolated organisms. Of the Gram-positive bacteria, *Staphylococcus aureus* and *Enterococcal* group B streptococci are most frequently reported.

### Epidemiology

Bacterial nosocomial infections occur world-wide. However, they have become recognized as a major cause of morbidity and mortality, particularly in the developed world. In the US, in 1975–76, it was estimated that nosocomial bacterial infection rates were approximately 5.7 per 100 hospital discharges or about 2.1 million infections annually in acute care hospitals. Estimates now, including all hospitals, equal at least two times these figures.

In the majority of instances, the reservoir of bacteria is the patient. Although hospital personnel may transmit bacteria and, indeed, certain medical or surgical equipment may be a source of infection at times, pathogenic bacteria of the genito-urinary tract, of the skin, and of the respiratory tract most frequently come from the patient. For UTIs the indwelling catheter most frequently introduces infection. For skin infections, staphylococci from the skin of the patient enter the incision site. For most lower respiratory tract infection

aspiration of respiratory secretions provides the most frequent mode of introduction of pathogens. Incubation periods of disease will vary tremendously according to the susceptibility and natural resistance of the patient, the mode of introduction of the organism, and the virulence and pathogenicity of the particular bacteria. However, because most infections tend to result from invasive procedures (indwelling catheters, surgery, mechanical methods for removing respiratory secretions) incubation periods tend to be short, usually hours to several days in length.

In general, nosocomial bacterial infections become communicable in an epidemic sense only when hospital staff inadvertently carry them from patient to patient or when equipment or instruments within the hospital are inadequately sterilized and transmit the organisms.

### Methods of control and prevention

Primary preventive and control programmes are based on intensive, active surveillance of bacterial infection in the hospital. Surveillance includes an active search for infections by regular examination of patients, by regular careful, review of hospital charts, and by a similar review of bacterial laboratory results. These duties are best performed by a specially designated full-time hospital epidemiologist who reviews these data daily, looking for clustering of disease, by time, place, or by organism, and frequently by antimicrobial susceptibility patterns of bacteria.

Careful attention should always be paid to proper sterilization and handling of hospital equipment, proper food handling, and careful housekeeping and laundry services.

## *Campylobacter* enteritis

### Clinical picture

*Campylobacter* enteritis is usually characterized by the abrupt onset of diarrhoea with fever, frank blood in the stools, and abdominal pain. Vomiting occurs somewhat less frequently. Most patients recover in less than a week, but up to 20 per cent of cases may relapse or have prolonged illness. Milder disease cannot be readily distinguished from other enteric bacterial infections.

### Agent

*Campylobacter jejuni* is a Gram-negative rod.

### Epidemiology

The organism is distributed world-wide and affects all age groups. Because stool cultures are not performed frequently and because physicians do not report, the incidence of disease is not really known. Some recent estimates, however, judge the occurrence of *Campylobacter* infection in the US to be equal to that of *Salmonella.* Common-source outbreaks have been reported usually associated with contaminated foods or unpasteurized milk. It is also an important cause of 'travellers diarrhoea'. Sporadic cases occur and are probably caused by faecal-oral transmission from contact with infected pets or domesticated animals. The incubation period is 2–10 days, and the period of communicability lasts for the duration of excretion of the organism. Chronic carriers are rare.

### Methods of prevention and control

Thorough cooking and preparation of foods derived from animal sources, particularly poultry. Pasteurization of milk.

## Chlamydial infections

### Clinical picture

The bacterial genus *Chlamydia* is comprised of two species, *Chlamydia psittaci* and *C. trachomatis*. The former is responsible for the pulmonary disease, psittacosis, and the latter for several rather specific clinical manifestations, including trachoma, inclusion conjunctivitis, lymphogranuloma venereum, infant pneumonia (sometimes called chlamydial pneumonia of infancy), and genito-urinary tract infections. The latter comprise the most important manifestation of chlamydial infections in the developed world in terms of incidence, prevalence, and morbidity. Genito-urinary tract infections with *C. trachomatis* in males may produce several different clinical presentations, including urethritis, epididymitis, prostatitis, and proctitis. *Chlamydia* urethritis in males, commonly called non-gonococcal urethritis (NGU), presents as urethral irritation, genital itching, or frank dysuria. Symptoms are less severe than gonococcal urethritis and are often accompanied by scanty or mucoid urethral discharge. If untreated, symptoms may persist for months or years. *C. trachomatis* infections in women resemble those of gonococcal infections with salpingitis, cervicitis, and sometimes urethritis. As with gonorrhoea, women may be completely asymptomatic, yet harbour the organism for months. Infertility is the most serious consequence of disease in both males and females.

### Agent

*Chlamydia trachomatis* is a small Gram-negative, spherical bacterium.

### Epidemiology

Although the organism is world-wide in distribution, the sexually transmitted disease has only recently become recognized as a very rapidly emerging problem in western Europe and the US. In both the US and Britain, chlamydial genito-urinary infections are estimated to be more than two times as frequent as gonorrhoea. *C. trachomatis* infection is transmitted by sexual contact when infected secretions come into contact with mucous membranes of the genito-urinary tract. The incubation period and duration of communicability have not been well established. Most patients, however, develop symptoms 1–3 weeks after sexual contact with an infected partner. Because the infection may last for several months or even appear following what appears to be a latent period, communicability may last for extended periods of time if the disease is untreated.

### Methods of prevention and control

Similar to those of syphilis and gonorrhoea.

## Gonorrhoea

### Clinical picture

Gonococcal infections may manifest themselves in a variety of clinical syndromes, including urethritis, epididymitis, cervicitis, salpingitis, conjunctivitis of the newborn, and more rarely bacteraemia with arthritis and endocarditis. The more frequent and important clinical manifestations of gonorrhoea infection are acute urethritis in the male with urethral discharge and pain upon urination, and pelvic inflammatory disease (PID) in women, with fever, abdominal pain, vaginal discharge, salpingitis, and endometritis. Gonococcal conjunctivitis of the newborn appears as an acute redness and swelling of the conjuctiva with a purulent discharge occurring usually within the first three weeks of life.

### Agent

*Neisseria gonorrhoeae* is a Gram-negative diplococcus.

### Epidemiology

The reservoir for *N. gonorrhoeae* is exclusively man. Almost one million cases were reported in the US in 1982, representing an estimated half of the true incidence. The disease is primarily transmitted by contact with exudates from mucous membranes of infected individuals almost always as a result of sexual contact. Gonococcal conjunctivitis of the newborn is transmitted by contact of the baby with the infected birth canal of a carrier of the organism. The incubation period is usually 2–7 days for sexually acquired gonorrhoea, approximately 1–5 days for gonorrhoeal conjunctivitis. Communicability of gonorrhoea varies but may last for months, particularly in asymptomatic females who can become chronic carriers. Susceptibility to the organism is general, and no immunity is developed following infection.

### Methods of control and prevention

Identical to those that apply to syphilis. However, prevention of gonococcal conjunctivitis in the newborn can be accomplished by immediate installation of appropriate doses of silver nitrate, tetracycline, or erythromycin into the eyes.

## Hemophilus influenza infection

### Clinical picture

*Hemophilus influenzae* causes two important clinical diseases, particularly in infants and children: meningitis and otitis media. Meningitis caused by this organism is usually sudden in onset with fever, vomiting, meningeal irritation, stiff neck, and frequently lethargy and coma. Otitis media, often a precursor of hemophilus meningitis is characterized by irritability, ear pain, and fever, usually following an upper respiratory infection.

### Agent

*Hemophilus influenzae* is a small pleomorphic Gram-negative coccobacillus. There are six antigenically distinct capsular types and other non-typable strains.

## Epidemiology

*Hemophilus influenzae* infection is world-wide in distribution and occurs most frequently in the age group of two months to three years. It accounts for approximately 25 per cent of cases of acute suppurative otitis media, a major cause of deafness. The reservoir is man; the source of the organism is the upper respiratory tract. Asymptomatic colonization is frequent, and person-to-person transmission occurs by droplet nuclei and discharges from the nose and throat during the infectious period. The incubation period is usually 2–4 days, and persons presumably remain communicable for as long as the organism remains in the upper respiratory tract. Immunity, as reflected by circulating antibody, follows infection with the specific capsular type.

## Method of prevention and control

There are no vaccines presently available for general use. Prevention measures centre primarily around the practice of good general, personal hygiene and education of parents regarding the risk of secondary cases in children less than six years of age.

## Pneumococcal infections

### Clinical picture

The most frequent clinical manifestations of pneumococcal disease are lobar pneumonia and otitis media. Pneumococcal pneumonia is an acute infection most severe in infants and the elderly characterized by the sudden onset of chills, fever, chest pain, difficulty breathing, and a productive cough. Acute otitis media commonly follows as a complication of viral upper respiratory disease and is characterized by fever, irritability, and pain in the ear.

### Agent

*Streptococcus pneumoniae* is a Gram-positive coccus which has more than 80 identifiable serotypes.

### Epidemiology

The pneumococci are ubiquitous organisms frequently present in the upper respiratory tract of normal carriers. The disease occurs world-wide, is usually sporadic in nature, but occasionally may occur in epidemics in closed populations such as schools or mental hospitals. The estimated range of cases occurring in the US is from 150 000 to 570 000 per year. The pneumococcus is responsible for approximately 40 per cent of cases of suppurative otitis media in the US. Pneumococcal diseases are more prevalent during the late winter and spring in temperate climate zones. Man is the only known reservoir, and the organisms are transmitted from person to person by direct contact or by droplet spread of respiratory secretions. The incubation period has been estimated to be between one and three days, but the period of communicability is unknown. Transmission probably can occur as long as the bacteria are present in the respiratory discharges. For most persons resistance is generally high, but factors regarding susceptibility are poorly understood. Immunity following infection with a specific capsular serotype, however, may last for years.

### Methods of control and prevention

In general, avoidance of crowded conditions, particularly in living quarters, may provide some method for prevention. However, a 14-valent pneumococcal vaccine is presently available in the US. Although currently available data show elevations in antibody titers 3–5 years after immunization, protection is variable and the duration of protection induced by this vaccine is still unknown.

## Salmonellosis

### Clinical picture

*Salmonella* infections may present as one or more of several different clinical manifestations including: gastroenteritis, enteric fever (including typhoid fever), bacteraemia, and certain focal infections of the meninges, the bones, and other organs. The most common form of salmonellosis is acute gastroenteritis with sudden onset of abdominal pain, diarrhoea, nausea, and sometimes vomiting, usually with fever often requiring hospitalization. The enteric fevers and bacteraemia are the most serious infections.

### Agent

*Salmonella* are Gram-negative rods of which there are more than 2200 serotypes. The most important human pathogens are *Salmonella typhimurium* and *S. enteritidis*. *Salmonella typhi*, though common in the developing world, is not an important *Salmonella* serotype in the industrialized countries. The prevalence of various serotypes vary from country to country.

### Epidemiology

*Salmonella* infections occur world-wide, and gastroenteritis occurs most frequently, particularly as small outbreaks. Larger outbreaks, however, occur in hospitals, institutions, and schools, and are usually related to contaminated food sources. Over two million cases of salmonellosis are estimated to occur in the US each year.

The principal reservoirs of non-typhoidal *Salmonellae* are animals, including poultry, livestock, and pets. *Salmonella typhi* is found only in man. Ill patients and convalescent carriers may also serve as reservoirs of the agent. Most infection is acquired by ingestion of food that has been contaminated by the faeces of an infected person or animal. Eating contaminated raw eggs and egg products as well as meat and poultry may result in disease. Transmission from person to person occurs by the faecal-oral route during acute diarrhoeal illness. The incubation period for salmonella gastroenteritis is 6–72 hours; however, for the enteric fevers the incubation period is usually 7–14 days. For gastroenteritis patients communicability extends throughout the course of infection, but infectiousness may vary considerably from days to weeks thereafter. For *S. typhosa* patients, a chronic carrier state may develop which can last literally for years.

## Methods of control and prevention

Careful preparation, thorough cooking, and adequate storage of foods that may be contaminated with the *Salmonella* organisms are important preventive measures. Education about handwashing, personal hygiene, and sanitary sewage disposal are also very important in prevention and control. For *S. typhosa* there is a vaccine which enhances resistance to infection, but the quality and duration of protection is limited. Only those persons with high risk of exposure, such as household contacts of typhoid carriers, travellers to highly endemic areas, and laboratory workers with frequent contact with this organism, should be considered for vaccination.

## Staphylococcal infections

### Clinical picture

The staphylococci can produce a wide variety of syndromes that range from the simplest of superficial skin infections to staphylococcal septicaemia and pneumonia. Staphylococcal enteritis and the most recently discovered clinical disease associated with this agent, toxic shock syndrome, represent totally different clinical manifestations of disease. The skin lesions, characterized as a single postule or impetigo, are usually self-limiting infections. However, they may progress into carbuncles, furuncles, or even cellulitis where systemic signs of fever and general malaise may be prominent. As referred to in the section on nosocomial infections, staphylococcal wound infections are an important cause of morbidity within the hospital setting. Staphylococcal pneumonia has been frequently recognized as a secondary pulmonary invader closely following influenza infection. The most common agent causing foodborne epidemics is the staphylococcus which, after incubating in certain foods, produces an enterotoxin that produces the characteristic explosive nausea, vomiting, and diarrhoea. The source of the organism is usually a food handler who is a carrier and who contaminates the food during handling and storage procedures.

Toxic shock syndrome, a relatively new disease, is believed to be caused by one or more toxins elaborated by certain strains of staphylococcus. The syndrome is characterized by the sudden onset of high fever, vomiting, diarrhoea, and muscle aches. This is often followed by a profound drop in blood pressure and is accompanied by an erythematous 'sunburn-like' rash often with desquamation, particularly of the palms and the soles.

### Agent

*Staphylococcus aureus* is a Gram-positive coccus.

### Epidemiology

The staphylococcus is a ubiquitous bacteria normally present on the skin and in the gastrointestinal tract, particularly prevalent where the use of soap and water is sub-optimal and people live in crowded accommodation. Infections occur sporadically but occasionally in small epidemics and, of most serious nature, as epidemics in paediatric wards.

Epidemics of foodborne staphylococcal gastroenteritis occur world-wide and are usually very focal in their occurrence.

Toxic shock syndrome, originally a very rare disease, associated primarily with children, became epidemic in scope in the US in 1980–81, appearing most frequently in menstruating women who were using tampons as a form of feminine hygiene.

Man is the only known reservoir of staphylococci, and the organisms are transmitted primarily from person to person by direct contact. Incubation periods are variable but range between 4–10 days. Persons remain communicable as long as their lesions continue to contain the bacteria. The carrier state is common, particularly carriage in the anterior nares or in the anogenital region without clinical signs or symptoms. Carriers can be important epidemiologically as common sources of infection, especially in hospitals. Susceptibility is universal, and no immunity is conferred following specific strain infection.

### Methods of prevention and control

Personal hygiene and frequent handwashing are the most effective ways of prevention of spread of staphylococcal disease. Proper preparation and storage of food is essential in prevention of staphylococcal foodborne outbreaks. Within the hospital setting, careful handwashing, cohorting of ill patients, and isolation may be necessary when highly resistant staphylococci cause nosocomial outbreaks.

## Streptococcal infections

### Clinical picture

Group A streptococci cause a variety of acute clinical diseases, the most important of which are acute tonsillitis/pharyngitis and certain skin infections such as impetigo and pyoderma. Other clinical infections include scarlet fever, which is simply a form of streptococcal infection with a characteristic skin rash; and erysipelas, an acute cellulitis with fever, localized redness, tenderness, and swelling of the skin where infection is located.

The most important aspect of streptococcal upper respiratory tract infection relates to the non-suppurative sequelae, namely, rheumatic fever and acute glomerulonephritis, both of which occur uncommonly after acute infection but which may cause permanent damage to the heart, the heart valves, and the kidneys.

Group B streptococci also produce human disease. In newborn children group B organisms are an important cause of septicaemia, pulmonary infection, and meningitis. During the perinatal period group B streptococci are also an important cause of endometritis, amnionitis, and urinary tract infection in women.

### Agent

Group A beta haemolytic streptococcus, *Streptococcus pyogenes*, comprises more than 70 serologically distinct types. Most of these strains can produce upper respiratory tract infection and subsequent rheumatic fever. However, only approximately a dozen serotypes have been associated with acute glomerulonephritis.

Group B streptococci comprise five serotypes, all of which can produce infections in newborns and adults.

## Epidemiology

Group A beta haemolytic pharyngitis is world-wide in occurrence and appears sporadically, particularly in the late winter and early spring in temperate climates. Explosive outbreaks may occur usually associated with food (especially milk and milk products) contaminated with the bacteria. Man is the primary reservoir of beta haemolytic streptococci although the agent may be isolated occasionally from domestic animals. The disease is transmitted by infected individuals by close, intimate contact. Rarely streptococci are transmitted via the airborne route from carriers to susceptibles. Pyoderma and impetigo are transmitted by close physical contact.

The incubation period of streptococcal tonsillitis/pharyngitis is between 2 and 5 days, and the period of communicability may last for weeks to months in chronic carriers of the disease. However, communicability of the organism is greatest during acute infection. Asymptomatic carriage of streptococci occurs in schoolchildren and may range as high as 20 per cent or more. Susceptibility to the streptococci is virtually universal although immunity develops after specific group A streptococcal infections that may last for many years.

Group B streptococcal infection is world-wide, and the organism resides commonly in the gastrointestinal tract and the female genital tract. Newborns acquire infection during passage through the birth canal, and those that become ill within the next several months probably acquire infection from the environment. The period of comminicability is not known but is presumed to last throughout colonization. The incubation period of early neonatal disease is less than three days. The incubation period of perinatal disease in the first few months of life is not known.

## Methods of control and prevention

For group A beta haemolytic streptococci, proper preparation and storage of food, particularly milk and eggs, is necessary to prevent foodborne outbreaks. Food handlers with skin lesions or respiratory illness should be excluded from work. For persons with recurrent streptococcal infection, long-term monthly injections of long-acting penicillin has proved very successful.

There are no routinely accepted measures for prevention of group B streptococcal infections.

## Syphilis

### Clinical picture

The venereal form of syphilis is characterized by acute, subacute, and chronic clinical manifestations. Clinical presentation may vary widely according to the predominant site of infection and the stage of disease. Characteristically, however, non-congenital syphilis is acquired by sexual contact and within about three weeks, a primary skin lesion appears as a papule, usually turning into a superficial chancre located most commonly on the genitalia. After 4–6 weeks, the initial lesion will disappear and often a secondary generalized skin rash will appear, sometimes with mild systemic symptoms. These skin lesions may disappear spontaneously within weeks or last for months when a latency period of infection takes place.

Latency may last for years before signs and symptoms of central nervous system disease or cardiovascular disease occur. The organism may also invade the bone, liver, and a variety of other organs late in the disease as well.

Syphilis is also acquired congenitally from an infected mother, secondary to placental infection. Congenital syphilis may result in liver disease, pneumonia, as acute manifestations of disease, or disease may appear much later with bone, cartilage, and central nervous system involvement.

### Agent

*Treponema pallidum*, a spirochete, is the bacteria responsible for venereal syphilis.

### Epidemiology

Syphilis is a disease of world-wide occurrence with a higher frequency in urban and highly populated areas. Although aproximately 33 000 cases were reported in the US in 1982, this represents approximately 50 per cent of the true incidence of disease and reflects a further increase in cases over the last five years. The reservoir is exclusively man, and disease is transmitted by direct contact with infectious exudates of lesions of primary or secondary stages of the disease. This contact takes place most frequently during sexual contact, rarely by kissing or other kinds of close exposures. Congenital syphilis is acquired by placental transfer of the bacteria. The incubation period varies anywhere from 10 to 90 days after exposure but is usually three weeks. Communicability may also vary considerably but is greatest during primary and secondary stages where there are open, highly infected lesions. Communicability, however, may last intermittently for 2–4 years. All ages are susceptible; however, disease occurs most frequently in the sexually active years. No immunity develops following infection.

### Methods of control and prevention

Primary methods for prevention and control centre about health and sex education, provision of facilities for early diagnosis and treatment, and rapid identification of contacts of known patients.

## Tuberculosis

### Clinical picture

Infection may manifest itself in a variety of ways, but usually it is a disease primarily of the lungs which very often goes unnoticed and heals spontaneously. However, when pulmonary disease does appear clinically, it usually starts by the gradual onset of low-grade fever, fatigue, weight loss, and a persistent cough, often with haemoptysis. Other forms of tuberculosis infection may affect organs outside of the lung, such as tuberculous meningitis, tuberculous infection of the lymph nodes, knees, bones, joints, larynx, and skin.

### Agent

The two most important species of mycobacteria causing human disease are *Mycobacterium tuberculosis* and *M. bovis*. Both species are rod-shaped bacilli that can often be identified in the sputum of infected individuals using special stains (the so-called 'acid fast' quality of these bacteria).

## Epidemiology

Tuberculosis is world-wide in distribution, but has been rapidly declining in the western world. The reservoir of infection is primarily man; *M. bovis* infection is considerably less important now as a clinical entity, but infected cattle still may serve as a source of infection for man. Tuberculosis is acquired by inhalation of the bacilli which are suspended as droplet nuclei in respiratory secretions of infected persons. Bovine tuberculosis usually results from ingestion of the bacillus present in unpasteurized milk or other dairy products. The incubation period varies considerably but usually ranges from between four and twelve weeks. Individuals will remain communicable as long as they are excreting any infectious bacilli in their respiratory secretions. All ages are susceptible to tuberculosis; however, those at greatest risk of developing disease are children under three years of age, and the most serious period for development of clinical disease is the first 6–12 months after infection. Latent infections may persist for many years. Although the US reported a record low case rate of 11.9 per 100 000 population in 1981, tuberculosis remains an important bacterial disease. Diagnosis, treatment, and follow-up are still costly and time consuming. Refugee populations often with higher incidence rates of disease have also added to health care costs.

## Methods of control and prevention

Patients actively excreting bacilli in the sputum can be rendered non-infectious by rapid, appropriate chemotherapy usually within several weeks. Treatment with isoniazid (INH) prevents progression of latent infection into active clinical disease in many individuals. Bacillus Calmette–Geurin (BCG) vaccine may be an important method of tuberculosis control in certain situations, but the degree of protection has been variable in different studies and locations.

## REFERENCES

Berkelman, R.L., Martin, D., Graham, D.R. *et al.* (1982). Streptococcal wound infections caused by a vaginal carrier. *JAMA* **247**, 2680.

Fraser, D.W., Tsai, T.R., Orenstein, W. *et al.* (1977). Legionnaires' disease. Description of an epidemic of pneumonia. *N. Engl. J. Med.* **297**, 1189.

Glick, T.H., Gregg, M.B., Berman, B. *et al.* (1978). Pontiac fever. An epidemic of unknown etiology in a health department: I. Clinical and epidemiologic aspects. *Am. J. Epidemiol.* **107**, 149.

Rosenberg, M.L., Hazlet, K.K., Schaefer, J. *et al.* (1976). Shigellosis from swimming. *JAMA* **236**, 1849.

Schlech, W.F. III, Lavigne, P.M., Bortobussi, R.A. *et al.* (1983). Epidemic listeriosis – evidence for transmission by food. *N. Engl. J. Med.* **308**, 203.

## FURTHER READING

American Academy of pediatrics (1982). *Report of the Committee on Infectious diseases.* American Academy of Pediatrics, Evanston, Ill.

Benenson, A.S. (ed.) (1981). *Control of communicable diseases in man,* 13th edn. The American Public Health Association, Washington, DC.

Bennett, J.V. and Brachman, P.S. (eds.) (1979). *Hospital infections.* Little, Brown and Company, Boston.

Christie, A.B. (1980). *Infectious diseases: epidemiology and clinical practice,* 3rd edn. Churchill Livingstone, New York.

Evans, A.S. and Feldman, H.A. (eds.) (1982). *Bacterial infections of humans. Epidemiology and control.* Plenum, New York.

Mandell, G.L., Douglas, R.G.,. Jr, and Bennett, J.E. (1979). *Principles and practice of infectious diseases* (2 vols). Wiley, New York.

Sanford, J.P. and Luby, J.P. (eds.) (1981). *The science and practice of clinical medicine,* Vol. 8. Grune and Stratton, New York.

Wehrle, P.F. and Top, F.H. Sr (eds.) (1981). *Communicable and infectious diseases.* Mosby, St. Louis.

# 18 Field investigations of air

Robert E. Waller*

## INTRODUCTION

During earlier centuries the proposition that adverse effects on health could be attributed to air pollutants originating from the combustion of fuels or industrial processes was considered many times. But it was difficult to distinguish such effects from those of microbial agents or of allergens of biological origin. Evelyn (1661) for example, in his classic treatise *Fumifugium*, said that 'New Castle Coale, as an expert physician affirms, causeth consumption, phthisicks and the indisposition of the lungs . . .' In the nineteenth century, the Registrar General (1845) expressed the opinion that smoke was injurious to health and one of the causes of death to which the inhabitants of towns were more exposed than those of the country. At that time he could not, however, detect short-term increases in mortality associated with high concentrations of smoke, as in London fogs. Such increases were observed later in the century and public and official concern was finally aroused by the large numbers of deaths associated with some notable episodes of fog during the present century, including that in the Meuse Valley in 1930 (Firket 1931), in Donora in 1948 (Schrenk *et al.* 1949), and in London in 1948 (Logan 1949) and in 1952 (Ministry of Health 1954).

While these incidents provided the most dramatic examples of adverse effects on health, the more insidious long-term effects on the development of respiratory disease were probably of much greater importance in the field of public health as a whole, but they were very difficult to demonstrate clearly. Thus while there has always been a relatively high death-rate from bronchitis in the highly polluted urban areas of the UK, it is only in the past few decades, during which time carefully designed prevalence surveys have been conducted, that it has become possible to determine the relative importance of air pollution along with that of other factors such as smoking and respiratory infections.

## AIR POLLUTANTS AND THEIR CHARACTERISTICS

The prime concern of the present discussion is with the health of the general public and interest centres, therefore, on pollutants that occur in the air of towns or other communities rather than in specific occupational environments. Such pollutants are derived mainly from the combustion of fuels for domestic heating or cooking purposes, for heating or power generation in industry, or for transport, though in some localities there may be additional pollutants from industrial process emissions. In most situations, therefore, there is a complex mixture of pollutants, which may also interact with one another, and in field (as opposed to laboratory) studies it is seldom possible to ascribe any adverse effects on health to one component in particular.

There are however two distinct types of mixture that occur widely throughout the world. One type is the traditional 'London smog' that is associated with smoke and/or sulphur dioxide from the burning of coal or heavy oil (Meetham *et al.* 1981). This type was responsible for most of the dramatic episodes cited above. The other is the 'Los Angeles smog' or photochemical oxidant type derived largely from the incomplete combustion of petrol in motor vehicles, together with emissions from refineries or associated chemical industry, interacting with other pollutants in the presence of sunlight to produce a lachrymatory haze (OECD 1975). The latter type creates a major nuisance for populations exposed to it, and it can damage horticultural crops, but there has not to date been any evidence of substantial effects on mortality or morbidity of the magnitude seen in association with the traditional pollutants.

Chemically speaking the two types have contrasting properties, the former being 'reducing' as a result of the sulphur dioxide present from the combustion of sulphur impurities in coal or heavy oil, and the latter 'oxidizing', due to the formation of ozone and organic oxidants in the photo-chemical process. While the two forms can co-exist, in a particular region and/or season of the year one type is often dominant, being associated with the characteristics of local sources and with climatic conditions. Thus, the most notable area of the world for photochemical pollution is the Los Angeles basin, where all the factors conducive to its formation are at a maximum. These conditions include a very high motor vehicle density, uninterrupted sunshine through much of the year, and a combination of topographical and meteorological factors that lead to light winds, frequent temperature inversions, and a very poor natural ventilation rate. Similarly, the most notable place in the world for traditional smoke/sulphur dioxide pollution at one time was London, due primarily to emissions from domestic open coal fires. The former London fogs (or 'smogs') were merely accumulations of coal smoke and other pollutants from the exceptionally inefficient combustion in such fires. Temperature inversions

*This contribution has been seen by colleagues in the DHSS: their comments and suggestions are gratefully acknowledged but the views expressed are the author's own and not necessarily those of the Department.

**Table 18.1.** *Some urban air pollutants and their effects on health*

| Traditional ('reducing') pollutants from coal/heavy oil combustion | | |
|---|---|---|
| SMOKE (SUSPENDED PARTICULATES) (Some contributions from diesel traffic also) | Can penetrate to lungs, some retained: possible long-term effects. May irritate bronchi also | LONDON SMOG COMPLEX |
| SO$_2$ | Readily absorbed on inhalation: irritation of bronchi, with possibility of bronchospasm | *Short-term effects:* Sudden increases in deaths, in hospital admissions, and in illness among bronchitic patients. Temporary reductions in lung function (patients and some normals) |
| H$_2$SO$_4$ (Mainly a secondary pollutant, formed from SO$_2$ in air) | Hygroscopic: highly irritant if impacted in upper respiratory tract. Acid absorbed on other fine particles may penetrate further to produce bronchospasm | *Long-term effects:* Increased frequency of respiratory infections (children). Increased prevalence of respiratory symptoms (adults and children). Higher death-rates from bronchitis in polluted areas |
| POLYCYCLIC AROMATIC HYDROCARBONS (Small contributions from traffic also) | Mainly absorbed onto smoke: can penetrate with it to lungs | *Possible carcinogenic effects:* May play some part in the higher incidence of lung cancer in urban areas |

| Photochemical ('oxidizing') pollutants from traffic sources, or other hydrocarbon emissions | | |
|---|---|---|
| HYDROCARBONS (Volatile: petrol etc.) | Non toxic at moderate concentrations | LOS ANGELES SMOG COMPLEX |
| NO | Capable of combining with Hb in blood, but no apparent effect in humans | *Short-term effects:* Primarily eye irritation. Reduced athletic performance. Possibly small changes in deaths, hospital admissions |
| NO$_2$ / O$_3$ — Mainly secondary pollutants formed in photochemical reactions | Neither gas is very soluble: some irritation of bronchi, but can penetrate to lungs to cause oedema (at high concentrations). Urban concentrations too low for such effects, but evidence of reduced resistance to infections in animals | *Longer-term effects:* Increased onsets of respiratory illnesses (children), increased asthma attacks (adults). No clear indication of increased bronchitis |
| Aldehydes, other partial oxidation products, PAN | Eye irritation, odour | |

| Others from traffic | | |
|---|---|---|
| CO (other sources contribute, and smoking an important one) | Combines with Hb in blood, reducing oxygen-carrying capacity | Possible effects on CNS (reversible unless concentrations very high). Some evidence of effects on perception and performance of fine tasks at moderate concentrations. Enhances onset of exercise angina in patients. Urban concentrations too low for specific effects |
| LEAD (some industrial sources contribute to air lead, and human intake often dominated by lead in food or drink) | Taken up in blood, distributed to soft tissues, and some to bone | Possible effects on CNS (longer time scale than in case of CO, and not necessarily reversible). Indications of neuropsychological effects on children within overall environmental exposure range, but role of traffic lead uncertain |

during cold, calm, clear periods in winter played an important part in causing episodes of high pollution. But London is not especially subject to such conditions and now that coal fires have been virtually outlawed under the Clean Air Act, London has proved to be a place particularly free from fog, since the 'heat island' effect (Chandler 1965) reduces the chance of natural wet fogs occurring. Although the use of open fires burning soft coal has been a particularly British habit, coal is still widely used in somewhat analogous ways for domestic heating and cooking in many parts of the world, with a risk of potentially harmful concentrations of smoke and sulphur dioxide arising in large, densely populated cities.

A summary of the principal pollutants from combustion sources together with an indication of possible effects on health is shown in Table 18.1. Methods of measuring concentrations in the air are detailed in other publications (BSI 1969; OECD 1964, 1975; WHO 1976) but, as a general introduction, the nature of the individual pollutants and approaches used in their determination are outlined below.

### Smoke, or suspended particulate matter

Though smoke is one of the most widespread components of urban air pollution, this is the one that leads to the most confusion in studies of effects on health. Smoke is not a chemical entity and in effect it is defined by the method of measurement. Thus, the term smoke is applied to the black suspended material in the air that is dominated by products of incomplete combustion. It is measured by its blackening power, usually by drawing a known volume of air through a white filter paper and measuring the reflectance of the resulting stain. National, or international, standard curves have been developed to convert the reflectance measurements to amounts of 'equivalent standard smoke', so that the final results can be quoted in units of $\mu g/m^3$. However, this is not necessarily equivalent to the actual amount of suspended particulate matter at the time. Thus Bailey and Clayton (1982) have shown that in many urban areas of the UK, standard smoke concentrations are now only about 40 per cent of the actual gravimetric suspended particle concentrations. However, all the material that is assessed in this way is within the respirable size range, since the sampling rate generally used is too low to collect particles much beyond 5 $\mu$m effective aerodynamic diameter, and the carbonaceous smoke aggregates that influence the result to a large extent are confined to an even smaller size range, the mass median diameters being around 1$\mu$m (Waller *et al.* 1963).

The alternative approach is to make direct gravimetric measurements of the suspended particulate matter, and when these are made with a high volume sampler, as in the standard US procedure, results are quoted as $\mu g/m^3$ total suspended particulates (TSP). The high sampling rate introduces a risk of including particles beyond the respirable range, should they be present (notably in dry windy climates, where soil and other non-combustion generated dust can become re-entrained), but cyclones or other elutriators are sometimes used to remove the larger particles.

There are many other developments in the field of gravimetric measurements. For example, dichotomous samplers are used, that collect a fine fraction (up to about 3.5 $\mu$m diameter) corresponding largely with combustion-generated material, being within the respirable size range, and a coarser fraction (to about 15 $\mu$m) that includes mechanically produced dusts likely to be of quite different composition from the other particulates and which would largely be retained in the upper respiratory tract if inhaled at all.

None of the routine methods of measurement characterizes the chemical composition of the material, which may vary widely from time to time and place to place, and since there is little indication as to which components might be responsible for adverse effects observed, much uncertainty remains as to which type of measurement is most appropriate in relation to health studies. The important point for the present purpose is to recognize that observations of smoke concentrations made by optical methods are quite distinct from gravimetric determinations of suspended particulates.

## Sulphur dioxide

This irritant gas is generally associated with smoke or suspended particulates, since it comes from the same sources, the burning of coal or heavy oil (the lighter distillates from oil, such as petrol, contain little sulphur). The routine method of measurement in the UK is coupled with that of smoke. The gas is collected in a bubbler beyond the smoke filter, sulphur dioxide concentration is determined by acidimetric titration, and the measurements related to 'net acid gas'. In many urban areas sulphur dioxide is the dominant influence, but in rural areas concentrations of ammonia may be of similar magnitude,

and corrections need to be made for this gas. More specific methods for sulphur dioxide are also quite widely used, including a pararosaniline colorimetric method (WHO 1976), and a thorin spectrophotometric method (BSI 1983).

## Sulphuric acid and sulphates

In some combustion processes a small proportion of sulphur in fuel is oxidized to sulphur trioxide rather than to sulphur dioxide, which is emitted as a fine sulphuric acid mist. Sulphur dioxide itself is also liable to react with other pollutants in the air to form further sulphuric acid of sulphates. Ammonia plays an important part in these reactions, the end-product being ammonium sulphate, but there are also photochemical processes involving hydrocarbons that promote the oxidation of sulphur dioxide. All the acid and sulphate is present in the particulate phase of the pollution, and is collected on filters as used for the determination of suspended particulates. The total sulphate content of samples can be determined by turbidimetric methods, but the separate assessment of sulphuric acid, which may be of greater relevance to effects on health is a more difficult task, and one that is not done on a routine basis. A procedure for the assessment of 'net particulate acid' (Commins 1963) has however been used regularly in London as an indicator of sulphuric acid in the air. This has shown very sharp increases during episodes of high pollution associated with increased morbidity and mortality.

## Oxides of nitrogen

Emissions of these gases to the air are derived largely from the fixation of atmospheric nitrogen in combustion processes, though in some cases there can be contributions from nitrogenous components of fuels (this is particularly true of vegetable products, such as tobacco). At the source, nitric oxide is generally the dominant oxide present, but there is some nitrogen dioxide, and in the air further nitric oxide is oxidized gradually to nitrogen dioxide, particularly in the photochemical oxidant cycle set up in the presence of volatile hydrocarbons. Only nitrogen dioxide is of possible concern in relation to health. The most satisfactory way of measuring it is with a continuous monitor based on the chemiluminescent principle that records nitric oxide and total oxides of nitrogen, displaying nitrogen dioxide as the difference between them. While large quantities of oxides of nitrogen are emitted from chimneys, emissions from motor vehicles tend to have the most influence on concentrations at ground level.

## Hydrocarbons

In the context of precursors of photochemical oxidant pollution, it is the volatile hydrocarbons emitted from motor vehicles or refineries that are of prime concern, notably the unsaturated aliphatic compounds. Routinely the total concentration of hydrocarbons, expressed as methane ($CH_4$), is monitored, but gas chromatographic techniques are required for more specific determinations. In general, these measurements are valuable as indicators of photochemical pollution problems, but at normal ambient concentrations these volatile hydrocarbons do not have any adverse effects on health. Some concern has been expressed recently about possible adverse effects of aromatic components, and in particular, benzene. Trace amounts can be present in streets either from the small proportion of benzene in petrol itself, or from the further amount produced on combustion, but few routine measurements have been made to date.

## Ozone and organic oxidants

In the photochemical process the main secondary pollutant produced is ozone which on inhalation has adverse effects due to its strong oxidizing properties. Since some hours are required for concentrations to build up to a peak (within the daylight hours) the maxima are not necessarily at the point of emission of hydrocarbon or oxides of nitrogen precursors. Concentrations of ozone and associated organic oxidants tend to be fairly uniform over whole regions, as illustrated in the occasional episodes of high oxidant pollution in the UK (Apling et al. 1977).

## Peroxyacetylnitrate

Many complex organic compounds produced in the photochemical pollution process contribute to its irritant and lachrymatory properties and to plant damage. Peroxyacetylnitrate (PAN) is one that has been identified and determined routinely in some areas. For practical purposes in studies of adverse effects of photochemical pollutants on health it is, however, generally sufficient to take ozone as an indicator of the complex as a whole. (However, episodes with high ozone concentrations that have occurred in the UK and Northern Europe, as cited above, have not been accompanied by the full range of products and effects as seen in Los Angeles, possibly because refinery and industrial sources of precursors have dominated, rather than emissions from motor vehicles.)

## Carbon monoxide

Emissions of this gas are common to a wide range of sources, including motor vehicles, most other combustion sources, and cigarettes. Ground level concentrations in city streets are affected most by motor vehicle emissions, and especially those from petrol engines, since the more efficient diesel engine produces little. The gas is relatively inert, and does not play any essential part in the photochemical process, but it is of interest in its own right since it is readily absorbed by blood, forming carboxyhaemoglobin (COHb). Concentrations in air are most conveniently measured by continuous instruments based on infra-red or electrochemical principles (WHO 1976).

## Lead

Lead compounds are dispersed into the atmosphere mainly as fine particulates. Contributions from coal or heavy oil burning are small, but in some localities there may be emissions from industrial sources such as lead smelters (either primary production from ore or secondary production from reclaimed materials) and battery works (making lead-acid batteries for motor vehicles). The most universal source in recent decades, however, has been petrol-engined vehicles, through the use of lead alkyls as anti-knock agents in the fuel. The organic lead is mainly burnt with the petrol to produce lead halides (through reactions with 'scavengers' in the additives) and other inorganic compounds such as lead oxides, carbonate, or sulphate. Samples collected for the routine determination of smoke or suspended particulates can be analysed for lead, but it is more satisfactory to collect the material specially on membrane or glassfibre filters for subsequent analysis by atomic absorption spectrophotometry or X-ray fluorescence methods. Since in general cars are the dominant sources, concentrations are highest close to busy roads, falling off sharply on moving away from them (DHSS 1980). Only a small proportion of the lead is present in the organic (vapour) form (Harrison and Perry 1977), and although the latter has more extreme toxic properties, for all practical purposes interest is confined to the inorganic particulate component.

## Polycyclic aromatic hydrocarbons

These products originate from the incomplete combustion of fossil fuels, wood, tobacco, or other organic material (referred to collectively as polycyclic or polynuclear aromatic hydrocarbons – PAHs). They mainly condense onto the particulate matter produced in the combustion process and are generally sampled on filter papers in much the same way as smoke or total suspended particulates, as described above. Some of the lower molecular weight compounds, such as phenanthrene, are fairly volatile and cannot be collected completely on filters, but, from the point of view of possible effects on health, interest is directed mainly towards higher molecular weight PAHs such as the five-ringed compound benzo(a)pyrene, which has carcinogenic properties. Even this compound has an appreciable vapour pressure at ambient temperatures so that collection may not be complete on filters. However, it is not easy to include vapour-phase collection in series with filters at the fairly high sampling rates (or extended sampling periods) generally required for determinations of the very small amounts present in urban air, and, to date, many of the studies have confined their attention to the particulate component. Samples are extracted with an organic solvent and the analytical methods now favoured are glass capillary gas chromatography combined with mass-spectrometry, or high-performance liquid chromatography (OECD 1983).

## HUMAN EXPOSURE

In most epidemiological studies on the effects of air pollution on health, advantage has generally been taken of observations made at existing monitoring sites. Sometimes these have been set up with the exposure of the general population in mind, but often there are other considerations, such as assessing the influence of local sources (factories, traffic, etc.) or effects on other aspects of the environment. The general principles to be considered in setting up a monitoring network have been discussed in a publication by WHO (1977) and a further one deals with the wider question of assessing human exposures to air pollution, using observations from networks or otherwise (WHO 1982). In general, for most air pollutants it is very difficult to assess the true exposure of individuals or the average exposure of groups, and what is sought is an index that in some way reflects contrasts in exposure. The situation compares poorly even with assessments of smoking, in which a smoker can at least give a fair estimate of the number of cigarettes smoked per day, and say when he or she started.

The simplest situation to consider is where an index of day-to-day variations in traditional pollutants such as smoke and sulphur dioxide in a single locality is required. As an example, Fig. 18.1 shows the set of monitoring stations in London selected for studies on short-term effects of pollution assessed by increases in daily deaths, in-hospital admissions, or exacerbations of illness among bronchitic patients. The population considered lived either within the boundary of the Greater London Council or within a slightly larger area defined by the circle. The seven sampling stations shown were originally set up by the (then) London County Council to be representative of the exposure of people living in the inner, more densely populated, part of the conurbation. There were eventually some 200 sampling stations in all in the London area, but these seven were sited close to ground level, in residential areas, and were operated in a consistent manner by a single authority from 1957 onwards, providing a virtually complete set of daily data throughout the subsequent years. They were adopted for studies in the wider area around London, on the precept that they still gave a reasonable indication of values experienced by the (adult) population as a whole in the places where they lived or worked. Whether or not the absolute values were different for people in the inner and outer areas, the important point was that day-to-day variations, being determined largely by meteorological variables, ran parallel with one another in all areas.

For studies in which area, rather than temporal, comparisons are being made it is more important to ensure that values are representative in an absolute sense. Further there is the added difficulty that such studies are often concerned with long-term effects, for which one might require an assessment of lifetime exposures, or possibly of exposures during a specific period earlier in life. It is then necessary to know something about the movements of the population concerned over the years and in what ways the pollution may have changed. Figure 18.2 illustrates the substantial changes in smoke and sulphur dioxide concentrations that have taken place in London over the past 25 years. This is sufficient to show at a glance that measurements made today would give little indication of possible exposure of the adult population earlier in their lives. In the case of London and some other large cities of the UK there are a few series of pollution measurements going back to the early years of the century. However, it is only in relatively recent years that extensive monitoring networks have been set up, and when earlier information is required it is sometimes necessary to resort to crude indirect indices, for example, ones based on coal consumption, as used by Daly (1959) and by Douglas and Waller (1966).

In some further respects the above is still a simplified discussion. It relates to pollutants such as smoke and sulphur dioxide as emitted from many thousands if not millions of chimneys serving solid fuel or oil fired heating installations in homes, offices, and factories. The chimneys effect varying degrees of dispersion, depending on their height and the temperature of the emissions, but the net result in a city such as London is to create an 'area' source in which there is a

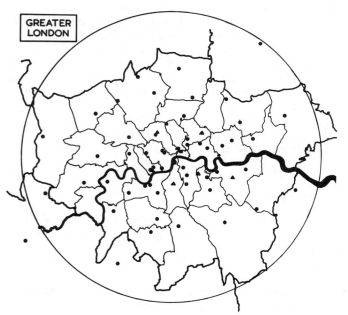

**Fig. 18.1.** Survey area as used in the 'diary' studies in London. ● – Chest Clinics and Hospitals through which subjects were recruited; ▲ – air pollution measuring sites.

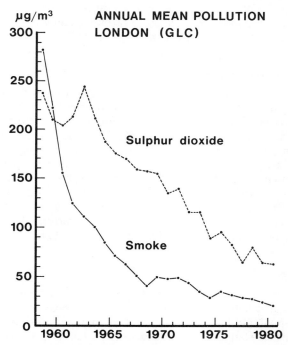

**Fig. 18.2.** Long-term trends in annual mean concentrations of smoke and sulphur dioxide in Greater London.

reasonable degree of mixing with the surrounding air before the emissions reach the inhabitants. In such circumstances exposures are not crucially dependent on the exact location of an individual, and concentrations do not vary wildly from one moment to another within the day. The situation is different when dealing with just a few point sources, as with power plants or other large industrial emitters situated in or close to residential areas where domestic sources make little or no contribution. Ideally such sources should have stacks high enough to ensure adequate dilution of the plume before it reaches ground level, even under the most adverse meteorological conditions. But, where there is a risk of inhabited areas being 'fumigated' by poorly dispersed plumes, great variations in concentration are to be expected over short distances and over brief intervals of time, depending on wind direction and speed. Smoke is not generally a problem with such sources, since combustion is usually complete and/or arrestors may be installed to remove particulates, but there may often be sulphur dioxide. Since short-term effects of that gas seem more likely to be related to peak values than to longer-term averages (Lawther *et al.* 1975), the monitoring of 24-hour mean values at just one or two sites may provide only a poor guide to the relevant exposure of individuals. It is in fact very difficult to make satisfactory estimates of the exposure of any group under study in those circumstances.

An equally difficult situation arises with traffic sources, since emissions occur within the breathing zone of people in the streets, who may momentarily experience high concentrations from passing vehicles before dilution has proceeded to the extent normally achieved with chimney emissions. The exact place and time of exposure then becomes of crucial importance again, and at least for primary pollutants such as carbon monoxide, hydrocarbons, nitric oxide, and lead, concentrations can be far higher within the confines of a busy street than in a quiet location say 50 metres away from traffic. Fortunately, each vehicle represents a small source relative to stationary combustion sources and the primary pollutants are not ones for which effects are dependent on transient peak vales rather than longer-term averages. Hence, the intermittent nature of exposure when moving around in a city does not create special problems. Nonetheless, much care is required when attempting to assess exposures to pollutants dominated by traffic sources and for these pollutants kerbside measuring sites are often set up that indicate the maximum values to which people may be exposed, supplemented by background sites away from traffic that indicate the minima. In the particular case of carbon monoxide the most satisfactory way of assessing exposure is through biological monitoring, on the population concerned. Since this gas is taken up by the blood and its effects are mediated in that way it is appropriate to measure carboxy-haemoglobin (COHb) directly on small blood samples (Commins and Lawther 1965). An alternative approach, avoiding the minor trauma of blood sampling, is to make observations on exhaled air samples (Stewart *et al.* 1976). The carbon monoxide content of alveolar air, sampled through the use of a double-bag arrangement allowing tidal air to be discarded first, is in equilibrium with that in the blood, and can be related to it via calibration experiments. Whether measurements of COHb are made directly or indirectly one

overwhelming problem is that the dominant contribution of carbon monoxide to the blood of people who smoke is their own smoking, so that in effect the part played by environmental sources can only be assessed in non-smokers (Lawther and Commins 1970). Exposure to traffic sources in streets cannot even be regarded as an added burden on top of smoking since the smoker who has a COHb level already above what would be in equilibrium with the concentration of carbon monoxide in the air at the time, will give out carbon monoxide to the street air rather than take more in.

A second traffic pollutant for which biological monitoring is possible is lead. Again direct observations on blood are practicable, and now widely used, but the attribution of the lead thus found to urban air rather than to other types of source is even more difficult than in the case of carbon monoxide. Smoking is not a major problem in this case, though it does have some effect (Pocock *et al.* 1983). The principal sources of lead are the ingestion of foods (part of that lead being via contamination by airborne lead) and water (via lead pipes). Direct human exposures to the airborne component are best assessed with personal samplers, or by calculating 'weighted weekly average' exposures based on measurements in the home, in the street, or at work, and a knowledge of activity patterns (WHO 1982). While in many countries the use of lead additives in petrol makes that the major contributor to airborne lead, industrial sources can be important in some localities. There have been some heroic attempts to determine the total contribution of petrol-lead (via inhalation or ingestion) to human uptake, by changing the type of lead used for the manufacture of additives used in a whole region (Facchetti and Geiss 1983), but such procedures are beyond the scope of most researchers.

Some secondary traffic pollutants are more uniformly distributed in space than the primary pollutants, but there can still be sharp variations with time, since the intensity of sunlight is important in their production and there is thus a marked diurnal variation, with a maximum in the late afternoon (Fig. 18.3).

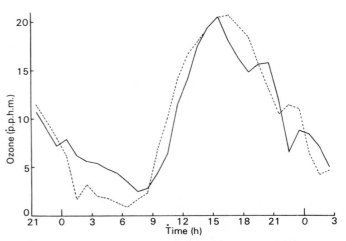

**Fig. 18.3.** Hourly mean concentrations of ozone in central London (solid line) and at a rural site outside London (dotted line) during an episode of photochemical pollution in the summer of 1976, showing typical diurnal pattern.

Much of the above discussion evades one particular problem – how to handle the major contrasts in exposures to pollutants indoors and outdoors. Reactive pollutants, such as sulphur dioxide and ozone, are readily lost on walls or other surfaces indoors, so that even at quite moderate ventilation rates concentrations indoors are generally less than those outside. The reverse can be true if there are sources indoors, and downdraughts in chimneys serving domestic coal fires can occasionally lead to occupants of a room being exposed briefly to extremely high concentrations of smoke and sulphur dioxide. In most epidemiological studies observations from routine (outdoor) monitoring stations have been used to provide indices of exposure of the populations concerned, even if they do not give a proper assessment of the absolute values or of the variations between individuals. This is reasonably satisfactory for studies within a region in which housing and general living conditions are similar throughout, but it would be unwise to extrapolate findings to other situations. Where there is a need to know more about the actual exposure of individuals in a study, then it may be necessary to resort to personal samplers. For most pollutants this is liable to increase costs and operating difficulties substantially, and the special problems of indoor air pollution are returned to in a later section in this chapter.

## STUDIES OF ACUTE EFFECTS

The response to exposure to high concentrations of urban air pollution is rapid and, as seen in the major London fogs, increased deaths occur among particularly susceptible sections of the population (notably the elderly and chronic sick) within 24 hours of onset of an episode. Thus records of deaths by exact day of occurrence are required to seek evidence of possible effects. Figure 18.4 shows day-to-day variations in deaths in Greater London during the winter of 1962–63 displayed as deviations from the 15 day moving average. This technique allows sudden increases lasting for only one or two days to be seen independently of the more gradual changes associated with influenza epidemics or other seasonal factors. The mortality data clearly show the impact of a period of high pollution lasting for several days in December 1962. This was the last occasion on which any substantial increase in deaths associated with air pollution was seen in London – the Clean Air Act of 1956 had not by then had its full impact, and concentrations of smoke as well as sulphur dioxide were still very high. Examination of a long series of data from London has indicated that increases in daily deaths became detectable when 24 hour mean concentrations of smoke and of sulphur dioxide both exceeded about 750 $\mu g/m^3$ (Holland *et al.* 1979). However, effects were related to the complex mixture of these pollutants from coal-burning and other sources, coupled with low temperatures and high relative humidity, and the same effects are not necessarily to be expected in other circumstances. Because there is usually much 'random noise' in daily mortality records, a further limitation to the above approach is that a population base of several million is required, concentrated in a single city with reasonably uniform pollution conditions throughout.

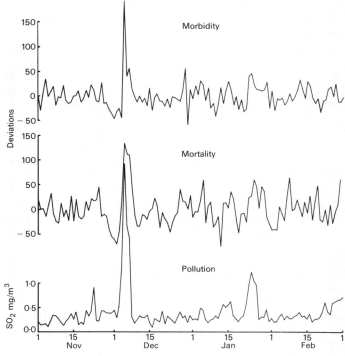

**Fig. 18.4.** Day-to-day variations in deaths in Greater London (mortality curve) and in emergency admissions to hospital (morbidity curve), both expressed as deviations from 15 day moving averages, and daily mean concentrations of sulphur dioxide. Winter 1962–63.

Some authors have applied multiple regression techniques to the analysis of daily records of deaths, pollution, and weather variables, to determine which of these factors have significant effects and to develop exposure-response curves. Thus Mazumdar *et al.* (1982), on re-examination of the London data, found a significant effect of smoke concentrations, but uncertainty remains about the form of the relationship.

A more sensitive measure of adverse effects can be provided by morbidity data, but these are rarely available on a routine basis. The index of morbidity displayed in Fig. 18.4 is based on hospital admissions data, provided by the London Emergency Bed Service that channels all requests for admission of patients who suddenly become ill through a central office, where daily records are maintained. Such data can be handled in an analogous manner to the daily deaths, calculating deviations from 15 day moving averages, though day-of-week corrections may be required first to eliminate biases arising from the more limited medical services operating at weekends.

More generally however special studies are required among selected subjects in order to relate exacerbations of illness to air pollution. A technique that proved effective in London was to collect information on self-assessed changes in condition among bronchitic patients (Lawther *et al.* 1970). The subjects were enrolled mainly at chest clinics, selecting ones who were fit enough to be out and about, but whose condition often deteriorated from time to time during the winter months. They simply noted in small pocket diaries whether they considered their breathing to be better, the same, or worse on each day, as compared with the previous one, and the answers were scored on a numerical scale (1, 2, or 3 respectively). The mean score was then calculated on a daily basis and with groups of patients as large as 1000 the random variation in this was small, allowing occasional peaks relating to adverse environmental conditions to stand out clearly. Figure 18.5 illustrates this for a winter (1959–60) in which there were several minor episodes of high pollution, and evidence of correlation with concentrations of both smoke and sulphur dioxide that was closer than with any of a number of weather variables examined. While this approach works best with dedicated subjects living in a large city where exposures are likely to rise and fall in unison throughout the area, analogous methods have been applied in other circumstances. Cohen *et al.* (1962), for example, used a relatively small group of asthmatic subjects for studies related to pollution around a large point source (a power plant). This, however, is a much more difficult type of situation to assess, since individuals within the group are likely to be subjected to highly variable exposures, with peak values occurring at different times as the plume moves in various directions with the wind.

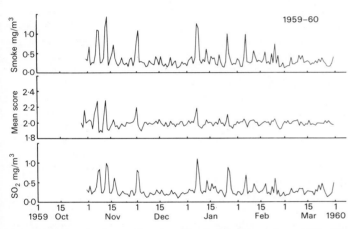

**Fig. 18.5.** Results from 'diary' studies in London, winter 1959–60, showing day-to-day variations in the illness score for bronchitic subjects together with mean daily concentrations of smoke and sulphur dioxide.

## ASSOCIATIONS WITH CHRONIC RESPIRATORY DISEASE

The high death rates from bronchitis in urban as compared with rural areas and the high overall rates in some countries (notably the UK), where there has been much air pollution, have long been taken as indicators of a role of pollution in the development of chronic respiratory disease. Studies of local or regional contrasts in death rates can provide leads concerning the existence of a problem, but because of uncertainties about diagnostic classifications and about the effects of other factors, such as smoking and occupational exposures to dust and fumes, it is difficult to draw firm conclusions in this way.

The most important development in pursuing this matter further during recent decades has been the use of standardized

questionnaires for enquiring into respiratory symptoms, so that their prevalence in defined populations can be related to a wide range of environmental and personal factors. Questionnaires of this form are discussed further in other chapters, but for studies on effects of air pollution the basic format commonly used is that of the Medical Research Council (MRC), successive versions of which were produced in 1960, 1966, and 1976 (MRC 1976). This was developed for clinical or survey use, and it sets out questions in a standardized manner on cough, phlegm production, breathlessness, wheezing, and history of respiratory illnesses. There are detailed enquiries into smoking habits, and opportunities to record occupational and residential histories, and other personal data, depending on the exact purpose of the study. Simple tests of ventilatory capacity are also commonly incorporated, such as forced vital capacity and forced expiratory volume in one second (FVC and $FEV_1$) or peak expiratory flow rate (PEFR).

While many of the studies based on respiratory symptoms questionnaires have been concerned with specific occupational risks, others have dealt with general population samples, so as to examine relationships between the prevalence of respiratory disease in areas of contrasting pollution levels. Van der Lende *et al.* (1973), for example, initially conducted a cross-sectional study in the Netherlands, but by repeating their surveys in the same areas every three years they were also able to look at changes in prevalence with time in relation to changes in pollution. To reduce the risk of differences in social class structure between areas affecting results, there are advantages in studying a single occupational group, providing it is not subject to special risks of respiratory disease itself. Thus telephone workers provided a suitable group among which to examine effects of pollution in urban and rural areas within and between Great Britain and the US (Holland *et al.* 1965).

Within all the studies reported to date the major factor affecting the prevalence of symptoms and lung function values has been smoking, which makes it difficult to isolate possible effects of air pollution. To circumvent this problem attention can be confined to schoolchildren although (regrettably) it is difficult to avoid effects of smoking altogether even then (Holland *et al.* 1969a). Other types of studies of children have related the frequency of acute respiratory illnesses to exposures to air pollution, and in some cases examined the same group of children repeatedly as they have grown up (Douglas and Waller 1966), even continuing this into adult life (Colley *et al.* 1973).

The various surveys discussed above suggest that exposure to air pollution is a relatively minor factor in the development of chronic respiratory disease compared with other factors. Long-term exposure stood out clearly only where there were quite large contrasts in exposure to pollution (usually expressed in terms of smoke and sulphur dioxide concentrations). Apart from smoking, one of the most important determinants of respiratory symptoms and deficits in lung function among adults is a history of acute respiratory illnesses earlier in life (Irvine *et al.* 1980). This may in turn reflect effects of urban air pollution or of parental smoking in the home (Holland *et al.* 1969b), but it underlines the point that the prevalence of chronic respiratory disease among adults cannot be related solely to the pollution (and other circumstances) at the time. Where pollution levels have changed substantially through the years, as they have in the UK in the wake of the Clean Air Act of 1956, it may be necessary to look back at former conditions when planning studies and interpreting findings. Because many adults have lived through periods of high pollution in the past there could still be a substantial backlog of effects of pollution detectable in surveys even where controls have now become effective. But the indications are that in populations exposed throughout their lives to only moderate levels of pollution, cross-sectional studies among sub-groups living in different areas are unlikely to yield much definite information of effects of pollution.

## LUNG CANCER AND AIR POLLUTION

Ever since a substantial increase in lung cancer mortality was first noted, in the 1930s, it has been apparent that death rates are generally higher in urban than in rural areas. A number of possible reasons for this have been considered through the years, including better opportunities for diagnosis in urban areas, and the presence of carcinogens such as benzo(a)pyrene and other polycyclic aromatic hydrocarbons (PAHs) in town air, suggesting that air pollution may play some role (Lawther and Waller 1976).

Investigations into this problem must, however, take into account effects of cigarette smoking which is the prime cause of lung cancer. Changes in smoking habits have been responsible for the long-term trends in lung cancer mortality seen in many countries, but it is less clear as to what effect they may have had on urban/rural differentials. In the UK there is now little difference in smoking habits between urban and rural areas, but there could well have been larger contrasts in the past that would affect the overall lifetime exposure of adults in the upper age ranges. Thus great care is required in interpreting findings based purely on death certification data, without any information on smoking. The situation in England and Wales is illustrated in Table 18.2, which contrasts death rates for one narrow age band in Greater London and the aggregate of rural districts throughout the country. While London rates were about twice those in rural districts for men born around 1891 who died in the early 1950s, this ratio is declining gradually and there may finally be little difference between the urban and rural rates. This could be interpreted as a direct effect of the reduction in pollution by coal smoke during the present

**Table 18.2.** *Lung cancer: age-specific death rates for males aged 60–64 in Greater London and in Rural Districts of England and Wales*

| Year of death | Year of birth | Deaths per 100 000 | |
| --- | --- | --- | --- |
| | | Greater London | Rural districts |
| 1951–55 | 1891 | 350 | 170 |
| 1956–60 | 1896 | 420 | 240 |
| 1961–65 | 1901 | 450 | 270 |
| 1966–70 | 1906 | 405 | 295 |
| 1973 | 1911 | 370 | 290 |

The death rates are approximate, being interpolated from tabulations in broader age aranges. Changes in the classification of rural districts limit this analysis beyond 1973, and data for the last quinquennium listed here are based on the single (mid) year only.

century, which gained much momentum after the Clean Air Act of 1956, but which had been going on more slowly for a long time in London. Measurements of benzo(a)pyrene have been made during the past few decades (Table 18.3) and these show a very sharp downward trend. The problem remains however that little is known of changes in the pattern of smoking habits within the various urban and rural areas, and it is conceivable that cigarette smoking was at one time more popular in large urban areas such as London than in rural districts and that the situation is gradually reversing.

**Table 18.3.** *Benzo(a)pyrene concentrations in the air of central London, 1949–81. All based on 24 h samples aggregated for yearly periods*

| Period | Sampling site | Benzo(a)pyrene ($\mu g/1000\ m^3$) |
| --- | --- | --- |
| 1949–51 | County Hall | 46 |
| 1953–56 | St. Bartholomew's Hospital | 17 |
| 1957–64 | County Hall | 14 |
| 1972–73 | St. Bartholomew's Medical College | 4 |
| 1974–81 | St. Bartholomew's Medical College | 1.6 |

Only epidemiological studies in which information on smoking habits, residential histories, and other relevant factors (including occupation), can resolve these matters. Two types have proved effective, at least for demonstrating the magnitude of smoking effects and secondarily, shedding some light on possible effects of air pollution. These are case-control studies in which enquiries are made among diagnosed cases of lung cancer and matched controls without the disease, and long-term prospective studies in which a defined population group is followed to death, gathering the required information on smoking and other factors at the outset, and at intervals of some 5 to 10 years thereafter (Doll and Peto 1976; Hammond *et al.* 1977). The outcome of most studies to date has however been that once smoking has been taken into account, the differential between urban and rural dwellers in the incidence of lung cancer is quite small. Clearly, to obtain any definitive results specifically on air pollution, large scale studies encompassing areas with substantial contrasts in some suspect component (for example, coal smoke) are required.

There has been some concern over the years that emissions from motor vehicles might have carcinogenic properties. There are traces of PAHs in the particulate components of both petrol and diesel engine exhausts, though in comparison with coal smoke the amounts are very small. Extracts of these particulates have however been shown to be active in short-term mutagenicity tests, and the activity does not appear to be related solely to their PAH content (currently nitro-derivatives of the PAHs are believed to contribute). While it is difficult to assess general population exposures specifically to vehicle pollutants and to identify groups with contrasting exposure, there have been some studies among occupational groups, particularly in relation to exposure to diesel fumes. One such study, among workers in bus garages subject to high concentrations of diesel smoke, has not revealed any appreciable difference in lung cancer death rates over a 25 year period, in comparison with other categories of London Transport workers without special exposure (Waller 1981).

# EFFECTS OF INHALED LEAD

A discussion on this topic is included as an example of problems that arise with a 'multi-media' pollutant. While relatively large exposures to lead, as in some occupational circumstances, can lead to a wide range of acute and chronic effects, the main concern in relation to more modest environmental exposures is with possible neuropsychological effects among young children (DHSS 1980). Sources of lead in air were discussed earlier. There is also lead in food, of which some results from contamination by air-lead and some natural or process sources, such as the solder in cans. In certain localities, where the drinking water supply is soft and acidic, and lead pipes are used, intake from that source becomes a major component. Children may also derive excessive amounts from a variety of adventitious sources such as old lead paint.

Thus studies on effects of lead must be related to environmental sources as a whole, and exposure is best assessed through biological measurements. Blood lead determinations are considered to be the best indicators of recent exposure. According to experimental studies reported by Chamberlain et al. (1978) the biological half-life of lead in the blood is of the order of 18 days, so that such measurements largely reflect uptake during the preceding few weeks. Other indirect indices of lead absorption have been used. The free erythrocyte protoporphyrin (FEP) assay was recommended by the Centers for Disease Control (1978) for initial screening purposes in large populations. It is more cost-effective than blood-lead screening (Berwick and Komaroff 1982), but the relationship with blood lead is not very close, so that the latter measurements are to be preferred from the start in epidemiological studies. Similarly, measurements of ALA-dehydratase activity have been used for some survey work (Secchi et al. 1973). There is an inverse relationship with blood-lead, but the method does not offer advantages in terms of reliability and specificity.

A much bigger question to consider is whether any measure of recent exposure is adequate in relation to anticipated effects. The model proposed as a result of follow-up studies of clinical lead poisoning cases among children coupled with information from biochemical and toxicological studies, is that elevated lead levels interfere with the development of the brain during infancy leading to adverse effects on cognitive function and/or behaviour that cannot in general be assessed until the primary school years are reached. There is no clear indication as to whether it is the average exposure during the early years or an acute episode within that period that is most critical, but there is some argument in favour of measurements relating to several years prior to the time when effects are assessed. It may sometimes be possible to organize a series of blood–lead measurements from birth onwards in longitudinal studies, but otherwise attention can be turned to lead in the longer-term storage compartments of the body. The major part of the body burden is relatively tightly bound in bone, and shed deciduous teeth of children provide one possibility for assessing average exposures, covering the period from the eruption of the tooth. The selection, preparation, and analysis of teeth is not easy, but it has been undertaken by research groups in several countries (Needleman et al. 1979; Smith et al. 1983; Winneke, 1983). As Smith et al. demonstrated, between-teeth differences within any child make it necessary to standardize the position of teeth being sampled. Analysis of hair samples has been put forward as an intermediate approach, reflecting exposures over a somewhat longer period than blood-lead, but it is difficult to separate external contamination from the intrinsic lead in the hair, and the method has not been widely adopted.

The assessment of effects is even more difficult than assessing exposure: carefully standardized and validated tests of the cognitive and behavioural effects considered are required and there are a great many confounding factors, related to family and social circumstances, that must be taken into account. Needleman et al. (1979), in their study in the US of dentine lead levels (the analysis being done on dentine rather than whole teeth), introduced teachers' assessments of behaviour in the classroom as well as standardized intelligence tests and others relating to visual motor function and motor co-ordination. The main comparisons made were between sub-sets at the high and low extremes of their dentine-lead distributions. For these subjects, information on a range of family factors such as mother's education, father's social class, and parental IQ were entered into the analysis of covariance used to evaluate the results. Significant differences in IQ were seen between the high and low dentine lead groups. Blood-lead data were also available for some of the children, as measured four or five years earlier, but results were not analysed directly in relation to them. Subsequently Yule et al. (1981), undertook a pilot study in the UK using a range of tests analogous with those used by Needleman et al. but linking findings with blood-lead measurements that had been made in a survey about a year earlier. Their results also indicated an association between attainment scores in several of the tests and the lead exposure indices (in this case blood-lead), after adjusting for social class. They did not, however, have much other information on family circumstances and in further work they planned to collect a wider range, including parental IQ tests.

As mentioned above tooth-lead determinations have been used in studies by Winneke (1983) in Germany, and by Smith et al. (1983), in the UK. These show further how important it is to control adequately for non-lead variables likely to be related to performance in the intelligence tests. Thus in the German work, associations were found between IQ and tooth-lead, but doubt was expressed as to whether they were truly causal, although some impairment of perceptual-motor integration was considered as being caused by lead. In the British study strong associations were reported between intelligence and other psychological measures, and the social factors that had been investigated. While there were significant differences for some of these tests between groups differing in tooth-lead levels, these became small and non-significant (though still in the same direction, with high lead levels related to deficits in attainment) once the main social factors were taken into account.

Not all problems in the field of air pollution epidemiology are surrounded by complications of multi-media sources, but most have analogous problems of non-specificity of effects and a wide range of confounding variables. The discussion above well illustrates the complexity and magnitude of the task in trying to reach conclusions firm enough for the guidance of public health policy.

## STUDIES ON INDOOR POLLUTION

Concern over possible effects of indoor air pollution has increased in recent years, as evidenced by the wide range of studies reported at a recent symposium on the topic (Spengler *et al.* 1982). Reasons for this include the improved control of pollutants outdoors, bringing into closer perspective those that remain indoors, the loss (in urban areas of the UK) of the open coal fire that used to induce high ventilation rates in rooms, removing other pollutants produced within them (though at times 'fumigating' the occupants with high concentrations of smoke and sulphur dioxide), and general efforts to increase the 'tightness' of buildings in the interests of fuel economy, often reducing ventilation well below the desirable level. In these circumstances odours and water vapour may in any case become a nuisance, but the main concern here is with some specific pollutants emitted from combustion sources or materials within the home.

Potentially the most dangerous pollutant is carbon monoxide, released from the incomplete combustion of fuels in unflued appliances or from faulty flues in other cases. Poor combustion coupled with limited ventilation can lead to lethal concentrations in these circumstances, and as Table 18.4 shows, about 100 deaths a year are currently attributed to accidental poisoning by carbon monoxide in the home in England and Wales (OPCS 1983). The higher figures up to the early 1970s are due to the presence of carbon monoxide in the town gas then supplied, leading to some direct toxic effects in the event of leaks, even without combustion. The

**Table 18.4.** *Deaths from accidental carbon monoxide poisoning in the home. England and Wales, 1968–81*

| Year | Number | Year | Number |
|------|--------|------|--------|
| 1968 | 469 | 1975 | 95 |
| 1969 | 357 | 1976 | 108 |
| 1970 | 303 | 1977 | 101 |
| 1971 | 226 | 1978 | 91 |
| 1972 | 150 | 1979 | 145 |
| 1973 | 139 | 1980 | 102 |
| 1974 | 103 | 1981 | 85 |

The figures relate to cause of death codes E870, 871, 872, and 874 (8th Revision) and E867, 868.0, 868.1, and 868.3 (9th Revision).

natural gas now supplied contains no carbon monoxide. With a number of deaths occurring from faulty combustion sources in the most extreme conditions, it is likely that some transient morbidity may also be associated with exposure to carbon monoxide in the home, but since the symptoms (lethargy, headaches, etc.) are ill-defined this problem is difficult to investigate satisfactorily. Surveys of carbon monoxide in blood or in exhaled air can help to identify cases, but as indicated earlier there is always, for this pollutant, the complicating factor of smoking.

An associated pollutant from combustion sources that has received particular attention in relation to health is nitrogen dioxide. In streets motor vehicles are the main sources (at least of its precursor, nitric oxide), but indoors any unflued combustion sources can lead to concentrations that are often substantially higher than in streets. In countries where gas cooking is widely used and (as in the UK) hoods for removing fumes from above the cooker are rare, that constitutes the commonest source. Concentrations are not likely to be sufficient to cause acute effects, but a number of studies have indicated possible associations between the occurrence of respiratory illnesses in children and the use of gas, as opposed to electric, cooking within the home. Sometimes it is difficult to exclude entirely social class or other factors that might also be related to risks of respiratory illness, but Melia *et al.* (1982), conducted a series of studies in an area of homogeneous housing, where gas and electric cooking was used to approximately equal extents, without any particular discrimination with respect to social class. In the homes, they measured nitrogen dioxide, using small diffusion-tube samplers that can be left in place in rooms without attention, and also air temperature and relative humidity. Despite an apparent association of respiratory illnesses in the (school-age) children with the presence of gas cookers in the home, in earlier phases of the work, no convincing evidence of a direct link with nitrogen dioxide concentrations was seen. A study done elsewhere among infants who had been followed from birth failed to reveal any association between respiratory illnesses and gas cooking (Melia *et al.* 1983). It is clear that in this field of indoor air pollution it is difficult to establish cause and effect relationships, one of the basic difficulties being to make adequate estimates of exposure to the suspect agents, bearing in mind the wide range of variations from house to house, room to room, and time to time.

In the last-mentioned study, one factor consistently associated with a high prevalence of respiratory illness in young children was parental smoking, and this feature has already been noted above in relation to earlier work (Holland *et al.* 1969*b*). Certainly cigarette smoke is a widespread problem in indoor environments, leading to odour, eye and throat irritation, and to more specific effects on respiratory illnesses and lung function, at least among young children.

A further indoor air pollutant that has gained some prominence in recent years, is formaldehyde, arising in some circumstances from the urea-formaldehyde foam used for insulating purposes in cavity walls (small amounts of formaldehyde being liberated more particularly within the first few days after installation) and from binding materials and adhesives used in chipboard furniture and some other materials around the home. The most obvious effects are eye and throat irritation and there are no indications at the present time that the concentrations liable to be encountered in the home lead to any longer-term effects.

Among other indoor pollutants of possible concern to health are various organic compounds arising from consumer products such as paints, polishes, wood preservatives and sprays, radon and its decay products that are derived from the soil and rocks beneath a house, as well as from the building materials, and asbestos that is used in some insulating and roofing materials (but more commonly in industrial and public buildings than in homes). Some of these are considered further in other chapters of this book, and often the clearest indications of possible effects on health come first from the more extreme occupational exposures, after which studies in the community at large might be considered.

## FUTURE PROSPECTS

Enough may have already been said within this chapter to indicate that a proper sense of perspective needs to be maintained in respect of effects of air pollution on health. The problems have been highlighted in developed countries where illness associated with communicable disease has often been well controlled, leaving effects of environmental conditions, together with excesses of eating, drinking, and smoking, of more concern. At the same time, where industry has developed and towns have grown up without due regard for the efficient use of fuel and proper control of pollution, as happened in Britain during the nineteenth century, severe problems have arisen. Many of the countries that were so badly polluted at one time have now taken steps to control the major pollutants, such as smoke (or suspended particulates) and sulphur dioxide, at least down to levels not expected, on the basis of previous experience, to have detectable adverse effects on health. In those circumstances there may be little more that can or need be done in the way of epidemiological studies of effects of air pollutants. As indicated in the preceding section however, attention may still be required to the 'micro-environments' in which people live, the difficulty then being that circumstances differ so widely and change so rapidly with time that the design and conduct of epidemiological studies to investigate possible effects becomes very complex.

The micro-environment can be of great importance also in developing countries, particularly where wood, coal, or other fuels are used for cooking inside primitive dwellings without any proper flue (Sofoluwe 1968). The smoke, carbon monoxide, oxides of nitrogen, sulphur dioxide, and partial combustion products such as aldehydes can exert a variety of adverse effects on occupants, and particularly on young children, who may sometimes be carried on their mothers' backs while cooking is in progress. In these cases epidemiological studies are hardly needed to recognize the obvious dangers. As far as urban growth and industrialization is concerned in developing countries, there are lessons from the past that might be learnt, but economic conditions and social pressures generally militate against their application, and serious problems of pollution still arise.

Vigilance is also required in relation to unforeseen problems. Photochemical pollution of the oxidant type is still relatively new and while there is no evidence that it is capable of exerting acute lethal effects on the scale of the traditional (smoke/sulphur dioxide) reducing type pollutants it may have some longer-term effects that are not fully recognized. The two types of pollution can co-exist, but relatively little is known as yet about adverse effects of such mixtures, and further changes in fuel usage or industrial processes could lead to other types of pollutants or different photochemical reactions. Epidemiological studies can help to resolve problems as they arise, though pointers from toxicological work or evidence from relatively extreme occupational exposures are often required before investigations in the general population become viable.

## REFERENCES

Apling, A.J., Sullivan, E.J., Williams, M.L. *et al.* (1977). Ozone concentrations in South East England during the summer heatwave of 1976. *Nature* **269**, 569.

Bailey, D.L.R. and Clayton, P. (1982). The measurement of suspended particle and total carbon concentrations in the atmosphere using standard smoke shade methods. *Atmospheric Environment* **16**, 2683.

Berwick, D.M. and Komaroff, A.L. (1982). Cost effectiveness of lead screening. *N. Engl. J. Med.* **306**, 1392.

BSI (1969). *Methods for the measurement of air pollution. BS 1747. Parts 2 and 3.* British Standards Institution, London.

BSI (1983). *Measurement of air pollution. BS 1747. Part 7.* British Standards Institution, London.

Centers for Disease Control (1978). *Preventing lead poisoning in young children: a statement by the Centers for Disease Control, Atlanta.* CDC, Atlanta.

Chamberlain, A.C., Heard, M.J., Little, P., Newton, D., Wells, A.C., and Wiffen, R.D. (1978). *Investigations into lead from motor vehicles.* AERE-R9198 United Kingdom Atomic Energy Authority, Harwell. HMSO, London.

Chandler, T.J. (1965). *The climate of London.* Hutchinson, London.

Colley, J.R.T., Douglas, J.W.B., and Reid, D.D. (1973). Respiratory disease in young adults: influence of early childhood lower respiratory tract illness, social class, air pollution and smoking. *Br. Med. J.* **iii**, 195.

Cohen, A.A., Bromberg, S., Buechley, R.W. *et al.* (1972). Asthma and air pollution from a coal fuelled power plant. *Am. J. Public Health,* **62**, 1181.

Commins, B.T. (1963). Determination of particulate acid in town air. *Analyst* **88**, 364.

Commins, B.T. and Lawther, P.J. (1965). A sensitive method for the determination of carboxyhaemoglobin in a finger-prick sample of blood. *Br. J. Ind. Med.* **22**, 139.

Daly, C. (1959). Air pollution and causes of death. *Br. J. Prev. Soc. Med.* **13**, 14.

DHSS (1980). *Lead and health.* HMSO, London.

Doll, R. and Peto, R. (1976). Mortality in relation to smoking: 20 years' observations on male British doctors. *Br. Med. J.* **ii**, 1525.

Douglas, J.W.B. and Waller, R.E. (1966). Air pollution and respiratory infection in children. *Br. J. Prev. Soc. Med.* **20**, 1.

Evelyn, J. (1661). *Fumifugium.* Reprinted 1961 by National Society for Clean Air, London.

Facchetti, S. and Geiss, F. (1983). *Isotopic lead experiment. Interim report.* Commission of the European Communities, Brussels.

Firket, J. (1936). Fog along the Meuse Valley. *Trans. Faraday Soc.* **32**, 1192.

Hammond, E.C., Garfinkel, L., Seidman, H., and Lew, E.A. (1977). Some recent findings concerning cigarette smoking. In *Origins of human cancer. Book A: Incidence of cancer in humans* (ed. H.H. Hiatt, J.D. Watson, and J.A. Winsten) p. 101. Cold Spring Harbor Laboratory, New York.

Harrison, R.M. and Perry, R. (1977). The analysis of tetra-ethyl lead compounds and their significance as urban air pollutants. *Atmospheric Environment* **11**, 847.

Holland, W.W., Bennett, A.E., Cameron, I.R. *et al.* (1979). Health effects of particulate pollution: re-appraising the evidence. *Am. J. Epidemiol.* **110**, 527.

Holland, W.W., Halil, T., Bennett, A.E. *et al.* (1969*a*). Factors influencing the onset of chronic respiratory disease. *Br. Med. J.* **11**, 205.

Holland, W.W., Kasap, H.S., Colley, J.R.T. *et al.* (1969*b*). Respiratory symptoms and ventilatory function: a family study. *Br. J. Prev. Soc. Med.* **23**, 77.

Holland, W.W., Reid, D.D., Seltzer, R. *et al.* (1965). Respiratory disease in England and the United States. Studies of comparative prevalence. *Arch. Environ. Health* **10**, 338.

Irvine, D., Brooks, A., and Waller, R.E. (1980). The role of air pollution, smoking and respiratory illnesses in childhood in the development of chronic bronchitis. *Chest* **77S**, 251S.

Lawther, P.J. and Commins, B.T. (1970). Cigarette smoking and exposure to carbon monoxide. *Ann. NY Acad. Sci.* **174**, 135.

Lawther, P.J. and Waller, R.E. (1976). Coal fires, industrial pollution and smoking. *INSERM Symposium Series* **52**, 27.

Lawther, P.J., Waller, R.E., and Henderson, M. (1970). Air pollution and exacerbations of bronchitis. *Thorax* **25**, 525.

Lawther, P.J., Macfarlane, A.J., Waller, R.E., and Brooks, A.G.F. (1975). Pulmonary function and sulphur dioxide: some preliminary findings. *Environ. Res.* **10**, 355.

Logan, W.P.D. (1949). Fog and mortality. *Lancet* **i**, 78.

Mazumdar, S., Schimmel, H., and Higgins, I.T.T. (1982). Relation of daily mortality to air pollution: an analysis of 14 London winters. *Arch. Environ. Health* **37**, 213.

Medical Research Council (1976). *Questionnaire on respiratory symptoms.* MRC, London.

Meetham, A.R., Bottom, D.W., Cayton, S., Henderson-Sellers, A., and Chambers, D. (1981). *Atmospheric pollution. Its history, origins and prevention,* 4th edn. Pergamon Press, Oxford.

Melia, J., Florey, C. du V., Sittampalam, Y., and Watkins, C. (1983). *The relation between respiratory illness in infants and gas cooking in the UK: a preliminary report.* Presented at 6th World Congress on Air Quality, Paris, May 1983.

Melia, R.J.W., Florey, C du V, Morris, R.W. *et al.* (1982). Childhood respiratory illness and nitrogen dioxide, temperature and relative humidity. *Int. J. Epidemiol.* **11**, 164.

Ministry of Health (1954). *Mortality and morbidity during the London fog of December 1952.* HMSO, London.

Needleman, H.L., Gunnoe, C., Leviton, A. *et al.* (1979). Deficits in psychologic and classroom performance of children with elevated dentine lead levels. *N. Engl. J. Med.* **300**, 689.

OECD (1964). *Methods of measuring air pollution.* Organization for Economic Co-Operation and Development, Paris.

OECD (1975). *Photochemical oxidant air pollution.* Organization for Economic Co-Operation and Development, Paris.

OECD (1983). *Polyclyclic aromatic hydrocarbons. Report of a Workshop held in Paris, October 1981.* Organization for Economic Co-Operation and Development, Paris.

OPCS (1983). *Mortality statistics, Series DH2 (Cause) and DH4 (Accidents and violence), for the year 1981 and earlier annual volumes.* HMSO, London.

Pocock, S.J., Shaper, A.G., Walker, M. *et al.* (1983). Effects of tap water lead, water hardness, alcohol and cigarettes on blood level concentrations. *J. Epidemiol. Community Health* **37**, 1.

Registrar General (1845). *5th Annual Report, for the year 1843,* 2nd edn. p. 415. HMSO, London.

Schrenk, H.H., Heimann, H., Clayton, C.D., Fafafer, W.M., and Wexler, H. (1949). *Air pollution in Donora, Pennsylvania.* US Public Health Service, Washington, DC.

Secchi, G.C., Alessio, L., Cambiaghi, G., and Andreoletti, F. (1973). ALA-dehydratase activity of erythrocytes and blood lead levels in 'critical' population groups. In *Environmental health aspects of lead,* p. 595. Commission of the European Communities, Luxembourg.

Smith, M., Delves, T., Lansdown, R., Clayton, B., and Graham, P. (1983). The effects of lead exposure on urban children: the Institute of Child Health Southampton study. *Dev. Med. Child Neurol.* Suppl. **47**, 1.

Sofoluwe, G.D. (1968). Smoke pollution in dwellings of infants with broncho-pneumonia. *Arch. Environ. Health,* **16**, 670.

Spengler, J., Hollowell. C., Moschandreas, D. and Fanger, O. (eds.) (1982). Indoor air pollution. *Environ. Int.* **8**, 1.

Stewart, R.D., Scot-Stewart, R., Stamm, W., and Seelen, R.P. (1976). Rapid estimation of carboxyhaemoglobin level in fire-fighters. *J. Am. Med. Assoc.* **235**, 390.

Van der Lende, R., Tammeling, G.J., Visser, B.F. *et al.* (1973). Epidemiological investigations in the Netherlands into the influence of smoking and atmospheric pollution on respiratory symptoms and lung function. *Pneumonologie* **149**, 119.

Waller, R.E. (1981). Trends in lung cancer in London in relation to exposure to diesel fumes. *Environ. Int.* **5**, 479.

Waller, R.E., Brooks, A.G.F., and Cartwright, J. (1963). An electron microscope study of particles in town air. *Int. J. Air Water Poll.* **7**, 779.

Winneke, G. (1983). Neurobehavioural and neuropsychological effects of lead. In *Lead versus health* (ed. M. Rutter, and R. Russell Jones) p. 249. J. Wiley, Chichester.

WHO (1976). *Selected methods of measuring air pollutants.* WHO Offset Publication No. 24, Geneva.

WHO (1977). *Air monitoring programme design for urban and industrial areas.* WHO Offset Publication No. 69., Geneva.

WHO (1982). *Estimating human exposure to air pollutants.* WHO Offset Publication No. 69., Geneva.

Yule, W., Lansdown, R., Millar, I.B., and Urbanowitz, M-A. (1981). The relationship between blood lead concentrations, intelligence and attainment in a school population: a pilot study. *Develp. Med. Child Neurol.* **23**, 567.

# 19 Field investigations of biological and chemical hazards of food and water

F. Fairweather

## INTRODUCTION

There is a constant need to monitor food and water for potential biological and chemical hazards. The media continually review these issues and both government departments and industry, sometimes separately, sometimes jointly, are endeavouring to solve the problem.

Identification of a hazard will eventually lead to a review of a problem that may have been outstanding for decades. It will also highlight the need for sound scientific evidence for the continued inclusion of microbiological or chemical contaminants in food and water and to ensure that they are safe for human consumption.

Field investigations play a vital role in identifying potential hazards, confirming links between outbreaks of disease and a particular element in the environment, and informing policy decisions on acceptable levels of contaminants of food and water. Field investigations of biological and chemical hazards relating to food and water call for co-operation between, among others, clinicians, epidemiologists, microbiologists, statisticians, and toxicologists, and access to toxicological services, microbiological and analytical laboratories.

Using food as an example, it must be stressed that the industry endeavours to ensure that its products are safe, carrying out both biological and chemical tests before marketing. The legislative requirements placed on the industry are stringent and demanding, and involve acute, subacute, and chronic studies in various animals to determine the toxicological, teratological or carcinogenic potential of the compounds included in the food. Rigid specifications are also laid down to ensure that raw material of the highest quality is used. Thus all food products are examined to ensure they meet toxicological, microbiological, and raw material standards and the factory process is subjected to safety surveillance. This is an important contribution to the reduction of hazard.

In the following section some general issues for field investigations of food and water-borne health hazards are discussed, before attention is given to the specific clinical conditions which may be encountered in man.

## GENERAL ISSUES

### Food

Food-borne health hazards have increased in importance following the centralization of food production, the increase in communal eating, and the development of international trade and tourism.

Food material in its natural state keeps sound and edible for only a comparatively short time. Seasonable production and poor distribution contribute to a wide disparity between production and need. As populations have become concentrated within towns and cities, the problem of the quality and supply of food has greatly intensified in some areas of the world since the consumer is moved away from the field of production. The greater handling time increases the wastage of food through contamination, its destruction by pests, inefficient utilization and spoilage. In industrial areas, there is less home-based eating, and many new preserved and processed foods are sold for convenience. Responsibility for the safety and wholesomeness of food has been moved away from the individual to industrialists and governments, creating a potential for large scale outbreaks of food-borne diseases.

### Water

Water quality contributes to the health and well-being of the individual and both biological and chemical hazards may be conveyed in this medium. In considering water both sewage and industrial effluents must also be taken into account.

Water-borne infectious diseases at one time were widespread and a serious problem. With advances in medical knowledge this hazard has receded in the economically developed countries, but with the growth of industry, chemical pollution of the aquatic environment is a growing concern for governments, scientists, and the, now well-informed, general public (Stevenson 1953; Diamant 1979).

### Surveillance of food-borne diseases

As the safety and keeping qualities of food are related to their microbial content, microbiological criteria have been

313

proposed for many varieties of food. Only those for pasteurized milk have been widely adopted.

Attempts to establish microbiological food standards are frequently arbitrary and may not be related to the microbiological status of the food. However, experience in many countries has shown that the establishment of microbiological standards leads to an improvement in the microbiological status of food, since food companies are encouraged to make improvements in plant hygiene and quality control.

Although low microbial counts do not guarantee its safety, foods that are consistently within established microbiological standards are probably less hazardous.

To establish a microbiological standard for a food or class of foods, the following technical and administrative aspects must be considered (WHO 1974):

1. The standard should be based on factual studies and serve one or more of the following objectives:
   (a) to determine the conditions of hygiene under which the food should be manufactured;
   (b) to minimize the hazards to public health;
   (c) to measure the keeping quality and storage potential of the food.
2. The standard should be attainable under practical commercial operating conditions and should not entail the use of excessive heat treatment or the addition of extra preservatives.
3. The standard should be determined after investigation of the processing operation.
4. The standard should be as simple and inexpensive to administer as possible – the number of tests being kept to a minimum.
5. Details of methods to be used for sampling, examining, and reporting should accompany all published microbiological standards.
6. In establishing tolerance levels for the permissible number of defective samples, allowance should be made for sampling and other variations due to differences in laboratory methods.

### Food hygiene control

Laws and regulations concerning food hygiene aim to protect the public against injury from the food they consume. The sale of foods that are unwholesome, contaminated or incorrectly processed is illegal under these laws.

All workers handling food should understand and receive instruction on the basic elements of food hygiene. This not only includes personal hygiene, but also factory design and all aspects of process safety.

Now, with widespread use of deep freezers and .products related to this, it is paramount that consumers are assured that products are free from infection. Therefore, all catering staff must be aware that their hair, and clothing as well as any open wounds or cuts can harbour bacteria that could cause disease.

### Refrigeration and cooking

Refrigeration and cooking play a part in preventing contamination of food. But, while refrigeration *retards* the increase in numbers of bacteria, it will *not* kill the bacteria. Cooking kills most pathogens, given a sufficiently long exposure time. Thus, cooking provides the easiest, most convenient method for controlling the quality of the food we consume.

Over the past two decades public health has grown in importance with respect to the consumer. More people eat out either for pleasure or because their place of work is too far away to conveniently return home for the midday meal. It is essential that they are assured of quality in both food and drink. For this reason the food manufacturer, the process operator, the caterer and retailer, have to assure themselves that they are providing food which is not infected or contaminated in any way. Public health authorities, at the same time, should exercise a constant vigil that premises and individuals work to the highest standards to ensure that the economic and social life of a country in no way suffers. It is sometimes forgotten that gastrointestinal disorders and the like are a major cause of sickness absence from work and thereby slow down production.

Food-borne hazards of the microbiological type are many and varied. Most are avoidable if correct procedures are adopted by the handler of the material and it is essential that these individuals adhere to strict sanitary techniques. Microbiological contamination of food can result in clinical short-term discomfort while at the other extreme it can have a very severe if not fatal, effect.

### Surveillance and control of water-borne hazards and diseases

Through advances in public health, medical knowledge, and water processing, water-borne diseases have largely been controlled. Windle-Taylor (1958) lists some of these measures as follows:

1. Advances in medical care and treatment, in particular the introduction of antibiotics and eradication of carriers.
2. Separation of water sources from sewerage contamination, for example, the siting of sewage outfalls downstream of water works river intakes.
3. Protection of water sources from pollution by surveillance, legislation, and legal action.
4. Treatment of water intended for human consumption by storage, chemical clarification, filtration, and disinfection. Many modifications and combinations of these basic purification processes are in use as well as special methods for specific purposes, such as iron elimination, water softening, taste and odour removal.
5. Prevention of external and accidental pollution of the water in the treatment plant and the distribution system to homes or factories. The latter is most important because, no matter how pure the water is when leaving the waterworks, if the distribution network of trunk mains, pipes, service reservoirs, and water towers is not hygienically sound, all efforts of purification will have been in vain.
6. Advanced treatment of sewerage. The treatment of waters for subsequent use requires physical, chemical, and biological processes. These will vary from plant to plant,

country to country but will usually include distillation, gas exchange, coagulation, flocculation, sedimentation, filtration, absorption, ion exchange, and disinfection.

During the course of this century, the incidence of infectious water-borne diseases in developed countries has steadily fallen and usually only occurs as a result of a technical breakdown or an accident. Direct contamination of water source by toxic waste figure in the news from time to time and chemical pollution is now one of the most important problems to be faced.

Classical examples of chemical pollution are the organic mercurial poisoning of Minamato Bay, Japan, and the incident where Canadian Indians suffered from tunnel vision following the consumption of fish heavily contaminated by mercury. Elsewhere, lead contamination of water represents a part of the whole-body burden of lead, and hence contributes to this potentially difficult clinical problem. Metals such as cadmium and lead have also been related to cancer although the data need to be interpreted with care.

Although generally the risk from water-borne infectious diseases has diminished considerably in developed countries, the large-scale use of swimming pools for recreational purposes, carries specific risks of various infections. These include skin, ear, eye, gastrointestinal, and respiratory infections, and amoebic meningoencephalitis (Galbraith 1980).

### Skin infections

The two most common water-borne infections are athletes foot, a fungal infection, and warts – a viral infection. The floor surface surrounding swimming pools becomes contaminated and the disease is spread by contact. Obviously cleanliness and disinfection of such areas are particularly important.

### Ear infections

Inflammation of the outer ear, a condition known as otitis externa, is caused by *Pseudomonas auruginosa* which can be present in the pool water.

### Eye infections

Most organisms which could cause eye infections and lead to conjunctivitis are easily controlled by adequate chlorination. However, at high concentrations, chlorine can cause inflammation and soreness.

### Gastrointestinal infections

Only very rarely, if swimming pools are contaminated with sewerage, can bacteria responsible for some gastrointestinal infections, cause disease. Poliomyelitis, which in the past has been linked with use of swimming pools, probably spread due to poor sanitation and over-crowding of the sanitary facilities.

### Primary amoebic meningoencephalitis

This is a fatal but rare disease, first recognized in the mid-1960s. Most cases were associated with swimming in lakes or thermal springs, in warm climates. An outbreak with 10 fatalities, in Czechoslovakia in the early 1960s was associated with a public swimming bath. Up to 10 years later patho-

genic amoebae were isolated from the swimming pool. Amoebae probably collected in areas which drain into the pool but are not disinfected (Cerva *et al.* 1968; Kadlec *et al.* 1978). The amoeba responsible, *Naegleria fowleri*, is found in warm water. Chlorination can prevent its growth.

## SPECIFIC FOOD- AND WATER-BORNE HAZARDS

Hazards associated with food and water can be classified into seven main types as shown in Table 19.1. The remainder of this chapter will discuss the clinical conditions that are encountered under these major categories.

**Table 19.1.** *Classification of food-borne and water-borne hazards*

(A) **Bacterial infections**
    (i) *Salmonella*
    (ii) *Shigella*
    (iii) *Streptococcal*
    (iv) *Escherichia coli*
    (v) Legionnaires' disease

(B) **Bacterial toxins**
    (i) *Staphylococci*
    (ii) Botulism

(C) **Viral infections**
    (i) Infectious hepatitis
    (ii) Lymphocytic choriomeningitis
    (iii) Haemorrhagic fever

(D) **Protozoan intestinal infections**
    (i) Amoebiasis

(E) **Parasitic diseases**
    (i) Trichinosis (roundworm)
    (ii) Cysticercosis (tapeworm)

(F) **Plant and fungal hazards**
    (i) Mycetismus
    (ii) Mytoxicosis – aflatoxins

(G) **Chemical hazards**
    (i) Cadmium
    (ii) Lead
    (iii) Polychlorinated biphenyls (PCBs)
    (iv) Pesticides
    (v) Antibiotics

## Bacterial

### Salmonella infections

In 1885, Dr S E Salmon first described a Gram-negative, rod-shaped bacillus now known as *Salmonella*. This causes a para-typhoid type of infection which in the acute form may produce a gastroenteritis, with a usual incubation period of 12–24 hours. In extreme cases this may extend to 48 hours. It is known that over 100 strains of salmonellae are pathogenic to man.

The group of organisms have similar fermentation and cultural reactions to the paratyphoid bacillae and specific identification of the organism has to be carried out using agglutination tests. The commonest organism known to cause human disease is *Salmonella typhimurium* and this causes typhoid fever. Other organisms seen from time to time are, *S.*

*enteriditis, S. heidelberg, S. newport,* and *S. montevideo.* Many salmonellae infect animals such as pigs, rats, and mice. The primary source of infection in most outbreaks is a farm animal, and secondary outbreaks arise from human carriers. Food such as eggs, poultry, meat, and meat products are usually involved in the spread of infection and man is always primarily responsible for the spread of salmonellosis. The onset of the clinical symptoms is usually abrupt, with headache and fever, followed by nausea, vomiting, and diarrhoea. Abdominal pain, which may be constant or colic-like in nature, is experienced and some patients may suffer great weakness and dehydration. The vomiting may continue for several days but usually ceases after about 48 hours. The diarrhoea is often severe and the stools are extremely offensive, and may contain mucus.

In approximately 10 per cent of patients septicaemia ensues, and some patients may develop complications such as meningitis, osteomyelitis, endocarditis, and pneumonia.

In view of this extremely severe clinical condition it is essential that all food-stuffs from animal sources are properly and correctly cooked, and the resulting material carefully handled. Legislation requires that all animals and meat should be inspected and checked for salmonellae, but an essential and important measure at this stage is that all people handling and involved in cooking should have a full knowledge of good hygiene practice.

Infected water may be responsible for salmonellae poisoning, and for this reason bacteriological checks should be made from time to time.

People making home-made products, such as ice-cream, should also guard against contamination of starting materials. Eggs, for example, can be contaminated with *S. typhimurium* (Gunn and Markakis 1978).

### Shigella

*Shigella* species cause a condition known as shigellosis in man. The commonly found species are *Sh. dysenteriae, Sh. flexneri,* and *Sh. sonnei,* and they are very easily grown from the faeces of man. Although individuals may show no symptoms at all, cases may present with acute diarrhoea, vomiting and stools streaked with blood, mucus, or pus. Because of the intense fluid loss in severe cases, there is marked dehydration and abdominal distention. The condition is most frequent in areas where malnutrition and poor sanitary conditions exist.

Infection may be spread through contamination of food or water with infected faecal material. Because of enormous progress in controlling water quality and sewerage treatment, dysentery has become very uncommon. However, elementary precautions such as keeping food covered to prevent contamination by flies is very important, particularly in developing countries (Gross *et al.* 1979).

### Streptococcal infections

There are two important food-borne streptococcal infections – α-haemolytic *Streptococcus faecalis* and the group A *Str. pyogenes. Streptococcus faecalis* causes a fairly mild form of gastroenteritis. The incubation period is usually 2–18 hours and the clinical picture is one of nausea, vomiting, diarrhoea, and abdominal pain. This organism has been reported as a contaminant of sausage, ham, and whipped cream.

The disease caused by *Str. pyogenes,* is usually confined to the respiratory system. Infection can be transmitted by the inhalation of droplets containing the bacterium or by ingestion of milk or other foods contaminated with it.

Following a 4 July celebration on an Indian reserve in Colorado, an increased incidence of sore throat and associated fever was noticed (McCormick *et al.* 1976). The Centres for Disease Control (CDC) was notified and advertisements were placed in local newspapers inviting those who had attended the picnic to fill in a questionnaire. Those who had attended the picnic and had developed a sore throat were called primary cases, those who had developed a sore throat after contact with a primary case but had not attended the picnic were secondary cases. Cases were compared with matched controls who had not attended the picnic and had not had any contact with primary or secondary cases.

Forty-eight per cent of those interviewed who had attended the picnic had a sore throat and the incubation period ranged from two to four days. Among those who had eaten potato salad at the picnic 59 per cent than developed a sore throat. This compared with 24 per cent of those who did not eat it. Sixty-three of the 139 from whom throat swabs were taken were positive for group A haemolytic *Streptococcus* and a culture from the potato salad also yielded this organism.

The 18-year-old son of one of the four who had prepared the food, had complained of a sore throat the previous day. The epidemiological and microbiological evidence showed the potato salad to be the infected foodstuff, but it was never proven how it became contaminated.

### Escherichia coli

There are two types of *E. coli* which may give rise to diarrhoea: (i) an invasive strain that primarily isolates itself in the colon causing symptoms which are very similar to *Shigella* infections; (ii) enterotoxic strain resulting in prostration and dehydration associated with watery stools. Meat packers are particularly vulnerable because of exposure to these strains of *E. coli.*

Usually food-borne and water-borne outbreaks of *E. coli* diarrhoea occur in areas with inadequate sanitation. Newborn babies, particularly premature ones, are extremely susceptible to this infection. Preventive measures include the sanitary disposal of human excreta, the boiling of milk and milk products, and adequate inspection of food manufacturing and serving areas.

### Legionnaires' disease

Legionnaires' disease is a bacterial infection which at its worst presents as a fatal form of pneumonia. Mild forms are known to occur, for example, pontiac fever, as well as many covert sub-clinical infections. It can occur as an epidemic and the name originates from an epidemic which occurred at a convention of American legionnaires in Philadelphia in 1976. There were 183 cases and 29 deaths (Lewis and Macrae 1977).

A survey carried out in hostels and hotels showed that the bacteria responsible, *Legionella pneumophila,* is not uncommon in water supplies within buildings. The source of the infection is not the mains water supply (Tobin *et al.* 1981) but water storage tanks and plumbing systems. In the USA, air conditioning systems have been shown to harbour the organism (Broome and Fraser 1979).

Tobin *et al.* (1981*b*), examined an outbreak of the disease among 58 workers from a commercial firm who took part in a golfing tournament. Four golfers went down with pneumonia after the tournament, two of whom required hospitalization. Blood tests revealed an increase in the antibody titre to *L. pneumophilia*. The third man also had a raised antibody level, but this was not shown in the fourth. When compared with an average antibody titre, the two men were confirmed to have Legionnaires' disease and the third man was also assumed to have the disease. All infected men had stayed at the same hotel. One employee at the hotel had a raised antibody level but had never exhibited any symptoms. The organism was later isolated from two storage tanks and shower outlets at the hotel.

### Bacterial toxins

#### Staphylococcus aureus

This enterotoxin-producing organism is found in skin lesions such as boils, and the nasal passages of carriers. Handlers of food who are carriers or have such lesions can contaminate food. Processed meats such as meat pies are a common source of such infections. The toxin is produced in the food before eating, and hence the incubation period is very short, usually 1–2 hours and never more than six hours after consuming contaminated food. The enterotoxin produced is heat stable, so heating contaminated foods will not prevent the ensuing food poisoning.

Nausea and vomiting of quick onset associated with upper abdominal pain are the major symptoms of this condition. At high concentrations toxin can cause prostration and hypotension, but recovery is usually complete within 48 hours. Confirmation of the diagnosis comes from culturing large numbers of organisms from vomit and, if available, the food.

Because of the potential of foods such as sliced meats, ham and bacon to produce this condition, it is of great importance that all such foods should receive prompt refrigeration to eliminate the reproduction of any toxin-producing staphylococci. Food handlers with pyogenic skin lesions and upper respiratory tract infections should be excluded from handling such products.

### Botulism

Botulism is a serious, but rare, clinical condition. It differs from other types of food poisoning in that the central nervous system is the prime area attacked and the gastrointestinal tract may only exhibit minor symptoms. This fatal form of food poisoning results from an exotoxin produced by *Clostridium botulinum,* which once absorbed by the gastrointestinal system acts on the central nervous system to cause widespread paralysis. *C. botulinum* is an anaerobic, spore-forming, Gram-positive bacillus. The disease in man is caused by the A, B or E type, each of which has a characteristic toxin. The exotoxin is usually formed under anaerobic conditions, in non-acid protein foods. The symptoms frequently appear up to 36 hours after ingestion of the toxin – this may be proceeded by vomiting, giddiness, and diplopia. Paralysis of cranial nerves is followed by difficulty in talking and swallowing. Paralysis spreads to the trunk and all limbs and is followed by death from respiratory failure.

In most cases food contaminated with *C. botulinum* and its toxin possess a characteristic sour odour and the taste of the food is altered. These properties should warn people that the food is spoiled and therefore should not be eaten. In field investigations it is important, where possible, to obtain the contaminated food to ascertain the type of toxin that has been released and hence to administer the correct polyvalent antitoxin.

It has always been accepted that *C. botulinum* does not grow in acidic conditions, a product marinated in vinegar would not be suspected as the source of an outbreak. However, Rigau-Perex *et al.* (1982) recently reported an outbreak of food-borne botulism in Puerto Rico in which marinated kingfish with a pH of less than 4.6 was the vehicle.

The first patient, a 46-year-old male Puerto Rican, was admitted to hospital on 10 August 1978. He was vomiting and complained of weakness and blurred vision. No sensory abnormalities were noted. As dysphagia developed a neurologist was consulted who diagnosed botulism. The physical examination on admission revealed an alert, distressed patient with sluggish responses, dry mouth, drooping eyelids, and difficulty in speaking and inability to extrude the tongue. The illness progressed and he died on 12 August. The second patient was a 24-year-old employee of the deceased. He was admitted to hospital on 8 August after four days of weakness. Examination showed similar symptoms to the first patient. By 10 August, when the diagnosis of botulism was made he was slightly improved and was not given antitoxin. He was discharged on 17 August, still feeling some weakness. A third patient, 16 years old, also an employee of the deceased, was admitted to hospital on 10 August with similar symptoms. The respiratory muscles became progressively weaker, and he was intubated and given ventilatory assistance. He was given botulinal antitoxin and discharged on 17 November, still weak, but walking without assistance.

An epidemiological investigation was begun on 10 August, with information obtained from the first patient and his wife. Attention was quickly drawn to home-made marinated kingfish that the patient had eaten the previous day. It was then determined that patient no. 2, who had already been sick for a few days, and patient no. 3 who was absent from work that day, had also eaten this fish. The food was confiscated and other persons who might have been exposed were traced and alerted.

The wife of patient no. 1 had prepared the fish on 22 July, frying the slices of fish and then marinating them in a mixture of oil, vinegar, onions, peppercorns, and bay leaves. She stored the fish in three large glass jars with screw caps and left them 'to cure' under a table in her husband's cafeteria-pizzeria business. The fish had been prepared for personal consumption and was never sold to the public. Patient no. 1 and his wife ate some of the fish the next week and gave some of it to neighbours who ate it on the same day. Patient no. 2 ate some of the fish on the 2nd, 3rd and 4th, and began feeling ill on 5

August. Patient no. 3 ate small amounts of the fish on 8 and 9 August and began feeling ill on 9 August. The father and two other employees of patient no. 1 tasted the fish on 4 and 9 August.

The contents of the three jars of marinated fish were examined by the Anaerobe Laboratory of the Centers for Disease Control, Atlanta. Type A *C. botulinium* was isolated from enrichment cultures of fish from two of the jars.

Prompt investigation of this incident after diagnosis of the first case of botulism led to rapid detection of the causative food and other possible cases.

The reason why this organism grew in the foodstuff was investigated. There was air in the jars, but a thick layer of oil between air and solution created a virtually anaerobic environment. The measured pH in all three jars was less than 4.5, a level at which there is little risk of botulism. The vinegar may not have completely or sufficiently quickly penetrated the fish, which would have left the interior pH high enough for spore germination, growth, and toxin production. This could not be proved, as too much time had elapsed between the preparation of the fish and its examination in the laboratory – equilibration would have taken place. The fact that some people ate the contaminated food and did not become ill would support the theory that the toxin was not equally spread throughout the fish.

This incident did not represent a widespread public health problem but shows how, under unusual circumstances, outbreaks of this kind can occur. It also stresses the need to monitor 'home-made' products and ensure education of the public to potential hazards. Insufficient attention has been given to this in the past.

## Viral infections

### Infectious hepatitis

The term hepatitis refers to an acute inflammatory disorder of the liver and the condition may be due to a variety of pathogenic agents. Two viruses are associated with viral hepatitis. Virus A, which gives rise to infectious hepatitis, is present in both the faeces and blood of the infected person and can be transmitted orally or parenterally. Virus B causes serum hepatitis, so called because it can only be transmitted parenterally. Virus A will be considered here as it is the form of the disease which is both food and water-borne (Follett and McMichael 1981; Orenstein *et al.* 1981). The disease is spread by person-to-person contact via the oral–faecal route and when populations are exposed to contaminated food, for example, milk or raw shellfish, an epidemic can result. It is common where conditions of hygiene are poor, and young people are particularly prone to the infection.

The disease has an incubation period of up to six weeks and the onset is usually acute with vomiting, headache, abdominal discomfort, and tenderness over the liver. Jaundice soon follows and hepatomegaly may be found on physical examination. To prevent such cases it is essential, that proper hygiene and good sanitation are practised. Sources of shellfish collected for consumption should be sited in areas free of sewage disposal. It is also advisable to immunize, with gamma-globulin, travellers who are visiting areas where the disease is endemic. Care must be exercised when using syringes and needles that have been used on an infected patient and in the handling of food given to and excreta from infected patients.

### Lymphocytic choriomeningitis

This form of meningitis is caused by an RNA virus, the natural host of which is the house mouse. Infection is transmitted via food contaminated with urine or faeces from an infected mouse. Mild infections not progressing to meningitis may occur. Illness may commence with an influenza-like attack 8–13 days after contaminated food is eaten. The patient either recovers completely, or 15–21 days after onset, signs of meningoencephalitis may appear. Recovery usually occurs within several weeks, although severe cases occasionally prove fatal. The disease can be prevented by rodent control and good food hygiene.

### Haemorrhagic fevers

The haemorrhagic fevers have been clinically diagnosed in the Far East for many years. They were first recognized during the Korean War, in which seasonal outbreaks occurred in American troops. The vectors in some haemorrhagic fevers have not yet been identified. It has been suggested that in some areas field rodents act as the reservoir.

## Protozoan intestinal infections

### Amoebiasis

Amoebiasis, originally confined to the tropics, is seen worldwide. It occurs where conditions of habitation are cramped and unhygienic, such as prisons, institutions, and refugee camps.

Amoebiasis, or as it is more commonly known, amoebic dysentry, is caused by a protozoan parasite invading the large intestine. Cysts of the protozoan can contaminate food or water. When consumed protozoa emerge from these cysts and invade the intestinal wall. If the gut wall is penetrated ulceration and abscess formation may occur. The amoebae may infect a person without giving any overt signs of infestation. Some diarrhoea may occur, but only sporadically. However, if amoebic dysentry sets in, blood-stained stools may be passed, but very few other symptoms exhibited. The disease can come and go, and this is quite a common sign of ingestation. Complications can set in, including peritonitis and, more rarely, liver abscesses.

The disease is easily spread by asymptomatic carriers, handling food or water, without taking due care of their own personal hygiene.

Eldin (1981) reported amoebiasis as the cause of death in a 71-year-old Scottish woman, taken into hospital after a 12-day history of diarrhoea. After various blood tests, including sodium, potassium, and blood urea, she was given a sigmoidoscopy and ulcerative colitis was diagnosed. Treatment was given, including tetracycline and pregnisilone, but her condition deteriorated until her death. No pathogens were isolated from the stools.

At post mortem, faecal peritonitis was evident. Diagnoses of tuberculous enteritis or amoebic colitis were considered. A frozen section of formalin-fixed tissue showed many *Entero-amoeba histolytica*, a type of amoeba widely present in healthy individuals, even in temperate climates. The case indicates that amoebiasis is always worthy of consideration when a patient presents with diarrhoea and bowel ulceration.

## Food- and water-borne parasitic helminths

Diseases caused by helminths, once largely confined to tropical areas, have spread with the increased mobility of populations, both for work and tourism. They are mainly found in young children in areas where standards of public health are poor.

Again, sanitation would go a long way to eliminating these disease, as many are spread in the faeces of the contaminated individual. There are many examples of such parasites which use man as one of its hosts. They include the namatodes (roundworms), cestodes (tapeworms), and the trematodes (flukes). The source of infection for these parasites include contaminated meat, such as pork and beef.

An outbreak of trichinosis occurred in Paris in January 1976 (Bourée *et al.* 1979). A large number of people presented with similar and severe symptoms including headache, fever, nausea, and, in some cases, periorbital odoema. The eosinophil counts were high. Very few parasites were isolated, but this was thought to be due to the fact that within the time of infection, the larvae had not yet become encysted. A biopsy taken from one patient 18 months later revealed a living larva, showing how long-lived the parasites can be. The disease was treated with anthelmintic drugs.

All the patients had consumed horse meat, bought from one particular butcher. The butcher and his family were infected. It was thought that the horses must have eaten hay contaminated with rodent droppings.

Tapeworms can be found in pork or beef. Infestation with pork tapeworm – cysticercosis – can be quite a serious condition and encystment can occur in organs other than the gut (Giri 1978). The larvae can develop in the subcutaneous tissues, the heart, eyes or central nervous system, where the condition often proves fatal. Again, infected faeces are the source of infection.

## Fungal hazards

### Toxic diseases associated with fungi

Many fungi, when ingested, are toxic to man. Fungal poisoning can be divided into two categories: (i) mycetismus – the disease caused by ingestion of the fungi; and (ii) mytoxicosis – ingestion of toxins produced by fungi.

### Mycetismus

There are many fatalities each year associated with the consumption of fungi – only an expert can distinguish safely one type from another. The cyclopeptides found in species of *Amanita* are some of the most toxic poisons contained in fungi. Consuming a single *Amanita phalloides* fruiting body can prove fatal (Wieland 1965).

Certain mushrooms when eaten in conjunction with other foodstuffs, such as alcohol, can give a violent reaction in some people. This is because they contain alcohol synergists, that in conjunction with alcohol block various enzyme pathways.

Some mushrooms contain muscarine, a chemical which exhibits a cholinergic effect in the body. The symptoms include sweating, salivation, and lacrimation. Other gastro-intestinal symptoms may develop with headache and visual effects. Atropine may be necessary but recovery is usually spontaneous.

Ergotism is a condition caused by the ingestion of the fungus *Claviceps purpurea* which grows on wheat, rye, and other cereal grains. It has a direct effect on the artery walls causing them to contract, leading to loss of circulation to the extremities. Gangrene sets in, often resulting in loss of fingers, toes, and even the ears and nose. In extreme cases, death occurs from neurological complications. Cereal crops are scrupulously monitored for the fungus and diseased grains destroyed (Abul-Haz *et al.* 1963).

### Mytoxicosis – aflatoxins

Common fungi, such as *Aspergillus flavus* and *A. parasiticus*, yield a group of compounds called aflatoxins. The term is also used for metabolites of aflatoxins that are formed in the body and are further identified by a letter. For instance, an aflatoxin currently of interest as a food contaminant is aflatoxin $M_1$, a metabolite of aflatoxin $B_1$ which is secreted into the milk of lactating animals. It is now possible to measure minute quantities of aflatoxin in foods. As a result there is a growing interest in their influence on public health. The $B_1$ aflatoxins are very toxic to animals and the manifestation is seen in the liver. Incidents have been reported of aflatoxicosis in man. In one outbreak 400 people from several villages in India, were affected and over 25 per cent of these died of fatal hepatic disease (Krishnamachie 1975).

A study in Swaziland (Peers *et al.* 1976), estimated aflatoxin ingestion over a period of one year, as judged by aflatoxin determination of food samples and related this to the incidence of primary liver cancer. It showed the importance of determining the levels of aflatoxin in the starting raw material, as ground nut is an important source of protein in Swaziland. It draws attention to the need in field operations of recording the storage and handling methods used in a particular country since this will help to judge the role of deterioration by fungi. At the same time it emphasizes the importance of having good, analytical facilities for measuring the levels of a contaminant and the need to create a team spirit amongst all workers, including clinicians, toxicologists, statisticians, epidemiologists, and microbiologists.

Aflatoxins were first isolated as contaminants of ground nuts and have since been found in maize. Inadequate drying of crops before storage and poor storage conditions lead to contamination by aflatoxin-producing fungi. Ground nut is commonly used in animal feeds and hence appropriate facilities must be provided for processing such raw materials to avoid contamination of products such as cows' milk with aflatoxin $M_1$.

A study by the Ministry of Agriculture Fisheries and Food

(MAFF Report 1980) showed that aflatoxin was present in nut products and milk and surveillance is continuing. Governments could ban the import of materials such as ground nuts but this would have serious implications for other countries. Aflatoxins will remain an important public health issue for many years to come and will become much more vexed in view of the excellent progress made by analytical chemists.

## Hazards association with plants and plant products

Many plants, vegetables, fruits, and nuts can cause illness or even death if ingested. Many are very familiar and form part of our everyday diet and environment. Some vegetables if cooked properly cause no problems, but if inadequately cooked will make people very ill. Potatoes, for example, under normal conditions, form a large and important part of many peoples' diet, but if they are eaten after they have turned green they contain quantities of toxic products which could make one quite ill. We will consider here some of these hazards.

### Enzyme inhibitors

*Trypsin inhibitors*: soya bean was the first crop to be recognized as containing a trypsin inhibitor. Since then trypsin inhibitors have also been isolated from potatoes, kidney beans, and haricot beans among others.

*Amylase inhibitors*: various amylase inhibitors have been found in wheat, beans, and unripe mango.

*Cholinesterase inhibitors*: solanine is a glycoalkaloid which is produced in the potato when it is exposed to light. A case of solanine poisoning was described by McMillan and Thompson in 1979, among schoolboys in south-east London. Seventy eight boys became ill, 7–19 hours after lunch at the beginning of the Autumn term and 17, of whom three were dangerously ill, required admission to hospital. Sickness began with headache, vomiting, abdominal pain, and diarrhoea. Fever was sometimes present and occasionally circulatory collapse. Prominent among the symptoms were neurological disturbances such as apathy, restlessness, drowsiness, mental confusion, rambling, incoherence, stupor, hallucinations, dizziness, trembling, and visual alterations. Most of the boys recovered in a day or two but others took 3–6 days. A thorough investigation of the cause of the outbreak was made. The epidemiological findings were complex but their interpretation was rendered easier by the fact that lunch had been served to two different sets of boys, and only one set was affected. Among the potatoes served to the latter group were some that had been left over from the Summer term. When peeled, these potatoes contained 33.3 mg of solanidine alkaloids per 100 g. Potato left over from the meal had very high anticholinesterase activity. The toxic dose of 20–25 mg could easily have been consumed in a normal helping.

### Phyto-haemagglutinins

These are plant proteins which clump or agglutinate red blood cells in a manner similar to antibodies. Sweet peas, lima beans, kidney beans, and soya beans, if eaten when insufficiently cooked, contain considerable amounts of the protein.

### Goitrogens

Goitrogens are natural products which cause hypothyroidism with an enlargement of the thyroid. In 1958 the incidence of goitre in Nigeria and Ceylon was such that the WHO was asked to make a survey of both countries (Wildon 1968). Incidence of goitre was linked to the amount of iodine in the soil, but this was only part of the story. In 1966 a new survey was carried out in Nigeria, following reports of a large number of cases in a part of the country where goitre had not been known to exist. There appeared to be no relationship between the mineral content of the soil or water, and the incidence of goitre. Examination of dietary habits of the local inhabitants showed that villages with a high incidence of goitre, consumed a large amount of unfermented cassava.

To determine whether cassava was goitrogenic, thyroid activity was studied in the rat. Those animals fed only cassava or equal parts of stock diet and cassava, showed enlarged thyroids when compared with animals fed only the stock ration.

The report concluded that for countries such as Nigeria and Ceylon, supplementation of some common food, such as salt, with an iodine compound was an urgent public health measure.

### Cyanogens and cyanogenetic glycosides

Several plant food stuffs in common use, particularly in the tropics, contain cyanide either in the form of glycosides or nitrites. Acute poisoning can occur, especially in conditions of economic stress. Chronic ill-effects from cyanide intoxication are thought to include degenerative tropical neuropathy, which has been found in African countries especially Nigeria. The main features of the fully developed 'ataxic syndrome' include optic atrophy, nerve deafness, and sensory spinal ataxia.

### Pressor amines

Certain naturally occurring phenylethylamine derivatives, such as tryptamine and dopamine cause a marked increase in blood pressure when administered intravenously to mammals. Amines including vasoactive ones are normally rapidly deaminated after they enter the body, a process that is catalysed by monoamine oxidase. Amines are present in numerous foods either because they are synthesized by certain plants or through microbial contamination or fermentation processes. Bananas contain large quantities of the amines, serotonin, noradrenaline, and tryptamine. Amines have been found in the following fruits and vegetables: tomato, red plum, avocado, potato, spinach, grape, orange, pineapple, lemons, and tea. Although little is known of the effects of these compounds, they are thought to be linked to migraine in man.

### Plant phenolics

Some plant phenolics present in human foods are toxic. Although anthraquinones in rhubarb are mainly found in the root high levels are also present in the leaves. Human poisoning occurs mainly from eating rhubarb leaves.

### Oxalates

Oxalates occur in all forms of living matter. Certain families and species of plant contain relatively large amounts of this substance, mainly as the soluble sodium or potassium salt. Some of the common plant foods containing appreciable oxalates are spinach, rhubarb, and cocoa. Ingestion of suficient oxalic acid can be fatal with associated corrosive gastroenteritis, shock, convulsive symptoms, and renal damage.

### Favism

Fava bean, a species of broad bean, is a staple part of the diet of Mediterranean countries. When ingested by persons who have previously been sensitized either by inhaling the pollen of this plant or by prior ingestion, severe illness may occur. The first green beans of the season are the most toxic. The toxicity is due to a nucleoside (vicine) that causes haemolysis when injected in rabbits (Noah *et al.* 1980).

The illness, known as favism, usually appears within one hour after ingestion, the patient complaining of dizziness, vomiting, diarrhoea, and severe prostration, followed by acute fevrile anaemia, jaundice, and haematuria. Treatment is symptomatic with replacement of electrolytes and blood transfusion in severe cases.

## Chemical

Fears are sometimes expressed that our food supply is contaminated by the addition of chemical compounds to ensure that a product is preserved correctly or kept wholesome. Today antioxidants, preservatives and sterile packaging have become part of our way of life, but all these compounds and processes must be tested to ensure safety, before being put into general use.

Governments and expert working parties have laid down rules for the use of such materials and the process of obtaining clearance is sometimes long and expensive because of the sophisticated toxicological work involved. The testing demanded include 90-day studies in animals to determine the 'no-effect level' in order to calculate the allowable daily intake for man, the determination of the metabolic pathway and the metabolites formed, and the teratogenic, mutagenic, and often the carcinogenic potential of these compounds. Such tests are also required on many materials deliberately added to water and there is constant surveillance to ensure the chemical, physical, and microbiological quality of water.

Whilst legislators and toxicologists can work together to ensure 'safety' of deliberately added chemicals, there are other uncontrolled ways in which chemicals may enter food and water. Inorganic or organic chemicals may inadvertently find their way into the food chain for example from soil, via both plants and animals. The microbial contamination of animal feeds was discussed above, but pesticides deserve consideration as potentially harmful chemicals that remain on foodstuffs because of inadequate washing.

Below a number of case studies are discussed that deal with specific chemicals and also provide general lessons for the conduct of field studies of water- and food-borne contaminants.

### Cadmium

In 1979, the findings of a nationwide survey of metal concentrations in streams in the UK suggested that concentrations of cadmium in the soil were unusually high in Shipham, Somerset. It was suggested that dust contamination of garden produce might put residents who consumed these products at high risk of cadmium poisoning. An enormous exercise was mounted to determine soil, dust, water, air, and food levels of cadmium and health checks were also carried out. Only a small proportion of the residents exceeded the intake of cadmium currently considered tolerable, and no-one in the study compared to controls showed any adverse health effects (Department of the Environment 1982). This example demonstrates how important it is to carry out studies of this nature only if a health risk is clearly defined and that it should not figure as a political issue.

### Lead

The possible health effects of lead have been the subject of debate for a long time. Food and water may become contaminated by exposure to lead solder in canning, by exposure to water, used for cooking and drinking, to lead in plumbing systems, by exposure to lead in air either directly, e.g. crops and food, or indirectly via contamination of soil. Lead-containing pesticides are also important since they increase directly the lead level in fruit and vegetables and if such compounds have been used for a long time, they increase the level in soil. The scientific data about this subject need to be tempered with a great deal of common sense. There are many different sources of exposure to lead but this problem is rarely considered in terms of the overall body burden. Contamination of vegetables due to combustion of lead-enriched petrol is one issue but this cannot be seen in isolation. Contaminated water supplies represent a bigger problem to residents in areas where lead-lined pipes have been installed for years, because of the constant use of lead-contaminated water for preparation and cooking of food, over a long period of time.

Mindus and Kolmodin-Hedman (1981) report the case of a 61-year-old housewife with a history of renal disease and calculus formation for more than 10 years, accompanied by impaired renal function. She was admitted to a urological ward with a very severe intermittent pain in the right lumbar region. In the past she had been diagnosed as having a parathyroid adenoma and treated. During the present admission she was found to be confused and one morning she was no longer able to move her arms. She was in a state of general mental confusion and her reflexes were weak. The symptoms were difficult to interpret but they seemed possibly to be of a psychogenic nature. After various examinations it was concluded that her symptoms could be due to some toxic effect. Laboratory tests revealed that she had a very high lead blood content. It was volunteered by the patient that she had been advised, 10 years previously by a urologist, to drink at least three litres of water every day and she had followed this recommendation conscientiously. Since she did not like cold water, she filled a one litre jug with half warm and half cold water three times a day. The jug was analysed and excluded as the lead source. However the source turned out to be a water boiler installed some 40 years previously and this had released very large quantities of lead.

### Polychlorinated biphenyls (PCBs)

Polychlorinated biphenyls are a complex mixture of chemicals known as chlorinated hydrocarbons. They are very widespread in the environment and are used in electrical equipment such as transformers. Over the past four to five decades they have been found in rivers, fish, and birds. They cause skin lesions and liver damage in man.

In Japan, food contaminated with PCBs has produced rashes, headache, nausea, diarrhoea, alopecia, loss of libido, and menstrual disorders. Exposure of women to PCBs during pregnancy can also harm the developing fetus. Mosher and Moyer (1981) described an incident where 13 children were born to women exposed to PCBs. Of these one fetus was still-born, four were small for their gestational age, ten possessed dark skin pigmentation, pigmented gums were present in four, eight had neonatal jaundice, and nine exhibited con-junctivitis.

A follow-up study on these children showed 'slight but clinically important neurological and developmental impairment'. PCBs can biologically accumulate, occurring in increasing concentrations at each step up the food chain.

### Pesticides

Insecticides have been employed for many years to improve the yeilds of agricultural produce and their use is governed by safety criteria and testing laid down by such bodies as the Pesticides Safety Precautions Scheme in the UK. In animal tests, many of these compounds were found to be both tera-togenic and carcinogenic and it therefore follows that extreme care must be exercised in the handling of these toxic chemicals. Furthermore, all such products should carry an adequate warning on the level of the materials. Contamination of food due to inadequate washing during the preparation of food is a major, and growing issue. People consuming such contaminated material may complain of headache, nausea, dizziness, confusion, and convulsions shortly after. In this area, adequate liaison with poison centres is essential in all field operations.

### Antibiotics

Certain antibiotics and hormones are used in preparing animals for meat production. Unfortunately, antibiotics in animal feeds have contributed to a growing number of anti-biotic-resistant bacteria.

### CONCLUSION

With the ever-growing need to monitor food and water with respect to contamination, it is essential that a multidisci-plinary approach is adopted to ensure wholesomeness of the product. The prevention and reduction of biological and chemical contamination can only be accomplised by public health authorities ensuring integration of the field operations as outlined in this chapter.

### REFERENCES

Abul-Haz, S.K., Ewald, R.A., and Kazyak, L. (1963). Fatal mushroom poisoning. Report of a case confirmed by toxicological analysis of tissue. *N. Engl. J. Med.* **269**, 223.

Bourée, P., Bouvier, J.B., Passeron, J., Galanaud, P., and Dormont, J. (1979). Outbreak of trichinosis near Paris. *Br. Med. J.* **i**, 1047.

Broome, C.V. and Fraser, D.W. (1979). Epidemiologic aspects of legionellosis. *Epidemiol. Rev.* **1**, 1.

Carruthers, M. and Smith, B. (1979). Evidence of cadmium toxicity in a population living in an zinc mining area. *Lancet* **i**, 845.

Cerva, L., Novak, K., and Cuthbertson, C.G. (1968). An outbreak of acute, fatal, amoebic meningoencephalitis. *Am. J. Epidemiol.* **88**, 436.

Department of the Environment Shipham Survey Committee (1982). *Final report to residents on metal contamination at Shipham. September 1982.* HMSO, London.

Diamant, B.Z. (1979). The role of environmental engineering in preventative control of water-borne diseases in developing countries. *R. Soc. Health J.* **3**, 120.

Eldin, G.P. (1981). Amoebiasis as a cause of death in a Scottish resident. *Scott. Med. J.* **26**, 350.

Fallett, E.A.C. and McMichael, S. (1981). Acute hepatitis. An infection in West Scotland. *Scott. Med. J.* **26**, 135.

Galbraith, N.S. (1980). Infections associated with swimming pools. *Environ. Health* **February**, 31.

Giri, I.W. (1978). Cysticercosis in Surabaya, Indonesia. *S.E. Asian J. Trop. Med. Public Health* **9**, 232.

Gross, R.J., Thomas, L.V., and Row, B. (1979). *Shigella dysenteriae, Sh. flexneri* and *Sh. boydii* infections in England and Wales: the importance of foreign travel. *Br. Med. J.* **ii**, 744.

Gunn, R.A. and Markakis, G. (1978). Salmonellosis associated with home-made ice cream. An outbreak report and summary of outbreaks in the United States in 1966 to 1976. *JAMA* **240**, 1885.

Kadlec, V., Cerva, A., and Skarova, J. (1978). Virulent *Naegleria fowleri* in an indoor swimming pool. *Science* **201**, 1025.

Krishnamachie, K.A.V.R. (1975). Hepatitis due to aflatoxicosis. An outbreak in Western India. *Lancet* **i**, 1061.

Lewis, M.J. and Macrae, A.D. (1977). Public Health Laboratory Service. Communicable Disease Report No. 45.

McCormick, J.B., Kay, D., Hayes, P., and Feldman, M.D. (1976). Epidemic streptococcal sore throat following a community picnic. *JAMA* **236**, 1039.

McMillan, M. and Thompson, J.G. (1979). An outbreak of suspected solanine poisoning in school boys. *Q. J. Med.* **48**, 227.

Mindus, P. and Kolmodin-Hedman, B. (1981). Told by her doctor to drink large amounts of water, suffered lead poisoning. *Acta Med. Scand.* **209**, 425.

Mosher, N.D. and Moyer, G. (1981). The PCB menace and breast milk. *Dangerous Properties of Industrial Materials Report.* **Nov/Dec.**

Noah, N.D., Bender, A.E., Raeidi, G.B., and Gilbert, R.J. (1980). Food poisoning from raw kidney beans. *Br. Med. J.* **ii**, 236.

Orenstein, W.A., Wu, E., Wilkins, J., Robinson, K., Francis, D.P., Timko, N., and Wayne, R. (1981). Hospital acquired hepatitis A. Report of an outbreak. *Pediatrics* **67**, 494.

Peers, F.G., Gilman, G.A., and Linsell, C.A. (1976). Dietary aflatoxins and human liver cancer. A Study in Swaziland. *Int. J. Cancer* **17**, 167.

Peers, F.G. and Linsell, C.A. (1973). Dietary aflatoxins and liver cancer – a population study in Kenya. *Br. J. Cancer* **27**, 473.

Plantanow, N.S., Funnell, H.S., Bullock, D.H., Amott, D.R., Saschenbrecker, P.W., and Grieve, D.G. (1971). Fate of poly-chlorinated biphenyls in dairy products processed from the milk of exposed cows. *J. Dairy Sci.* **54**, 1305.

Rigou-Peréz, J.G., Hatheway, C.L., and Vatentin, V. (1982).

Botulism from acidic food: first cases of botulinic paralysis in Puerto Rico. *J. Infect. Dis.* **145**, 783.

Riverside County Department of Health (1971). Collaborative study from Riverside County Department of Health, Riverside, California. A water-borne epidemic of salmonellosis in Riverside California 1965. Epidemiologic aspects. *Am. J. Epidemiol.* **93**, 33.

Stevenson, A.H. (1953). Studies of bathing water quality and health. *Am. J. Public Health* **43**, 529.

Tobin, J. O'H., Swann, R.A., and Bartlett, C.L.R. (1981*a*). Isolation of *Legionella pneumophila* from water systems: methods and preliminary results. *Br. Med. J.* **282**, 515.

Tobin, J.O'H., Bartlett, C.L.R., Watkins, S.A. *et al.* (1981*b*). Legionnaires' disease: further evidence to implicate water storage and distribution systems as sources. *Br. Med. J.* **282**, 573.

Wieland, O. (1965). Changes in liver metabolism induced by the poisons of *Amantia phalloides. Clin. Chem.* **11** Suppl., 323.

Wilson, D.C. (1968). Goitre among the Ceylonese and Nigerians. *Nutr. Rev.* **26**, 77.

Windle Taylor, E. (1958). *The examination of waters and water supplies,* 7th edn. Churchill, London.

## FURTHER READING

*Clean catering. A handbook on hygiene in catering establishments.* HMSO, London.

*Drinking-water and sanitation 1981–1990. A way to health.* WHO, Geneva (1981).

*International standards for drinking water,* 3rd edn. WHO, Geneva (1971).

*Re-use of effluents: methods of waste water treatment and heath safeguards. Report of a WHO meeting of experts.* WHO Technical Report Series no. 517, Geneva (1973).

*Food-borne disease: methods of sampling and examination in surveillance programmes. Report of a WHO study group.* WHO Technical Report series no. 543, Geneva (1974).

*Reports on public health and medical subjects No. 71. The bacteriological examination of water supplies.* HMSO, London (1969).

*Food Hygiene Codes of Practice 10: The canning of low acid foods.* HMSO, London (1981).

*Lead and health. Report of a DHSS Working Party on Lead in the Environment.* HMSO, London (1980).

E.G. Knox (1977). *Foods and diseases. Br. J. Prev. Soc. Med.* **31**, 71.

National Research Council (1973). *Toxicants occurring naturally in foods,* 2nd ed. National Academy of Sciences, Washington, DC.

*Survey of Mycotoxins in the United Kingdom. The fourth report of the Steering Group on Food Surveillance. The Working Party on Mycotoxins.* MAFF. Food Surveillance Paper No. 4, London (1980).

# 20 Radiation

## A.P. Brown and †J.A. Reissland

## INTRODUCTION

Radiological protection is probably the most elaborate and comprehensive system yet devised to safeguard the health of the public from the hazards associated with an environmental agent. Since ionizing radiation from cosmic rays and from primordial radionuclides in the earth's crust is a ubiquitous factor common to all life on this planet, protection cannot be achieved by eradication of the hazard, as with say smallpox. Indeed, as man has evolved against a more or less constant level of radiation, its presence up to a certain level may be beneficial (Luckey 1982) and positive claims have been made for 'radiation hormesis' (Hickey *et al.* 1983). Concern about possible harmful effects began to emerge shortly after the discovery of artificial sources of radiation in the last decade of the nineteenth century (Upton 1982). In 1928, the International Commission on Radiological Protection (ICRP) was first established to collate information and to make recommendations so that patients and radiological staff should not be exposed to unnecessary risks. Since that time an enormous literature about the effects of radiation has been generated, and this is continuously reviewed by national and international bodies of scientists in order to derive numerical estimates of the risks to man. Risk coefficients are needed for the following reasons:

1. To provide a logical basis for radiological protection so that the health of people exposed to radiation for medical purposes, from their occupation, or as a result of living in an area of high natural background radiation, is adequately safeguarded.

2. To calculate as accurately as possible the likely public health impact of the nuclear power industry at all its stages from uranium mining to the eventual disposal of radioactive waste.

3. To assess the probability that a particular cancer that has developed in a person previously exposed to radiation either occupationally or in the course of atomic weapons testing, is radiation induced so that appropriate monetary compensation can be made.

The calculation of risk coefficients from epidemiological surveys of human populations exposed to relatively high levels of radiation and their use in current radiological protection will be examined in the final section of the chapter. However, the evaluation of risk is a much more complex process than just the consideration of a numerical probability. A Royal Society

Study Group (1983) acknowledged that 'the public not infrequently have a different perception of events from those suggested by the objective statistical assessments made by scientists or other experts'. This is certainly true for radiation and the nuclear industry, and several plausible reasons have been suggested as to why this should be. Perhaps the two anxieties of overriding importance in this context are the perceived associations with nuclear warfare and the dread nature of the possible harm, namely cancer and genetic effects. More attention has been paid to the public's attitudes towards nuclear power than any other safety issue to date, although other industries and technologies are not exempt from similar scrutiny (Kletz 1971; Lowrence 1976), and psychological research continues into the public's perception of hazards.

## SOURCES OF IONIZING RADIATION

Numerous surveys have been made of the sources and levels of radiation in the environment to which human populations are exposed. A comprehensive summary of this work is contained in the most recent report of the United Nations Scientific Committee on the Effects of Atomic Radiation (UNSCEAR 1982). In order to allow for the different biological effectiveness of various forms of radiation and the varying sensitivity of different human organs and tissues, a concept known as effective dose equivalent is employed. This calculated quantity is expressed in units called sieverts (Sv) and has great utility in radiological protection, not least as the currency for administrative dose limits (see pp. 330–2).

The overall annual effective dose equivalent to an 'average' member of the UK population is shown in Fig. 20.1. Of the total of about 2.4 millisieverts (mSv), natural radiation contributes almost 80 per cent and medical usage is the predominant man-made component. For sound pragmatic reasons, natural radiation has been of little or no concern to bodies like ICRP until relatively recently. Indeed, since natural radiation remains remarkably constant over time it provides a convenient yardstick by which the magnitude of artificial radiation can be judged, particularly when the geographical differences in the background levels as a result of local geology seem to be acceptable to society.

However, within the last few years there has been a growing awareness internationally that indoor levels of radon gas and its radioactive decay products can reach concentrations where control measures might be deemed advisable on public health

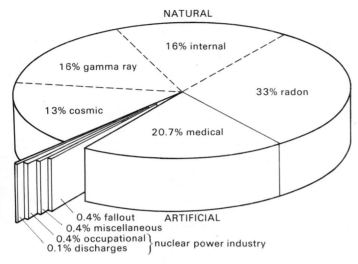

NATURAL

16% internal

16% gamma ray

33% radon

13% cosmic

20.7% medical

0.4% fallout    ARTIFICIAL
0.4% miscellaneous
0.4% occupational } nuclear power industry
0.1% discharges

**Fig. 20.1.** Average annual radiation dose to the population of the UK.

## SOURCES OF INFORMATION ON LATE EFFECTS OF RADIATION EXPOSURES

Late effects on the health of those exposed to ionizing radiation fall into two types, somatic (see pp. 327–8) and genetic (see pp. 328–9). The most important of the somatic effects and the only one which will be discussed here is the induction of malignancies. It has not been established that low levels of exposure to ionizing radiation will produce an excess in the number of malignancies above that expected in a population. However, it is presumed that effects observed at higher dose levels will occur at lower doses, although maybe at such low rates that they are difficult to detect. The effects of radiation on biological tissue can be investigated in three ways: (i) animal or cellular experiments; (ii) theoretical modelling of the basic mechanisms involved; (iii) epidemiologically.

Laboratory experiments on cells or on other animal species at best only provide guidance to the possible effects of human exposures. They are valuable as a means of indicating potential hazards and cause–effect relationships but give little quantitative evidence of relevance to man. Once a cause and effect have been related, as is the case with ionizing radiation, theoretical studies play an important role in understanding how to interpret the results of observations. However, by themselves they can provide no estimate of the magnitude of the biological effects in man associated with a particular dose of radiation. Epidemiological studies are the only way of providing direct quantitative estimates of the risks associated with exposure to different levels of radiation. By their very nature these are limited to observations of statistically calculated excesses of the number of effects in an exposed population compared with that expected in the same population had it not been exposed.

Since in the developed world approximately one in five (20 per cent) of all deaths are caused by malignant neoplasia, any group studied will produce deaths from these causes. Malignant tumours that might have been induced by ionizing radiation cannot be distinguished histologically from those that occur for other reasons. Therefore, when evaluating the induction rates of malignancies due to radiation by observing extra malignancies in an exposed population, the excess ones have to be resolved from the background or 'naturally' occurring cancers in that population. The expected number is not a well-defined quantity and may have a large variance associated with it. Land (1980) has estimated that to detect the effect of an absorbed dose of 1 gray* per person would require 1000 persons to be exposed at that level. Since the population size required to detect an effect is inversely proportional to the square of the excess risk, the detection of the effect of 0.1 gray requires an exposed population of 100 000 and to detect the effect of 0.01 gray requires ten million. Thus, it is very much easier to carry out an epidemiological study on a population exposed at doses of around 1 or 2 gray. However, although this provides a way of directly observing the effects, those that are of interest may be incurred by individuals exposed to much lower levels.

Those who incur exposures to radiation occupationally may accumulate doses of around 1 gray over a lifetime but more

grounds (O'Riordan *et al.* 1983). Radon ($^{222}$Rn) is a chemically inert but radioactive gas that is part of the main uranium decay series. Its immediate predecessor in that series is radium and the concentration of radium in soil or rock determines the amount of radon generated at a particular site. Since rock, soil, and building materials containing radium are porous to some extent, the radon gas produced within them will tend to diffuse out. Usually the bulk of radon in buildings enters from the subjacent ground with a smaller fraction diffusing out of the building materials and its indoor concentration tends to build up because of limited ventilation. In certain situations, mainly because of local geology, indoor radon concentrations have been shown to be unacceptably high. Remedial cleaning up operations have been necessary in Colorado and Ontario where dwellings had been unwittingly constructed on sites containing tailings from uranium mills. The most extensive problem has occurred in Sweden where, because of the widespread use of alum shale that is rich in uranium as a building material, there are 40 000 dwellings in which the dose from radon exceeds the provisional limit of 25 mSv a year set by the Swedish Radon Commission in 1980. The National Radiological Protection Board (NRPB) is carrying out a survey to monitor radon levels in UK houses and has suggested that control measures might be considered for a small number of households so that their occupants do not continue to receive relatively high doses.

The association between radon exposure and lung cancer was established in uranium miners who received very high doses (Myers 1982; BEIR 1980) and it seems unlikely that any direct epidemiological evidence will ever be obtained for domestic dwellings, at least in the UK. Nevertheless, as will be seen later, radiological protection in occupational settings is now based on extrapolation from observations made at much higher dose levels.

*A gray (Gy) is the unit of dose and represents the absorption of 1 joule of energy per kilogram of tissue (1 gray = 100 rads).

typically would accumulate a few tenths of a gray. Doses to the general population other than from medical applications are unlikely to exceed a few hundredths of a gray. Therefore, the direct observation of late somatic effects of radiation at exposure levels of interest requires unrealistically large populations. The current radiation protection standards (see pp. 330–2) are based on observations of populations exposed to radiation doses in excess of 1 gray. The data that exist on populations exposed at such levels come from the intensive studies of those who survived the atomic bombs at Hiroshima and Nagasaki in 1945, and from studies of various groups of patients exposed to doses of radiation for medical purposes. There is some difficulty in the use of all these data both from the epidemiological point of view and from the assessment of the doses actually received by those studied. Nevertheless, they represent the best source of information from which to derive numerical risk estimates and a summary of the most important radiation induced cancers is given in Table 20.1.

**Table 20.1.** *Examples of human cancers that have been shown to be radiation induced*

| Neoplasm | Main groups of people studied |
| --- | --- |
| Leukaemia (except chronic lymphatic leukaemia which has not been observed in excess) | Atom bomb survivors Irradiated ankylosing spondylitis patients Irradiated menorrhagia patients |
| Thyroid cancer (well-differentiated) | Atom bomb survivors Children irradiated for *Tinea capitis* (ringworm) and supposed thymic enlargement |
| Breast cancer | Atom bomb survivors Women irradiated for post-partum mastitis Multiple fluoroscopies for TB |
| Lung cancer | Atom bomb survivors Miners exposed to radon decay produced in uranium and fluorspar mines |
| Bone, sarcomas | Dial painters who ingested radium Patients given radium injections for ankylosing spondylitis or tuberculosis |
| Multiple myeloma | Atom bomb survivors |
| Skin | Early X-ray workers |
| Stomach, colon | Atom bomb survivors |

To apply these risks estimates at the lower doses of interest requires an assumption about how the rates of induced effects vary with dose. Since these data are to be used to extrapolate to much lower doses, uncertainties in the way in which the effect depends on dose may be crucial. Theoretical considerations suggest that for X- and $\gamma$-rays a linear extrapolation may overestimate the effect at the low doses (see pp. 327–8). For high neutrons and $\alpha$-particles a linear extrapolation, that is assuming that the risk per unit dose is the same at high and low dose, is believed to be a good representation of dose response.

The most comprehensive discussion of the scientific data on the biological effects of radiation is given in the UNSCEAR publications (1977, 1982) and these are the sources used by ICRP to arrive at its judgement of the risks involved. Technical evaluation of risks from the collated data has to be supplemented by professional judgement in weighting the validity of different contributions to the evidence, and inevitably there is controversy over the values which emerge. There is no evidence to disprove the low dose risk factors given by ICRP; however, neither is there direct evidence to verify them. Until recently, it was widely accepted that linear extrapolations from high-dose effects to zero dose resulted in radiation protection standards that were conservative, that is, that they gave additional safety margins by overstating the risk per unit dose of low doses. Despite the current controversy, this is probably still true for low linear energy transfer (see p. 327) radiations since: (i) lower doses delivered at lower dose rates give more opportunity for repair mechanisms to operate; (ii) the dose-response curve is probably the sum of a square and a linear term, therefore extrapolation from the same data points using only a linear term will predict higher effects.

In the US in 1980, the BEIR (Biological Effects of Low Levels of Ionizing Radiations) committee published a detailed review of the state of knowledge on the effects of radiation. It also speculated on the wide range of possible numerical estimates implied by the uncertainties in the evidence. More helpfully, the committee draw some qualitative conclusions which are useful to the epidemiologist. Leukaemia and cancer of the thyroid were identified as being particularly susceptible to induction by radiation with the female breast only slightly less so. Female breast cancer has a high spontaneous incidence while leukaemia occurs in unirradiated populations with only moderate frequency, and thyroid cancer occurs with low frequency. Clearly, there is a greater chance of observing an excess of a cancer with a high induction rate but low spontaneous incidence than that of observing excesses of more common cancers. Some types of cancer seem to be particularly insensitive to induction by radiation. The BEIR report lists eight types of malignant disease for which there is no positive evidence for induction by radiation in man. Among these is chronic lymphatic leukaemia and therefore it is strictly necessary to distinguish between different types of leukaemia when considering any influence of radiation.

Another important factor in considering the inference of numerical risks by epidemiological techniques, is the time between exposure and an induced disease becoming recognizable, that is the latent period. This is not a well-defined time interval and there is a wide range in the latent period for any given tumour type that has been observed following radiation. For many solid cancers the mean latent period is 20 years or more, and until the Japanese bomb survivors have been followed up well into the next century, it will be uncertain how long after exposure an excess of cancers might still be seen in people who were young at the time of irradiation. Leukaemia seems to differ from other cancers induced by radiation in that the mean latent period is about 10 years and after 30 years the risk of excess cases is relatively small (Kato and Schull 1982).

Despite the uncertainties inherent in the data available for the estimation of numerical values of malignancy induction rates by radiation, it is informative to have some idea of the magnitudes of the effect which may occur. Any numerical values quoted to describe the effects of radiation are inevitably over-simplifications. Those used in radiological protection ignore differences in susceptibility of individuals, largely ignore variations in susceptibility with age, and have usually been inferred from observations on groups exposed at dose levels which may be very different from those for which the risk estimates are required. However, with these cautionary remarks in mind Table 20.2 summarizes the current values in use by ICRP.

**Table 20.2.** *Risk factors for fatal cancers used by ICRP for radiation protection purposes.*

| Tissue or organ | Risk factor per Sv |
|---|---|
| Gonads (hereditary)* | $4.00 \times 10^{-3}$ |
| Breast | $2.50 \times 10^{-3}$ |
| Red bone marrow | $2.00 \times 10^{-3}$ |
| Lung | $2.00 \times 10^{-3}$ |
| Thyroid | $5.00 \times 10^{-4}$ |
| Bone surfaces | $5.00 \times 10^{-4}$ |
| Remainder | $5.00 \times 10^{-3}$ |
| *Total risk* | $1.65 \times 10^{-2}$ |

*Risk of serious hereditary defects being induced in the first two generations due to irradiation of the gonads.

Source. ICRP (1977*b*).

## BIOLOGICAL EFFECTS OF IONIZING RADIATION AND RADIATION CARCINOGENESIS

The processes which ensue from the interaction of radiation with living tissue are so complex that it is not possible with present knowledge to trace a chain of events leading from the absorption of energy to the production of a radiation induced disease. Much experimental radiobiology has concentrated on the lethal action of radiation on living cells, and the scientific understanding of the more subtle and prolonged mechanisms that lead insidiously to cancer is scant. Nevertheless, certain important principles have been established over the last 30 years or so, and an attempt is made to summarize those that are pertinent to the interpretation of epidemiological data.

Ionization, the removal of electrons from the atoms of irradiated tissue, is the major physicochemical process underlying the biological changes due to radiation (Hall 1978; Kellerer and Rossi 1982). Ionizations occur mainly along the tracks of individual charged particles and the pattern of ionization depends on physical properties – for example, charge, velocity – of the particles involved. High-speed electrons are generated when X- and $\gamma$-rays are absorbed in tissue, and the distribution of ionizing events along the paths of these electrons tends to be sparse. By contrast, heavy charged particles such as $\alpha$-particles produce a dense pattern of ionizations along their tracks. These differences between various forms of radiation are denoted by the term 'linear energy transfer' (LET). X-rays are low-LET radiation (about 2 keV/$\mu$m), $\alpha$-particles are high-LET (about 100 keV/$\mu$m), and neutrons occupy an intermediate position (although they are usually classed as high LET). Linear energy transfer is an important factor in determining the biological effectiveness of different types of ionizing radiations. High-LET radiations have a greater biological effect on higher organ-

isms, including man, than X- and $\gamma$-rays when absorbed in equal doses – that is, 1 gray of neutrons is more biologically damaging than 1 gray of $\gamma$-rays. This is because the biological outcome depends on the localized deposition of energy in certain crucial sites. It seems probable that DNA in the cell nucleus is the critical structure that is damaged directly or indirectly by ionizing radiation. The nature of the DNA damage then determines whether the cell will die prematurely when it next attempts mitotic division, or whether a non-lethal change or mutation occurs in its coded information which is then incorporated in its daughter cells and future progeny, eventually resulting in a malignant tumour. If germ cells are affected, the DNA damage could result in sterility (if sufficient cells are killed) or genetic abnormalities in any subsequent offspring.

The hypothesis that DNA mutation by radiation or other carcinogenic agents can lead to the malignant transformation of cells is supported by much clinical and experimental evidence (Hall 1978; Coggle 1983). The exact nature of the damage that is necessary for malignant transformation is unknown, but recent observations on human oncogenes (Logan and Cairns 1982; Krontiris 1983; Rowley 1983) suggest that almost imperceptible point mutations in DNA might be significant. On a microscopic rather than molecular level, chromosome aberrations due to radiation have been studied for over 40 years and these led to the first mathematical formulations relating biological effects to radiation dose. More recently biochemists have been able to detect radiation-induced breaks in one or both strands of a DNA molecule (single- or double-strand breaks), and double-strand breaks may be responsible for the well recognized chromosome aberrations.

For low-LET radiation the yield ($y$) of chromosome aberrations following a dose $D$ can best be described by a linear-quadratic relationship:

$$y = \alpha D + \beta D^2$$

where $\alpha$ and $\beta$ are constants. It has also been postulated that double strand breaks obey the same equation although direct experimental verification has proved more difficult. The biophysical interpretation of this linear-quadratic formula is that the necessary breaks in both strands of the DNA molecule can either result from the passage of a single ionizing particle ($\alpha D$) or from the separate tracks of two particles ($\beta D^2$). Similar formulations also describe quite successfully cell killing, and there is a close correlation between the presence of chromosome aberrations and the number of cells dying at mitosis.

These tantalizing similarities have led to attempts to devise general models or theories of radiation biology (for example, Chadwick and Leenhouts 1981; Kellerer and Rossi 1972) in which DNA lesions and carcinogenesis are also described by mathematical formulae. Thus, the linear-quadratic dose-response relationship has been applied to the epidemiological data for radiation-induced cancer (see pp. 326–7), in order to assess the risks at low levels of dose. Not surprisingly, such far reaching theories have not met with universal acceptance (Goodhead 1982) and they have been criticized on conceptual and empirical grounds. Alternative theories (Alper 1977) stress the importance of active DNA repair after radiation damage and suggest that repair processes themselves might be dose dependent, being saturated at high levels. Earlier radiobiology experiments demonstrated that low-dose rates or fractionation of dosage reduced cell killing, implying that some degree of effective repair could take place under certain circumstances. However, positive evidence of DNA repair by enzymes has been accumulating rapidly in the last few years.

Even though it is very plausible that DNA damage can predetermine malignant change, albeit with an unknown efficiency, there are many other relevant factors, both constitutional and environmental, which may influence the outcome in any individual case. There are limited data from epidemiological studies on the interaction of radiation with some of the more obvious variables which might affect the carcinogenic process. The main factor examined has been age at the time of irradiation and some fascinating evidence has emerged from the continuing study of Japanese A-bomb survivors (Kato and Schull 1982). In general, cancer is predominantly a disease of the elderly and is uncommon in the first three or four decades of life. With the passage of years, survivors who were children or teenagers at the time of the bomb are now reaching the ages at which malignant diseases are more commonly seen in any population, and it is only now that they are showing an excess of certain solid cancers, known to be radiation induced. This has been most striking in the case of breast cancer where an excess in Japanese women who were less than 10 years of age when exposed to radiation in 1945 was detected for the first time in 1982 by Tokunaga et al. (1982). Since then there has been corroboration from a study among American women who received radiation treatment in infancy for supposed enlargement of the thymus gland (Hildreth et al. 1983); curiously the youngest age at diagnosis for both groups was 29 years. Similar patterns have been observed for lung and stomach cancers in the Japanese survivors and, for these tumours at least, the latent period from the time of radiation exposure to the overt expression of a cancer is longer the younger the age at the time of the bomb. In chemical carcinogenesis a two-stage process of tumour induction and promotion has often been demonstrated, and these age effects in radiation carcinogenesis may to a large extent reflect the contributions of endocrine stimulation and co-carcinogenic factors such as smoking. It is not clear whether or not risks of lung cancer from radiation and smoking are additive (Kato and Schull 1982; Edling and Axelson 1983).

These observations for lung, stomach, and breast cancers lend support to the 'relative risk' model which predicts that following a latent period after exposure the risk of radiation induced cancers will be proportional to the natural age-specific cancer risk for that population. The alternative, and administratively simpler theory, is the 'absolute risk' model which assumes that all the excess cases will, after a latent period, be expressed within a certain period of years, the risk of excess cancers then becoming zero. Leukaemia due to external radiation and osteosarcomas due to treatment with injections of radium-224, both seem to follow the latter pattern, but the general applicability of the two models will not be established until an exposed population has been followed to extinction. The implications of the two models for the prediction of the lifetime risk of excess cancers in an exposed population were considered in detail by Myers (1982).

## GENETIC EFFECTS

It is generally estimated that about one person in ten suffers from an inherited genetic defect which will lead to a clinically detectable disease at some stage during their life (UNSCEAR 1982). Genetic defects include aberrations in chromosome structure, variations in the number of chromosomes per cell, and point mutations or changes in the genetic information of the DNA within the chromosomes. As discussed above, radiation can produce chromosomal aberrations and gene mutations and so if germ cells (oocytes or spermatozoa) are irradiated there must be a risk of producing hereditary effects. If the genetic diseases resulting from radiation are dominant or X-linked they would start to appear in the first generation of children and the number of cases would be directly proportional to the rate of mutations. If diseases of multifactorial or recessive aetiologies were involved, the apparent excess in the first generation would be much lower and might continue undetected for many succeeding generations. Also, in these types of disease, the relationship between incidence and the underlying mutational rate would not be straightforward.

Since life has evolved against a continuous background of radiation, one would not expect exposure to artificial radiation to cause any new genetic diseases, but rather to increase the rate of genetic mutations that occur spontaneously. As many spontaneous genetic diseases in humans are of the multifactorial type, it is perhaps not surprising that no epidemiological study to date has convincingly demonstrated any genetic effects of radiation in man. The most recent review by Schull et al. (1981) of data collected since 1946 on the offspring of the atom bomb survivors in Hiroshima and Nagasaki again does not identify any statistically significant genetic effects. There has been no emergence of an otherwise rare genetic disorder comparable with leukaemia in the study of radiation-induced malignancies. However, for the biological indicators studied (which ranged from stillbirth to rare electrophoretic variants of plasma proteins), the observed effects were compatible with the hypothesis that the survivors of the bombings sustained some genetic damage. Schull et al. (1981) used these data to make calculations of the genetic risk in man.

Despite the lack of empirical evidence, there is no reason to suppose that humans are not prone to genetic effects from radiation in the same way as other living organisms. With the exception of the Japanese study, the genetic risk in man has been estimated only by extrapolation from other organisms used in experiments.

The first experiments, in the 1920s and 1930s, used the fruit fly, *Drosophila*. The frequency of gene mutations was found to be linearly related to radiation dose and there was no threshold level below which mutations were not seen. Furthermore, the genetic effects of a given total dose were the same whether it was delivered almost instantaneously or slowly over a period of time: there appeared to be no biological repair of genetic damage. These findings when extrapolated to man led to the belief, widely held for 30 years, that genetic effects were the most important long-term consequence of radiation.

Experiments initiated after the Second World War, using millions of mice studied over several generations, have radically altered these views (see Hall 1978). Perhaps the most important conclusion has been that repair processes do indeed operate between the primary induction of genetic damage and its final expression. There is a substantial dose-rate effect so that extending the period over which radiation is given, greatly reduces the genetic consequences. It also follows that by postponing conception for a period following irradiation the likelihood of transmitting genetic damage is lessened. The length of time necessary for genetic repair in humans is unknown, but following significant gonadal dose medical advice is usually to delay for 6–12 months before a planned conception.

Two main methods of extrapolation have been used to try to scale the genetic risks of radiation from mouse to man (UNSCEAR 1982). The direct method depends on multiplying the risk of a gene mutation per unit of dose in mice by the corresponding number of genes in man. This method has limited application and subsumes enormous uncertainties. The second method employs the doubling dose: that dose of radiation required to double the rate of spontaneous genetic mutations in humans. After reviewing all the available data the Genetic Committee of UNSCEAR assumed a doubling dose of 1 Gy for all genetic effects which was then applied to the natural frequencies of the various categories of human genetic disease in order to estimate the excess that might be expected from radiation. Their most recent estimate for a population continuously exposed to low-LET radiation at a 'low' dose rate of 1 Gy per generation (although a dose of 1 Gy is not low in environmental terms) is that there would be about 2200 extra cases of genetic diseases in the first generation of one million liveborn progeny. This radiation increment is calculated on a natural or spontaneous incidence of approximately 106 000 cases per million liveborn. If time is allowed for all the genetic diseases to be expressed over future generations such that a new equilibrium is reached with an elevated incidence rate for the population, the total increment is predicted to be about 15 000 cases per million progeny. These estimates are slightly lower than the corresponding UNSCEAR figures of five years previously and the genetic risks of radiation have been steadily downgraded by the various scientific review bodies since the early 1960s.

If one accepts and uses the above risk estimates despite the many inherent uncertainties, it should be realized that they apply to doses absorbed by the gonads before or during the reproductive period, that is, all the dose is genetically significant. Therefore, when considering the genetic consequences for a population following its exposure to radiation, some estimate has to be made of the average child expectancy per person on the basis of the age and sex characteristics of the population. A concept that has been used to represent the risk of hereditary radiation damage to a population is the genetically significant dose (GSD): this is defined as that dose which, if given to every member of a population, would produce the same genetic harm as the actual doses received by the various individuals who have been exposed. In the UK it is believed that about 90 per cent of the total GSD to the population from all artificial sources of radiation derives from diagnostic radiology. A survey carried out in NHS hospitals by Darby et al. (1980) estimated the GSD from diagnostic radiology to be $113 \pm 12$ $\mu$Sv. Although the GSD from diagnostic radiology had not increased significantly over the previous 20 years, it was suggested that simple improvements in operational techniques could lead to a substantial reduction. The average annual gonadal dose from natural background radiation is nearly 1000 $\mu$Sv.

Just as different malignant diseases differ in their mortality rates, genetic diseases vary in severity, time of onset, etc., and therefore in their impact on the individual, his or her family, and society at large. UNSCEAR (1982) and ICRP (1977a) have both made preliminary suggestions as to how these seemingly imponderable matters might be quantified and used in developing new standards. In the meantime, many scientists have taken the pragmatic view that the genetic diseases and cancers from radiation are roughly equivalent in importance.

## NON-STOCHASTIC EFFECTS OF RADIATION

Both cancer induction and the genetic effects of radiation have been classified as stochastic effects by ICRP (1977b). That is to say, the probability of such an effect occurring is a function of radiation dose but the severity of the effect does not depend on the dose. By contrast all other biological effects of radiation can be considered as non-stochastic in that their severity varies with the dose. Such effects depend on large numbers of cells being killed by irradiation to the extent that there is some impairment of organ function, either directly or as a result of tissue repair by fibrosis (see Berdjis 1971). There may therefore be a threshold or critical dose below which no effect is seen, whereas no threshold can be assumed for the stochastic processes which are thought to depend on changes within a single cell. One of the aims of radiological protection is to prevent non-stochastic effects by ensuring that an individual cannot approach the threshold dose for any organ. The non-stochastic effects are of great practical importance in radiotherapy where the tolerance of normal tissue is often critical in determining the exact treatment that will be given.

There are three well-recognized acute syndromes that occur in man following exposure to very high, whole-body radiation doses. Two of these syndromes, involving the central nervous system and gut, are uniformly fatal, whereas the bone-marrow syndrome occurs at doses close to the $LD_{50}$ or dose that would be fatal in 50 per cent of people. The value of the $LD_{50}$ for man is not accurately known but is probably in the region of 4 gy for low-LET radiation. At doses of about 5–6 gy survival is very unlikely, although patients have survived up to about 10 gy with intensive medical care including bone marrow transplantation (Barrett 1982).

## COUNTERMEASURES AFTER RADIATION ACCIDENTS

There is a clear distinction between therapeutic measures that might be taken in the case of an individual who has been accidentally exposed to high levels of radiation that are considered to be life threatening, and the steps that might be taken following, for example, the accidental release of radioactive material from a nuclear power station, where a large number of people may receive small doses of radiation. In the former case intensive medical care might be necessary and this would have to be supervised by specialist clinicians. Such treatment could be offered in only a few centres, and it would probably change the outcome in only a small proportion of cases. In the event of a nuclear war it seems probable that no such medical services would be available although casualties from blast and burns would substantially exceed those resulting from radiation (BMA 1983).

Effective public health measures are certainly feasible following the unlikely event of a serious accident at a nuclear power station. Each civil nuclear installation in the UK has a prepared emergency plan that details the appropriate courses of action following an accident. The National Radiological Protection Board has specified Emergency Reference Levels (ERLs) of dose at which certain countermeasures such as sheltering indoors or evacuation should be considered, and these levels have been incorporated into the emergency sites plans. The provision, for example, of stable iodine tablets in order to block uptake by the thyroid gland of radioactive iodine has proved a contentious matter, particularly in the USA (von Hippel 1982; Yallow 1982). In the UK, the NRPB has recommended that tablets be issued to prevent projected thyroid dose equivalents above 250 mSv and that distribution be considered once it appears likely that thyroid doses will reach 50 mSv. If a population of 10 000 people received an average dose of 250 mSv, the ICRP risk estimate suggests there would be about one extra fatality from thyroid cancer.

Although NRPB does not think the very low risk associated with dose equivalents less than 50 mSv justifies the costs of stockpiling and distributing the tablets, the US Food and Drug Administration has advocated just such a policy. In the case of New York City, it has been calculated that an expenditure of approximately $13 million would be necessary to purchase enough tablets for the general population (Simon and Shils 1983). This proposal has been rejected by the local Committee on Public Health. For this public health issue to be resolved within the USA as a whole, one or more of the federal agencies involved will have to modify their views.

## PRINCIPLES OF RADIOLOGICAL PROTECTION

Radiological protection in most developed countries is based on the recommendations of the International Commission on Radiological Protection. The approach is to control doses of radiation which workers or members of the public may receive by requiring that any activity meets the following conditions:

1. No practice shall be adopted unless its introduction produces a positive net benefit, that is, *justification.*
2. All exposures shall be kept as low as reasonably achievable, economic and social factors being taken into account, that is, *optimization.*
3. The dose equivalent to individuals shall not exceed the limits recommended for the appropriate circumstances by the Commission, that is, *dose limitation.*

This three-stage system of dose limitation must be taken as a whole when considering the effectiveness of the protection it provides. Point 1 requires that if humans are to be exposed to radiation by any activity then that activity will result in a gain judged by society to be desirable. If the outcome cannot be so described then the exposure of humans to radiation cannot be justified and should not take place. Point 2 takes account of practical consideratons that no benefits are achievable without some cost. The reduction of the possible effects of the hazard (in this case radiation) can usually be achieved by greater expenditure on safety features. Clearly no society operates with unlimited financial resources so it is necessary to optimize expenditure on the reduction of any hazard. This point is explicit in recommending that such considerations should be taken into account. The methods by which risks, benefits, and costs can be optimized range from professional judgement to sophisticated mathematical theories. Point 3 comes into force whatever points 1 and 2 permit. Whatever the justification or economic argument in support of a particular activity, no normal or routine operation should result in a worker or a member of the public being exposed at or above the dose limit. Emergencies and very special operations are dealt with under separate arrangements.

Dose limits are specified to restrict the risk to those exposed to an acceptable level. These 'primary' dose limits are specified as the amount of radiation to be received in one year. The way in which this dose is to be assessed is described below. In addition to these primary dose limits which have been related to the risk and set at a level by reference to other industrial hazards, a system of secondary and derived dose limits have been devised. Secondary dose limits are quantities related to the source of the exposure and expressed in terms of the actual quantity to be restricted to a level such that the primary dose limits will not be exceeded. In practical situations it is often not possible to measure quantities directly related to the primary or secondary limits and further quantities called 'derived' limits are defined. These are expressed directly in terms of quantities which can be measured. Examples of all three types of limits are discussed below.

The amount of radiation received by a man is described in terms of two quantities; absorbed dose and dose equivalent. The absorbed dose is the amount of energy deposited per unit mass of tissue. Absorbed dose is measured in units of gray where 1 gray is equal to 1 joule absorbed in 1 kilogram. The absorbed energy is not uniformly distributed on a microscopic scale. In particular, different types of radiation will deposit their energies in different ways (see pp. 327–8). This gives rise to different effectiveness of different radiations in producing tissue damage for the same amount of absorbed energy. The quantity dose equivalent is defined in order to take this into account and to avoid the need for different numerical limits for different types of radiation. Dose equivalent is related to absorbed dose by a factor which is dependent on the type of radiation. This factor is complex and energy dependent but for radiological protection purposes is usually simplified by specifying one factor to be applied to each quality of radiation. The product of this quality factor and the absorbed dose is called dose equivalent and is expressed in units of sieverts (in previous units 1 gray (Gy) is equivalent to 100 rads and 1 sievert (Sv) is equivalent to 100 rem).

**Table 20.3.** *ICRP weighting factors for use in calculating the effective whole-body dose equivalent when the body is non-uniformly irradiated. These weighting factors are the fractional contributions of the risk factors for each organ given in Table 20.2*

| Tissue or organ | Risk factor per Sv |
| --- | --- |
| Gonads | 0.25 |
| Breast | 0.15 |
| Red bone marrow | 0.12 |
| Lung | 0.12 |
| Thyroid | 0.03 |
| Bone surfaces | 0.03 |
| Remainder | 0.30 |
| Whole body | 1.00 |

Most radiation exposures result in non-uniform deposition of energy within the body. The organs of the body have different sensitivities to radiation and for general purposes a combined quantity called the effective dose equivalent has been defined. The effective dose equivalent is the sum of the dose equivalent received by each organ multiplied by a weighting factor to take account of the different sensitivities of the organs. Table 20.3 shows the values of these weighting factors proposed by ICRP. The intention behind the use of this quantity is to limit the total risk associated with a non-uniform exposure to the risk which would result from the whole body being irradiated uniformly at the numerical value of the dose limit. The recommended value for this limit is 50 mSv per year. In the case of highly non-uniform radiation where a few organs may be selectively irradiated, a limit which overrides the effective dose equivalent limit is imposed. This limit specifies that no organ shall be irradiated such that it receives a dose equivalent of 500 mSv in any year and the eye shall not receive more than 300 mSv in any year. These are called non-stochastic limits, that is they are designed to prevent non-stochastic effects, such as fibrosis, occurring (see p. 329). Dose limits for members of the public are restricted to levels of a factor of 10 smaller than these.

A particular example of radiation exposures which result in non-uniform radiation of the body organs is from radioactive material taken into the body by inhalation, ingestion, or through a wound into the blood. A special ICRP committee deals with internal irradiation and has published recommendations that give limits on intakes of radioactive materials that will meet the requirements of the primary dose limits (ICRP 1979). The secondary dose limits are called annual limits on intake (ALI). The ALI of a radioactive material depends on a number of factors: (i) the radioactive nuclide present; (ii) the chemical form in which the radioactive nuclide is bound; (iii) the physical characteristics of the intake, such as the particle size and the solubility of the material; (iv) the metabolic behaviour of the element to which the radionuclide belongs; (v) any differences in individuals in terms of age, size, or sex which may influence the metabolic behaviour of material in the body.

Radioactive nuclides with a long physical half-life which belong to elements which either have a long biological half-time in the body or are retained in particular organs, will continue to irradiate the body organs for periods longer than one year. This means that intakes of radioactive material in subsequent years will be added to those from earlier years. To take this into account in restricting the annual effective dose equivalent another quantity is defined called the committed effective dose equivalent. The committed effective dose equivalent is the effective dose equivalent integrated over 50 years following the intake. The ALI is defined as that intake which will result in a committed effective dose equivalent equal to the annual effective dose equivalent limit, namely 50 mSv for workers and 5 mSv for members of the public. The limits to prevent the occurrence of non-stochastic effects override these limtis and for some nuclides will determine the ALI. The ALI is expressed in terms of activity which has units of becquerel (1 becquerel (Bq) is an activity of 1 radioactive disintegration per second – in previous units 1 curie $= 3.7 \times 10^{10}$ Bq). Because of the many factors which affect the value of the ALI, the tables which give these values for all the important nuclides run into several volumes (ICRP 1979, 1980, 1981, 1982).

Intakes of radioactive materials cannot be measured except in the case of deliberate medical administrations. Therefore, control on intakes must act through derived quantities. In the case of inhaled material, control is exercised by monitoring the air concentration and a quantity the 'derived air concentration' (DAC) is defined. The DAC is that concentration which will result in an intake of one ALI by a standard man working in that concentration for 2000 hours. Thus, the DAC is determined by standard breathing rates and the value of the ALI. Values of the DAC for workers are given along with the values of ALI in ICRP tables (1979–1982). Correspondingly, for ingestion the derived quantity is the amount of activity in unit mass of food or drink. Other derived quantities include the amount of contamination per unit area on surfaces and equipment.

Since doses per unit intake of radioactive material will depend on metabolic behaviour and organ sizes, the ALIs to protect members of the public may not be simply a factor of 10 smaller to achieve a factor of 10 less dose. In particular, infants and children among the general population may need to be taken into account explicitly for particular nuclides which may behave significantly differently in young persons. The derived quantities will also be affected, for example, by the considerably higher intake of milk by infants than that for other members of the population. The ICRP has not published ALIs for all these different situations but advice on the most appropriate value to use may be obtained from the National Radiological Protection Board.

A group of workers for whom special protection may be necessary is women of reproductive capacity because deleterious effects such as microcephaly and mental retardation have been shown to result in humans as a result of exposure to moderate or high doses of radiation *in utero* (BEIR 1980). The ICRP believes that the normal dose limits for workers will provide appropriate protection during the essential period of organogenesis, since it is unlikely that any embryo could receive more than 5 mSv during the first two months of pregnancy provided that the exposures are at a fairly uniform rate. Once a women is known to be pregnant, the ICRP recommends that arrangements should be made to ensure that the woman works only under conditions where she is most unlikely to receive more than three-tenths of the dose equivalent limits. It is probable that the next set of ionizing radiation regulations to be adopted in the UK (HSC 1982) will specify separate dose limits for the abdomen for women of child-bearing age and will also recommend special measures to restrict the exposure of pregnant women arising from dispersible radioactive substances.

Situations may arise in plant operations where planned special exposures higher than the normal dose limits may be justified. The ICRP recommends that in these circumstances, whether the exposures result from external radiation or from intakes of radioactive material, a worker does not exceed twice the relevant annual limit on any single occasion and that the sum of such doses over the lifetime of the worker should not exceed five times the limit. They emphasize that such exposures can be considered justified only when alternative techniques cannot be used.

Crucial to the radiological control of the working environment and for protection of members of the public is a system of monitoring and measurement of radiation levels. Unless it is extremely unlikely that workers will reach three-tenths of the annual dose limits, the individual monitoring of workers is recommended. Workers wear a personal dosemeter which measures the dose of radiation accumulated during the monitoring period. These dosemeters are based on the exposure of a film, a thermoluminescent material or some other device which integrates the amount of radiation received. The length of the monitoring period varies according to the level of the radiation expected in the working environment. Where the levels may become very high direct reading or alarm dosemeters are used in addition to the passive integrating devices. The most typical monitoring period in current use in one month. Monitoring of the working environment consists usually of dose rate measurements for external radiation and air sampling for measurements of radioactivity in the atmosphere. Operators of nuclear plant are also responsible for monitoring the general environment in the neighbourhood of their plant. Routine air sampling measurements are made at reference points in the neighbourhood. These serve to ensure the efficacy of the on-site safety precautions and are available should any unplanned release of radioactive materials into the environment take place. These measurements must form part of the comprehensive monitoring programme that is designed to meet clearly defined objectives. The ICRP recommends periodic review of the monitoring programmes, particularly when there has been any major modification to the installation or to the type of operations carried out by the plant. Each plant must meet certain conditions laid down when they are awarded a licence to operate, and the monitoring programme must ensure that these conditions are met.

## SUMMARY

Ionizing radiation as a potential cause of cancer and genetic defects is an important subject for public health. Radiological protection as a discipline has to encompass events on a timescale that stretches from less than a microsecond (when the interaction between radiation and biological tissues is being considered) to the next generation and beyond (when trying to predict possible genetic effects). There is considerable knowledge about many of the processes involved although they are so numerous and complex that our understanding is likely to remain imperfect and incomplete. Nevertheless safety standards have been greatly improved by various national and international bodies so that the risks to workers and the general public from the medical and industrial uses of radiation are now extremely low and compare favourably with the accepted risks from many other environmental hazards. Despite this, fear of radiation remains widespread and is difficult to assuage without sounding complacent.

## REFERENCES

Alper, T. (1977). Hypothesis. Elkind recovery and 'sub-lethal damage' a misleading association? *Br. J. Radiol.* **50**, 459.

Barrett, A. (1982). Total body irradiation (TBI) before bone marrow transplantation in leukaemia: a co-operative study from the European Group for Bone Marrow Transplantations. *Br. J. Radiol.* **55**, 562.

BEIR–Committee on the Biological Effects of Ionizing Radiations, National Academy of Sciences (1980). *The effects on population of effects to low levels of ionising radiations.* National Academy Press, Washington, DC.

Berdjis, C.C. (1971). *Pathology of irradiation.* Williams and Wilkins, Baltimore.

British Medical Association (Board of Science and Education) (1983). *The medical effects of nuclear war.* Wiley, Chichester.

Chadwick, K.H. and Leenhouts, H.P. (1981). *The molecular theory of radiation biology.* Springer, Berlin.

Coggle, J.E. (1983). *Biological effects of radiation.* Taylor and Francis, London.

Darby, S.C., Kendall, G.M., Rae, S., and Wall, B.F. (1980). *The genetically significant dose from diagnostic radiology in Great Britain in 1977.* NRPB-R106. HMSO, London.

Edling, C. and Axelson, O. (1983). Quantitative aspects of radon daughter exposure and lung cancer in underground miners. *Br. J. Ind. Med.* **40**, 182.

Goodhead, D.T. (1982). An assessment of the role of microdosimetry in radiobiology. *Radiation Res.* **91**, 45.

Hall, E.J. (1978). *Radiobiology for the radiologist.* Harper and Row, New York.

Health and Safety Commission (HSC) (1982). *The ionising radiations regulations 1982. Consultative document.* HMSO, London.

Hickey, R.J., Bowers, E.J., and Clelland, R.C. (1983). Radiation hormesis, public health and public policy: a commentary. *Health Physics* **44**, 207.

Hildreth, N.G., Shore, R.E., and Hempelmann, L.H. (1983). Risk of breast cancer among women receiving radiation treatment in infancy for thymic enlargement. *Lancet* ii, 273.

ICRP (1977a) *Problems involved in developing an index of harm,* Annals of the ICEP Publication 27. Pergamon Press, Oxford.

ICRP (1977b). *Recommendations of the International Commission on Radiological Protection.* Annals of the ICRP Publication 26. Pergamon Press, Oxford.

ICRP (1979). *Limits for intakes of radionuclides by workers.* Annals of the ICRP Publication 30, Part 1. Pergamon Press, Oxford.

ICRP (1980, 1981, 1982). Limits for intakes of radionuclides by workers. Publication 30 Parts 1, 2 and 3. Pergamon Press, Oxford.

Kato, H. and Schull, W.J. (1982). Studies of the mortality of A-bomb survivors (cancer mortality 1950–1978). *Radiat. Res.* **90**, 395.

Kellerer, A.M. and Rossi, H.H. (1972). The theory of dual radiation action. *Curr. Top. Radiat. Res. Q.* **8**, 85.

Kellerer, A.M. and Rossi, H.H. (1982). Biophysical aspects of radiation. In *Carcinogenesis in cancer: a comprehensive treatise,* Vol. I (ed. F.F. Becker) p. 569. Plenum Press, New York.

Kletz, T.A. (1971). *Hazard analysis—a quantitative approach to safety* (Symposium series No. 34). Institution of Chemical Engineers, London.

Krontiris, T.G. (1983). The emerging genetics of human cancer. *N. Engl. J. Med.* **309**, 404.

Land, C.E. (1980). Estimating cancer risks from low doses of ionising radiation. *Science* **209**, 1197.

Lowrance, W. (1976). *Of acceptable risk: science and the determination of safety.* W. Kaufman, Los Altos, California.

Logan, J. and Cairns, J. (1982). The secrets of cancer. *Nature* **300**, 104.

Luckey, T.D. (1982). Physiological benefits from low-level ionizing radiation. *Health Physics* **43**, 771.

Myers, D.K. (1982). *Low-level radiation: a review of current estimates of hazards to human populations.* Chalk River Nuclear Laboratories, Chalk River, Ontario.

O'Riordan, M.C., James, A.C., Rae, S., and Wrixon, A.D. (1983). *Human exposure to radon decay products inside dwellings in the United Kingdom.* NRPB-R152. HMSO, London.

Rowley, J.D. (1983). Human oncogene locations and chromosome aberrations. *Nature* **301**, 290.

Royal Society Study Group (1983). *Report—risk assessment.* Royal Society, London.

Schull, W.J., Otake, M., and Neel, J.V. (1981). Genetic effects of the atomic bombs: a reappraisal. *Science* **213**, 1220.

Simon, N. and Shils, M.E. (1983). Potassium iodide: policy in New York. *Science* **221**, 318.

Tokunaga, M., Land, C.E., Yamamoto, T. *et al.* (1982). Breast cancer in Japanese A-bomb survivors. *Lancet* **ii**, 924.

UNSCEAR (1977). *Sources and effects of ionising radiation. Report to the General Assembly, with annexes.* United Nations, E77.IX.1. New York.

UNSCEAR (1982). *Ionising radiation: sources and biological effects. Report to the General Assembly, with annexes.* United Nations E82.IX.8. New York.

Upton, A.C. (1982). Physical carcinogenesis: radiation-history and sources. In *Cancer: a comprehensive treatise,* Vol. 1 (ed. F.F. Becker). p. 551. Plenum Press, New York.

von Hippel, F. (1982). Potassium iodide policy. *Science* **218**, 6.

Yallow, R.S. (1982). Potassium iodide: effectiveness after nuclear accidents. *Science* **218**, 742.

# 21 Iatrogenic hazards

William H.W. Inman

## INTRODUCTION

Fifty years ago the British Pharmacopoeia listed a mere 36 synthetic drugs (Wells 1980). With very few exceptions, the cure or control of serious diseases was virtually beyond the reach of most patients, and doctors could offer only reassurance and palliatives. In the 1930s, however, the health of our society began to be transformed by the dramatic achievements of a rapidly expanding pharmaceutical industry. Sulphonamides in the 1930s, penicillin, tetracycline, and other chemotherapeutic agents in the 1940s, poliomyelitis vaccine in the 1950s, and many other similar discoveries removed much of the fear of early death from infectious disease. With the introduction of streptomycin and para-aminosalicylic acid, the mortality from tuberculosis fell from about 550 per million in 1946 to 12 per million in 1980. Diphtheria virtually disappeared in the 1950s, together with epidemic poliomyelitis, and pneumonia or other infections became a comparatively uncommon cause of death except in the very old or debilitated.

From the 1950s, major advances were also achieved in the treatment of chronic diseases such as hypertension and as a result of the introduction of powerful psychotropic agents there were large reductions in mental hospital admissions.

Longevity and well-being, shorter periods of illness, relief of symptoms, greater mobility, and huge savings in the cost of health care have been achieved at remarkably little cost in terms of the drugs themselves. In 1978, for example, it was estimated that the per capita expenditure on drugs was about £13, compared with an average of £135 spent on alcohol and £320 spent on food (Wells 1980).

Progress, however, cannot be achieved without risk. All effective medicines are toxic to some individuals, and some major disasters have occurred, although fortunately they have been rare.

Some of the earliest organized attempts to enquire into drug toxicity have been reviewed by Wade (1970). Frequently there was a long interval between the introduction of a drug and the recognition of its dangers. For example, sudden deaths attributed to chloroform, which was discovered in 1831, were first investigated by the British Medical Association in 1877, and this drug was not replaced by the much safer agent, halothane, for more than a century. Agranulocytosis was attributed to amidopyrine in 1933, 44 years after its first use as an analgesic and antipyretic. A number of serious accidents have occurred with vaccines: 191 shipyard workers in Bremen developed jaundice after smallpox vaccinations in 1883, 12 children died from contaminated diphtheria antitoxin in Bundaberg, Australia, in 1928, and more than 50 infants died from virulent tuberculosis after a faulty batch of BCG had been used in Lubeck in 1930. A batch of Salk polio vaccine produced by Cutter Laboratories in the USA in 1955, was responsible for paralytic poliomyelitis in several hundred vaccinated children or their contacts.

Disasters caused by the faulty manufacture of synthetic drugs have been relatively infrequent. In 1937, 107 deaths occurred when diethylene glycol was used as a solvent in a sulphanilamide mixture, in spite of the fact that its toxic properties had been recognized at least 16 years earlier (Geiling and Cannon 1938). In 1954, a pharmacist in a small town near Paris prepared an organic tin preparation for the treatment of boils, poisoning 217 people of whom 100 died.

None of these accidents, however, rival the thalidomide experience of 1961, in bringing to public attention the problem of unexpected drug toxicity, and stimulating governments to regulate drug production and to set up systems for monitoring adverse drug reactions. Approximately 6000 abnormal babies were born in Germany, 500 in Great Britain, and smaller numbers in other countries. In Great Britain, the Committee on Safety of Drugs (Dunlop Committee) was established in 1964, and a Medicines' Act, to control the licensing of drugs was passed in 1968. In 1971, this Act became effective and the work of the Dunlop Committee was continued by a reconstituted Committee on Safety of Medicines (CSM). The main responsibility for monitoring the effects of marketed drugs rested on a Subcommittee on Adverse Reactions, whose activities from 1964 to 1980 have been reviewed by Inman (1980). From January 1982 this body merged with other subcommittees under the new title of Safety Efficacy and Adverse Reactions (SEAR). To a considerable extent, the identification of hazards has depended on the collection of anecdotal accounts of adverse drug reactions (ADRs). Similar bodies have been established in more than 20 countries, and the World Health Organization (WHO) has a central collecting office for reports derived from many national centres, currently located in Uppsala.

The arrangements which have been made to monitor drug safety after the thalidomide affair have not prevented further accidents entirely. The two most notable examples are the outbreak of subacute myelo-optic neuropathy (SMON), affecting several thousand patients, mostly Japanese, who used clioquinol as an antidiarrhoeal agent (Kono 1978), and the delayed recognition of the adverse effects of practolol, used to treat heart disorders and hypertension, in many patients in Great Britain and other countries. This latest accident led to a general recognition of the need to develop improved methods of post-marketing surveillance (PMS), and to the establishment, in 1980, of a national scheme for PMS by the Drug Surveillance Research Unit at Southampton University (Inman 1981*a, b*).

## ADVERSE DRUG REACTIONS

Most pharmacologists recognize two kinds of adverse drug reactions (ADRs), sometimes described as type A and type B reactions. Type A reactions may be explained by the pharmacological properties of the drug; they are often dose-dependent, and should be identified during the course of the early laboratory and clinical studies of a new product. Type B reactions are unrelated to the drug's pharmacology and are not usually detectable during the normal pharmacological screening process. They tend to be rare and are often more serious than reactions of the first type. Type B reactions are not usually dose-dependent but they tend to occur in certain types of individuals with acquired, or genetically determined, susceptibility. They are occasionally caused not by the drug itself, but by excipients, such as colouring agents, included in the finished medicine.

Although the above distinction is generally satisfactory, there is almost certainly a need for a third category – type C reactions – to describe events which cannot be distinguished clinically, pathologically, or in laboratory tests from diseases or symptoms which can occur spontaneously in the absence of drug treatment. These reactions may be identified because of an increase in the incidence of a disease after the introduction of a new drug. Thrombosis in women using oral contraceptives is a classic example of a type C event.

To some extent, the method of study required to identify and measure the incidence of adverse reactions is linked to this classification. Type A reactions tend to be common and mild, and should be detected in relatively small numbers of patients during the course of clinical trials. Type B reactions may be very serious, but because of their rarity may only be brought to light in very large studies or by spontaneous anecdotal reporting. Type C events invariably require epidemiological methods for their evaluation.

## POST-MARKETING SURVEILLANCE

In order to secure a licence for marketing, a new drug has to pass a series of rigorous toxicity tests in laboratory animals. It has to be formulated in such a way that it is suitable for use in human patients, and it has to satisfy exhaustive pharmaceutical quality assurance requirements. It is then subjected to clinical pharmacological investigations which include dose-ranging studies, screening for toxic effects, and the study of its metabolism and excretion. This work is frequently done in human volunteers. Later it is tested in clinical trials among patients suffering from the disease for which therapeutic benefit is expected. Later still, if the results are promising, the trials are expanded, and the new drug may be compared with established products in order to determine its relative efficacy and safety and to provide a platform for subsequent commercial development. If the results of laboratory and clinical studies are deemed by the national drug regulatory agency (DRA) to be satisfactory, a licence is granted, and the new drug is marketed.

The whole procedure of laboratory and clinical testing may take as long as 10 years, and only a very small proportion of the new chemical entities prepared by pharmaceutical chemists actually find their way on to the market. Laboratory animals frequently fail to predict toxic effects, which appear later in human trials, or they may identify dangers which preclude subsequent experimentation in man. It is possible that a number of potentially useful medicines are rejected because of toxicity in animals which would not occur in humans. The clinical trials, usually in a few hundred patients, will enable the drug's efficacy to be assessed, but there are severe limitations to their ability to reveal any but the most common side-effects or adverse reactions. If, for example, the true incidence of a particular side-effect is one in 1000, the chance of encountering a single case in a trial of 100 patiens is only 1 in 10. Even if we encountered one case during 10 trials of this size, it is more than likely that we would fail to recognize it as a drug effect. All we can reasonably assume when a new drug is first marketed, is that no unacceptable hazard has been identified during its pre-marketing study. There can be no assurance that serious effects will not occur once the drug is used on a wide scale. This uncertainty arises partly because the number of patients that it is practicable to include in a clinical trial is small, partly because the trial is usually of a limited duration, and partly because the trial may have deliberately excluded certain types of patient who might be unduly sensitive to the drug – for example, pregnant women, children, or the elderly.

Post-marketing surveillance is thus essential for all new drugs. Post-marketing surveillance uses a wide variety of techniques ranging from spontaneous reporting of individual drug experiences to highly organized intensive studies in which both the numerator – for example, adverse reactions – and the denominator – number of patients – can be estimated.

The various methods of PMS which have been developed may be listed as follows: (i) non-systematic reporting; (ii) spontaneous reporting systems; (iii) retrospective studies; and (iv) prospective studies. All these methods are non-experimental in the sense that, once a drug has been marketed, randomization of treatments is not usually possible, as it often is during the clinical trial stage.

Many classifications have been used and there is frequent confusion in terminology. It is believed, however, that all the monitoring systems that have been described can be fitted fairly easily into one or other of these four categories.

### Non-systematic reporting

Many suspected adverse drug reactions have been reported for the first time in the correspondence columns of medical journals. Most frequently these take the form of brief accounts of clinical observations. These reports are frequently incorporated in the Register of Adverse Reactions compiled by the Committee on Safety of Medicines (CSM), as if they had been reported spontaneously to the Committee. They account for approximately 0.5 per cent of the information held on the Register. Indeed, many of them have also been reported to the Committee who have suggested that they should be submitted to a journal in order to stimulate other doctors to report similar observations.

There is no doubt that journal reports are valuable, but the individual case reports are often of doubtful reliability. Once published they cannot be removed, and they are often given undue weight by the popular press. Great care is, therefore, needed before they are used as the basis for regulatory decisions or medicolegal actions. Before publication journal editors sometimes refer anecdotal reports to monitoring centres and to manufacturers for expert opinion.

## Spontaneous reporting systems

A number of the industrialized nations operate spontaneous reporting systems. Doctors are invited to submit reports of suspected adverse drug reactions to a national register, usually organized by a government health department. Many manufacturers also keep their own registers, and in some countries special registers have been set up to deal with certain types of reactions. For example, in 1975, a National Register of Drug-Induced Ocular Side-Effects was funded by the Food and Drug Administration and established at the University of Arkansas and a File of Adverse Reactions to the Skin was established in 1977 at the Free University of Amsterdam (Inman 1980).

In the United Kingdom, the 'yellow card' system was set up by the Committee on Safety of Drugs (later Medicines) in 1964, and its Register of Adverse Reactions now contains more than 100 000 individual reports. The reports are sent to the Committee on the understanding that they will be treated with complete professional confidence and that they will never be used for disciplinary purposes or for enquiries about prescribing costs. Doctors are requested to report their suspicions rather than restrict their reports to reactions which they are reasonably certain were caused by drugs, the motto being 'when in doubt, report' (Committee on Safety of Drugs 1968).

Spontaneous reporting systems are an effective method for generating hypotheses but rarely provide material for testing them. 'Signals' are recognized either because reports of a particular reaction seem to be unexpectedly frequent or because they are of a very serious or unusual nature. The numerator (number of ADRs) is always incomplete because of under-reporting and the denominator (number of patients being treated) is usually unknown. A secondary denominator obtained from estimates of tablet sales, is often available, however, and a rough approximation of the true denominator may sometimes be derived by dividing the number of tablets by the average daily dose and then by the average number of days' treatment most patients receive. Other valuable clues may be obtained by observing the concurrence of two or more reactions – for example, rash and leucopenia – in the same patient, or the receipt of a cluster of reports of a condition which is normally thought to be very rare. Once the reports have been processed, it is also possible to use simple analytical

techniques which greatly increase the sensitivity of the system. Probably the most useful of these techniques is the ADR profile.

### Adverse drug reaction profiles

Lists of reactions that have been reported to a number of therapeutically related drugs are grouped according to the systems affected – for example, skin, gastrointestinal, vascular, and so on. The sum of the reactions in each group is expressed as a percentage of the total number of reports for the drug. The group percentages are then compared, one drug with another. This procedure takes care of the fact that the actual number of ADRs reported may differ widely for different drugs, and it also enables the profiles or patterns of reactions to be compared in the absence of precise estimates of the denominator (Inman 1972).

Prepared in this way, the data may be set out most conveniently in the form of histograms, so that the profiles of therapeutically related drugs may be compared and contrasted.

As Fig. 21.1 shows, some of the profiles for non-steroidal anti-inflammatory agents (NSAIs) reveal similarities between chemically related drugs and some reveal marked differences in the pattern of reactions. For example, it can be seen that the profiles for phenylbutazone and oxyphenbutazone are remarkably similar, with a large relative excess of blood disorders (which appear to be uncommon with the other 14 drugs). With fenbufen, benoxaprofen, alclofenac, and fenclofenac skin reactions predominate, although with diclofenac, a close relative of the last two, the proportion of skin reactions is low. Gastrointestinal disturbances, on the other hand, appear to be prominent with nearly all these drugs, though in some cases they are overshadowed by other types of reaction, and particularly skin reactions.

### Use of spontaneous adverse drug reaction reports

Thromboembolism and the contraceptive pill

The first reports of thrombosis associated with oral contraceptives reached the Committee in May 1964 and, by the end of December that year, the total number of reports was 29 (Inman 1970). By 31 August 1965, 16 fatal and 95 non-fatal cases with thrombosis or embolism had been reported. At this time it was estimated that some 400 000 women, aged between 15 and 44 years were using oral contraceptives. Table 21.1 shows how this number of reports would compare with the number expected in a population of women of this size, based on the Registrar General's report and on the data derived from the hospital in-patient enquiry (Inman and Vessey 1968). There are no large differences between the number of cases reported to the Committe on Safety of Drugs and the number that would have been expected. If it could have been assumed that every case of thromboembolism in a contraceptive pill user had been reported, then the contraceptive pill was probably not a cause of thrombosis, but little confidence could be placed in this assumption. It seemed probable that the reports, particularly of pulmonary embolism, represented a relative excess of mobidity and mortality in oral contraceptive users. This prompted the Adverse Reactions Sub-Committee to

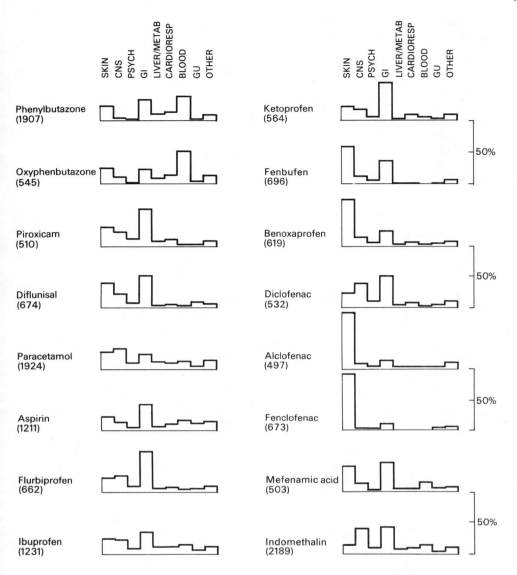

**Fig. 21.1.** Adverse drug reaction profiles of 16 non-steroidal anti-inflammatory drugs. (Source: Committee on Safety of Medicines 1981. Number of patients in parentheses.)

**Table 21.1.** *Observed and expected cases of thromboembolism disease in women using oral contraceptives (Reports to the Committee on Safety of Drugs for year ending 31 August 1965)* *

| Diagnosis | Non-fatal Observed | Expected † | Fatal Observed | Expected ‡ |
|---|---|---|---|---|
| Pulmonary embolism | 46 | 25 | 8 | 2 |
| Cerebral thrombosis | 32 | 16 | 2 | 2 |
| Myocardial infarction | 15 | 16 | 5 | 9 |
| Mesenteric thrombosis | 2 | 1 | 1 | – |
| All reports | 95 | 58 | 16 | 13 |

*Based on estimated population of 400 000 women aged 15–44 years using oral contraceptives.

†Derived from estimates from the Hospital In-Patient Enquiry.

‡Derived from the Registrar General's annual report.

conduct the first case-controlled study which produced statistically significant evidence that the contraceptive pill probably was a cause of thrombosis. This case-control study was based on all deaths of women of childbearing age in England and Wales occurring during 1966. By September, a statistically significant excess had been noted among contraceptive pill users dying from pulmonary embolism. In order to avoid causing public alarm, publication of this evidence was deferred for nearly two years until these results had been repeated in two other studies – one small study of venous thrombosis by the Royal College of General Practitioners set up in September 1966, and a study of hospital patients by the Medical Research Council set up in December of that year. A joint publication by the three groups appeared in 1967 (Medical Research Council 1967; Royal College of General Practitioners 1967; Inman and Vessey 1968; Vessey and Doll 1968). The Committee on Safety of Drugs was probably not given the credit it deserved for this first demonstration of a significant effect of oral contraceptives on the incidence of thromboembolism, but it is worth noting that the yellow card system had produced the strongest of the early signals and that the CSD had not only set up the first of the case-control studies, but produced the earliest statistically valid evidence obtained in any study throughout the world. Moreover, it was largely because of the Committee's work that the other groups were encouraged to investigate this problem.

We have already seen how adverse reaction profiles may be constructed for the various drugs. It is also possible to construct drug profiles for the various reactions. In August 1966, one month before statistical evidence of an association between the contraceptive pill and thrombosis appeared in the report of the Committee's case-control study, an examination of the yellow cards had revealed an unexpected distribution of the reports of thrombosis associated with various brands of oral contraceptive preparations. By that time, some 940 reports of adverse reactions had been received, and of a total of 88 reports of pulmonary embolism, 63 (72 per cent) were associated with products containing mestranol, while only 25 (28 per cent) were associated with products containing ethinyloestradiol. The share of the UK market for the two types of oral contraceptive was roughly equal (Table 21.2), and, provided there were no differences between the two hormones, it would have been reasonable to expect that adverse reaction reports would be distributed in more or less the same way. Remarkably, when all other reactions were compared, their distribution was identical to that of the two hormones in the oral contraceptive market.

**Table 21.2.** *Reports of pulmonary embolism in women using different oestrogens*

| | Products containing mestranol | Products containing ethinyloestradiol |
|---|---|---|
| Share of UK market (per cent) | 52 | 48 |
| Number of reports of pulmonary embolism (per cent) | 63 (72) | 25 (28) |
| Number of other suspected reactions (per cent) | 441 (52) | 413 (48) |

It was appreciated that products containing mestranol generally contained larger doses than those containing ethinyloestradiol. But, because mestranol was a weaker oestrogen, it was thought at this stage that the association with thromboembolic disease might be attributable to some subtle chemical difference between the two forms of oestrogen.

Since no clear evidence of thrombogenicity had at that time been obtained, no further action was taken until considerably more data had been accumulated, a process which took three years. In addition to reports accumulated by the Committee on Safety of Drugs, the Swedish and Danish Government drug monitoring centres provided data from their national registers, together with estimates of sales in those countries. In November 1969, an analysis of reports of thrombosis associated with the use of a large number of different oral contraceptive preparations, revealed that there was a highly significant trend in relative risks, related, not to the two individual oestrogens, but to the total dose of oestrogen contained in each tablet. These data are shown in Table 21.3, in which the estimates of relative risk are shown for each dose level, with 50 μg taken as the unit dose for comparative purposes (Inman *et al.* 1970). Later work on cases reported to the Committee has suggested that the dose of progestogens may also be a factor contributing to the risk (Meade *et al.* 1980).

**Table 21.3.** *Relative risks of thromboembolism related to oestrogen dose-levels*

| Oestrogen | Mestranol | | | | Ethinyl-oestradiol | | Number of reports |
|---|---|---|---|---|---|---|---|
| Dose (μg) | 150 | 100 | 75–80 | 50 | 100 | 50 | |
| Venous thromboembolism | 2.4 | 1.6 | 1.2 | 1.5 | 2.5 | 1.0 | 780 |
| Cerebral thrombosis | 3.9* | 1.4 | 0.8* | 0.6* | – | 1.0 | 79 |
| Coronary thrombosis | 3.0* | 1.4 | 0.3* | 1.3* | 2.1* | 1.0 | 61 |

*Values based on less than 10 reports.

## Halothane jaundice

While it had been recognized for several years that patients receiving halothane on more than one occasion might have a greater risk of developing postoperative jaundice, many anaesthetists assumed that this was simply because such a high proportion of the population had been anaesthetized with this agent. Close examination of the cases reported to the Committee confirmed beyond reasonable doubt that many were caused by halothane, although the true incidence of this complication has not been measured (Inman and Mushin 1974, 1978). The majority of cases had indeed been exposed to halothane more than once and the mortality rate tended to increase with the number of exposures (Table 21.4). The most important observation, however, was that the interval between the latest exposure to halothane and the onset of jaundice was significantly shorter in those patients who had been exposed most frequently. This effect was particularly striking in the subgroup of patients in whom the two most recent exposures had been within a period of less than 28 days.

**Table 21.4.** *Relation between number and timing of exposures to halothane and the onset of jaundice*

| Number of exposures | Days between last 2 exposures | Mean interval between onset of jaundice and last exposure (days) |
|---|---|---|
| **Single exposure** | — | 11.4 (20)* |
| **Multiple exposures** | | |
| Two | >28 | 10.5 (19) |
| | <28 | 5.6 (67) |
| Three | >28 | 7.4 (11) |
| | <28 | 4.6 (40) |
| Four | >28 | 5.5 (8) |
| | <28 | 3.4 (17) |

*Number of cases in parentheses.

The events that followed the publication of these results were somewhat traumatic to the Committee on Safety of Medicines. At least 17 anaesthetists wrote to medical journals to complain about the publication. Several doubted, even at this stage, that halothane was a significant cause of jaundice. Others attacked the Committee for publishing these results on the grounds that an anaesthetist who continued to use halothane might be held responsible if jaundice did develop. Others again suggested that, although a small but definite risk seemed to have been demonstrated, other anaesthetic agents carried a greater risk than halothane which is pleasant for the patient during recovery phase, easy to handle, and very safe even in relatively inexperienced hands.

Eventually, a group of anaesthetists, which included some of the most severe critics of the jaundice hypothesis, collected another series of 203 patients. Each history was examined by a panel of hepatologists. A reduction of the latent interval – between exposure and the onset of jaundice – was found, and the authors conceded that their results confirmed the earlier findings of Inman and Mushin (Walton *et al.* 1976).

## Practolol and the oculomucocutaneous syndrome

The CSM's experience with the spontaneous reporting of adverse reactions to practolol contrasts strongly with the two previous examples. The yellow card system totally failed to identify the serious adverse effects of practolol. This led to an examination of the reasons why adverse events are not always reported and to a reappraisal of the need to develop new methods which did not rely on spontaneous reporting.

In June 1970, after four years of pre-marketing study, the cardioselective beta-blocking agent practolol – used mainly for the treatment of angina and arrythmias – was marketed by ICI under the trade name of *Eraldin*. During the next few years a small number of reports of skin reactions resembling lupus erythmatosus were received by the CSM together with two reports of psoriasis and a single report of conjunctivitis. By the end of 1973, there had been a number of reports of 'exfoliative dermatitis' which would normally be regarded as a very sinister reaction carrying a high mortality. In a letter to the *British Medical Journal* in May 1974, Felix *et al.* drew attention to patients who had developed a rash resembling psoriasis, and they later published a full account of 21 patients (Felix *et al.* 1974). In six patients the rash had developed within one month of starting treatment with practolol, and in the remaining 15 patients it had developed during periods ranging up to 26 months. Three patients had also developed ocular symptoms, including one with bilateral corneal ulceration requiring grafting. One other patient had pleural and pericardial effusions.

In June 1974, Wright, in another letter to the *British Medical Journal*, described a number of patients who had developed ocular symptoms. He subsequently published a full report on 27 patients with eye reactions, 19 of whom had also developed skin reactions similar to those described earlier. He identified this complex of reactions to practolol as the oculomucocutaneous syndrome (Wright 1975). The eye symptoms had developed after periods ranging from six months to four years, and in a number of cases the patients had also complained of deafness and tinnitus. Characteristic of the eye symptoms were diminished tear secretion leading to conjunctival damage and, in some cases, serious fibrotic destruction of the lacrimal apparatus. Five eyes perforated but most cases showed improvement once the drug had been stopped.

A third manifestation, known as sclerosing peritonitis, was reported by Brown *et al.* (1974). Three patients had developed peritoneal thickening and adhesions leading to abdominal symptoms and had required surgery to relieve obstruction.

Up to the time of Wright's original communication, the number of reports of eye problems received by the CSM remained at one. The yellow card system had thus failed to identify the oculomucocutaneous syndrome. This failure resulted not from any defect in the mechanism for reporting adverse reactions but from the fact that doctors had not used the system. Once the syndrome had been described in the *British Medical Journal,* the yellow cards became extremely useful; very large numbers of reports were received and this gave a complete picture of the extent of the tragedy. About 100 000 patients had been exposed to practolol for various periods, and the Committee received nearly 2500 reports. More than 600 reports had mentioned diminished tear secretion, and more than 1000 had other ocular signs, including about 400 patients with corneal ulceration, a small number of whom lost their sight. There were more than 200 reports of sclerosing peritonitis, including 23 deaths, and 370 reports of deafness. The reporting of suspected reactions to practolol, which was almost entirely retrospective, suggested that important side-effects were occurring in at least 2 per cent of the patients. The real tragedy is that the yellow cards were not used very much earlier, as soon as these events occurred.

## *Advantages and disadvantages of spontaneous reporting*

Spontaneous reporting to a central registry is potentially the most efficient and rapid method of detecting problems with drugs and, over the years, has generated very large numbers of hypotheses. It does, however, say very little about actual patients except that their doctor suspects an adverse event to be caused by a drug. The greatest defect in the system is under-reporting and this occurs for two main reasons – doctors may fail to recognize events as adverse reactions or to report those that they have recognized. The first reason is excusable in many cases because many drug effects are indistinguishable from events which occur spontaneously in the absence of treatment. This is particularly true of common events (described earlier as type C reactions) and also of reactions to drugs which have been consumed by the patient without the doctor's knowledge.

The various reasons for the failure to report recognized adverse drug reactions were described in 1976 as the 'seven deadly sins' (Inman 1978). They are: (i) *complacency* – the belief that only safe drugs are allowed on the market; (ii) *fear* of involvement of litigation; (iii) *guilt* because a patient has been harmed by a doctor's prescription; (iv) *ambition* to collect and publish a series of cases; (v) *ignorance* of the requirements for reporting; (vi) *diffidence* about reporting mere suspicions; and (vii) *lethargy.*

In spite of these defects, voluntary reporting has proved its worth on many occasions. The action that is taken by the CSM or other similar bodies is usually undramatic, amounting to little more than the modification of manufacturers' literature or the curtailment of certain indications. Occasionally, a drug has been withdrawn from the market because of the spontaneous reports. Notable examples of this more radical action were benziodarone, a drug used for the treatment of angina, and ibufenac, both of which produced a number of reports of jaundice within a few weeks of their first marketing.

Brief reports on yellow cards can be the starting point for much more detailed investigations of an individual case. The CSM employs around 100 medically qualified field workers who can arrange interviews with reporting doctors and obtain much more detailed information. The same team has been used on a number of occasions to conduct a variety of epidemiological studies.

## Retrospective studies

Retrospective or case-control studies normally start with the identification of patients who have developed the disease of interest and controls who have not. Enquiries are then made retrospectively into drugs that may have been taken and which might have been responsible for the disease. They are thus distinguished from prospective studies in which groups of exposed and unexposed patients are compared and the events which occur are recorded months or even years later. In the three examples of retrospective studies which follow the first two were designed to test a specific hypothesis and the third to generate new hypotheses.

### Thromboembolism and the contraceptive pill

In this study, already referred to briefly on pp. 336–7, transcripts of 499 death certificates of women aged between 20 and 44 years, who died in England, Wales, and Northern Ireland during 1966, were used to identify cases of pulmonary, cerebral, or coronary thrombosis or embolism. Eighteen certificates indicated that the thrombosis was part of a terminal illness such as cancer. Of the remaining 481 patients, 385 were successfully investigated by medically qualified field officers. After follow-up, 51 cases were excluded for various reasons, mainly because cause of death could not be confirmed. Thirty-five medical field officers took part in the study and at each interview with a general practitioner, the records of living women in the same practice were examined to determine whether or not they had been using oral contraceptives. The very simple procedure for obtaining controls was to locate the position in the doctor's file which would have been occupied by the dead women's notes and then work alternately forwards and backwards in the file until an appropriate number of controls of the right age had been selected. Nine hundred and ninety-eight satisfactory controls were available for comparison with the 334 deaths finally available for study, a ratio of almost exactly three controls for every case.

Because the controls had been obtained in the same practices in which a death had occurred, their use of oral contraceptives up to the time of death of the index case was considered to be truly representative of the population in which the index cases had occurred. The death of the index case could not have influenced doctors' prescribing for other women in his practice before that death had occurred, but in order to exclude the possibility that more oral contraceptive users had conditions which would predispose to thromboembolism, cases were further subdivided into three classes. Class A patients had no identifiable predisposing condition, class B had predisposing conditions such as hypertension or diabetes, and class C patients were pregnant or had been delivered during the month before the terminal episode. All the case histories were reviewed by three independent assessors who did not know which women were oral contraceptive users, and it was found that there was close agreement about the presence or absence of predisposing conditions.

The use of oral contraceptives by control patients was closely linked with parity, rising from 5 per cent in nulliparous controls, to 27 per cent in controls who had had four or more babies. Twenty one per cent of 591 controls under the age of 34 years had been using oral contraceptives, compared with only 11.5 per cent of 407 women aged 35 to 44 years.

The observed and expected deaths in class A, for each of the three diagnostic groups, are shown in Table 21.5. Although the number of patients without predisposing conditions is small, it can be seen that there was a highly significant excess of oral contraceptive use by women dying of pulmonary embolism, and a significant excess in the small number of women dying of cerebral thrombosis. The excess in women dying from coronary thrombosis did not quite reach statistical significance.

**Table 21.5.** *Observed and expected deaths of patients with no known predisposing conditions (class A)*

| Diagnosis | Observed deaths | Expected deaths | $p$ |
|---|---|---|---|
| Pulmonary embolism | 16 | 4.2 | < 0.001 |
| Coronary thrombosis | 18 | 11.4 | 0.06 |
| Cerebral thrombosis | 5 | 1.5 | < 0.01 |

With the help of independent estimates of oral contraceptive use, supplied by a market research company, and with data obtained from the Registrar General on the non-pregnant female population of England, Wales, and Northern Ireland in the appropriate age group (5.7 million), it was possible first to check that the oral contraceptive use by control patients was consistent with oral contraceptive sales. Secondly, it was possible to calculate the relative and the attributable mortality in oral contraceptive users and non-users. In women aged between 20 and 34 years, the relative risk was 7.5 and in those aged between 35 and 44 years the relative risk was 7.8. In absolute terms, the attributable mortality was very much lower among those aged 20–34 years, the excess mortality being 2.2 per 100 000 users aged 20–34 years and 4.5 per 100 000 users aged 35–44 years. The statistical technique employed in this particular study has been used by Bradford Hill to illustrate a general application of the principle of standardized death rates in epidemiological studies (Bradford Hill 1971).

### Fatal subarachnoid haemorrhage and the contraceptive pill

In October 1977, the Royal College of General Practitioners published evidence from their long-term study which suggested that oral contraceptives might be strongly associated with fatal cerebrovascular disease (Royal College of General Practitioners 1977). The trial included some 43 000 women. Ten of those who had used the contraceptive pill at any time during the eight years of the study had died from cerebrovascular disease compared with only three control subjects. Of those 10, nine had died from subarachnoid haemorrhage compared with none in the control group. These results caused considerable alarm among oral contraceptive users. A relative risk of this size in at least three million women using oral contraceptives should have produced a considerable increase in the annual mortality from subarachnoid haemorrhage. During the 20 years, 1957–76, the death rate in women of child-bearing age from this cause had remained remarkably constant at about three deaths per 10 000 per annum (Office of Population Censuses and Surveys 1959–78).

In order to resolve this apparent discrepancy, a case-control study was set up along almost the same lines as the study of thromboembolic disease. Death entries for women aged 15–44 years who died from subarachnoid haemorrhage in England and Wales in 1976 were provided by the Office of Population Censuses and Surveys (Inman 1979). To keep the numbers within reasonable bounds, all entries for women aged 15–34 years and alternative entries for women aged 35–44 years were selected for further study. As in the previous investigation, women living in the same practice areas were selected as control subjects. Allowing for failure to make contact with general practitioners and other losses for administrative reasons, this procedure yielded a total of 134 practice-matched case-control pairs for analysis. Although the matching was based only on age, it was found that, in other respects, the case and control populations were closely similar.

In 63 per cent of the cases, the diagnosis had been confirmed at necropsy. Among the remainder, it had been confirmed by angiography or computer tomography, or was considered most likely on clinical grounds. Fifty cases had a history of hypertension with or without renal disease, or of pre-eclamptic toxaemia, in contrast with only 21 control subjects.

Although many doctors had records of prescriptions for oral contraceptives, some were uncertain whether they were in use at the time of death. Current use of oral contraceptives was known definitely in 109 of the 134 matched pairs, and the diagnosis was certain in 77 of the 109. Because of the obvious importance of hypertension in the aetiology of subarachnoid haemorrhage, the data have been arranged in Table 21.6 so that like may be compared with like. The relative risk for diagnostically proved cases was 1.22 (95 per cent confidence limits 0.46 to 3.33). It was concluded that, while a few patients might have developed hypertension as a result of oral contraception, subarachnoid haemorrhage was not a serious cause of concern in healthy non-hypertensive women using the contraceptive pill.

**Table 21.6.** *Current use of oral contraceptives by 77 women with proven subarachnoid haemorrhage and their practice-matched controls in relation to hypertension*

| Hypertension in | Oral contraceptives currently in use by | | | | Total number of pairs |
|---|---|---|---|---|---|
| | Case and control | Case only | Control only | Neither | |
| Case and control | 0 | 0 | 1 | 2 | 3 |
| Case only | 0 | 2 | 2 | 18 | 22 |
| Control only | 0 | 0 | 0 | 1 | 1 |
| Neither member of pair | 8 | 11 | 9 | 23 | 51 |
| Total number of pairs | 8 | 13 | 12 | 44 | 77 |

The discrepancy between the RCGP results and those from other studies suggests that the apparently strong association between oral contraceptives and subarachnoid haemorrhage was likely to have arisen either from chance or from some unidentified confounding factor.

### Congenital abnormalities

The two preceding accounts show how the case-control approach was used to test the hypotheses that oral contraceptives might be a cause of thromboembolism or subarachnoid haemorrhage. In 1969, the Committee on Safety of Medicines started an investigation of the drug-histories during pregnancy of women who had given birth to children with a variety of types of congenital abnormality (Greenberg *et al.* 1979). It was appreciated that, although the voluntary reporting system was working well, it would be most unlikely to identify teratogens. The long gap between exposure during early pregnancy and the delivery of the baby, and the absence of information about normal pregnancies, made it extremely doubtful that sufficient reports would be received to alert the Committee to this type of hazard. Once again the case-control approach was used, but this study was designed to generate rather than test hypotheses. The selection of children was based on the register of abnormal births maintained by the Office of Population Censuses and Surveys (OPCS). The mothers' general practitioners were identified with the help of local community physicians, and then interviewed by the Committee's medical field workers. At each interview a healthy 'control' baby, who had been born within three months of the index case, was selected from practice records. This ensured that, even if the abnormal birth had modified the doctor's subsequent prescribing, the change could not have affected first trimester prescriptions for the mother of the control baby.

Eight hundred and thirty-six case-control pairs which met these requirements were available for analysis. They were 'practice matched' and the matching was also very close with regard to maternal age, parity, and past history of miscarriage. Fourteen per cent of the index cases and only 3 per cent of the control group, however, had a history of congenital abnormality. Eleven of the index cases were members of twin pairs and in three the twin was also abnormal (but not included in the study). One pair of conjoined twins was treated as a single individual. Neural-tube defects were found in 189 (23 per cent) of the index cases, 412 (49 per cent) had oral clefts, 59 (7 per cent) limb reduction deformities or other defects, and 176 (21 per cent) other abnormalities.

The distribution of some of the drugs used by the mothers is shown in Table 21.7. A surprising finding was a significant excess of exposure to hormonal pregnancy diagnosis tests by index mothers. Although the numbers were small, there was also a significant excess of use of barbiturates, mostly as anticonvulsants. When case-control pairs with a family history of abnormality were removed, the ratio of discordant pairs remaining was 2.0, which was not significant. In view of political pressures in the UK after a court decision in the USA against the manufacturer of the anti-emetic *Bendectin* (subsequently reversed after a retrial), the negative relative risk for the similar product *Debendox* is of considerable interest.

As a result of this study, the Committee recommended that, since non-invasive methods for testing were freely available, and since even a small risk was unacceptable, the hormonal test should no longer be used. This study was widely interpreted by the press and consumer activists as providing firm evidence that hormone therapy was teratogenic. More than 100 papers have

**Table 21.7.** *Use of drugs during early pregnancy by mothers of 836 abnormal babies and 836 normal control babies*

| Class of drug | Case and control | Case only | Control only | Neither | Total number of pairs | Discord- ant pairs only |
|---|---|---|---|---|---|---|
| Hormonal pregnancy test | 20 | 73 | 35 | 708 | 836 | 2.09* |
| Hormonal support of pregnancy | 2 | 17 | 10 | 807 | 836 | 1.70 |
| Oral contraceptive | 0 | 11 | 10 | 815 | 836 | 1.10 |
| Doxylamine† | 13 | 63 | 75 | 685 | 836 | 0.84 |
| Promethazine‡ | 4 | 41 | 37 | 754 | 836 | 1.11 |
| Meclozine‡ | 6 | 28 | 35 | 767 | 836 | 0.80 |
| Benzodiazepines | 2 | 60 | 42 | 732 | 836 | 1.43 |
| Antibiotics | 2 | 60 | 42 | 732 | 836 | 1.43 |
| Barbiturates | 1 | 27 | 12 | 796 | 836 | 2.25** |

\* $p < 0.01$ $\chi^2 = 5.03$.
\*\* $p < 0.05$ $\chi^2 = 12.68$.
† One component of Debendox.
‡ Components of other anti-emetics.

appeared on the role of sex hormones in congenital abnormality, but the overall balance of the evidence appears to be strongly against this hypothesis. Test cases against the manufacturers of one of the preparations have recently been withdrawn after counsel for the plaintiffs had examined the testimony of more than 20 expert witnesses who had independently examined all these papers in preparation for the defence.

Studies of this type are liable to many forms of bias. Since the interviews with doctors were necessarily lengthy, they were unpopular with both the interviewers and the general practitioners concerned. At the start of each interview, both parties knew which baby was abnormal. Consequently, less effort may have been made to ascertain control histories. There had been earlier publicity about this problem which could have led to biased selection of mothers. There was no suggestion of any effect on a specific organ. Cases and control subjects were not matched for social class. There was no record of the reasons why patients required a pregnancy test and no details about what attempts, if any, the women might have taken to terminate unwanted pregnancies.

Case-control studies designed to generate hypotheses are of great value, provided their limitations with regard to proving causal relationships are clearly recognized. Public action should rarely be taken on the results of a single case-control study. Experience has also shown that studies in which the total number of discordant pairs is small – that is, less than 100 – or in which the relative risk is small – that is, less than 5 – call for exceptional care in interpretation. Confounding factors are often responsible for statistically significant differences, especially confounding by diagnosis, selection, or observer bias. Moreover, in many studies, as was probably the case in this example, it is usually impossible to identify all the biases.

**Prospective studies**

Cohorts of patients for a prospective study may be assembled in several ways. They may be groups of patients sharing certain demographic characteristics, such as married women of child-bearing age, or patients suffering from certain diseases, such as diabetes or hypertension, or patients taking a particular drug.

Some epidemiologists believe that the prospective approach is preferable because it may be possible to eliminate the concealed biases which often confound retrospective studies. Certainly, prospective studies have the advantage that more than one beneficial or harmful effect may be studied simultaneously. They also enable both relative and absolute risks to be determined. They also, however, suffer from certain major disadvantages. The number of patients required to enable infrequent or rare events to be detected and measured may be very large and thus a study may be very expensive. Sometimes a prospective study has to be very prolonged in order to yield answers to the questions asked. Prospective studies of carcinogenicity may take 25 years, for example, and may thus be an unattractive proposition for a worker who expects to retire from active research before the study is completed. Except in situations in which treatment can be randomized – that is, experimental studies – and where those who observe or record the observations are unaware of which treatment is being used, even the well-known sources of bias cannot be eliminated. In a study of 46 000 women, which was started by the RCGP in 1968, for example, it seems probable that some of the differences in the incidence of diseases occurring in users of oral contraceptives and control subjects who never used them, may be the result of differences between these groups of women which were present before entry into the trial. The actual decision a woman takes on whether or not to use the contraceptive pill could well be related to aspects of her constitution or outlook on life which might be reflected later in the study and attributed incorrectly to the use of oral contraceptives.

In spite of these differences, non-experimental prospective observational studies can be of considerable value in post-marketing surveillance, especially as a means of generating hypotheses. In western society, nearly all patients with important signs or symptoms of disease receive some form of treatment, and untreated control subjects are hard if not impossible to find. Nearly all judgments are based on relative rather than absolute differences between groups of patients receiving various types of treatment.

A new and very promising technique, known as prescription-event monitoring (PEM), will be discussed in some detail because of its potential for studying, at relatively low cost, substantial cohorts of patients treated with most of the new drugs marketed for use in general practice. It is a prospective method in which the treatment cohorts are identified shortly after the drug has been administered for the first time.

*Prescription-event monitoring*

Prescription-event monitoring (PEM) is a modification of the concept of recorded release, first proposed in 1976 (Inman 1978). The earlier proposal was that certain medicines should be designated as 'recorded drugs' and their use limited to prescription by doctors who agreed to participate in the recorded release scheme. Each doctor would be issued with a specially prepared prescription form. Using pressure-sensitive paper, two copies would be made of the initial prescription.

The first copy would be posted immediately to a monitoring centre, and the second copy retained in the patient's notes so that significant events which occurred subsequently would be recorded. On receipt of fist copy, the monitoring centre would issue the doctor with a pad of prescriptions, personalized for the individual patient, which would be used each time the patient returned to the surgery for a further prescription. The recorded. On receipt of first copy, the monitoring centre would on Safety of Medicines, but it was generally felt to be too complicated, and a further variant, known as the Retrospective Assessment of Drug Safety (RADS), was also turned down by the authorities, mainly on economic grounds. In anticipation of this decision, a Drug Surveillance Research Unit (DSRU) was set up at the University of Southampton in 1980.

All prescriptions written by GPs in the UK are processed centrally by the Prescription Pricing Authority (PPA) so that chemists may be remunerated for the prescriptions they dispense. Up to 300 million prescriptions are processed each year, originating in the 90 Family Practitioner Committee Areas of England. Each prescription identifies a doctor, a patient, and one or more drugs that have been prescribed. Prescription-event monitoring is restricted to England, for reasons which at first sight may appear rather curious. Many prescriptions do not include the full name of the patient or the complete address. Nevertheless, the patient's surname and initials are usually sufficient to allow a GP to locate the appropriate medical records rapidly. In Wales and Scotland, however, an individual practitioner may have on his list a comparatively large number of patients with an identical surname – for example, Jones, McDonald and so on. This would make it difficult for the practitioner to retrieve the correct notes rapidly and, indeed, with a frequently used drug, it is probable that he will have prescribed it for a number of patients with the same surname and even the same first name.

The number of patients required in the screening programme depends on the magnitude of the risks which it is intended to detect. To be 95 per cent certain of detecting a unique event affecting one per cent of a population would require a minimum of 300 observations. Detection of a risk of 0.1 per cent requires a minimum of 3000 observations. Since it seemed unlikely that all doctors would respond to the questionnaires, and because some medical records would be incomplete or patients impossible to trace, it was decided that the basic cohort should comprise the first 10 000 patients who receive a new medicine.

The Prescription Pricing Authority (PPA) employs approximately 2000 pricing clerks each of whom processes an average of 150 000 prescriptions in one year. They can memorize the names of up to four drugs at a time, and while carrying out the pricing procedure, they temporarily isolate all prescriptions for these four drugs so that they can be photocopied before returning them to the main pricing stream. The photocopies are then posted in regional batches to the DSRU. The batches are then sorted into sub-batches for individual doctors. More than one doctor in the same general practice may have prescribed for the patient over a period of time. The patient's name and an abbreviated address, and the date of the prescription are entered on microcomputer disks and, as each subsequent batch of prescriptions is received, they are checked against the prescriptions previously identified in the same practice. In this way, it is possible to build up a complete month-by-month record of prescribing for individual patients. In the case of new drugs, assuming that PEM has been initiated at the point of first marketing, all treatments may be identified from the moment they start. In the case of drugs which may be used for control purposes, however, it is not possible in the first batch to determine which patients are starting treatment and which may have been on treatment for some time. In order to obtain suitable contemporary control subjects for patients treated with new drugs, it is possible to identify new treatments with older drugs by following the prescriptions for several months and selecting, as control subjects, those patients who appear to be new to the system after PEM has been running for a few months.

Once adequate numbers of patients have been assembled, the identifying information and certain details, such as the date of the prescription, are transferred automatically on to the Drug Surveillance Research Unit's (DSRU) green forms (see Fig. 21.2). These forms are extremely simple, asking the doctor merely to provide information about the indication for treatment, whether or not treatment has been continued, and any event that may have occurred. Each form carries a definition of an event and includes a simple example, which

Fig. 21.2. Drug Surveillance Unit green form for prescription-event monitoring.

seems to have been proved to be an extremely effective way of defining events; 'a broken leg is an event; if more fractures were associated with this drug they could have been due to hypotension, CNS effects, or metabolic bone changes'.

Events include any new diagnosis, any reason for referral to a consultant, or admission to hospital – for example, operation, accidents, or pregnancy – any unexpected deterioration (or improvement) in current illness, any suspected drug reaction, and any other complaint which was considered of sufficient importance to enter into the patient's notes. ·

Subsequent green forms will include a request to provide the patient's national health registration number so that, if necessary, the record may be 'flagged'. When the patient dies, the National Health Service Central Register can notify the DSRU of the date and cause of death. This procedure could facilitate long-term monitoring for effects of drugs on the incidence of disease and might also be helpful in comparing the efficacy of drugs. It is possible, for example, that patients treated with one drug, survive longer than those treated with a different drug and that fewer patients treated with the first died from the effects of the disease that was being treated.

From the general practitioners' point of view, the procedure is very simple. Having located the notes, they need only to insert the indication for the drug in the appropriate position on the form and then list any events which have come to their attention using 'key words' copied from their own notes. They do not need to give opinions as to whether the events are related to the use of the drug.

Event-reporting requires no medical judgment, and it is perfectly feasible for a practice nurse or secretary to abstract the case notes and provide the essential information. Since the doctor need not comment on causality, there is less medicolegal risk than in the reporting of a suspected adverse reaction, which implies admission that the drug prescribed may have been responsible for damage to the patient. If practolol had been studied by PEM it is almost certain that the syndrome it caused would have been identified long before 100 000 patients had been exposed to risk. Records of psoriasis or conjunctivitis would have alerted the DSRU because they would have occurred much more frequently than with another beta-blocking drug used as a control.

From 1 January 1981, the DSRU started to collect prescriptions for four drugs and, by mid-1982, a total of 10 drugs were being processed. They included two non-steroidal anti-inflammatory agents (NSAI), three hypotensive drugs, three antibiotics, and two drugs used for the treatment of peptic ulceration. The first follow-up exercise was started in January 1982, using the two NSAIs to test the system. In order to avoid the possibility of any bias which might modify doctors' prescribing habits, neither the general practitioners nor the manufacturers of the drugs were informed about which drugs had been chosen until the collection of prescriptions had been completed. Since the first experiment was designed primarily to test the system rather than the drugs, the two NSAIs were selected entirely on the basis of sales forecasts, and in the hope that approximately 10 000 prescriptions would be obtained during the first month. Heavy promotion of one of the two products, *Opren* (benoxaprofen), greatly increased its use in early 1981. Instead of the predicted 10 000 prescriptions for

January, the DSRU received more than 70 000, and the prescriptions for the second drug *Lederfen* (fenbufen) were reduced to about 5000 prescriptions. All the prescriptions for fenbufen and approximately one in every six of those for benoxaprofen were selected for the first experiment. Nine days before dispatching the questionnaires, the Director of the Unit wrote to all 23 000 GPs in England, describing the scheme and enclosing reprints of two papers which had been published nine months earlier (Inman 1981*a, b*). Within a few days, completed green forms started to be returned and, although most of the green forms were received within the first four weeks, small numbers of forms continued to be returned over the next six months. A total of 6130 (52.6 per cent) of the *Opren* forms were returned together with 2137 (52.0 per cent) of the *Lederfen* forms. Of these 3.2 per cent of the *Opren* forms and 3.3 per cent of the *Lederfen* forms were void, usually because the notes were unobtainable, sometimes because the patient had left the practice or the doctor had retired or died. This left slightly less than 50 per cent of the forms available for analysis. Two thousand six hundred and ninety seven of the *Opren* forms and 873 *Lederfen* forms described one or more events.

Earlier in this chapter, the technique of adverse reaction profile analysis was described. Adverse event profiles can be constructed in exactly the same way, and the profile of events of various types is shown in Fig. 21.3. Reports of photosensitivity, together with thickening and loosening of the finger nails (onycholysis), account for most of the difference, and in almost all the other body systems there was no appreciable difference in the frequency of events. Table 21.8 shows the results in more detail. The ratio of forms returned was 2.9 in favour of *Opren* and, with certain exceptions, the ratio of events was similar or even sometimes identical to this figure.

While photosensitivity and onycholysis were unique to *Opren*, the ratio of all other skin reactions was precisely what would be expected if no difference between the drugs existed.

**Table 21.8.** *Some results of prescription-event monitoring of two non-steroidal anti-inflammatory agents*

|  | Opren (benoxaprofen) | Lederfen (fenbufen) | Ratio Opren Lederfen |
|---|---|---|---|
| Green forms dispatched | 11 646 | 4113 | 2.8 |
| Green forms returned | 6130 (52.6%) | 2137 (52.0%) | 2.9 |
| Green forms void | 367 ( 3.2%) | 134 ( 3.3%) | – |
| Green forms available for analysis | 5763 (49.5%) | 2003 (48.7%) | 2.9 |
| Number of events recorded |  |  |  |
|   Photosensitivity | 252 | 0 | – |
|   Onycholysis | 90 | 0 | – |
|   Other skin events | 389 | 134 | 2.9 |
|   CNS and psychiatric | 362 | 130 | 2.8 |
|   Ocular and auditory | 168 | 56 | 3.0 |
|   Gastrointestinal | 622 | 216 | 2.9 |
|   Respiratory | 326 | 108 | 3.0 |
|   Cardiovascular | 314 | 101 | 3.1 |
|   Cystitis, dysuria, frequency | 104 | 20 | 5.2 |
|   Other genitourinary | 136 | 51 | 2.7 |
|   Other events* | 496 | 188 | 2.6 |
| All deaths | 171 | 56 | 3.1 |

*A large number of·events linked with the arthritic conditions being treated are not included in this Table.

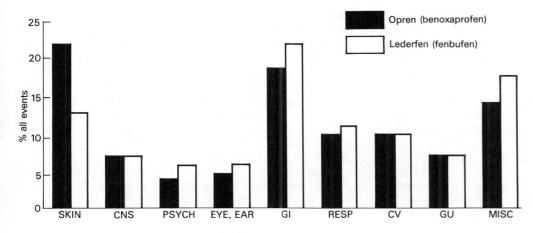

**Fig. 21.3.** Event profiles for benoxaprofen and fenbufen.

This was also true for central nervous, gastrointestinal, respiratory, and cardiovascular events. There was a marked excess of reports of cystitis, dysuria, and frequency in the *Opren* group. This has been attributed to the fact that the drug and its metabolites are acidic and probably cause chemical irritation of the bladder. Only three of eight cases of jaundice in the *Opren* group were thought to have been possibly attributed to it.

## SOME GENERAL CONSIDERATIONS

### Complementary roles of spontaneous reporting and prescription-event monitoring

Of the many methods which have been developed, mostly since the thalidomide disaster, voluntary reporting systems and various types of intensive monitoring in hospital patients have been the most successful. Individual pharmaceutical companies have undertaken post-marketing clinical trials but, however well these may have been done, the fact that many of them are promotional has tended to diminish their credibility. Another important limitation is that they are very often uncontrolled because a competitor is unlikely to agree to the use of its product for what may turn out to be an adverse comparison. Drug company post-marketing surveillance tends to be expensive, because participants are paid to collaborate, but the quality and quantity of information can be very substantial. Prescription-event monitoring conducted on a national scale, by an independent, non-governmental, and non-regulatory agency, may well prove to be the most effective of all the PMS methods so far developed. It should complement rather than replace voluntary reporting systems, and has the advantage of being considerably less expensive.

Prescription-event monitoring, unlike voluntary reporting, cannot be applied to all drugs at the same time, nor can it be expected to provide information about adverse reactions during the earliest months of marketing. Spontaneous reporting of the earliest clinical experiences is vital, but because of the publicity it attracts, it may sometimes give a distorted impression of apparent dangers. The post-marketing experience with benoxaprofen is an example of this. During its second year of use in general practice, a cluster of anecdotal reports of cholestatic jaundice appeared in the UK medical journals. Between April and June 1982, about 18 months after the drug was first marketed, 14 cases, 11 of them fatal, had been described in six letters to the *British Medical Journal* or the *Lancet*. Remarkably, 11 of the 14 cases originated in Northern Ireland or Scotland, and only three in England. All but one of the patients were women and all were extremely elderly (average age 77 years). About half had been treated concurrently with diuretics. One doctor in Northern Ireland had reported that all six of the patients he had treated had died, an experience that was quite out of line with that of other doctors who, by that time, had probably prescribed the drug for at least half a million patients. This report, and a few other letters describing similar cases, caused considerable concern. Support from a number of doctors who had found the drug to be valuable and who had not encountered cases of jaundice followed, but the Department of Health and Social Security decided to suspend the licence for the drug on 3 August 1982.

Although intended to test the method rather than the drug, the first experience with PEM which happened to include benoxaprofen, tended to put its toxicity into perspective. Jaundice in elderly patients taking diuretics was identified by PEM, but the signal was very weak, depending on, at most, three very doubtful histories. It was certainly not sufficient to justify special mention in the preliminary report that had been circulated in February 1982. What the journal letters, the CSM reports, and the PEM results had in fact identified was a subgroup of patients with impaired renal function taking large doses of benoxaprofen. During the preliminary analysis of the PEM data on the drug it had been noted that about 40 per cent of the original cohort of patients treated, mostly for the first time, in January 1981, were still taking the drug in January 1982. Photosensitivity had led some to interrupt treatment temporarily, while others had continued to take the drug in spite of it because of the benefit they were experiencing. Suspension of the licence for benoxaprofen, undoubtedly an effective means of preventing future toxicity – however rare it might be – also precluded use by a small but important population of patients of a drug which many had found to have unique advantages in pain relief and prevention of further joint destruction.

The only two clear-cut examples of the use of voluntary reports to test a hypothesis (thromboembolism and oestrogen content of the contraceptive pill and halothane jaundice) have already been quoted in this chapter. Voluntary reporting is mainly of use as a means of generating hypotheses. Prescription-event monitoring, on the other hand, can do both. New hypotheses will emerge during routine PEM, and the ability to collect and store very large numbers of prescriptions, each of which identifies a doctor, a patient, and a drug, should prove to be of great value as an insurance against difficulties that may be experienced in identifying suitable cohorts for future epidemiological studies.

Both voluntary reporting and PEM will tend to generate more hypotheses than can be tested by those operating these two types of system. Both groups need to encourage others to test their hypotheses using large-scale intensive surveys in hospital or general practice, extended clinical trials, or small-scale laboratory or pharmacological investigations into the aetiology of possible associations between drugs and events. Both groups, together with those who are subsequently involved, need to be protected against the effects of irresponsible reporting by the media, or premature decisions that may be forced on regulatory agencies for the same reason.

### Use of brand names

Prescription-event monitoring depends on the ability of prescription pricing clerks to memorize the names of drugs that are to be selected. Four names seem to be a manageable number at any one time, and all prescriptions bearing these four names can be extracted and copied for the DSRU. There has been some criticism over the use of brand rather than generic names, but it should be pointed out that the increasing tendency to encourage doctors to use generic names will adversely affect not only PEM, but other forms of post-marketing surveillance which are of direct benefit to patients.

Widespread use of generic names for unique branded products would involve the pricing clerks in the selection of prescriptions written in both ways, and this would reduce by half the number of drugs that could be studied at any one time. Fortunately, most doctors use the brand name, especially when prescribing a new drug for the first time.

Prescription-event monitoring is not the only scheme that would suffer if the use of generic names became widespread. In any monitoring system it is always desirable to be able to identify precisely the source of supply of the material. Subtle differences in formulation or bioavailability may have profound effects on the patient's response to treatment. Frequently, a brand name is the only means of identifying a complex mixture. The relative excess of reports of thrombosis with certain brands of oral contraceptives has already been referred to. After publication of this observation, and on the basis of other studies which had confirmed an association between the use of oral contraceptives and thrombosis, brands containing the larger doses of oestrogen were abandoned, and many thousands of lives may have been saved. These observations were only possible because doctors had used the brand names when completing their yellow cards.

There are a number of other disadvantages of using generic names in prescribing, both for patients and for drug epidemiologists investigating possible safety hazards. Brand names are selected so that they can be remembered easily, by both doctor and patient, and this is helpful when examining case notes, particularly when the examination is carried out by people who are not expert in drug terminology. The drug epidemiologist frequently benefits from the expert technical advice available from the manufacturers of branded products and can make use of their library facilities. Finally, from the patients' point of view, the prescription of a generic product may diminish their chances of compensation in the event of an accident. Humanitarian, out-of-court settlements on damaged patients are unlikely if the source of supply is the Far East or a communist-bloc country in Europe.

### Establishing cause and effect

While it is quite easy to generate hypotheses, either by astute observation of individual patients, or by recording a signal during PMS, it is often quite another matter to prove a causal link between drug and event. If a patient collapses within seconds of an injection of a drug such as penicillin, to which he is known to have reacted on an earlier occasion, it may be reasonable to attribute his collapse to the drug. Much more frequently, however, classes of events are clinically indistinguishable from processes which can occur spontaneously without apparent cause, such as cancer, congenital abnormalities, heart disease, or diabetes. Thus it is almost always necessary to conduct epidemiological studies which measure the frequency of the event in treated or untreated populations, and to examine the data carefully to exclude confounding factors. Even if a statistically significant relationship between a drug and an event is demonstrated, it may still be impossible to distinguish those individuals among the drug-treated groups who suffered from taking the drug, and those who could have suffered the event without it. This difficulty is of considerable legal as well as scientific importance, since drug epidemiologists are increasingly drawn into the courts. In practice we can only be reasonably certain of causality in the individual when patients treated with the drug suffer the event very commonly, while those who are not treated develop the event very rarely. When dealing with emotive topics, such as congenital abnormality or thrombosis and the contraceptive pill, it is important to remember that both types of event are common in the general population and that it is never possible to apportion blame in an individual case.

### Bias

An extensive review of the biases which may affect post-marketing epidemiological studies is beyond the scope of this chapter, but it is worth highlighting some of the biases particularly likely to interfere with drug-safety studies. Possibly the most important barrier to effective PMS is that created by premature publicity. Not only may this harm patients by causing them to lose confidence in a treatment which is generally safe, it may also make it almost impossible to set up or complete the studies required to establish safety. Occasionally, as a result of adverse publicity, the drug disappears before there is time to decide if the publicity was justified. Publicity affects patients, prescribers, and investigators, and may introduce bias at almost every phase in the development and surveillance of a drug.

Three classes of bias are particularly likely to influence investigations of drug safety. The first is *diagnostic bias* (closely related to referral bias). The question has often been asked whether or not women taking the contraceptive pill are more likely to be diagnosed as suffering from deep venous thrombosis if they are known to be using oral contraceptives, or are more likely to be admitted to hospital with somewhat less severe symptoms than would otherwise justify such a diagnosis or referral. Is a contraceptive pill user more anxious about the possible consequences and is she more likely to put pressure on her doctor to investigate her symptoms? Alternatively, a condition might be masked by treatment and therefore underdiagnosed. An example of this might be the early symptoms of gastric cancer, masked by the administration of cimetidine used to treat what was thought to be a simple peptic ulcer. Cancers could be unmasked after patients had been accepted into a trial of this drug, and it is even possible that the drug might be blamed.

The second type of bias, which is particularly difficult to allow for in case-control (retrospective) studies, is *investigator bias* brought about by previous knowledge of what treatment has been given or what abnormality has occurred. Ideally, the investigator should not be aware of whether the patient is an index case or a control, and should approach the interview or case-records of either type of patient with equal vigour. Often this is impossible because, for example, the index case may be dead and the control subject living, or it may be obvious from a cursory inspection of the notes what treatment had been taken or what abnormality occurred. Conversely, the patient's doctor may go to more trouble to provide the required information if he knows that a particular patient may be of special interest to the investigator.

The third, and possibly most important, bias is *recall bias*. It is especially likely to influence the results of studies which depend on patient interviews and, if the topic of interest has been the subject of publicity, it often rules out the possibility of drawing valid conclusions from the study. The mother of a baby with a congenital abnormality, for example, who has read in the papers that a possible explanation has been offered, will be more likely to recall exposure to the suspect drug than one who has borne a healthy infant.

All three sources of bias may be exaggerated by the fact that sick patients seek and receive more attention than fit ones. Sick patients will be attended by the doctor more frequently and their notes are therefore likely to be more comprehensive. They will be more knowledgeable about their diseases and therefore better able to recall important factors of past history or investigations. Both patients and doctor will be more likely to help the investigator if they know what drug or what possible complication is involved.

It is doubtful if any epidemiological study has ever been free from one or more biases of this type, but the risk of false conclusions may be substantially reduced by the application of one simple rule. Wherever possible conclusions should be based exclusively on observations that have been recorded in the patient's records *before* the event occurred. To this may be added 'beware of conclusions based on what the patient or the attendants think they remember after the event, especially if the event itself has been publicized'.

In the unlikely event that all these biases could be taken care of, there is still the major problem of *confounding bias* which may make it impossible to distinguish events caused by the disease which is being treated from those caused by the treatment itself. Congenital heart disease, for example, has been associated with the use of insulin, but is the true cause of the defect the mothers' diabetes? Women with abnormal vaginal bleeding are more likely to be admitted to hospital, more likely to be treated with sex hormones, and more likely to deliver abnormal babies. The last statement is true also when no treatment is given.

## ADVERSE DRUG PUBLICITY

We have already seen how adverse drug publicity may damage or even destroy our attempts to draw scientific conclusions from epidemiological studies. Good news about a drug's efficacy rarely attracts the same attention as bad news about its alleged toxicity. The contraceptive pill, congenital abnormalities, and fear of cancer are particularly emotive topics and there can be little doubt that much harm has been done from time to time by inaccurate and irresponsible reporting. Gillie (see Inman 1980) has admitted that while the scientist aims for 100 per cent of the truth, 'if a journalist is able to capture 75 per cent of the truth then he reckons he has done well'.

Fortunately, the effects of adverse publicity are often as ephemeral as the journalist's interest in the subject. When challenged about the accuracy of an article in a Sunday newspaper, the journalist's classic reply is 'Ah, that was yesterday's story. Now I am working on something else'. But the consequences of inaccurate publicity can be very harmful. Death or unnecessary suffering on sudden cessation of treatment after reading a news story, pregnancies after the latest contraceptive pill scare, and false hopes of compensation leading to prolonged misery and sometimes substantial loss of savings by members of patient action groups, are but a few of the results of our failure to find a satisfactory method of communicating information about drug safety and efficacy.

It is not only the journalists who get it wrong. Doctors and editors of medical journals will tend to publish accounts of rare and interesting events, while undramatic accounts of efficacy or non-toxicity may not be submitted for publication or may not be published. This is termed *positive results bias* by Sackett (1979) or, if the topic is emotive, *'hot stuff bias'*. Review articles are often one-sided simply because a reviewer does not have access to the unpublished data.

Another very influential group are the consumer activists and politicians who have tended to promote the notion that allegedly drug-damaged people are an elite, demanding extraordinary care and astronomical sums in compensation. All too often they seem to take advice from laymen, especially the so-called investigative journalists, ignoring or even failing to seek that of the researchers who are familiar with the data and their limitations.

Finally, we have the 'septic poltergeists who hover around the beds of those who have suffered adversity and make a good living from the pickings' (Inman 1981c). Although an unpopular view in the eyes of the legal profession, insurance rather than litigation would seem to be the best solution to the injured patient's problems. Whatever the cause of the injury, whether it be a spontaneous illness, a physical accident, or the result of unexpected drug toxicity, the injured person deserves the highest standard of care that society can provide. This must be instantly available and not the result of many years of struggle for compensation.

Clearly, people have a right to know about the dangers of the drugs they consume. They have an equal right, however, to expect that the information that they acquire from their doctors, the drug industry, and the media is accurate and understandable. Fear of the unknown and inability to appreciate the significance of risk-estimates are probably the most important factors. The risks of cigarette smoking, crossing the street, or defective electrical appliances are well known but frequently ignored. A sevenfold increase in risk of death from thromboembolism in a young woman using the contraceptive pill, where the baseline mortality is only two per million, is headlines. Many women have abandoned the use of oral contraceptives after reading such statistics. Yet the same women accept the advice of a surgeon without qualms although, as may have been explained to them, the mortality of an operation may be measured in whole numbers per thousand.

An essential preliminary to the release of information is peer review by experts. The role of the expert journal referee and editor is also vital in this respect. Unfortunately, there is little sense of corporate responsibility among lay journalists. Patients do suffer as a result of medical mistakes and doctors who make mistakes may get sued. But journalists, like members of parliament and some consumer activitists, enjoy the immunity provided by a free press.

Clearly, no one can deny that thalidomide was an appalling tragedy, no one suggests that the public should not be informed, no one would doubt the right of a patient, a doctor, a journalist, or a politician to question established practices, and no one would wish to delay responsible warnings about drug toxicity. In many situations, however, adverse reported drug publicity has had far more damaging consequences than the adverse drug reactions themselves. We must not forget the benefits which the development of drugs has brought in the last 50 years.

## REFERENCES

Bradford Hill, A. (1971). *Principles of medical statistics*, 9th edn. The Lancet Ltd, London.

Brown, P., Baddeley, H., Read, A. E., Davies, J.D., and McGarry, J. (1974). Sclerosing peritonitis, and unusual reaction to a β-adrenergic-blocking drug (practolol) *Lancet* ii, 1477.

Committee on Safety of Drugs (1968). *When in doubt—report adverse reactions.* Series No. 7. HMSO, London. (Unpublished document printed for DHSS.)

Felix, R.H., Ive, F.A., and Dahl, M.G.C. (1974). Cutaneous and ocular reactions to practolol. *Br. Med. J.* iv, 321.

Geiling, E.M.K. and Cannon, P.R. (1948). Pathogenic effects of elixir of sulfanilamide (diethylene glycol) poisoning. *JAMA* 111, 919.

Greenberg, G., Inman, W.H.W., Weatherall, J.A.C., Adelstein, A.M., and Haskey, J.C. (1977). Maternal drug histories and congenital abnormalities. *Br. Med. J.* ii, 853.

Inman, W.H.W. (1970). Role of drug-reaction monitoring in the investigation of thrombosis and 'the pill'. *Br. Med. Bull.* 26, 248.

Inman, W.H.W. (1972). Monitoring by voluntary reporting at national level. In *Adverse drug reactions: their prediction, detection and assessment* (ed. D.J. Richards and R.K. Rondel) p. 86. Churchill Livingstone, Edinburgh.

Inman, W.H.W. (1978). Detection and investigation of drug safety problems. In *Epidemiological issues in reported drug induced illness. Honolulu* 1976 (ed. M. Gent and I. Shigematsu) p. 17. McMaster University Library Press, Hamilton, Ontario.

Inman, W.H.W. (1979). Oral contraceptives and fatal subarachnoid haemorrhage. *Br. Med. J.* ii, 1468.

Inman, W.H.W. (1980). *Monitoring for drug safety.* MTP Press, Lancaster.

Inman, W.H.W. (1981a). Post-marketing surveillance of adverse drug reactions in general practice. 1: Search for new methods. *Br. Med. J.* 282, 1131.

Inman, W.H.W. (1981b). Post-marketing surveillance of adverse drug reactions in general practice. II: Prescription-event monitoring at the University of Southampton. *Br. Med. J.* 282, 1216.

Inman, W.H.W. (1981c). Post-marketing drug surveillance. In *Risk-benefit analysis in drug research. Proceedings of an International Symposium, University of Kent, Canterbury, 27th March 1980* (ed. J.F. Cavalla) p. 147. MTP Press, Lancaster.

Inman, W.H.W. and Mushin, W.W. (1974). Jaundice after repeated exposure to halothane. *Br. Med. J.* i, 5.

Inman, W.H.W. and Mushin, W.W. (1978). Jaundice after halothane: a further analysis. *Br. Med. J.* ii, 1455.

Inman, W.H.W. and Price Evans, D.A. (1972). Evaluation of spontaneous reports on adverse reactions to drugs. *Br. Med. J.* iii, 746.

Inman, W.H.W. and Vessey, M.P. (1968). Investigation of deaths from pulmonary, coronary and cerebral thrombosis and embolism in women of childbearing age. *Br. Med. J.* ii, 193.

Inman, W.H.W., Vessey, M.P., Westerholm, B., and Engelund, A. (1970). Thromboembolic disease and the steroidal content of oral contraceptives. *Br. Med. J.* ii, 203.

Kono, R. (1978). A Review of S.M.O.N. studies in Japan. In *Epidemiological issues in reported drug-induced illness—SMON and other examples* (ed. M. Gent and I. Shigematsu) p. 121. McMaster University Library Press, Hamilton, Ontario.

Meade, T.W., Greenberg, G., and Thompson, S.G. (1980). Progestogens and cardiovascular reactions associated with oral contraceptives and a comparison of the safety of 50- and 30-μg oestrogen preparations. *Br. Med. J.* i, 1157.

Medical Research Council (1967). Risk of thromboembolic disease in women taking oral contraceptives. *Br. Med. J.* ii, 355.

Office of Population Censuses and Surveys (1959–78). *Mortality statistics 1957–1976.* HMSO, London.

Royal College of General Practitioners (1967). Oral contraception and thrombo-embolic disease. *J. Coll. Gen. Pract.* 13, 267.

Royal College of General Practitioners (1977). Mortality among oral contraceptive users. *Lancet* ii, 727.

Sackett, D.L. (1979). Bias in analytic research. *J. Chronic Dis.* 32, 51.

Taggart, M.Mc.A. and Alderdice, J.M. (1982). Fatal cholestatic jaundice in elderly patients taking benoxaprofen. *Br. Med. J.* 284, 1372.

Vessey, M.P. and Doll, R. (1968). Investigation of relation between use of oral contraceptives and thromboembolic disease. *Br. Med. J.* **ii**, 199.

Wade, O.L. (1970). *Adverse reactions to drugs*. Heineman, London.

Walton, B., Simpson, B.R., Strunin, L., Doniach, D., Perrin, J., and Appleyard, A.J. (1976). Unexplained hepatitis following halothane. *Br. Med. J.* **i**, 1171.

Wells, N. (1980). *Medicines: 50 years of progress, 1930–1980.* Office of Health Economics, London.

Wright, P. (1975). Untoward effects associated with practolol administration: oculomucutaneous syndrome. *Br. Med. J.* **i**, 595.

# 22 Field investigations of noise hazards

M. van der Venne

## INTRODUCTION

The damaging effects of noise on health present a complex problem. Exposure to noise can impair the hearing function or can produce non-auditory effects ranging from disturbance of the circulatory or neurological systems, to causing or contributing to stress, psychological, and sociological disorders.

In any investigation of health effects, the considerable variation in individual sensitivities to noise (in both the physiological and psychological fields) which, for the moment at least, cannot be predicted, must be borne in mind. Reference is thus generally made to a 'normal situation', as observed in a given population and often described in terms of statistical distribution. The choice of an appropriate reference group must be made considering carefully the relevant contributing factors.

A fruitful concept in the limitation of hazards to health relies on dose-effect relationships which can be used as one objective element in assessing the acceptability of a given risk and provide information to decision-makers in health policies. In establishing such relationships the agent (in this case the noise) and its effects on human health have to be quantified.

This chapter will be restricted to a consideration of the problems of field measurements specific to noise and two main points will be covered – measurement of noise, and determination of the hearing capacity. In both cases, it is essential to determine clearly the purposes for which the results will be used, as this fixes the parameters to be measured and governs the choice of method. Discrepancies and misunderstandings have in the past resulted from inappropriate use of a given set of results, or invalid comparisons.

Besides the two aspects mentioned above, many other factors can be involved. The evaluation of physiological (e.g. blood pressure or components) or behavioural functions (e.g. performance rating, acceptability of a noisy situation), or data collecting (e.g. occurrence of gastric ulcer, accident statistics) are all relevant to the study of noise but will not be considered here.

## MEASUREMENT OF NOISE

Noise is defined as any disagreeable or undesired sound (IEC 1960). Thus measuring noise means measuring sounds, and in the overwhelming majority of health-related cases, airborne sounds.

For the physicist, sound is the propagation of a disturbance in an elastic medium – that is, a pressure wave in air. For the physiologist, sound is the sensation of hearing excited by that phenomenon. We must thus consider both aspects of sound – physical properties and resulting perception.

### Physical aspects of noise measurement*

A noise source radiating in air induces minute fluctuations around the ambient air pressure and these fluctuations constitute the sound pressure. This is the basic quantity measured by sound monitoring equipment and is expressed, unless otherwise stated, as its root mean square (RMS) value ($\bar{p}$) in pascals (Pa). The propagation of those fluctuations of the air pressure results in sound waves which, like all waves, transport a flux of energy. The sound intensity ($I$), expressed in watts per square metre (Wm$^{-2}$), is defined as the rate of flow of sound energy through a unit area normal to the direction of propagation. Let us look at the relation between sound pressure and sound intensity for a progressive plane sound wave:

$$I = \frac{\bar{p}^2}{\varrho c} \tag{22.1}$$

where $I$ = sound intensity in W m$^{-2}$; $\bar{p}$ = RMS sound pressure in Pa; $\varrho$ = density of air in kg m$^{-3}$; $c$ = velocity of sound in air in m s$^{-1}$.

The range of values met in acoustics is very large. At 1000 Hz, the average of the threshold of hearing for young people with otologically normal ears corresponds to a sound pressure of $2 \times 10^{-5}$ Pa, while the threshold of pain is in the range of 100–200 Pa. On the other hand, our ear perceives noise according to the logarithm of its intensity. For various reasons, therefore, it is customary to express acoustic measurements as their ratio to an arbitrary value, using a logarithmic scale. Applying this to sound intensities, eqn 22.1 leads to eqn 22.2:

$$10 \log\left(\frac{I}{I_0}\right) = 10 \log\left(\frac{\bar{p}^2}{I_0 \varrho c}\right) = 10 \log\left(\frac{\bar{p}}{p_0}\right)^2 \tag{22.2}$$

where $I_0$ = reference sound intensity and $p_0 = I_0 \sqrt{\varrho c}$ = reference sound pressure.

The reference terms $p_0$ and $I_0$ are not independent, and either of them can be used to fix a scale. For practical reasons, the sound pressure (the quantity usually measured) is considered first, and its reference value has been set at

*A summary of the definitions, symbols, relationships, and dimensions of the units used, which belong to the Systeme International d'Unités (SI) can be found in the appendix to this Chapter.

$p_0 = 2 \times 10^{-5}$ Pa (see above for its physiological meaning) giving the familiar sound pressure level ($L_p$) in decibels (dB) defined as

$$L_p = 20 \log \left( \frac{\bar{p}}{p_0} \right). \qquad (22.3)$$

The validity of determining the sound intensity by measuring the sound pressure level is, strictly speaking, restricted to specific ambient conditions. Eqn 22.1 shows that for a given sound pressure, the sound intensity depends, through the acoustic impedance ($\varrho c$), on the temperature and pressure of the air. Using the values in prevailing room conditions as a guide, the acoustic impedance has been estimated as $\varrho c = 400$ SI units; with the chosen value of $p_0$, this leads to a reference sound intensity $I_0 = 10^{-12}$ W . m$^{-2}$. The error is a fraction of dB for normal barometric pressure and air temperatures around 20°C, but it becomes more important in other conditions. However, these restrictions are of practical importance only if accurate power calculations are requested, and for health purposes sound pressure generally is an appropriate measure for noise intensity (eqn 22.3).

The use of a logarithmic scale in relation to noise is convenient, but it must be clear that the figures so obtained are not additive. Each doubling of sound intensity adds about 3 dB to the value of the sound pressure level ($L_p$), the addition becoming 10 dB for a tenfold increase in intensity. Even more care must be taken when dealing with values of sound pressure – a tenfold increase in sound pressure, leading to a 100-fold increase in sound intensity increases the reading of a sound-level meter by 20 dB. So inadvertent guessing can be misleading. To determine the combined noise resulting from various sources, the decibel values must be converted into (linear) intensities. These must then be added and the results reconverted to decibels. Apart from the simple examples given above, this can be done using tables and graphs which relate sound intensity (or sound pressure) ratios with decibels. However, the wide availability of pocket calculators makes it easy to apply the formula

$$L_p = 10 \log \left( \sum_{i=1}^{n} 10^{0.1 L_i} \right) \qquad (22.4)$$

where $L_p$ = total sound pressure level, in dB; $L_i$ = value of sound pressure level resulting from noise source $i$ alone, in dB; $N$ = number of sources contributing to noise.

The sound power level of a source is also used (total noise emitted). This is a characteristic of the source, and not of direct concern to us, since the effects of noise depend on its intensity at a given point. This in turn will vary with distance from the source and conditions of transmission such as, direction, reflection, and absorption. Knowledge of the total noise emitted by noisy equipment provides useful information for predicting its effects on man. Here again, a logarithmic scale is used, and the sound power level $L_w$ in dB is defined as

$$L_w = 10 \log \frac{w}{w_0} \qquad (22.5)$$

where $w$ = mean power emitted in W; $w_0$ = reference power equal to $10^{-12}$ W. Other values for the reference power are

sometimes used, and it is good practice to specify which one was chosen.

Care must be taken in using acoustic power levels, as their numerical values may differ considerably from those of sound pressure levels at a distance of practical interest. In the case of an isotropic source radiating in a sphere of radius $r$ and whose geometric dimensions are small compared to $r$, the relation is

$$L_p = L_w - 10 \log 4 \pi r^2. \qquad (22.6)$$

To give a practical example, an air compressor having a sound power level $L_w = 101$ dB(A)/1 $pw$, situated on a hard reflecting plane, free from obstructions – for example, on a concrete base in open air – will result in a sound pressure level around 80 dB(A) at a distance of five metres.

Besides its intensity, a sound is also characterized by its frequency spectrum which can range from very simple (puretone sine sound wave) to very complex (broad-band random noise). The frequency is expressed in Hertz (units: s$^{-1}$) and its distribution for a given noise is analysed with more or less refinement according to the needs of the specific problem.

The description of a noise at a given moment must consist of the sound pressure level as well as the frequencies at which the measurement has been made. This is done either by giving the limits – for example, dB linear from 50 to 20 000 Hz, or dB for a given octave-band – or by specifying the frequency weighting used – for example dB (A).

If the noise is not steady, the fluctuations in time of the sound intensity must also be known so that the effects on health can be established. Here again, the amount of information needed depends on the specific problem. It can range from a simple averaging of the sound pressure levels to a full description of the statistical distribution of noise levels during time, and we will return to this later in the chapter.

One special case must be mentioned, the so-called 'impulse and impact' noise. There is no generally acceptable current definition for or standardized description of the essential characteristics of this type of noise. It consists of noise burst(s) of short duration rising sharply. Parameters recorded include the peak sound pressure, the onset time, the decay rate, the form of the pressure wave. It is advisable for impulse noise to express the peak sound pressure values in pascals. It is always possible to convert these values to the dB scale (re 20$\mu$Pa), but it must then be made clear that we are dealing with an instantaneous (instead of RMS) value, and that very short times are involved – an impulse noise with a peak sound pressure of 65 Pa falling down to 20 Pa in 50 milliseconds is not uncommon. The (peak value) and 120 dB (after 50 ms). A steady noise of 130 dB (A) – for example, the take-off of a jet heard at about 50 m – is quite a different matter with a much more serious potential effect on health.

### Perceptive aspects of noise measurement and evaluation

The sensation of hearing induced by a sound wave depends on its intensity and its frequency. It varies from one person to another and follows generally the Weber–Fechner law (logarithmic pattern). Sounds are perceived only in a limited range of frequencies – for man from about 16 Hz to 20 000 Hz. Other frequencies give infra- or ultra-sounds.

The use of electrophysiological techniques to determine hearing is uncommon in field studies of noise effects on man. Data are normally obtained by collecting the subjective reactions of a suitably selected population sample, and averaging the individual responses according to classical statistics. Such techniques have been used to determine the loudness of sounds with various physical characteristics, for example, or noise reduction provided by ear protectors, as well as the annoyance rating of different noises. This method is time-consuming and efforts have been made to substitute objective determination of the physical parameters of noise. A number of correlations have been standardized. For example, the average sensitivity of the human ear has been determined, leading to the isosonic curves, and to the standardization of the phone, the unit of loudness level.

The mere sensation of hearing is not sufficient to account for all the perceived effects or hazards involved in exposure to noise, and the data obtained by sound measurements must be further processed in order to assess damaging or annoying effects. Some knowledge of the frequency spectrum is generally requested, and this can be obtained by specifying standardized weightings produced by incorporating filter networks in the measuring equipment. The A, B, and C curves approximate the isosonic curves passing respectively by 40, 70, and 100 dB for 1000 Hz and are broadly used despite their restricted physical significance. Most widely used is the A-weighting, as the data so obtained correlate surprisingly well with rather different effects of noise. For instance, the hearing loss induced by industrial noise, or the community response to environmental noise, are predicted, by broad agreement, using measurements expressed in dB(A). If information on the spectrum of noise is sought, the difference in readings between the C- and A-weighted values gives an indication of the relative importance of low-frequency components and is simple to perform. D-weighting has been standardized to assess the annoyance of aircraft noise. It is an approximation of the subjective 'isoannoying' curve passing by 40 dB at 1000 Hz, a process similar to the approximation of an isosonic curve by the A-weighting.

There are, however, cases where a fixed frequency weighting does not fulfil the needs of the investigator, and a frequency analysis must then be performed. This gives the sound pressure level over a band of specified width, usually one octave or one-third octave, but sometimes down to one Hz. Obviously, the narrower the band, the more information is available on the spectrum. Examples of problems which require the use of frequency analysis include the noise abatement of rotating machines where almost pure tones are generated, the quantitative study of the interaction of noise with communication (Articulation Index, Speech Interference Level), the evaluation of the annoyance caused by specific noise sources – for example, in the acoustic certification of aircraft (Perceived Noise Level, Total Noise Exposure Level) – and the rating of ear protectors.

The variations of sound intensity with time must also be monitored, and here again efforts have been made to simplify and standardize the measurements. The problem may be formulated as finding by how much the intensity of a given noise must be reduced to result in the same effect when the exposure duration is doubled. This implies an assumption about the factor which controls that effect. If the effect – for example, a given hearing loss – depends on the total energy received, doubling the time of exposure would involve halving the intensity, and the corresponding sound pressure level must be 3 dB lower to give the same result. But if the sound pressure is assumed to be the determining factor and must thus be halved, the sound pressure level, as shown by eqn 22.3 should be 6 dB lower when doubling the exposure duration. The value of the 'halving factor' (termed $q$ and, in this example equal to 3 or 6 dB respectively) must be determined for each specific application. Much consideration has been given to the case where $q = 3$, corresponding to the total energy assumption, and a number of quantities have been derived, which can be regarded as a measure of either the noise dose or the dose-rate, or, with due regard to acoustic impedance (see eqn 22.2 and text hereafter – p. 350), the energy or power involved. One of the most used ones is the equivalent continuous sound pressure level over a given time period ($L_{eq,T}$), which is the constant sound pressure level which would, in the course of that time period, cause the same sound energy to be received as that arising from the considered noise. In terms of energy, it is a mean value, defined in dB as

$$L_{eq,T} = 10 \log \frac{1}{T} \int_0^T \left( \frac{p(t)}{P_0} \right)^2 dt \qquad (22.7)$$

where $p(t) =$ time-varying value of sound pressure in Pa; $p_0 =$ reference sound pressure of $2 \times 10^{-5}$ Pa; $T =$ total time period considered.

It is common practice to use the A-weighting for sound pressures, resulting in $L_{Aeq,T}$. Two values of the time period have been normalized: one second for the single event noise exposure level ($L_{AX}$), and eight hours for occupational purposes ($L_{Aeq,8h}$). Similar expressions have been defined for the total amount of noise received, and one finds the noise immission level (NIL), defined in dB (A) as

$$\text{NIL} = L_{Aeq,8h} + 10 \log \frac{T}{T_0} \qquad (22.8)$$

where $T =$ duration of exposure in years and $T_0 =$ reference period of one year.

The values of NIL will increase with the duration of exposure for a given fixed value of $L_{Aeq,8h}$, and this is not always taken into account. For example, an exposure of 40 years to $L_{Aeq,8h}$ of 90 dB (A), in line with the 1972 Code of Practice (HSE 1972), yields a NIL of 105 dB (A).

Recently, another quantity has been introduced (ISO 1982), the noise exposure level, defined in dB (A) as

$$L_{EX,T} = 10 \log \frac{E_T}{E_0} \qquad (22.9)$$

where $E_T = \int_0^T p_A^2(t) \, dt$; $E_0 =$ reference value of $1.15 \times 10^{-5}$ Pa²s; and $T =$ total time period considered.

It has appeared desirable to choose $E_0$ so that for a given eight-hour exposure $L_{EX}$ is numerically equal to $L_{Aeq,8h}$. If it is more relevant to use another exposure period $T$, such as a working week of 40 hours, and keep equal numerical values for $L_{EX}$ and $L_{Aeq,T}$, then another value must be chosen for $E_0$.

The noise exposure level and the equivalent continuous sound pressure level are related by the formula

$$L_{EX,T} = L_{Aeq,T} + 10 \log \frac{T}{T_0} \qquad (22.10)$$

where $T_0$ = reference duration of 8 h or $28.8 \times 10^3$ s.

The values of $L_{Aeq,T}$ and $L_{EX,T}$ can be determined from measurements made during fractional exposure periods by the relations

$$L_{EX} = 10 \log \left[ \sum_{i=1}^{N} 10^{0.1 L_{EX,i}} \right] \qquad (22.11)$$

$$L_{Aeq,T} = 10 \log \left[ \frac{1}{N} \sum_{i=1}^{N} 10^{0.1 L_{Aeq,i}} \right] \qquad (22.12)$$

where $L_{EX,i}$ = value of $L_{EX,T}$ over the fractional period of time $T_i$; $L_{Aeq,i}$ value of $L_{Aeq,T_i}$ over the fractional period of time $T_i$; $T = \Sigma T_i$; and $N$ = total number of fractional periods of time.

Another trend which is also apparent involves the use, especially for occupational exposure, of a linear scale, which is more intuitive than the (logarithmic) dB scale and easier to understand for large numbers of unspecialized users. This has resulted in the calibration of exposure meters in pascal-squared-hours, or in fractional exposure; in this last case the base exposure must be known – for example $L_{EX} = 90$ dB (A).

All the above-mentioned quantities, by definition, rely on the 'equal-energy' concept. Similar ones can be derived using other assumptions, and an example can be given by the occupational exposure regulation in force in the US (OSHA or Walsh-Healey regulation – OSHA 1983) where the time-weighted average sound level is calculated by permitting a 5 dB increase in level for each halving of duration of exposure ($q = 5$).

The terminology and quantities used are in a state of change, and standardization is far from complete. It is essential to use all those quantities properly, and to be aware of the assumptions underlying the time-intensity conversion factor.

As we have already seen the intensity of impulse noise varies very rapidly (in industry, rise times shorter than 1 milli-second can occur), and this has previously demanded rather intricate equipment and measurement techniques such as photography of the trace left on an oscilloscope unsuitable for broad field use. Here again, simplification was desirable. Sound level meters have been equipped with a special time-weighting characteristic, featuring a short rise time and a much longer decay time which can show, using simple apparatus, whether impulse noise is present or not. Unfortunately, the measurements do not apply equally well over the broad range of impulse and impact noises met in practice. As the sound pressure signal is frequency-weighted before being fed into the asymmetrical detector–indicator, the resulting indication could be expected to vary with the exact characteristics of the noise, and empirical relations, each valid over a limited set of conditions, have to be developed. As an example, DIN 45641 (a German standard for determining the rating-level of noise at the workplace) requests additional measurements with the C-weighting, if the value obtained with the A-weighting and the characteristic 'Impuls' exceeds 100 dB (A). Great care should be taken when measuring with the Impuls characteristic, and fortunately the development of modern electronics has led to a new generation of instruments which overcome that limitation.

As was the case with frequencies, some problems require a detailed knowledge of the variation of sound intensity versus time, and a statistical analysis must then be performed. This gives the noise levels (expressed according to the specific problem) which have been exceeded for a given fraction of the time, or which have occurred during a certain period, for example, at night.

In any evaluation of the effects of noise on health, therefore, the intensity, the frequency, and the fluctuations of the noise in question must be considered, and attempts have been made to combine the three factors. A simple example of this is the expression of the occupational exposure for hearing conservation purposes as A-weighted noise exposure level ($L_{EX}$). The situation rapidly becomes more complex, however, when the annoyance must also be rated. The large number of indices and methods proposed to predict community responses to noise (see, for example, WHO 1980) is an indication that our knowledge of the governing factors is far from satisfactory.

## Measurement methods

Measurement of airborne noise involves measuring a time-fluctuating pressure, and this is done with a microphone, the electrical signal of which is suitably processed. A range of microphones is available to suit the individual needs of sensitivity, frequency response, interaction with the noise field, and environmental conditions.

Whenever possible, the microphone is coupled to a sound level meter which incorporates an amplifier (with various levels of gain, in order to cover a broad measuring range), one or more frequency weighting networks, a logarithmic detector, and an indicating device. We have seen that sound intensity is related to the root mean square value of the instantaneous pressure, and the reading of the sound pressure level will vary according to the duration of the averaging process, if the sound intensity is not constant. The standardized (IEC 1979a) sound level meters use a detector giving RMS values with two time weightings: 'F' (time constant 125 ms) and 'S' (time constant 1000 ms). The characteristic 'I' is also available, in which case the averaging circuit (time constant 35 ms) is followed by a peak detector (decay time constant 1500 ms). These standardized sound level meters are specified in four degrees of precision: type 0 intended as a laboratory reference standard; type 1 for laboratory use; type 2 suitable for general field use; type 3 primarily for field noise survey applications. The instruments may also have a 'peak hold' feature, allowing the peak value to be read.

In addition, instruments have been developed which integrate the signal during the measurement time, and display (often in digital form) a normalized function of the time-integrated sound pressure or its logarithmic transform, or calculate its mean value over a given time-interval. It is essential to identify the assumptions on which the instrument is based – time-intensity relationship, values (if any) of the reference noise dose or dose rate, and of the averaging time-interval. According to their size and function, they are generally called noise dose meters (small individual instruments with tolerances corresponding to class 2 or 3 sound level meters), or integrating sound level meters (which perform the integration besides the RMS detection in a class 1 apparatus). These instruments, thus, indicate some form of the noise dose or dose-rate, and since the integration is carried out directly on the pressure signal (suitably processed for intensity-time trade-off and frequency weighting), the values displayed are independent of the time constants and response limits of the indicator. This means, for instance that, within the capabilities of the microphone and electronic circuits, even impulse noise is normally integrated. The use of such measuring instruments certainly eases the task of the field investigator when some function of the total energy is relevant, and the noise pattern is not a simple one: industrial noise exposure is a typical example.

Where a frequency distribution or a time-dependent statistical analysis is requested, the microphone may be connected to a measuring amplifier, and the signal fed into an appropriate system which performs the necessary analysis. Portable octave-band analysers are available, but the constraints of field investigations limit the possibility of installing sophisticated instruments. It is then common practice to use a high grade tape recorder, and to play the tape back in a laboratory with the necessary equipment.

Estimation of the noise attenuation afforded by hearing protectors provides an example of applying frequency analysis to a practical problem (Sutton and Robinson 1981). Three methods are compared. The most complete method involves an octave-band analysis of the noise actually experienced. For each band, the attenuation given by that protector (as measured by a standardized subjective method) is then subtracted, and A-weighting characteristic applied to determine the partial exposure relevant to that band; a summing of all those contributions according to Eqn 22.4 yields the total A-weighted sound level received by a wearer.

The second and simpler method uses the difference between measurements of the noise under consideration with different frequency weightings (usually the A and C curves) as information on the spectrum of that noise. Typically, an overall attenuation factor previously determined by an octave-band technique for a reference noise – for example, a pink noise – and that protector, is subtracted from the measured C-level of the prevailing noise. The result provides a good approximation of the A-level received by the wearer.

The third possibility is simply to subtract a suitable overall attenuation factor (which will generally be lower than the one used in the previous method) from the A-weighted sound pressure level of the noise, obtaining a value of the A-weighted exposure of the wearer.

These three methods have different measurement requirements, but they correspond to different levels of knowledge of the noise to be protected against. For a specific protector and a given level of protection (the noise reduction computed for that protector must be reached or exceeded in say 95 per cent of the cases), it is to be expected that the last procedure will result in a lower attenuation factor. The larger uncertainty on the noise characteristics results in a necessary increase of the safety margin, thus overprotecting in more cases. This is the price that must be paid for lack of knowledge of the frequency spectrum involved in the actual noise to be protected against.

When performing sound measurements, care should be taken to site the microphone properly to limit the disturbance of the noise field. There may, however, be conflicting requirements, as in the measurement of individual exposures with portable equipment; when hearing protection is the objective, the noise should be determined as close as possible to the external ear canal but the head and body interact with the acoustic waves in a manner which varies with the frequency. When the effects of the reflecting surfaces, such as skin and clothes, are also taken into account, a complex interference pattern can be experienced (Redwood 1977), so the conditions for measurement are frequently specified in standards.

The statistical aspects of noise measurement should not be overlooked, as they may play an important role in the selection of the instruments to be used. As for other physical variables, a confidence interval can be assigned to the measured values of a randomly variable noise; when $n$ measurements are made, yielding an arithmetic mean $m$ and a standard deviation $d$, the true value of the parameter belongs, with a given probability $p$ to the interval

$$m \pm t(p) \cdot \frac{d}{n}$$

where $t(p)$ is a statistical variable (Student distribution).

A specific case of practical importance occurs when it must be ascertained whether the noise exceeds a limit value or not; assuming that at least six short-time (say 15 s) measurements are made, the following relation will hold with a probability of 95 per cent at least

$$L \leqslant \frac{1}{n}\sum_{i=1}^{n} L_i + 2 \sqrt{\left[\frac{\sum_{i=1}^{n}\left(L_i - \frac{1}{n}\sum_{i=1}^{n} L_i\right)^2}{n(n-1)}\right]} \quad (22.13)$$

where $L$ = true value of the investigated parameter; $L_i$ = individual measured value of $L$; and $n$ = number of measurements.

In the conditions defined by the standard DIN 45645/2, the mean of the measured values must be lower than the limit value, by a quantity which depends on the instrument: 3 dB for class 2, and 6 dB for class 3 (Hübner 1983). This allows the calculation of the minimum number of measurements to be made, considering the equipment used, the level of the noise, its variations during time, and how close it is to the specified limit. When that number of measurements exceeds two digits, automatic reading becomes attractive, with the possibilities of recording or processing the data. An integrating sound-level meter, which is even simpler, would yield a direct reading of the integrated quantity (for example, $L_{Aeq}$). Performances of two such typical instruments (as advertised) are a measuring time exceeding 24 hours with a resolution of 0.1 dB, or a measuring time of one hour with a resolution of 0.5 dB.

## MEASUREMENT OF HEARING

One important consequence of a hearing impairment, often the first to be noticed, is a difficulty in understanding normal conversation. This is not simple to measure, however, so here again, an approximation has been sought, and pure-tone subjective audiometry is broadly used. This consists in presenting to the subject pure tones of different frequencies and intensities, and noting the faintest one which can still be heard. Other methods do exist, such as speech audiometry or detection of hearing response through electrophysiological functions, but they are outside the normal scope of field investigations.

The basic technique presents sounds of the specified frequencies and intensities to each of the ears through earphones, allowing the determination of the air-conduction threshold of hearing. As in many subjective measurements, the procedure is repeated for those intensities which bracket the hearing threshold of the subject, in order to reduce the range of uncertainty. There is no particular problem in generating an electrical sine-wave signal of the desired frequency and amplitude; the ear phones must however be of high quality so that reproducible sound pressure levels result, and they must match the generator. The audiometers (IEC 1979b) used in industrial practice can be either manual, in which case the signal selection and presentation as well as the recording of the results are performed by an operator, or automatic, where the whole process is implemented automatically (they are also called 'Bekesy audiometers').

Thus an audiogram expresses the variation of hearing as a function of frequency, and it gives an indication of the subject's 'quality of hearing'. The hearing level is expressed in the familiar dB system, with the reference values chosen to represent the average threshold of hearing for a population of otologically normal young people (ISO 1975).

Audiometry is not a very accurate method. Besides variations in individual hearing levels, it is also affected by the technique used, the training of both the audiometrist and the subject, and the psychological and physiological condition of the subject. More obvious factors, such as the background noise level (which can obscure very faint signals) or the temporary reduction of threshold hearing levels by pathological conditions or recent exposure to noise can also influence results. Many industrially used audiometers change sound intensities by steps of 5 dB, and this may give an indication of the uncertainty to be expected. When accuracy and reproducibility are very important, standardized procedures should be followed as closely as is practicable. For hearing conservation purposes, such a method has been described (ISO 1981a), and specifies the apparatus, the operating procedures, the maximum ambient noise, the preparation and instruction of subjects, and the presentation of the resulting audiogram.

Simplified procedures can, however, be used for solving specific problems, mainly where large numbers of people are involved. The screening of industrial workers on a 'pass–no pass' basis, with a limited number of frequency-intensity combinations, is a typical example. Another helpful practice consists in assigning the subjects to special categories according to their hearing loss. Rossi (1981) has presented an overall view of industrial audiometric practice.

This leads us to the point of assessing the consequences of a given hearing impairment, or 'translating' an audiogram into handicap. Very often, values of the hearing threshold level measured at specified frequencies are combined into a 'fence' threshold (above which a hearing handicap is deemed to exist). The rules used to make this conversion are established according to the aim which has been fixed, and there are many of them in use. The social handicap resulting from a lack of understanding of speech can be expressed, for example, as a function of the arithmetic mean value of hearing threshold levels at 1000, 2000, and 3000 Hz. In Belgium 55 dB is the value which opens the right to compensation for industrial disease, while in the United Kingdom such a right starts at 50 dB. The British Standard BS 5330 admits that 30 dB represents a social handicap (difficulty in understanding speech). If interference with speech is considered not only in a quiet environment, but in more noisy situations, a social handicap is already noticeable for a 15 dB loss (Smoorenburg 1982).

Ageing is another factor which interferes with the limit values specified for the hearing threshold levels. Some rulings substract the part of hearing impairment associated with ageing – for example, those which aim at compensating for damage caused by occupational exposure and assign the corresponding expenses to the employer. But when the objective is to limit the number of handicapped, the effect of ageing is not given special consideration. In that case the cause of the hearing impairment (and its consequence) is immaterial, so no allowance for ageing will be made.

The effect of age on hearing intensifies the uncertainty of what 'normal' hearing is, and makes it more difficult to quantify impairment caused by extraneous factors. In an attempt to restrict the corresponding range, the hearing threshold level of otologically normal populations has been standardized for groups of men and of women, ranging from young people (18–30 years old) up to the age of 65 years (ISO 1981b). However it must always be ascertained that the group taken as a control has been chosen properly for the specific problem.

## CONCLUSION

Field investigations specific to noise rely on rather simple principles but their application may be intricate. It is essential that the objectives to be met are carefully analysed and the questions to be answered by the measurement are clearly formulated. The effects of fluctuations and uncertainty must be considered, particularly when the result must err on the safe side, as for example in checking compliance with regulations.

When considering the measurement of noise, the choice of the apparatus should be given thought, as it may ease considerably the procedure. The technology is changing rapidly and a new generation of instruments, which rely on electronic processing of the primary signal is appearing. However they have not yet been fully standardized or their use (and advantages) incorporated into the rules governing the measurement and control of noise levels.

## APPENDIX

A number of basic units are used in this chapter along with some derived units. They are defined as follows.

### Basic units

#### Unit of length

The metre (m) is the length of 1 650 763. 73 wavelengths in the vacuum of the radiation corresponding to the transition between the levels 2 $p_{10}$ and 5 $d_5$ of the atom Kr-86.

#### Unit of mass

The kilogramme (kg) is equal to the mass of the international prototype.

#### Unit of time

The second (s) is the duration of 9 192 631 770 periods of the radiation corresponding to the transition between the two hyperfine levels of the fundamental state of the atom Cs-133.

### Derived units

#### Frequency

The hertz (Hz) is a frequency of one complete cycle per second.

#### Area

The unit of area is equal to one square metre ($m^2$).

#### Volume

The unit of volume is equal to one cubic metre ($m^3$).

#### Velocity

The unit of velocity is equal to one metre per second ($m.s^{-1}$).

#### Density

The unit of density is one kilogramme per cubic metre ($m^{-3}.kg$).

#### Force

The newton (N) is the force which accelerates a mass of one kilogramme at a rate of 1 metre per second per second ($m.kg.s^{-2}$).

#### Energy or work

The joule (J) is the work produced by a force of one newton which moves a body over a distance of one metre in the direction of that force ($N.m = m^2.kg.s^{-2}$).

#### Power

The watt (W) is the power of a source producing one joule per second ($J.s^{-1} = m^2.kg.s^{-3}$).

#### Pressure

The pascal (Pa) is the pressure produced by a force of one newton per square metre ($N.m^{-2} = m^{-1}.kg.s^{-2}$).

### Note

To realize the magnitude of the forces and pressures involved in acoustics, it is useful to remember that the force exerted by the standard gravity on a mass of one kilogramme is approximately equal to 9.81 newtons; in standardized conditions (0°C and 760 mm of mercury), the atmospheric pressure has a value of $1.01325 \times 10^5$ Pa = 1.01325 bar. The reference pressure of $2 \times 10^{-5}$ Pa is thus about five billion times smaller than the standard atmospheric pressure.

## REFERENCES

Burns, W. (1973). *Noise and man,* 2nd edn. Murray, London.

Burns, W. and Robinson, D.W. (1970). *Hearing and noise in industry.* HMSO, London.

Glorig, A. (1965). *Audiometry, principles and practice.* Williams and Wilkins, Baltimore.

Health and Safety Executive (1972). *Code of practice for reducing the exposure of employed persons to Noise.* HMSO, London.

Hübner, G. (1983). *Correlation between hearing impairment risk and exposure to noise.* EUR 7874. Office for Official Publications of the European Communities, Luxembourg.

IEC (1960). *International electrotechnical vocabulary,* 2nd edn. Bureau Central de la Commission Electrotechnique Internationale, Geneva.

IEC (1979a). *Soundlevel meters.* IEC Publication 691. Geneva.

IEC (1979b). *Audiometers.* IEC Publication 645. Geneva.

ISO (1975). *Standard reference zero for the calibration of pure-tone audiometers.* ISO 389, Geneva.

ISO (1981a). *Pure tone air-conduction threshold audiometry for hearing conservation purposes.* ISO/DIS 6189, Geneva.

ISO (1981b). *Threshold of hearing by air conduction as a function of age and sex for otologically normal persons.* ISO/DIS 7029, Geneva.

ISO (1982). *Determination of occupational noise exposure and estimation of noise-induced hearing impairment.* ISO/DIS 1999, Geneva.

Kryter, K.D. (1970). *The effects of noise on man.* Academic Press, New York.

Martin, R. (1981). Fachgebiete in Jahresübersichten: Geräuschmessung, Geräuschbeurteilung. *VDI-zeitung* **123**, 553.

OSHA (1983). Occupational Safety and Health Administration 29cFR Part 1910. *Federal Register* **48**, 9738. Washington DC.

Redwood, R.A. (1977). Investigation of the errors in noise dose measurements caused by wearing the microphone. M.Sc. dissertation. Institute of Sound and Vibration Research, University of Southampton.

Rossi, G. (1981). Stato attuale dello screening audiometrico nell'industria. (Paper presented at XVII Congresso Nazionale della Società Italiana di Audiologia, Torino, 14–16 October 1981): Edizioni Luigi Pozzi, Rome.

Smoorenburg, G.F., de Laat, J.A.P.M., and Plomp, R. (1982). The effect of noise-induced hearing loss on the intelligibility of speech in noise. *Scand. Audiol.* Suppl. **16**, 123.

Sutton, G.J., and Robinson, D.W. (1981). An appraisal of methods for estimating effectiveness of hearing protectors. *J. Sound Vibration* **77**, 79.

WHO (1980). *Environmental health criteria 12, Noise.* WHO, Geneva.

## FURTHER READING

Numerous publications present a general outline of the physical characteristics of noise and of its various effects on human health; the interested reader can choose according to his needs and the degree of specialization requested.

Examples of classic texts are Burns 1973, Burns and Robinson 1970, Glorig 1965, Kryter 1970; periodic reviews of the literature are also published – for example, Martin 1981. A convenient way of searching for specific publications is to use one of the many data-banks actually available, for example CIS (the International Occupational Safety and Health Information Center operated by the International Labour Office in Geneva), ENVIROLINE, MEDLARS, or MEDLINE.

# Research and development of health promotion services

# 23 Research into sociomedical problems: an example in the field of alcohol abuse

Mildred Blaxter

## INTRODUCTION

Medicine, and especially public health or community medicine, increasingly acquires responsibility for problems in which social, behavioural, and medical components are inextricably mixed. This is partly a reflection of the historical trend towards whole person medicine – the linking of social and physical health in the individual – and partly a result of the success of scientific medicine and public health in dealing with the old scourges of health in the community. Attention can now be turned to epidemics associated with behaviour which are in some ways more difficult to tackle – smoking, accidents, the abuse of drugs and alcohol.

The focus in sociomedical problems may be on prevention and education or on services for control, care, or management. In either case, before priorities can be decided and resources allocated, some description and quantification of the specific problem to be examined is necessary.

The questions which public health asks are the following. How many people suffer from a particular problem? Who are they? How serious is the problem? How does this geographical area compare with another? To whom should health education programmes be directed in this instance? What services does the community need and are the services which are provided efficient and reaching those for whom they are intended?

While the answers to these questions should be based on ascertained facts and not on individual value judgments, they cannot be entirely value-free. It is society as a whole, or a section of it, which defines a particular problem for which services, treatments, or controls should be provided, and different groups may define the problem differently. The nature of the problem of old age, for example, depends not only on its context within particular family structures, but also on the viewpoints of different caring professions or administrative departments. Descriptive statistics which are used for resource allocation and policy making are themselves a product of the value judgments which identify the people who ought to be counted.

Those who have responsibility for health education of the public, or for providing or evaluating services in the community, must base effective action on results of research into the nature and extent of health or social problems. The study described in this chapter provides an example of the sociological approach to a particular sociomedical problem, alcohol abuse. First, however, some general questions on this type of research will be reviewed.

## PROBLEMS OF MEASUREMENT

The first and basic question concerns prevalence – how many people have a specific problem? – and it is unfortunately common for estimates of prevalence to vary wildly. Estimates of the number of alcoholics to be found in England and Wales are shown in Table 23.1, and some rates of alcoholism or problem drinking found in community surveys in different parts of Britain in Table 23.2. Since early surveys, the estimated numbers have tended to rise steeply, and this represents, to some extent, a true rise. On the other hand, it is obvious that such a steep rise, and such differing figures, must indicate some differences in definition or case-finding.

**Table 23.1.** *Estimates of the number of alcoholics or alcohol abusers in England and Wales*

| Source | Number |
|---|---|
| Admissions to psychiatric hospitals with a diagnosis of alcoholism or alcoholic cirrhosis, 1975 | 18 900 |
| Royal College of Psychiatrists, 1975 | 300 000 |
| Based on formula employing the connection between liver cirrhosis and alcoholism, 1976 | 350 000 |
| Department of Health and Social Security, 1975 | 400 000 |
| Central Policy Review Staff, 1979* | 640 000 |

*Quoted by Brun (1982).

Similarly, Table 23.3 gives some suggested prevalence rates of a different sort of sociomedical problem, physical or mental disability. The studies from which these rates were derived did not necessarily define disability in the same way, survey exactly the same age-group, or use the same method. A change in wording in the General Household Survey (a regular sample survey of households in Great Britain), for instance, between 1976 and 1977 altered considerably the number of people declaring that they had an impairment or chronic illness. Nevertheless, this type of estimate (like the estimate of alcoholism) is frequently used as though it were precise. Table 23.4 gives some examples of prevalence rates of disability found in surveys conducted by local authorities in

**Table 23.2.**  *Rates of alcoholism or problem drinking reported in community surveys in Great Britain*

| Survey | Definition used | Rate/1000 Male | Female | Reference |
|---|---|---|---|---|
| 480 general practices | Alcoholics | 1.7 | 0.8 | Parr (1954) |
| Cambridgeshire | Alcoholics known to agencies | 6.2 | 1.4 | Moss and Beresford Davies (1966) |
| 279 employers in London | Problem drinkers in employment | 3.54 | 0.09 | Hawker *et al.* (1976) |
| London | Abnormal drinkers | 5.0 | 1.7 | Hensman *et al.* (1968) |
| Highlands and Islands, Scotland | Alcoholics | 11.1 | 1.5 | Whittet (1970) |
| London | Alcoholics | 6.0 | 1.3 | Pollack (1971) |
| London | Having a notable drinking problem | | | |
| | known to GPs | 1.2 | 0.7 | Edwards *et al.* (1973) |
| | Known to 16 agencies | 8.6 | 1.3 | |
| | Identified by survey | 31.3 | | |
| Manchester, 192 general practices | Problem drinkers | 3.36 | | Wilkins and Hore (1976) |
| | Alcohol addicts | 1.35 | | |
| Manchester, one general practice | Alcoholics | 28.6 | 5.7 | Wilkins (1974) |
| | Abnormal drinkers | 42.2 | 12.4 | |
| London | Excessive drinkers | 21.0 | | Cartwright *et al.* (1975) |
| | Problem drinkers | 35.0 | | |

**Table 23.3.**  *National estimates of the prevalence of disability in Great Britain*

| Definition | Rate/1000 population Male | Female | Reference |
|---|---|---|---|
| Handicapped and impaired | 67 | 88 | Harris (1971) |
| Disablement condition limiting activities | 99 | 143 | Townsend (1979) |
| Self-declared limiting long-standing sickness | 153 | 170 | General Household Survey (1976) |
| Self-declared chronic health problem | 670 | 710 | General Household Survey (1977) |
| Estimated frequency of major classes of impairment | 343 | | Wood and Badley (1978) |

**Table 23.4.**  *Examples of variation in the results of surveys of the prevalence of disability conducted by local authorities in England*

| | Rate/1000 population |
|---|---|
| Northwich | 21 |
| Salford | 20 |
| Essex | 19 |
| Leeds | 85 |
| Cumberland | 68 |
| Kingston | 72 |

Collated and standardized by Knight and Warren (1978).

England in compliance with their duty, under the 1970 Chronically Sick and Disabled Persons Act, to make themselves aware of the numbers and needs of disabled people in their area. Again, though some geographical differences may be expected, such wide variations are difficult to reconcile.

An obvious starting-point is to consider official statistics. There are, however, many reasons why such figures are unlikely to be very useful. Administrative statistics of sociomedical problems are likely to be descriptions of services supplied rather than accurate prevalence rates. Each probably measures only one aspect of a problem, and each is collected for a particular purpose. It is, for instance, obvious that the

**Table 23.5.**  *Numbers of registered blind and deaf people, England and Wales, 1975*

| | Number (thousands) |
|---|---|
| Blind | 106.7 |
| Partially sighted | 44.2 |
| Deaf | 26.9 |
| Hard of hearing | 21.3 |

18 900 alcoholics who had been admitted for psychiatric treatment (Table 23.1) cannot be a total count of all those who might have been so labelled, had they ever come to the attention of a psychiatrist. Again, if one wished to consult routine statistics of disability, those available – persons registered under the Disabled Persons (Employment) Act, or registered with local authorities – would offer only special groups, identified in complex and not always obvious ways. This is illustrated in Table 23.5. Blindness and partial sight, deafness and partial hearing, are two disabilities for which objective clinical categories exist, with precise modes of measurement. They ought, therefore, to offer the most reliable categories. Yet the proportions of people registered in these categories in Britain seem to suggest that there are more than twice as many people who are blind as there are with partial sight, and that the hard-of-hearing are outnumbered by the totally deaf. This is obviously untrue, and an artefact of the way in which people can come to be registered. Registration takes place only if it has some purpose – in this case, if services or concessions are being allotted. Close examination of these processes may show that, since the benefits of registration are few for the partially-sighted, there is little incentive to register, and since professionals wish to achieve the maximum benefits for their clients, the category assessed as blind in fact includes many with partial sight. A category such as hard-of-hearing is potentially so large, especially among the elderly, that there is no point in attempting an accurate administrative count: services could not be provided for so many. Another example might be the prevalence of mental retardation in a community. Again, it might seem that accurate statistics

ought to be available since this is another disability for which standards (even if arbitrary) are set down. The statistically normal intelligence can be quantitatively described. Yet, the author of one eight-year study of a sample of 7000 subnormal people in an American city concluded that the questions: 'Who is really mentally retarded? What is the true prevalence rate?'

. . . are nonsense questions, which cannot be answered. Individuals have no name and belong to no class until they are assigned to one. The definer determines the terms of his definition and sets the boundaries for his classes. He constructs the model and prescribes the operations he will use to organise the world according to his categories (Mercer 1973).

## Reliability and completeness of case-finding

Many sociomedical problems concern behaviour which is considered unsatisfactory or damaging – at least by those who wish to alter it, or have to deal with its medical consequences – or even illegal. It may also be behaviour which is entirely private: schoolboys may intoxicate themselves with glue behind the shed, and the housewife may drink an excess of vodka behind closed doors. Thus it is not surprising that true prevalences are difficult to ascertain. Sometimes population surveys asking people about their own behaviour are the only possible method, but their results must always be suspect. In the survey *Drinking in England and Wales* (OPCS 1981), the admitted consumption of alcohol was equivalent to only 53 per cent of the total consumption according to the figures held by Customs and Excise, and comparable results of 40–60 per cent have been found in many countries. In surveys of youthful smoking or soft drug consumption, adolescent bravado on the one hand and guilty concealment on the other confound the results.

Completeness of case-finding is equally problematic if professionals are used as informants about their patients, clients, or pupils. It is not simply that problems may be concealed and unknown. Professionals may (without intentional exaggeration) overemphasize a problem that they wish to have brought to attention, or (more commonly, and again with no suggestion of deliberate concealment) may deny that a problem exists within their own sphere of responsibility. To admit that a particular problem is very prevalent suggests, after all, that they should have done something about it. There are many studies demonstrating that primary care doctors may be blind to alcohol problems in their patients, and that alcohol problems are rarely identified in hospital patients even though they may be very relevant to the illness which has brought them to the hospital. The low rates reported by general practitioners in Table 23.2 may be noted. If other agencies are included, the rates may be increased, as the studies of Edwards *et al.* (1973) and Cartwright *et al.* (1975) showed, but the completeness of case-finding must still remain problematic.

## Validity and the meaning of categories

As Table 23.2 demonstrates, however, it is not simply the reliability or completeness of surveys that is in question. These surveys are measuring different things. So what is it, in assessing the prevalence of sociomedical problems, that we wish to measure? In the case of alcoholism, it is obviously not simply those alcoholics who have come to the attention of psychiatric services, and been labelled by them. Even if there were absolute agreement within psychiatry about the criteria for a diagnosis of alcoholism, and even if all who fitted these criteria were identified, these are by no means the only people who constitute a problem. And it has been amply demonstrated that the precise definition of the meaning of 'alcoholic' differs among members of the public, among the medical profession, and among psychiatrists. As Orford and Edwards (1977) noted

That one should have to admit such loose usage of a key word is unsatisfactory but inevitable – perhaps more positively one should accept that this term's looseness of meaning is in accord with society's need for a very elastic word to describe such extremely variable happenings, and clusters of happenings, as may constitute the adverse consequences of excessive drinking.

A solution is sought by substituting the words problem drinking or excessive drinking for alcoholism. But what is excessive drinking? And do we mean that there are problems for the drinker or problems for society? Just as it is possible for an individual to have, or to create for others, problems because of his use of alcohol, without in any sense fitting the criteria for diagnosis as alcoholic, so it is possible for a dependent alcoholic to drink quietly by himself or herself, and create no problems for anyone else.

There are particular difficulties where the problem concerned is not a dichotomous one. If a substance is completely prohibited, or a type of behaviour is always injurious to health, then both control and health education are in principle simplified. If people with a certain disability will always need a specific service, then knowledge of prevalence will produce accurate requirements for planning. When, however, it is a matter of abuse rather than use or a matter of degree, then the social and contextual definitions of the boundaries become relevant. Normal drinking, and abuse, are socially defined: they depend upon the individual who is doing the drinking, the context in which the drinking occurs, and the customs of the society. In a society or group which condemns all alcohol, then any drinking at all may constitute a problem. On the other hand, even very heavy drinking, if it has no medical or social consequences in a particular individual, may not be relevant as a problem. Different standards apply to young workmen and old ladies. It may not be the drinking, but the context in which it occurs which is the problem: not how much alcohol has been consumed, but whether the drinker then drives a car. The form which alcohol-associated problems may take depends upon the way of life in a particular environment.

In practice, the problem is often defined in terms of those who need services. *All* the elderly cannot possibly be a problem, but the frail and elderly who have no-one to care for them are. *All* drinkers are not a problem but those identified as alcoholic are. *All* very youthful childbearing is not a problem, but unintended children born to very young mothers are. This may seem to simplify matters, since the definition and identification of special groups with special needs is easier. But it is a circular definition, since the problem has to be identified, and need for services perceived, before the potential clients can be numbered.

## What is the problem and to whom?

This is not to suggest that research into the extent of the sociomedical problems which concern public health is impossible or fruitless. Those who have responsibility for services need to respond to problems which are manifestly troubling a community, and need information on which preventive programmes may be based or services evaluated.

What is suggested is that the simplest epidemiological model – define precisely what it is that you are counting, and then count it as accurately as possible, in relation to a defined population – may not be appropriate. Nor may the usual model of evaluation – define precisely the objectives and clientele of this service and measure its efficiency. To impose definitions – for example, people who are housebound are disabled; people who consume more than 25 pints of beer a week are excessive drinkers – may be useful for some specific purpose, but will be useless for others. Evaluation is complicated by the fact that the total system of services for sociomedical problems is made up of a multitude of professions, who may each have different aims and different concepts of the problem.

Sociomedical problems rise to the top of the agenda, present themelves to doctors in the community for solution or alleviation or management, in varied and complex ways. There may be true increases in the behaviour involved, epidemics which demand control. Sometimes, however, it is not so much a real increase which has caused concern, but rather a change – for example, in the visibility of the problem, or in the composition of the group of the population involved. It is when a problem becomes difficult to manage, when there are no services available, or when the appropriate services are flooded, that voices are raised. Changes in the ideas about their own role held by professions may change the visibility or the apparent nature of a problem. It could be argued that the contemporary concern about the extent of a problem of alcohol abuse has been affected not only by a real increase in the number of excessive drinkers, but also by the fact that the disease model of alcoholism is less favoured. Since conventional psychiatric in-patient treatment has not been conspicuously successful, the problem moves out into community treatment and becomes a task for community agencies. All these processes have to be borne in mind in attempting to quantify a sociomedical problem.

Instead of asking – How much of this problem exists? – the relevant questions may be – Why is this a problem, and to whom?

## RESEARCH STUDY

The study to be described is offered as a more extended illustration of some of the above points. It was an attempt to describe and measure the problem of alcohol abuse in one community, the Western Isles of Scotland. The detailed results cannot, of course, be applied to any other community. As argued above, however, sociomedical poblems are specific to social contexts and must ultimately be studied at community level. The advantage of this particular geographical area as an example is that it is small enough and sufficiently clearly defined for a detailed examination which may demonstrate the issues involved.

The study was conducted at the request of the Social Work Department of the local authority (the equivalent in Scotland of Social Service Departments in England) and the Council of the Islands. It was thought that a problem of alcohol abuse did exist in this community, and that some quantification and description would be useful. The response of the sociologists involved was to suggest that a study focusing upon *alcohol problems,* however manifested, would be appropriate, rather than one which attempted to produce a prevalence of alcoholism. The research questions which were addressed were as follows.

1. What is the nature of the problem as presented to those who have to deal with its consequences – principally social workers and doctors, but also nurses, teachers, clergy, police, publicans, and others?

2. How much of the time of social workers or doctors is taken up with these problems? In what ways do they or other professional groups feel that they have difficulties in helping, controlling, or educating drinkers, and what solutions does each group suggest? In what ways are people referred to helping services?

3. What are the views of the general public? Do they match those of professionals or community spokesmen?

4. What is the level of drinking in this population? Does it appear to be true that the use and abuse of alcohol is increasing?

5. In what different ways can the prevalence of problem drinkers be quantified, and what is the relationship between the different measures?

## Method

A four-pronged method was adopted, focusing on the questions in four different ways, and using for each part of the study the method most appropriate for obtaining the sort of information required.

1. A random-sample questionnaire survey of the population (aged 18 years and over) was conducted by a team of interviewers. The object of this was not to ask people about their alcohol consumption in detail, in part because of the problems of reliability and in part because of a desire not to offend the population by asking questions they might not have wished to answer. Rather, they were asked about their drinking habits in general, their views on what constituted normal and heavy drinking, their descriptions of drinking patterns among their friends and the people of their district, and their views and attitudes on a variety of associated issues. Several of the qustions and attitudinal measures were designed to be comparable with a survey on drinking habits in Scotland undertaken by the Office of Population Censuses and Surveys (OPCS 1980). In a sample of 1000 respondents (about 5 per cent of the population) a 90 per cent response rate was achieved.

2. Interviews were conducted with as many social workers, doctors, and other community professionals and spokesmen as possible (in all 113), to obtain their accounts of the extent

of the problem, its causes and nature, its relevance to their own work, and opinions about its solution.

3. In order to set these views beside actual practice, and estimate the actual work-load associated with alcohol abuse, work-load diaries were obtained from representative samples of social workers (nine) and primary care doctors (11). Each social worker or doctor was asked to fill in diary sheets for seven days, noting the characteristics of all patients or clients (without identification by name) and the nature of the work performed for them. Special note was made of any involvement of alcohol abuse in the problem of the patient or client, and these cases were afterwards discussed with a research worker.

4. Nine social workers and four general practitioners undertook the considerable work of a survey of patients/clients. Each went through their entire list of patients or clients and filled in a detailed form for each individual for whom they had evidence of a medical or social problem associated with the consumption of alcohol. No definition of a problem was imposed since the objective was to derive from the forms the professionals' own definitions of what constituted an alcohol problem, and to compare the definitions used by each group of professionals, or by each individual. At the same time, many more restricted groups of alcohol abusers defined by various criteria can be identified with some reliability from these returns – for example, alcoholics so diagnosed by a psychiatrist, or people with physical illness which is diagnosed by their doctor as the result of alcohol abuse, or drinkers known to the social work department because of concern about the welfare of children, and so on. The doctors' returns, in this section of the study, can be compared with another area of the Scottish Highlands and Islands, Shetland, where all the general practitioners took part in an identical survey (Blaxter 1981).

## Results

The detailed results of this study are given elsewhere (Blaxter *et al.* 1982). Here, a selection of findings is presented, chosen to illustrate the issues which have been discussed.

### Incidence of heavy drinking

There is no doubt that some very heavy drinking does occur in this community. The evidence for this can only be the accounts of both professionals and public, but these accounts were unanimous. Some indirect evidence can be derived from the question in the survey of the public: 'How much would someone have to drink in a week before you would call them a heavy drinker?' The answer was usually in terms of bottles of whisky per week, and if not was converted into this measure. Table 23.6 shows that the amount suggested – an average of two and a half bottles – was conspicuously higher than the amount suggested by the Scottish population as a whole in the survey *Scottish drinking habits* (OPCS 1980). Even more clearly than in that survey, the definition of heavy drinking was more liberal for those who themselves drank.

Another question asked in the survey was 'Of the men (women) you know, how many would you say are heavy drinkers?' Twenty two per cent of men said that at least half

**Table 23.6.** *Definition of heavy drinking in the Western Isles. Number of bottles whisky/week which constitutes heavy drinking*

|  | Western Isles | | Scotland* | |
|  | M | F | M | F |
| --- | --- | --- | --- | --- |
| All | 2.5 | 2.4 | 2.2 | 2.2 |
| By own drinking habits: | | | | |
|   Teetotal | 1.9 | 2.1 | 2.1 | 2.1 |
|   Occasional drinker | 2.3 | 2.6 | 2.1 | 2.2 |
|   More regular drinker | 2.8 | 2.6 | 2.3 | 2.2 |

*OPCS (1980).

of the men they knew were heavy drinkers, though only 6 per cent said that at least half the women they knew were heavy drinkers.

Against this, however, must be set the evidence of self-declared drinking habits. As already noted, no attempt was made to ascertain the quantity of alcohol which people claimed to drink, but they were asked about the occasions when they (or 'people you know') drank, and were asked to place themselves in the crude categories illustrated in Table 23.7. Some who were heavy drinkers may have preferred to conceal the fact. It seems unlikely, however, that many would claim to be teetotal if this were not true. By comparison with the population of Scotland as a whole, and with England and Wales, there were very many *more* non-drinkers in this community. Analysis by age indicated that the non-drinkers, especially among women, were likely to be older: among men over 50 years, 55 per cent admitted to more than very occasional drinking, and among women over 50 years only 9 per cent. This matched well with the data obtained in the similar community of Shetland, using the knowledge which general practitioners had of their patients in small rural practices.

**Table 23.7.** *Distribution of self-declared drinking habits, per cent, in the Western Isles compared with Scotland and England*

|  | Western Isles | | Scotland* | | England and Wales † | |
|  | M | F | M | F | M | F |
| --- | --- | --- | --- | --- | --- | --- |
| Teetotal | 17 | 39 | 5 | 12 | 6 | 11 |
| Occasional drinker | 21 | 41 | 22 | 42 | 18 | 31 |
| More regular drinker | 62 | 20 | 74 | 46 | 76 | 58 |
| (Sample *N*) | (405) | (495) | (1618) | (1887) | (931) | (1003) |

*OPCS (1980).
†OPCS (1981).

Thus, it appeared that the *overall* amount of drinking in this community was, in fact, probably less than in Scotland as a whole. The problem begins to emerge as one of sharp divisions within the community, with some heavy drinking set beside a high level of abstinence.

These divisions are illuminated by an analysis by area and by religious adherence of self-declared drinking habits, or of opinions about the extent of a problem of alcohol abuse, or of answers to attitudinal questions. This is a community in which religion has great importance, and in which adherence to different churches is strongly associated with area of residence. Some of the most striking contrasts are illustrated in Table 23.8.

**Table 23.8.** *Extremes of difference, by area and by religious adherence, in the answers to various questions in a population survey of the Western Isles*

| | Per cent | |
|---|---|---|
| **People holding the view that heavy drinking is a special problem in this area** | | |
| Town | 64 | |
| One rural area in North of Isles | 39 | |
| One rural area in South of Isles | 24 | |
| Church of Scotland | 37 | |
| Free Church of Scotland | 47 | |
| Roman Catholic | 18 | |
| No religious adherence | 44 | |
| **Self-declared regular drinkers** | M | F |
| Town | 55 | 18 |
| One rural area in North of Isles | 62 | 12 |
| One rural area in South of Isles | 75 | 40 |
| Church of Scotland | | 34 |
| Free Church of Scotland | | 28 |
| Roman Catholic | | 55 |
| No religious adherence | | 64 |
| **People expressing agreement with the statement 'There is nothing wrong in having a few drinks'** | | |
| Town | 45 | |
| One rural area in South of Isles | 90 | |
| **People agreeing with the statement 'People drink because it is the polite thing to do'** | | |
| Town | 80 | |
| One rural area in North of Isles | 21 | |
| **People expressing agreement with the statement 'Doctors shouldn't waste time on alcoholics'** | | |
| One rural area in North of Isles | 13 | |
| One rural area in South of Isles | 38 | |

Other conflicts, besides these obvious ones of religion, area, and the urban/rural dimension, emerged from the population survey and from the interview data. It was frequently suggested that it was the incomers rather than the indigenous population who perceived a problem of drinking, and so in a sense created it, because they did not understand the culture of the Islands. Some heavy drinking on specified and almost ritual occasions was the norm, and the offering of alcoholic drink was bound up with traditions of hospitality. Some slight evidence of this incomers-versus-locals conflict was found in the population survey, where 40 per cent of those who were locally born agreed that drinking was a special problem in the area, and 44 per cent of those who had been born elsewhere in Scotland, compared with 61 per cent of the rather small number born in England or other countries.

In noting these contradictions within the community, however, mention must be made of one conflict that was absent.

Unusually in alcohol studies, social class was not an important variable in any analysis. There were some occupations where drinking appeared to be more common – for example, fishermen – or less common – for example, crofters – but there appeared to be little difference by socio-economic status in the amount of alcohol drunk or in attitudes and opinions.

*Attitudes to drinking problems*

Further evidence about the nature of the problem was obtained from the parts of the study involving professional workers and community spokesmen. Various objective indicators all suggested that the level of alcohol-related problems was, in fact, rather less than on the mainland of Scotland. Formal statistics of alcohol-associated crime, vandalism, violence, delinquency, broken homes, underage drinking, or drinking and driving offences, were all relatively low. It was notable that every spokesman *thought* they were high, except the particular agency responsible. That is, both the public and the community spokesmen thought that drinking and driving was a serious and growing problem, but the police statistics showed low rates and modest growth. High rates of liver disease were generally postulated, but hospitals showed low figures. Every informant thought that drinking at work was a problem, except employers; juvenile drinking was generally stressed, except by the schools, which saw it as a minor and easily contained problem, and by the system of juvenile justice, which saw few cases.

The explanation for this may lie in the processes by which these deviants are officially identified in this particular society. Employers might be unusually tolerant of drinking workers, or the police of drinking and driving. The public's opinion was that, to some extent, this might be true. The social and geographical environment, with its many scattered rural communities, and relative absence of industrial work, must also be taken into account. This is a society in which violence and crime are in general very low. However, whether these rates are real or the product of particular identification processes, there is a sense in which behaviour, seen as deviant in other communities, is not a problem if it is seen as normal or without serious consequences in this community. If these formal indicators are low, by Scottish standards, then the problem of drinking is perhaps not one of high rates of alcohol-associated public offences, just as it is not one of overly high general consumption, but rather one of attitudes.

The less structured parts of the survey of the public, and all the interview data, made it very clear that alcohol has special meanings in this society. The tradition of almost ritual and ceremonial occasions for heavy drinking was stressed, and the association of drinking with manliness. Social and economic changes were being imposed upon this culture: women were drinking publicly, which was once taboo; young people could afford to drink more. The custom of social drinking had been imported from the Scottish mainland, but it combined uneasily with the older tradition of special-occasion drinking. It was, in fact, their perception of *change* which identified a problem in the public mind. The age-distribution of women among self-declared drinkers was one indication that this perception was accurate.

At the same time, it became clear that there was another

conflict associated with attitudes to drinking which was characteristic of this particular community, compared with Scotland as a whole. Drinking was associated with hospitality and celebration: but at the same time, the regular drinking of individuals (especially privately) was associated with negative emotions, with depression, loneliness, frustration, inadequacy, and guilt. In the population survey, and in the interviews with community spokesmen, increasing incomes and imported life-styles were frequently offered as reasons why the problem was growing. As one member of the public said: 'it's affluence – changing from relative poverty to relative affluence very quickly with no time to adapt and keep a sense of true values'.

The isolation of the Islands, unemployment, and lack of prospects for the young, were equally favoured as explanations for heavy drinking. In the population survey many people made thoughtful suggestions such as: 'Precarious employment – the uncertainties of fishing and crofting, the problems of loneliness, especially among the old'; 'It's shy people – their common characteristic is inferiority, inhibition, those without the character or sense to withstand social pressures to continue drinking'.

More structured data were obtained, in the population survey, by the administration of groups of attitudinal questions repeated from *Scottish drinking habits* (OPCS 1980). A few examples of the results are illustrated in Table 23.9. In the Scottish survey, there had been moderate agreement with many anti-drinking statements, but also agreement with pro-drinking statements. Drink could be both good and bad. In the Western Isles, however, attitudes were conspicuously different. Although a majority of men were drinkers, most still expressed attitudes which were strongly against drink although they were not less sympathetic towards alcoholics (Table 23.9). Similarly, in a set of questions about motivation for drinking (where the results are not entirely

**Table 23.9.** *Attitudes to drinking: the Western Isles compared with the Scottish population*

| | Per cent of respondents agreeing | | | |
| | Western Isles | | Scotland* | |
| Examples of statements | M | F | M | F |
|---|---|---|---|---|
| **Examples of anti-drinking statements:** | | | | |
| Drink brings out the worse in people | 73 | 80 | 47 | 49 |
| Drink is one of the main causes of immoral behaviour | 80 | 85 | 65 | 76 |
| **Examples of pro-drinking statements:** | | | | |
| Having a drink is one of the pleasures of life | 46 | 28 | 79 | 57 |
| A drink makes people more sociable | 60 | 43 | 87 | 82 |
| **Examples of attitudes to alcoholics statements:** | | | | |
| People who become alcoholics have only themselves to blame | 62 | 61 | 51 | 42 |
| Alcoholics can never reach the point where they stop drinking for good | 23 | 22 | 29 | 27 |

*OPCS (1980).

**Table 23.10.** *Reasons for drinking: the Western Isles compared with the Scottish population*

| | Per cent of respondents agreeing | | | |
| | Western Isles | | Scotland* | |
| Examples of statements | M | F | M | F |
|---|---|---|---|---|
| To give them confidence | 78 | 87 | 10 | 9 |
| To forget their worries | 76 | 76 | 9 | 5 |
| Because it makes them feel at ease | 73 | 80 | 21 | 18 |
| Because it is the polite thing to do | 63 | 66 | 39 | 42 |
| Because they enjoy the taste | 36 | 37 | 51 | 27 |

*OPCS (1980).

comparable with *Scottish drinking habits,* since a slightly different form of words was used) the emphasis on drinking to give oneself confidence, forget one's worries, or for other psychological reasons, rather than because it was intrinsically pleasurable, was very notable. In Table 23.10, only those who are drinkers themselves are included. In the other attitudinal measures a difference might, of course, be expected between drinkers and non-drinkers. This difference was apparent (as it was in the Scottish survey) but was less than the associated difference between religious adherences and area of residence. In many other parts of the survey, opinions similar to those of the Scottish population had been expressed, and it was only in these attitudinal questions that major differences emerged. It seemed obvious that the ambivalences and contradictions with which the subject of drink was surrounded were a major cause of the problem.

*Prevalence rates based on information from doctors and social workers*

The second and third components of the study – the surveys of patients/clients and the workload studies – provided different ways of measuring and describing alcohol abuse. From the information gathered in these studies, the number of problem drinkers in the population could be estimated. Table 23.11 shows some of the prevalence rates that could be derived, depending upon the definition used. It demonstrates clearly not only that the prevalence of a problem depends upon the way it is defined, but offers examples of all the factors of reliability and validity discussed earlier.

The general practitioners, by going through their records and filling in a form for each patient whom they thought to have a problem of alcohol abuse, produced prevalence figures which are very high, especially for males. They may be compared, for instance, with some of the rates produced in general practice shown in Table 23.2. It happened that they were almost identical with the rates produced in the similar but more complete survey in general practice in Shetland. However, there is no way of knowing without further replication whether this indicates that rates are truly similar, or whether application of the same method among the same group of professionals is likely to produce similar rates.

These high rates in both studies may simply be the result of the greater knowledge that these doctors may have of their patients, especially in rural areas and in practices which are

**Table 23.11.** *Problem drinkers in the Western Isles defined in different ways. Population rates per 1000, aged 18 years and over*

| Definition | M | F |
|---|---|---|
| Known to doctors | 63 | 12 |
| Known to social workers | 10 | 5 |
| Psychiatrically-diagnosed alcoholic | 17 | 6 |
| Drinkers with symptoms of dependence | 39 | 10 |
| Drinkers with illnesses associated with alcohol abuse | 38 | 7 |
| Drinkers known to doctors with: | | |
|   Family problems | 41 | 10 |
|   Employment problems | 40 | 6 |
|   Care of children causing concern | 7 | 3 |
|   Drink-associated crimes and offences | 17 | 2 |
| Drinkers known to social workers with: | | |
|   Family problems | 9 | 4 |
|   Employment problems | 7 | 1 |
|   Care of children causing concern | 5 | 2 |
|   Drink-associated crimes and offences | 7 | < 1 |
| Categorized by doctor as: | | |
|   Alcoholic | 20 | 7 |
|   Problem drinker/bout drinker | 22 | 2 |
|   Heavy drinker with (only) medical problems | 4 | < 1 |
|   Heavy drinker with no known problems | 6 | < 1 |
|   Alcoholic at present abstinent | 11 | 2 |
| Self-defined problem drinkers: | | |
|   Who have sought help from doctors | 28 | 5 |
|   Who have sought help from social workers | 1 | < 1 |

Bases for rates: doctors' records, knowledge, or opinions in four general prctices, totalling 4486 people; knowledge and opinions of seven social workers, covering a population of approximately 13 560 people.

relatively small. The high rate of self-defined problem drinkers seeking help from their doctor (again, almost identical in Shetland) is unusual, and must represent a particular relationship in these communities. In the survey conducted by Wilkins (1974), in comparison, only eight out of 155 problem drinkers identified had themselves consulted about their drinking. Examination of the returns of different doctors showed clearly that this must in part be a function of the doctor's style of practice and interests, for there was great variation between them. The likelihood that patients will identify themselves to him is only one of many factors – length of time in the community, stability of the population – which will obviously affect the rate at which an individual doctor can identify problem drinkers.

The derivation of a population rate from the knowledge of social workers is even less legitimate. Social workers do not, of course, have defined practice populations in the way that doctors do. In Table 23.11, an assumption, only partly warranted, is made that an area and its population belong in equal proportions to all the social workers working in it. Equivalences between social workers and the population they serve are straightforward where there is only one worker in a defined area, but where teams are operating (as in the town) different workers may have different interests, and it cannot be assumed that all are equally likely to have problem drinking clients. Since those who took part in the survey were more

likely than others to have this interest, the rates derived from their returns may be exaggerated.

The rates produced by social workers are in any case very much lower than those obtained from the doctors. It could be argued that the drinking clients of social workers are, by definition, drinkers with problems, whereas the doctors may know many more who abuse alcohol but have no problems, or only medical problems. Yet, as Table 23.11 shows, these categories were very small among the doctors' patients, and the doctors knew that a high proportion of their patients were experiencing social problems. The only category where the knowledge of the doctors and the social workers produces similar rates is that of drinkers where the care of children is causing concern.

Despite this, social workers, in interview, emphasized the serious problem of alcohol abuse in the community rather more than doctors. Why this should be so is illustrated in Table 23.12. Although the doctors knew many alcohol-abusing patients, their daily work contained only a small proportion of alcohol-related cases. For the social workers, on the other hand, alcohol abuse caused or contributed to over a third of their daily tasks, and it was only to be expected that they would stress its prevalence.

**Table 23.12.** *Prevalence of alcohol problems in the Western Isles expressed as proportions of the work of doctors and social workers*

| | Per cent |
|---|---|
| Proportion of consulations which were alcohol-related (work of 11 doctors during one week, diary sheets) | 5 |
| Proportion of cases which were alcohol-related (work of nine social workers during one week, diary sheets) | 35 |

*Characteristics of drinkers identified by doctors and social workers*

Table 23.13 shows some distributions, by social variables, of the problem drinkers identified by doctors and by social workers. It becomes obvious that each is identifying a group which must be to some extent different. Compared with the problem drinking patients of doctors, the problem drinkers known to social workers (whether as clients, or as family members of clients) are more likely to be female, and to be younger, though there may also be a small group of elderly widows who are not known to their doctors as drinkers. Some of the differences in Table 23.13 doubtless result from the different information available to each profession. Social workers may be more likely to know, for instance, that the problem drinker is unemployed. Others, however, obviously represent the different types of problem presented to each profession. Doctors are likely to become aware of alcohol abuse when it has medical consequences, which may take some years to develop. For social workers, it was the existence of young families, or sometimes the problems of old people, which focused their attention on alcohol abuse.

**Table 23.13.** *Distribution by some social variables of the problem drinkers identified by doctors and by social workers in the Western Isles*

| | Per cent of all problem drinkers of this sex | | | |
| | Identified by doctors | | Identified by social workers | |
| | M | F | M | F |
|---|---|---|---|---|
| Under 40 years of age | 35 | 30 | 41 | 57 |
| 60 years of age and over | 21 | 7 | 19 | 12 |
| Widowed | 5 | 7 | 5 | 24 |
| Divorced/separated | 5 | 15 | 19 | 21 |
| Fisherman or Merchant Navy | 23 | – | 8 | – |
| Unemployed | 3 | – | 29 | – |
| Spouse known to be also problem drinker | 11 | 33 | 12 | 41 |

The doctors identified more people (an average for each participating doctor of 41, compared with 12 for each social worker). To what extent, however, were the two professions selecting the same individuals? This can be answered only in a few medical practices where it is possible to define equivalent client populations for the social workers. Also, individuals cannot be identified with absolute certainty, since confidentiality was retained with regard to names and the matching has to rely on the detailed personal data on the returns.

The meaning of 'identified' may, of course, vary. The two professions may actually know different individuals, or they may be defining a problem drinker in different ways. If a heavy-drinking person was identified by his doctor but not recorded by a social worker, it may be that the social worker did not have any knowledge of him, or did not define this drinking as a problem.

The two areas used in this analysis are one small rural island population, and two general practices in the town. In the town, the question 'How many of the social workers' problem drinkers were also known to doctors?' cannot be answered, since these clients might be patients of other doctors.

The notable finding of this matching exercise was how few of the problem drinkers were jointly identified, especially in the town (Table 23.14). Of the 114 problem drinkers known to the three doctors involved, only 13 were identified by social workers. Those who were jointly identified were not, as might be expected, disproportionately female.

There were some obvious reasons why many of the 101 drinkers identified only by doctors might not be known to

**Table 23.14.** *Doctors' problem drinkers, identified and not identified by social workers*

| | No of problem drinkers | | |
| | Returned by doctor only | Returned by both | Returned by social worker only |
|---|---|---|---|
| One rural practice | 32 | 8 | 5 |
| Two town practices | 69 | 5 | NA |

social workers. Seventeen were described as seamen, drinking heavily only when they came ashore, the majority of whom were single men. Social workers would be unlikely to see these as potential clients. Another 19 of the males (but no females) were described by the doctors as sober alcoholics. To the social workers, a man who was no longer drinking was not likely to be identified as a problem. To the doctors, however, 'alcoholic' was a diagnosis of a condition which could not be reversed, even after years of abstinence – in any list of problem drinkers such a person must still be included. Another characteristic of the problem drinkers identified only by doctors was their likelihood of having professional or other non-manual occupations. Eight of the 14 women were from non-manual families, and 20 of the 87 men. Six of these were among the cured alcoholics. Since the social class distribution of the total list identified by social workers did not differ greatly from that of the doctors, the conclusion would appear to be, not that social workers have no involvement with non-manual families (in this community), but that doctors are less likely to *refer* such families to them. There were also 11 cases where the patient was described as a secret or solitary drinker who would not admit to any problem, so that any formal referral to another agency would have been difficult or inappropriate.

For the remainder of drinkers identified only by doctors, there were no obvious reasons why they should not be known to social workers. Nine of the women, and 28 of the men, had been psychiatrically diagnosed as alcoholic. It was not true that drinkers whose problems were *only* medical formed a significant proportion of the group. Indeed, only six were identified on the grounds of health problems alone, even if health is defined as including accidents, symptoms of addiction, or suicide attempts. Thirty-seven of the men were described by the doctors as having no health problems whatsoever, being identified only on the grounds of their heavy drinking and its social consequences. Fixty-six were known by the doctor to have employment problems and 14 drink-associated criminal offences. Perhaps more relevantly, 42 of the men (20 with dependent children) were believed by the doctor to have problems of marital relationships, child care, or family functioning.

Thus the conclusion must be that these two professions are, in part, seeing different *versions* of this problem: there are groups known to doctors whom social workers would be unlikely to be in contact with. But also, in part, they can identify different *individuals* within very similar groups: practical contingencies, the actions and choices of the drinker or his family, the particular consequences of the drinking behaviour, might determine whether the problem was presented to this professional or that, but the essential nature of the problem could be the same.

*Drinkers known to both doctors and social workers*

These people, though so few in number, were of considerable interest. Comparison of the returns in each case demonstrated, first, how problematic the concept of referral from one professional to another may be. Each described how the drinker had come to his attention, and there was little coincidence between the accounts. In some cases, for instance, the doctor believed that it was he who had referred the problem to the social worker, while the social worker said the case had come from quite other sources such as the police. It was obvious that family members – sometimes the same family member and sometimes different individuals – were consulting doctors and social workers independently. Sometimes drinkers themselves had sought help from both.

Secondly, this comparison demonstrated how differently professionals might view the same situation (or, perhaps, how different the presentations of the individual concerned might be to different professionals). Of one patient, for instance, the doctor noted that 'He maintains that he can control his drinking' and there were no social problems. The social worker involved in the case had been consulted by the wife because she wished to leave her husband, listed many social problems, and commented 'He has no wish to control his drinking, accepts that it is self-destructive but does not care'. It was social workers rather than doctors who gave psychologically-oriented descriptions of a problem. For instance, the doctors' verdict of 'antisocial behaviour' in one case became, for the social worker, 'immature personality rejecting his role as husband and father'.

Both doctors and social workers demonstrated concern about their patients/clients, and both had a great deal of detailed knowledge about the families involved. In many instances, however, they were seeing the case in quite different ways. If it had been possible to ask others who knew problem drinkers on an individual basis – the police, for example, or Alcoholics Anonymous – to describe the same people, there is no doubt that their perceptions of each problem would have been different again.

### Prevalence of alcoholism

Table 23.11 also illustrates the problematic nature of administrative statistics of alcoholism. The category of 'psychiatrically-diagnosed as alcoholic' is likely to be reliably counted. There may have been patients whose psychiatric history was unknown to their doctors, but only very few. At the same time, it is obvious that this is a very selected category, for there were more than twice as many men (but a smaller proportion of women) whom the doctors knew to have symptoms (tremors, amnesia, withdrawal symptoms, and so on) suggestive of dependence, who might equally have merited the diagnosis.

The variables by which people may be selected for psychiatric referral, or diagnosed as alcoholic, are of several different sorts. The doctors' individual attitudes may be crucial, and this was demonstrated in both the Western Isles and Shetland by a wide practice variation in rates. Characteristics of the patient may also be relevant: comparison of all those with dependence symptoms with those who had been diagnosed as alcoholic suggested that, other things being equal, women were more likely to be referred for treatment than men, non-manual workers slightly more likely than manual workers, and the divorced and separated particularly likely. There is no way of telling from these data, of course, the direction of any causal relationship between the diagnosis and marital breakdown. A third type of variable affecting referral rates must be the provision of services. Here, as in Shetland, there appeared to be some community resistance to accepting treatment in a psychiatric hospital, and some reluctance on the part of doctors to suggest it, since in-patient treatment meant leaving the Islands.

### The categories used by professionals

No definition of alcoholic or problem drinker was imposed on the doctors or social workers, since the objective was to study the interpretations which the professionals themselves put upon these labels. For each patient whom they identified, they were asked to provide a summary categorization representing their opinion of the appropriate diagnosis.

Few of the social workers were prepared to categorize clients in this way. They preferred to think in terms of problems, rather than categories of clients, and to view each individually. Most felt that it was not their function to offer a diagnosis of alcoholism, nor did they feel that the category was a particularly useful one.

The categorizations of the doctors, however, provided an interesting analysis. In interview, there was little consistency between them, for many different interpretations of the word alcoholic were offered, and several doctors queried whether the term was at all meaningful. There were a few differences in the returns of individual doctors. Some, for instance, tended to include very youthful heavy drinkers among their problem drinkers even though they knew of no problems caused by their drinking, while others required evidence of medical or social damage before they would identify a problem.

However, the returns demonstrated that there was a much greater measure of agreement in practice than had appeared in interview. As shown in Table 23.11, the doctors categorized many more people (especially men) as alcoholics, past or present, than had been given a formal psychiatric diagnosis. Alcoholics were likely to be those with known symptoms suggesting dependence, daily or continuous drinkers, who had themselves consulted the doctor about their drinking or about whom others had consulted. Those who were called problem drinker rather than alcoholic were likely to be weekend or bout drinkers, and more likely to be beer than spirit drinkers. Three-quarters of the small number of women identified were called alcoholic, but only half of the men. This and other evidence suggested that, for the doctors, the consequences of drinking had to be rather more serious for women than for men before they would be known about, or perhaps that doctors were more unwilling to label women without very good cause. Known social problems were not relevant to the distinction between alcoholic and problem drinker for either sex.

### Professional work and the perception of a problem

The sample-in-time of the day-to-day work of doctors and of social workers showed that their perceptions of their own workload and normal practices, which they had described in interviews, were not always accurate. Descriptions of the mechanisms by which clients were usually referred to the Social Work Department, or of the referrals to other agencies that were made on their behalf, were not entirely substantiated in the week – presumed to be typical – during which work was actually monitored. In the week's consultations reviewed the doctors were found, in about half the cases, to be treating the presenting medical symptoms or giving a certificate for absence from work, without any discussion of the alcohol problem. With the majority of the rest, the doctor discussed the problem or advised the patient to drink less, but in this sample of time it was rare for any other action to be taken.

This is not to suggest that, in talking about the problem, either profession was being misleading. Few people have a totally accurate impression of how they spend their working time, and quantification of time does not necessarily bear any relation to the salience of working problems. The point to be made is the danger of relying for information on rules-in-theory – that is, all people who come into this category are dealt with thus, and so may be found within these administrative statistics – which, though perfectly honestly held, may differ for many reasons from rules-in-practice.

The workload studies, together with the patient/client surveys and the interview material, demonstrated that problems of alcohol abuse presented many difficulties for the professionals involved. These include the inherently intractable nature of alcohol problems, uncertainty about professional functions, and the perceived lack of varied and appropriate specialist services to which problem drinkers could be referred. Concealment and denial made the treatment of an unwilling patient or client impossible. Certain of the attitudes identified as particular to the community – the association of drinking with manliness, traditional patterns of consumption, the conflicts in the community about alcohol – compounded their difficulties. There was reluctance to tackle alcohol-abusing patients and clients, because no very effective cures could be offered. This work was worrying, time-consuming, and often unrewarding. Cases in which it was the spouse or other relative of the drinker who was seeking help from a doctor, or in which it was another person's drinking which was causing problems for the social worker's client, were particularly troubling.

People in other occupations where drinking problems were relevant – publicans in their discussions of under-age drinking, for instance, or some of those responsible for health education of young people – were equally eloquent about the very real problems that their work presented them with. As far as the service-providers in the community were concerned, it was often ambiguity about their responsibilities, and a felt lack of specialist help and advice, that was at the core of their concern. To this extent, it was the service-providers who were creating the problem.

## CONCLUSIONS

There were, of course, many other topics of the study which have been described, related to the structure of cure or control in the particular community, the interrelation of services, and the views of public and professionals on the practical measures which might be taken, which are less relevant here. Any study, and especially one which relies on the good will and co-operation of professional people, ought to attempt to be of practical use.

The following is a summary of the most important *general* points about the description of a sociomedical problem which have been illustrated.

1. Formal statistics of a problem are created by complex processes, and are likely to be misleading unless they are recognized to be statistics of services provided, in categories chosen as appropriate by the providers.

2. Attitudes and the social environment create sociomedical problems in ways which are particular to specific communities, and close examination is likely to show that even a small and culturally distinct area (such as the Western Isles) cannot be thought of as one community. The lesson might be that since the same problem is differently caused in different communities, it ought to be differently managed. Health education or any other programme directed at the alleviation of a problem must be based on a knowledge of its specific nature in a specific environment.

3. Problems are closely associated with the perception of social change. It may not be so much a true increase in a problem that is troubling a community, as a change in its nature or in the group of the population affected, seen to be associated with general social changes about which there is ambivalence.

4. Problems are to some degree created by professionals. That is, it is their own problems in dealing with the cases they are presented with which highlight the extent of the problem. When this occurs, it suggests that there are some uncertainties about professional functions, or services are inadequate in scale, or perhaps that there are different sorts of services which should be provided.

5. Different professionals, dealing ostensibly with the same problem, are likely to be dealing with different aspects of it and different populations. For many, the problem will be seen as occurring somewhere else, for in their own sphere of responsibility they will have developed routines for dealing with it, so that it ceases to be a problem of any magnitude. Because sociomedical problems are rarely amenable to precise, clinical, or objective definition, even individuals within the same profession may vary greatly, not only in their knowledge about the people they deal with, but also in the way that they define the problem.

6. Thus, although it is essential that the quantification of a problem should be based on the perceptions of those who, in practice, define the problems in the community in question, there is unlikely to be a single source of information that will cover all the manifestations of the problem. Sociomedical problems, by definition, involve a variety of social and medical agencies.

7. An informed concern about sociomedical problems implies a very special relationship between those who work in public health or community medicine, and their community. Of course, the causes and cures of these problems very frequently lie outside individual behaviour. Even when a type of behaviour is clearly implicated – as in the case of alcohol abuse – the root causes of sickness may be structural, and as much to do with a society's attitudes, environment, and economic condition as with the individual. Attempts to exert influence upon the societal and structural causes of illness have not always been seen as the traditional sphere of medicine. It is within public health, however, that the responsibility to look clearly at the relationship between medical and social ills traditionally lies.

*Acknowledgements*

The research study from which these data were extracted, *Problems of alcohol abuse in the Western Isles,* was supported jointly by the Chief Scientist Organisation of the Scottish Home and Health Department, and the Social Work Department and Health Board of the Western Isles.

## REFERENCES

Blaxter, M. (1981). *Survey of problem drinking in Shetland,* Shetland Isles Health Board, Lerwick.

Blaxter, M., Mullen, K., and Dyer, S. (1982). *Problems of alcohol abuse in the Western Isles: a community study.* Scottish Health Service Studies No. 44, Scottish Home and Health Department, Edinburgh.

Brun, K. (1982). *Alcohol policies in the United Kingdom.* Sociologiska Institutionen, Stockholm.

Cartwright, A.K.J., Shaw, S.J., and Spratley, T.A. (1975). *Designing a comprehensive community response to problems of alcohol abuse.* Maudsley Alcohol Pilot Project, London.

Edwards, G., Hawker, A., Hensman, C., Peto, J., and Williamson, V. (1973). Alcoholics known or unknown to agencies: epidemiological studies in a London suburb. *Br. J. Psychiatry* **123**, 169.

Harris, A.I. (1971). *Handicapped and Impaired in Great Britain, Part 1.* OPCS Social Survey Division, HMSO, London.

Hawker, A., Edwards, G., and Hensman, C. (1967). Problem drinkers on the payroll. *Med. Officer* **118**, 313.

Hensman, C., Edwards, G., Hawker, A., and Williamson, V. (1968). Identifying abnormal drinkers: prevalence estimates by general practitioners and clergymen. *Med. Officer* **120**, 215.

Knight, R. and Warren, M.D. (1978). *Physically disabled people living at home: a study of numbers and needs.* DHSS, Report on Health and Social Subjects No. 13. HMSO, London.

Kreitman, N. (1977). Three themes in the epidemiology of alcoholism. In *Alcoholism: new knowledge and new responses* (ed. G. Edwards and M. Grant), p. 48. Croom Helm, London.

Mercer, J.R. (1973). *Labelling the mentally retarded.* University of California Press, London.

Moss, E.C. and Beresford Davies, E. (1967). *A survey of alcoholism in an English county.* Geigy (UK) Ltd., Cambridge.

OPCS Social Survey Division (1980). *Scottish drinking habits* (S.E. Dight). HMSO, London.

OPCS Social Survey Division (1981). *Drinking in England and Wales* (P. Wilson). HMSO, London.

Parr, D. (1954). Alcoholism in general practice. *Br. J. Addict.* **54**, 25.

Pollack, B. (1971). Prevalence of alcoholism in a London practice. *Practitioner* **206**, 531.

Royal College of Psychiatrists (1979). *Alcohol and alcoholism.* Tavistock Publications, London.

Whittet, M.M. (1970). Epidemiology of alcoholism in the Highlands and Islands. *Health Bull.* **28**, 4.

Wilkins, R.H. and Hore, B.D. (1977). A general practitioner study of the estimated prevalence of alcoholism in the Greater Manchester area. *Br. J. Addict.* **72**, 198.

Wilkins, R.H. (1974). *The hidden alcoholic in general practice.* Elek Books, London.

Wood, P.H.N. and Badley, E.M. (1978). Setting disablement in perspective. *Int. Rehabil. Med.* **1**, 32.

# 24 Research and development of health promotion services – screening

M. L. Burr and P. C. Elwood

## INTRODUCTION

It sometimes happens that a patient first becomes aware of a disease when it is already too late for it to be successfully treated. A man is found to have inoperable cancer of the lung: if only he had been diagnosed earlier, an operation might have been successful. An apparently healthy person has a stroke and is found to have high blood pressure: if only this had been detected earlier, the stroke might have been prevented. Such occasions suggest the desirability of detecting these diseases before the patient is aware of them while they may still be curable. There are other conditions which are treatable when they present spontaneously and yet may with advantage be detected at an earlier stage. Thus it is best to detect visual defects in schoolchildren as early as possible rather than to wait until they complain that they cannot see the blackboard, by which time their education may have suffered.

The detection of diseases before patients are aware of them is termed *screening*, which has been defined as 'the presumptive identification of unrecognized disease or defects by the application of tests, examinations or other procedures which can be applied rapidly' (Commission on Chronic Illness 1957). That is, screening sorts a population of subjects who are apparently well into those who probably have a disease, without knowing it, and those who probably have not. In this context a test is not necessarily diagnostic but only points to a presumptive diagnosis, and persons with a positive result have to be referred for further examination to confirm whether or not the disease is present. While in ordinary clinical practice the patient presents with symptoms, in a screening programme the subject is either symptomless or does not recognize the importance of the symptoms he or she has. If screening is undertaken it is assumed that early diagnosis is better than late diagnosis.

Some screening tests are directed at the risks of acquiring a disease rather than to the undiagnosed disease itself. An example might be the estimation of serum cholestrol to discriminate between subjects with different levels of risk of developing ischaemic heart disease. To justify such a screening procedure it is assumed that prevention of the disease is still possible when the tests are performed.

The assumptions implicit in screening need to be carefully tested. Any proposed screening procedure should be very carefully evaluated before it is introduced and monitored afterwards, not only for ethical and economic reasons but also for purely practical reasons. If a screening procedure is commenced without sufficient planning and evaluation, it may either run out of momentum and be abandoned, or else be adopted as a public health measure which it is impolitic to abandon and impossible to evaluate.

## ETHICAL ASPECTS OF SCREENING

In normal clinical practice a doctor or a health worker is approached by a patient who believes him or herself to be ill and who wishes to have whatever investigative and treatment procedures the doctor judges to be appropriate. Both patient and doctor realize that what is available has limited effectiveness and usually accept that almost every procedure carries some risk of undesirable side-effects.

In screening, a doctor or a health worker approaches subjects who do not consider themselves ill. A screening procedure is offered, perhaps very persuasively. The clear implication is that there is effective treatment available for those who have the disease, and that there will be no harm to those who have not.

No treatment is fully effective and few tests are without dangers. It is incumbent therefore on those who would promote a screening procedure first to assure themselves that the test that is to be used is reliable and that an effective treatment exists which will be readily available to those detected with the disease. Secondly, it must be clear that it is worthwhile for subjects to co-operate, that is, that the sum of the benefits of the procedure to the population screened is likely to outweigh all the disadvantages.

This leads to an unfortunate aspect of screening when high-risk subjects are identified to whom preventive measures can be applied. 'High-risk' does not imply certainty of developing disease, and amongst those to whom the preventive measure is applied only a proportion, and usually only a small proportion, would have developed the disease anyway. People are understandably sensitive to the inconvenience and side-effects of treatment designed to reduce the risk of something that may never happen. So compliance with a given type of treatment will be lower if it is perceived as preventive rather than curative. A similar difficulty arises in interpreting the results of preventive screening. Some of those who participate will be protected by the preventive measures advised following screening, and these might be termed 'successes' for the programme. But they cannot be distinguished from the other 'high-risk' subjects who complied unnecessarily with the preventive measure. On the other hand, 'failures', that is, the 'high-risk' subjects who are given the preventive measure and later develop the disease, together with those who suffer undesirable side-effects from the preventive measure, or from the further investigation required, do become known, and may well bring the whole procedure into disrepute.

This is a feature of most forms of preventive medicine, and may be illustrated by the drug treatment of asymptomatic mild hypertension. Out of a group of patients being treated in this way, a few will thereby avoid a stroke in the next five years. But they will be indistinguishable from the majority who would not have had a stroke anyway – that is, the successes cannot be identified. On the other hand the patients who will have a stroke despite antihypertensive therapy, together with those who complain of side-effects from the treatment, will certainly become known to doctors and probably to other patients as well. Prevention carries little glamour and can lead to misunderstanding.

## A SUITABLE DISEASE

The following criteria should be taken into account in assessing whether or not a disease is suitable for screening.

1. *The prevalence of the disease.* Other things being equal, it is obviously more worthwhile to screen for a disease that is common rather than for one that is rare. Thus screening for phenylketonuria is worthwhile in a European but not in an African or an Oriental population, since in these races the incidence of the disease is about a tenth of that in people of European descent. The usefulness of screening may be increased by selecting groups at special risk. Some preliminary selection is inherent in any screening procedure since it will not be equally appropriate to everyone. The measurement of blood pressure might be offered only to subjects over, say, 40 years of age since hypertension is very rare in younger people. Still more selective invitations might be issued to high-risk groups in which the condition is particularly common – for example, blood lead tests might be offered to the children of lead workers, or an estimation of faecal proto- and copro-porphyrins might be offered to relatives of a patient who has suffered an attack of acute intermittent porphyria. Clearly the greater the selection the more the cost-benefit balance is improved although it is still desirable that careful costing and monitoring is undertaken.

2. *Its seriousness.* This may be considered in relation to prevalence of the condition, in that the lower the prevalence the more serious the disease would have to be to justify screening for it. Thus screening for anaemia in the general population is not worthwhile because mild anaemia, though common, has little health risk, while severe anaemia is rare.

3. *Its natural history.* Ideally there should be a fairly long presymptomatic period during which the disease can be detected. Obviously the natural history of the condition will determine the frequency with which individuals need to be re-examined. This presents a difficulty in screening for certain cancers, in that the most malignant tumours spend less time in the presymptomatic phase and are unlikely to be picked up unless persons are re-screened at unreasonably short intervals. Yet these are the tumours with the highest mortality for which early detection might be most beneficial.

## A SUITABLE TEST

The test must be able to detect the condition before it is otherwise apparent. The test must satisfy certain criteria:

1. *It must be simple and capable of rapid application to large numbers of subjects.* Thus urine glucose estimation is suitable in this regard as a screening test for diabetes whereas a full glucose tolerance test is not.

2. *It must be acceptable to the subject with regard to inconvenience, discomfort, and risks of side-effects.* Sigmoid-oscopy is not acceptable as a screening test for bowel cancer in Britain, although it seems to be in the US.

3. *It should be reproducible.* Many tests (for example, serum cholesterol) which are acceptable in clinical practice show wide variation in the hands of different observers or in the same subject over a period of time.

4. *The validity of the test must be known.* This is probably the most important criterion and is usually considered in two respects: the 'sensitivity' denotes the ability of a test to detect all cases of a disease, while its 'specificity' is its ability to identify correctly those persons who are free from it. Another way of expressing validity is the proportion of false-negatives among those who really have the disease and the false-positives among those who really do not. By defining these terms as the test's performance among diseased and non-diseased groups respectively they are made independent of the prevalence of the condition. Table 24.1 summarizes these definitions. Sensitivity and specificity are inversely related, so that greater efforts to detect every case (that is to achieve fewer false-negatives) produce more false-positives. If these exceed a certain proportion the expense and anxiety that will be generated may cause the whole screening programme to break down.

**Table 24.1.** *The validity of a screening test*

| Screening test | Further evidence | |
| | Disease present | Disease absent |
| --- | --- | --- |
| positive | agreement (a) | false-positives (b) |
| negative | false-negatives (c) | agreement (d) |

Sensitivity: the proportion of diseased subjects in whom the screening test is positive, i.e. $a/(a + c)$.

Specificity: the proportion of subjects without the disease in whom the test is negative, i.e. $d/(b + d)$.

## SUITABLE TREATMENT

Obviously there is no point in screening for a condition which cannot be treated. For screening to be justified, there must be an advantage in treating the disease earlier than at the stage when it would present spontaneously. This advantage may take various forms:

1. *In reducing mortality or disability from the disease.* In the case of screening to detect healthy subjects at high risk of developing a disease there should be good evidence that the prophylactic measure that will be recommended does substantially reduce the incidence of the disease. Where screening aims at early identification of disease, there should be good evidence that early diagnosis reduces morbidity or mortality. There are some diseases (for example, lung cancer) with a high fatality even at an early stage, while other conditions can be easily and effectively treated, and the stage at which they are treated may matter little.

2. *In offering less radical treatment than would be necessary when the disease has progressed further.* A familiar example is in screening for dental caries by regular inspection of the teeth.

3. *In relieving a disability for which the patient might never seek help:* for example, visual defects in schoolchildren.

4. *In preventing the condition from being a risk to others.* Thus train-drivers are screened for colour-blindness, and the treatment is to divert them to other employment.

## EVALUATION OF THE TEST

The test itself should be carefully evaluated. Its acceptability needs to be considered in relation to the community in which it will be used. It sometimes happens that a test which is perfectly acceptable in one culture is not in another. The test may be more acceptable to some sections of the population than to others, and this must be considered in relation to the relative frequency of the disease in the people concerned. Evidence about acceptability can be obtained by means of a pilot study in a population which is representative of that in which it will ultimately be used.

The reproducibility of the test is established by repeating it at intervals within the same subjects or in the hands of different observers. If there are wide variations in the results, the reason should be investigated. For example, changes in blood-pressure readings may be partly due to changes occurring within the subjects. These can be reduced by standardizing the conditions in which blood pressure is measured, for example, with the subject seated at rest in a quiet room. Variations due to the observer's own inconsistencies can be minimized by training, which also reduces inter-observer error, but it is wise to assume that this may still occur and therefore to monitor it from time to time.

The validity of the test is investigated in a pilot study conducted in circumstances similar to those in which it will ultimately be used. All those who are positive to the test are referred for a definitive diagnostic procedure so as to distinguish between the true and the false-positives. Ascertainment of the false-negatives is more difficult, but an attempt should be made to estimate how many occur so as to estimate the sensitivity of the test. In some circumstances they will reveal themselves – for example open spina bifida that has been missed by ante-natal screening. But for many conditions (for example, cancer of the cervix) the disease will need careful

monitoring if newly-diagnosed cases are to be linked with the results of the screening test, and even then it may be difficult to be sure whether the condition was present at the time of the test or has developed since. Some false-negatives may be found by re-applying the screening test (although it may consistently miss the same cases) or by referring a random sample of negatives for the definitive diagnostic procedure (which is not always feasible). For some conditions the sensitivity can be assessed by applying the screening test to a representative group of patients with the disease. But if the object is early detection of a progressive condition, the test may not produce the same results in the presymptomatic and the symptomatic stages of the disease.

## EFFECTIVENESS OF THE SCREENING PROCEDURE

Determining the value of the whole procedure is a separate exercise. This is the more important issue and even more difficult to assess. The benefit of certain screening procedures is self-evident, such as the discovery of deafness in a schoolchild whose inattention has been attributed to stupidity, or the detection of amblyopia before it has become irreversible. But many screening procedures require careful investigation to see whether they are really worthwhile.

Screening has been recommended for a very large number of conditions. A textbook on paediatric screening tests (Frankenburg and Camp 1975) lists 32 conditions recommended in the US and to this could be added at least an equal number of conditions which have been recommended for screening in adults or in the elderly. Wilson and Jungner (1968) list over 50 'common procedures and tests that have been applied ... in screening surveys in a population'. Many of these tests have never been evaluated and are almost certainly not justifiable as performed at present. The evidence that can be collected about the value of a test needs to be examined carefully. For example, it has been stated that the five-year survival of bowel-cancer patients detected by screening is twice that occurring when patients present spontaneously. But the people attending such a screening clinic are unlikely to be typical of the general population. The tumours picked up by screening will tend to be the less malignant lesions since they grow more slowly and spend a longer time in the presymptomatic stage. And, in any case, earlier diagnosis gives an apparent lengthening of survival (the 'lead-time') even if the patient dies at the same time that he would have done anyway.

The ideal method of evaluating a screening programme is by means of a randomized controlled trial. In theory, this is very simple. The trial can take one of two forms. The more sensitive approach is to screen a community and refer a random half of the 'positives' for treatment (for example, persons found to have mild hypertension). But for some diseases (for example breast cancer) it is unethical to withhold treatment once the condition has been detected. The best course then is to offer the screening procedure to a random half of a defined population and compare the eventual outcome in the two halves. An example of this approach is the HIP breast cancer study described below.

But matters are often not as simple as this. The first type of trial is seldom possible, while the second type presents formidable logistic difficulties, especially if the condition is at all uncommon. A very large number of subjects must be identified, randomized and followed up, and the follow-up must be equal in the two groups. Persons allocated to the screened group must be analysed as a whole whether or not they actually accepted the screening test and the consequent investigation and treatment, since only at the point of randomization are the two groups comparable. But the defaulters will probably be more difficult to trace than those who comply, and if they are at all numerous they may obscure a real effect of the screening programme. And sometimes a controlled trial cannot be conducted because public opinion demands a screening service without waiting the requisite number of years for a definitive evaluation.

In these circumstances, evidence of various other kinds can be considered. If the object of the screening programme is to reduce mortality from a certain disease, then the death-rates for that disease can be monitored to see whether the introduction of screening is followed by a decline in mortality. But there may be an underlying change in the death-rates that would have occurred anyway, due to changes in incidence or in treatment. Furthermore, it may not be known with certainty how long should elapse before screening produces a detectable change in death-rates owing to uncertainties about the natural history of the condition (for example, cervical cancer). It is likely that screening will have been introduced in different areas at different times, and comparisons between such areas may provide further clues. Changes in the incidence and prevalence of the condition may require special monitoring. In some cases the screening programme itself should increase the apparent incidence, at least when it is introduced, by finding cases that would not have come to light until later. But if the object is to reduce the prevalence of a condition, periodic surveys should be undertaken to ensure that its prevalence does eventually decline.

Sometimes a compromise between the observational and experimental design can be used. It may be possible to introduce screening in one area or grouping (such as a factory or a school) and not in another, comparing the outcome in the two places. The results from this kind of study will not be as conclusive as those from a trial where the individual subjects are randomly allocated, since there may be unsuspected differences between the two groups.

This type of study can be greatly improved by increasing the number of groupings and then allocating them at random to receive screening or not. If the number is sufficient the study will be for practical purposes as conclusive as a randomized trial of individuals. For example, Brett (1968) randomly divided 119 factories into two groups. The men in one group were offered a chest X-ray initially and again after three years, while those in the other group were offered chest X-rays every six months as a screen for lung cancer. The death rates from lung cancer were 0.7 per 1000 per annum in the screened group and 0.8 in the unscreened group, so that the screening did not produce a significant reduction in mortality.

The retrospective approach can also be used. Cases of the disease or events which the screening programme should have prevented can be investigated to see whether they were screened and if so with what result. A case-control enquiry will show whether they were less likely to have been screened than similar persons without the disease. These methods have the weakness that the persons who decline screening differ from those who accept it in ways which may, independently of screening, affect their risk of disease. But by appropriate matching for confounding variables it may be possible to obtain evidence which strongly suggests that the screening is or is not having its desired effect.

Even if the value of screening has been shown in a controlled trial, it is still desirable to monitor its effectiveness by means of observational studies. It may be that in the circumstances of the trial the programme functioned more effectively than when it is a routine service offered to the public. There are several screening procedures (for example, cervical cytology) which operate very much more satisfactorily in some countries than in others. And the incidence or the distribution of the disease may change unexpectedly in ways that alter the usefulness of the screening programme.

## EFFICIENCY OF THE SCREENING PROCEDURE

Even if the screening procedure confers undoubted benefit, that benefit has to be considered in relation to the costs of the procedure. The resources available to health services are always likely to be limited, and less than the potential demands upon them, so some way must be found of deciding how they shall be used. It is therefore necessary to assess the efficiency of a proposed service so as to determine how the benefits deriving from it compare with those that would derive from an alternative use of the same money.

There is virtually no limit to the number of screening tests that might be used if effectiveness were the only criterion. For example, Cochrane and Holland (1971) pointed out that population screening for porphyria variegata would undoubtedly benefit the small number of persons who have the condition. They estimated that the cost of saving a life in this way would be about £250 000 in 1971, and suggested that, since screening for this disease has never been tried, it is implicitly recognized that this is too much to pay.

The actual calculation of costs and benefits is not easy. A simpler exercise is to rank alternative screening procedures in order of efficiency. It is obviously more efficient to screen a group where a disease is common than one where it is rare. But sometimes a decision has to be taken which requires some balance of costs and benefits to be drawn up. Should we continue to screen for pulmonary tuberculosis in a country where the incidence has become much lower than it was when the screening service was set up? How do we decide when to stop? What should be the lower age limit for cervical cytology screening, bearing in mind that death from cervical cancer is very rare in young women, but when it does occur it is especially tragic? If breast cancer screening saves some lives, ought it to be offered to the public?

Since these and similar questions have to be answered somehow, it is clearly better that decisions are made on the basis of objective facts rather than by taking the line of least resistance. The principles of cost-benefit analysis have been worked out by economists in recent years, so that an attempt can be made to balance the costs and benefits of screening. The cost of the screening procedure can be ascertained and compared with the cost of not doing it in terms of the treatment and care that would be required if the disease runs its usual course. At first sight many screening procedures seem obviously worthwhile, in that their cost is less than that of treating the disease they are designed to prevent. But the issues are usually much more complex than this. Various hidden costs are involved in the screening test, such as the publicity and the expense of attending for screening and treatment. Similar hidden extras, together with medical uncertainties about the value of the procedure, make it difficult to estimate the benefit. And the relationship between cost and benefit is complicated by 'discounting', in that a pound saved in a year's time is not as valuable as a pound now, which could be invested to produce more than a pound by that time. This has a profound effect on the economics of screening, since the benefits are in the future, sometimes many years ahead. For these reasons Drummond (1980) considers that, 'by and large, screening programmes are not likely to be justified merely by their impact on health service resource use. It is usually necessary to calculate a wider set of costs and benefits'.

A cost-benefit analysis of screening for spina bifida was conducted by Hagard et al. (1976). They took account of a wide range of direct and indirect costs to the families and the public services for the screening test and its benefits (that is, the cost of supporting children with spina bifida). They concluded that, on economic grounds, screening may be worthwhile only in populations with a high incidence of spina bifida. A still wider range of costs and benefits was used in a similar analysis by Henderson (1982). He considered the discounted costs and benefits of a replacement cohort, since it might be assumed that after screening and abortion many parents would embark on another pregnancy. He concluded that the tangible benefits of screening probably outweigh the tangible costs by a substantial amount. The intangible psychological costs and benefits are more difficult to estimate but the balance is likely to be greatly in favour of screening.

Many screening tests involve measuring a continuously-distributed biological variable, part of whose distribution is considered to constitute a disease (for example, haemoglobin concentration and anaemia, blood pressure and hypertension). In order to determine the point in the distribution beyond which the persons concerned should be treated, evidence is needed not only that treatment for that part of the range is likely to confer some benefit but also that the benefit will outweigh the costs and disadvantages. And these may be substantial, both in financial and in non-financial terms. A small change in the level of the variate which defines the illness (say 0.5 g/100 ml haemoglobin or 5 mm Hg diastolic pressure) automatically transfers a large number of persons into the category of the diseased. If a controlled trial is sufficiently large it may be possible to show a small benefit of treating these persons, but this may well be outweighed by the costs and side-effects of treatment and the consequences of labelling them as sick.

The over-diagnosis of disease carries its own morbidity.

This is particularly true in regard to cardiac disease in children owing to the detection of 'benign murmurs'. Bergman and Stamm (1967) reported that 81 per cent of schoolchildren with a diagnosis of a heart condition actually had no detectable disease. Of these 'false-positives', 40 per cent were restricted in some way, including 8 per cent whose activities were severely restricted. The authors concluded that disability from cardiac non-disease in children was greater than that from actual heart disease. Perhaps the risk of cardiac non-disease has declined with a greater awareness of its dangers, but it illustrates the importance of balancing the benefit and the harm of a screening procedure.

Other cost-benefit issues arise in cancer screening. There is a certain degree of public resistance to screening for cancer, expressed in the remark 'I would rather not know'. This is not necessarily as irrational as it seems. In any cancer-screening programme, the cases detected will fall into three groups. First, there are those who are curable when detected and who would not have been curable had they been left to present spontaneously. It is for their benefit that screening is undertaken. Secondly, some will be curable at screening who would still have been curable when they presented spontaneously. They benefit from screening only if early diagnosis enables the treatment to be less severe; otherwise they are worse off, since they spend more of their lives in the shadow of the disease and its treatment. Thirdly, some are already incurable when screening detects their condition. They are very much worse off for having been screened, since they now have a longer period of distress and ineffective treatment before they die. This illustrates a non-financial form of discounting, in that an unpleasant diagnosis and its equally unpleasant treatment are worse the earlier they occur in a person's lifetime. It is therefore important to know the relative likelihood of falling into the three groups and not merely to discover whether the first group has any members at all.

## ORGANIZATION AND ADMINISTRATION

The success of a screening programme depends on the way it is organized as well as on its inherent properties. The varying effectiveness of the same screening procedure in different places shows how important it is to plan and administer it carefully. Screening involves the testing of large numbers of persons who initially are presumed to be healthy. Contacting the right subjects at the right time may be difficult; it is much easier to screen people who are already in contact with health services than those who have to take the initiative of applying for the test.

Thus the routine screening of pregnant women for hypertension and rhesus incompatibility is fairly easy, since they are usually attending antenatal clinics during the period when the screening tests need to be performed. But serological screening for neural-tube defects should take place between the sixteenth and eighteenth weeks, and some women do not attend the clinic at that time. The success of this screening procedure thus requires a degree of public education which may not be easily achieved.

Screening at birth is easy to organize and detects various congenital abnormalities. The neonatal period is also easy to monitor, but thereafter it becomes more difficult to trace and examine infants. The difference between the effectiveness of screening for phenylketonuria and congenital dislocation of the hip is very instructive in this regard, and will be considered in more detail below.

School entry, at about five years of age in the UK, is another point at which it is easy to screen. A readily-defined cohort of children is examined for various conditions, and a variety of defects are picked up. Thereafter, schoolchildren form a captive population who are conveniently screened for conditions ranging from headlice to plantar warts, although truancy reduces the completeness of these surveys during adolescence. In view of the ease with which controlled trials might be done to evaluate these various activities it is remarkable how few have actually been conducted.

During adult life the organization of screening depends on the type of procedure. Large offices and factories can arrange for their staff to be offered a screening service, sometimes in relation to the particular hazards of the industry. Thus, persons who work with lead are screened regularly for high blood lead levels so that lead poisoning can be avoided. It is obviously important to discuss all such schemes with the trades unions or other representatives of the workers. Issues of confidentiality and compensation for industrial disease must be carefully considered. In view of the long latent period of some industrial toxins, it may be appropriate to screen persons at intervals after they have left an occupation which involved exposure to certain substances.

But the screening of adults outside the large office or factory presents special difficulties. A high level of public awareness of a disease will promote the success of a screening procedure – thus a high prevalence of pulmonary tuberculosis favours the success of a mass miniature radiography programme. Education of the public has a rather uneven effect and influences the upper social classes selectively, as may be seen in 'well-women' clinics. There are marked differences between the way in which different cultures and nationalities respond to invitations to be screened. The multiphasic screen or health check is utilized more readily in North America than in Britain, although whether the Americans derive any benefit from their propensity to screening is doubtful. When it is intended to screen a cross-section of British adults of a given age-group (for example, for bowel cancer by means of occult blood detection), an age-sex register of patients registered with general practitioners is an invaluable aid. Screening for hypertension is most easily carried out by general practitioners at consultations for other matters, since nearly everyone consults a doctor at least once every five years.

In general, it may be said that screening programmes work best when they do not depend on the initiative of the subjects in seeking them. They are more effective when administered by a single unified organization than by a multitude of bodies (see the example of cervical cytology below) and their completeness may be improved by computerization.

## EXAMPLES OF SCREENING PROCEDURES

A selection of screening programmes will now be reviewed in more detail to illustrate the various issues that have been discussed.

### Neural-tube defects

Pregnant women are screened for serological evidence of alpha-fetoprotein (AFP) at about 16 weeks. Those whose AFP values are above a certain limit are referred for ultrasonography and amniocentesis, by means of which nearly all cases of neural-tube defect can be detected and referred for abortion. The first problem about this proceudre is that it is most effective at 16–18 weeks gestation; but a substantial proportion of pregnant women do not book until after this time. Secondly, there is no fixed level of AFP above which the test may be regarded as positive. The usual practice is to take a percentile determined by balancing the numbers of false-positives and false-negatives that will result. Thus if the ninetieth percentile is selected, about 80 per cent of all affected infants will be detected (84 per cent of those with anencephalus and 77 per cent with open spina bifida) and 20 per cent will be missed (Roberts *et al.* 1983); but about 10 per cent of normal pregnancies will be referred unnecessarily. The third problem is that there is no ideal diagnostic test. Ultrasound does not always detect abnormalities, while amniocentesis sometimes produces 'borderline' results which are difficult to interpret. It also entails a small risk of abortion to a healthy fetus. The fourth problem is that the treatment which is ultimately offered – abortion of the affected fetus – is by no means universally acceptable to the mothers. It may therefore be advisable to offer the screening service only to those who would agree to abortion if a neural-tube defect were detected and so avoid unnecessary anxiety and mental turmoil to women who would not be happy to have their pregnancies artificially terminated.

In one such screening programme it was found that the proportion of open neural-tube defects in the population which were detected and terminated as a result of serum AFP testing was only 56 per cent (the efficacy of the procedure). The authors concluded that 'given present practices and knowledge we doubt whether overall efficacy levels above 60–65 per cent for open spina bifida could be achieved under normal service conditions' (Roberts *et al.* 1983). This conclusion arose partly from the problems outlined already and partly from the sheer complexity of the screening process, which provides many opportunities for clinical and administrative error. Technical improvements, especially in the sensitivity of ultrasonography, may well lead to a substantial rise in efficacy. But the difficulty of ensuring early screening and the organization of a complex referral procedure within a short period of time will make a really high degree of success unlikely.

### Phenylketonuria

Screening for phenylketonuria was introduced in Britain during the 1950s. At that time the screening test in common use was the Phenistix ferric chloride urine test. Treatment was by means of a diet low in phenylalanine, and follow-up of the patients revealed a good intellectual development if the diet was started early, in contrast to those who were not given the diet. From 1964, a national register of children with phenylketonuria has been maintained, the MRC/DHSS Phenylketonuria Register, which lists all patients with the disease who have been born since 1964. Checks are made on the completeness of the register by periodic enquiries made to paediatricians, and the records have been computerized.

The Phenistix nappy test was found to produce an unacceptable proportion of false-negatives. Since 1969, it has been replaced by the Guthrie test, which depends on blood phenylalanine concentration. A heel-prick specimen of blood is obtained between the infant's sixth and fourteenth day of life, absorbed on to a special card and sent to one of a small number of laboratories for analysis.

The results of this programme are shown in Fig. 24.1 (taken from the report of the MRC Steering Committee 1981). A few cases of phenylketonuria born before 1969 are still coming to light because of mental retardation. This under-diagnosis of the condition in the earlier years presumably explained the slight apparent rise in incidence, which was 6.7, 8.7, and 10.4 per 100 000 live births in 1964–8, 1969–73, and 1974–8 respectively. It is clear that the number of missed cases has fallen to a remarkable degree, due equally to the high sensitivity of the test and to the near-complete coverage of the population at risk. The latter achievement is attributed to a 1969 circular from the Ministry of Health which recommended that: (i) the senior administrative medical officer in each region should be responsible for ensuring that a specimen is obtained from every infant in the area; (ii) the test should be performed between the sixth and fourteenth day of life; (iii) it should depend on the blood concentration of phenylalanine; and (iv) it should be processed in a central laboratory. The effectiveness of the treatment is witnessed by the near-disappearance of phenylketonuria as a cause of mental retardation in children.

This success story illustrates the effect of a good test, good treatment, and good organization. The test is applied when the baby is being statutorily visited by the midwife, a designated individual in each region is responsible to see that it is done, it is processed at a central laboratory, and the results are monitored by means of a single national register.

The same blood specimen can be used for a screening test for congenital hypothyroidism. As this condition is twice as common as phenylketonuria and can also be detected and treated satisfactorily, it would seem to be highly efficient to combine the two procedures (Hulse *et al.* 1980; New England Congenital Hypothyroidism Collaborative 1981; Hulse *et al.* 1982).

### Congenital dislocation of the hip

Congenital dislocation of the hip is a fairly common disorder, affecting two to three infants per 1000 live births. It is liable to cause permanent disability unless it is diagnosed and treated before the child begins to walk. For many years newborn infants have been routinely examined for this condition, the screening test being the abduction of both hips when a palpable click may occur if it is present. But the condition is not always detectable at birth, and re-screening at the age of three months has been recommended. This could be undertaken when the infant is seen for immunization.

Despite a general impression that screening for hip dislocation is satisfactory, evidence is available to suggest that this is far from true. In Southampton a register of cases has been maintained for many years and its completeness checked with Hospital Activity Analysis. A study based on this register shows a rising incidence of congenital hip dislocation untreated by one year (Catford *et al.* 1982). The authors conclude that 'despite the introduction of neonatal screening . . . we have failed to make a substantial impact on avoiding the late diagnosis of cases'. The situation is complicated by an apparent rise in the underlying incidence of the condition, which has been reported from other countries and is unexplained.

These conclusions are confirmed by a retrospective study of 56 children in whom the diagnosis was first made after the age of six months (David *et al.* 1983). The parents were interviewed and the neonatal hospital records were examined. Other information was obtained from clinic records. In 13 cases (23 per cent) the hips had not apparently been examined at birth, and in seven an abnormality was noted at birth but not followed up. In 27 cases (48 per cent) there was no record of a routine hip check after three months. The mean age at which parents first noticed an abnormality was 11 months, but the mean age at diagnosis was 26 months, the delay being partly due to the parents' failure to report symptoms and partly to the health visitors' and doctors' failures to act on them.

Both these studies point to a serious failure in the screening programme. The initial screening test is sometimes omitted; it produces many false-negatives, partly because it is performed by newly-qualified doctors whose technique is unsatisfactory. Re-screening is recognized to be necessary in order to pick up cases not detectable at birth, but no one person is responsible so in many cases it is never done. It is widely believed that screening is carried out successfully for this condition, and this belief probably induces a false sense of security in doctors and health visitors who fail to consider the possibility that a child with relevant symptoms has an undiagnosed dislocation.

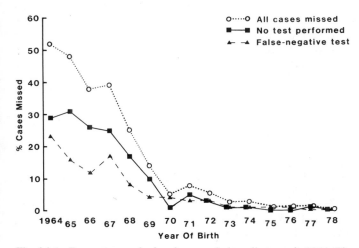

**Fig. 24.1.** Percentages of missed cases of phenylketonuria 1964–78.

The contrast with phenylketonuria screening is very striking, and points to the importance of monitoring the effect of a screening programme in order to reveal its shortcomings.

## Developmental screening

During the first few years of life children rapidly acquire various skills, which seem to develop according to an approximate time-table. At any given age it is therefore possible to compare a child with his or her peers to see whether his or her progress is unusual in any way. Delayed development can be the first or most obvious sign of a wide variety of medical and social disorders (for example, chronic urinary infection, parental ill-treatment), and since some of these are treatable it seems worthwhile finding them. Other conditions (for example, mental retardation) may require special facilities for the child's education which can be arranged in advance if the abnormality is detected.

It has therefore been advocated that children should be screened at various intervals by doctors, health visitors or other personnel, with the object of detecting delayed or abnormal development. A great variety of screening tests are available, ranging from a simple interview to a sophisticated battery of tests such as the Denver Developmental Screening Test (DDST), which has been formulated and standardized in large numbers of children.

The value of such screening has, however, still to be established. In an Australian study the use of DDST was assessed by comparing it with a detailed clinical examination conducted by a paediatrician (Carmichael and Williams 1981). With regard to major delays in development the test was effective but largely unnecessary, in that the majority of infants detected were already under surveillance for their condition. For minor delays, where the likelihood of spontaneous discovery was less, the test was very insensitive. Furthermore, the authors pointed out that 'many conditions being screened for are inadequately understood, their natural history unknown and the need for intervention and treatment unproven'.

Ellenberg and Nelson (1981) set up a study to investigate the early detection of infants with cerebral palsy. This took the form of a classic prospective study. A cohort of about 40 000 unselected infants was neurologically examined at four months and followed up; more than 32 000 of them were again examined at seven years of age without reference to the original findings. Of those considered neurologically 'normal' at four months, 0.1 per cent had cerebral palsy by seven years; of those considered 'suspect' and 'definitely abnormal' the percentages who later had cerebral palsy were 1.0 per cent and 14.1 per cent respectively. If 'suspect' and 'abnormal' are both considered as positive tests, the sensitivity was 64 per cent and the specificity 89 per cent. But, unfortunately there is little evidence that early detection of cerebral palsy is beneficial owing to the lack of any treatment which has been shown to alter the natural history of the condition (Pearson 1982). Furthermore, the large number of false-positives represent a very great potential for harm – a mistaken suggestion that a child may be 'spastic' causes profound anxiety and distress to the parents and may affect the child in later years since such

labels tend to stick. Screening for mental retardation may similarly produce damage to the false-positives which far outweighs any benefit to the true-positives. Developmental screening needs very careful evaluation and monitoring to ensure that it does more good than harm.

## Cervical cancer

There are over 2000 deaths from cancer of the cervix uteri in England and Wales each year. The detection of this cancer in a pre-invasive stage, when it is presumably curable, is an attractive prospect. Examination of a smear of cells taken from the cervix has therefore become a very widespread screening procedure and in the UK over two million smears are taken annually. About five per 1000 women are found to have cancer-like cellular changes, without evidence of invasion, the so-called carcinoma-in-situ; and these lesions are removed, either by cone biopsy, or, more recently, by cryosurgery or by laser.

Cervical smears were introduced in the late 1940s and their availability became widespread throughout the UK by the middle 1950s. Unfortunately a randomized controlled trial was not done in the early years when the procedure was being developed and was too scarce to be offered to every woman. Difficulties arise therefore in evaluating cervical cytology because the natural history of the condition is not known. The proportion of invasive carcinomas which go through a pre-invasive phase and the proportion of cases with these 'pre-cancerous' changes which go on to cancer is unknown. Nor is the incubation period of the condition known, though all the available evidence, which is of necessity indirect, suggests that the pre-invasive changes first occur on average about 20 years before invasive cancer develops. These gaps in our knowledge mean that estimates of the likely effectiveness of the screening procedure cannot be made. Furthermore, the wide availability of screening means that no 'control' population is available for comparison, and any effect of screening will be confounded with secular changes in incidence and case-fatality.

Despite the absence of a controlled trial, there is a body of evidence suggesting that cervical cytology is beneficial. Screening was introduced in British Columbia before the rest of Canada, and there seems to have been an associated fall in deaths from cervical cancer (Miller et al. 1976). A similar decline has occurred in the US, again related to the degree of screening (Cramer 1974). In Scotland screening started in the Grampian region in the early 1960s and has been followed by a decline in mortality especially in women aged 55–64 years, for whom no decline has occurred in the rest of Scotland (MacGregor and Teper 1978). Similar supportive evidence has been found in Finland (Hakama and Rasanen-Virtanen 1976) and Iceland (Johannesson et al. 1978). A case-control study of individual patients with cervical cancer has also been conducted (Clarke and Anderson 1979), in which 212 cases of invasive cervical cancer were compared with 1060 age-matched neighbourhood controls. The cases were far less likely to have been screened during the previous five years than the controls, and the difference was not explained by a variety of potential confounding variables, although of course some relevant characteristics may have been overlooked.

One aspect of cervical cytology certainly militates strongly against its being anything like as effective as it might be. While the overall response to an invitation to be screened is about 50–60 per cent, the response rate falls off sharply with increasing age and with lower social class and increasing family size. Yet it is the older women and those of lower social class who have the highest mortality from cervical cancer. Women in the population who are at greater risk of carcinoma of the cervix uteri are therefore least likely to present for screening, while those least at risk show the most ready response (Editorial Committee of the Cardiff Cervical Cytology Study 1980).

Another aspect of cervical cytology which is of relevance to the ultimate value of screening is the validity of the test. The false-negative rate is believed to be around 20 per cent, based on studies of women screened a second time after a very short interval. This implies a rather poor sensitivity of the test and has led some to recommend that women aged over 35 years with a first negative test should be re-screened within a year (Spriggs and Husain 1977).

Perhaps the greatest handicap, so far as Britain is concerned, is the lack of a unified screening service. Cervical smears are taken by general practitioners, local authority clinics, family planning clinics, hospital out-patient departments and other clinics. The records are not linked, and although a summary form is submitted by pathology laboratories to the Department of Health it does not distinguish between first and other smears, so that the numbers of women screened are quite unknown. A national recall scheme was operated by the National Health Service Register, but some laboratories did not participate in the scheme and it is being discontinued, to be replaced by local recall schemes. In any case, only women who had attended already could be recalled; there was no mechanism for detecting and inviting women who had never been screened. The Working Party set up to consider the matter concluded that the relative failure of the British screening service is due to the lack of a co-ordinated mechanism for its development and management (Draper 1982). It is instructive to compare this state of affairs with the situation in Finland, where a national computerized system operates under the aegis of the Finnish Cancer Registry. Women are automatically invited to attend for screening every five years and the system is not limited to the recall of those who have already been screened.

Thus cervical cytology illustrates again the importance of good organization, together with the need to ensure that the service is reaching those who are most at risk.

## Breast cancer

Carcinoma of the breast is a common condition which carries a substantial mortality. It is therefore especially interesting to note that screening for breast cancer has been evaluated by means of a randomized controlled trial. The HIP study in New York (Shapiro 1977) involved the random allocation of 62 000 women into two groups, one of which was offered annual screening tests (palpation and mammography) while the other was left unscreened. After nine years, 91 deaths due to breast cancer had occurred in the group offered screening and 128 in the other group. No reduction in mortality occurred in women under 50 years of age, and in them the small risk of radiation exposure due to mammography was thought to be a potential hazard. It is highly desirable that this study should be replicated in another area, and a similar trial has been set up in Sweden (Linell et al. 1980). The main problem in breast cancer screening is one of logistics; there are not at present the personnel in the UK for such a procedure to be made generally available as a service if the screening is undertaken by surgeons and radiologists. But George et al. (1980a,b) have shown that nurses and radiographers can be trained to examine breasts and read mammograms just as well as doctors, and that the additional surgical workload becomes quite manageable by the third year of the screening service.

Another alternative is to teach women to palpate their own breasts, so that they apply a screening test to themselves. It has been shown that a high percentage of women can be taught this technique, and the tumours found in this way carry a lower mortality than breast cancers in general (Gastrin 1980). But this observation has the same weakness as that discussed earlier in relation to bowel cancer; the lead-time of breast cancer may be a year, and the less malignant tumours are more likely to be found by screening. Furthermore, there are reasons for suspecting that there is some histological overdiagnosis of cancer in breast lumps (Lancet 1981). These factors may confer a spuriously lower mortality on cancers discovered by screening, and it has to be acknowledged that self-palpation has not been properly evaluated.

## Tuberculosis

Until the middle of this century tuberculosis was one of the major public-health problems of the western world. Two screening procedures have been used as part of the control of this disease. One is the tuberculin testing of schoolchildren, by means of the Mantoux or the Heaf test: children with negative results are given BCG vaccination to protect them against infection. This is a paradoxical screening test in that a negative result indicates the lack of naturally-acquired resistance, and in screening theory this constitutes a positive test identifying an unrecognized defect. The other screening procedure is mass miniature radiography, which detects the disease before it presents spontaneously.

The incidence of the disease has declined dramatically, and it has ceased to be a major cause of death in most western countries. This is probably due largely to improvements in nutritional and housing conditions together with the advent of effective chemotherapy. Screening also played a part in protecting children and in detecting unrecognized cases who would otherwise have been a source of infection for other people. It may also have been the case that when chemotherapy was first introduced it was more effective in the early stages detected by mass radiography than in established cases. Now chemotherapy is effective at virtually all stages of the disease, and the question arises as to whether screening should be continued. By 1970 the cost of detecting a case of tuberculosis in Britain probably exceeded the cost of allowing it to present spontaneously (Cochrane and Holland 1971), and mass radiography is no longer advocated for the population at large. Similarly the cost of prevention by tuberculin testing and BCG vaccination probably exceeds the cost of treating the cases that would otherwise occur, and when the inconvenience of vaccination is taken into account it becomes questionable whether the scheme should continue.

But in certain sections of the population it may well be worthwhile to maintain screening services. Surveys of tuberculosis notifications in England and Wales show a considerable excess of cases among the immigrant communities (British Thoracic and Tuberculosis Association 1973; MRC Tuberculosis and Chest Diseases Unit 1980). The incidence is particularly high in those who originated from the Indian subcontinent; in 1978 these persons formed only 1.6 per cent of the population but accounted for 35 per cent of all notifications. In the Asian community the notification rate was highest among young women, and it was also very high among children, both those who have entered the country and (to a somewhat lesser extent) those born to Asian parents in Britain. These high rates are attributable to the greater prevalence of tuberculosis in India, Pakistan, and Bangladesh, together with the tendency for these immigrants to live in rather overcrowded conditions. It would therefore seem reasonable to screen new immigrants as they enter the country and to offer a screening service to Asian communities in Britain.

### Cardiovascular disease

Ischaemic heart disease is now the largest single cause of death in the western world, and both this and cerebrovascular disease are most important causes of disability, particularly in older subjects. Possible screening procedures for early disease, or for subjects at increased risk, must be very carefully examined.

The case for screening for cardiovascular disease breaks down on a number of issues. First, the sensitivity and specificity of the available screening tests are poor. The Framingham study (Keys et al. 1972) showed that only one-third of the new events of cardiovascular disease occurred in the quarter of the men with the highest cholesterol levels and only half of the new events occurred in the quarter of the men with the highest blood pressures. Moreover, of the men with the highest cholesterol levels and those with the highest blood pressures only 27 per cent and 26 per cent respectively died or developed cardiovascular disease. Put more succinctly, the sensitivity of a cholesterol level is 38 per cent and its specificity 75 per cent, and for blood pressure these estimates are 46 per cent and 69 per cent.

Secondly, the available treatment for high-risk individuals or patients with early disease is not known to be very effective in reducing morbidity or mortality. Correction of a number of 'risk factors' (such as raised serum cholesterol, raised low-density lipoprotein cholesterol, inadequate physical activity, and obesity) is possible, and although for lipoproteins the evidence is suggestive, in no case has clinical efficacy, in terms of a reduction of disease or death, been established beyond reasonable doubt. Cessation of cigarette smoking is almost certainly beneficial, but here screening is virtually unnecessary and what is needed is some way of promoting action on the part of subjects. Whyte (1975) has summarized the likely situation in relation to screening for serum cholesterol level. If 100 subjects aged 35 years were found in a screening programme to have a high serum cholesterol level (over 260 mg/100 ml) and if they were all advised to go on a low-fat diet, then over the next 20 years, assuming that they all maintained dietary control for this period, six would probably avoid a heart attack, 94 would reap no benefit and of these probably about eight would still get a heart attack despite the diet. While the benefits from cessation of smoking are probably larger than this, those from weight reduction or increased physical activity are likely to be less.

The exception to this rather gloomy picture relates to blood pressure. The burden of death and disability which can be attributed either directly or indirectly to hypertension is enormous. Clearly, screening must be considered carefully.

The measurement of blood pressure is simple, cheap, fairly reliable, and acceptable. The disease is not easily defined, but if a diastolic pressure over, say, 95 mm Hg is taken to indicate a need for further investigation (since it carries an increased risk of death and disability), then the condition is relatively common. A diastolic pressure of 105 mm Hg or more implies a substantial risk, and drug therapy has been shown to be beneficial in carefully controlled trials (Hamilton et al. 1964; Veterans Administration Co-operative Study Group 1967, 1970). Screening may easily be undertaken by general practitioners seeing patients in ordinary consultations about other matters (Hart 1970).

For a realistic evaluation of screening the likely benefits must be quantified. Severe hypertension carries a high risk but is rather rare in the community. Less severely affected subjects have a lower risk so that the proportion who can benefit from long-term treatment is lower. The law of diminishing returns operates, and one either screens out a very small number of subjects with markedly raised pressures, many of whom will benefit from treatment, or one identifies a large number of mildly affected subjects, very few of whom will benefit from treatment, but many of whom will subsequently regard themselves as ill and will perhaps curtail their activities unnecessarily, while enduring various side-effects from the drugs. However, compliance with treatment is generally poor, and retrospective studies have shown that the main problem is not the identification of subjects who will benefit, but the monitoring and sustained treatment of those who have been identified (Beevers et al. 1973).

Before screening is started a very careful judgement must be made of the value of subjecting large numbers of persons to regular measurement of blood pressure, and of subsequently advising a proportion of them to take powerful drugs for the rest of their lives. While a few extra years of life are undoubtedly very precious to those subjects who benefit, adequate cost-benefit estimates must take account of the total procedure, including the lifelong treatment of many subjects, without benefit, but with all the disadvantages and undesirable side effects of the treatment.

## Anaemia

Anaemia, or a reduced concentration of circulating haemoglobin, is relatively common and is easily, cheaply and reliably detected. Further investigation to discriminate between the different causes of anaemia is relatively simple, and for all the common causes treatment is available which will markedly raise haemoglobin levels.

Anaemia would therefore appear to be a most suitable disease for screening. Difficulties arise however in relation to the clinical importance of the condition. The World Health Organization (1972) and other bodies have defined anaemia as a reduction in circulating haemoglobin below 13 g per 100 ml in males or below 12 g per 100 ml in adult non-pregnant females. Recent surveys show that around 1 per cent of males and about 5–10 per cent of females in western communities are below these limits. But these standards are little more than arbitrary, and most attempts to define the level of circulating haemoglobin below which there are effects which are harmful and which can be removed by treatment suggest that realistic standards should be much lower (Elwood 1973, 1974). One therefore has a condition which, in western countries at any rate, is defined in such a way that it is common but unimportant, and if more reasonable standards are set, it is important but rare.

Few would therefore promote screening for anaemia in western communities except in persons being screened for another purpose or in special groups (for example, patients about to undergo surgery). In some developing countries, however, the occurrence of clinically significant anaemia is probably very much higher and the possible benefits from treatment may be greater. But in many of these countries a high prevalence of anaemia is evidence that the whole community has an inadequate intake of iron and probably of many other nutrients. An increase in dietary iron, perhaps by a food fortification programme, may be the appropriate prophylaxis but any such programme must be adequately evaluated. In such communities the identification of certain individuals by a screening process followed by their treatment by a short course of iron therapy, which will probably only have a transient effect, is quite inadequate.

## SUMMARY AND CONCLUSION

1. Screening forms an important part of public-health practice. It enables diseases, or their more serious effects, to be prevented, and therefore can offer great benefits to the community as a whole as well as to the individuals who participate.

2. Screening represents a major departure from ordinary clinical practice, in that people are being persuaded to accept tests and treatment that they are initially unaware that they need. It is therefore incumbent on the screener to evaluate the procedure very carefully indeed, both as regard its effectiveness and its possible drawbacks.

3. The criteria by which screening tests should be judged have been well worked out. Many screening procedures fail because the tests are unacceptable to those who most need them or are insufficiently sensitive.

4. The screening procedure as a whole should be evaluated to ensure that it is effective. This involves all the classic epidemiological methods, viz. cross-sectional, prospective, and retrospective studies, but the most reliable evidence is provided by randomized controlled trials.

5. Because the effectiveness of a screening procedure has been demonstrated in one set of circumstances it should not be assumed that it will apply in other circumstances or at other times. All screening procedures should be monitored to ensure their continued effectiveness.

6. A careful cost-benefit analysis is necessary to assess the efficiency of screening. Since neither the costs, the benefits nor the relationship between them are wholly self-evident, this is a difficult exercise. It should take into account hidden expenses, costs to society at large as well as to health services, and non-economic factors.

7. The administration of a screening programme is just as important as the tests and treatment that comprise it. Several potentially useful screening procedures yield disappointing results because they are not adequately organized.

## REFERENCES

Beevers, D.G., Fairman, M.J., Hamilton, M., and Harpur, J.E. (1973). The influence of antihypertensive treatment over the incidence of cerebral vascular disease. *Postgrad. Med. J.* **49**, 905.

Bergman, A.B. and Stamm, S.J. (1967). The morbidity of cardiac nondisease in schoolchildren. *N. Eng. J. Med.* **276**, 1008.

Brett, G.Z. (1968). The value of lung cancer detection by six-monthly chest radiographs. *Thorax* **23**, 414.

British Thoracic and Tuberculosis Association (1973). A tuberculosis survey in England and Wales 1971. *Tubercle* **54**, 249.

Carmichael, A. and Williams, H.E. (1981). Developmental screening in infancy – a critical appraisal of its value. *Aust. Paediatr. J.* **17**, 20.

Catford, J.C., Bennet, G.C., and Wilkinson, J.A. (1982). Congenital hip dislocation: an increasing and still uncontrolled disability? *Br. Med. J.* **285**, 1527.

Clarke, E.A. and Anderson, T.W. (1979). Does screening by 'Pap' smears help prevent cervical cancer? *Lancet* **ii**, 1.

Cochrane, A.L. and Holland, W.W. (1971). Validation of screening procedures. *Br. Med. Bull.* **27**, 3.

Commission on Chronic Illness (1957). *Chronic illness in the United States,* Vol. 1. Harvard University Press, Cambridge, Mass.

Cramer, D.W. (1974). The role of cervical cytology in the declining morbidity and mortality of cervical cancer. *Cancer* **34**, 2018.

David, T.J., Parris, M.R., Poynor, M.V. *et al.* (1983). Reasons for late detection of hip dislocation in childhood. *Lancet* **ii**, 147.

Draper, G.J. (1982). Screening for cervical cancer: revised policy. The recommendations of the DHSS Committee on Gynaecological Cytology. *Health Trends* **14**, 37.

Drummond, M.F. (1980). *Principles of economic appraisal in health care.* Oxford University Press.

Ellenberg, J.H. and Nelson, K.B. (1981). Early recognition of infants at high risk for cerebral palsy: examination at age four months. *Dev. Med. Child Neurol.* **23**, 705.

Elwood, P.C. (1973). Evaluation of the clinical importance of anaemia. *Am. J. Clin. Nutr.* **26**, 958.

Elwood, P.C. (1974). The clinical evaluation of circulating haemoglobin levels. *Clin. Haematol.* **3**, 705.

Editorial committee of the Cardiff Cervical Cytology Study (1980). The Cardiff Cervical Cytology Study. *J. Epidemiol. Community Health* **34**, 9.

Frankenburg, W.K. and Camp, B.W. (1975). *Pediatric screening tests*. C.C. Thomas, Springfield, Ill.

Gastrin, G. (1980). Programme to encourage self-examination for breast cancer. *Br. Med. J.* **281**, 193.

George, W.D., Sellwood, R.A., Asbury, D., and Hartley, G. (1980*a*). Role of non-medical staff in screening for breast cancer. *Br. Med. J.* **280**, 147.

George, W.D., Sellwood, R.A., Asbury, D., and Hartley, G. (1980*b*). Hospital work load produced by breast-cancer screening programme run by trained non-medical staff. *Br. Med. J.* **281**, 653.

Hagard, S., Carter, F., and Milne, R.G. (1976). Screening for spina bifida cystica: a cost-benefit analysis. *Br. J. Prev. Soc. Med.* **30**, 40.

Hakama, M. and Rasanen-Virtanen, V. (1976). Effect of a mass screening programme on the risk of cervical cancer. *Am. J. Epidemiol.* **103**, 512.

Hamilton, M., Thompson, E.N., and Wisniewski, T.K.M. (1964). The role of blood pressure control in preventing complications of hypertension. *Lancet* i, 235.

Hart, J.T. (1970). Semicontinuous screening of a whole community for hypertension. *Lancet* ii, 223.

Henderson, J.B. (1982). Measuring the benefit of screening for open neural tube defects. *J. Epidemiol. Community Health* **36**, 214.

Hulse, J.A., Grant, D.B., Clayton, B.E. *et al.* (1980). Population screening for congenital hypothyroidism. *Br. Med. J.* **280**, 675.

Hulse, J.A., Grant, D.B., Jackson, D., and Clayton, B.E. (1982). Growth, development and reassessment of hypothyroid infants diagnosed by screening. *Br. Med. J.* **284**, 1435.

Johannesson, G., Geirsson, G., and Day, N. (1978). The effect of mass screening in Iceland, 1965–74, on the incidence and mortality of cervical carcinoma. *Int. J. Cancer* **21**, 418.

Keys, A., Aravanis, C., Blackburn, H. *et al.* (1972). Probability of middle-aged men developing coronary heart disease in five years. *Circulation* **45**, 815.

*Lancet* (1981). Early diagnosis and survival in breast cancer (Editorial.) *Lancet* ii, 785.

Linell, F., Ljungberg, O., and Andersson, I. (1980). Breast carcinoma. *Acta Pathol. Microbiol. Scand. (A) Suppl. 272.*

MacGregor, J.E. and Teper, S. (1978). Mortality from carcinoma of cervix uteri in Britain. *Lancet* ii, 774.

Medical Research Council Steering Committee for the MRC/DHSS Phenylketonuria Register (1981). Routine neonatal screening for phenylketonuria in the United Kingdom 1964–78. *Br. Med. J.* **282**, 1680.

Medical Research Council Tuberculosis and Chest Diseases Unit (1980). National survey of tuberculosis notifications in England and Wales 1978–1979. *Br. Med. J.* **281**, 895.

Miller, A.B., Lindsay, J., and Hill, G.B. (1976). Mortality from cancer of the uterus in Canada and its relationship to screening for cancer of the cervix. *Int. J. Cancer* **17**, 602.

New England Congenital Hypothyroidism Collaborative (1981). Effects of neonatal screening for hypothyroidism: prevention of mental retardation before clinical manifestations. *Lancet* ii, 1095.

Pearson, P.H. (1982). 'The results of treatment'; the horns of our dilemma. *Dev. Med. Child Neurol.* **24**, 417.

Roberts, C.J., Hibbard, B.M., Elder, G.H. *et al.* (1983). The efficacy of a serum screening service for neural-tube defects: the South Wales experience. *Lancet* i, 1315.

Shapiro, S. (1977). Evidence on screening for breast cancer from a randomized trial. *Cancer* **39**, 2772.

Spriggs, A.I. and Husain, O.A.N. (1977). Cervical smears. *Br. Med. J.* i, 1516.

Veterans Administration Co-operative Study Group (1967). Effects of treatment on morbidity in hypertension I. Results in patients with diastolic blood pressure averaging 115 through 129 mm Hg. *JAMA* **202**, 1028.

Veterans Administration Co-operative Study Group (1970). Effects of treatment on morbidity in hypertension II: Results in patients with diastolic blood pressure averaging 90 through 114 mm Hg. *JAMA* **213**, 1143.

Whyte, H.M. (1975). Potential effect on coronary heart disease morbidity of lowering the blood cholesterol. *Lancet* i, 906.

Wilson, J.M.G. and Jungner, G. (1968). *Principles and practice of screening for disease*. World Health Organization, Geneva.

World Health Organization (1972). *Nutritional anaemias: report of a WHO scientific group*. World Health Organization Technical Report Series No. 503. Geneva.

# 25 Setting nationwide objectives in disease prevention and health promotion: the United States experience

J.M. McGinnis

## INTRODUCTION

Of the broad range of governmental responsibilities in public health, perhaps none is more fundamental than the obligation to provide perspective and direction to guide health programmes along a productive course – the agenda-setting function. For governments with a strong central planning focus, setting the agenda determines the distribution of national resources. For others, its importance stems at least as much from the ability of nationally identified goals to motivate and recruit the commitment of local and private resources.

Recently in the US, effort has been directed towards the establishment of measurable national goals in disease prevention and health promotion. The process is described in this chapter as a case study on the experience of setting nationwide objectives in disease prevention and health promotion.

Periodic reviews of the charge to the US public health community date back to the work in New England of the Reverend Edward Wigglesworth in 1789, who provided the first American mortality tables, and the 1850 *Report of a general plan for the promotion of public and personal health,* presented to the Massachusetts Legislature by Lemuel Shattuck (Williams 1976). The most recent, and most comprehensive, review was initiated in 1979 with the publication of *Healthy people,* the first Surgeon General's report on health promotion and disease prevention (DHHS 1979). In the report the following five national public health goals were announced for enhancing the health of the US population at the five major life stages:

1. To continue to improve infant health, and, by 1990, to reduce infant mortality by at least 35 per cent, to fewer than nine deaths per 1000 live births.

2. To improve child health, foster optimal childhood development, and, by 1990, reduce deaths among children aged 1 to 14 years by at least 20 per cent, to fewer than 34 per 100 000.

3. To improve the health and health habits of adolescents and young adults, and, by 1990, to reduce deaths among people aged 15 to 24 years by at least 20 per cent, to fewer than 93 per 100 000.

4. To improve the health of adults, and, by 1990, to reduce deaths among people aged 15 to 64 years by at least 25 per cent, to fewer than 400 per 100 000.

5. To improve the health and quality of life for older adults and, by 1990, to reduce the average annual number of days of restricted activity due to acute and chronic conditions by 20 per cent, to fewer than 30 days per year for people aged 65 years and older.

These goals were based on an assessment of the recent historical trends combined with an estimate of the extent to which concerted and strategic intervention might accelerate potential gains. Special emphasis was given to two problems, expressed as subgoals, for each life stage. For infants, particular attention was given to the problems of low-weight births and birth defects; for children, factors in childhood growth and development as well as childhood accidents and injuries; for adolescents and young adults, fatal motor vehicle accidents and misuse of alcohol and drugs; for adults, heart attacks, strokes, and cancers; and for the elderly, increasing functional independence and reducing premature death from influenza and pneumonia.

Fifteen priority areas, were also identified as the objects of intervention programmes necessary for achieving overall health status goals. These activities were grouped as below into three categories – preventive health services, health protection, and health promotion – as a structure for planning national health strategies:

(a) *Preventive Health services*
 – High blood pressure control
 – Family planning
 – Pregnancy and infant care
 – Immunizations
 – Sexually transmitted diseases services
(b) *Health Protection*
 – Toxic agent control
 – Occupational safety and health

− Accidental injury control
− Fluoridation of community water supplies
− Infectious agent control
(c) *Health Promotion*
− Smoking cessation
− Reducing misuse of alcohol and drugs
− Improved nutrition
− Exercise and fitness
− Stress control

Following the identification of these priority areas, broad specific and measurable decade-long objectives were developed for each of the 15 areas (DHHS 1980*a*). The strategy was presented in the form of 226 objectives, with measurable end-points targeted to 1990. The development of these health objectives was undertaken in response to three perceived needs: (i) to clarify national opportunities and intentions; (ii) to establish benchmarks to which federal programmes could be addressed, and by which they could be assessed; and (iii) to establish a process which, while national in character, could be adapted to facilitate the development of local programmes. The result was a reasonably straightforward application of the management by objectives concept to the public health arena. This effort is discussed in the context of the procedural rationale, international experience, and some specific applications.

## MANAGING BY OBJECTIVES

Though the term 'management by objectives' was introduced only in the last generation (Drucker 1954), the concept has been emerging for some time. The notion refers to a set of procedures directed to identifying the individual steps and targets necessary to achieve common goals. The underlying assumption is that it is possible to specify common goals that, when explicitly identified, will yield efforts which are more focused, efficient, and consonant with the prevailing consensus about desired outcomes. A related assumption is that people closest to a particular problem or issue have an advantage in identifying management opportunities, given certain broad parameters. This concept has been applied widely to a number of management enterprises, public and private, in which the intent is to reach some usually quantifiable or measurable goal (Odiorne 1972).

Management by objectives has been a sporadic feature of governmental decision making and implementation since the 1930s, but the private sector has generally been recognized as its most vigorous proponent. More recently, however, as the complexity of governmental activities has grown, management by objectives has appeared with increasing frequency in the public lexicon.

The benefits from this approach are derived both in terms of the objectives and of management. Applying the concept of management by objectives results in a number of revelations about the objectives themselves. First, it makes clear whether an agency actually has objectives or merely good intentions. Setting an objective establishes the framework for its attainment. Hence a programme objective must lead naturally to the component tasks and the assignment of those

tasks. Second, its application reveals that equally valid objectives may be mutually inconsistent or even incompatible and that often risky efforts at balancing and tradeoffs are required in decision-making. Priorities must be set, and these will involve postponing some actions in favour of others. Furthermore, even within the context of a single goal, a choice will have to be made among various strategies. Third, the systematic appraisal of services and activities will identify candidates for abandonment – programmes that are obsolete or non-productive. Fourth, the management by objectives process will help clarify whether or not the objectives are realistic in terms of specific targets, timetables, strategies, and resource allocation. In other words, whether or not a plan can be implemented. Finally, it will establish a measurement standard. Without objective means of assessing outcomes, a programme cannot have easily discernible accomplishments, only expenditures of resources. Defining measurements makes it possible to organize the feedback from results and to systematically review and revise objectives, roles, priorities, and allocation of resources (Drucker 1981).

A number of features of public sector activities make management by objectives especially applicable to government. The sheer size of government makes it more likely that organizational motives and goals will be diffused by the complexity of the tasks and functions. For example, the personnel branch, the grants and contracts branch, the public affairs branch, and the various programme branches of a government agency may each be motivated by different forces which relate in very different ways to an organization's overall mission. This complexity has inherent within it the potential for conflicting objectives. A focus of the personnel branch on employee privileges may run directly counter to the interest of a programme manager who wishes to streamline certain employee functions. Or the needs of a programme manager may conflict with the procedures of a contracts branch charged with safeguarding against system abuses. Furthermore, in public sector activities much of the energy and discussion within an organization may be focused on issues which in fact bear little relation to actual performance relative to the organization's mission. Budgetary allocations offer an example of this phenomenon. In government, because the intended inputs and outputs are not things but people and identifiable social improvement in some discrete sphere, the direction programmes ought to take may not be inherent in the activities. Indeed rules, regulations and smooth functioning can be mistaken for real accomplishment (Drucker 1981).

The complexities are readily apparent in the health arena. The overall aim of health policy is of course to improve health. But an elaboration on the focus and means for improving health reveals some of the tensions and uncertainties. Does this mean building more sanitation facilities? Does it mean better inspection to ensure a safe food supply? Does it mean supporting research to improve the knowledge base upon which action can be taken? Perhaps it means a prohibition of smoking or the growing of tobacco. Should the focus be on physicians – training them, licensing them and reimbursing them? Or should it be on other people, the clients of physicians – ensuring the delivery of basic health services?

If so, to all the people or only certain vulnerable subsets? And, which ones? What is the proper mix of activities? What are the priorities? What ought to be reasonably achievable, given resources and constraints?

The full set of issues contains multiple strategies which are often conflicting and it may be impossible to address them all simultaneously. These are the sorts of issues which management by objectives ought to be helpful in resolving. Because its central utility is in reducing broad aspirations to concrete programme actions, it is much more than a way to implement decisions. It is the process by which those decisions are made. Assuming that objectives stated in measurable terms are actually measures of performance – not just efforts – the process of arriving at each objective is, in effect, a policy decision.

Some general prerequisites pertain to the successful application of the process of setting objectives, whether in a commercial or a social context. They include the ability to define a problem clearly, the existence of a discrete constituency, the availability of an effective intervention methodology, the social acceptability of that methodology, and a means to track the progress.

Assuming these prerequisites, several types of objectives can be developed and applied to a management process: outcome objectives, strategy objectives, marketing objectives, productivity objectives, and innovation objectives. In fact, stating the outcome objectives (for example, profits) may be superfluous, for desirable outcomes should be viewed as requirements, not as objectives, for the process.

Table 25.1 compares the application of the various objective classes to a business and a health context. In these examples, the final outcome sought for the business sector is profits and for the health sector it is reduced morbidity and mortality. Because these are the requirements or goals of the enterprise, they need not be explicitly stated, except perhaps as broader goals or predictions. For the purpose of tailoring organizational activities to achieve the component goals, the most important objectives are those directed to programme processes which will yield the intended outcome – that is those related to strategy, marketing, productivity, and innovation.

A strategy objective, in the business setting might be the charge set for a particular product. In the health setting, it might be which risk factors to try to affect. In seeking to reduce heart disease, for example, what changes might be reasonably sought with respect to smoking, high blood pressure, or blood cholesterol levels? A marketing objective in the business setting might refer to the changes sought in client attitudes and awareness, hence how much effort to devote to advertising and which audiences to target for certain behaviour change. In health, marketing objectives might be tailored to changing the level of awareness of certain population groups, for example, the awareness of pregnant women about special controllable hazards to the fetus, or of teenagers about risks of alcohol or drug misuse, or even the awareness of primary care physicians about the preventable problems over which they might have some influence.

Productivity objectives in the business setting relate to the targeting of certain levels of product output for a given labour, capital, or technical input. And in the health care setting these kinds of objectives relate to the number of people reached with certain services, or to the scope and intensity of health protection efforts for various population groups. Innovation objectives for business include the extent to which they invest in laboratories and quality control. For health, the innovation objectives relate both to efforts to monitor progress with surveillance systems and to efforts aimed at developing new intervention methodologies through research.

Although the most widely recognized proponents of management by objectives have come from the corporate world, the applications to health are expanding rapidly. Examples include the efforts undertaken to gauge the productivity of health care institutions in terms of bed utilization rates, laboratory capacity or patient visits per unit of time. Some efforts have been more explicitly relevant to health gains. The WHO's smallpox eradication programme, especially in its later phases, provides perhaps the best example of an effort deploying locally derived objectives on both process and outcome to assist in the global elimination of the disease. The US National Childhood Immunization Initiative, implemented between 1977 and 1979 by the Department of Health and Human Services, provides a good example of successful application of the concept on a national basis. Both will be discussed more fully below, as will other examples indicating that the management by objectives process can work not only with major perceived threats, but also with routine public health programmes.

## INTERNATIONAL CONTEXT

Establishing targets in public health as a national effort has been undertaken by many countries, particularly in recent years. Especially as research has unveiled more opportunities, population growth and industrialization have created more problems, and the exigencies of economic pressures have offered more constraints, many leaders have felt the need to clarify national directions in health. An additional force compelling such exercises has been the realization that efforts to improve health must be linked to other efforts aimed at improving social and economic conditions, the complexity of the task requiring careful integration and planning.

Several such efforts have been undertaken recently. In 1971, the Federal Republic of Germany issued a planning document which noted the importance of linking health

**Table 25.1.** *Application of the management by objectives concept*

| Objective classes | Business applications | Health applications |
|---|---|---|
| Outcome | Profits | Morbidity and mortality reduction |
| Strategy | Product type and mix | Risk factors |
| Productivity | Labour/capital mix | Scope of services |
| Marketing | Client attitudes and awareness | Public/professional attitudes and awareness |
| Innovation | Product improvement | Surveillance, evaluation, and research |

policy with economic policy, cultural attitudes, and political values. Special emphasis in the document was given to prevention, health maintenance, and care of the sick and handicapped. The Soviet Five-Year Plan for Public Health 1971–75, also took a broad view, calling for a general improvement in mental and physical health and a lowering of the prominent sources of morbidity and mortality. Problems emphasized were infectious diseases, and those of children and the elderly. Tools to be particularly employed were sanitary measures and epidemiological analysis. In 1972 the 10-Year Plan for the Americas (1971–80) was issued by the Pan American Health Organization (PAHO). That plan noted the importance of health generally to national development, and offered goals on health services, maternal and child health, and infectious diseases, with special attention to the emerging chronic diseases. Among the quantified targets was a two-year increase in life expectancy over the decade for those countries with personal life expectancies in the range 65 to 69 years. In 1973, the Swedish National Board of Health and Welfare issued a planning document addressing the future organization of health, emphasizing service integration and long-term care, and offering a plan for the establishment of local health centres. It also proposed a three-cycle planning process focusing on 5-, 15- and 30-year plans. In 1974, the Mexican Health Plan was issued which included 10-year goals in health to be integrated with other aspects of overall national development, and calling for emphases including health education, nutrition, sanitation, worker's health,

maternal and child health, and infectious diseases. Also in 1974, the Minister of National Health and Welfare in Canada issued *A new perspective on the health of Canadians* which called for a five-pronged health strategy with renewed emphasis on health promotion, regulatory protection, research, efficiency of health care services, and goal setting. In 1976, England's Department of Health and Social Services released a document on priorities for health and personal social services which emphasized care and preventive services. A special focus was placed on vulnerable populations – the elderly, children, the handicapped, and the mentally ill. Table 25.2 displays some of the areas of special interest to 48 nations whose activities of the last 15 years have been reviewed (DHEW 1977).

There is wide variety in both the structure and the focus of these goal-setting efforts. This reflects the fact that each of the countries sponsoring the work has different needs and different uses to which the goal-setting process might be put. While the major problems in certain countries relate to infectious diseases, those in others may be driven by industrial pollution or life-style factors. Whereas some countries need only general indicators of national problems and priorities, others need specific direction on the allocation of national budgets. Accordingly, the goal statements reflect the disparate uses to which they will be put. For some countries they are couched more as national hopes and aspirations than attainable goals. For others they reflect more the utility of the process in consensus building than in predicting an achievable

**Table 25.2.** *National health goals* *

| Goal statements by goal dimensions | Numbers of countries incorporating goal statement | | | | | | | |
|---|---|---|---|---|---|---|---|---|
| | Total (n=48) | West Europe (n=8) | East Europe (n=4) | Western Hemp. (n=12) | Medit. (n=5) | Africa (n=11) | SE Asia (n=4) | West Pacific (n=3) |
| **Health status** | | | | | | | | |
| Reduce communicable disease | 23 | 2 | 1 | 12 | 1 | 5 | 2 | – |
| Reduce infant mortality | 14 | 1 | 2 | 8 | – | 2 | 1 | – |
| Reduce mental illness | 8 | 2 | – | 5 | 1 | – | – | – |
| Reduce accidental deaths | 7 | 1 | – | 5 | – | – | – | 1 |
| **Health promotion** | | | | | | | | |
| Improve sanitation and environmental conditions | 20 | – | 1 | 10 | 3 | 3 | 3 | – |
| Extend health consciousness | 20 | 5 | 1 | 6 | 3 | 3 | 2 | – |
| Improve access to safe drinking water | 11 | – | – | 6 | 2 | 1 | 1 | 1 |
| Improve availability of adequate diet | 8 | 1 | 1 | 4 | 1 | – | 1 | – |
| Reduce environmental pollution | 7 | 1 | 1 | 4 | – | – | – | 1 |
| **Health services** | | | | | | | | |
| Increase access in rural and urban areas | 25 | 2 | 4 | 9 | 2 | 5 | 2 | 1 |
| Increase number of providers | 18 | 3 | 1 | – | 1 | 8 | 3 | 2 |
| Increase number of facilities | 23 | 5 | 1 | 4 | 5 | 4 | 3 | 1 |
| Improve maternal and child health services | 20 | 2 | 1 | 6 | 4 | 3 | 3 | 1 |
| Increase in-service training | 13 | 3 | – | 4 | 3 | 2 | 1 | – |
| Develop comprehensive services | 12 | 3 | 2 | 2 | 1 | 2 | 1 | 1 |
| Improve health care for mentally, physically handicapped | 6 | 4 | – | 1 | – | – | – | 1 |
| Improve services to elderly | 5 | 5 | – | – | – | – | – | – |
| Improve management | 8 | – | – | 5 | – | – | – | – |
| **Innovation** | | | | | | | | |
| Increase research efforts | 6 | – | 1 | 2 | 1 | 1 | – | 1 |
| **Data** | | | | | | | | |
| Improve data systems | 11 | 1 | – | 7 | 2 | 1 | – | – |

*20 goals most frequently found in national health plans, by goal dimensions and numbers of countries incorporating such statements, world-wide and by geographical regions.
Source: DHEW (1977).

end-point. In other cases, stated goals may be tailored by perceptions of what potential institutional or international grant-giving bodies might want to see. Only rarely is the principal motivation for such activities related directly to programme management.

## UNITED STATES MODEL

### The context

A more detailed examination of the recent US experience in objective setting may be instructive with respect to both the prospects and the problems of the process. First a review of the context. In the US, a number of factors have converged to foster the development and implementation of an agenda setting process. Possibly the most significant of these was the development of a fuller understanding of the factors which affect health status and a sense of confidence with respect to our ability to control those factors.

The health of Americans has improved steadily even without a system to identify health objectives explicitly. For example, the provisional age-adjusted death rate for all Americans in 1980 was only about one-third the rate in 1900 (Table 25.3). Most of the improvement in health status is assigned to gains against infectious diseases, but the precise nature of factors contributing to this gain remains debatable. Indeed, given the progress that apparently occurred well before widespread application of any of the major interventions of vaccination and antibiotics, a good case has been made for the contribution of fundamental improvements in socio-economic status with concomitant improvements in nutrition and sanitary conditions (McKeown 1976).

Perhaps most remarkable have been gains in the survival of infants and children. Indeed, as Table 25.4 shows, by 1980, the provisional death rate for infants had dropped to less than one-tenth of the level at the turn of the century, and for children up to age 15 years, to one-twentieth of the level in 1900.

During the decade 1970–80, life expectancy at birth increased by some 2.8 years, an increase greater than that for the previous two decades combined (Table 25.5). Overall life expectancy at birth has increased by 24 years since 1900 (from 49.2 years in 1900 to 73.6 years in 1980). During the same period, however, the life expectancy gain for a 45-year-old American was only 7.3 years (from 24.8 years in 1900 to 32.1 years in 1980).

Impressive health gains for the adult population however, have been realized in recent years, at least as measured by mortality figures. The expected additional years of life for a 45-year-old person have amounted to about 2.0 years during the last decade, a striking 6.6 per cent increase. This gain for adults – substantially attributable to declines in the death rates from heart attacks and strokes of 25 per cent and 40 per cent, respectively – is proportionately greater than the 4.0 per cent increase in life expectancy at birth for the same period (McGinnis 1982).

Many factors are involved in these gains in ways not yet fully understood. Certainly the growth in the knowledge base has provided considerable impetus. As noted in Table 25.6, the improvement in our understanding of the factors involved in various diseases has been impressive.

But with the development of our enhanced understanding, as well as the improvements in health status, a number of issues have been raised related to the US public health agenda. Although the recent trends cited certainly offer cause for encouragement, questions must be answered about the extent to which health gains have occurred 'at the margin' – that is among the persons most easy to reach or to convert to a more healthy life-style rather than among the highest cost users of health care. Could more carefully targeted and monitored efforts help facilitate gains for the most vulnerable groups?

### The model

Against the backdrop of health gains, reinforced by the prospects of even greater gains, an interest has developed in the clarification of national goals and objectives in health. Consequently, out of efforts to analyse the risk factors from the leading causes of morbidity and mortality in the US, has

**Table 25.3.** *Age-adjusted death rates per 100 000 population for leading causes, 1900 and 1980*

| 1900 | | | 1980* | | |
|---|---|---|---|---|---|
| Cause | Rate | Per cent of total † | Cause | Rate | Per cent of total † |
| Influenza and pneumonia | 210 | 12 | Heart disease | 205.3 | 34.6 |
| Tuberculosis | 199 | 11 | Cancer | 134.2 | 22.6 |
| Heart disease | 167 | 9 | Stroke | 41.5 | 7.0 |
| Stroke | 134 | 8 | Accidents | 43.4 | 7.3 |
| Diarrhoea and related diseases | 113 | 6 | Influenza and pneumonia | 12.6 | 2.1 |
| Cancer | 81 | 5 | Cirrhosis/chronic liver disease | 12.6 | 2.1 |
| Accidents | 76 | 4 | Suicide | 12.2 | 2.1 |
| Diabetes | 13 | 2 | Diabetes | 10.1 | 1.9 |
| Suicide | 11 | 1 | Homicide | 11.4 | 1.9 |
| Homicide | 1 | 1 | Tuberculosis | 0.5 | 0.1 |
| All other causes | 775 | 44 | Diarrhoea | 0.7 ‡ | 0.1 ‡ |
| | | | All other causes | 109.6 | 18.4 |
| All causes | 1779 | 100 | All causes | 594.1 | 100.0 |

Sources: Annual Summary of Births, Deaths, Marriages, and Divorces: United States, 1930, Monthly Vital Statistics Report, Nol. 29, No. 13, 17 Sept. 1961; and unpublished data. National Center for Health Statistics.

* Provisional data.
†Percentages do not add to 100 or 100.0 because of rounding.
‡Figure is for 1978. Not available for 1980.

**Table 25.4.** *Mortality rates by age group*

| Age group | Deaths per 100 000 population | |
| --- | --- | --- |
| | 1900 | 1980* |
| Infants | 16 244.8 | 1310.7 |
| Children (ages 1–14) | 866.3 | 40.7 |
| Adolescents and young adults (ages 15–24) | 585.5 | 118.8 |
| Adults (ages 25–64) | 1270.2 | 506.9 |
| Older adults (ages 65 and over) | 8225.8 | 5290.8 |

*Provisional data.
Source: National Center for Health Statistics.

**Table 25.5** *Changes in life expectancy in the United States*

| Year* | Life expectancy at birth in years | Percentage gain in decade | Life expectancy at age 45 in years | Percentage gain in decade |
| --- | --- | --- | --- | --- |
| 1900 | 49.2 | – | 24.8 | – |
| 1910 | 51.5 | 4.7 | 24.5 | –1.2 |
| 1920 | 56.4 | 9.5 | 26.3 | 7.3 |
| 1930 | 59.2 | 5.0 | 25.8 | –1.9 |
| 1940 | 63.6 | 7.4 | 26.9 | 4.3 |
| 1950 | 68.1 | 7.1 | 28.5 | 5.9 |
| 1960 | 69.9 | 2.6 | 29.5 | 3.5 |
| 1970 | 70.8 | 1.3 | 30.1 | 2.0 |
| 1980 ‡ | 73.6 | 4.0 | 32.1 | 6.6 |

*Except for 1980, the numbers given are based on data for three-year periods. For example: figures for 1970 are based on data for 1979–71.
‡Provisional data.
Source: National Center for Health Statistics.

**Table 25.6.** *Risk factors for leading causes of years of potential life lost (ages 1–74)*

| Cause | Risk factors |
| --- | --- |
| Heart disease | Smoking, high blood pressure, elevated serum cholesterol, diabetes, obesity, lack of exercise, coronary-prone behaviour |
| Cancers | Smoking, alcohol, diet, sexual behaviour, solar radiation, ionizing radiation, worksite hazards, environmental contaminants, certain medications, infectious agents |
| Motor vehicle accidents | Alcohol, no safety restraints, speed, automobile design, roadway design |
| All other accidents | Alcohol, smoking (fires), product design, home hazards, handgun availability |
| Suicide | Handgun availability, alcohol and drug misuse, stress |
| Homicide | Handgun availability, alcohol, stress |
| Stroke | High blood pressure |
| Cirrhosis of liver | Alcohol |
| Influenza/pneumonia | Vaccination status, smoking |
| Diabetes | Obesity (for adult-onset disease) |

grown the development of the 1979 Surgeon General's Report on Health Promotion and Disease Prevention and the 1980 report which identified the health objectives for the decade. The conceptual underpinning for those efforts is noted in Fig. 25.1, which portrays the various factors which go into determining the health status profile of a particular population group (McGinnis 1983). Health status is determined by a variety of biological, behavioural, environmental, and social risk factors. Biological risk factors are those individual physiological and structural features – often genetically endowed – which

determine special propensities, susceptibilities, or immunities in various circumstances. Behavioural risk factors are those specific behaviours that may put an individual at increased or decreased risk, and which may be engaged in with some knowledge of potential consequences. Environmental risk factors are those potentially hazardous agents or factors in the environment, both manmade or natural, which affect the risk for disease or disability. Social risk factors include a host of exogenous influences over which an individual may have only marginal control, such as, economic status, educational level, geographical isolation, access to health services, and nature of the food supply.

These risk factors can in turn be influenced by the presence or absence of various programmes. The types of service programmes will include general health services, that is, those medical and surgical interventions offered by health providers

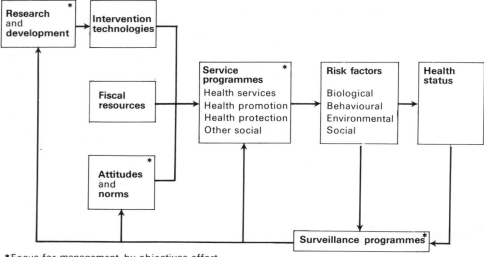

*Focus for management by objectives effort

**Fig. 25.1.** Factors determining health status.

to remedy a biological or behavioural condition endangering health status. But they also include health promotion programmes which include educational and motivational services to enhance health behaviour, as well as health protection efforts which evoke statutory and regulatory measures to facilitate the health of a population group. Other relevant social programmes that may influence health status range from income supports and unemployment benefits to meals for the aged, day care, and farm policies.

The availability of services is determined by the existence of appropriate intervention technologies, hospitable fiscal conditions, and receptive attitudes and norms. An effective research and development capability is necessary to the production of innovative intervention technologies. Surveillance programmes provide information about health status and risk factor prevalence which can be used to shape the character of services, public and professional attitudes and norms, and research and development efforts.

## The process

In the US experience, management by objectives has been applied to enhance the work of a national health agency seeking to influence various pressure points in this scheme in such a way that progress can be directed and facilitated. The Department of Health and Human Services identified a number of loci as appropriate targets for setting objectives – the service programmes, attitudes and norms, surveillance programmes, and research and demonstration projects. In 1979 and 1980 attention was focused on the development of objectives in these areas. Objectives were also stated for improved health status and reduced risk factors – both outcome measures – but were included more as an indication of where the US might reasonably be expected to emerge, in terms of national health status, if the stated process objectives were attained.

The process of developing the objectives themselves had several stages. This together with the process of implementation and review is illustrated in Fig. 25.2. The process was initiated with the decision to set quantified health status goals in *Healthy people,* as noted above in the introduction (DHHS 1979). The 15 general strategy targets were simultaneously identified by assessing the risk factors involved in the leading sources of morbidity and mortality for each age group, and determining those for which the health-care system might reasonably accept responsibility. It was then decided that a broad-ranged public and private effort would be the best vehicle for establishing a national consensus on quantifiable objectives within each of the strategy categories. Motivating the collective approach was the knowledge that developing and implementing a national strategy for prevention, not merely a federal one, required the co-operation of many public service organizations from federal, state, and local governments, and from the private sector.

To initiate the formulation of the objectives, a governmental planning group was assembled and agencies within the US Public Health Service were assigned responsibility for developing background documentation, which reviewed the major challenges in each of the 15 areas, noted the programme

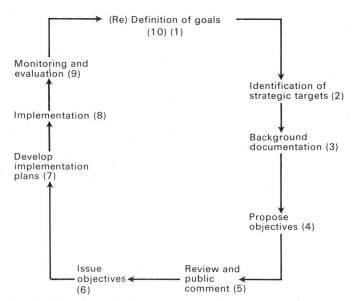

**Fig. 25.2.** Setting objectives – a process schematic.

opportunities, and postulated a number of feasible objectives for the respective areas. These papers were then provided to the participants in a 1979 conference which brought together 167 invited experts from outside the government who were organized into 15 working groups and charged with developing the first public drafts of objectives for the 15 areas. Participants were selected for their insight into some aspect of risk reduction in a particular area and represented a variety of institutional perspectives, including providers, academic centres, state and local health agencies, and voluntary health associations (DHHS 1980a). In addition to the invited experts, approximately 50 representatives of interested federal agencies attended the various working group sessions as observers.

The priorities for each category were generally arrived at through a consensus process, drawing baseline and background information both from the individual expertise of the participating authorities, and the papers which had been prepared for the use of the conferees. The process involved first identifying the most serious problems in each of the respective areas, giving attention not only to aggregate national data, but also to what was known about high risk groups, then matching up those problems with what the knowledge base offered as the most viable opportunities for intervention against those problems. The last step in the process required assessing the various objectives which had been developed, for balance between the objective categories – Was there an imbalance between risk factor objectives versus awareness objectives versus services objectives? If so, was it justifiable, or was something being overlooked?

In some cases there was a temptation in the working groups to let the ease of establishing a specific number drive the priority. That is to say, if a well-known data set related to a particular area was available, and if there was some confidence that those data would also be available in 1990, and if the relevant programme activity seemed to be relatively easily implemented, there was a temptation to identify automatically that activity as a priority objective category. Though pragmatism compelled a certain tolerance for this inclination, working groups were generally urged to search carefully for opportunities for legitimate, sustained and meaningful change, rather than yield to the course of least resistance.

The development of the numbers themselves for each of the objectives varied with the particular objective. Some were linear extrapolations of the current trend, as was the case, for example, with the infant mortality objective. In other cases, particularly in those like polio incidence where progress had already been substantial and similar gains could not be expected, the projected number represented maintenance of the *status quo*. But some objectives targeted a quantum improvement in the situation, for example, the objective that the proportion of women in any county, or racial, or ethnic group, who obtained no prenatal care during the first trimester of pregnancy should not exceed 10 per cent (versus the 40 to 45 per cent currently prevalent for some ethnic groups).

In each of the work group discussions on quantification there was a lively exchange over the merits of establishing as the target a figure which would represent: (i) a societal tolerance level for a particular condition (in which case politics would demand that the number be set very low), or (ii) a figure representing what society ought practically to be able to achieve within the requisite period of time, given reasonably likely resources. But the element of quantification was placed as paramount. For every objective category, except the surveillance and evaluation objectives, working groups were urged to establish a specific objective which was quantifiable and which could theoretically be tracked. Broad non-numerical statements of good intentions were not considered acceptable.

Finally, each working group was asked to identify the principal assumption on which its projection was based. What resources were anticipated for accomplishing the goal? Was any change foreseen in the technology available or in societal attitudes and norms?

The papers developed out of the working group efforts were then edited within the Department of Health and Human Services to format as uniformly as possible, their availability was published in the *Federal Register*, and they were circulated to more than 2000 groups and individuals nationally for review and comment. Revisions were made based on the comments received, circulated within the government for a final review, and issued in 1980.

## The objectives

A few items deserve special emphasis. First, although the objectives were printed by the US Government and subjected to the review process normally required of positions developed by the US Government, they did not necessarily reflect a federal perspective. The objectives themselves were intended to be national, not federal. In effect they are national guidelines to be used as reference points for the broad range of national organizations and institutions responsible for actually achieving the health gains which are possible in the US. Secondly, they reflect arbitration and consensus, and as a result represent a curious *mélange* of values and perspectives. Hence some are imperfect statements of the actual potential

involved. On the other hand, an effort was made to minimize such problems through the provision of some general guidelines. Specifically, participants were directed to confine the objectives developed to what might feasibly be attained during the decade of the 1980s, assuming neither major breakthroughs in prevention technology nor large infusions of new federal monies. The interest was in focusing on the possible. A good example of this perspective is offered by the goal for infant health which is to reduce the infant mortality rate to no more than nine deaths per 1000 live births in 1990. Because several areas in western Europe, and certain locales within the States have already achieved rates of five deaths per 1000 live births, theoretically the US should be able to do much better than this. Yet, because there exist substantial disparities between the risks experienced by some population groups within the US, it was judged prudent to set a realistic target (DHHS 1980a).

The distribution of the objectives by area is noted in Table 25.7. The range is from nine objectives for high blood pressure to 20 objectives each for toxic agent control and occupational safety and health. Within each area, the objectives are grouped into five categories: improved health status; reduced risk factors; improved public and professional awareness; improved services and protection; and improved surveillance and evaluation. Table 25.8 indicates the number of objectives grouped into each of these categories. The objectives on improved health status and reduced risk represent statements

**Table 25.7.** *Number of objectives by area*

| | |
|---|---|
| **Preventive services** | |
| High blood pressure control | 9† |
| Family planning | 10 |
| Pregnancy and infant health | 19* |
| Immunization | 18* |
| Sexually transmitted diseases | 11 |
| **Health protection** | |
| Toxic agent control | 20 |
| Occupational safety and health | 20 |
| Accident prevention and injury control | 17 |
| Fluoridation and dental health | 12 |
| Surveillance and control of infectious diseases | 12* |
| **Health promotion** | |
| Smoking and health | 17 |
| Misuse of alcohol and drugs | 19* |
| Nutrition | 17† |
| Physical fitness and exercise | 11 |
| Control of stress and violent behaviour | 14 |
| | 226‡ |

*One duplicate.
†Two duplicates.
‡Accounting for duplicates, discrete objectives total 222.

**Table 25.8.** *Number of objectives by category*

| | |
|---|---|
| Improved health status | 58* |
| Reduced risk factors | 47† |
| Increased public/professional awareness | 38* |
| Improved services/protection | 51 |
| Improved surveillance/evaluation systems | 32 |
| | 226 |

*One duplicate
†Two duplicates.

of anticipation and intent, rather than management enterprises. While they are important indicators of overall national policy, they do not offer, in and of themselves, the core principles necessary for management decisions. Rather, the directions for these decisions are found more substantially in the three objective categories that relate to improved public/professional awareness, improved services/protection, and improved surveillance/evaluation.

Table 25.9 reproduces the full list of objectives for high blood pressure control as an example of the kinds of objectives developed for each of the major categories. In this example, one objective is stated for improved health status, and two objectives for each of the other four categories. The improved health status objective – better control among an expanded portion of the hypertensive population – is straightforward. The objectives related to reduced risk factor include reducing the average daily sodium intake, salt being a prominent risk factor for hypertension in certain population groups, and reducing the prevalence of obesity, since this is also a prominent risk factor. The awareness objectives focus on two dimensions of the issue: awareness by individuals that hypertension is a prominent component of a broader range of risk factors for heart disease and awareness by individuals of their actual blood pressure levels. Both provide important programme guidance since they can serve as rallying points for a variety of activities. For other conditions, for example, sexually transmitted diseases, health professionals as well as the general public are the target of awareness objectives.

The two objectives listed for improved services and protection also relate to important approaches to controlling high blood pressure. The first is the provision of an effective service delivery system accessible to all sections of the US population, and the second relates to the provision of a mechanism to facilitate individual decisions with respect to dietary factors which might influence high blood pressure, that is caloric or sodium intake. No statement is made as to the extent to which regulations may be involved in obtaining this objective, thereby leaving the issue of voluntary versus mandatory labelling policies open to agency judgment. The objectives related to improved surveillance and evaluation are to refine our understanding of high blood pressure's incidence and sequelae, including development of a taxonomy that facilitates categorization.

Establishment of the objectives was based on certain assumptions about the anticipated scope of programme activity, the level of financial support, the range of participants involved, the state of the science base, and so forth. It was presumed that if major disjunctures occurred with respect to one or more of the assumptions, certain of the objectives would require amendment. Table 25.10 presents the principal assumptions underlying the high blood pressure control objectives.

**Table 25.9.** *High blood pressure control objectives*

**Improved health status**
  (a) By 1990, at least 60 per cent of the estimated population having definite high blood pressure (160/95) should have attained successful long-term blood pressure control, i.e. blood pressure at or below 140/90 for two or more years

**Reduced risk factors**
 *(b) By 1990, the average daily sodium ingestion (as measured by excretion) for adults should be reduced at least to the 3–6 g range

 *(c) By 1990, the prevalence of significant overweight (120 per cent of 'desired' weight) among the US adult population should be decreased to 10 per cent of men and 17 per cent of women, without nutritional impairment

**Increased public/professional awareness**
  (d) By 1990, at least 50 per cent of adults should be able to state the principal risk factors for coronary heart disease and stroke, i.e. high blood pressure, cigarette smoking, elevated blood cholesterol levels, diabetes

  (e) By 1990, at least 90 per cent of adults should be able to state whether their current blood pressure is normal (below 140/90) or elevated, based on a reading taken at the most recent visit to a medical or dental professional or other trained reader

**Improved services/protection**
  (f) By 1990, no geopolitical area of the United States should be without an effective public programme to identify persons with high blood pressure and to follow up on their treatment

  (g) By 1985, at least 50 per cent of processed food sold in grocery stores should be labelled to inform the consumer of sodium and caloric content, employing understandable, standardized, quantitative terms

**Improved surveillance/evaluation systems**
  (h) By 1985, a system should be developed to determine the incidence of high blood pressure, coronary heart disease, congestive heart failure and haemorrhagic and occlusive strokes. After demonstrated feasibility, by 1990 ongoing sets of these data should be developed.

  (i) By 1985, a methodology should be developed to assess categories of high blood pressure control, and a national baseline study of this status should be completed. Five categories are suggested: (i) unaware; (ii) aware, not under care; (iii) aware, under care, not controlled; (iv) aware, under care, controlled; and (v) aware, monitored without therapy

*Same objectives as for nutrition.

**Table 25.10.** *Principal assumptions for high blood pressure objectives*

• The aetiology of high blood pressure is multifactorial and no research breakthrough will eliminate it as a public health problem in the next decade

• The basic components of successful control programmes will continue to be detection, evaluation, treatment and/or changes in life-style, and follow-up

• While there are still some uncertainties about the quantitative relationship between sodium ingestion and high blood pressure, it is important to begin moving in the direction suggested by the data

• While there is not yet a true consensus as to what constitutes dangerous levels of overweight for the population as a whole, the stated targets provide the pattern for a productive trend

• Governmental efforts to control high blood pressure will be continued and expanded

• Voluntary and private sector efforts to control high blood pressure will be continued and expanded

• Health Systems Agencies will give high priority to high blood pressure detection, treatment, and control

• Implementation of the smoking, nutrition, and physical activity recommendations (see appropriate sections) will have a favourable impact on the prevention and control of high blood pressure

## Implementation

Once the objectives were published in 1980, the government's task was twofold: to tailor its own agenda to achieving the objectives and to stimulate activity in the non-federal sector as well. Several steps were initiated to develop the federal agenda. Each of 15 areas was assigned to one or another of the Public Health Service agencies with responsible programme activity in the area (Table 25.11), and that agency was directed to lead in planning the federal contribution to obtaining the objectives. The designated lead agency then assumed the obligation to develop an implementation plan

**Table 25.11.** *Lead US agencies for objectives*

| Category | DHHS agency/Office |
|---|---|
| **Preventive services** | |
| High blood pressure control | National Institutes of Health |
| Family planning | Health Resources and Services Administration |
| Pregnancy and infant health | Health Resources and Services Administration |
| Immunizations | Centers for Disease Control |
| Sexually transmitted diseases | Centers for Disease Control |
| **Health protection** | |
| Toxic agent control | Senior Advisor for Environmental Health |
| Occupational safety and health | Centers for Disease Control |
| Accident prevention and injury control | Centers for Disease Control |
| Fluoridation and dental health | Centers for Disease Control |
| Surveillance and control of infectious diseases | Centers for Disease Control |
| **Health promotion** | |
| Smoking and health | Office on Smoking and Health |
| Misuse of alcohol and drugs | Alcohol, Drug Abuse, and Mental Health Administration |
| Nutrition | Food and Drug Administration |
| Physical fitness and exercise | President's Council on Physical Fitness and Sports |
| Control of stress and violent behaviour | Alcohol, Drug Abuse, and Mental Health Administration |

that reflected not only its potential contribution, but that of its sister agencies as well, in achieving the set of objectives for a particular area. In doing so, the lead agencies were asked to convene working panels involving the other agencies to identify those objectives which were the highest priority from the federal perspective, to develop implementation plans which reflected the available and potential programme activity to meet these objectives, and to identify the non-DHHS governmental and private sector participants whose co-operation in the process might be required. Once these implementation plans were developed they were again circulated within the government to various interested parties and revised accordingly. They were published in 1983 in a special supplement of *Public Health Reports* (DHHS 1983*b*).

A system of monthly progress reviews was established. Each month a session has been scheduled to assess the progress toward the objectives in one or another of the 15 areas. Consequently, in the course of a little over a year each of the priority areas will have had one progress review to

identify relevant activities, accomplishments, and needs. At these progress review sessions, the lead agencies gather together with other co-operative agencies and present to the Secretary their programme of activities. At that time the potential shortfalls are noted, problems are raised and suggestions made for revision of either the objectives or the implementation plans, based on progress and experience to date. Summaries of the progress reviews are published in *Public Health Reports* to provide broader dissemination of the activities.

In addition to the federal activities to implement progress in each of the objective categories – including individual agency work to involve the private and voluntary sectors – a broad effort directed at catalysing state and local efforts to tailor the objectives to their needs is overseen by the US Public Health Service's Centers for Disease Control in Atlanta, Georgia. Here the intent is to encourage states and localities to take the model provided by the nationwide objectives and apply it to local conditions, based on their own assessment. A volume to assist in this effort has been prepared and published through the Centers for Disease Control, *Model standards for community preventive health services*. This manual was a co-operative effort of the federal government, the American Public Health Association, and the Association of State and Territorial Health Officers. Several States have already attempted to tailor the process to their own needs and it is anticipated that involvement of this sort will be broadened in the future.

## Monitoring

The task of monitoring progress on a national basis is among the most challenging faced in the process. When the objectives were first published the data sources then available were listed for each of the 15 areas. Unfortunately, the data necessary to track progress must come from a variety of different data sources and baseline data are not always available for the objectives that have been established. For example, of the 190 objectives outside the surveillance and evaluation category, only 112 have extant data sources. The greatest share of those which are currently measurable are in the health status category – about 89 per cent of which are measurable – while only about 10 per cent of the objectives related to public and professional awareness are measurable with current sources.

There is a wide range of possible systems which can be drawn upon to provide these data. They include (i) data systems based on records, such as those in the US Vital Statistics System; (ii) population based surveys, such as those periodically undertaken by various health agencies to determine the prevalence of various health habits; (iii) surveillance and monitoring systems, such as those established to monitor infectious disease prevalence; and (iv) regulatory reporting systems established to monitor compliance with statutes or regulations (Green *et al.*, in press). The agency which generates the data sets with broadest applicability to the objectives is the US Public Health Service's National Center for Health Statistics, which sponsors surveys such as the National Health Interview Survey, the National Health and Nutrition

Examination Survey, the National Ambulatory Medical Care Survey, the National Hospital Discharge Survey, the National Natality and Fetal Mortality Surveys, the National Survey of Family Growth, and the National Vital Registration System.

In spite of the considerable resources made available by these surveys, the various agencies overseeing implementation of the objectives must draw upon more than 40 agencies as data sources, and more data are still needed to track progress adequately. The problems for monitoring are obvious. Many of the surveys employed are one-time only surveys, hence will not provide data on a longitudinal basis. Furthermore, the fact that so many different sources are involved in generating the data used for monitoring raises problems of comparability of sampling techniques, thereby limiting the generalizability of the findings.

To address the monitoring problem, a formal data working group has been established which is carefully reviewing the requirements to make recommendations for federal action in this respect, including consideration of the parameters for a broad information management system. A sound monitoring system is an essential for future effectiveness of the effort to manage national progress through objectives.

## CASE EXAMPLES

Use of the management by objectives process, explicitly or implicitly, to direct health progress is certainly not without precedent nationally or internationally. Several examples of its application to health related issues are presented below. They indicate the extent to which a systematic approach of this sort can be successful in facilitating attainment of certain goals. Many of the examples – smallpox eradication,

childhood immunization, and lead poisoning control – illustrate the use of quantified objectives. High blood pressure control and smoking cessation are included as examples in which objectives are not quantified.

### Smallpox eradication

The WHO's global smallpox eradication programme, which formally began in 1967 and achieved eradication of the disease in 1977 (Fig. 25.3), offers one of the most spectacular examples of successful targeting in health. Its latter phases are particularly instructive with respect to the utility of quantified objectives for programme management.

Efforts to eliminate smallpox as a global scourge slowly increased and expanded following Edward Jenner's discovery in 1796 that cowpox infection would confer protection against the smallpox virus. Formal vaccination programmes followed shortly with Austria leading the way in 1799, and the Grand Duchy of Hesse developing the first legislation making vaccination compulsory in 1807. Thereafter, vaccination legislation was passed by various countries around the world. By the 1920s, the problem had become an international issue. In 1926 the health section of the League of Nations initiated publication of a weekly bulletin on disease prevalence in various countries and smallpox was made a reportable disease. The Pan American Sanitary Bureau – now the WHO Regional Office for the Americas – began an active involvement in smallpox control in the 1940s and 50s, and by 1959 smallpox had been effectively eliminated in the Americas with the exception of outbreaks in Argentina, Brazil, Bolivia, Colombia, and Equador.

In 1966, noting the success of certain control programmes

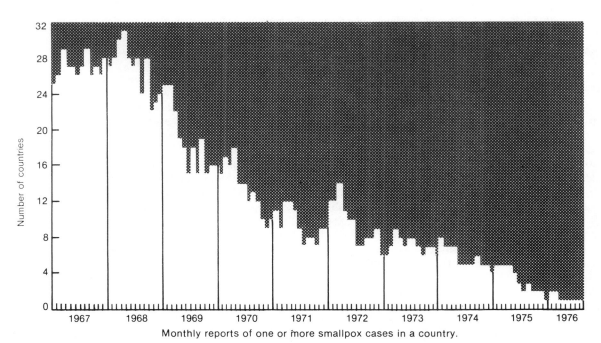

**Fig. 25.3.** Smallpox reports. Source: Henderson (1976).

of various countries around the world, the World Health Assembly authorized a programme to eradicate the disease, to commence 1 January 1967. At the time smallpox was endemic in 33 countries with major reservoirs in three general areas: South Asia, SubSaharan Africa, and Indonesia (WHO 1972).

The overall goal of the WHO was to eliminate the disease globally by the end of 1976. To accomplish this, several specific objectives were established from the outset: standardization of vaccines; simplification of vaccination techniques; improvement of the reporting systems; and initiation of national mass vaccination programmes. Other objectives were added after the programme had been in operation for a period: the focal concentration of programme efforts around outbreaks; the initiation of active surveillance techniques; and expansion of public awareness of and involvement with the programme.

One of the first tasks undertaken was the standardization of vaccines through the establishment of two reference centres which could work on vaccine improvement. By 1970, all of the vaccine used in the programme met the accepted international standards (Henderson 1976). In addition, an efficient mechanism was needed for delivering the vaccine doses. The scratch technique, which had been used for some years, proved both inefficient and wasteful. For a period mechanical injection via a jet injector, which had been developed by the US Army, was deployed but complications arose due to the breakdown of these injectors and the difficulty of repairing them. Finally, a major technological breakthrough by Wyeth Laboratories – the bifurcated needle – made it possible to deliver a drop of vaccine efficiently via a puncture technique.

To improve reporting, efforts were made to strengthen the capability of various national governments to retrieve accurate and regular reports from the field through special surveillance teams. This need was prompted by an early recognition that the disease was vastly under-reported and unreliably reported, thereby making the targeting of control efforts more difficult.

The control measures were initially designed as two-to-three year efforts toward mass vaccination of a national populous. It was felt that if 80 per cent of the population could be vaccinated smallpox incidence would be substantially reduced (Henderson 1976). As the campaign proceeded, and indeed relatively early in its course, several strategic enhancements were implemented. First, as a result of work in Nigeria· to focus scarce vaccine resources around identified outbreaks, it was discovered that the initiation of focal containment efforts could be highly successful in eliminating broader scale transmission of the disease. Consequently, the strategy of mass vaccination was shifted to one of surveillance and containment, which included improved search and detection, isolation of the affected cases, and vaccination of suspected or potential contacts around the identified cases. During the course of the various efforts, as the resources could be concentrated even further with the declining incidence of the disease, containment included posted watch guards outside the houses of contaminated visitors to insure vaccination of all contacts and intensive vaccination efforts of all exposed populations in a one mile radius around a case.

Similarly, surveillance became much more active. Rather than relying on a passive reporting system sent in from districts, states and regions, in 1973 in India a system of weekly active searches was established. Smallpox workers around the country were pulled together and mobilized for a week-long village-to-village and house-to-house search for cases. Again, as resources became more readily available with the declining disease incidence, greater emphasis was placed on any village with a reported case and individuals were posted in those villages to watch for the occurrence of new cases and to initiate new containment procedures. Ultimately, teams were posted in these villages for periods of up to six weeks after the last case had occurred to insure that no new cases were in fact occurring.

As part of active surveillance, an intensive effort was undertaken to expand the level of public involvement through efforts to inform the public about the nature and importance of the disease. A reward was offered for reporting of the disease and, in the Indian programme, the availability of the reward was posted prominently in each village with vulnerability to a smallpox outbreak. The reward eventually grew to a sizeable amount, as the disease declined in incidence and the importance of these reports by the public became more prominent.

In the very last stage of the programme – as for example in the last year of the programme in India – the explicit use of management by objectives became a prominent programme feature. Target levels were set both for disease incidence and for surveillance efforts, by state, region, and district. Active searches of large regions were held on a monthly basis and detailed reports made to central state and national officials. Regular statewide and national reviews were held on the progress in meeting the stated objectives. Detailed discussions were held on reasons for success or failure, and programme activity or the objectives were revised accordingly.

By October of 1977 the last field case of smallpox occurred in Merka, Somalia, and in May of 1979 the World Health Assembly officially declared smallpox eradicated.

## Childhood immunization

Childhood immunization is another infectious disease control effort illustrative of the successful application of the management by objectives process. In 1977 in the US, a major national immunization initiative was launched to immunize children under the age of 15 years for the seven most common preventable childhood diseases: polio, measles, rubella, pertussis, tetanus, diphtheria, and mumps. At that point nearly 20 million of the 52 million children in the country were not adequately immunized against these diseases and the incidence of several was beginning to increase (Fig. 25.4). For example, the incidence of measles had increased consistently since 1974 with the number of cases in 1977 running some 50 per cent higher than the preceding year. More importantly, the disease was being reported more frequently in older age groups – among junior high school, senior high school, and even college students – and these cases were accompanied by the increased risk and severity of complications which frequently characterize the occurrence of childhood diseases in young adults.

The national immunization initiative was begun in May 1977 with two basic goals: first, by October of 1979 to raise

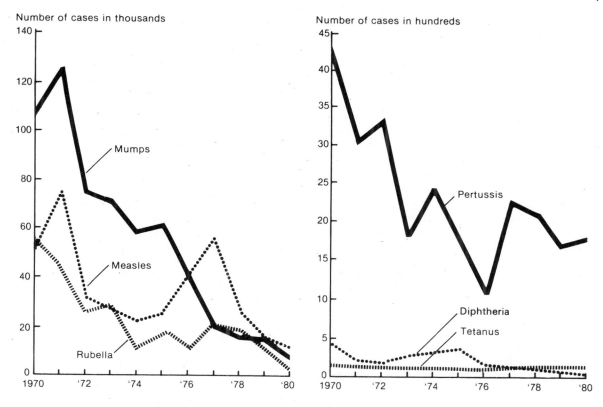

**Fig. 25.4.** Reported cases of measles, mumps, rubella, diphtheria, pertusis, and tetanus – 1970–80. Source: Centers for Disease Control.

immunization levels above 90 per cent for all children under age 15 years; and second, to establish a permanent mechanism to provide comprehensive immunization services to virtually all of the newborns in the US every year.

To meet these goals several specific objectives were established: improving awareness of the general public about the importance of childhood immunization; encouraging the interest and involvement of both public and private health care providers in immunization services delivery; creation of a broad network of volunteer programmes as participants in the effort to identify children in need of immunization and deliver services to those children; involvement of business, industry and organized labour as full partners in the immunization effort; establishment of a special focus on individuals and organizations with access to urban inner-city areas and pockets of rural poverty; and full participation by state health and education authorities in the effort with special emphasis on enactment and enforcement of school entry laws requiring immunization for all school children.

To implement the stated objectives, a special unit was established by the Secretary of Health and Human Services (then Health, Education, and Welfare) under the leadership of the US Public Health Service's Centers for Disease Control and directives were issued by the Secretary to all relevant departmental units to offer full co-operation with the effort. Special immunization liaisons were identified in the service delivery

programmes which had special access to children, such as, the federally operated community health centres around the country, the Head Start/Day Care facilities operated through the national Office of Human Development Services, the education units involved in the establishment of school policies and especially school health policies, the health care financing efforts which paid for services offered to low-income children. Liaisons were also established with other federal agencies important to implementing the effort such as the Department of Defense which had a large dependant population (not to mention the recruit population) in need of immunization services, the Community Services Administration with community programmes oriented towards youth, the Department of Agriculture which operated a large network of agricultural extension agents at the local level who could be employed in raising the awareness of the needs for immunization activities. Liaisons were also established with the voluntary organizations such as the Parent Teachers Association, the National League for Nursing, and a host of other voluntary organizations with resources to be used at the local level.

For those agencies within the Department of Health and Human Services which had direct access and responsibility for a client population (that is the community health centres, the Indian Health Service, the Head Start programmes, the Medicaid programme) specific targets were set for immunization doses delivered, share of the population immunized, and implementation of surveillance activities. Both quarterly and annual targets were established, and quarterly review sessions were held, chaired by the Secretary, to review progress of each of the agencies in meeting their targets. Where short-falls were noted, full explanations were required; where new opportunities existed, strategies were developed to take advantage of those opportunities.

By the fall of 1979, the goal was largely attained for children entering school, with immunization rates of 94 per cent for measles, 93 per cent for rubella, 93 per cent for DPT (diph-theria, pertussis, and tetanus), 93 per cent for poliomyelitis, and 86 per cent for mumps. More importantly, in 1980 the number of cases of measles, mumps, rubella, tetanus, and diphtheria was at an all-time low (Fig. 25.4). Indeed, the nation has now achieved a level of control sufficient to warrant the expectation that measles can be eliminated as an indigenous problem in the US within a short time. This success is attributable to a programme that sought to achieve a speci-fied set of objectives in a very structured way.

### Control of environmental lead levels

Whereas the previous two examples recount efforts which were for the most part administratively derived, the efforts which have been undertaken in the US to control the toxic effects of lead exposure have an additional dimension – prominent involvement of the legislature. None the less, the experience is also instructive for its success in establishing quantified targets as a means of focusing national energies towards specific endpoints.

Lead has no known useful function in the body and exerts adverse effects in both adults and children. Young children are much more susceptible to the effects of lead exposure than adults because of the increased vulnerability of the developing brain and increased intestinal absorption of lead. Lead pri-marily affects three systems in man: the nervous system, the kidney, and red blood cell synthesis (Leah 1976). Lead is a metallic element that occurs naturally in extremely small concentrations but is highly toxic in a slow-acting manner. Lead poisoning can result from exposure to either inorganic or organic lead compounds taken into the body by ingestion, inhalation, or absorption through the skin. Some of the major sources include exposure to organic forms of lead such as tetraethyl and tetramethyl lead which are used in 'antiknock' ingredients in petrol, and inorganic lead compounds used as pigments in corrosion-resistant paints.

Though instances of lead poisoning have been recorded for centuries, even millenia, with the advent of the industrial age lead and its compounds have found many applications in industrial processes. Along with those applications, incidences have increased in which people have had harmful health effects as a result of exposure to lead poisoning. As a result of expanded awareness of these illnesses, concern about the problem has grown. Consequently, the federal government has taken a number of actions during the past several years to limit the exposure of Americans to lead residues. These actions have included limits on the allowable lead content in low-dose sources such as water, ambient air, and processed food in addition to the high-dose exposure sources of paint and petrol.

Several statutes are relevant. Each has the goal of reducing exposure of the US population to lead and lead compounds, and requires the responsible agencies to establish quantifiable objectives to that end. In 1971 the lead based paint Poisoning Prevention Act (P.L. 91-695) and subsequent amendments in 1973 and 1976 gave the US Department of Housing and Urban Development a broad mandate to conduct research and demonstrations related to lead paint hazards. Specifically, the Secretary of the Department was instructed to develop and carry out research to determine the nature and extent of the problem of lead-based poisoning in the US, particularly in urban areas, and the method by which lead-based paint can most effectively be removed from interior and exterior surfaces. The original and subsequent amendments further instructed the Department of Health, Education, and Welfare to fund local programmes for lead paint poisoning control, which have been carried out through the US Public Health Service's Centers for Disease Control.

In 1971, the Food and Drug Administration issued a standard that lead based paints could contain no more than 0.5 per cent of lead by weight. In 1973, the newly created Consumer Product Safety Commission was instructed in P.L. 93-151 to conduct appropriate research in lead-based paint in order to ascertain the safe level of lead in residential paint products. Although the study caused the Commission to uphold the standard of 0.5 per cent of lead by weight as a safe level, the results were disputed by Congress which considered the imposition of legislation requiring much more stringent standards. Ultimately, regulations were adopted by the Consumer Product Safety Commission which lowered the lead standard for paint to 0.06 per cent by weight.

In the Clean Air Act of 1970, as amended, Congress also initiated vigorous action with respect to ambient air standards for lead emissions. It required the Environmental Protection Agency (EPA) to set standards for any pollutant that might endanger the public's health and welfare. As a result, EPA has promulgated regulations specifying a schedule for reducing the lead content of petrol. Two sets of regulations were issued, one requiring the sale of 'unleaded' petrol (less than 0.05 g/gal) and another reducing the content of leaded grades of petrol. The schedule initially established by the EPA was subsequently altered as a result of a combination of factors including court decisions, administration deregulatory emphases, and the prospect of petrol shortages. Even though the schedule for phasing down the level of lead content was delayed, the overall lead content has dropped substantially and accordingly the public's exposure has diminished. During the 1976 to 1980 period the amount of lead used in gasoline production fell from 53 000 to 24 000 tons per quarter year (DHHS 1983a).

Meanwhile, the results on exposure to the general public of all these factors has been substantial. Figure 25.5 shows the drop which has occurred in the average blood lead levels in the US population ages six months to 74 years. The results of the US National Health and Nutrition Examination Survey (NHANES) between 1976 and 1980 indicates that there has been a decrease over these years of the mean blood lead level

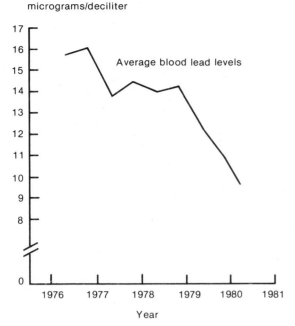

micrograms/deciliter

Average blood lead levels

Year

**Fig. 25.5.** Mean blood levels of population six months–74 years: United States, February 1976–February 1980. Source: DHHS (1982).

from 15.8 micrograms per decilitre to 10.0 micrograms per decilitre. This represents a 37 per cent reduction in these blood lead levels (DHHS 1982). One estimate suggests that during the period of 1976 to 1980 an estimated 46 per cent of the blood lead of the average American was due to petrol lead emissions, indicating the importance of controlling emission in the past and prospective gains (ICF Incorporated 1982).

In addition, since the inception of a childhood lead-based paint poisoning prevention programme in 1973, nearly four million children have been screened and 6.1 per cent were found with lead toxicity. For 1981–82, approximately 500 000 children were screened and only 4.1 per cent had lead toxicity, the lowest figure ever (CDC 1982).

In spite of the substantial gains which have been achieved there are still formidable problems for certain population groups. Specifically, black children have higher blood lead levels than older blacks or whites as a result of exposure to the same levels of petrol lead emissions. The NHANES II showed that 18.6 per cent of black children living in inner-cities or urban areas of one million or more population had unacceptably high blood lead levels. Comparable figures for other groups include: white inner-city children, 4.5 per cent; children from smaller urban areas (that is less than one million population) 3.5 per cent; and children from rural areas 2.1 per cent (NCHS 1981). The challenges for more rigorous implementation of these objectives are apparent.

### Non-quantified targeting

The fact that these three examples manifest impressive success in the use of quantified targets to achieve health gains does not imply that targeting which does not include the *a priori*

establishment of measurable objectives – non-quantified targeting – is unimportant. Indeed, quite the contrary is true. Many more broadly and less specifically quantified efforts have been successful in the past. The national reduction in infant mortality has already been noted. High blood pressure control and smoking cessation are also good illustrations of the success of programmes with a broad focus.

In 1972, the National High Blood Pressure Education Program (NHBPEP), co-ordinated by the National Heart, Lung, and Blood Institute (NHLBI) at the National Institutes of Health, was begun as a government and private sector partnership to reduce cardiovascular deaths by detecting and controlling high blood pressure. The NHBPEP is a coalition of about 15 federal agencies, 150 major national organizations, 50 state health departments, 2000 organized community control programmes, and a variety of other facilitating groups. The federal role in the process is that of a catalyst – helping in the design of intervention methods, identifying target groups, and stimulating the activities of a number of resourceful participants around the country. As Table 25.12 shows, the results of the NHBPEP have been dramatic. Between 1971–72 and 1974–75, the share of people with diastolic blood pressure greater than or equal to 105 mm Hg, but whose hypertension was never diagnosed, declined 30 per cent for the population as a whole. The decline was greater for blacks (43.8 per cent) than for whites (17.2 per cent).

**Table 25.12.** *High blood pressure control*

| Group | Per cent with diastolic blood pressure 105 mm Hg or more but never diagnosed | | |
| | 1971–72 | 1974–75 | Per cent change |
| --- | --- | --- | --- |
| Total population | 45.6 | 31.9 | −30.0 |
| Whites | 48.8 | 35.0 | −17.2 |
| Blacks | 40.4 | 22.7 | −43.8 |

Source: National Health and Nutrition Examination Survey I, 1971–75, National Center for Health Statistics.

Surveys also indicate that public knowledge about high blood pressure has substantially improved over the last eight years, that first visits to physicians for hypertensive disease (not including referrals) increased by 45 per cent between 1971 and 1976, and as noted earlier, that stroke deaths have declined markedly (NHLBI 1978).

National efforts aimed at reducing cigarette smoking have also had notable successes. Reports about the health hazards of cigarette smoking began making their way into the public press in the early 1950s. In response to these reports, there were occasional transient downturns in smoking behaviour. But it was in 1964, with the publication of *Smoking and health*, the report of the Advisory Committee to the Surgeon General, and the intitiation of a vigorous anti-smoking programme, that the increase in per caput cigarette consumption began to be checked over a sustained period (DHEW 1964). A recent regression analysis of cigarette demand has suggested that in the absence of an anti-smoking campaign, consumption of cigarettes in 1980 would have been about 41.5 per cent greater than that which actually occurred (Fig. 25.6). Per caput consumption of cigarettes has fallen

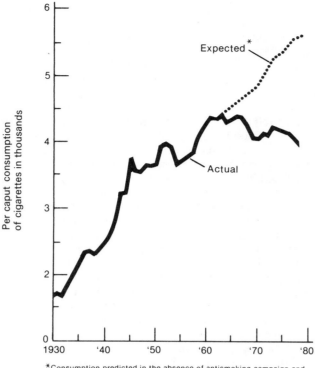

*Consumption predicted in the absence of antismoking campaign and with assumed price constancy.

**Fig. 25.6.** Trends in cigarette consumption. *Consumption predicted in the absence of antismoking campaign and with assumed price constancy. Adapted from Warner, 1981 (p. 730) – copyrighted 1981 by the American Association for the Advancement of Science.

approximately 1 per cent per year since 1973 (Warner 1981). The proportion of all males who smoked in 1979 was about 37 per cent versus 53 per cent in 1964; in females, the proportion was about 28 per cent compared with 42 per cent in 1964 (DHHS 1980*b*). Even for teenagers, among whom the problem has been the greatest recently, current trends are encouraging. Though there was an increase in smoking by teenagers from about 12 per cent in 1968 to 16 per cent in 1974, the proportion of persons between the ages of 12 and 18 years who smoked regularly had dropped again by 1979 to below 12 per cent (Green 1979).

With the stimulus provided by the 1964 report, a broad range of contributors have pooled their scientific, legal, and marketing talent to establish programmes successfully targeted to specific populations. The impressive results obtained reflect an effective partnership between public programmes and private efforts such as those of the American Cancer Society, American Lung Association, and American Heart Association.

Yet even these general national efforts to reduce smoking and high blood pressure encompass important elements of targeting and monitoring. Each has fostered directed efforts to identify and reach vulnerable population groups, to enroll a wide variety of service agencies, and to stimulate the monitoring of programmes not only at the national, but also at the local level. The local focus of activities has in fact been a prominent feature of the work.

## CAVEATS AND CONCLUSIONS

The prospects for wider application of these models to a broad set of health problems – that is, the prospects for achieving the targets set forth in *Promoting health/preventing disease: objectives for the nation* – are as disparate as the objectives themselves. In spite of the merit and utility of the management by objectives approach, there are certainly constraints.

The targets with the best prospects are probably those that depend more on technical interventions and less on behavioural change, those that offer the potential for greater economic returns or at least fewer economic losses to industry or society, and those that appear to be most socially neutral. Accordingly, a few important caveats must be considered.

First, the amount of support that can be drawn from the science base for use in the formulation of objectives varies considerably in the five categories. For example, among the health status objectives, a specific objective for reduction of caries can feasibly be established based on the anticipated provision of fluoridated water supplies, because the protective nature of fluoride against dental caries is well defined. On the other hand, understanding of the relationship between a number of toxic agents and various disease outcomes is still emerging, so that qualitative – not to mention quantitative – estimation of the potential for improved health status is difficult. Among the objectives related to reducing risk factors, setting up a target on exposure to the risks of smoking is much easier than setting up one on exposure to atmospheric sulphates, or even one on the adoption of certain exercise levels (levels that people frequently misreport). Action based on the information available is none the less required.

Second, even when quantified objectives are established, state and local interest in, and the capacity for, such evaluative efforts vary substantially. Yet, since the purpose of setting objectives is to encourage programme evaluation and adaptation of the objectives at the local level, progress depends on that interest and those efforts. This link between federal and state and local efforts is particularly needed as the distribution of federal funds emphasizes the mechanism of block grants, which provide for greater state and local discretion in setting priorities and allocating resources.

Third, progress depends upon the continued development of data systems. Yet at this time data collection is especially vulnerable because of financial constraints. Although data-gathering capabilities in the US surpass those of many other countries, some prominent geographical and substantive deficiences still exist in these data sets. Possibly, the most limiting is the paucity of data available at the state and local levels. Beyond these geographical constraints are the limits in information relation to certain categories of objectives, especially those related to improving public and professional awareness of the various prevention areas. An apparent lack of interest in assessing such awareness suggests that people are assumed to be passive participants in the protection of their own health – an attitude that presents a compelling programme challenge. The gains that will be most difficult to achieve will be in health promotion and behaviour enhancement; facilitation of the gains made in those areas will depend upon adequate data to track progress.

Fourth, though much of the progress of the future will depend upon how effectively people can be motivated, understanding of both the potential and the constraints of the behavioural and communications sciences remains limited. Although considerable numbers of people apparently have been improving their life-styles as better information has become available about the links of life-style to ill health, there is still scant evidence to offer tested ways of accelerating societal response to this information.

Fifth, if this goal-oriented approach is to succeed, a social will must exist to support its various components. Though uniform agreement is not required on the priorities to be assigned to activities, some commitment is needed to the process of establishing targets, measuring progress, and realigning activities. This commitment requires not only consensus, but a considerable amount of will at a variety of levels.

Caveats notwithstanding, the establishment of measurable health objectives holds promise for enhancing health gains. One of the more significant features of this process is the extent to which the effort reflects progress in the development of consensus about our health goals and about some of the means for attaining them. The broad and elaborate review that was undertaken in the course of drafting and revising the health objectives for the US nation has ensured a thorough discussion of the issues. Consensus, however, does not denote unanimity. Diversity and compromise are prominent components of consensus development, and the product that emerges is inevitably more conservative than many participants would have urged. But the degree of consensus about appropriate directions for prevention is considerable, given the scope of the objectives and the number of participants in the process.

Setting objectives is in effect only a starting point. This process reveals the need also for a commitment, which must be met by realigning activities and resources – tasks that can be onerous, particularly for those at the state and local level. Although difficult, a deliberate review of priorities and the targeting of activities can improve the allocation of resources – chores that are even more critical during times of fiscal constraint. If targeting progress in health helps set the sights more specifically, a nation should be better able to register its successes and detect its failures – and perhaps even, in time, correct its course. The potential for gain seems well worth the effort.

## REFERENCES

Centers for Disease Control (1982). Surveillance of childhood lead poisoning – United States, *Morbidity Mortality Weekly Rep.* **31**, 118.

Department of Health and Human Services (1980a). *Promoting health/preventing disease—objectives for the nation.* DHEW (PHS) Publication No. 79-55071. US Government Printing Office, Washington, DC.

Department of Health and Human Services (1980b). *The health consequences of smoking for women: a report of the Surgeon General.* Office on Smoking and Health, Public Health Service, Rockville, Md.

Department of Health and Human Services (1982). *Blood lead levels for persons 6 months–74 years of age—United States 1976–80, NCHS Advance Data* **79**, 2.

Department of Health and Human Services (1983a). Drop in blood lead levels found in US population. *Public Health Reports* **98**, 524.

Department of Health and Human Services (1983b). Public Health Service implementation plans for attaining the objectives for the nation. *Public Health Reports,* **September–October** Suppl.

Department of Health, Education, and Welfare (1964). *Smoking and health. Report of the Advisory Committee to the Surgeon General.* PHS Publication No. 1103. Centers for Disease Control, Public Health Service, US Government Printing Office, Washington, DC.

Department of Health, Education, and Welfare (1977). *Baselines for setting health goals and standards,* DHEW Publication No. (HRA) 77-640. US Government Printing Office, Washington, DC.

Department of Health, Education, and Welfare (1979). *Healthy people—the Surgeon General's report on health promotion and disease prevention.* DHEW Publication No. (PHS) 79-55071, US Government Printing Office, Washington, DC.

Drucker, P.F. (1954). *The practice of management.* Harper and Row, New York.

Drucker, P.F. (1981). *Toward the next economics and other essays.* Harper and Row, New York.

Green, D.E. (1979). *Tennage smoking: immediate and long-term patterns.* National Institute of Education, Department of Health, Education, and Welfare, Washington, DC.

Green, L.W., Wilson, R.W., and Bauers, K.G. Data requirements to measure progress on the objectives for the nation in health promotion and disease prevention. *Am. J. Public Health.* [In press.]

Henderson, D.A. (1976). The eradication of smallpox. *Sci. Am.* **235**, 28.

ICF Incorporated (1982). *The relationship between gasoline lead emissions and lead poisoning in Americans.* ICF Incorporated, Contract No. 68-01-5845. Washington, DC.

Leah, T.D. (1976). *The production, use and distribution of lead in Canada.* Environmental Contaminents Inventory Study No. 3, Report Series No. 41. Cat. No. En 36-508/41. Environmental Canada, Ottawa.

McGinnis, J.M. (1982). Recent health gains for adults. *N. Engl. J. Med.* **306**, 671.

McGinnis, J.M. (1983). Tracking the national prevention objectives. In *Proceedings of the Annual Meeting on Health Statistics,* National Center for Health Statistics. US Government Printing Office, Washington, DC.

McKeown, T. (1976). *The role of medicine.* Nuffield Provincial Hospitals Trust, London.

National Center for Health Statistics (1981). *Plan and operation of the second national health and nutrition examination survey, 1970–1980. Vital Health Statistics.* (PHS pub. No. 81-1317. series 1, no. 15). US Government Printing Office, Washington, DC.

National Heart, Lung, and Blood Institute (1978). *Progress report on high blood pressure control in the United States.* National Institutes of Health, Bethesda, Md.

Odiorne, G.S. (1972). *Management by objectives.* Pitman, New York.

Warner, K.E. (1981). Cigarette smoking in the 1970s: the impact of the anti-smoking campaign on consumption. *Science* **211**, 729.

Williams, G. (1976). Schools of public health – their doing and undoing. *Milbank Mem. Fund. Q.* **S4**, 493.

World Health Organization (1972). *WHO Expert Committee on Smallpox Eradication—Second report. WHO Technical Report Series,* No. 493, Geneva.

# 26 Initiating and supporting public health research – United Kingdom

M. Ashley-Miller and Andrew Watt Kay

## INTRODUCTION

Following legislation separate autonomous National Health Services were established in 1948, in England and Wales, Northern Ireland, and Scotland (HMSO 1978). And yet it is only in the past 15 years or so that research into the UK health services has developed significantly. This late development of health service research probably stemmed from the belief of many of the founders of the National Health Service (NHS) that expenditure on health services would diminish because the introduction of free and universally available services would improve the health of the population and therefore over time lead to a diminution in demand. However, this was not borne out in practice. Since 1948 there has been a steady rise in the demand for services and in the expectations of consumers, and a considerable growth in the number of health service staff and in the deployment of medical technology. This increasing cost and complexity of health care provision has been further exacerbated by the maintenance of the concept of 'clinical freedom' and the desirability of establishing equality both in provision and in access. These factors, combined with the realization that a major investment in personal health services has substantial limitations in improving the health and well-being of people, have focused attention on the need for the development of health services research aimed at evaluating the effectiveness of services (both existing and new), in increasing the efficient use of existing resources, and containing costs whilst continuing to attempt to develop and improve the Service. In this respect Maxwell (1981) distinguished between the largely successful efforts of western governments in recent years to control total public-sector health expenditure and what he called 'tomorrow's problem' of getting value for money in health services. The need for research was emphatically endorsed by the Royal Commission on the National Health Service in their Report (1979): 'Research is vital to improve standards of patient care. It increases knowledge and fosters a critical attitude to existing patterns of care and treatment.'

In the UK, prime responsibility for funding and developing health services research has rested with the central government Health Departments, although significant and valuable contributions have been made by the Research Councils, certain Foundations, and voluntary agencies. In 1973, following publication of a Government Report entitled *Framework for Government Research and Development* (Civil Service Department 1972), the rather disparate activities undertaken in this field by the Health Departments in Scotland and in England and Wales became co-ordinated and formalized by the establishment of Chief Scientist Organisations (CSO) under the leadership of Chief Scientists. This chapter is based on the experiences of the CSO of the Scottish Home and Health Department gained since 1973. The relative smallness of the Organisation and the authors' direct involvement with its development during the initial nine years of its existence has provided the opportunity to review and assess the problems facing a central government Health Department in organizing and supporting research relevant to its needs and those of the NHS.

## THE ORGANIZATION AND DEVELOPMENT OF A RESEARCH AGENCY WITHIN A GOVERNMENT DEPARTMENT

At the outset, it is important to distinguish between two functions of a research funding agency. The first is a mainly *passive* function, namely, receiving, assessing, and supporting unsolicited applications for research funds. Provided that the agency has a clear remit as to the type of research and development that it is willing to support, then this function can be met by a sound and relatively small administrative structure and the scientific assessment forum: the former to handle applications and control its financial position, and the latter to advise on the relative quality of the applications received, so that these may be ranked against the funds available for disbursement. The progress of supported research is monitored on the basis of interim progress reports from researchers and these are also assessed by the scientific advisers.

However, this *passive* function alone is usually inadequate if a new research field is to be developed rapidly in order to study urgent problems. A fully developed and effective research agency must, therefore, exercise a second and *active* role which entails a positive approach to the definition of problems and the development of research policies and strategies within its field of interest. This involves determining research and development capable of making a contribution to the solution of defined problems, seeking out and fostering researchers capable and willing to undertake such research and development, the placing of contracts, the monitoring of progress of such commissioned research and, in the case of health services research, persuading and encouraging those responsible for running the Service to implement useful research findings. For example, one of the major difficulties encountered in the support and development of health service research has been the relative scarcity of experienced research workers, and in particular, research teams. A significant proportion of the Scottish CSO's resources have therefore been positively devoted to developing a number of Health Service Research Units where expertise could be built up and researchers trained for the future. It is in respect of this *active* function that particular skills are required.

An *active* research agency is an organization comprising interdependent secretarial, clerical, administrative, and professional staff. The head of the agency is usually professionally qualified and, although not personally involved in day-to-day research work, it is of prime importance that he or she should have management skills to co-ordinate the scientific role of the agency with the administrative, financial and personnel roles. This role of *controller* is distinct and separate from that of the Chief Scientist which is described later.

For the scientific aspects of their work research managers within the agency – usually in practice, the professional staff – need to be able to assimilate rapidly and assess information from a number of sources so that they can arrive at a critical understanding of a particular topic and appreciate its significance, importance, and the relevance of research to its furtherance. They also need empathy to enable them to work closely with colleagues – who may be from different disciplines – and to communicate with research workers, administrators, and practitioners within particular fields. In their information collection and handling role, research managers need extensive knowledge about experts in certain scientific fields and a range of personal contacts from whom views can be sought informally, and if necessary, in confidence. Finally, they must have the skills to prepare for and conduct the committee/working party meetings upon which an *active* agency is so dependent for advice both in assessing applications and in developing research policies. It will be appreciated from the foregoing that an active research agency requires whole-time research managers of skill and experience who must be offered a career structure.

The overall remit given to the CSO in Scotland was to identify, encourage, promote, and support research and development relevant to the improvement of the NHS in Scotland. The Organisation, led by and supporting the Chief Scientist, comprises an executive Office and a standing advisory machinery. The Office or agency is responsible for the award of grants and for financial control. It is headed by a Director (Controller) and comprises professional (medical, scientific, and nursing), administrative, and secretarial staff. The standing advisory machinery consists of an overall research policy committee chaired by the Chief Scientist which co-ordinates the advice of specialist research committees, assesses the relative research priorities, advises on broad financial allocations, and ensures that an appropriate balance is maintained within the overall research portfolio. The number of supporting specialist committees reflects the broad span of research and development relevant to the NHS. These are concerned with: health services research; applied biomedical research; computer research related to medicine; research into prosthetics and orthotics; and equipment research. As required, *ad hoc* expert and working groups have been established to undertake particular tasks and reviews of problems and research needs; these are always disbanded on completion of their work.

Membership of the advisory committees and expert groups has four components: research management (the Chief Scientist and the Office), academic disciplines concerned directly and indirectly with the health service, senior administrators from the Health Department and the Health Authorities, and health service practitioners. Through bringing together the different interests in this way, the academic scientists, all of whom engage in research, have become more aware of the problems and needs of the Health Service and are thus encouraged to orientate their research efforts to finding solutions to its problems and needs. Equally, the administrators have derived benefit from the illumination of their problems in discussion, and have become more aware of the difficulties of undertaking research in some areas and the contribution – and the limitations of this contribution – which properly directed research can make towards improving the Service.

The specialist committees are responsible for acting as peer groups in considering spontaneous applications for research support – the *passive* research agency role. But in pursuance of the *active* role they have increasingly, particularly in the case of the Health Services Research Committee, been seeking to develop research policies and programmes to meet Departmental needs, reviewing problems in the light of the information available to them on planning policies, defining research requirements, and arranging for relevant research to be undertaken. The latter functions are normally exercised through specialist sub-committees or working groups appointed *ad hoc* to consider a problem area identified by the main Committee.

The Chief Scientist of the Health Department in Scotland holds a part-time appointment, the holder being also an active and distinguished academic research worker. The role has developed over the years and can now be seen to have three main components. The first is as a scientific leader and adviser to the agency, dealing with specific research issues and advising and deciding upon the handling of research policy developments: for example in the final determination of areas to be reviewed and the manner of review, and the establishment of research units. The second component is the selection of members and overseeing the proper functioning of the main research policy committee, of the specialist advisory committees, and of working groups; and leading the assessment teams which visit research units and major research programmes to review progress. The influence of the Chief Scientist is of vital importance in obtaining both the ready assistance of the scientific community as advisers to the agency and also the trust of fellow researchers that the assessment of their work and their research applications will be dealt with in a careful, considered, and fair manner. Thirdly, the Chief Scientist is involved at the top level of the Department in general policy considerations and discussions concerning the NHS. The importance of this latter role was emphasized by the House of Lords Select Committee on Science and Technology (1981) which stated in their report: 'the starting point for good policy related science is not in fact science but the policy problems it attacks. . . . The Chief Scientist must not only advise on gaps in knowledge but also develop research programmes from an understanding and involvement in policy making.' This is no less true for research managers who, at their level, must also have close contact with administrators in the Department and the Service.

## POLICIES AND PRIORITIES FOR THE SERVICE: PROBLEMS FOR RESEARCH

The NHS is a very complex organization in terms of its management, the relations between the various tiers of administration, its very large and multidisciplinary workforce and its inter-relationship with other agencies such as local authorities. Not surprisingly, there are many areas of the Service where it has not been thought necessary to have specific policy guidance, and others where the policies that do exist have evolved either symbiotically, through discussions and jointly agreed actions between central Departments and health authorities, or simply in a reactive form to developments in the Service. Indeed, it was not until 1976 that the first comprehensive general policy document for the NHS in Scotland entitled *The Way Ahead* (Scottish Home and Health Department 1976) was published and in the following year the comparable document *The Way Forward* for England and Wales (DHSS 1977). Successor documents entitled *Scottish Health Authorities Priorities for the 80s* (Scottish Home and Health Department 1980) and *Care in Action* (DHSS 1981) followed four years later. It is probably fair to say that the desire of successive Governments to ensure that the NHS should operate in a highly delegated way, and the concentration in the early years on measures to remedy perceived deficiencies and inequalities in provision, combined to delay the introduction of broadly-based forward planning for the NHS. As late as 1979, the Royal Commission on the National Health Service (1979) commented upon the absence of objective criteria for setting health priorities and the need to consider the influence upon and relations between health and other services. Illsley (1980) also criticized the processes by which health policy is formulated.

These complexities pose formidable problems both for the determination and the undertaking of health services research, and make it essential that senior administrators with responsibility for developing and implementing Departmental policies for the Service be directly involved in decisions about the need for research in particular areas and whether the outcome of that research can be implemented. Indeed, the key criterion for consideration in developing research into the health services must be whether or not there are immutable barriers to the implementation of findings posed by organizational factors. Scarce resources should not be deployed for research into areas where change cannot be effected however

apparently desirable such research may be. It is for this reason that major health-service research agencies should be sited within central government Departments with policy responsibilities for the Service and where such advice is available. However, this involvement of senior administrators may pose further difficulties for the agency if by the nature of their background and training they lack sympathy towards research and an understanding of its potential contribution to the solution of problems. This widespread lack of scientific and technological understanding amongst the Civil Service was criticized by the House of Lords Select Committee on Science and Technology (1981).

As mentioned, much of practice and policy in the NHS has developed in an *ad hoc* reactive manner as a result of new discoveries, new practices, or the efforts of pressure groups. A number of developments were not adequately researched nor evaluated due to their late recognition and the failure to mount effective research that could at least have provided information to assist in decision making, even if it could not have provided definitive answers in the time-scale allowed. From the standpoint of the Health Departments therefore, it is vital for the future that discoveries and developments likely to have significant import for the Service are recognized at a very early stage, and that appropriate research is mounted in order to provide information on which the best possible decisions can be taken within a realistic time-scale. In this respect it is encouraging that carefully planned research into the benefits and problems associated with screening, such as that for breast cancer and for the detection of spina bifida and anencephaly, has been put in train before generalized screening for these conditions is adopted as standard practice within the NHS. The recent adoption of national screening for hypothyroidism followed a similar detailed appraisal of effectiveness, organization, and costs. The research agency and its research managers have an important role to play in assisting administrators by appraising them of developments of which they become aware, drawing their attention to the significance of those coming to the notice of the agency, and discussing and, if necessary and possible, organizing research to assist in their evaluation.

The Royal Commission (1979) recognized 'that health service research is a complex process in which continuity is essential, embracing many disciplines including epidemiology, statistics, sociology, psychology and economics. The activities range over wide and disparate topics such as demand for health care, needs of client groups, organization of services and their cost effectiveness, the ordering of priorities, manpower and industrial relations and the efficient and effective use of resources.' Similarly, Opit and Holland (1983) consider health service research to be concerned with examining some or all of the following factors; quality, distribution, access to, outcome or effectiveness of health care services provided by professional health care providers or by some alternative mechanism such as self-care or public health measures.

It is the relative newness of the discipline, the huge range of the field, the lack of trained research workers and established methodologies, together with the requirement for many disciplines to work together, the long-term nature of much of the research, and the difficulty of applying research findings, that distinguish health service research from biomedical and clinical research. Furthermore, by its nature health service research must always have a relevance to Service problems and the potential for application from the outset.

As a relative newcomer to the triad of the health sciences, health service research needs careful fostering and patience; it cannot match the speed of its recognition with achievement. Furthermore, its successful development will depend upon policy direction from sources other than research and the establishment of a career structure for workers. The latter has particular importance for younger researchers working as members of multidisciplinary teams on long-term programmes, since individuals within teams may find it difficult to establish and gain recognition within their parent discipline. Again, in contradistinction to biomedical research where useful findings are published and if confirmed are often rapidly adopted by other workers, a different community in the shape of administrators and lay committees will determine the implementation of health service research findings. This can result in long delays in the recognition of successful research which in turn may have a repressive effect upon the workers concerned, thus affecting their future contribution to the field. Later on we refer to ways in which these difficulties can be diminished

## THE CONTRIBUTION OF HEALTH SERVICE RESEARCH

So far we have attempted to illuminate the difficulties facing health services research – and the agencies concerned with its support and development – in the context of its growth as a relatively new multidisciplinary applied science concerned with one of the most complex of organizations, namely the NHS. Before proceeding to describe and illustrate the ways in which requirements can be ordered and determined and research commissioned, we next attempt to analyse from Scottish experience and achievements to date, the likely orientation and development of health services research in the foreseeable future. In our view, future NHS developments and policies will occur broadly in the following ways:

### Major NHS policy developments

By these we refer to such issues as reorganization of the NHS management structure; the positive development of community care versus hospital care; increased resources and services for certain large client groups, such as the disabled; the provision of major new services by the NHS, for example, family planning services. Major policy decisions of this nature may originate from different sources, but are essentially political decisions; and indeed their fulfilment can only be attained by political wish, decision, and direction. To date, research has had little direct influence or bearing on such developments or decisions and is unlikely to do so in the foreseeable future. But research can contribute significantly to a deeper understanding of the implications, options, and requirements involved in attaining such policies.

### Services and their development

This broad area embraces existing services or practices, and new developments and potential services. It is here that health services research has made and will increasingly play a significant and influential role in assessing the benefits, costs, and organization. The importance of this role has been emphasized by Cochrane (1971). With regard to existing practices and services, attention has focused on the costs and effectiveness of 'demand' services such as ambulance, general practice, pathology, radiology, accident and emergency; or clinical conditions for which there are several treatments of apparently equal benefit but of differing costs, such as those for varicose veins (Chant et al. 1972; Piachaud and Weddell 1972); or where the efficacy of certain treatments has been questioned and there are wide variations in the rates of treatment between different health authorities, as for example tonsillectomy (Mawson et al. 1967). In the case of new developments, the need for such assessments frequently stems from biomedical, technical, or clinical research discoveries which are assumed to be beneficial and desirable providing they are cost-effective. Examples are: the examination of the costs, advantages, and organization for screening procedures, such as those for general multi-phasic screening (South-east London Screening Study Group 1977) and the screening for breast cancer; the assessment of the benefits of specialist care services such as coronary care (Mather et al. 1971) and stroke units (Garraway et al. 1980); and the feasibility of alternative forms of care and treatment such as that for day-care surgery (Ruckley et al. 1978) or domiciliary care for the elderly with acute illnesses (Currie et al. 1980). It is here that particular skills of the research agency are required if proper and useful assessments of significant new developments are to be made before such developments are widely adopted ad hoc on a disparate basis by the NHS. It is much easier to introduce a new service into the NHS than to discontinue it even if subsequent evaluation shows it to be of little value – this is particularly so if major capital investments have been made.

### Short-term immediate problems

The third broad category is concerned with shorter-term circumscribed projects, not necessarily of small cost, to examine specific problems concerned with facets of the whole range of the NHS activities. Examples of this kind of research range from evaluations of new local developments (day hospitals, nursing homes, special clinics), the development and application of techniques and treatments, to the evaluation of new equipment. In some instances, research of this nature is required within a very short time span either to illuminate a problem or to meet concerns of administrators or politicians; or to provide some, albeit far from definitive, information to better assist policy decisions. This type of 'incomplete' research is not particularly attractive either to research workers or research managers, but it can make an important contribution to decisions which have to be taken within a short time-scale.

There will be a continuing and expanding need for this 'project-type' research across the whole range of service activities but this will inevitably be controlled largely by the perceived relative importance and immediacy of the work and the availability of research funding.

The difficulties in 'preventing' the adoption of unevaluated but initially attractive new developments into the NHS are considerable. Even if practitioners, politicians, and administrators are willing to delay on the basis that a careful assessment is being carried out, frequently the time-scale in which research can be completed is unacceptably long and during this time other more formidable and less resistable pressures may develop. Furthermore, it is in this area, perhaps, that the distinction between practitioners wishing to offer individual patients what they believe to be the best and most advanced available services, and administrators wishing to evaluate overall benefits for populations, is most sharply drawn. It is imperative, therefore, that developments with significant potential for the NHS be appreciated, examined, and assessed at the earliest opportunity so that, if necessary, appropriately timed research evaluation can be mounted. At present, this need is perhaps most acute for careful overall evaluations of new costly high technology before demands arise for installation in inappropriate locations. The key here is anticipation of needs and problems so that research may be given sufficient lead time to provide information to assist in effective and carefully considered policy development.

## THE APPROACH OF A GOVERNMENT HEALTH DEPARTMENT TO DEVELOPING POLICIES AND PROGRAMMES FOR HEALTH SERVICE RESEARCH: COMMISSIONING OF RESEARCH

Against the background of the formidable complexity of the NHS, a research agency of a Health Department with responsibility for developing and supporting health service research is posed with its own particular problems in determining approaches and policies within its research budget. First, the agency must attempt to balance short-term work with longer-term research and, as an important corollary, it must attempt to balance between long-term support for specified research programmes and support for research units examining problems on a broader front and within which additional training and educational activities can be undertaken. Secondly, the agency must balance resources devoted to its own commissioned work whilst retaining the ability to fund unsolicited applications arising spontaneously from researchers and practitioners with original proposals often stemming from local situations and opportunities for collaboration. Thirdly, in 'investing' for the future, the agency must consider the development of certain disciplines and, if necessary, supplement the training opportunities offered to junior workers supported by grants, and within units, by means of research fellowships and studentships (in Scotland, special fellowships in nursing and computing research are offered, together with a medical student vacation training scheme). Finally, the agency must regularly review its existing overall policies and specific research strategies against those for the Service, determine new ones, and assess the balance of its

support between broad fields and areas within these. Account must also be taken of developments and opportunities for research that exist or arise, against new problems and new requirements in the Service. Throughout, contact and liaison must be maintained with other relevant research agencies in order to avoid unnecessary duplication, but also to develop jointly supported ventures if appropriate.

The use of the word 'priority' has been deliberately avoided in the foregoing, since in our experience it is not productive to place research fields and activities in rank order. Whether the problems of the elderly are more important than those of the mentally handicapped can only be a subjective decision. In Scotland, therefore, a designation of Service problems into broad categories of major, intermediate, and minor, was adopted and 'priority' is given to components of all those in the major category. A similar but more sophisticated approach involving the assessment of five components of the burden of diseases upon the Service was described by Black and Pole (1975). It will be appreciated that research cannot always be undertaken in every area, since it will depend upon the availability of skilled workers, methodologies, and opportunities.

Over the years of its existence, the CSO has steadily developed the *active* role as a research agency and has determined and supported major new research initiatives (ranging from the provision of multiple short-term grants, through programme grants, to the establishment of research units) in fields covering family planning (Illsley 1975), alcoholism (Ashley-Miller 1976), dental disease (Ashley-Miller 1977), mental handicap (Chief Scientist Organisation 1979), ischaemic heart disease (Forbes 1979a), breast screening (Forbes 1979b), care of the elderly (Isaacs 1975; Chief Scientist Organisation 1980), health and behavioural change (Chief Scientist Organisation 1981) – less major initiatives were also undertaken in incontinence, rheumatism and arthritis, head injuries, and respiratory diseases (Chief Scientist Organisation 1978). The commissioning of applied health services research is complex and difficult. It takes much time and requires considerable skills and close co-operation between the various parties involved.

In our experience commissioning involves the following steps (though in the actual process these steps are not necessarily discrete ones).

### Identification of problem areas

In Scotland the CSO has used a variety of approaches towards problem identification which include: ideas generated from within the agency itself; preparation and analysis of morbidity, mortality, and health service data by the Information Services Division of the NHS; seeking the views of the Administrative Divisions and Medical Groups in the Health Department on problems within their spheres of responsibility; seeking and receiving views of NHS administrators, members of the health care professions, and of the scientific community; seeking and receiving views from advisory committees; and in more recent times taking account of the views and work of the Scottish Health Service Planning Council and its various committees.

## Problem definition

This is probably the key step in commissioning research and in our experience takes the most time. Without adequate definition of problems, or their components, an effective dialogue with research workers and the careful preparation of research proposals likely to provide relevant results is well nigh impossible. Apart from ensuring that views are sought from an appropriate span of personnel with knowledge and understanding of the problem, appropriate relevant data must be available: these may have to be obtained and collated from various sources or, in some instances, collected especially for the purpose.

## Identification of research likely to contribute towards solution or elucidation of defined problems: assessment of feasibility of determined research

After the problem(s) has been defined, the next stage is the planning of relevant research. Where several lines of research are proposed, it will be necessary to assess their inter-relationship and relevant contribution to the major problem. At this stage, some assessment of resources required for the various approaches defined should be made, so that when considered against the budget available for the commission an indication of priority in terms of relevance and cost can be attached to the research approaches formulated. Consideration of feasibility involves a knowledge of existing techniques and methodologies; and of those workers or groups of workers possessing the necessary capacity and interest for undertaking or developing the identified research needs.

## Discussion with selected research workers

Various approaches can be adopted in relation to 'commissioning'. The simplest is for the research agency to inform the scientific community by various means avilable to it (journals, etc.) that they have identified a problem(s) – and research needs relating to this in general terms – and would be interested in receiving and would give special consideration to specific relevant research proposals. A more specific approach is to invite one or more selected contractors (individual workers or university departments) to submit outline research proposals, relevant to the problem and research needs in so far as the agency has been able to define them, together with an indication of the kind and level of support considered appropriate. These would then be discussed and refined together by the agency, as the customer, and the researchers, as contractor, before a decision is taken on the final commission on the basis of a jointly agreed research strategy and proposal. The most advanced step, normally considered to constitute a 'specific' commission, is when the customer or agency has defined a research proposal in complete detail and invites tenders from a contractor(s) to undertake this specified research in which no variation is allowed from the stated protocol.

To date the majority of important commissions have been negotiated by the CSO using variations of the second approach described above.

## Placing of contract and monitoring of work

Because commissioned research is of special importance and relevance to the Service, careful consideration must be given to the approved research contract and to the monitoring of progress to ensure that the work is prosecuted to maximum effect. In some cases, particularly where new methodologies have to be developed, it is useful to set up an advisory group to assess progress and to proffer advice when required. Again, assessment of progress is important if there is a need to change the direction of the research; and also so that dissemination of results and possible implementation of successful findings into a service context can be anticipated within a realistic time-scale.

In Scotland, various procedures have been adopted for monitoring research supported from Departmental funds, whether or not commissioned. In general, small short-term grants are formally monitored by the relevant specialist committee which advised originally upon the award of the grant on the basis of brief interim progress reports or, because of the care taken in assessment at the time of award, reports may only be required on completion of the project. In the case of special or larger research projects or programmes, monitoring may be undertaken on the basis of progress reports and regular visits to the researcher(s) by appropriately constituted sub-committees. The progress of major programmes and research units is routinely monitored at intervals of two to three years by both the specialist committees and the main research policy committee on the basis of a full progress report from the research director and a detailed report from a visiting sub-committee. The visiting sub-committees are always led by the Chief Scientist and spend a day assessing the Unit on the basis of presentations by staff about the work and detailed discussions about problems, opportunities, and future plans. Like the specialist advisory committees (see p. 403), the visiting sub-committees comprise research managers, health service administrators and practitioners, and research workers so that the programme and its components can be assessed against the twin criteria of scientific merit and Service importance and relevance. In our experience, this difficult procedure has not in fact posed problems in permitting such groups to reach agreed assessments. Adequate time and great care must be devoted to these assessments, for on occasion it may be necessary to reorientate the work or even to close a unit which is failing in its remit, and such a serious action must be above reproach.

Apart from these formal assessments, the research managers maintain a general oversight of all work in progress through direct and continuing contacts with the researchers.

## Dissemination of research results

Because there is a wide variety of journals in which health service research can be published, research findings are not always brought to the attention of relevant NHS personnel. It is necessary, therefore, for the agency to ensure that such personnel are directly informed about the initiation, progress, and findings of research specifically related to their interests and responsibilities.

## Implementation of successful research findings

Implementation of research findings in a health service context is rarely easily or quickly achieved and, unfortunately, very rarely solely on the basis of a report of findings. In our experience it is necessary to ensure that some personnel capable of influencing the adoption of successful findings are involved from the outset in confirming the importance and relevance of the research, and, in its definition and progress so that there is not only interest but a potential commitment to assist with the adoption of the findings in their area of responsibility. In effect this means involving appropriate NHS decision-makers in the entire commissioning process. A successful practical innovation by one health authority is likely to prove a potent stimulus for others to follow suit.

The commissioning process is difficult and complex; it requires considerable effort and skilled advice from information services, Departmental and health service administrators, relevant service and scientific research personnel as well as research management. The time-scale is long – the average time taken from identification of a problem to placing a major contract is two years and research findings may not be available for a further three to four years. Rarely is it possible for the customer to say precisely what he wants; even more rarely for the contractor to be able to meet this requirement fully.

## SUMMARY

Health services research has expanded considerably in the UK during the past 15 years and a number of studies have had considerable influence on the NHS. Continued expansion and further contributions are highly desirable if the Service is to develop in a climate of necessary cost-containment. The difficulties in carrying out this relatively new type of research are, and will remain, formidable, although approaches and methodologies are steadily being developed. The main challenges in the immediate future are for the Health Departments, as the prime research funding agencies, to further develop expertise in research management; to secure long-term funding for major research teams; and to establish a career structure for younger research workers prepared to devote their research careers to the field.

## REFERENCES

Ashley-Miller, M. (1976). The problems of alcohol. *Health Bull.* **34**, 299.

Ashley-Miller, M. (1977). Dental research. *Health Bull.* **35**, 46.

Black, D.A.K. and Pole, J.D. (1975). Priorities in biomedical research: indices of burden. *Br. J. Prev. Soc. Med.* **29**, 222.

Chant, A.D.B., Jones, H.O., and Weddell, J.M. (1972). Varicose veins: a comparison of surgery and injection/compression sclerotherapy. *Lancet* **ii**, 1188.

Chief Scientist Organisation (1978). Respiratory disease: a major service problem. *Health Bull.* **36**, 318.

Chief Scientist Organisation (1979). Mental handicap. *Health Bull.* **37**, 279.

Chief Scientist Organisation (1980). Report of the Working Party on Care of the Elderly. *Health Bull.* **38**, 252.

Chief Scientist Organisation (1981). Health and behavioural change: report of a Working Party. *Health Bull.* **39**, 182.

Civil Service Department (1972). *Framework for government research and development.* Cmnd 5046. HMSO, London.

Cochrane, A.L. (1971). Effectiveness and efficiency: random reflections on health services. (Rock Carling Fellowship.) Oxford University Press for Nuffield Provincial Hospitals Trust, London.

Currie, C.T., Burley, L.E., Doull, C., Ravetz, C., Smith, R.G., and Williamson, J. (1980). A scheme of augmented home care for acutely and sub-acutely ill elderly patients: pilot study. *Age Ageing* **9**, 173.

Department of Health and Social Security (1977). *The way forward: priorities in the health and social services in England.* HMSO, London.

Department of Health and Social Security (1981). *Care in action: a handbook of policies and priorities for the health and personal social services in England.* HMSO, London.

Forbes, W. (1979a). Ischaemic heart disease (IHD) in Scotland. *Health Bull.* **37**, 226.

Forbes, W. (1979b). Screening for breast cancer. *Health Bull.* **37**, 185.

Garraway, W.M., Akhtar, A.J., Prescott, R.J., and Hockey, L. (1980). Management of acute stroke in the elderly. *Br. Med. J.* **280**, 1040.

House of Lords Select Committee on Science and Technology (1981). *Science and government.* HMSO, London.

Illsley, R. (1980). *Professional or public health?: sociology in health and medicine.* (Rock Carling Fellowship.) Nuffield Provincial Hospitals Trust, London.

Isaacs, B. (1975). Working Party on Research into the Health Problems of the Elderly. *Health Bull.* **33**, 266.

Mather, H.G., Pearson, W.G., Reid, K.L.Q. *et al.* (1971). Acute myocardial infarction: home and hospital treatment. *Br. Med. J.* **iii**, 334.

Mawson, S.R., Adlington, P., and Evans, M. (1967). A controlled study evaluation of adeno-tonsillectomy in children. *J. Laryngol.* **81**, 777.

Maxwell, R.J. (1981). *Health and wealth.* Lexington Books for Sandoz Institute for Health and Socio-economic studies, Lexington, Ma.

Opit, L.J. and Holland, W.W. (1983). *Health services research.* Department of Community Medicine, St Thomas's Campus, United Medical Schools of Guy's and St Thomas' Hospitals, London.

Piachaud, D. and Weddell, J.M. (1972). Cost of treating varicose veins. *Lancet* **ii**, 1191.

Royal Commission on the National Health Service (1979). *Report.* Cmnd 7615. HMSO, London.

Ruckley, C.V., Cuthbertson, C., Fenwick, N., Prescott, R.J., and Garraway, W.M. (1978). Day care after operations for hernia or varicose veins: a controlled trial. *Br. J. Surg.* **65**, 456.

Scottish Home and Health Department (1976). *The way ahead: the health service in Scotland.* HMSO, Edinburgh.

Scottish Home and Health Department (1978). *The National Health Service in Scotland 1948–78.* HMSO, Edinburgh.

Scottish Home and Health Department (1980). *Scottish Health Authorities priorities for the eighties.* HMSO, Edinburgh.

South-east London Screening Group (1977). A controlled trial of multiphasic screening in middle age: results of the South-east London Screening Study. *Int. J. Epidemiol.* **6**, 357.

# 27 The initiation and support of public health research in the United States

Jay Moskowitz and David M. Robinson

## INTRODUCTION

How was the work done, when things turned out well? Is there any sort of regular, predictable pattern discernible in highly successful biomedical research, so that it might be codified and duplicated to speed up the process in the problems still to be solved? If so, the pattern remains obscure; all that can be said with certainty is that you need much more time than anyone could have anticipated, plus hard work by some extremely bright and imaginative people. The time span can be shortened, perhaps, but this requires more people, more effort, and a certain element of luck (US Department of Health, Education and Welfare 1976).

Public health research is complex in its subject matter because it deals with the complete biological hierarchy. For example, at the same time that it must relate to the individual patient and to entire populations, it must also examine the smallest separable biological phenomenon or molecular structure of a disease. Planning for public health research, therefore, must be comprehensive in its approach. Both planning and research must span the entire biomedical spectrum from the acquisition of new and basic information, through the validation and testing of existing information, to the application of proven information towards the goal of maintaining, protecting, improving, and promoting the health of a people through an organized community effort involving both the private and public sectors (Fig. 27.1).

Planning for public health and the research itself have been effective: as we enter the decade of the 1980s, the health of the population of the US has never been better. During the twentieth century, life-threatening infections and communicable diseases have been remarkably reduced; no longer are such epidemics the major cause of death (Fig. 27.2). Since 1900, the annual death rate in the US has decreased from 17 per 1000 persons to less than 9 per 1000. In other words, if the mortality from certain diseases prevailed today, as it did at the beginning of the century, almost 400 000 Americans would die from tuberculosis; another 300 000 from gastroenteritis; about 55 000 from poliomyelitis; and 80 000 from diphtheria (US Department of Health, Education and Welfare 1979). Instead, because of fundamental and clinical advances, the toll from all four of these diseases was less than 10 000 lives in 1982. Advances in public health are further illustrated by vital statistics on births and life expectancy. Between 1950 and 1977, the mortality rate for children between the ages of 1 and 14 years fell by a half; in fact, in 1977 a record low of 14 infant

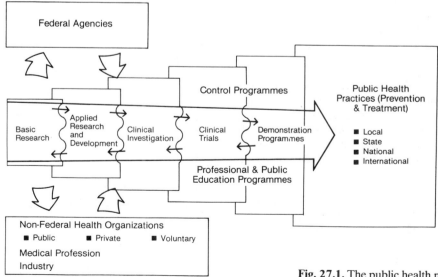

**Fig. 27.1.** The public health research spectrum in the US.

409

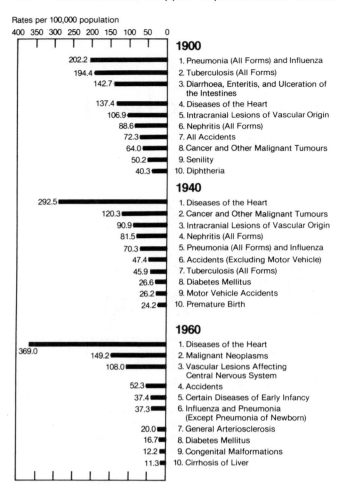

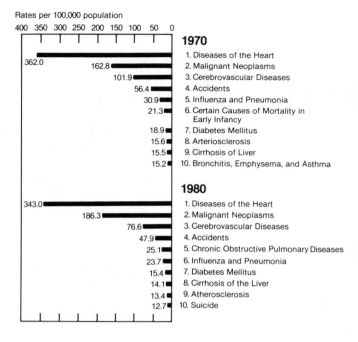

Rates per 100,000 population

400 350 300 250 200 150 100 50 0

**1900**
| | |
|---|---|
| 202.2 | 1. Pneumonia (All Forms) and Influenza |
| 194.4 | 2. Tuberculosis (All Forms) |
| 142.7 | 3. Diarrhoea, Enteritis, and Ulceration of the Intestines |
| 137.4 | 4. Diseases of the Heart |
| 106.9 | 5. Intracranial Lesions of Vascular Origin |
| 88.6 | 6. Nephritis (All Forms) |
| 72.3 | 7. All Accidents |
| 64.0 | 8. Cancer and Other Malignant Tumours |
| 50.2 | 9. Senility |
| 40.3 | 10. Diphtheria |

**1940**
| | |
|---|---|
| 292.5 | 1. Diseases of the Heart |
| 120.3 | 2. Cancer and Other Malignant Tumours |
| 90.9 | 3. Intracranial Lesions of Vascular Origin |
| 81.5 | 4. Nephritis (All Forms) |
| 70.3 | 5. Pneumonia (All Forms) and Influenza |
| 47.4 | 6. Accidents (Excluding Motor Vehicle) |
| 45.9 | 7. Tuberculosis (All Forms) |
| 26.6 | 8. Diabetes Mellitus |
| 26.2 | 9. Motor Vehicle Accidents |
| 24.2 | 10. Premature Birth |

**1960**
| | |
|---|---|
| 369.0 | 1. Diseases of the Heart |
| 149.2 | 2. Malignant Neoplasms |
| 108.0 | 3. Vascular Lesions Affecting Central Nervous System |
| 52.3 | 4. Accidents |
| 37.4 | 5. Certain Diseases of Early Infancy |
| 37.3 | 6. Influenza and Pneumonia (Except Pneumonia of Newborn) |
| 20.0 | 7. General Arteriosclerosis |
| 16.7 | 8. Diabetes Mellitus |
| 12.2 | 9. Congenital Malformations |
| 11.3 | 10. Cirrhosis of Liver |

Rates per 100,000 population

400 350 300 250 200 150 100 50 0

**1970**
| | |
|---|---|
| 362.0 | 1. Diseases of the Heart |
| 162.8 | 2. Malignant Neoplasms |
| 101.9 | 3. Cerebrovascular Diseases |
| 56.4 | 4. Accidents |
| 30.9 | 5. Influenza and Pneumonia |
| 21.3 | 6. Certain Causes of Mortality in Early Infancy |
| 18.9 | 7. Diabetes Mellitus |
| 15.6 | 8. Arteriosclerosis |
| 15.5 | 9. Cirrhosis of Liver |
| 15.2 | 10. Bronchitis, Emphysema, and Asthma |

**1980**
| | |
|---|---|
| 343.0 | 1. Diseases of the Heart |
| 186.3 | 2. Malignant Neoplasms |
| 76.6 | 3. Cerebrovascular Diseases |
| 47.9 | 4. Accidents |
| 25.1 | 5. Chronic Obstructive Pulmonary Diseases |
| 23.7 | 6. Influenza and Pneumonia |
| 15.4 | 7. Diabetes Mellitus |
| 14.1 | 8. Cirrhosis of the Liver |
| 13.4 | 9. Atherosclerosis |
| 12.7 | 10. Suicide |

**Fig. 27.2.** The ten leading causes of death in the US, 1900–80.

deaths per 1000 live births was achieved. A baby born in the US today can be expected to live on average for 73 years whereas a baby born in 1900 could only be expected to live 47 years (US Department of Health, Education and Welfare 1979). During the past decade, the expected life span for Americans has increased by 2.7 years in contrast to the 1960s, when it increased by only one year (Fig. 27.3) (Levy 1978). Much of the credit for these accomplishments must be attributed to disease prevention efforts, for example, immunization, based on knowledge gained through research in the past few decades. But changes in society, especially the increased affluence associated with industrialization, have led to improvements in sanitation and nutrition which, in turn, have helped defeat even such once great killers as tuberculosis and typhoid fever.

Nevertheless, the health picture is not totally bright. Currently, nearly 75 per cent of deaths in the US are caused by degenerative diseases such as heart disease, cancer, and stroke. Of the two million Americans who died of all causes in 1980, one million died of cardiovascular diseases, and more than 400 000 of cancer (US National Heart, Lung, and Blood Institute 1981). However, cardiovascular mortality has

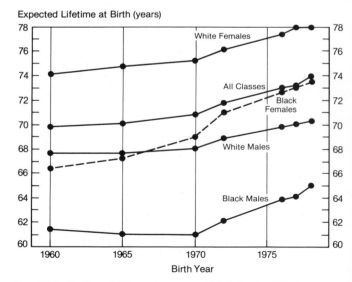

**Fig. 27.3.** Projected life expectancy at birth in the US, by year of birth, 1960–78. (Source: National Center for Health Statistics.)

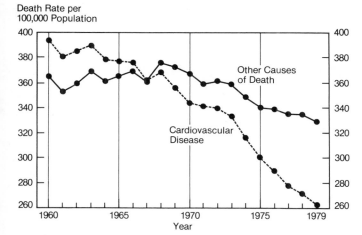

**Fig. 27.4.** Cardiovascular and non-cardiovascular mortality rates in the USA, 1960–79. (Excludes congenital heart disease. Death rate age-adjusted to US population, 1940.)

decreased more than 30 per cent in the last 30 years (Fig. 27.4). Although important insights into the prevention of these conditions have become apparent recently, unfortunately the promise of progress is currently threatened in the US by a rapid increase in health expenditures, particularly in hospital charges. Health expenditures increased by 15 per cent during the fiscal year ending in June 1981, by comparison with the previous year, and amounted to some 9.5 per cent of the gross national product, with only a small percentage of the rise attributable to population growth (US Health Care Financing Administration 1982). This financial threat challenges but may also limit the ability of policy-makers to direct health resources effectively.

The degenerative nature of today's diseases and the costs of treating them will provide a perspective on public health in the 1980s with an unprecedented impact in the US. This perspective was expressed by Joseph Califano Jr, former Secretary of

Health, Education and Welfare, in 1979: 'You, the individual, can do more for your own health and well-being than any doctor, any hospital and drug, any exotic medical device' (US Department of Health, Education and Welfare 1979). Califano was referring to the control an individual has over personal behaviour and habits which can promote health and discourage disease. Millions of Americans are already heeding this advice; for example, more Americans are having their blood pressures checked, cigarette smoking is on the decline, and enthusiasm is growing for exercise, prudent eating habits, and relaxation. However, most Americans still rely on the traditional formula of placing the responsibility for health on the medical system when crises occur (US National Heart, Lung, and Blood Institute 1981; Levy and Moskowitz 1982).

Accompanying such changes in personal habits has come an increased perception of the importance of the applied science of clinical immunology as a cornerstone of successful public health practice. Not only do new, effective vaccines, such as that for hepatitis B, promise eradication of infections, but also the development of monoclonal antibodies from hybridomas and the application of recombinant DNA techniques to the production of 'synthetic' vaccines all predispose the next generation for a new public health revolution. Just what kind of research is most appropriate becomes an increasingly difficult question. To that end, the mechanisms by which the federal and private sectors initiate research leading to improvements in public health are described in this chapter.

## INITIATING AND SUPPORTING PUBLIC HEALTH RESEARCH

### Magnitude of the support of public health research in the US

During the decade of the 1970s, the total support of health research and development in the US rose fourfold to $8.5 billion in 1981 (Fig. 27.5 and Table 27.1). Of this, $300 million came from non-profit organizations such as foundations and

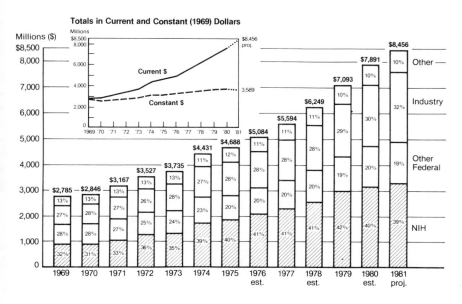

**Fig. 27.5.** National support for health research and development in the US by source, 1969–81. (Constant dollars based on biomedical R and D price index, 1969–80. For 1981, based on percentage increase in estimated GNP implicit price deflator. Projected biomedical R and D price index: 235.6.)

**Table 27.1.** *National support for health research and development by source or performer, 1970–81*
(millions of dollars)

| Sector | 1970 | 1971 | 1972 | 1973 | 1974 | 1975 | 1976 (est.) | 1977 | 1978 (est.) | 1979 | 1980 (est.) | 1981 (est.) |
|---|---|---|---|---|---|---|---|---|---|---|---|---|
| **Total of A or B ($)** | **2846** | **3167** | **3527** | **3735** | **4431** | **4688** | **5084** | **5594** | **6249** | **7093** | **7891** | **8456** |
| **A. By source of funds** | | | | | | | | | | | | |
| Government | 1836 | 2074 | 2375 | 2470 | 3008 | 3118 | 3371 | 3734 | 4197 | 4736 | 5178 | 5414 |
| Federal | 1667 | 1877 | 2147 | 2225 | 2754 | 2832 | 3059 | 3396 | 3811 | 4321 | 4723 | 4932 |
| **NIH** | **873** | **1039** | **1271** | **1323** | **1737** | **1880** | **2060** | **2280** | **2581** | **2953** | **3182** | **3328** |
| State and local | 169 | 197 | 228 | 245 | 254 | 286 | 312 | 338 | 386 | 415 | 455 | 482 |
| Industry | 795 | 860 | 925 | 1033 | 1171 | 1306 | 1446 | 1587 | 1770 | 2055 | 2391 | 2703 |
| Private non-profit | 215 | 233 | 227 | 232 | 252 | 264 | 267 | 273 | 282 | 302 | 322 | 339 |
| Foundations | 69 | 83 | 77 | 75 | 79 | 86 | 76 | 71 | 65 | 63 | 60 | 56 |
| Voluntary health agencies | 61 | 63 | 63 | 70 | 84 | 85 | 94 | 102 | 113 | 131 | 144 | 158 |
| Other | 85 | 87 | 87 | 87 | 89 | 93 | 97 | 100 | 104 | 108 | 118 | 125 |
| **B. By performer** | | | | | | | | | | | | |
| Government | 590 | 676 | 730 | 772 | 826 | 843 | 904 | 1003 | 1163 | 1264 | 1399 | 1468 |
| Federal* | 489 | 568 | 609 | 629 | 668 | 715 | 780 | 867 | 1032 | 1120 | 1233 | 1295 |
| State and local | 101 | 108 | 121 | 143 | 158 | 128 | 124 | 136 | 131 | 144 | 166 | 173 |
| Industry | 826 | 888 | 964 | 1043 | 1207 | 1334 | 1483 | 1546 | 1680 | 1932 | 2251 | 2556 |
| Private non-profit | 1349 | 1499 | 1724 | 1772 | 2203 | 2301 | 2461 | 2769 | 3099 | 3532 | 3809 | 3985 |
| Higher education | 1050 | 1172 | 1365 | 1396 | 1725 | 1808 | 1945 | 2177 | 2459 | 2820 | 3063 | 3208 |
| Other | 299 | 327 | 359 | 376 | 478 | 493 | 516 | 592 | 640 | 712 | 746 | 777 |
| Foreign | 81 | 104 | 109 | 148 | 195 | 210 | 236 | 276 | 307 | 365 | 432 | 477 |

*Includes programme management and direct operations attributable to health research and development in addition to intramural research.

voluntary health agencies, $2.7 billion came from industry, and the balance of $5.5 billion from federal, state, and local governments. Of the government funds, $3.3 billion was disbursed by the National Institutes of Health (by far the largest single source of health research support in the US), with 68 per cent in the form of research project grants to investigators at universities and other non-profit institutions, 15 per cent as contracts to universities and the profit-making industrial sector, and the balance for interagency agreements and intramural research at the NIH (National Institutes of Health 1981).

Unlike industrial research funds, 80 per cent of which were consumed by industry itself on such projects as drug development, more than 50 per cent of federal research funds went to institutions of higher education, largely in the form of support for individual, investigator-initiated research projects, with many for basic biomedical research. In this sense, the federal government is the principal means in the US for sustaining an essential base of biological science at an advanced level to produce fundamental breakthroughs crucial to all fields of medicine, including public health.

### The role of private foundations

Private philanthropy, through foundations, supports about 4.5 per cent or less of the total expenditures for health care in the US (Robert Wood Johnson Foundation 1980). To a large extent, foundations that provide funding in the health care area support demonstration programmes that have research or evaluation objectives which vary according to the interests of individual foundations. These interests range broadly and include, for example, improving access to personal health care for underserved population groups; helping people maintain or regain maximum attainable function in their everyday lives;

assuring the quality of health services; developing projects related to health promotion, disease prevention, and public health; developing improved contraceptive technology; understanding mental health and the psychological and behavioural aspects of health and rehabilitation, developmental processes across the life span, and state of consciousness and of unconscious processes.

Two of the most active foundations in public health are the Robert Wood Johnson Foundation and the Kellogg Foundation, each awarding approximately $50 million a year in grants. Other foundations that have provided grants in the health area are the Rockefeller, John D. and Catherine I. MacArthur, Andrew W. Mellon, and Ford Foundations. The Rockefeller, Mellon, and Ford Foundations have entered into an informal collaborative arrangement for review of proposals in specified areas of research in the reproductive sciences. The three foundations have had longstanding interests in population problems, including the need to develop additional safe and effective contraceptive methods for people, both in the US and overseas. The goal of the collaboration is to accelerate the progress of selected research areas and to assess, as soon as possible, their potential application to the regulation of fertility.

Within the framework of a general philosophy established by their founders, the private foundations nevertheless retain sufficient flexibility to enable them to support work in areas not well covered by federal or industrial funds. For example, since the mid-1950s, the John A. Hartford Foundation has contributed more than $200 million to biomedical research and has helped in the establishment of some of the more innovative medical technologies presently being applied to patient care. Just prior to the 1980s, the Foundation directed part of its resources to the more efficient use and less costly applications of these technologies. In 1979 the Foundation established a new granting programme for research approaches to improve the organization and financing of health care within the US. This programme was based on evidence that many of the problems of cost, quality, and accessibility of health care in America result from methods of reimbursement of physicians and health care institutions.

Changes in the US health care financing system are clearly necessary if the present medical care capabilities are to be maintained. It was clear to the trustees and staff of the Hartford Foundation that better methods to pay for medical care are available, and that such approaches would produce more efficient health care without sacrificing quality. At first the Foundation made awards of $3.5 million to 11 institutions conducting experiments and demonstrations to develop better health care financing systems. Their activities have expanded considerably since that time and support has more than tripled.

Several principles have guided the implementation of the programme. 'First ours is a large and diverse country, and we do not advocate any particular model. Health Maintenance Organizations may be right for Minneapolis or Salt Lake City, while a community-wide hospital budget approach may work best for Rochester. Second, we concentrate on supporting local initiatives, since we are convinced that most answers lie with the innovative practitioners and individuals responsible for running health care institutions – not in the offices of policy analysts or regulators. Third, we try to work with private institutions, to help them handle the problems they face with public and private third-party payers and regulators' (John A. Hartford Foundation 1980). The Hartford Foundation views this work and similar efforts undertaken by others as laying the foundation for a health care system that will ultimately rely more on competitive market forces and will be more responsible to local needs. In this sense the private foundations tend to provide support for work in areas apparently neglected by federal or industrial programmes.

## The role of the universities and academies

### The universities

That the universities provide the principal focus for biomedical research in the US is self-evident. They are also, of course, the source of the highly trained specialists who perform this research. In this sense, scientific investigation goes hand-in-glove with graduate education and postdoctoral training, with the support of manpower development an essential component of the total picture of public health and other biomedical research. The federal agencies provide the greater share of training and career-development awards; however, the same pressures and constraints that are felt on research grant programmes are also found to apply to training programmes. In the case of environmental health problems in particular, public concern has increased consistently during the past decade, with considerable influence on the opportunities available for professional development. This concern is shown by the amount of new legislation passed into law in the 1970s, including the Occupational Health and Safety Act, the Safe Drinking Water Act, the Toxic Substances Control Act and the

Clean Air Act. These actions by the US Congress led to sharp increases in the demand for trained professionals, including scientific staff, for new environmental health research programmes. A survey of 157 such university programmes in the US including such areas as radiation protection, toxicology, epidemiology and occupational health, showed that during the 10-year period from 1967 to 1976, the number of people completing graduate studies as MS, PhD, or postdoctoral students actually doubled (Moeller *et al.* 1979). This study showed that financial support for university-based environmental health research rose during the period, although the sources of support began to change, with the contribution of the US Department of Health, Education and Welfare (DHEW) – now Health and Human Services – remaining constant, whilst the funds provided by industry and other federal agencies increased. Interestingly, although the support for environmental health training rose significantly at first, by 1971 these funds reached a plateau, where they remained until the end of the period in question, in 1976. During this latter phase the support provided by DHEW remained constant, but funds provided by the Environmental Protection Agency decreased by 50 per cent. The only reason that total support of training remained constant was that the universities themselves provided a threefold increase in support of trainees from their own resources.

Although the universities were able to sustain their commitment to established programmes even in the face of declining federal support, this degree of flexibility is becoming increasingly difficult to provide in the 1980s. A problem remains, in that legislation providing mandates for practices requiring increases in professional manpower, in some instances, may not provide for this very increase. However, the Clean Air Act Amendments of 1977, provide specific authority to assure a proper level of appropriate personnel (Moeller *et al.* 1979). Without assurances, such as this, the universities of the 1980s will be unable to meet the changing demands of society for well-trained professionals.

### The National Academy of Sciences and the National Research Council

The National Academy of Sciences (NAS) is a private, non-profit, self-governing corporation, established by Act of Congress in 1863 for 'the furtherance of science and technology'. The NAS is required to advise the federal government, on request, within its areas of competence. The NAS has since established two subsidiary organizations within the framework of its charter, these are the National Academy of Engineering and the Institute of Medicine. In addition, the National Research Council was formed in 1916 to become the principal operating agency of the National Academy of Sciences, the National Academy of Engineering, and the Institute of Medicine.

In the conduct of its operations, the National Research Council uses four assemblies and four commissions, each with its own area of concern (for example, there is an Assembly of Life Sciences and a Commission on Human Resources). In the field of health, the Council of the Institute of Medicine serves as an additional Commission. Assemblies and Commissions are responsible for the content and conduct of their programmes, and for the appointment of the committees that implement these programmes.

Typically, the Academy's process begins, often by request from an agency of the federal government, with the identification of a specific topic for examination in depth by an appointed committee of unbiased experts. The committee prepares a report – a typical example would be *Drinking water and health* – which is reviewed by informed individuals who were not involved in the report's preparation. Subsequently, appropriate adjustments may be made before final publication of the report. The support of the work is often by cost-reimbursable contracts with the US Federal Government. In this way, the Academy and the National Research Council use federal funds to further knowledge in science, including some aspects of public health research, especially when reports identify areas likely to benefit from further study.

### The role of industry

In the private sector, industry invested more than $2 billion in health research and development in 1978 (Table 27.1). Of that, $1.3 billion was invested by the 135 members of the Pharmaceutical Manufacturers Association, which includes some non-drug manufacturers. Another $475 million was invested in health research and development by the more than 2000 firms that produce medical devices and instruments (Banta 1981). Industrial research and development is conducted largely in company-owned research laboratories, although industry also makes arrangements with outside researchers, including those in the universities. However, direct industry support for university-based research is small compared to funds coming from the federal government and non-profit organizations. In 1978, only 2.7 per cent of the total expenditures for basic research came from the industrial sector (Fig. 27.6). Nevertheless, industrial support for research at universities is twice the

amount allocated to basic research from all sources (US National Commission on Research 1980).

Industry has also become involved in public health research from the perspective of the health of their employees, primarily through preventive programmes. Escalating health-care costs have convinced many companies to establish health-maintenance programmes. The objectives of these programmes are not only to increase productivity but also to decrease absenteeism and to help prevent the loss of valuable personnel by death or disability (Kubiak 1980). These comprehensive workplace programmes are mushrooming throughout the country. The Ford Motor Company, Campbell Soup Company, Metropolitan Life Insurance Company, and Kimberly-Clark Corporation have all developed a comprehensive approach to cardiovascular risk reduction and health promotion (US Department of Health and Human Services 1981). An example is the Johnson and Johnson Company's 'Live for Life' programme (Anon. 1981) which is a health promotion effort intended ultimately for all Johnson and Johnson employees world-wide. The objectives of the programme include improvements in health, knowledge, nutrition, fitness, and weight control, smoking cessation, and stress management. It is anticipated that these improvements will lead to positive changes at the worksite including morale, company perception, job satisfaction, productivity, and reduction in absenteeism, accidents, and total health-care costs. The company will carefully evaluate the programme in terms of its impact on employee health and its overall corporate cost-benefit.

### The role of state governments

Traditionally, state governments have not invested substantial resources in public health research, but rather in providing health services. Consistent with this priority, they tend to support applied studies in public health, with a focus on making services more efficient and cost-effective. For example, topics preferred by state governments include the allocation of funds by geographical area and by the requirements of particular population groups, the assessment of needs for health services, evaluations of the feasibility and efficacy of alternative approaches to the delivery of health services, and evaluations of the cost-effectiveness of management procedures and systems. Under the currently proposed federal block grant programme, the states will assume greater responsibility for decisions about the support of different types of health services delivery programmes. Given this responsibility, it can be expected that the commitment of the states to health services research will increase despite limited resources. Two specific projects illustrate the nature of public health research activities supported by state governments. In South Carolina a monitoring system has been established to collect information on the incidence of low-birth-weight deliveries. The system has enabled state officials to identify areas with relatively greater needs for services and to direct resources to meet these needs. New York State recently began a demonstration project to evaluate the feasibility of using incentives to encourage the elderly and the disabled to select alternatives to nursing homes for daily health care and support. Both of these projects

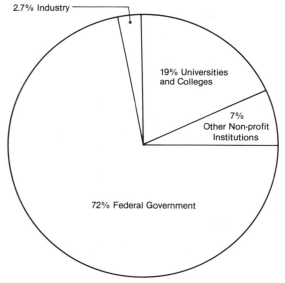

**Fig. 27.6.** Total 1978 expenditures for basic research in United States universities.

exemplify the intent of the National Health Planning Program (US Health Resources Administration 1980).

## The role of federal agencies

### The origin and development of the US Public Health Service

Government support for public health research in the US evolved directly from the development of the US Public Health Service (PHS), which had its origins in the Marine Hospital Service established in 1798 by the 'Act for the Relief of Sick and Disabled Seamen'. The law created, in effect, a payroll deduction plan for the medical care of a group of citizens most obviously exposed to environmental hazards to health, especially the great infectious pestilences of that time: yellow fever and smallpox. Soon a number of institutions were established where clinical care was provided, and by 1804 the Marine Hospital at Boston had begun to admit the first patients. However, more than 80 years elapsed before the work of Pasteur and Koch made it evident to American physicians that microorganisms were the cause of these epidemics. The earliest bacteriological laboratory in the US was established at the Staten Island Marine Hospital in 1887; others were soon established by the Service and by state and local authorities and were given an organizational basis by the State Boards of Health, which had been instituted during the 1870s and 1880s (Bordley and Harvey 1976).

Such facilities represented the first formal recognition by government in the US of the need for the practice of public health medicine; however, the federal government played virtually no part in these developments, other than to provide the facilities of the Marine Hospitals, which were the subject of such neglect and administrative incompetence that their reorganization became imperative. By 1902, with added responsibilities superimposed by the Quarantine Act of 1890, the Marine Hospital Service was renamed the 'Public Health and Marine Hospital Service' and necessary changes in administration began to take place resulting in efficient operations and real progress. At the same time, the federal 'Hygienic Laboratory' – the precursor of the National Institutes of Health – came into being, initially to control interstate commerce in sera, toxins, and similar products, but later, with the formation of a Biologics Control Commission, to test and guarantee the safety and effectiveness of vaccines and other biologicals under development. This stage represents the first, albeit rudimentary, organized support of public health research by the federal government. It became formalized, in 1912, in an Act that created the current designation 'United States Public Health Service' and provided for the basic activities of the Service, to include 'investigation and research'.

The Act gave considerable impetus to work on the causes of epidemic and endemic diseases. For example, in 1914, the new PHS assigned a physician-investigator, Joseph Goldberger, to search for the causative agent of pellagra, a disease then endemic in the US and assumed to be infectious. By careful application of sound scientific principles, Goldberger identified the cause of pellagra to be a dietary deficiency of niacin, thereby opening the way to eliminating the disease. Similarly,

but sometime later, the prevention of goitre was made possible by the introduction of iodized table salt, and of rickets by dietary supplementation with vitamin D. This type of success notwithstanding, the early work of the Hygienic Laboratory was most often confined to microbiology and communicable diseases, until in 1910, a profound change in emphasis occurred when the PHS became concerned with cancer. In 1922, the PHS provided support for a small laboratory at Harvard Medical School for the study of malignant disease and total expenditure on cancer research by the PHS rose to slightly more than $10 000 per year (it was believed at the time that federal expenditures on cancer research would never rise above a ceiling of $25 000 per year). By the late 1920s, PHS support of research on chronic, non-infectious disease had increased dramatically, with heart disease and mental illness now included. In response to heightened public awareness of these activities, the Randsell Act was passed in 1930 'to establish and operate a National Institute of Health, and to authorize the government to accept donations for use in ascertaining the cause, prevention and cure of disease affecting human beings, and for other purposes'. The Act also provided $750 000 for new buildings for the Institute. The present NIH property in Bethesda, Maryland, was acquired and the Institute was created by transfer of the staff and activities of the former Hygienic Laboratory to new buildings at this location. Further funds were provided by the Congress in the Social Security Act of 1935, and in 1937, in response to overwhelming public support, an additional $700 000 was appropriated for a National Cancer Institute at Bethesda.

To encourage national participation in biomedical research, the Institute began to solicit applications for grants-in-aid from the scientific community, and during 1938–40, 33 awards were made from 137 applications, for a total of $220 000. Here began the substantial support of extramural biomedical research that so typifies the activities of the US Public Health Service today and that was formalized in the Public Health Service Act of 1944, which gave the PHS authority to 'pay for research to be performed by laboratories, hospitals, universities and other public or private institutions, specifically by grants to individuals if necessary'.

By the mid-1930s more than 120 agencies of the federal government were engaged in or supporting research in various fields, with total expenditures around $125 million per year. Of these funds, $82 million was allocated to natural science and technology, including medicine. By 1947 the national expenditure on medicine alone had reached $85 million, of which $26 million, or about 30 per cent, came from federal funds. Although such sums appear paltry by current standards, they do represent a profound change in the role of the federal government in the internal affairs of the US: for the first time, the federal government accepted major responsibility for the health and welfare of the American citizen. The current federal commitment for health research and development is calculated by agency in Table 27.2.

### Missions of agencies of the Federal Government

The numerous agencies of the PHS are illustrated in Fig. 27.7. Those having a significant role in initiating and supporting public health research, in addition to the National Science

**Table 27.2.** *Federal obligations for health research and development by source or performer, fiscal years 1970–80*
(millions of dollars)

| | 1970 | 1971 | 1972 | 1973 | 1974 | 1975 | 1976 (est.) | 1977 | 1978 (est.) | 1979 | 1980 (est.) |
|---|---|---|---|---|---|---|---|---|---|---|---|
| **Total of A or B ($)** | **1666.6** | **1876.6** | **2147.3** | **2225.3** | **2753.6** | **2831.7** | **3058.7** | **3395.9** | **3811.2** | **4321.2** | **4723.4** |
| **A. By source of funds*** | | | | | | | | | | | |
| HHS (HEW) | 1177.0 | 1316.0 | 1584.3 | 1609.9 | 2092.2 | 2196.6 | 2382.7 | 2651.5 | 3012.6 | 3450.7 | 3694.7 |
| NIH | 873.3 | 1038.9 | 1271.3 | 1323.2 | 1736.8 | 1879.9 | 2060.2 | 2279.9 | 2580.9 | 2953.1 | 3181.9 |
| Other PHS | 270.0 | 247.6 | 275.8 | 254.7 | 315.2 | 278.5 | 287.7 | 308.4 | 364.3 | 419.9 | 458.6 |
| Other HHS (HEW) | 33.8 | 29.4 | 37.1 | 32.0 | 40.2 | 38.2 | 34.8 | 63.2 | 67.5 | 77.6 | 54.3 |
| OTHER AGENCIES | 489.5 | 560.6 | 563.1 | 615.4 | 661.4 | 635.1 | 675.9 | 744.4 | 798.6 | 870.5 | 1028.6 |
| Agriculture | 50.1 | 60.3 | 67.3 | 61.1 | 59.7 | 61.4 | 61.7 | 85.6 | 96.5 | 112.4 | 147.3 |
| Defence | 124.9 | 124.2 | 126.0 | 126.6 | 119.0 | 115.9 | 120.6 | 150.5 | 164.4 | 186.4 | 211.0 |
| Education† | – | – | – | – | – | – | – | – | – | – | 32.1 |
| Energy (ERDA, AEC) | 104.2 | 104.9 | 102.7 | 110.6 | 121.4 | 163.9 | 167.9 | 181.2 | 193.2 | 191.8 | 210.9 |
| Environmental protection | – | 13.1 | 14.5 | 20.3 | 18.8 | 38.1 | 63.0 | 56.2 | 56.6 | 67.2 | 78.1 |
| Int'l Dev Coop Agency (AID) | 10.8 | 15.2 | 15.1 | 16.3 | 10.3 | 6.4 | 8.8 | 23.7 | 17.2 | 20.2 | 13.4 |
| Aeronautics and space | 85.9 | 74.9 | 50.3 | 42.3 | 80.1 | 74.9 | 72.9 | 47.8 | 56.6 | 41.4 | 71.8 |
| National science foundation | 29.0 | 34.3 | 37.2 | 45.5 | 47.0 | 44.7 | 51.8 | 55.4 | 65.3 | 73.8 | 75.7 |
| Veterans | 58.7 | 62.7 | 68.9 | 74.2 | 84.0 | 94.8 | 97.7 | 107.0 | 114.0 | 127.0 | 133.4 |
| Other | 27.0 | 71.1 | 81.0 | 118.6 | 121.2 | 35.0 | 31.5 | 37.0 | 34.9 | 50.3 | 54.9 |
| **B. By performer** | | | | | | | | | | | |
| Federal laboratories | 488.3 | 566.5 | 608.2 | 627.3 | 667.9 | 714.2 | 779.3 | 865.9 | 1031.0 | 1119.1 | 1232.5 |
| Non-federal laboratories | 1178.3 | 1310.1 | 1539.1 | 1598.0 | 2085.8 | 2117.4 | 2279.3 | 2529.9 | 2780.2 | 3202.2 | 3490.9 |

*As organized in year specified.
†Office of Handicapped Research, formerly part of 'Other HHS (HEW)'.

Foundation, the Department of Defense, and the Veterans Administration, all provide funds within the framework of specific mandates, or missions, which limit the scope of their support.

The mission of the *National Institutes of Health* is to improve the health of the nation by increasing the understanding of processes underlying human health, disability, and disease; advancing knowledge about the health effects of interactions between humans and the environment; and developing and improving methods of preventing, detecting, diagnosing, and treating disease. The NIH accomplishes this mission through support of research in universities, hospitals, and research institutions in the US and abroad; conduct of research in its own laboratories and clinics; support of training for promising young researchers; development and maintenance of research resources; identification of research advances that have significant potential for clinical application, and the facilitation of the transfer of such advances to the health care system; and promotion of effective ways to communicate biomedical information to scientists, health practitioners, and the public.

The mission of the *Centers for Disease Control* (CDC) is to prevent unnecessary morbidity and mortality by assisting state and local health authorities and other health-related organizations in stemming the spread of communicable diseases; protecting against other diseases or conditions; providing protection from certain environmental hazards; and improving occupational health and safety. The CDC accomplishes this mission through a multifaceted programme of basic preventive health activities; health incentive grants, disease-risk-reduction demonstrations, and health education; targeted disease prevention programmes for states and communities including venereal disease control, childhood disease immunization programmes, influenza immunization programmes, fluoridation programmes, control of infectious and chronic disease, and prevention of environmental hazards such as lead-based paint poisoning; providing support to state authorities by investigations of epidemics and analyses of disease problems and trends; promotion of occupational safety and health; laboratory services and improvements; and international health co-operation.

Industrial efforts are encouraged by studies done and data collected by the *National Institute of Occupational Safety and Health* (NIOSH), a component of the Centers for Disease Control. The NIOSH mission is to identify and control harmful substances and work practices, and to establish remedial measures in occupational health. It produces 'criteria documents' in which all available information is analysed in recommending standards for safe levels of exposure to chemical and physical agents in the workplace. NIOSH also conducts studies on the effect of long-term exposure to processes and conditions that may cause illness or disability. Resources and personnel are provided to educational centres throughout the US to act as focal points for expertise in occupational health and safety. Research grants in occupational health are awarded by the Division of Safety Research.

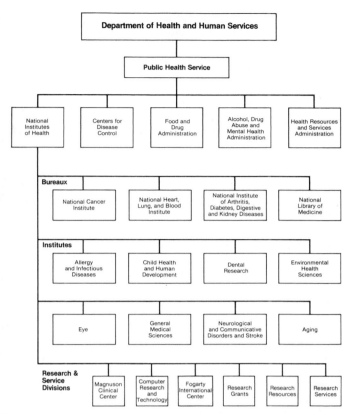

**Fig. 27.7.** Organization of the US National Institutes of Health within the public health service, 1982.

The *Food and Drug Administration* (FDA) aims to ensure that food is safe and wholesome; that drugs, biological products, therapeutic devices and diagnostic products are safe and effective; that cosmetics are safe; that the use of radiological products does not result in unnecessary exposure to radiation; and that products are honestly labelled. Most FDA regulatory actions require information generated through laboratory research and through evaluations conducted by well-trained agency scientists. Regulatory actions of the FDA reflect some of the most important public health decisions made in the federal government, and many such actions impose substantial economic burdens on society. Scientific research is, therefore, important both for the general improvement of regulatory decision-making and as a key national resource when serious health problems require special attention. Indeed, the degree to which regulatory decisions gain credibility and merit the support of the public and the scientific community, depends on the extent to which they reflect the best available scientific knowledge.

The *Alcohol, Drug Abuse, and Mental Health Administration* (ADAMHA) was established by Congress as the principal federal agency to prevent, control, and treat alcoholism, drug abuse, and mental illness, and to promote mental health. The three ADAMHA institutes – the National Institute on Alcohol Abuse and Alcoholism, the National Institute on Drug Abuse, and the National Institute of Mental Health – are the main sources of support for research on these public health problems affecting millions of Americans. As part of its mission, ADAMHA supports a broad spectrum of research aimed at expanding knowledge of aetiological factors, intervention, and prevention, and at training researchers, treatment and prevention staff, and other workers. To carry out its research, ADAMHA provides grants to state and local agencies, laboratories, other public and non-profit organizations, and individuals; supports a wide variety of research on improved methods of diagnosis, care, treatment, and rehabilitation of the mentally ill and those abusing or addicted to alcohol or drugs; conducts research in these areas in its own intramural facilities; provides funds for training of researchers; and disseminates emerging research information to researchers and practitioners.

As recently as 1982, two agencies, the Health Services Administration (HSA) and the Health Resources Administration (HRA), were merged to form the *Health Resources and Services Administration* (HRSA). The HRSA mission is to provide leadership and direction in the provision of health services to the nation, and in the development of resources for the health care system of the future. This includes the aims of the former HSA, to address the gaps and inequities in the nation's health care system, more specifically, to improve the organization and efficiency of health care delivery, to build and maintain primary health care capacity in underserved areas, to promote effective and equitable public health and preventive services, and to provide high-quality comprehensive health services to federal beneficiaries. The former HRA mission was to identify health care resource problems and to maintain or strengthen the distribution, supply, utilization, quality, and cost-effectiveness of these resources to improve the health care system and promote personal health. Major objectives included the development of a national health planning capability to promote access to quality health care for all at a reasonable cost, the design of innovative strategies, and targeted development of manpower, facilities, and other resources required for an effective health care system.

The *National Science Foundation* (NSF) was established as an independent agency of the federal government in 1980 to 'promote and advance scientific progress in the United States'. The NSF does this largely by sponsoring research and science education. Proposals are accepted for review in any field of science and engineering, including the biological and social sciences and interdisciplinary areas. No clinical research is supported, however, nor is work using animal models of disease, or the development or testing of drugs or other forms of treatment. The policy-making body of the NSF is the National Science Board, composed of 25 members appointed by the President of the US. The Board also approves all new programmes, grants, and contracts requiring a total commitment in excess of $2 million, or $500 000 annually. In deciding which proposals to fund, the NSF relies on advisory committees and outside reviewers, including scientists from universities, non-profit organizations, and the federal government. Awards are based on the competency of the researcher, the intrinsic merit of the proposed research, the utility or relevance to solving societal problems, and the effect on the national infrastructure of science. The NSF accepts proposals from commercial organizations and encourages collaboration amongst universities, industries, and state and local governments. Awards are made both for solicited and unsolicited proposals, in the latter case most often on a cost-sharing basis.

The *Department of Defense* (DOD) is concerned with national defence and security, which embrace a very wide range of activities. From the standpoint of public health, several aspects of the DOD programmes are relevant, and the support of research in this area although not predominant is certainly apparent. The three services, Army, Navy and Air Force, all offer grant and contract funds by which they support research at universities and other non-profit institutions, and each service maintains its own laboratories. A large part of the external support provided by the DOD is in the form of contracts, which means that the work to be supported will be expected to result in some form of service or product. In other words, the contract mechanism tends to support applied research or development, rather than basic science.

The Office of Naval Research, which pioneered the idea of the university research contract, has in its mission several issues of importance to public health, including behavioural studies on group living and stress caused by separation from home and family; noise reduction (designed to protect submariners) and a substantial blood research programme. The Air Force Office of Scientific Research provides extramural support in basic life sciences that clearly relates to public health, and the office encourages awards that involve partial support to encourage co-operation between outside investigators and Air Force scientists. The Army Research Office also sponsors basic research in the life sciences, including physiological responses to climatic extremes, but also in areas like helicopter noise control that will obviously have an ultimate environmental health impact. In addition, the Army has extensive programmes in the behavioural and social sciences as well as medicine. At one time, the Army supported a substantial programme in biological warfare defence that resulted in much new knowledge about the detection of, and the protection against, a large variety of pathogens. The containment facility at Fort Detrick in Maryland, built to allow this research, has now passed into the hands of the National Cancer Institute, where work on the causes, diagnosis, prevention and treatment of cancer is presently proceeding.

The *Veterans Administration* (VA) through its Department of Medicine and Surgery, provides health care to patients having previously served in the armed forces. Its mission is served by a research and development programme designed to provide new knowledge, techniques or products leading to improved prevention, diagnosis, treatment and control of disease, as well as correction or compensation of disabilities. Clearly, such work benefits far more than just the veterans, and significant amounts of VA research concerns problems in public health. However, unlike the case with most other federal agencies, the VA supports only that research which is performed by its own staff in its own hospitals and laboratories, a network of which extends over the US. One effective mechanism employed by the VA is the Cooperative Study Program, in which investigators at a number of VA medical centres investigate a given problem in a uniform manner under a common protocol. Whilst the majority of these studies emphasize therapy, some are classical public health research, for example, those studies concerning vaccines.

## PLANNING FOR PUBLIC HEALTH RESEARCH IN THE US FEDERAL GOVERNMENT

Just as the scientific method itself has become a type of planning mechanism that has resulted in real progress, so too has the allocation of limited federal resources to the support of public health research become a method with an effective life of its own. Ideally, the process of planning the support of research includes five integrated functions:

1. *Analysis:* the review of a topic and the identification of relevant problems, with possible solutions. The available resources are determined and recommendations for action are made.

2. *Formulation:* the establishment of objectives and the allocation of appropriate resources. Due consideration is given to policies, constraints, and priorities. The result is a feasible, but generalized, plan.

3. *Implementation:* the specification of schedules and timetables, together with details of staff, materials, and operating procedures. The plan is then put into effect.

4. *Evaluation:* the collation and analysis of the results of the planned activities. On the basis of the evaluation, the formulation or implementation stages of the process are modified if necessary and the process continues.

5. *Assessment:* the determination of the success or failure of the planned activities, together with an appreciation of their influence on future strategy.

During planning, not all of these steps are discrete; nevertheless, each does tend to become the responsibility of a specific group, particularly when the planned activities will receive federal support.

An important basis for understanding where the responsibilities for planning will fall is the distinction between basic and applied research. The best basic research comes not from consideration of global issues, or of relevancy or expediency, but rather from sharply focused, extremely well-informed recognition of those areas most likely to benefit from very detailed investigation using the scientific method. Planning for basic research, therefore, tends to be concentrated in the formulation, implementation, and evaluation phases, with the last-mentioned being applied rigorously. Federal support of basic research is provided largely by grants-in-aid of individual projects, initiated by the individual investigator. Federal administrators generally allocate such funds to broad 'programme' areas, in amounts that tend to reflect current scientific demands and, rarely, political or economic pressures. The functions of analysis and assessment, as defined, are thus generally outside the scope of plans for basic research made by the individual investigator, for basic research deals essentially with what seem to be discrete and isolated questions. The basic scientist examines small, defined, separable phenomena. Applied research, on the other hand, is more oriented to practical ends and has a tendency to involve collaboration between groups of investigators. The investigator is usually caught up in concerns which include all five phases of the planning process. A large-scale clinical trial of a new vaccine, for example, involving the expenditure of relatively large sums of money, will be set up only after a careful and detailed diagnosis of the situation, often by a team that includes administrators and investigators. The final assessment of such a trial will again involve not only the practitioners who have been engaged in the research, but also the managers of health care delivery and may lead to significant changes in national health practices.

The American system is characterized by a great deal of independence on the part of the scientific investigator, and a relative lack of centralization on the part of the agencies providing support for research. Undoubtedly this creates a small amount of duplication of effort and a degree of redundancy. In addition, the coordination of research becomes more a matter for advice and persuasion than for imperative. Nevertheless, the checks and balances created by this very independence tend to make it unlikely that gross errors of judgment will prevail.

### Factors influencing research planning

The federal government has had a long-standing involvement and commitment to health science research, with an especially high concentration of support in the Department of Health and Human Services. Placing most of the US health research budget in a single Department has facilitated co-ordination of information and programmes towards the solution of public health problems. The future will require even more co-ordination. Changes in needs, in national economics, and in scientific institutions have brought demands for review and adaptation of the national commitment to health research.

For example, special demands on public health researchers have been created by the recent changes in a population that is becoming ever more urban and industrialized. The regulatory agencies, burdened with health mandates, appeal for information which in some cases may be beyond the capabilities of the research laboratories. In some research areas an imbalance seems to exist between programmes whose goals are the acquisition of more basic knowledge and the application of knowledge to very specific problems. Undoubtedly prevailing influences can result in a disproportionate amount of support for one particular aspect of a problem, resulting in an imbalance. One current example is in the area of therapeutic apheresis, a technique that is burgeoning. The removal from blood of immune complexes, toxins or agents believed to be implicated in the progression of disease has led to a large increase in the number of patients being treated by apheresis, for a host of disorders, including haematological, nephrological, neurological, and the rheumatological conditions. The use of apheresis is considered experimental in many of these cases, but the research being conducted amounts largely to observations of clinical progress in small groups of patients in non-randomized, unblinded, and uncontrolled trials. What is really needed, however, may be an examination of the basic underlying physiological changes that accompany apheresis, in health and disease, using animal models at first, and the use of large-scale controlled clinical trials to examine the effects of apheresis in specific diseases, where the data acquired have statistical validity.

The direction which biomedical programmes, including public health research, should take is one of the most difficult subjects presented to the US Congress. The Senate Committee on Appropriations stated in 1973 that it 'is convinced that the time has come when the health research resources of our nation must be better organized and address themselves to problems at hand in a more systematic manner. . . The NIH must make a more determined effort to attain a proper balance between applied and basic research in biomedicine' (US Senate 1973). Greater accountability is possible in the field of health, and the Committee expected all of the NIH to formulate 'blueprints' or health research strategies. In the past few years, contention has arisen among the federal supporters of the sciences concerning the proper loci of certain kinds of research, notably nutrition, biological effects of ionizing radiation, and toxicology. And changes in governmental organization of research including efforts to facilitate co-ordination are becoming more common.

Numerous factors outside the Public Health Service affect research planning at the NIH; their degree of influence, and the manner in which they are considered in each planning process may vary. In general, these factors are the following:

*State of knowledge:* All research planning proceeds from what is known about a health problem, life process, or disease and results in the identification of scientific opportunities, gaps, and needs; rapidly advancing areas of research; potential interventions ready for clinical testing; and changes in direction, approaches, or emphasis required to advance knowledge.

*Health priorities and policies for the Assistant Secretary:* Each year early in the planning process, the Assistant Secretary for Health meets with the NIH Director to discuss health research priorities and to identify planning issues to be examined during the year. These are reflected in planning documents and progress reports provided periodically.

*Congressional actions:* Authorizing legislation, mandates, directives, and appropriations all directly influence research planning. Samples of such actions are the establishment of new institutes, changes in research training legislation, contracts for small business set-aside, mandates to allocate a proportion of resources to a particular disease area, directions to develop a national plan, and interest in providing greater support to an identified area of research or specific mandated study.

*Input from constituency groups:* Interest groups, professional societies and organizations, lay individuals, and the biomedical research community all play a part in the research planning process. Their input can be expressed in a variety of ways, ranging from structured activities such as advice from the National Advisory Councils and the Director's Advisory Committee, planning subcommittees of these bodies and special groups or task forces convened to consider a specific health research area, to less-structured interaction with representatives of these groups about specific issues.

*Social and economic burden of illness:* Incidence, prevalence, morbidity, mortality, and health costs are all factors to be balanced with scientific opportunity in planning directions and changes in programmes and in developing priorities.

*Budget decisions:* Decisions made at the PHS level on the NIH budget throughout the course of the budget development process directly affect research planning. As resource levels change or emphasis shifts, research planning must respond.

*Existence of adequate research resources:* Trained manpower, adequate facilities, and modern equipment and instrumentation are essential to implementing and continuing a high-quality research programme. Constant attention must be given to such resources during the planning process to ensure their availability.

*Other PHS agencies:* When major changes occur in other PHS agencies, such as occurred with the dissolution of the Office of International Health, the NIH research planning process must accommodate and provide for these events. In addition, budget reductions or shifts in priorities in other PHS agencies can affect NIH research planning to the extent that jointly sponsored activities (such as the National Toxicology Program) are involved.

*Other factors:* The Department of Health and Human Services (DHHS) and White House priorities, directives from the Office of Management and Budget, reports of special commissions and task forces, and media reports, are all factors which affect research planning.

### Evolution of major events in planning for public health research

#### Initiation of the National Institutes of Health

The National Institutes of Health, founded in 1930, were incorporated into the Public Health Service with the passage of the Public Health Service Act in 1944 (P.L. 78–410). This landmark legislation revised and consolidated all laws relating to the Public Health Service, and Section 301 (A) gave broad authorization to the Surgeon General to conduct and support research into human diseases:

The Secretary shall conduct in the service, and encourage, cooperate with, and render assistance to other appropriate public authorities, scientific institutions, and scientists in the conduct of, and promote the coordination of, research, investigations, experiments, demonstrations, and studies relating to the causes, diagnosis, treatment, control, and prevention of physical and mental diseases and impairments of man, including water purification, sewage treatment, and pollution of lakes and streams.

#### Creation of the research institutes and co-ordination 1937–48

With the creation of the National Cancer Institute (NCI) in 1937, the Congress launched the first of several federal research programmes, the purpose of which was to establish the means of controlling major human chronic and debilitating diseases. The NCI was the first federal health agency assigned to categorical disease research and it became a prototype of the institutes now under the administration of the NIH. Supporting the 1937 legislation, Senator Bone commented that the funding for cancer research was a '. . . lopsided sort of a picture. There is no specific direction to it. There is not any challenge to the men who are engaged in research work. It is just a condition that seems to have grown up . . . I find almost everywhere a feeling that there is not a direction to the expenditures nor any direction to the efforts of those engaged in research work which would permit any

sort of coordination . . .' (Bone 1937). Senator Bone perceived the need for co-ordinating scientific knowledge.

In 1948, the National Heart Act (P.L. 80-655) as an amendment to the Public Health Act, established the National Heart Institute. Representative Wolverton gave the following supportive rationale: 'An essential step toward reducing the ravages of these diseases is the stimulation of large-scale research into the causes, treatment, and methods of prevention of cardiovascular conditions. The current level of funds from all sources for cardiovascular research is far short of that available for other diseases of less significance as killers and disablers of man' (Wolverton 1948). He described research facilities and funds for cardiovascular diseases as 'pitifully inadequate'. To apply the results of basic research widely and quickly, the national need was (first) to strengthen and expand clinical facilities and to increase the trained personnel available in the various communities. Mr Wolverton stated that 'these community programs should be primarily the responsibility of State and local government bodies working with the Federal Government in a relationship similar to that which has proved so successful in the tuberculosis, venereal diseases, cancer, mental health, and other programs of the Public Health Service'.

#### The seventies: blueprints and accountability

The purpose of the National Cancer Act of 1971 was to 'enlarge the authorities of the National Cancer Institute (NCI) and the National Institutes of Health in order to advance the national effort against cancer'. The law simultaneously created the National Cancer Program (NCP) and assigned responsibility for its development and management to the Director of the NCI. The two major components of the cancer eradication effort are research and control, and the greatest share of the financial support for research comes from the federal government. The goal of these efforts is to develop the knowledge and techniques needed to control or eliminate cancer. The control activities include rapidly disseminating new knowledge and techniques, applying the available knowledge to the population at risk, evaluating the impact of the application of knowledge and techniques, and feeding back the results of the evaluation so that all the components of the research and control process can be adapted or changed as required. As shown in Fig. 27.8, national programmes such as that for cancer, and the National Heart, Blood Vessel, Lung and Blood Program described below, provide funds to a number of groups and organizations for conducting research, control, and support activities. The relationships amongst the major scientific and technical activities conducted within the National Cancer Program and the public health care delivery system are illustrated in Fig. 27.9 (US National Cancer Institute 1975).

The planning activities conducted to support the NCP involve extensive participation of representatives of the scientific community. Participants include laboratory scientists, research physicians, practising physicians, cancer specialists and other specialists, allied health professionals, social scientists, third-party payers, fiduciaries, cancer health care consumers, and the public at large.

Recognizing its responsibility to act decisively in the face of a mounting problem of death and disability from cardiovascular

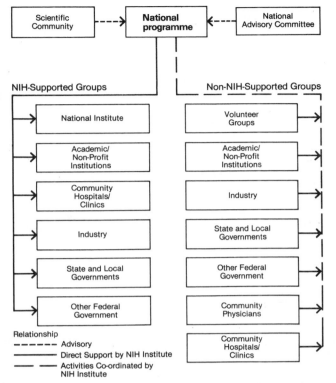

**Fig. 27.8.** Inter-relationships in a typical national research programme at the US National Institutes of Health.

disease, the US Congress had established the National Heart Institute. In the years since, the Congress has expanded the scope of the Institute's activities to the extent that the present National Heart, Lung and Blood Institute (NHLBI) is responsible for a comprehensive and co-ordinated research plan, formulated as the National Heart, Blood Vessel, Lung and Blood Program. This programme was formally established in 1972 by act of law following the development of a cycle of planning activities illustrated in Fig. 27.10.

To ensure that the NHLBI would carry out these broadened responsibilities most effectively, the Congress required the Director of the Institute to develop, with the advice of the National Heart, Lung, and Blood Advisory Council, a national plan within 180 days of the enactment of the law. A thorough review was undertaken of the state of scientific research in heart, lung, and blood diseases, and a plan was outlined for a comprehensive national programme responsive to the requirements of the law. In the 1976 amendments to the Public Health Service Act, Congress further strengthened its commitment to blood diseases and resources in particular, and the NHLBI assumed its present name. The national programme continues to be the foundation of the activities of the Institute and is reviewed every year (US National Heart, Lung and Blood Institute 1978).

### The President's Biomedical Research Panel

The President's Biomedical Research Panel was established in January 1975 (P.L. 93-352) to review and assess the support policy and management of biomedical and behavioural research conducted through programmes of the National Institutes of Health and the Alcohol, Drug Abuse, and Mental Health Administration. The panel assessed the state of knowledge, especially in relation to health care; heard testimony at public hearings from public and private sector witnesses with diverse interests about issues and problems in need of review; commissioned studies on the impact of federal funding on research in institutions of higher learning, on the dissemination of research findings, and on methods of developing policy options for funding; conducted interviews with officials from NIH and DHEW, Congressional staffs, the Office of Management and Budget, other federal agencies, professional and special interest groups; and collected information through correspondence, staff research, and surveys (Fig. 27.11).

### Health research principles

In April 1978, HEW Secretary Joseph Califano Jr initiated a major review and reappraisal of departmental health research activities. The review reflected his concern about the future of federal support for health research at a time when national resources were insufficient to meet all competing demands, and careful balancing of the options was critical. The purposes of this initiative were to broaden the context for planning health research, to view highly varying applications of the scientific method by different disciplines within a common structure, and to develop criteria for examining the health research activities of the DHEW. The result was a set of principles issued in July 1979 for formulating a plan for health research in the DHEW (US Department of Health, Education and Welfare 1978). The review provided data for a limited but useful description of the distribution of the DHEW total research resources of $4 billion. To the extent that categories now used

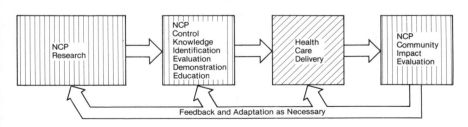

**Fig. 27.9.** Major components of the US National Cancer Program.

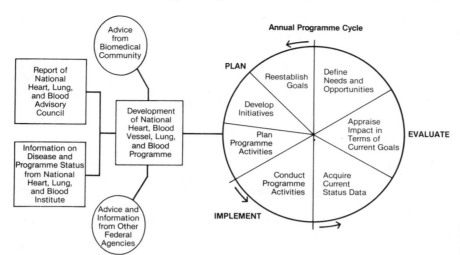

**Fig. 27.10.** Origin and annual planning cycle of the US National Heart, Blood vessel, Lung and Blood Program.

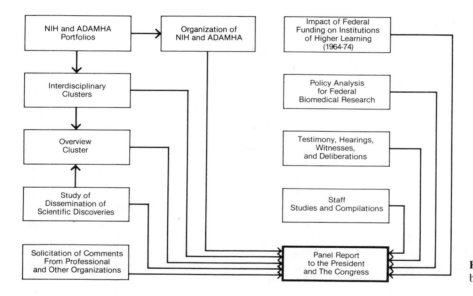

**Fig. 27.11.** Strategy in the development of initiatives by the US President's Biomedical Research Panel.

by NIH are applicable to other agencies, it appears that approximately 75 per cent of the DHEW health research money is spent on activities primarily aimed at increasing scientific knowledge. From 10 per cent to 15 per cent of the total supports the application of knowledge at highly practical levels. About 6 per cent is used to disseminate the results of field tests: to demonstrate or otherwise transfer new technology derived from research. The remaining 6 per cent supports training of research scientists. Two agencies – the Health Care Financing Administration and the Office of Health Research, Statistics, and Technology – did not find the analytical categories adaptable to their health services research (amounting to about 2 per cent of the total) so this was not included in the review. These data are considered useful as a starting base for projections and for future deliberations by the Department, the Executive Branch, the Congress, and all others who have an interest in this matter.

During the review, a number of issues emerged that reflect differences in approach between general-purpose research agencies and mission-oriented agencies. The scientific activities of the Department are not fully interchangeable units; they derive from and are responsive to the unique mission of each of the separate agencies that carry them out. One function of HEW health research planning is to comprehend the magnitude and complexity of the enterprise and to strive for orderly and productive relationships amongst the components. Progressive integration of complementary agency research programmes has occurred during the past few years; however, it has been the continuing DHEW policy that co-operative research activities should not automatically override other research priorities of individual agencies.

*Health Research Amendments 1982*

Of the actions taken by the 97th US Congress in the area of public health, the major one has been to transfer several health programmes from federal control to the states, returning programme initiatives in the form of block grants. The states will determine which programme to emphasize. Four health block grants were established which consolidated 19 categorical health programmes, these are: Maternal and Child Health, Preventive Health Services, Alcohol, Drug Abuse and Mental Health Services, and Primary Care.

In addition to the block grant strategy, the US Senate is assuming an important role of oversight of biomedical research. As stated by Senator Hatch in his opening remarks at the 31 March 1982 hearing of the Senate Labor and Human Resources Committee on the Biomedical Research, Training, and Medical Library Assistance Amendments of 1982: 'I support our government's commitment to biomedical research . . . we as elected officials . . . are obliged to serve as advocates for our citizens by ensuring that their money and tax dollars are spent efficiently and properly. The budget of the NIH . . . has grown by leaps and bounds. . . . This grand scale investment requires effective and ongoing Congressional oversight. As long as I am Chairman of this Committee, this will be done' (Hatch 1982).

The US House of Representatives is also leaning towards more accountability of government health programmes. In Chairman Waxman's opening statement at the 29 March 1982 Hearing of the Subcommittee on Health and the Environment on the Health Research Act of 1982, he stated his concern for the future of biomedical research: 'The "Health Research Act of 1982" accords the National Institutes of Health the distinction and recognition that it deserves as the world's foremost biomedical research body. Our task . . . is not to devise shortsighted strategies to enable NIH to make do with less, but rather to chart a course for future research priorities that will enhanced the mission of NIH, not only in the current fiscal year but in the decade ahead' (Waxman 1982).

Biomedical and public health research will be the subject of more accountability and oversight in the 1980s. Future research priorities will need more justification and thorough and precise planning will become the rule rather than the exception in federally supported research. Now is a good time to take inventory of the products of basic research and apply them to the community, but it is also a time to re-examine this corpus of knowledge in order to extract the innovative areas which need nurturing.

### Planning approaches at NIH

Each Institute at the NIH plans in its own particular way. One illustration is that of a large NIH Bureau, the National Heart, Lung, and Blood Institute.

#### The National Heart, Lung, and Blood Institute planning process

A major juncture in the development of a formal planning process at the NHLBI was the passage, in 1972, of the National Heart, Blood Vessel, Lung, and Blood Act (P.L. 92-423) which provided for expanded, intensified, and co-ordinated efforts against heart, blood vessel, lung, and blood diseases. The resulting National Program of research, prevention, educa-

tion, and control provides a planned institutional focus on these diseases. In 1976, legislation extended and expanded that authority. As a result, research related to cardiovascular, lung, and blood diseases, and blood resources is supported by three major extramural divisions with a total of 20 programme elements.

The NHLBI uses an integrated and continuous process to plan, implement, and evaluate its National Program. This process was established to ensure responsiveness to legislative mandates, identification and pursuit of the most promising opportunities, and the effective use of resources. The planning, implementation, and evaluation process takes place in a yearly cycle which involves a continuous flow of information from the public, the medical community, other federal agencies, and non-federal organizations. The Institute is responsible for co-ordinating this flow and converting and channelling it into timely, worthwhile programmes. The scientific community plays a prominent role through participation on various advisory and review groups, task forces, and working groups involved in assessing progress and determining future directions of the programme.

The process can be characterized as systematic and disciplined, while dynamic and varied in terms of specific approaches (Fig. 27.12). It is designed to ensure a thorough

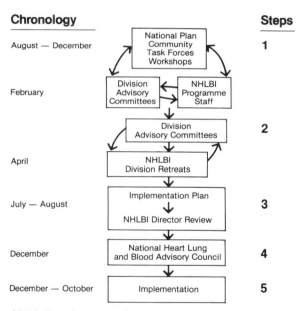

**Fig. 27.12.** Development of the annual implementation plan at the US National Heart, Lung and Blood Institute.

review of the entire programme as well as the implementation of new initiatives and the expansion, modification, or discontinuation of existing programmes. This process involves five steps as follows:

1. *Review, assessment, evaluation, and initial planning* of programmes is effected by a review of the goals, objectives, and progress of the five-year National Program Plan with respect to the state of knowledge, as well as the impact of the programme on medical care and the health of the public. This is

accomplished with the participation of the NHLBI programme staff, scientific advisory committees, and members of the general scientific community through workshops, task forces, and technical working groups convened to reach consensus on future directions for the programme. The results of special evaluation studies provide important information at this step. The end products are a review and modification of the most current five year plan and a preliminary list of initiatives and recommended directions for future years, together with revised objectives where appropriate.

2. *Priority setting* is the second step in the process, in which proposed new initiatives for implementation in the next year are ranked according to goals and objectives of the National Program; to the results, progress, and potential impact of current programmes; and financial and time constraints. This is accomplished jointly by the staff of the NHLBI divisions and appropriate advisory committees. The product of this step is a set of further defined initiatives, ranked by priority within major programme categories.

3. *Implementation planning* constitutes the third step, in which the staff of the division and the office of the Director convert the ranked initiatives into specific plans including justification, management and fiscal plans, and funding mechanisms. The end product of this step is the preliminary NHLBI Implementation Plan and Program Budget which reflects available resources, legislative mandates and intent, as well as inter-institute and inter-agency responsibilities.

4. *Advisory Council review* consists of a thorough review of the Implementation Plan by the full National Heart, Lung, and Blood Advisory Council. Council advice and recommendations are solicited and considered in developing the final NHLBI Implementation Plan and Program Budget.

5. *Programme implementation* consists of translating specific mandates and approved initiatives contained in the Implementation Plan into operational projects. This is a complex process requiring the availability and application of scientific knowledge and resources of all kinds, including scientific manpower, facilities, equipment, and funds. Implementation is carried out through various types of grants and contracts, intramural research, collaboration with other federal agencies through inter-agency agreements, as well as jointly supported international activities.

The NHLBI uses these major processes and systems to provide for expedient and effective planning and implementation of the programme. These systems help to ensure appropriate utilization of new knowledge and provide for scientific validation of new techniques of prevention and treatment. The results of these processes are applied in the implementation of the programme and are disseminated to the health care community as a whole.

The majority (70 per cent) of funds that NHLBI uses to support its programme initiatives are allocated to research grants (US National Heart, Lung, and Blood Institute 1981). Awards of these grant funds are subject to the formalized NIH peer review process.

### NIH peer review process

The National Institutes of Health is an important, unique interface between American academic institutions and their public health researchers, medical scientists, and physicians. Through its support of training and fellowship programmes, NIH has a direct line to those individuals who will be preparing the future research programmes. To ensure that public funds for health-related research are allocated wisely and in the public interest, the government has set up a procedure for reviewing applications for funding. A large number of scientists can thereby compete for the limited research funds by having the merits of their prospective projects judged by a peer review system.

When a grant application is submitted to NIH, it goes to the Division of Research Grants (DRG) where staff scientists read the application and assign it to one of the NIH Institutes or other awarding units in the Public Health Service with responsibility for supporting scientific research in that specific area (Eaves 1972). The first review of the application is for scientific merit and is made by a study section. The second review is by one of the national advisory councils of the Institutes (Fig. 27.13).

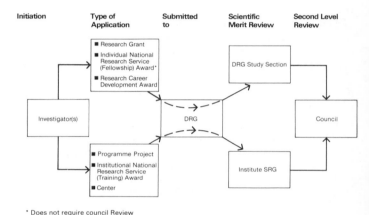

**Fig. 27.13.** Initiation and review of a grant application made to the US National Institutes of Health.

Study sections, or scientific review groups (SRG) are advisory committees of ten to fifteen consultants from the scientific community. Members of these committees serve limited terms and are selected on the basis of recognized competence and achievements in the research fields in the purview of a committee. During formal meetings, the study sections discuss each application individually. The study sections review the applications on the basis of scientific merit, including the importance of the proposed research problem, the originality of the approach, the training experience and research competence or promise of the investigators, the adequacy of the experimental design, the suitability of the facilities, and the appropriateness of the requested budget to accomplish the proposed work. A majority vote of the members makes the final recommendations of approval, disapproval, or deferral for future examination. Each study section member scores the approved applications for scientific merit. After the meeting, these scores are averaged, authenticated and entered into a computer system. The composite score is known as the priority score of that grant; it is a guide to national advisory councils and the awarding units in deciding the order in which approved applications can be funded.

The second review is by advisory council (Fig. 27.14). Each Institute or division that awards grants has an advisory council or equivalent group which is mandated by law to recommend approval before a grant can be awarded. These councils consist of more than sixteen scientists or physicians from the academic community who are leaders in the respective fields of the institutes, together with representatives of the general public. A National Advisory Council receives the study section recommendations on applications and reviews the proposals against the needs of NIH and the mission of the individual Institutes, the total pattern of research in universities and other institutions, and need for the initiation of research in new areas. The councils usually accept the study section appraisal of scientific merit, but may modify the recommendation in relation to the other relevant factors.

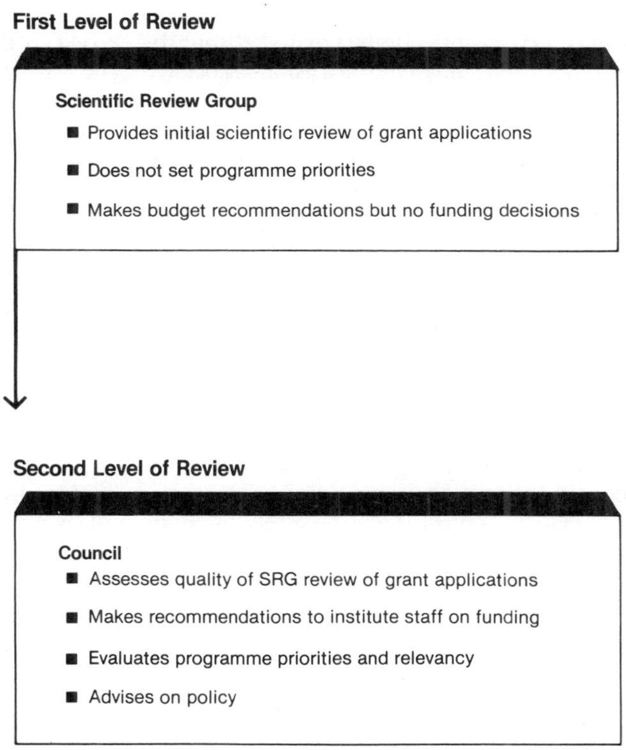

**First Level of Review**

**Scientific Review Group**

■ Provides initial scientific review of grant applications

■ Does not set programme priorities

■ Makes budget recommendations but no funding decisions

**Second Level of Review**

**Council**

■ Assesses quality of SRG review of grant applications

■ Makes recommendations to institute staff on funding

■ Evaluates programme priorities and relevancy

■ Advises on policy

**Fig. 27.14.** Dual review system for grant applications made to the National Institutes of Health.

## COMMENTS

The support of public health research in the US is essentially pluralistic, with funds being provided by numbers of different organizations, each with its own mission and motivation. It might be thought that such an apparent lack of cohesion would be disadvantageous, there being no central control and no overall plan, and that national aspirations might be met in a somewhat haphazard fashion. In fact, the system is most effective, with significant advances coming from many quarters of a highly diversified research effort. It is often said

that if a strictly centrally organized and massive federal 'war on poliomyelitis' had been mounted in the 1940s, the likelihood is that most funds would have been directed to the development of more and better iron lungs. As it happened, however, in the absence of such specific direction, the safe and effective Salk and Sabin vaccines arose as a result of the development of the techniques of tissue culture, an area at that time quite unrelated to poliomyelitis research.

However, good as the system is, mistakes are sometimes made. A classical example of failure by the federal establishment to respond appropriately to a public health problem is that of the 'swine flu affair' (Neustadt and Fineberg 1978). The National Influenza Immunization Program, the official title for a mass immunization programme against a new strain of influenza virus, was launched by President Gerald Ford in March, 1976. One year later the programme was set aside by HEW Secretary Joseph Califano Jr. As a full-scale operation, it lasted only two months. The aim was to innoculate every American against what some believed was the threat of pandemic influenza with the potential to cause one million deaths. The first doses of a new vaccine were given in October 1976, but over a two-month period, in which several millions received it, deaths from Guillian–Barré syndrome, apparently related to the vaccine, were reported. The programme was halted in December 1976, to assess the significance of this dangerous side-effect, and indeed, it was never restarted. Nor did the influenza epidemic come. The fact that it was believed probable, indicates how little the experts really understood influenza, and how equivocal and damaging a hastily mounted initiative in public health can be. Neustadt and Fineberg (1978) included in their characterization of the decision-making process in the swine flu affair, overconfidence by specialists in theories spun from meagre evidence, zeal by health professionals to force their lay superiors into certain actions, insufficient questioning of the possible outcome of the implementation of mass immunization, and failure to recognize the power of the press or the credibility of various institutions. This experience brought questions that typically challenge officials at the high policy levels of government. HEW Secretary Joseph Califano Jr has asked (Neustadt and Fineberg 1978):

First, how shall top lay officials, who are not themselves expert, deal with fundamental policy questions that are based, in part, on highly technical and complex expert knowledge – especially when that knowledge is speculative, or hotly debated, or when 'the facts' are so uncertain? When such questions arise, with how much deference and how much skepticism should those whose business is doing things and making policy view those whose business is knowing things – the scientists and the experts?

How should policy makers – and their expert advisers – seek to involve and to educate the public and relevant parties on such complicated and technical issues? To what extent can there be informed and robust public debate before the decision is reached?

On the other hand, the planning process can work well. In the case of research into the control of hypertension, the National High Blood Pressure Education Research Program (NHBPERP) mounted under the leadership of the National Heart, Lung, and Blood Institute, has been a particularly effective operation, and premature death and illness from diseases associated with high blood pressure have declined dramatically since the programme began.

The objectives, when the programme was initiated early in the 1970s, were first to support investigators working to develop instruments for gathering information – prior to any intervention – in the areas of knowledge of, and attitudes towards, hypertension, of demographic characteristics, of adherence behaviour if a medical regimen for hypertension had been previously prescribed, and of such special characteristics as the perception held by the patient of his or her illness, the forces affecting that illness, any related behaviour, the attitude of his or her physician, etc. Following this, educational intervention to enhance or develop adherence to treatment was to be instituted. Finally, any changes in knowledge, attitudes, adherence behaviour and other special characteristics were to be documented. On the basis of these findings, the most effective strategy of intervention was to be developed and applied.

The magnitude and complexity of hypertension as a public health problem meant that the NHBPERP had to be comprehensive in its attempts to mobilize and co-ordinate the resources and energies of all interested groups in government and the private sector. Under the leadership of the National Heart, Lung, and Blood Institute, the joint national effort now includes numerous federal agencies, virtually all state health departments, and more than 150 private sector organizations, such as professional societies, voluntary health associations, certifying and accrediting bodies, pharmaceutical companies, labour and management groups, and insurance companies. Hundreds of community efforts are also allied with the Program and are involved in every facet of high blood pressure control.

Progress is being made towards this goal. Recent surveys indicate improved public understanding of the condition and increased attention being paid to the disease by health care providers at all levels. Continued progress depends on maintaining current activities while also responding to evolving needs. Programmes at all levels are developing the resources to make comprehensive high blood pressure control services a permanent function of the health care system.

In recent years, perhaps as a consequence of the swine flu affair, new problems in American public health are being addressed with a great deal less guesswork and a good deal more caution. For example, despite the virtual elimination of hepatitis type-B virus from the national blood supply, post-transfusion hepatitis still remains, with the causative agent(s) being the elusive non-A, non-B (NANB) virus(es). The Transfusion Transmitted Viruses Study, supported by the National Heart, Lung, and Blood Institute (Aach et al. 1981) indicated a strong correlation between elevated levels in the blood of the liver enzyme alanine aminotransferase (ALT) and the presence of active NANB hepatitis. Wholesale introduction of ALT testing of blood donors would theoretically have had the effect of dramatically reducing post-transfusion hepatitis, yet at a considerable cost in ethical as well as financial terms. The enzyme is elevated in blood for many other reasons than NANB hepatitis. There is great variation in 'normal' blood levels of ALT depending on a variety of demographic factors. At what level of blood ALT should donors be told that their blood is unacceptable? What should they be told about their condition, since they may or may not be ill? For these and similar reasons, the precipitous and widespread introduction of ALT testing has not been advocated, rather, resources and energies are being directed to the identification of specific serological markers for NANB virus(es), so that the eventual elimination of post-transfusion hepatitis may be achieved by more precise and effective means.

Finally, as this chapter is being written, the US is facing what appears to be a serious new epidemic, unprecedented in its morbidity and mortality and with alarming possibilities. This is acquired immune deficiency syndrome (AIDS), first apparent amongst male homosexuals, but now including other groups evidently at high risk. The syndrome is one of an imbalance in T-helper/T-suppressor lymphocyte function, with the compromised cellular immune system allowing a multiplicity of opportunistic infections, and certain neoplasms, particularly Kaposi's sarcoma (Macek 1982). Recent evidence involving haemophiliacs and others (US Centers for Disease Control 1982) clearly indicates the possibility that this condition is produced by an infectious agent that may be carried in the blood, and thus may be transfusion-associated. The response of the federal government has so far been prompt, but measured. Epidemiological studies have been initiated in several population groups thought to be at risk, so as to verify the risk factors and question the transfusion association. Testing for T-lymphocyte function has been augmented by the Centers for Disease Control. The HHS Assistant Secretary is advised on AIDS by a select committee of experts. Funds are being diverted to planned research on the nature and aetiology of AIDS. Such reasoned planning for appropriate public health research holds promise that AIDS will be documented expeditiously, and the epidemic contained.

However, the ability to react to urgent developments in the field of public health requires the continuing availability of well-trained, research-oriented scientists and physicians, with access to the best equipment and instruments available. And the ability to prevent disease – surely the main aim of public health research – will come ultimately from the results of investigations performed by this same cadre of workers.

## APPENDIX – RESOURCES ON GRANTS AND FUNDING

*(Compiled by the John Vinten Dahlgren Memorial Library, Georgetown University)*

### I. Reference sources (non-government)

*Annual Register of Grant Support, 1981–82.* 15th edn. Marquis, Chicago (1981).
The annual volume includes grant support programmes of government agencies, public and private foundations, corporations, community trusts, unions, educational and professional associations, and special interest organizations. More than 2000 agencies are described.

*Corporate 500: The Directory of Corporate Philanthropy.* Public Management Institute, San Francisco (1980).
Information on 500 national philanthropic corporations has been collected from the companies' annual reports, special

publications, and tax returns. The top 500 corporations are determined by categories from *Forbes Magazine*. First edition.

*Directory of European Associations,* Part 2. National Learned, Scientific and Technical Societies. Gale Research, Detroit (1979).
Covers national associations in continental Europe in all fields of activity. Text is in English, French and German.

*Directory of Federal Health/Medicine Grants and Contacts Programs.* Science and Health Publications, Bethesda, MD (1979).
Grants, fellowships, scholarships, and other forms of financial assistance are listed according to the issuing agency with detailed information on how and where to apply.

*Directory of Research Grants, 1981.* Edited by William K. Wilson and Betty L. Wilson. Oryx Press, Phoenix (1981).
Over 2000 grant programmes are listed, from both government and private sources. The directory includes an excellent bibliography on proposal writing and methods for developing grants.

*The Foundation Center Source Book, 1975/76.* Edited by Terry-Diane Beck and Alexis Teitz Gersumsky, 2 vols. The Foundation Center, New York (1975).
Detailed information on the larger grant-making foundations in the US. There is a profile of activities for each foundation.

*The Foundation Directory,* 8th edn. Edited by Mariana O. Lewis and Alexis Teitz Gersumsky. The Foundation Center, New York (1981).
This biennial publication gives information on non-governmental grant-making foundations in the United States. Included are private foundations with assets of $1 million or more or which gave $100 000 or more in the year of record.

*The Foundation 500.* Edited by David M. Lawson. Douglas M. Lawson Associates, New York (1978).
A loose-leaf volume which gives information on the nation's top 500 foundations and where and to what programmes they give their money.

*The Foundation Grants Index, 1980.* The Foundation Center, New York (1980).
An annual publication which lists grants of $5000 or more awarded to non-profit organizations by major US foundations.

*Foundation Grants to Individuals.* Edited by Carol M. Kurtzig. St Martin's Press, New York (1980).
Scholarships, fellowships, company-sponsored foundations, and employee fund foundations which go directly to individuals and are not channeled through a research institution or non-profit organization.

*The Grant Register, 1981–83.* Edited by Graig Alan Lerner. St Martin's Press, New York (1980).
Intended for students at the graduate and post-doctoral levels

and lists assistance from government agencies and from international, national, and private organizations. Published every two years.

*The International Foundation Directory,* 2nd edn rev. and enl. Consultant Editor, H. V. Hodson. Gale Research, Detroit (1979).
Over 600 foundations divided by country with a subject index.

*McGraw-Hill's Guide to Health Grants and Contracts.* McGraw-Hill, Washington, DC (1978).
A loose-leaf binder, covering 13 broad areas and describing in detail 211 federal programmes.

*Taft Corporate Directory.* 1982 edn completely rev. and updated. Yvette Henry, Editor-in-Chief. Taft Corporation, Washington, DC (1981).
Includes detailed information on 350 corporation foundation files. Updated by a newsletter, *Corporate Updates.*

White, V. *Grants: How to Find Them and What to do Next.* Plenum Press, New York (1975).
An excellent source of information on the grant application process. Includes basic definitions of grants, contracts, fellowships, etc.; sources of information (general); government and foundation grants; how to write a proposal; the application and finding process; follow-up.

*Yearbook of Higher Education, 1981–82.* 13th edn. Marquis, Chicago (1981).
Includes a section on resources, which deals with government funding for student aid and student loans and lists all education-related associations and councils.

## II. Reference sources (government)

*BHPr Support FY 79: Directory of Grants, Awards and Loans.* US Department of Health and Human Services, Public Health Service, Health Resources Administration, Bureau of Health Professions, Bethesda, MD (1981).
Provides detailed information on all support programmes administered by the Bureau of Health Professions. BHPr supports education and training in medicine, nursing, allied health professions, osteopathy, dentistry, optometry, pharmacy, podiatry, veterinary medicine, and public health. Funding is in the form of institutional support, special projects, student loans, scholarships, and research training.

*Catalog of Federal Domestic Assistance.* The office of Management and Budget, Washington, DC (1981).
An annually updated loose-leaf binder covering federal assistance for health programmes in the form of loans, grants, and training. The programmes are listed by agency, with subject and categorical indexes.

*NIH Grants for Training, Construction, Cancer Control, and Medical Libraries.* US Department of Health and Human Services, Public Health Service, National Institutes of Health,

Division of Research Grants, Bethesda, Md (1981). (Fiscal Year 1980 Funds.)
Grants are listed by state with area of training, grant number, and dollar amount.

*NIH Research and Development Contracts,* US Department of Health and Human Services, Public Health Service, National Institutes of Health, Division of Research Grants, Bethesda, Md (1981). (Fiscal Year 1980 Funds.)
Listed by state, with project director, purpose of contract, contract number, and dollar amount.

*NIH Research Grants.* US Department of Health and Human Services, Public Health Service, National Institutes of Health, Division of Research Grants, Bethesda, Md (1980). (Fiscal Year 1980 Funds.)
Grants are listed by geographic area, with information on the awardee (individual and institution), project title, and grant number. Only NIH grants are included, not funds awarded by other Public Health Service agencies.

*Public Health Service Grants and Awards.* US Department of Health. Education and Welfare, Public Health Service, National Institutes of Health, Rockville, Md (1976–77). (Fiscal Year 1976–77 Funds.)
Three volumes cover: Research grants; training, health manpower education, construction and medical libraries; health planning and services grants.

*Research Awards Index, Fiscal Year 1980.* US Department of Health and Human Services, Public Health Service, National Institutes of Health, Division of Research Grants, Bethesda, Md (1980).
A source of information on health research currently conducted by non-federal institutions and supported by the Department of Health and Human Services.

## III. Newsletters

*Corporate Giving Watch/Corporate Updates*
This is amonthly newsletter, put out by the Taft Corporate Information System, which updates the Taft Corporate Directory, giving information on new foundations or foundations which have undergone significant changes since the last publication of the *Directory.* Each issue includes articles which highlight particular corporations and their giving programmes.

*Grantsmanship Center News*
This is a bimonthly newsletter, produced by the Grantsmanship Center, which gives information on non-profit and public agencies, foundations, and corporations.

## IV. Online Databases

CANCERPROJ
Available through the US National Library of Medicine (NLM); produced by the International Cancer Research Data Bank. This database consists of summaries of federally funded cancer research projects and covers the current three fiscal years. The hard copy form, *Special Listing of Current Cancer Research Projects,* is available through the reference Department.

FOUNDATIONS
Available through Lockheed/DIALOG; produced by the Foundation Center. This is the online database that is used to generate three publications: the *Foundation Directory, Foundation Grants Index,* and *National Foundations.* It provides information on the grants awarded by non-governmental and non-profit foundations.

RPROJ (a subfile of TOXLINE)
Available through NLM; produced by the Smithsonian Science Information Exchange.
This is a file of current Toxicology/Epidemiology Research Projects for which the information is supplied by SSIE. It covers federally funded projects from 1979 to 1982, but because the funds for SSIE have been cut, no new information will be added to the file.

SSIE
Available through BRS; produced by the Smithsonian Science Information Exchange. The file gives information on current federally funded research projects in the areas of life, physical, social, behavioural, and engineering sciences. It covers the current three fiscal years; however, as of February 1982, the funding for SSIE was cut and the database will probably be phased out.

USGCA (US Government Contract Awards)
Available through SDC/ORBIT; produced by Washington Representative Services. This covers contract awards that are announced in the *Commerce Business Daily* in the general areas of conservation and energy; education and human development; urban and rural systems; health; safety, regulation and justice; and defense.

## V. Organizations and Agencies (for further information)

THE FOUNDATION CENTER
888 Seventh Avenue
New York, NY 10106

Foundation Center Washington Library
1001 Connecticut Avenue, NY
Washington, DC
(202) 331-1400

The Foundation Center is a non-profit organization which was established to collect information on foundations and the grants they award. In addition to establishing libraries and offices in four cities, the Center puts out several publications including the *Foundation Grants Index Annual, Foundation Grants to Individuals,* and *The Foundation Directory.*

THE GRANTSMANSHIP CENTER
1031 S Grand Avenue
Los Angeles, California 90015
(800) 421-9512

Also a non-profit organization, the purpose of this institution is to train staff members of public and private agencies in fund-raising and grantsmanship through training programmes and seminars. The Grantsmanship Center produces *Grantsmanship Center News*.

TAFT CORPORATE INFORMATION SYSTEM
5125 MacArthur Boulevard
Washington, DC 20016
(202) 966-7086

This is a research company intended to help non-profit organization leaders learn about corporate giving. The Taft Corporate Information System produces the *Taft Corporate Directory, Corporate Updates,* and *Corporate Giving Watch*.

US PUBLIC HEALTH SERVICE,
NATIONAL INSTITUTES OF HEALTH,
DIVISION OF RESEARCH GRANTS
Westwood Building, Room 3A03
Bethesda, Maryland 20014
(301) 496-4000

This is the central office for initial review of scientific grants and for receipt, assignment, and awarding of NIH grants and training programs. The Division of Research Grants also has a storage and retrieval system for NIH grant and contract programmes.

## REFERENCES

Aach, R.D., Szmuness, W., Mosley, J.W., Hollinger, F.B. *et al.* (1981). Serum alanine aminotransferase of donors in relation to the risk of non-A, non-B hepatitis in recipients. The Transfusion-Transmitted Viruses Study. *N. Engl. J. Med.* **304**, 989.

Anon. (1981). Johnson and Johnson offers employees healthy product: live for life. *Health Educ. Rep.* **3**, 3.

Banta, H.D. (1981). Major issues facing biomedical innovation. In *Biomedical innovation* (ed. E.B. Roberts, R.I. Levy, S.N. Finkelstein, J. Moskowitz, and E.J. Sondik) p. 352. MIT Press, Cambridge, MA.

Bone, H.T. (1937). Joint hearing before a Subcommittee of the Committee on Commerce, United States Senate, and a Subcommittee of the Committee on Interstate and Foreign Commerce, United States House of Representatives July 8, 1973. In *Hearing book,* p. 7. Government Printing Office, Washington, DC.

Bordley, J. and Harvey, A.M. (1976). *Two centuries of American medicine, 1776–1976.* Saunders, Philadelphia.

Eaves, G.N. (1972). Who reads your Project-Grant application to the National Institutes of Health? *Fed. Proc.* **31**, 2.

Hatch, O. (1982). Hearing before the Committee on Labor and Human Resources, United States Senate, on the reauthorization of Health Legislation, March 31, 1982. *Hearing book,* p. 2. Government Printing Office, Washington, DC.

John A. Hartford Foundation (1980). *Annual Report.* Hartford Foundation, New York.

Kubiak, M.K. (1980). Coronary risk factor screening in an industrial health management program in Wisconsin. *Wisconsin Med. J.* **79**, 23.

Levy, R.I. (1978). Progress in prevention of cardiovascular disease. *Prev. Med.* **7**, 464.

Levy, R.I. and Moskowitz, J. (1982). Cardiovascular research: decades of progress, a decade of promise. *Science* **217**, 121.

Macek, C. (1982). Acquired immune deficiency syndrome cause(s) still elusive. *JAMA* **248**, 1423.

Moeller, D.W., Pahl, H.B. and Hammond, P.B. (1979). Trends in university environmental health research and training. *Am. J. Publ. Health* **69**, 125.

Neustadt, R.E. and Fineberg, H.V. (1978). *The swine flu affair.* DHEW Pub. No. 017-000-0021-4. Government Printing Office, Washington, DC.

Robert Wood Johnson Foundation (1980). *Annual Report.* Johnson Foundation, Princeton, NJ.

US Centers for Disease Control (1982*a*). Update on acquired immune deficiency syndrome (AIDS) among patients with hemophilia A. *Morbid. Mortal. Weekly Rep.* **31**, 644.

US Centers for Disease Control (1982*b*). Possible transfusion-associated acquired immune deficiency syndrome (AIDS) – California. *Morbid. Mortal. Weekly Rep.* **31**, 652.

US Department of Health and Human Services (1981). *Cardiovascular primer for the workplace.* DHHS Pub. No. (NIH) 81–2210. Government Printing Office, Washignton, DC.

US Department of Health, Education and Welfare (1976). *Report of the President's Biomedical Research Panel, Appendix A. The place of biomedical science in medicine and the state of science.* DHEW Pub. No. (OS) 76-501. Government Printing Office, Washington, DC.

US Department of Health, Education, and Welfare (1978). *DHEW Health Research Principles.* DHEW Pub. No. (NIH) 79-1890. Government Printing Office, Washington, DC.

US Department of Health, Education, and Welfare (1979). *Healthy People: The Surgeon General's Report on Health Promotion and Disease Prevention.* DHEW Pub. No. (PHS) 79-55071. Government Printing Office, Washington, DC.

US Health Care Financing Administration (1982). *Health care financing trends.* HCFA Pub. No. 03140. Government Printing Office, Washington, DC.

US Health Resources Administration (1980). *The Health Planning Program: Citizens Planning for Local Needs.* DHHS Pub. No. (HRA) 80-14018. Government Printing Office, Washington, DC.

US National Cancer Institute (1975). *National Cancer Program Operational Plan, Fy 1976–1980.* I/1-X/30. DHEW Pub. No. (NIH) 75-777. Government Printing Office, Washington, DC.

US National Commission on Research (1980). *Industry and the Universities: Developing Cooperative Research Relationships in the National Interest.* National Commission on Research, Washington, DC.

US National Heart, Lung, and Blood Institute (1978). *Fifth Report of the Director.* DHEW Pub. No. (NIH) 78-1415. Government Printing Office, Washington, DC.

US National Heart, Lung, and Blood Institute (1981). Report of the Working Group on Arteriosclerosis. DHHS Pub. No. (NIH) 81–2034. Government Printing Office, Washington, DC.

US National Institutes of Health (1981). *Basic Data relating to the National Institutes of Health.* DHHS Pub. No. (NIH) 81-1261. Government Printing Office, Washington, DC.

US Senate (1973). *Department of Labor, and Health, Education, and Welfare, and Related Agencies Appropriation Bill.* Senate Rep. No. 92-894. Government Printing Office, Washington, DC.

Waxman, H. (1982). Hearing before the Subcommittee on Health and the Environment of the Committee on Energy and Commerce, United States House of Representatives, on the Health Research Act of 1982, March 29, 1982. In *Hearing book,* p. 267. Government Printing Office, Washington, DC.

Wolverton, C.A. (1948). Comment made on the floor of the United States House of Representatives, June 8, 1948. In *Congressional Record (House),* p. 7405. Government Printing Office, Washington, DC.

# 28 Planning and managing a health service in the United Kingdom

A.H. Snaith

## THE NATIONAL HEALTH SERVICE

Health services in the UK National Health Service (NHS) are governed chiefly by three factors: the historical legacy, the influence of the medical profession, and the level of finance allocated by government.

Both the standards and the volume of hospital provision inherited by the NHS when it was introduced in 1948 varied considerably in different parts of the country. The north and the midlands were relatively disadvantaged compared with London and the south of England. For the first 25 years the chief aim in the hospital sector was to achieve equality of clinical standards throughout the country. Each provincial region had a medical school in its major city. Great emphasis was placed on training hospital specialists in the teaching hospitals and their satellites, under the close supervision of university and associated clinical teachers. Since the financial rewards and the quality of medical and social life were not less attractive away from the main centres, in due course the peripheral hospitals acquired staff of high quality. The general practitioner specialist became a thing of the past and universally accepted standards of hospital care were obtained throughout the country. The medical profession, encouraged by government, played the main part in this transformation, which of course took place during a time of rapid technical advance in medicine. The Royal Colleges (including some that were newly created), represented the different specialties. As well as providing for professional and technical exchange among senior members of the profession, they had the key role in higher specialist training. The medical profession was a radical force in the NHS and the hospital consultant corps its most important asset.

However, although equality of standards was achieved the large variations in the volume of hospital provision continued. This was partly because a government plan for a network of new hospitals was never implemented and partly because pressure for resources from the medical profession has always been exerted at least as effectively in the better provided parts of the country as in the less well provided. The outcome was that growth in each region was at about the same rate, so that although the NHS doubled in size, in parallel with the increase in the GNP, the geographical differences in volume remained.

## NHS management

In 1974 the NHS was reorganized, with a further modification in 1982. The public health departments (which previously had remained under local government) were amalgamated with the hospital service. The present structure is based on the creation of health districts serving defined populations of about 200–400 thousand in most cases. Previously only the public health departments had a responsibility for a population as such; hospitals and general practitioners simply served patients. Each district is governed by a district health authority (DHA) and is managed by a district management team (DMT) of six members: an administrator, a treasurer, a nurse, a community physician, and two active clinicians (one a hospital consultant, one a general practitioner) who serve part-time, normally for two years. A recent NHS Management Inquiry has, however, recommended the appointment of general managers at all levels (Griffiths 1983). Each DHA determines its own management infrastructure for the various units. This includes apparatus to provide advice from the medical, nursing, and other health professions. A statutory Community Health Council for each district represents the consumer interest. Each district has an acute hospital (the district general hospital) and further hospital provision for obstetrics, psychiatry, geriatrics, and mental handicap, together with a medley of small community hospitals, day hospitals, health centres, clinics, and community health staff. The general practitioner service is a branch of the NHS but has remained essentially independent, though in each district it is closely associated with the district health authority.

## Finance

There is no charge to patients for hospital services and virtually the whole of NHS finance is provided by central government from taxation. In 1977 the UK ranked 12th in a list of 15 developed countries in the percentage of GNP it spent on health services. Expenditure per head of population (which has fluctuated between 4 and 6 per cent of the GNP) is about one-third to one-half of that in West Germany, France, Belgium, the Netherlands, and Scandinavia and about the same as in Italy, Austria, and Japan (Maxwell 1981).

At the time of the 1974 reorganization the government

adopted a new financial policy, based on differential allocations to regions according to provision and need. Although the NHS inherited fewer hospitals in the midlands and the north, morbidity and mortality were higher there, so that the previous financial policy was not merely inequitable but perverse. Social class composition is less favourable in the north, the nature of employment is different and the people still bear the physical stigmata of the harsh conditions of earlier times. To take just one example, women are shorter in the north and this influences perinatal mortality rates adversely. A formula was devised to measure need in each region, based on the size of the population, its age and sex structure (which have a major influence on hospital admissions) and on standardized mortality ratios (which were made to serve as a proxy for morbidity). Previously, financial allocations directly reflected provision; the more hospitals and staff in a locality the more money it received to maintain them. The effect of the new method of computation based on population characteristics meant that quite different figures for allocation were derived, not related to current provision. In some regions these figures were higher than current allocations, in other regions, lower. The new figures were therefore identified as targets.

In practice, the historical financial allocations were retained, so that hospitals could continue to function, but a policy of differential growth of income applied, the poorer health authorities receiving more growth than the rich, with the objective of achieving equality, according to need as defined in the formula, over a number of years. The policy is one of levelling up, exactly as had occurred during the first phase of the NHS with respect to clinical standards.

Therefore the position in the NHS now is that each health district has a defined population for which a district health authority is responsible and for which it is financed. Patients move freely across district boundaries according to the hospitals they are referred to by their general practitioners. Since districts frequently provide certain specialist services on behalf of others, cross boundary patient flow is inevitable and financial adjustments are made (some two years in arrear), to reflect net patient imports or exports. Financial growth depends on the relation between the current allocations and the financial target, reset each year, established by the needs formula. While government is responsible for the total volume of finance allocated to the NHS and for national terms and conditions of service for staff, it has little direct influence on the health services given to the public by the districts or on the developments they make. The same three influences are paramount, namely the inheritance, the influence of the medical profession, and the finance available for developments. All three represent the resource approach to health services policy.

## The NHS and planning

When the NHS was created medicine was dominated by advances in technology. Morbid conditions and therapeutic methods were studied exhaustively and the results communicated through the learned societies and the medical literature. It followed that each new advance had to be incorporated

into the provision of services made available to the public, either as an addition or as a replacement for obsolescent methods. The net price of the total change each year represented, in the clinicians mind, the growth required in his or her locality to maintain a modern service. The origins of the 'resource' philosophy lie in the piecemeal development of health services in earlier times. It amounts to identifying priorities for the expenditure of the available new money according to the sectional interests of the local patient populations, as perceived by the district management team, which is influenced predominantly by the medical profession in its district.

The medical profession is an extremely sensitive and effective instrument for determining what developments in health services should take place, to the extent that it endeavours to take into account the scientific issues, seeks to advance along the whole front, and is highly committed to the decision making process in the national health service. (In the UK there is relatively little private practice.) Its methods are rooted in the British tradition of pragmatism, which seeks to avoid the huge mistakes to which macro planning is susceptible. The problem is that medical practitioners are not equipped to evaluate policy issues except in terms of the individual patient, or at most, groups of patients with particular clinical conditions. Social perspectives and indeed, the public interest, do not come within its competence. To adopt a policy of providing the most advanced technical treatment and extended care for every patient considered as an individual, is the medical equivalent of the religious ethic of the western world, which (rightly) counts a single life as valuable as an infinite number. This principle is in direct contradiction with the interests of the body politic, interests which in the medical sphere find expression through epidemiology, in numbers.

The public and its elected representatives have become increasingly aware that, over time, the improved health of the population has largely been due to economic factors rather than to health services. The objective of curing the acutely ill by modern techniques does not have quite the importance in the public mind that it had when the NHS was established. On the other hand, the chronically ill, the elderly, the mentally ill and the handicapped are felt to be an increasing burden by their families, who therefore look more to the NHS and other social services for support. Thus there is a conflict for resources between the kind of developments in high-technology medicine favoured by most hospital doctors, in which the overriding concern is the individual, and public pressure for services which provide for the care of large numbers of dependant people.

There are, of course, a number of different approaches to health services policy. Resource planning is restricted to the provision of finance, staff, and facilities. There are however greater variations in outputs than in resources among the English regions. The information systems used by the NHS are currently under review, presumably with the object of influencing all authorities to achieve the same efficiency, in output terms, as those which are most cost-effective. More important still is outcome planning, based on the assessment of needs and the evaluation of the benefits of medical interventions and of health care. Both output and outcome planning involve consideration of the population as a whole, precisely what the new structure of the NHS is designed to facilitate. Unfortunately, despite the increasing interest among epidemiologists, social scientists, health economists and others, in the delivery and effectiveness of health services (health services research), many studies in the non-acute care sector of medicine have relied on the construction of artificial criteria of needs or benefit. These disguise value judgements not less subjective than those of clinicians who press for investment in their own specialties. A major example of this is the *Report on inequalities in health,* 'the Black Report' (DHSS 1981), which, from a review of the literature, was able to demonstrate unequivocally that greater mortality and morbidity rates obtain among people in the lower socio-economic classes of the population. However, the remedies proposed by the authors of the Report, chiefly redistribution of income through taxation in favour of families with young children, together with better services for pregnant women, children, the elderly and the handicapped, merely reflect their personal views. No convincing evidence was presented (or was available) that such measures would influence the observed mortality rates.

The chief impediment to the rational planning of health services lies not in the structure of the NHS and its management, as politicians have supposed, but in lack of knowledge about the influence of health services on the health of the population as a whole and subgroups within it. The fundamental work on provision, needs and outcomes remains to be done. For this reason district management teams are not able to advance beyond the use of information about average provision throughout the country – the so called norms – as a guide to investment policy, together with general policy documents issued by the DHSS or the professional bodies, all of which are simply advisory in character and apt to express a neutral position on issues about which there is more than one clinical view. The decisions of a district management team remain overwhelmingly under the influence of the attitudes of doctors in its district.

### The community physician

The community physician was a new creation at the time of the reorganization of the management of the NHS in 1974. Hospital medical administrators, medical officers of health from the previous public health service and epidemiologists in universities and research units united to form a new specialty, with its own higher qualifications granted by a new Faculty of Community Medicine of the Royal Colleges of Physicians. Training is based on epidemiology, health services administration and the social sciences. Every DHA must employ one community physician as a member of its management team, usually supported by several others. The first responsibility placed on community physicians is to 'keep under review the health care needs of the population and initiate special studies and research' (DHSS 1972). Their primary function is to plan health services, taking into account not only clinical issues but the broader public interest, including epidemiological and social perspectives of health, prevention, health education, and problems arising from the implementation of health

policies in a locality because of professional and public pressures. Thus, community physicians working in the NHS are uniquely placed, because of their role in management, to ensure that the outcome of an investigation is not just a report or the publication of a paper, but effective action. Given the absence of an established methodology for health service planning, however, it is difficult to adopt an epidemiological approach to planning and to avoid lapsing into routine institutional administration, which in practice may be more concerned with the competing claims for resources of clinicians in the different branches of medicine than with the functional performance of the service as it affects the public. In Bristol the aim of the community physicians has been to contribute to management functions not just by resource planning but by undertaking studies on outputs, needs and outcomes. These studies include collaboration with consultants and other health staff in a variety of trials. If health authorities generally adopt this approach it seems reasonable to expect a corpus of knowledge to emerge about investment in health services and the effects of this on the health of populations. The next section describes some of the work of the Bristol unit.

### THE BRISTOL COMMUNITY MEDICINE UNIT: AN EXAMPLE OF A PLANNING INSTRUMENT

The staff of the Bristol unit was the normal complement provided by the NHS, but the opportunity was taken to ensure the appointment to community medicine posts, or associated administrative posts, of those who had relevant experience of health services research. In addition, one or two research assistants were appointed on short-term contracts with soft money, so that on average there were about a dozen graduate staff: four community physicians, two or three trainee registrars, two administrative staff with PhD or similar qualifications in the social sciences, a computer manager, and the research assistants. Given this level of staffing plus active support and encouragement from administrative, finance, and nursing colleagues, it is difficult to accept that community physicians in the NHS lack the necessary capability to undertake the R & D function. Too often management thinking in the NHS is limited to the concept of buying expertise from outside, from universities or government funded research units, or choosing between advice from different groups of experts. This philosophy underlies the resource approach to planning, i.e. acceptance by management that its function is simply to provide resources, while leaving outputs and outcomes to clinicians without regard to an overall strategy. The Bristol community medicine unit has endeavoured to undertake studies, in collaboration with clinicians, which would examine the merits of different policies and influence management decisions accordingly. There is a categorical imperative for community physicians to give a lead here both to their management and their clinical colleagues. Resource, output, and outcome planning are all required if the best use is to be made of the resources we have and developments of services no longer based on the expectation of continued growth.

## Studies

The key problem in health services planning is the difference in approach between doctors, who tackle specific clinical problems, predominantly at the level of the individual patient, and that of the health authorities and their mangers, who must make decisions about resource allocation between different sectors of health care in accordance with what is felt to be the public interest – and who should therefore attempt to take output and outcome issues into account. The aim of the unit has been to try to bridge this gap and the studies described below are examples of initiatives taken by the unit with this object. At the same time, resource planning has proceeded as in any other health authority. On the one hand services have been reconstructed on general policy grounds, e.g. improvement of community services with a reduction in the numbers of hospital residents in the long-stay sector; on the other hand, every opportunity has been taken to collaborate with clinicians in a wide variety of investigations. These include the involvement of the unit's epidemiologists in work of interest to them but somewhat distinct from health services research strictly defined. For example, a longitudinal study is being conducted of aetiological factors in coronary thrombosis, based on observations made during the surveillance of an unselected population in a clinic which provides health checks for its surrounding community and acts as a population laboratory (Bainton et al. 1982; Baker et al. 1982). Another group of studies on immunization levels in the child population is carried out with the National Institute of Biological Standards and Control (Bainton et al. 1979). But chiefly, collaborative studies with clinicians have attempted to find a rationale for services and their development, in both clinical and resource terms. Some have been concerned with precise clinical issues, others with ascertaining needs, the outcome of surveillance systems, or the quality of care.

The following account of some of the studies undertaken in the unit illustrates different categories of activity.

## STUDIES OF PROVISION

### Surgical operations

The most publicized problem in the NHS is the length of the queue and the waiting time for admission to hospital. The official figures relate almost exclusively to cold surgery. All acute surgical patients, about half the total number of surgical patients, are admitted immediately. They include major surgical catastrophies, accidents, cancer, and similarly urgent cases. There is no waiting list for acute medicine but geriatric, psychiatric, and chronically disabled patients do have difficulty in obtaining all the services they require.

A study of the provision of cold surgery in England found that waiting was associated with one variable and two constants (Buttery and Snaith 1979). The size of the overall national queue varied directly, not inversely, with the number of surgeons employed. Between 1959 and 1976 the numbers of surgeons increased by 49 per cent and the numbers in the queue increased by 43 per cent. The waiting list size per surgeon, on average, was a constant, $145 \pm 7$. Waiting time

was also a constant; in the different regions 59–69 per cent of patients were operated on within three months of being put on the waiting list for admission, 77–87 per cent within six months and 89–96 per cent within one year.

It is evident from this information that waiting lists cannot be reduced by simple increase in provision. (If they could the belief attributed to the founders of the NHS, that health problems would gradually diminish if treatment was provided free to the population, would be true.) It was calculated that theoretically waiting time in Bristol could be halved by an increase in the provision of operations of 9.5 per cent. Such an objective could be reached in five years simply by increasing the number of operations pro-rata with average financial growth. In fact this would not happen because the number of patients coming forward for surgery would more than keep pace with increasing provision. Health service managers have to come to terms with a system which is not static, a finite volume of morbidity being addressed by an inadequate volume of resources, but dynamic, as in an economic model, supply and demand being related, albeit directly, not inversely.

Further analysis showed that the supply of operations per unit of population in the different specialties varied between regions by a factor of about two, a ratio which dwarfs apparent shortfalls in provision. The numbers of surgeons employed and the numbers of operations each did on average, also varied to a similar degree, with little relation between finance and output in terms of numbers of operations. When output figures were compared with finance (allocated in accordance with 'needs' by the finance formula) it was possible to ascertain whether a region was providing more or less operations than its revenue could sustain. Thus an objective basis for planning was elucidated – not as a determinator of resource allocation, for it is not suggested that this should exactly reflect financial provision, but as a point of departure for rational planning (Buttery and Snaith 1980).

### Psychotropic drug prescribing in general practice

Psychotropic drugs are one of the most frequently prescribed classes of drugs and there is increasing concern about their abuse and misuse. They account for 20 per cent of all prescriptions in the NHS and are taken by some 15 per cent of the population. It must be questioned whether the net effect of this therapeutic activity is beneficial or whether the most important consequence is iatrogenic drug dependency.

In collaboration with the University of Bristol Department of Mental Health and an inner city general practice, a register of patients who were receiving prescriptions for psychotropic drugs was established. A random sample of patients receiving these drugs was then interviewed together with a group of age and sex matched controls. The third stage of the project was the evaluation of alternative (i.e. non-drug) forms of management for this group of patients as a way of helping them, without resorting to the use of psychotropic drugs.

Both 'hard' and 'soft' data were combined to answer questions about who received scripts of this type, the pattern of the prescribing, and the reasons given by both patients and doctors. No attempt was made to look at compliance and 'script' receiving is the term used rather than drug taking.

## Quantitative data

A register of patients receiving prescriptions for antidepressants, hypnotics, and tranquillizers was created by means of carbons attached to all the prescriptions written by the general practitioners. These were sorted into psychotropic and other drugs, and the prescriptions coded in some detail. Two complete years of this information was collected so that prescribing could be examined against the background of the age/sex file of the practice. This updated file provides denominators which make possible a number of calculations.

Thus second and subsequent prescriptions can be related to the individual and sex and age specific rates derived for those who received this group of drugs, 'incident' cases defined, seasonal fluctuations in prescribing followed and so on.

The register therefore provides a basis for initiating methods of intervention and for evaluating the outcome of such intervention.

## Qualitative data

The collection of this information was based on an ethnography of patients receiving this group of drugs. In-depth interviews were designed to explore patients' perceptions of their medication, and their explanations for beginning and continuing their drug-taking careers. Their views of the doctors and of themselves was explored. Typologies of reasons for drug taking have been produced from these data with a view to providing sufficient understanding of the relevant factors to generate hypotheses which might be tested by appropriate interventions directed to reducing drug dependency.

Sixty patients were interviewed at home by two interviewers. Thirty respondents were chosen by random sample from the register of script receivers and the other half were sampled according to various criteria, stratifying for factors such as age, sex, and length of time of drug taking. The use of ethnography to explore the meaning to the patients of drug taking was adopted after a pilot study using structured interviews with a questionnaire had been tried. This was found to provide a less complete account of why people began getting these drugs and why they continued to seek them. For looking at reported behaviour and beliefs about drugs, the ethnography approach seemed more flexible and effective. Data collected in this way on reported behaviour augments the data on behaviour observed by means of the register.

The other aspect of the qualitative method looked at prescribing practices. Interviews with the general practice personnel included seven general practitioners, the community psychiatric nurse, the practice receptionists, and the health visitors. Attempts were made to elicit the attitudes of the staff towards emotional problems, 'mental illness', and drug use. These data were compared with the patients' accounts and the drug register.

The issue of psychotropic drug prescribing and receiving defies a simplistic research method. A dual research strategy was therefore employed in an attempt to deal with the complex behaviour of the patients; that is, observing what drugs were prescribed, on the one hand; on the other hand, enquiring into what was said to be happening by both the prescribers and the patients.

## STUDIES OF NEEDS

### Functional limitations in the elderly

In this study an estimate is being made of functional limitations in men and women aged 75 years or more, with a view to assessing the services they require and the extent to which these are being met at the present time. The emphasis is on functional limitation in daily life as distinct from physical disability or disease as ascertained in the clinic. The population chosen was that of a local government district.

The majority of elderly people in the study area live in their own homes; some live in local authority provided elderly person's housing (EPH), a proportion of which are supervised by a resident warden although most are unsupervised; and some live in residential care accommodation. All elderly people, irrespective of domicile, have access through the NHS to the whole range of community health services, including general practitioners and home nurses. Home help, meals-on-wheels, and similar provision is made by the local authority social services department or by voluntary bodies. However, the provision of services depends on needs, demand and availability which fluctuate over time, and about which information is rarely available to service providers in a consistent form.

### Objectives of the study

These were to describe: the functional ability of a representative sample of people aged 75 years and over who live in the community, in terms of mobility, self care, and domestic activities; the health and social services that are provided to that sample; the effects, as far as possible, of health and social services in influencing the functional ability of the sample; and to estimate the resources required to make good any shortfall in provision and the feasibility of applying a standardized assessment procedure to ascertain requirements and guide service provision.

The study population consists of the following samples of the population residing in the district.

1. A randomly drawn sample of 188 people aged 75 years and over who live at home and are on the lists of one of the 40 general practitioners in the district. The sampling frame is the Family Practitioner Committee (FPC) age/sex register.

2. A randomly drawn sample of 188 people aged 75 years and over living in EPHs run by the local authority housing department and which have no wardens.

3. An exactly similar sample from EPHs with wardens.

4. All those aged 75 years and over, 110 in number, who live in the three local authority old people's homes (Part III homes) in the district.

The total study population numbers 600. It was necessary to stratify the samples so that sufficient males were selected to allow sex comparisons.

### The questionnaire

The main instrument, that which measures functional limitation, is derived from the St. Thomas's Hospital Health Services Research Unit Services for the Elderly Questionnaire (Dunt *et al.* 1980). There are two important features:

1. It measures actual function (asking 'do you, e.g. walk indoors) rather than possible performance ('can you, etc.').

2. It uses two trichotomous scales ( (i)–(iii) and a–c) as shown in Table 28.1.

It can therfore be determined whether the use of aids to daily living and personal services (a home help perhaps, or a relative) improves the functional ability of any respondent. The figures in Table 28.1 relate to the proportion of the

**Table 28.1.** *Example of the format of questions in the functional limitations questionnaire*

| Question | Results (from development study) |
|---|---|
| 'Do you, e.g. walk indoors?' | |
| (i) Unassisted | |
| (a) with no difficulty | 61.3% |
| (b) with difficulty or sometimes | 16.1% |
| (c) completely unable | 22.6% |
| (ii) Using an aid | |
| (a) with no difficulty | 74.2% |
| (b) with difficulty or sometimes | 19.4% |
| (c) completely unable | 6.4% |
| (iii) With help from another person | |
| (a) with no difficulty | 75.3% |
| (b) with difficulty or sometimes | 22.6% |
| (c) completely unable | 2.2% |

sample who co-operated in the pilot study of the questionnaire, who actually walked indoors. It will be seen that 22.6 per cent did not walk if unassisted, 6.4 per cent did not even with an aid and that 2.2 per cent did not when helped. However, even with help, 22.6 per cent had difficulty. This spectrum can be reported both for the whole study population and for sub-groups.

The instrument has been piloted on a sample of the elderly and is known to have acceptable repeatability. In addition, concurrent validity was established by comparing the responses with assessment made by service providers (a general practitioner and a health visitor) who knew the respondents. The two data sets closely corresponded for the mobility functions but were less concordant for the domestic functions. However, the questionnaire enquires about actual performance not (as in the assessments) what the respondents should be doing. In terms of daily life, this is perhaps more relevant.

A further factor which is important in the description of dependency levels among the elderly is that of mental state. The Cape Cognitive Assessment Scale (Pattie and Gilleard 1976), which is known to be reliable and is quick and easy to administer, is used in addition to the main questionnaire.

*Method*

The analysis has concentrated on summary statistics of functional ability and service provision to the elderly in the district; the relationship between functional ability and provision of services, both formal and informal, among the elderly in each of the four living settings; a comparison of the effect of different types of formal services provision on functional ability, controlling for various factors such as the

extent and quality of informal assistance, type of dwelling, etc.; and estimates of resources used by the elderly in the district both at the time of the study and in the event of any future shift in the overall degree of dependency of people living in each of the four living settings.

## EVALUATION OF A TREATMENT OR INSTRUMENT

### The management of acute head injury

Studies on the current use of computerized tomography in relation to head injuries in different hospitals in England and Wales and the prognosis of head injuries admitted to a regional neurosurgery unit are being undertaken with neurosurgeons (Baker 1982). Severe head injuries may result in death, vegetative states, severe disability, and lesser forms of disability. Surgical intervention may in some cases only sustain life at a vegetative or severly disabled level. This presents not just a tragic problem for the patients and their families but long-term nursing problems for the health service. The ability to predict the probable outcome from the presenting characteristics of the injured patient may assist management. While substantial research has been carried out on this, the characteristics employed in studies have been those existing at least six hours post-injury. However, the decision to ventilate and thereby sustain a patient for a considerable period has often been taken shortly after presentation at the hospital.

*Prospective study*

The basic objectives of studies in Bristol, in collaboration with the neurosurgeons, is to decrease mortality without an increase in the number of patients left in a vegetative state or otherwise very severely disabled; to decrease existing levels of vegetative or otherwise severe disability; and to compare outcomes with other centres. In developing a new policy, a prospective study was chosen giving consideration to the following points:

● cases should be selected for the main range of outcomes of interest, e.g. low on the Glasgow Coma Scale;

● the timing of assessment: the earlier the assessment, the greater the difficulty in predicting future outcome, but if decisions over ventilation are taken early, assessment will have to be early;

● the characteristics of cases to be assessed with emphasis on those variables demonstrated in other studies as being the main predictors of outcome states, together with additional variables present on earlier assessment;

● outcome assessment should be made in a standardized manner after three months and six months;

● the need for an estimation of the numbers of cases required for predictions of outcome to be possible in accordance with the conventional limits of statistical confidence.

Such an approach should give some indication of the possibility of predicting certain outcome states on the basis of different assessment characteristics and the order of error in the predictions. Existing studies suggest the possibility of predicting outcomes correctly in about 70 per cent of fairly severe head injuries, with an error within these predictions of about 10 per cent. The limitations on predicting outcomes should influence how far it is possible to adopt a particular policy for ventilation.

### Retrospective study

While predictive associations for outcomes of head injury are best established from prospective studies of unselected patients, such studies are time-consuming. A retrospective approach may therefore be adopted, using consecutive cases of admissions, if information has been recorded in a comprehensive and standardized manner and outcomes are known. A small feasibility study is being undertaken to determine whether such a retrospective approach will be possible for head injury admissions.

The procedure is to obtain from hospital activity analysis data (HAA) routinely recorded, a listing of consecutive head injury admissions for one year, under the relevant ICD rubrics, together with a copy of each patient's record. These records will make it possible to determine the frequency with which the coma scale, pupil reactions, eye movements, reflexes and power in limbs, are used as indicators by clinicians to monitor patients in the first 24 hours after admission. The frequency with which alcohol or other drugs contributed to the initial characteristics on presentation, and the time and levels of earliest BP, haematocrit, $P_{O_2}$ and $P_{CO_2}$ recordings, will be ascertained. An assessment will be made as to whether the initial clinical examination is the 'best' or 'worst' state of the patient in comparison with subsequent examinations within the first 24 hours.

So also will the outcome at three and six months or at date of last entry into the clinical notes, that is, death; vegetative state (total dependence); severe disability (independent for basic functions); or full recovery. If such information has been reliably recorded in the clinical notes and the records required are available, it should be possible to estimate predictive associations between entry characteristics of patients and outcomes.

### Photorefractive vision screening in infants

The importance of identifying vision defects in pre-school children is well recognized and vision screening programmes are implemented to this end. Traditional ophthalmic testing is geared to the communicative and co-operative child who thus needs to be about three years of age for reliable results. It is only at this age or when overt vision defects present, that they are being detected.

Strabismus and amblyopia are the commonest visual disorders in early childhood and estimates of prevalence in the pre-school years vary between 4 per cent and 14 per cent (Oliver and Nawratzki 1971). Scientific and clinical evidence on the plasticity of the visual system suggest that these disorders should be identified and treated as early as possible, to prevent a reduction in visual acuity and binocular function.

Early hypermetropia and severe astigmatism appear to persist up to the age of three years and these early refractive errors correlate with the development of squint or amblyopia 2-3 years later (Ingram *et al.* 1979).

A new simple and rapid technique – isotropic photorefraction – has been developed initially in an academic setting as a research tool by Atkinson and Braddick in Cambridge (Atkinson and Braddick 1971; Braddick *et al.* 1979). It can be applied to children of any age and therefore offers the possibility of large-scale screening of infants for refractive errors. In this technique three flash photographs of the infant's eyes taken from a distance of 75 cm give an estimate of refraction. Trials of photorefraction, alongside an ophthalmologist's and an optician's retinoscopic infant refractions, have shown a consistent relationship between photorefractive and retinoscopic measures.

Two kinds of questions must be answered before any screening programme could be considered for widespread adoption. First, how well does the photorefractive screening work in the field, in the sense of being a valid, reliable, and economic procedure to pick out infants with significant refractive errors? Secondly, what benefit is there in picking out such infants at an early age?

A study was set up by the Bristol unit in collaboration with the Cambridge workers in 1980, to answer the first question. It was based on the original research of Drs J. Atkinson and O.J. Braddick in Cambridge. With their assistance and that of orthoptists and ophthalmologists at Bristol Eye Hospital the study was undertaken in four health centres in Bristol. Three aspects of the screening procedure were tested:

1. The proportion of a total population who would attend for screening.

2. The feasibility of the procedure being carried out in the field by non-research personnel, i.e. orthoptists.

3. The consistency of the relationship between photorefractive and ophthalmological retinoscopy carried out by different personnel.

### Evaluation of the technique as an early screening procedure on a total population

The community medicine unit's child health computer was used to estimate numbers of the study population attached to various health centres. Four health centres were then selected which had appropriate numbers to facilitate an adequate total sample size for the feasibility and pilot study to be carried out over a twelve-month period. All six-month-old infants attached to those health centres were identified from the computer register and invited to attend for vision screening. The programming was carried out by the child-health-services computer personnel. It was anticipated, and has subsequently been proven, in the pilot study, that the attendance rate at this early age would be approximately 90–95 per cent, whereas at a later age of 3.5 years the attendance may be only 40 per cent.

The benefits of initiating such a project from a unit of community medicine within the NHS, include easy access to the child-health-services computer as a data base for initial estimates of numbers, for the actual programming and call up to be undertaken, and co-operation and support for the project from administrative and clinical staff.

Community orthoptists, already in posts within the NHS, were trained to carry out the technique. Written protocols and instructions were provided on the use of equipment and the procedure to be adopted and the research personnel from

Cambridge undertook individual training at the initial screening sessions. Orthoptists need only a few sessions to master the necessary skills and have subsequently trained a further three community orthoptists to carry out the technique.

The orthoptists were also trained to interpret results and to pick out infants with refractive errors according to criteria previously agreed with the ophthalmologists. Again a few initial training sessions were all that were required for orthoptists to recognize the major visual disorders, and concordance between those identified by the independant observers (i.e. orthoptists in Bristol and research personnel in Cambridge) on a double-masked approach has been extremely good.

The categories of infants with visual disorders identified by the technique include hypermetropes, myopes, anisometropes, astigmats, and any physical defects (e.g. cataracts and congenital squint), all selected according to prescribed criteria. A group of infants with no defects were also selected at random. All these categories of infants were called for orthoptic testing and ophthalmological retinoscopy, and the concordance between the class of anomaly detected by photorefraction and that by retinoscopy were in close agreement. From these data the specificity and sensitivity of the screening method can be measured.

Any infant requiring immediate treatment has received this; others are being followed to ascertain the natural history of the various visual problems detected in a sample of children of adequate size to produce statistically valid results. This will require follow-up until traditional ophthalmic testing can estimate the infants' visual acuity accurately (usually aged about three years).

The second question, evidence of benefit, must also be answered and the longer term aim is to investigate the predictability of strabismus and amblyopia from hypermetropic and anisometropic infants. An intervention study is being set up, in the form of a randomized controlled trial, to test the hypothesis that spectacle correction in hypermetropic infants can prevent the development of strabismus and amblyopia in the pre-school years.

The project thus has two interlocked purposes. Early vision screening is only of value if the disorders detected can be treated and are better treated at an early age: this depends on the answer to the scientific question of whether refractive corrections can prevent strabismus and amblyopia. Conversely, this scientific question can only be answered by instituting a trial vision screening programme, in order to detect the children believed to be at risk. The study will also aid the evaluation of the optimal approach to vision screening in the pre-school years.

## Ultrasound and peripheral artery disease

In the community screening programme an unselected adult population is screened routinely by a system of health checks. Screening is organized in such a way that longitudinal studies can be carried out to establish the value of the surveillance of the health of adults and of the clinical techniques employed, and at the same time enable measurements of value in clinical medicine to be established in a normal population.

In this study the unit has been able to assist research being undertaken on peripheral artery disease by Bristol University Department of Surgery and the University Hospital Department of Medical Physics. The object is to measure arterial stiffness by an ultrasound method. The tests were carried out on unselected subjects attending for health checks to determine normal values. Some of the subjects present with arterial disease while others develop symptoms or signs over time and are identified at subsequent health checks. Over 1500 subjects have been tested in this longitudinal study.

## EVALUATION OF A SERVICE

### Urinary incontinence

Urinary incontinence in women is a common clinical problem particularly in those aged 65 years and over. For many women in this age group active procedures may be inappropriate and an integral part of the conservative management of such patients includes the use of a pant and pad system as a way of keeping the patient dry. Comparisons of the effectiveness of different types of pants and pads are few and have been carried out in a laboratory setting or for short-term periods in a hospital ward. In collaboration with the incontinence research unit directed by Mr R.C.L. Feneley a comparative trial was therefore carried out in a domiciliary setting of two types of pants and pads, with the object of making it possible to offer patients the most acceptable and economic system (Bainton *et al.* 1982).

### Method

The trial design was of a 'cross-over' type where each patient was asked to wear one particular pant/pad combination for four weeks, after which she tried the second 'system' for a further four weeks. The sequence of the two types of pants and pads for an individual was determined on a random basis.

A questionnaire was administered to all patients at the end of the fourth and the eighth week. This sought patients' answers to questions about the effectiveness of the pants and pads to keep them dry and also their views on the comfort and acceptability of the products. A five-point scale of answers was offered for a series of questions. Also, in an attempt to provide at least a partial check in the consistency of answers offered by the patients, a final question asked them to show their overall opinion of the pants and pads by placing an X on a 10 cm line, whose poles were recorded as the extremes of satisfaction and dissatisfaction. Distances were then measured from one pole, and within-patient distances compared for the different pants and pads. The problem of inter-patient variation, for example, in thresholds of comfort, were overcome by making use of the comparisons of the ranked statements for the different pants and pads on a within-patient basis, and by the use of a 10 cm line analogue to provide supportive data to the answers obtained for the ranked statements.

Many of the judgements made by patients in this study were inevitably subjective. However, patients perceptions, together with their expectations, are likely to determine their satisfaction with medical care – the crucial issue in a complaint like incontinence.

### Incontinence in elderly persons homes

A related project is investigating the allegedly high prevalence of urinary incontinence in elderly persons homes provided by social services departments. A study has been carried out with the object of confirming or refuting that prevalance rates in the homes are high. Every episode of incontinence was logged in a defined census week.

In conjunction with this, senior care officers and a one-in-two random sample of care staff were interviewed to determine their understanding and perceptions of incontinence. The intention is to use this information as a basis for devising an intervention strategy.

### Speech therapy for acquired aphasia

Speech therapy belongs to those specialties, ancillary to medicine, in which the therapies employed may not have a securely established scientific basis. Chiropody and occupational therapy are other examples. Nevertheless, speech therapists are employed in substantial numbers in NHS hospitals. Attempts to evaluate speech therapy have had methodological weaknesses, e.g. selection of patients, lack of controls, unrealistic amounts of treatment, or the use of non-comparable control and treatment groups.

In this study (David et al. 1982) the question posed was whether any improvement associated with speech therapy for stroke patients was the result of the specific skill and experience a speech therapist has acquired, or was a consequence of the general stimulation and support most therapeutic relationships provide. To this end the outcome in two groups of patients was compared; one group received conventional speech therapy from trained therapists, the other stimulation and support from untrained volunteers.

A test of repeatability of the outcome measures employed was first undertaken, followed by a six months pilot trial to test the feasibility of a randomized controlled trial. The pilot gave no evidence to suggest that patients allocated to a volunteer therapist were at a disadvantage.

To obtain sufficient numbers of cases multicentre collaboration was essential. A total of 14 centres were recruited to participate with Bristol hospitals in the trial and the study ran for three years.

All patients referred for speech therapy with a clinical diagnosis of stroke complicated by aphasia were eligible for the study and were entered three weeks after the stroke to allow for spontaneous recovery.

Assessments to determine the severity of the initial aphasia, the prognosis of the patient within treatment (by either group), and the post-treatment outcome, were all carried out using the Functional Communication Profile. Scores in five different areas of communicative function were recorded, weighted and converted to an overall percentage of the patient's estimated previous communicative ability. The assessing therapist was never the treating therapist.

### Development delay in infants

At the beginning of the century, serious concern about the health and education of the population was expressed in the UK. This was due to the discovery that a high percentage of young men were unfit for service in the armed forces. The consequence was the introduction of maternity and infant welfare clinics for the whole population, directed particularly at the industrial poor.

Health authorities still provide surveillance systems for infants, even though the introduction of the national health service provides every family with a practitioner whose services are free. The cost of this service is perhaps £200 million per annum or roughly 2 per cent of the cost of the NHS and the problem, as so often in preventive medicine in particular, is to demonstrate evidence of positive benefit. Over the last two decades efforts have been made to rest the case for infant surveillance systems on the premise that their purpose is the early detection of delay in physical or mental development, with the object of providing remedial medical and educational intervention, including support and reassurance for the parents.

An appropriate test of the effectiveness of early detection and treatment of developmental delay is the influence therapeutic intervention has on subsequent educational attainment. A prospective study is therefore in progress which aims to assess the association between developmental delay and behaviour disorders in 3½-year-old children with subsequent persistant poor performance in the school years. A screening instrument employed and used in a standard manner by the clinic doctors has been constructed and piloted. Reliability is tested by arranging for a number of infants to be examined twice, on two separate occasions by two different doctors, with a two-week interval. The concurrent validity of the screening is established by comparing the results obtained in a population sample screened in the infant surveillance clinics, with the results obtained by a paediatrician, speech therapist, and a nursery school teacher. Children with developmental delay or behavioural disturbance, together with a similar number matched for age and sex and judged not to have a problem, are examined by these specialists to enable their results to be compared with those obtained in the surveillance clinics.

The assessment contains four developmental sections – physical, play, language and social – together with a behavioural assessment. Development and behaviour are scored by the specialist on a four-point scale, to determine the level of true and false positive and negative associations with the scores obtained in the clinics.

If the screening has acceptable validity, the prevalence of developmental delay and behavioural problems in the population sample will become available. Subsequent steps will include cohort follow-up for predictive association with educational or social disadvantage; ascertainment of the efficiency of screening (i.e. effectiveness and compliance); and intervention studies aimed at cure, or care and containment, of language or behaviour problems and other difficulties. Assessments of the infants when they reach school age will be made by teachers and other staff employed by the education authority.

## HEALTH POLICY AND RESEARCH AND DEVELOPMENT

In Bristol, as elsewhere in the NHS, a ten-year strategic plan and a series of three-year rolling operational plans were devised in collaboration with administrator, finance, and nurse colleagues and in part implemented. These plans were concerned chiefly with resources and were of local interest. They have not been described here. Management will never advance, by planning of that kind, beyond a resource relationship with clinicians – 'give them the tools and they will do the job'. The two important questions are: what levels of resources will optimize outputs?; and what should investment be in the different sectors of health care? Special studies are required to address these questions. No one health authority or community medicine unit can provide all the answers and a variety of solutions may have equal validity. The work of the units must find expression in the policies their authorities adopt so that the effectiveness of different policies can be compared. While the contribution of university and DHSS-funded health services research is of course important, far more emphasis should be put on output and outcome planning by the health authorities themselves. Not just community physicians but health economists, statisticians, and social scientists should be employed by them to work on these problems together with clinicians and health service managers. A methodology for the R & D function in the NHS has yet to be worked out.

Projects generated jointly by management staff and clinicians will comprise a spectrum, clinical at one pole, managerial at the other, but mostly mixed in character. Unless community physicians are prepared to become immersed in clinical problems they cannot expect their clinical colleagues to take an interest in investment problems – which they must if they are to remain a radical force in the NHS and not withdraw into technological ivory towers. In Bristol the community medicine unit originated some projects, clinicians others, but, in nearly all, the unit had the major responsibility for research design and research management. The two studies concerned with provision examined national outputs (surgical operations) in the one case and local practice (psychotropic drugs) in the other. The study of the needs of the elderly may provide some general lessons but it was essentially of interest to those responsible for designing local services. Probably it should be replicated by each authority. The evaluation projects were of both general and local interest; not least important was the influence they had in bringing the clinicians and the community physicians into working relationships, so that they could begin to appreciate each others perspectives. The projects which were concerned with the evaluation of a service demonstrate that services cannot simply be left to clinicians to organize; other skills are required and other values are involved than those associated with clinical practice.

Hitherto, NHS policy has been concerned with levelling up – first clinician standards, subsequently volumes of provision. In future, the NHS will not be dominated, as it has been in the past, by the inheritance it obtained in 1948. With the restructuring of the management of the service in 1974 and in 1982, the scene is set for an attack on the objectives of health services in evaluative terms. The problem is how to replace the incremental extension of services that has previously dominated NHS policy by the implementation by health authorities of identified levels of provision for their populations, and in such a way that the effects of different policies by different authorities can be compared. The R & D function is the means by which this transformation can be brought about and it means health authorities taking an active interest in applied research. This is the next stage in the development of the national health service.

*Acknowledgements*

I should like to thank the following for accounts of projects undertaken in the unit: Sue Atkinson, I.A. Baker, D. Bainton, A.C. Brown, R.B. Buttery, Rachel David, Pam Enderby, R.C.L. Feneley, Lesley Jones, A.R. Maw, H.G. Morgan, and K.F.H. Morgan.

## REFERENCES

Atkinson, J. and Braddick, O.J. (1979). New techniques for assessing vision in infants and young children. *Child Care Health Dev.* **5**, 389.

Bainton, D., Blannin, J.B., and Sheppard, A.M. (1982). Pads and pants for urinary incontinence. *Br. Med. J.* **285**, 419.

Bainton, D., Freeman, M., Magrath, D.I., Sheffield, E., and Smith, J.W.G. (1979). Immunity of children to diphtheria, tetanus and poliomyelitis. *Br. Med. J.* **i**, 854.

Bainton, D., Burns-Cox, C.J., Elwood, P.C., Lewis, B., Miller, N.E., Morgan, K., and Sweetnam, P.M. (1982). Prevalence of ischaemic heart disease and associations with serum lipoproteins in subjects aged 45–64 years – the Speedwell study. *Br. Heart J.* **47**, 483.

Baker, I.A. (1982). Availability of computerised tomography for the management of head injuries in England and Wales. *Br. Med. J.* **285**, 487.

Baker, I.A., Eastham, R., Elwood, P.C., Etherington, M., O'Brien, J.R., and Sweetnam, P.M. (1982). Haemostatic factors associated with ischaemic heart disease in men aged 45–64 years – the Speedwell study. *Br. Heart J.* **47**, 490.

Braddick, O.J., Atkinson, J., Howland, H.C., and French, J. (1979). A photorefractive study of infant accommodation. *Vis. Res.* **19**, 1319.

Buttery, R. B. and Snaith, A.H. (1979). Waiting for surgery. *Br. Med. J.* **ii**, 403.

Buttery, R.B. and Snaith, A.H. (1980). Surgical provision, waiting times and waiting lists. *Health Trends* **12**, 57.

David, R., Enderby, P., and Bainton, D. (1982). Treatment of acquired aphasia: speech therapists and volunteers compared. *J. Neurol. Neurosurg. Psychiat.* **45**, 957.

DHSS (1972). Management arrangements for the reorganised health service. HMSO, London.

DHSS (1981). *Inequalities in health.* Report of a research working group. Department of Health and Social Security, London.

Dunt, D.R., Kaufert, J.M., Corkhill, R., Creese, A.L., Green, S., and Locker, D. (1980). A technique for precisely measuring activities of daily living. *Community Health* **2**, 120.

Griffiths, E.R. (1983), *NHS management inquiry.* DHSS, London.

Ingram, R.M., Trayner, M.J., Walker, C., and Wilson, J.M. (1979). Screening for refractive errors at one year of age: a pilot study. *Br. J. Ophthal.* **63**, 243.

Maxwell, R.J. (1981). *Health and wealth.* Published for Sandoz Institute for Health and Socio-Economic Studies by Lexington Books, Lexington.

Oliver, M. and Nawratzki, I. (1971). Screening of pre-school children for ocular anomalies. *Br. J. Ophthal.* **55**, 462.

Pattie, A.H. and Gilleard, C.J. (1976). The Clifton assessment schedule – further validation of psycho-geriatric assessment schedule. *Br. J. Psychiatry* **129**, 68.

Snaith, A.H. (1982). Health service administration and health services research. *Br. Med. J.* **284**, 1722.

# 29 The environment of health policy implementation: the Ontario, Canada example

Raisa B. Deber and Eugene Vayda

Glendower: I can call spirits from the vasty deep.
Hotspur:    Why, so can I, or so can any man;
            But will they come when you do call for them?
                                        *William Shakespeare*
                                        *King Henry IV, Part I*
                                        *Act III, Scene i*

## INTRODUCTION

By the mid 1970s, Canada was spending almost 12 billion dollars on its publicly-funded universal health insurance programme. Since nearly three-quarters of the public expenditures for health care were for institutional and physician services, these sectors of the health care system came under increasing government scrutiny. The institutional sector was particularly vulnerable because it alone accounted for over half of the government paid health care expenditures, with an annual rate of increase above inflation.

A series of planning documents in the 1960s and 1970s had suggested changes which emphasized alternatives to institutional care. Provincial Ministries of Health, which had constitutional authority for health care in Canada, then began to formulate policies which would de-emphasize institutional care. In many discussions of planning, analysis culminates with the policy decision. In this chapter, we will *begin* with the decision to achieve a policy goal, and concentrate on the efforts to implement it.

To understand fully the framework of policy implementation, one must appreciate the complexities and constraints of the political/bureaucratic system within which policymakers must operate. Accordingly, we will first briefly describe the Canadian political system and the Canadian health care system. We will then concentrate on a case study of one Canadian province, Ontario, and the efforts made by its government to implement its planners' goals.

## THE POLITICAL SYSTEM OF CANADA AND ONTARIO

Canada, the largest country in the Western Hemisphere and the second largest in the world, is sparsely populated. In 1976, its population was only 23 million; its population density of 2.5 persons per square kilometre is among the lowest in the world. However, over 75 per cent of the population is found in urban centres within 150 kilometres of the US border. Two vast northern territories are virtually unpopulated, with densities of 0.04 persons per square kilometre or less (*Canada Year Book 1978–79*).

Canada was founded as a partnership between English and French cultures but there has since been sizeable immigration, particularly from Europe, Asia, and the Caribbean. Cultural differences are supported and encouraged by government. Ottawa, the capital of Canada, is located in the most populous province, Ontario.

Any political system must strike a balance between two desirable characteristics – the ability of the government to take action and the need for the people to restrain their leaders from taking action. An excess of freedom of action can lead to arbitrariness, a lack of accountability, and even dictatorship; an excess of restraint can lead to paralysis. The perfect balance has remained an elusive goal.

In Canada, government is modelled on British parliamentary tradition. The executive and legislature are closely related, and the political philosophy is based on the necessity for the leaders to be able to carry out their programmes. Officially, all power resides in the sovereign or his/her representative (a governor general federally, lieutenant governors in the provinces). In fact, the sovereign acts only through, and on the advice of, an executive – the Cabinet – which is selected from members of the elected legislature. The judiciary has had a more circumscribed role than is the case in US tradition – it upholds the law, but has not claimed the power of judicial review of the merits of public policy (Van Loon and Wittington 1981). This may change in view of the new Charter of Rights in the new Canadian Constitution, but the precise role the judiciary will play awaits the development of case law.

The Ontario electoral system, like that of the national government, is based on single-member constituencies in which the candidate with the most votes wins. The party with the most seats is then asked by the sovereign's representative to form the government. If the winning party holds more than half the seats, it is termed a 'majority government'. If it holds fewer than half the seats, and thus could be defeated in the legislature by a coalition of opposition members, it is termed a 'minority government'.

The leader of the party winning the most seats becomes the

Premier (provincially) or Prime Minister (federally). In practice, he/she is the executive head of government. This individual then selects an executive council called the Cabinet from among his/her party's elected members in the legislature. The selection takes into account geographical balance, political standing, experience, and ability. Each Cabinet Minister is assigned responsibility for a portfolio (department or ministry) of government. Although Ministers are rarely chosen for their knowledge of a policy area and indeed are usually moved about among portfolios too rapidly for profound knowledge to be a realistic expectation, there was a historical tendency for the Minister of Health to be associated with the health care field. More recently, as the role of government in health care has changed from bill paying to more active management of the system, Ministers of Health have been far less likely to possess a health care background.

The understanding that the government should remain in power only as long as it 'retains the confidence' of a majority of the legislature means that elections are not held at fixed time intervals. Instead, they are called whenever the government requires or wishes a new mandate – either because it has lost the confidence of the legislature, or because it feels it is likely to win. By convention, a government serves a maximum term of five years; however, the defeat of any major piece of legislation which the government had supported can be considered to be a 'vote of non-confidence', warranting the dissolution of the legislature. Elections are held soon after the election call. There are two consequences of the non-fixed term. First, the government generally can control the timing of an election, and thus orchestrate its policy initiatives to maximize opportunities for re-election. Second, the fact that defeat on one bill can precipitate the defeat of the government acts as a strong incentive for party loyalty. There are few modifications of legislation sufficiently important to an elected representative of the party in power to cause him/her to risk the defeat of the government (or, conversely, to cause an opposition member to support a government which might be defeated). Accordingly, most party members almost always vote in blocs. The individual member of the legislature thus has little influence on legislation, and will rarely be approached by groups wishing to modify policy. Pressure groups can be most effective before a bill has been introduced – either with the Minister and/or the civil service while policy is being formulated, or within the Cabinet. Once a bill has been introduced and enjoys the continued backing of a majority government, it is virtually assured of becoming law.

A minority government, however, must be more circumspect. It is aware that the opposition parties can select any potentially winning issue, defeat a government bill, and precipitate an election. Under minority government far more effort must be taken by the party in power to anticipate reactions before legislation is introduced.

Although Cabinet ministers are in charge of their departments, a convention of the Canadian political system is that the full Cabinet is responsible for the activities of government ('Cabinet solidarity'). All policy decisions must be approved by the full Cabinet before being introduced into the legislature.

Cabinet secrecy is a long-standing Canadian tradition. The federal and provincial governments operate within stringent security conventions arising from the principles of the confidentiality of Cabinet discussions. This assures that few details of policy deliberations will become known. In the absence of publicly available draft proposals, minority government provides one of the few opportunities to see policy being made. During these times, governments often find it necessary to modify original proposals (often presented as 'tentative plans') in the light of reactions from the public and from the opposition parties, lest a non-confidence vote result.

An understanding of Canadian politics is further complicated by the federal nature of the country. Canada is a loose confederation of 10 provinces and two territories, as established by the British North America (BNA) Act of 1867. This Act set up an organizational structure for the new nation, and divided powers between the provincial governments and the new national (federal) government in Ottawa. The Act assigned all matters of national concern, plus those endeavours likely to be costly, to the federal government, which had the broadest tax base; Ottawa was given jurisdiction over such items as railways, canals, coinage, and, in the health area, quarantine, marine hospitals, and health services for native peoples and the armed forces. The provinces were given authority for those local concerns which were unlikely to be costly – including roads, education, and 'the Establishment, Maintenance and Management of Hospitals, Asylums, Charities, and Eleemosynary Institutions in and for the Province, other than Marine Hospitals'. Municipal governments have only such powers as are delegated to them by the provinces.

In retrospect, the Fathers of Canadian Confederation proved poor prophets. The resulting imbalance between fiscal resources and constitutional responsibilities has made the primary concern of Canadian politics 'federal-provincial relations'. These issues have tended to be 'resolved' at endless conferences between the relevant federal and provincial Ministers and bureaucrats, their respective legislatures generally having little choice but to ratify the resulting agreements. Simeon (1972) has described these interactions as 'federal-provincial diplomacy', much like the relationships between heads of sovereign states.

Health care has been seen as a natural extension of 'hospitals' and as such an undisputedly provincial responsibility. However, the disparities in provincial wealth soon involved the federal government in financing health services; Ottawa can therefore exert an influence on health policy despite its lack of constitutional authority. Historically, Canadians have been accepting of government intervention in social programmes (Van Loon and Wittington 1981; MacDonald 1980) and have welcomed government sponsorship of health care programmes.

## THE CANADIAN HEALTH CARE SYSTEM

Although universal health insurance was first proposed in 1919, it was not enacted until much later. Local governments, industries and voluntary agencies instead developed a variety of prepayment plans, which inevitably left some services not covered and some people not insured.

Following the Second World War, the bureaucratic energies in Ottawa which had been directed towards winning the war turned towards domestic matters. A Federal-Provincial Conference convened in 1945 to consider programmes of social reform proposed universal health insurance with federal-provincial cost sharing. The Conference also produced a model draft health care bill for the provinces, indirectly modelled on the UK National Health Service proposals. These proposals, although viewed favourably by both the public and key professional groups including the Canadian Medical Association, ultimately failed to be enacted because they were viewed as federal incursions into provincial jurisdiction. None the less hospital facilities were perceived to be insufficient in number, inadequate, and outdated; governmental inaction was not seen as an appropriate policy. In lieu of a full health insurance programme, the federal government made grants for planning and hospital construction available to the provinces. This marked the first acceptance of the concept of federal-provincial cost sharing for health services, a principle which has been the foundation of all subsequent health policy in Canada (Taylor 1978).

Hospitals and hospital care in Canada had previously been financed by municipal governments, religious groups, voluntary insurance programmes, and patient payments. As facilities were built and modernized with government help, this funding base became increasingly inadequate and the financial problems of hospitals worsened. By 1955, five provinces had enacted universal hospital insurance plans to rescue their hospitals. These plans, although politically popular, proved expensive. The five provinces soon pressed the federal government to honour its 1945 hospital insurance cost-sharing offer by enacting nation-wide universal hospital insurance. Financial incentives in the ensuing Hospital Insurance and Diagnostic Services Act induced all provinces to adopt this programme by 1961. Under this Act, services were insured and eligible for 50 per cent federal cost sharing only when provided in a hospital; there were no incentives to use less expensive sites. Proposals to cover home care, for example, were not adopted. In consequence, hospital-based patterns of practice were solidified, leading to some of the current financial problems.

Hospital construction continued; between 1961 and 1971 the number of hospital beds in Canada increased twice as rapidly as the population (33 per cent versus 18 per cent). Bed occupancy, which tends to correlate with bed availability, remained at about 80 per cent (Vayda *et al.* 1979). Thus, per caput utilization was also increasing. Moreover, although universal hospital insurance in Canada provided *payment* to hospitals, it did not mandate an organizational framework to increase efficiency or prevent duplication of services. With '50 per cent dollars' for hospital care, and no federal subsidies for non-hospital services, there was an incentive for provincial health care systems to become hospital-intensive.

With hospital expenditures covered, public pressure grew for coverage of medical-care costs. In 1961, a Royal Commission (the 'Hall Commission') (Royal Commission on Health

Services 1964, 1965) was appointed to study health services in Canada. While it was deliberating, the Western province of Saskatchewan unilaterally enacted universal medical care insurance. That programme survived a 21-day doctors' strike to become both popular and successful. In 1964, the Hall Commission delivered its lengthy report. Among its recommendations was that the federal government cost-share a universal medical insurance programme based on the Saskatchewan model. The resulting Medical Care Act of 1968 incorporated some of Hall's recommendations; however, it did not include his suggested reorganization of medical services delivery.

The Medical Care Act, like the previous Hospital Insurance and Diagnostic Services Act, removed financial barriers to medical services, but entrenched the most expensive means of delivering services; this time federal-provincial cost sharing was allowed for those medical services provided by physicians.

Because the federal government had no jurisdiction in health care, both the hospital and medical care insurance programmes were co-operative and voluntary. To qualify for federal-provincial cost sharing, the provincial programmes had only to meet certain requirements:

1. Universal coverage on uniform terms and conditions 'that does not impede, or preclude, either directly or indirectly whether by charges made to insured persons or otherwise, reasonable access to insured services by insured persons' (95 per cent of the population, without exclusions, had to be covered within two years of provincial adoption of the plan).
2. Portability of benefits from province to province.
3. Insurance for all medically necessary services.
4. A publicly administered non-profit programme.

Despite the reluctance of some provinces to adopt public medical insurance, it was politically difficult for a province to justify having its citizens' federal tax dollars going to support such programmes in other provinces while it failed to adopt such a programme itself. By 1971, even the most resistant province had adopted universal medical care insurance.

The economy was buoyant, and governments appeared to believe that it would continue to be so. In later years, much policy making would concentrate on how to retrench from the commitments made during this expansive period.

Not only did federal-provincial cost sharing stimulate the provinces to adopt health insurance programmes, it also served as a means of income redistribution between the wealthier and poorer provinces. The 50 per cent federal share was distributed as follows: each province was paid 25 per cent of the per caput costs it incurred for hospital in-patient services plus 25 per cent of the national average per caput cost; this sum was then multiplied by the province's population. For medical insurance, each province received 50 per cent of the average national per caput medical care expenditure multiplied by its population (Soderstrom 1978). As a result, the wealthier provinces that spent more would receive less than 50 per cent of their costs. The differentials were especially apparent for medical care cost sharing, which was entirely based on national rates. For example, in 1973–74, Ontario received 49.4 per cent of its hospital costs and 44.8 per cent of its medical care costs from federal contributions;

at the other end of the spectrum, the poor Atlantic province of Newfoundland received 57.6 per cent of its hospital and 81.5 per cent of its medical care costs from the federal government (Andreopoulos 1975).

It was soon evident that the federal government had no control over the total amounts expended by the provinces and received no political credit for its contributions. After initial unilateral attempts by the federal government to limit its contributions without otherwise altering the programme, the federal and provincial governments settled on a new fiscal formula in 1977. Bill C-37 (Federal-Provincial Fiscal Arrangements and Established Programs Financing Act) reduced the direct federal contribution for health care to 25 per cent of total 1975–76 expenditures and tied any subsequent increases in federal payments to the growth of the gross national product (GNP) after 1975. To compensate, federal income and corporate taxes were decreased in order to create 'tax room' for the provinces, which could (and did) increase their tax rates to balance the federal reductions without increasing total taxation levels (Soderstrom 1978; Vayda *et al.* 1979). Additional revenues required to meet any cost increases in excess of growth in the GNP would be primarily the responsibility of the provinces rather than, as in previous years, a responsibility shared with the federal government. Cost control was thereby shifted to the provinces, where both the constitutional authority for health care and the management of health-care services rest. Similar treatment was given to post-secondary education, another expensive and formerly open-ended cost-shared programme under provincial jurisdiction.

Bill C-37 retained the four requirements for provincial health insurance programmes. However, the federal contributions for health care and post-secondary education were no longer earmarked, but became part of general provincial revenues and now had to compete for dollars with other provincially-funded programmes. Some federal ability to 'steer' provincial programmes was retained through a series of additional per caput grants (for example, to develop potentially less costly services like home care and extended care), but the overall federal steering effect was substantially reduced. Recently, the federal government has announced its intention to alter the agreements to further reduce its financial commitments while increasing its ability to set health policy.

As a result of Bill C-37, the provinces have greater flexibility and fewer reporting requirements, but greater fiscal responsibility. It should be recognized that Canada has never had 'a health care system'; it has ten provincial health care systems, plus two in the northern territories (where the federal government plays a more direct role). Although Bill C-37 accentuated differences among provinces as the federal role decreased, essential similarities across provinces do exist. For example, virtually every Canadian has comprehensive medical and hospital insurance. Most hospitals are paid by provincial governments on the basis of negotiated budgets. Physicians are paid through a fee-for-service system on the basis of provincially negotiated fee schedules.

Although the details vary from province to province, all physicians have the choice of 'opting in' or 'opting out' of the provincial plan. For opted in services, the physician accepts the negotiated fee as full payment and is paid directly by the provincial government; the patient pays nothing and receives no bill. In all provinces except Quebec, an opted out physician may bill the patient above the provincial fee schedule ('extra billing'). The plan still pays its portion, either to the patient or the physician, and the patient pays the remainder, if any, of the fee. 'Opting in' is attractive to physicians, given a reasonable fee schedule, since it eliminates bad debts and reduces administrative costs. Presently, the number of opted out physicians varies from a low of less than 1 per cent in Quebec (where the plan does not reimburse either patient or physician when the physician is opted out) to about 15 per cent in Ontario. 'Opting out' has been employed primarily by specialists, by groups of physicians in a few geographical areas in which most doctors decided to 'opt out' and by those philosophically opposed to 'socialized medicine'. Some provinces (like Ontario) have not actively discouraged the continuation of 'opting out', as this practice enables unhappy physicians to receive additional money without the necessity of raising fee schedules. However, a fine balance has to be maintained so that too much opting out does not occur and tip the balance of the system (Badgley and Smith 1979; Barer *et al.* 1979; Wolfson and Tuohy 1980).

Taxes and premiums collected by federal and provincial governments finance the publicly funded health-care system. Although public administration was mandated from the outset of universal hospital insurance, the medical insurance plans allowed for a brief transition period during which private health insurance companies continued to operate. Now, private health insurance plays almost no part in the universal plan, covering only supplemental benefits (such as semi-private accommodation and other amenities). By regulation, private insurance cannot pay the 'extra billing' charges payable to opted out physicians; this policy has succeeded, as intended, in discouraging 'opting out'.

Initially, most provinces administered the programmes with quasi-public medical care and/or hospital commissions. In recent years, most of these provincial hospital and medical care commissions have been eliminated and their functions assumed by the provincial ministries of health.

The primarily French-speaking province of Quebec has a far more interventionist, planned, and state-controlled system than do the other provinces (Boivin-Lesage 1982). Quebec's innovations have as yet had little effect on the other provinces. This may be due in part to cultural differences and the language barrier.

## HEALTH CARE COSTS

In 1965, the total cost of all health care services in Canada was $3.3 billion; in 1970, $6 billion; and in 1975, more than $11 billion. Of the total health care expenditures in 1975, 54 per cent went to institutional care and 16 per cent to physician services (Health and Welfare 1979). Health care costs make up 10 per cent of federal expenditures and 30 per cent of Ontario spending, sums that must be raised by taxes or premiums. The magnitude of these expenditures and the rate of their increase have captured the attention and concern of politicians.

Following the introduction of hospital insurance, health expenditures in Canada rose rapidly, both in absolute terms and as a percentage of GNP. Gross national product expenditures on health care rose from 5.5 per cent in 1960 to 7.3 per cent in 1971 and actual expenditures from 2 billion to 7 billion dollars (250 per cent increase) (Health and Welfare 1979; Hatcher 1981). The introduction of medical care insurance had less effect. Between 1971 and 1975 expenditures rose again (from 7 billion to almost 12 billion) but the percentage of GNP spent on health care remained constant at about 7 per cent and continued at that level until the late 1970s. (Unpublished data indicate that currently it has reached 8 per cent.) However, because of government insurance, public sector funding of health care rose from 43 to 75 per cent of costs; actual government spending thus increased from about $1 billion in 1960, to $5 billion in 1971, $9 billion in 1975 (Health and Welfare 1979), and 13 billion in 1978–79 (Hall 1980). The magnitude of health care expenditures became more visible once governments started paying most of the bill.

In the period before universal hospital and medical care insurance the private sector had covered some hospital and physician care. At present over 90 per cent of the costs of hospital and physician services are paid by the public sector. Private payments are now limited primarily to nursing homes (40 per cent of costs), dental care (90 per cent of costs), and drugs and prostheses (75 per cent of costs) (Health and Welfare 1979).

Hospital use and its attendant costs were particularly vulnerable to examination in Canada because, compared to many countries and particularly to the US, Canada had high bed to population and bed use to population ratios. The elderly were particularly high users of institutional care, and the 65 years and older population was projected to increase from almost 9 per cent in 1976 to 12 per cent of the total population in 2001 (Gross and Schwenger 1981). While a small portion of the higher Canadian bed use could be explained by its remote and isolated north, which was served by many small hospitals, some appeared to be a reflection of increased bed supply. By 1971, Canada had 23 per cent more hospital beds than the US and used 30 per cent more hospital days per caput (Vayda et al. 1979).

Between 1965 and 1975, per caput expenditures for health care services in Ontario were the highest in Canada. They rose from $188 per person in 1965, of which $92 per person came from the public sector, to $556 per caput ($405 from the public sector) in 1975. Thus, over the 10 year period, Ontario's total per caput expenditures on health care increased 200 per cent, but public sector expenditures increased 340 per cent (Health and Wealth 1979; Ontario Ministry of Treasury and Economics 1981). As a result, Ontario had a major stake in cost containment. This interest was magnified as a result of the renegotiated cost-sharing agreements (Bill C-37), which had shifted most of the responsibility for meeting cost increases to the Ontario government.

## PLANNING REPORTS

Concern that health care expenditures were increasing above inflation was reflected in a number of official planning reports, commissioned both by the national (Task Force 1969; Hastings 1973; Lalonde 1975) and provincial (Commission of Inquiry on Health and Social Services 1970; Department of Health and Social Development 1972; Foulkes 1973) governments. These reports identified rising expenditures and stressed the need for greater efficiency and the provision of less expensive forms of health services delivery. Their goals were not necessarily to cut costs, but rather to contain their rate of increase. They were influenced by a strong body of expert opinion calling for improvements in efficiency and containment of the costs of the health care system through such measures as shifting from in-patient to out-patient care, reducing the number of hospital beds, and promoting paramedical workers and community health (and social service) centres. This emphasis was further justified by the work of Illich (1975), Fuchs (1974), and McKeown (1979), who challenged both the efficacy and the marginal benefits of further increases in health care expenditures in developed countries. In Ontario, the Report of the Committee on the Healing Arts in 1970, the 1974 report of the Health Planning Task Force (the Mustard Report) and the 1976 Health Report of the Ontario Economic Council, all identified increased cost, excessive use of hospital services and the control and deployment of medical and health manpower as key issues, and included rationalization, regionalization, and deinstitutionalization among their remedies. Although most of these recommendations have not been implemented, the ideas contained within the reports have had a major influence on thinking and planning for Canadian health policy.

## ONTARIO

Ontario, the second largest province in Canada, is the most industrialized and the most populous of the provinces. Much of its population of 8.5 million (one-third of the population of Canada) is located in the urbanized corridor stretching along the US border. Ontario contains both the national capital (Ottawa) and the country's major English-speaking city (Toronto). Its older British-descended population has been augmented by heavy and recent immigration, particularly to Toronto. The province also contains farming areas, and a large, resource-rich, sparsely-populated north to which services must be provided. Like the states of the US northeast which border it (such as New York, Pennsylvania, and Michigan), it must now cope with an ageing industrial infrastructure and the recent plant closures affecting that region. Ontario voters are said to prefer order, stability, and continuity, with a touch of reform when the times demand it (MacDonald 1980).

Since 1943, Ontario has been governed by successive leaders of the Progressive Conservative (PC or Tory) party. The party's name illustrates its ideology – conservatism and cautious reform. The party has combined a perceived capacity to manage the system effectively (of crucial importance to the stable Ontario electorate) with a capacity for maintaining a seemingly equitable balance among the principal interests in the province.

This electoral success can be attributed to three factors.

First, the Conservatives have shown an ability to modify their policies in keeping with public opinion. Second, neither of the two opposition parties, the Liberals and the New Democratic Party (NDP), has been able to become the sole, or even the most evident, alternative to the government. Third, the geographical distribution of party support tends to favour the Progressive Conservatives. Although they have not won a majority of the popular vote in any of the twelve elections since 1943, they have formed nine majority governments. In their best showing, in 1951, they translated 48 per cent of the votes into 88 per cent of the seats in the legislature (MacDonald 1980).

Ideologically, the three parties follow a spectrum from moderately conservative to moderately social democratic; with the possible exception of the trade union influenced NDP, voters perceive little ideological difference among them. In 1968 and 1977 public opinion surveys, there was almost no issue on which mass opinions varied as a function of party affiliation. To the electorate, the Progressive Conservatives were seen as 'dull but competent' – stable, efficient, experienced, but also complacent, untrustworthy, profligate spenders, and too closely aligned with big business (MacDonald 1980).

## Structure of the Ontario government

The growth of the Ontario health bureaucracy was haphazard and fragmented. As befitted a conservative government in a stable society, the Ontario provincial government tended to see its role as one of regulation rather than of control. As previously noted, most health policy initiatives had emanated from the federal government, with the provinces induced to join through cost-sharing incentives. When Ontario became involved in the universal plans, it defined its role as one of administrative supervision to ensure a greater access to 'high quality' health care services. Decisions about how the money was to be spent were made by 'experts' – health care professionals and other providers. The administrative questions were often removed from 'political interference' and assigned to semi-autonomous agencies, boards and commissions which tended to be dominated by providers. Thus, the administration of hospital insurance was carried out through one semi-autonomous agency – the Ontario Hospital Services Commission. Other semi-autonomous agencies were involved at various times in administering the medical insurance programmes. Although semi-autonomous agencies were designed to defuse issues by raising them above partisan politics, the Cabinet appointed their members and retained the ability to veto their decisions. The Ministry of Health was left with the residual programmes, including traditional public health activities.

The semi-autonomous agencies were highly acceptable to the providers, who felt they were involved in a 'partnership' with the government to ensure the continuing well-being of the hospitals. However, the status quo was less acceptable to the government, which soon realized that it had neither priorities nor mechanisms for arriving at them. The then Deputy Minister of Health of Ontario summarized the problem: 'These special interests have resulted in a fragmen-

tation of health services to a degree that interferes with the effective use of available resources . . . Planning is done more or less independently within each programme area, and consists largely of adding on new services'. 'Bureaucratic capture' meant that most branches spent their time fighting for 'their' programmes, with little regard to overall government priorities.

In 1972, a major re-organization of the entire Ontario government was undertaken with the aim of improving government productivity and policy formation, and allowing political control to be exerted in all policy fields. The Department of Health was transformed and most of the services formerly run by semi-autonomous agencies were incorporated into the new Ministry of Health. The reorganization was justified in terms of the need to provide a single integrated policy focus, cut costs, reduce bureaucracy, and allow for the introduction of innovations.

Although individual government ministries have undergone frequent re-organizations in subsequent years, such that any organizational chart more than six months old is outdated, the general framework of policy making in Ontario still retains the 1972 structure.

The 1972 reforms acted to centralize policy formation through the setting up of a system of Cabinet committees, as shown in Fig. 29.1. The most powerful committee of Cabinet

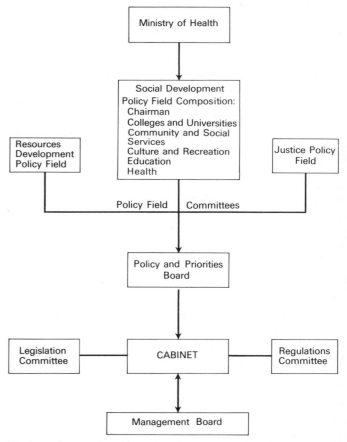

**Fig. 29.1.** The Ontario Cabinet Committee structure: health policy development process.

is the Policy and Priorities Board, which develops, reviews, co-ordinates, and advises the full Cabinet on political and financial policies and priorities. The Management Board is an administrative committee, in charge of monitoring programme implementation and controlling expenditures of public money. Its staff are also involved in approving organizational procedures. Two 'housekeeping' committees – the Legislation Committee and Regulations Committee – screen proposed laws and regulations before they are introduced. The most notable reform of 1972 was the introduction of three co-ordinating committees called Policy Field Committees, in which policies in closely related Ministries were to be reconciled. The Chairman of each Policy Field Committee, originally termed a 'super Minister', is a member of the Policy and Priorities Board. Co-ordination difficulties still arise, particularly with respect to issues which span policy fields. Housing, labour and the environment, for example, all fall into the Resources Development Policy Field; health has been placed in the Social Development Policy Field. As a result, the Policy Field mechanism could not be used for policy co-ordination in the areas of occupational and environmental health. Co-ordination was achieved ultimately by moving responsibility for occupational health programmes from the jurisdiction of the Ministry of Health to the Ministry of Labour.

The official Ministry process of developing policies is as follows: once a policy issue is recognized, policy alternatives are developed, usually within the concerned Ministry. The brief is then presented to the appropriate Policy Field Committee for evaluation and recommendations. If the proposal is approved at this stage, it is often sent first to the Policy and Priorities Board to ensure that it conforms with general government policy and priorities before going to full Cabinet. Under unusual circumstances, some of these steps may be omitted; however, by the time a proposal has come to Cabinet, at least one-third of the Ministers have usually scrutinized it. The proposal may then receive approval in principle by the full Cabinet. At this point, the implementation procedure begins: the proposal is sent back to the concerned Ministry for any required modification, and then sent to the Management Board for a review of resource requirements and administrative, financial, organizational, revenue and other implications. It is then returned to Cabinet, along with the recommendations of the Management Board, for final approval. Only after these reviews are completed will the policy be approved and implemented (MacDonald 1980).

### The Ontario Ministry of Health

The Ministry of Health, like other government Ministries, is organized hierarchically. Its chief executive officer is the Deputy Minister, who must balance the dual roles of senior advisor to the Minister and senior manager of the Ministry. The Deputy is appointed by the Premier (not by the Minister), and inter-departmental reassignments of Deputy Ministers are common. Between 1972 and 1982 the Ministry of Health has had five Deputy Ministers. The Deputy is in turn aided by a number of Assistant Deputy Ministers (ADMs), each with responsibility for one segment of the department. Below the

ADMs are a series of Executive Directors and/or General Managers, each with responsibility for two or more branches. The next level of the hierarchy includes the Branch Directors, with responsibility for the operational management of programmes. Minor variations on this pattern are possible. For example, some Ministries contain Associate Deputy Ministers, who may marginally outrank the Assistants. Some branches may report directly to the Deputy, bypassing middle levels of the hierarchy. Semi-independent agencies, commissions, or advisory committees may report directly to the Minister (Ontario Ministry of Health 1972–82).

Although frequent adjustments to the structure of the Ministry were made during the period under analysis, the organization of the Ontario Ministry of Health resembled Fig. 29.2. There were three ADMs, one each for Institutional Health Services, Community Health Services, and Administration and Health Insurance. Principal planning activities were located in several places, which can be categorized as follows: (a) *Semi-autonomous sources of long-term advice*, such as the Ontario Council of Health (a senior advisory body to the Minister selected so as to provide 'a reasonable balance of public interest, expert knowledge, experience and geographic distribution', and hence usually reflecting the key interest groups) and various *ad hoc* advisory committees on particular areas. Their input has varying degrees of influence; (b) *Internal sources of planning (long and medium range)*. The Strategic Planning and Research Branch, of particular relevance here, reported directly to the Deputy Minister and was given responsibility for 'the development of medium- and long-term economic and financial planning strategies, and consideration of the implications of these strategies for the health system'. It was this Branch, along with appropriate Assistant Deputy Ministers, which developed many of the strategies employed by the Ministry in the chronology that follows. In 1978–79, it was merged with the Policy Coordination Secretariat and the Manpower Planning and Development group to form a Policy Development and Research Branch. (c) *Sources of short-range, operational planning* were also available within constituent Divisions (Fig. 29.2).

Despite the availability of planning and planners, there was a perception that health policy making in the province was *ad hoc* and responded to political necessities. Despite frequent (and continuing) re-organizations this *ad hoc* tendency appears to have persisted. Further, the many stages of overview from Cabinet committees mean that Ministry recommendations are likely to be altered to reflect more global (or more political) considerations.

### Funding mechanisms

The Ministry of Health funds about 95 per cent of hospital operating costs from revenue which includes federal contributions under Bill C-37, as noted previously (Ontario Ministry of Health 1972–82). The hospitals also obtain limited funds from other sources (e.g. the government operated Workman's Compensation Board, payments for services rendered to patients from other provinces and countries, extra payments for semi-private and private hospital rooms and other amenities).

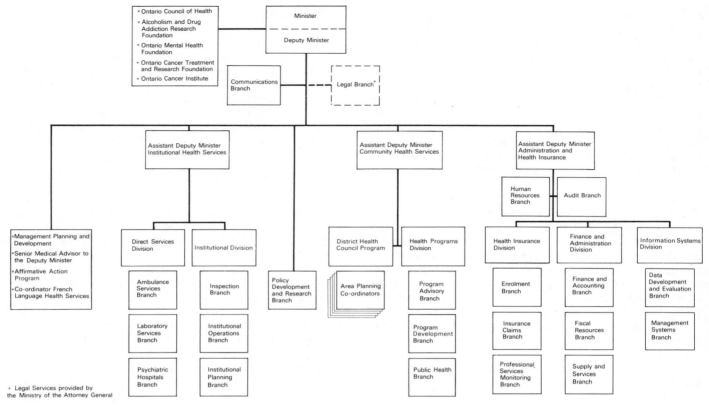

**Fig. 29.2.** Organization of the Ontario Ministry of Health. Source: Ontario Ministry of Health *Annual Report 1978/79.*

Prior to 1969, hospital budgets were negotiated individually between hospitals and the Ontario Ministry of Health on a 'line-by-line' basis. Since 1969, they have been determined centrally by prospective global budgeting on the basis of a percentage-increase formula. Annual increases are based on Ministry forecasts of expected rises of prices of such items as fuel, food, capital goods, and wages. A uniform percentage increase in the 'base budget' of provincially reimbursed operating revenues to all hospitals is then announced; it reflects the amount required to maintain hospital services at their current level, and is referred to as 'Part A' of the budget (Detsky *et al.* 1983).

Based on this percentage increase, individual hospitals develop budgets, which must be reviewed and approved by the Ministry. An appeal process exists whereby individual hospitals can negotiate with the Ministry for adjustments in base budgets and/or higher percentage increases. In addition to these individual adjustments, province-wide adjustments may occur if the Ministry's forecasts of price increases prove to be incorrect (for example, if unions receive higher wage settlements than predicted).

New and special programmes are funded in a separate section of the hospital budget known as 'Part B'. These funds establish government reimbursement for operating costs of 'new and expanded' programmes not yet covered under the base budget. Since 1979, certain special programmes (for example neo-natal intensive care, dialysis, cardiac pacemaker

units, total parenteral nutrition, or chemotherapy units) are also funded outside the global budget because their cost increases were not viewed as being 'controllable' by the hospitals (Detsky *et al.* 1983).

The Ministry, with advice from District Health Councils, must also approve all capital building projects, and all major new items of equipment. The Ministry of Health funds all approved capital works for the province's teaching hospitals, two-thirds of capital construction costs for all community hospitals in Southern Ontario, and five-sixths of capital construction costs for all community hospitals in Northern Ontario. The hospitals (and their communities) are responsible for raising the remaining funds. Recently, the Ministry has permitted hospitals to proceed at their own expense on new projects which the Ministry has approved but is unable to fund because of financial constraints.

## CONSEQUENCES FOR IMPLEMENTING POLICY

The Ontario political system described above has a number of consequences which affect the ability of a government to implement desired policies.

1. The provincial governments have clear constitutional authority in the health area. Beyond its powers over minor aspects such as quarantine, the federal government has only the indirect (although substantial) power resulting from its

role in financing health programmes; municipal governments have no independent role at all.

2. The tradition of parliamentary supremacy has ensured that the province could act with few controls within its areas of jurisdiction. Courts have ruled that the judiciary should not interfere with government's ability to make policy. Party solidarity has ensured that the policy of a majority government will be supported in the legislature. Cabinet secrecy has meant that policy alternatives could be debated internally and consensus reached, without the risk of embarrassment to the government through public disclosure. The tradition of Cabinet solidarity has meant that policies, once adopted, were likely to be supported by the government. (The future impact of Canada's new Constitution and Charter of Rights on parliamentary supremacy is unclear; over time, it is likely to increase the relative power of the courts, but it has as yet had little effect.)

3. The Cabinet Committee system described previously incorporates mechanisms for ensuring that all policy decisions from within individual Ministries conform to governmental priorities.

4. Non-fixed terms of office give the party in power great control over the timing of elections. Since a majority government can be considered to have the two years following its election basically free from electoral constraints, policy initiatives can be manipulated accordingly. Tough measures may be taken early in the term, to be followed by potentially vote-winning policies in the later years.

5. Under universal health insurance and the current cost-sharing arrangements, the provincial government is both the budgetary authority, and the financially responsible party. Owing to the absence of private insurance for the bulk of hospital and physician costs, Canadian authorities do not have the problems with fragmented fiscal authority which plague US attempts to introduce cost control. There is essentially one paymaster for hospitals and physicians. In addition, the provinces dispense the funds to post-secondary educational institutions and therefore have the potential for considerable control over the supply (although *not* the distribution) of health manpower.

6. The provincial government sets hospital budgets (through direct negotiations) and negotiates fee schedules with the physicians. It thus has access to much financial information about providers.

7. Public opinion provides only a partial constraint. Universal health insurance is perhaps the most popular programme of government; accordingly, the province must be careful not to 'threaten' it. However, the Canadian political culture has traditionally been strongly deferential to authority and accepting of government activity and intervention in the economy. With the exception of physicians, there is virtually no dispute about the 'right' of government to intervene in health care, as long as the public believes that the government will ensure the maintenance of a good universal health care system.

8. In Ontario, one party has been in power since 1943. Thus, there is a degree of understanding between civil servants and politicians which would be unlikely in a jurisdiction in which there had been frequent changes in the party in power. In theory, the party and the bureaucrats could afford to take a 'longer view' in confidence that they would both continue to be in office. The Progressive Conservative party tends to be pragmatic, and open to policy proposals which promise to be popular.

None the less, as will become evident, the Ontario government, in the mid 1970s, was also subject to a number of constraints in implementing policy decisions.

1. They were not beginning with a blank slate. Ontario had an existing system of public hospitals, a large number of physicians, and a funding system under universal health insurance which ensured that both would be paid. The 'ideal solutions' thus might be neither possible nor cost-effective, given the system already in place. Planning thus was pushed towards incremental rather than radical solutions.

2. The existing system of health care was very popular with the public, who tended to be supportive of the institutional sector and of physicians. Governments would risk their re-election if they were seen to be 'dismantling' the current system 'merely' to save money, particularly if the savings were used for less popular programmes. This constraint was heightened during periods of minority government, since both opposition parties were eager to come to the defence of the health care system.

3. Ontario's geography presented difficulties in health care delivery. The governing party would have to be alert to distributional implications of policy changes, particularly in Northern Ontario and in electorally marginal constituencies where a small number of votes could change the outcome of an election.

4. Cost containment in the health care sector had been previously aided by the traditional underpayment of health care workers. This era had ended, and was replaced by one of labour militancy. The emergence of province-wide bargaining units meant that strikes might shut down the health care sector if cuts were stringent.

5. The federal government was attempting to change some of the ground rules. It was particularly interested in limiting the growth of federal funds to the provinces; beyond that, it wished to gain more credit for itself and, for ideological reasons, to eliminate certain practices (such as balanced billing, user charges, and the use of premiums) which the provinces had been employing to reduce their financial responsibility.

6. Proximity to the US meant that American examples would influence Canadian opinion. Much of the physician militancy, for example, sprang from the fact that average physician incomes in the US were higher than in Canada.

7. Because the economy was not growing, no additional money was available. The easiest way to change the system, by adding dollars for new programmes, was thus foreclosed.

8. Finally, like all governments, the Progressive Conservatives wished to remain in office. This understandable desire would influence both their reaction to external constraints and their willingness to delegate authority to other (for example regional) bodies.

On balance, the advantages detailed above would mean that, once a policy direction was accepted, Ontario would find it easier than most governments to implement its plans.

As long as the only policy was for 'more and better' services and the economy was buoyant, the government and providers had the enviable task of devising technical solutions to satisfy all participants. However, the policy of universal access to quality health care regardless of cost could not persist over the long-term. Demand for health care is both 'elastic' (in economic terms) and virtually limitless; public funds are not. Ultimately, as other programmes compete for the same resources, some controls or constraints are inevitable.

Canadian economists such as R.G. Evans (1982) have observed that health care is noteworthy for the failure of market mechanisms, under a universal system, to function as an acceptable way of balancing supply and demand for services. If access to health care is determined on the basis of need, rather than on ability to pay, over-servicing of the wealthy and under-servicing of the poor are unacceptable. But there are always more health care services that could be provided. Allowing providers to determine the appropriate level of supply may thus resemble handing over a blank cheque. In retrospect, it was therefore inevitable that the partnership which had developed between providers and Ministry officials was disrupted and some policy control given to decision makers with a broader view of overall (including non-health) priorities. As the biggest spenders, the hospitals could be expected to bear the brunt of any control activities.

## THE DIRECT APPROACH TO COST CONTAINMENT

The hospital 'cutbacks' – rates of growth in spending less than desired by providers – began in 1973. The Minister of Health announced a freeze on government funding of capital construction projects, a 5 per cent ceiling on annual increases in operating costs, and an arbitrary closing of between 1200 and 1500 active treatment beds. Compared to most developed countries, Ontario (like the rest of Canada) had a relatively high active treatment bed to population ratio. The Ministry announced they hoped, in the long term, to reduce Ontario's current ratio of 5.0 beds per 1000 population to 4.0 per 1000 (4.5 in the North), with an interim goal of 4.5 per 1000.

Although the increase in hospital expenditures in 1973–74 was limited to 5 per cent over the previous year, the ceiling did not stay on. Constraint since 1970 had been aided by relatively modest salary increases for hospital workers, which in turn aided in the unionization of that sector. A series of labour actions resulted, including the beginning of centralized province-wide negotiations between the hospitals and their workers. In 1974, the government intervened to halt a threatened strike of non-medical employees by promising the money to give hospital service workers a 48 per cent raise. A similar settlement was awarded, by arbitration, to nurses in an Ottawa hospital. Since over three-quarters of Ontario's hospitals had at least one union certification, these settlements had a 'ripple effect' throughout the province and led to a 50 per cent increase in the wage and salary bill. Total hospital expenditures in 1974–75 jumped nearly 29 per cent over the previous year, whereas other provincial programmes were getting increases of only 10 per cent. The province did

not wish to increase taxes, and felt that it could not borrow any more money without damaging its excellent credit rating. The seeds of future difficulty had been sown.

The Ministry's generous settlements to hospital workers may have been related to the fact that 1975 was an election year. In that election, the Progressive Conservatives dropped to 36 per cent of the vote, and won only 43 per cent of the seats in the legislature. The Liberals were close behind them, with 34 per cent of the popular vote. Owing to their geographical distribution of support, however, they won only 26 per cent of the seats, and the New Democratic Party, with 30 per cent of the seats, formed the official opposition. Both opposition parties intermittently expected that they might do even better in the next election, and thus sporadically appeared willing to precipitate one through a vote of non-confidence. They also sensed that 'health care' might prove to be a compelling election issue, and gave particular scrutiny to activities in the area. All health policy over the next two years was thus played against the imminent threat of a new election.

None the less, the bed reduction policy had had some impact. About 1500 beds were closed in the province between 1973 and 1975. Hospitals closing beds reported decreased lengths of stay, increased waiting lists, increased percentage occupancy, increased out-patient utilization, and reduced costs. However, it appeared that much of the 'savings' was allotted to other activities within each hospital. Ministry planning groups began to formulate plans to achieve more realizable savings.

In 1975, a further complication was introduced by the federal government. With the downturn in the economy, they announced that they would unilaterally seek to terminate the existing Hospital Insurance and Diagnostic Services Act as soon as this was permitted under law and proposed a new formula that would restrain increases in federal contributions, preferably to amounts below the rate of cost increases. The threat of reduced federal contributions reinforced a desire within the Ontario government to 'get its own financial house in order'. This intention was backed, strongly, by the then Minister of Health, Frank Miller, who believed in balanced budgets.

### The hospital closure policy

In October, 1975, Mr Miller warned the Ontario Hospital Association Convention that 'the many problems of cost related to health care delivery have been building to a point where unpleasant, caustic action may be called for'. Although the quality of health care would be maintained 'The seriousness of our present dollar challenge must take precedence over local feelings of pride or convenience . . . There is a lot of ground between hardship and inconvenience.' He added that rationalizing services would be a governmental priority.

The Ministry had projected that merely maintaining existing services at the present level, with no allowances for new programmes, would require an annual budget increase of over 16 per cent. The province had made a commitment to hold its increase in spending to 10 per cent, so health's spending would increase by 'only' $300 million. The Ontario Ministry of Health set the goal of cutting $50 million from its budget in 1976 (from a total projected budget of $3.3 billion dollars, of which over half was allocated to hospitals).

This determination to achieve cost efficiencies was accompanied by a new 'streamlining' of the Ministry organization. Some bureaucrats identified with provider interests were replaced. The old relationships between the bureaucracy and the dominant pressure groups were thus breaking down; from the perspective of the field, the new managers appeared to see their jobs as emphasizing cost-containment and cost-effectiveness, rather than as increasing 'quality' care. An adversarial relationship was beginning to appear.

On 1 December 1975, a memo was sent to all hospitals in the province announcing a three-phase programme. Phase 1 was an immediate freeze on all planned expansion, new services and programmes (as well as on the salaries of senior administrators), an increase in semi- and private room rates, and limitations on increases in hospital costs. It was announced that phases two (specific spending guidelines in line with the federal government's wage and price control regulations) and three (specific constraints on individual hospitals) would follow in mid-January. The Ministery subsequently explained that the necessary budget reduction ($50 million) might be achieved through a reduction of up to 3000 hospital beds, and up to 5000 hospital staff. However, he felt that the reduction could be accompanied by an increase in the overall quality of health services through disease prevention and health promotion. He gave as examples the new law requiring drivers to wear seat belts and legislation against drinking drivers. Ontario's 242 public hospitals were asked not to submit their 1976 budgets until phases two and three had been clarified.

In addition to a number of other economies, the newly appointed Deputy Minister, who had been an architect of the cost cutting programme, stated that he intended to reduce the beds staffed and in operation from the current level of 4.8 beds per 1000 population (itself a reduction from 1973) to the provincial guideline of 4.0 per 1000 (4.5 in the North). It was stated that 6000 of the previous 40 000 hospital beds were 'surplus' and that twenty hospitals, all with occupancy rates considerably lower than their peers, would be potential candidates for closure. Reaction to the notice of intention was remarkably restrained at first, but would change once the details were revealed.

The concern about bed numbers was further intensified because the number of nursing home beds had been increasing, from 19 000 in 1970 to 26 000 by early 1976. To prevent the 'new' nursing home beds from becoming 'add ons', it would be necessary to reduce available active treatment beds.

It was soon made known that the Ministry had been working for more than two years towards a plan for closing hospitals. Criteria for closure had been identified: proximity of alternative (and available) hospital facilities; low occupancy rates; status of the hospital's physical plant; and potential requirements for capital improvements. In the three months following the Minister's phase one announcement, a confidential list of at least 25 hospitals which were candidates for closure (referred to in the press as 'the hit list') had been prepared. This list was never publicly revealed.

A final selection of ten hospitals to be closed before 1 April 1976 was made. Only the Minister of Health, high ranking civil servants in his Ministry, and the Cabinet knew the identity of these hospitals. However, the Minister decided that all hospitals to be closed should be notified by him in person. The press therefore maintained representatives outside his office and followed him on his appointed rounds. Media coverage was to remain significant throughout.

The hospitals selected included eight rural hospitals, each under 100 beds, plus a chronic hospital in a medium sized city (soon removed from the list) and a 319 bed community hospital in Toronto. Together, they contained over 700 beds, with estimated annual operating costs of perhaps $20 million dollars (of which the Ministry estimated perhaps $10 million would be saved). They employed about 1300 staff. In addition, responsibility for the two previously closed psychiatric facilities would be transferred to the Ministry of Community and Social Services, where they would be used as mental health resource centres, with savings to the Health Department budget (although perhaps not to the government) of $7.5 million.

Following the hospital closures, the Ministry planned to close down 1212 beds (in units of 20–30 bed wards) in 36 hospitals around the province (projected savings – about $15 million) and make line-by-line budget cuts to another 47 hospitals (savings target $4 million). The hospitals' approved budgets were derived by Ministry staff from a series of regression analyses which had been used to guide policy formation. Hospitals were grouped by size and type into eight categories and compared for efficiency on the basis of paid staff hours against indices of hospital activity (such as patient days, laundry, radiology exams, and housekeeping). 'Overstaffing' was thus statistically identified. This over-reliance on statistical arguments, which would prove to be vulnerable to rebuttals from provider groups and opposition critics reanalysing the same data, served to dampen trust in the Ministry. Over the next few years disputes over general principles would often degenerate into abstruse methodological arguments or contrary approaches to data gathering or analysis. Statistics could be, and were, used to prove anything; the government rarely ended up with advantageous public relations.

Following Mr Miller's announcement, the hospitals selected for closure reacted immediately and strongly. On the Minister's visit to the small community of Durham, he was met by an angry, placard-bearing crowd who threw snowballs and eggs at him. The terms 'Miller the Killer' and 'executioner' were used by other hospitals. Two hospitals refused to close on the appointed dates, and hired lawyers to bring their cases to court – an almost unprecedented action for a Canadian hospital.

A particularly strong attack was mounted by the Doctors Hospital in central Toronto, a community hospital situated near the University of Toronto and near four of the University's teaching hospitals. Over the years, the hospital had made a special effort to accommodate the needs of the surrounding ethnic community which included many recent immigrants to Canada. Indeed, many of the physicians who had privileges at Doctors Hospital were themselves immigrants who would have had difficulty gaining admitting privileges to other hospitals. The hospital's district was represented in the legislature by Larry Grossman, a young Progressive Conservative in his first term of office.

Doctors Hospital first learned that it was on the 'hit list' on 8 February 1976, when the Minister called the Executive Director and asked him to get the hospital's Board of Trustees together for a meeting the next day. The hospital mounted a counter-attack remarkable for its thoroughness; it mobilized the community and made the continued operation of the hospital a reflection of ethnic pride. A co-ordinating committee was linked with a Save Our Hospital Committee; public demonstrations, local canvassing, and petition signing were combined with the mobilization of prominent supporters. The Mayor gave his 'full support' to the institution; one of the city's Archbishops toured the institution and commented that, although he did not understand the political background, he 'would like to see this hospital live'. The hospital pressed for 'more statistical evidence' to support the closure, and stressed that their average cost per patient day was about half that at the teaching hospitals.

Despite the agitation, the hospital closure policy could probably have been sustained. The Ontario Hospital Association (OHA) remained low key in its response, simply issuing a statement that more time would be required for the orderly closing of hospitals. However, the government was in a minority position, and the opposition was considering precipitating an election. Within two days the opposition parties in the legislature began attacking the government's plan to close Doctors Hospital. In particular, the New Democrats chose to make health care an overriding issue; the party already had a strong basis of support among the urban ethnic groups and wished to consolidate it by supporting the 'ethnic hospital'. They would not be allowed to claim the ethnic vote without a fight from the Progressive Conservative backbencher representing the constituency. On 9 February, the same day the closing was announced, Mr Grossman challenged the government's projected savings from closing the institution. He continued his support of the hospital in the legislature; such opposition by a legislator to the policy of his own government was (and remains) unusual in Canadian politics. Owing to the party's desire to keep its foothold in ethnic Toronto, however, no adverse consequences fell to Mr Grossman. He has retained his seat, was subsequently appointed to the Cabinet, served as Minister of Health, and currently holds the post of Treasurer of Ontario and Minister of Economics.

By 4 March, the New Democratic Party had toured the hospital, and promised to introduce a non-confidence motion is the hospital were closed. The following day, the Canadian Union of Public Employees (CUPE), a union including non-medical workers in hospitals, threatened an illegal strike if any of the four hospitals with closure orders ceased operation. Doctors Hospital continued to host 'Open Houses' and tours for all interested parties, including community leaders, church officials, the local public, the press, and representa-

tives from all major political parties. Mr Grossman persisted with his 'embarrassing questions' to the Minister, and the New Democratic Party health critic continued his attack.

On 12 March, the Lieutenant-Governor delivered the 'Speech from the Throne', in which government lays out its policy initiatives for the coming year. A slight change in tone was noticeable; the government proposed a new role for 'doomed' institutions, converting the facilities into chronic-care health centres. However, on the same day, Doctors Hospital received a letter from the Deputy Minister of Health confirming that the facility would be closed as scheduled. Hospital supporters now openly called for the resignation of the Minister, Deputy Minister, and the civil servants in the Institutional Division responsible for formulating the closure policy. During the Throne Speech debate which began 15 March, the New Democratic Party leader supported the call for mass resignations. An amendment was introduced to require the government to change its policy on hospital closures; defeat of the government's position would be considered to be a vote of non-confidence which would require the government to resign and call for an election. The Liberal leader announced that he would support the New Democrats. The vote was scheduled for 5 April. Mr Grossman again addressed the legislature, questioning the government's reasons for selecting Doctors Hospital to be closed. The Opposition members vocally applauded his questioning. The Minister of Health left his seat in the Legislature without comment.

The Cabinet was now in a difficult position. By convention, they were bound to support the Minister in a policy to which they had all agreed and to which he remained committed. They were also concerned about government deficits and resentful that the high costs of the Ministry of Health not only reduced their ability to implement their own Ministries' new projects, but even required budget cuts. However, the government was now faced with the likelihood of having to fight an election on the unpopular grounds of defending hospital closures in communities for which hospitals represented both a source of employment and one of pride.

On the evening of 16 March 1976, while playing hockey with friends, Mr Miller suffered a heart attack and was admitted to hospital. In the morning, Dr Bette Stephenson, a physician member of the legislature, was appointed acting Minister of Health. Meetings between the acting Minister, the Premier, and top representatives from the Doctors Hospital commenced. On 30 March, the acting Minister announced publicly that a new target date would be set for hospital closures if legal appeals were initiated. She set up a special committee in the Institutional Services Division of the Ministry of Health to examine alternatives to the complete closure of Doctors Hospital. She further announced that there had evidently been a misunderstanding; the Ministry had never intended to leave the hospital as 'an empty shell'. A series of contradictory announcements came out over the next month, depending upon which group within government had prepared the press release. In May, a unanimous court decision was handed down from the Provincial Supreme Court that the Ministry could not use the authority of the Public Hospitals Act to *close* hospitals for financial or budgetary considerations. However, the court decision did not specify that the Ministry was required to *fund* all hospitals.

Responses to the court decision varied. Dr Stephenson, the acting Minister, declined to comment. The Hospital celebrated. Mr Miller (still recovering from his heart attack) and his Deputy Minister both publicly stated that they were firmly convinced that the Minister had the jurisdiction to close hospitals.

Several courses of action were available to the government. The Court judgement might have been appealed; the Minister might have withdrawn all government funds from the threatened hospitals (clearly legal under the Public Hospitals Act); the government might have introduced amendments to the Act to empower the Ministry to close hospitals. None of these measures was taken. The deadline for appeals of the judgment was allowed to come and go. A low profile was kept, as befitted a minority government. Mr Miller recovered and returned to his post. In March 1977, the Premier announced a Cabinet shuffle. Mr Miller was moved from Health to another Cabinet position, and was replaced by Dennis Timbrell. Of the ten hospitals on the 'hit list', only four had been closed as of 1981. All were small private hospitals; the largest had 38 beds. In three of the hospitals, 5, 6, and 18 beds were converted from acute care to chronic care, although the hospitals retained other acute care beds. In some, reductions in beds and staff occurred (as in many other Ontario hospitals). Using the figures in the Canadian Hospital Association Directories for 1976 and 1981, for all ten 'hit list' hospitals, there was a net reduction of 174 beds (153 acute care) and 250 staff between the two time periods. The budgets for the six hospitals remaining open was about $4 million higher by 1981 than the budget for all ten hospitals in 1976. Doctors Hospital remained an acute care hospital, decreased in size by only 16 beds, and saw its budget increase by over $3 million dollars. Ultimately, of the total $48 million Mr Miller had hoped to save in the closure programme, a saving of only $26 million was realized. Overall, hospital budgets rose an average of 13.4 per cent in 1976 as compared to 1975 (which had increased by about 20 per cent over 1974).

The direct approach was abandoned as a policy failure, to be followed by a series of indirect attempts to achieve the same results. Why had this direct attack been unsuccessful?

The court ruling, although inconvenient, could have been handled by the government. An appeal might have overturned it; new legislation could certainly have overridden it. The failure of the policy sprang instead from two interrelated elements; the constraints of minority government and the power of community-based hospital boards. Toronto hospitals accounted for more than one-third of the operating costs of the Ontario hospital system. Not only were they close to each other, but transportation in the city was good. A case could have been made for closing down, consolidating, and/or converting some Toronto hospitals to chronic care or community health centres. However, most hospitals select as members of their boards powerful community figures, many with strong links to political leaders. In consequence, a hospital with a strong board has an ally whenever funds must be raised or when it is in conflict with government policy. The

hospitals selected as most vulnerable to closure on the basis of 'rational planning' – due to deteriorating physical plants, proximity to other more up to date hospitals, and so on – thus turned out to be small rural hospitals or community hospitals with an ethnic clientele. Although they were important to their communities as major employers, as a source of status, and/or as an attractor of physicians, they tended to have weaker boards, and less powerful allies.

One might thus infer that one reason Doctors Hospital, rather than one of Toronto's downtown teaching hospitals, was selected for closure was the relative power of their boards. Both the need for Doctors to conduct a public, community-based campaign and the fact that it lacked prior warning of its possible demise were evidence of its lack of power. Indeed, one of the first actions taken by the Hospital after its 'stay of execution' was to recruit a number of influential community and political figures, including Mr Grossman, to its board.

It is conceivable that the government could have chosen to take the 'political heat' from the public and persisted in closing those hospitals with less powerful boards. However, it is unlikely that any government would wish to fight (and probably lose) an election based on hospital closures. Most probably, a majority government early in its term could have followed through on this policy; minority governments must be more cautious.

**Interim activities**

While the government was recovering from its direct assault on hospital costs, it took two initiatives. First, a time honoured method – the committee of inquiry – was employed to remove political heat. In July 1977, the Premier authorized a joint committee of the Ontario Government and the Ontario Medical Association, chaired by a trust company executive, to study the health care field and to recommend cost-control possibilities. As might be expected based on its composition, the committee was essentially supportive of cost containment within the context of the status quo (Joint Advisory Committee 1977).

Second, the government attempted to end the difficulties of accommodating opposition parties by dissolving the legislature and calling an election. Its only issue was the 'need for strong majority government'. The public was unconvinced. Results were virtually identical to those before dissolution – the Progressive Conservatives formed a new minority government with 46 per cent of the seats. Although both opposition parties lost slightly in proportions of the popular vote, the geographical distribution of their support resulted in a slight gain for the Liberals and a decline for the New Democrats; the Liberals (with 27 per cent of the House) now formed the official opposition; the New Democratic Party, with 26 per cent, was close behind.

However, the atmosphere in the new legislature differed from that of the previous two years. This election was seen as having taught the lesson that the public disliked 'unnecessary elections'; all parties were therefore anxious to avoid precipitating one in the near future. In addition, both opposition parties had changed their leaders. The new leader of the New

Democratic Party was less appealing than his charismatic predecessor, and his party was reluctant to risk the loss of seats. Accordingly, despite its minority position, the government would have more breathing space. Their minority government lasted four years, far longer than is customary. (In the next election, March 1981, the New Democratic Party would suffer substantial losses and drop to 17 per cent of the seats, while the Progressive Conservatives would be rewarded for their responsiveness to the electorate during the past years of minority government with 44 per cent of the votes, 56 per cent of the seats, and a new majority government.)

## THE INDIRECT APPROACH TO COST CONTAINMENT

In late 1977, the new Minister of Health, Mr Timbrell, outlined a new plan for his department. It contained a four-pronged attack on health-care costs: deinstitutionalization, decentralization, health promotion, and disease prevention. For the next four years, cost containment was pursued through a series of simultaneous indirect measures aimed at both supply of and demand for institutional health services. The policies pursued will be analysed within the following categories: demand reduction and shifting within the universal system; supply reduction; buffering; and demand reduction by shifting payment and resources outside the universal system, including an expanded role for the private sector.

### Demand reduction and shifting within the universal system

Although the chief Ministry activities occurred in the areas of supply limitation, some demand reduction within the context of a universal system was also undertaken.

As indicated earlier, the Ministry was aware of the limitations of health care services, which had been noted by such critics as Fuchs (1974), the Lalonde Report (1975), and McKeown (1979). Pollution, occupational health hazards, life-style, and economic well-being were recognized as important determinants of health status, and hence of the subsequent need for medical resources and expenditures. Thus, one prong of the Ministry's new programme was to 'reduce and redirect' the need and demand for care. Public education programmes were devised to 'heighten public awareness of personal responsibility for health', and 'to sell people on the benefits of healthier lifestyles'. Government campaigns stressed exercise, the use of seat belts, non-smoking, and moderation in the use of alcohol. In 1981, an advertising campaign was conducted around the theme 'Health Begins at Home'. Resources devoted to disease prevention and public health programmes were increased. Funding for public health units tripled over 10 years, although their budget ($70.5 million in 1981–82) was still small compared to hospital and medical care spending. In addition, the Ministry emphasized provision of alternatives to institutional care. At any one time, 15–20 per cent of acute-care beds in Ontario are occupied by persons who do not need this level of care, but must remain in hospital beds until they can be transferred to more appropriate facilities such as

chronic-care institutions or nursing homes. The average per diem cost in a chronic hospital was approximately half that in a community hospital, and about one-third that in a teaching hospital. A logical solution might be the transfer of patients to more appropriate, less costly types of care. Acute care beds, thus released, could either be closed or used to eliminate the necessity for new construction. Substantial savings might then occur without negative political consequences. The Ministry's efforts to achieve this movement of patients took several directions.

In 1979–80, hospitals were given financial incentives to expand their out-patient services (and thereby reduce in-patient admissions). Day surgery services were encouraged and became more available. Additional incentives were given to convert acute care hospital beds to chronic, convalescent, or rehabilitation care, and the construction of new nursing home beds was approved. In 1980, the Minister of Health stated that, over the past five years, 3600 'surplus' active treatment beds had been eliminated in the province, but 6700 long-term beds had been added. It was none the less soon apparent that the potential demand for non-acute institutional care was too large to be met through such new construction. Ontario already institutionalized a higher percentage of its elderly population than most jurisdictions. Emphasis thus turned towards providing home-care services.

In theory, one cost-effective way of replacing institutional care would be to include chronic home care as an integral part of the health care system. This service would permit the maintenance of the semi-independent elderly in their homes by providing them with the necessary professional and support services. Public responsibility for their care could thus be shared with family members.

Politically, a programme which would be equally (or more) effective, more humane, more popular, and less expensive than the status quo had great attraction for the government, and the concept of home care received Cabinet approval. The 1980 Throne Speech made the extension of chronic home-care programmes throughout Ontario a provincial priority. By the end of the 1980 fiscal year, the Ministry of Health's seven existing chronic programmes had been joined by another eighteen (covering 50 per cent of the province's population), and full provincial coverage was expected to be in place by early 1982. The 1980 home care budget was $34 800 000, and provided nearly 3 million days of care. Jurisdictional difficulties between the 'free' insured services provided by the Ministry of Health and the home-care services partially financed by means tested user fees offered by the Ministry of Community and Social Services are being resolved as of this writing. Although home care had been proposed as a cost-effective substitution for institutional care, there was a strong likelihood that many clients would be served under new programmes who previously had been under-served, or not served at all. Chronic home care might thus act to improve quality of care; without careful definition of eligibility, however, it would probably be a more expensive service. Indeed, home care costs doubled between 1978–79 and 1979–80 as the programmes were extended to new sections of the province. In addition, there was a risk that extending chronic home care would act as an 'outreach' programme, and lead to increased demands on institutional care. Since homes for the aged – the 'first line' of institutional care – at present have relatively low provincial funding, chronic home care has the potential to increase health care costs if public pressure were to build up for continuing public assistance for patients who require transfer from home-care programmes into homes for the aged.

## Supply reduction

Although a detailed discussion is beyond the scope of this chapter, the Ministry has taken some initial steps to reduce the supply of physician manpower. Population to physician ratios have been steadily declining since the mid-1960s as Ontario's (and Canada's) stock of physicians has increased. Policy initiatives have included federal immigration restrictions of foreign physicians and, in Ontario, reductions in the permitted number of medical and surgical residency posts. However, more innovative measures have not as yet been taken.

During the period under examination, the major thrust of the Ministry's policy continued to be a reduction in the supply of hospital resources on the theory that, as Milton Roemer (1961) has stated, 'need expands into supply'. The first step was a further alteration in the bed guidelines.

As of 1 April 1980, the bed guideline used in Ministry planning was reduced by 0.25 beds per 1000 population with an additional reduction of 0.25 to take effect by 1 April 1981. By that date, the province would fund hospitals for only 3.5 beds per 1000 population in Southern Ontario, and 4.0 per 1000 in Northern Ontario. Because of the adverse reactions to their previous attempts to close small hospitals, the Ministry modified its policy to permit hospitals with 100 or fewer active treatment beds to retain up to ten beds above the figure authorized by the guidelines before their budget base would be reduced. When a hospital of less than 50 active treatment beds was the only one in a community, it was exempted from the guidelines altogether. Unless they qualified for the above exemptions, hospitals would have their budgets reduced by $12 000 for each active treatment bed kept open above those permitted by the guidelines.

From a policy standpoint, five things were notable about the Ministry's actions. First, publicly available formula was used to compile allowable beds, dispelling accusations of favouritism. Second, the formula was based on the demographic characteristics of the populations served; thus, hospitals in regions with a high proportion of elderly would have this factor recognized in bed allocations. Third, the formula was based on current patterns of utilization by demographic group, and thus enshrined them. Fourth, there was no explicit justification for the bed to population ratios selected. Last, the $12 000 per excess bed penalty was very effective in ensuring the success of this policy.

To enable bed reductions to be implemented without sacrificing quality of care, the Ministry had suggested improving occupancy (for example through improved scheduling) and reducing length of stay. These measures have managed to keep hospital utilization roughly steady; occupancy rates have fluctuated between 81 per cent and 84 per cent between 1976 and 1981.

A more precise evaluation of the success or failure of government policy is complicated by the tendency of the Ministry to revise the way in which they define and present data. In consequence, it is almost impossible to construct consistent and accurate time series. For example, an analysis of the success of bed reductions would demand an examination of bed numbers and how they have changed over time. The annual hospital statistics published by the Ontario Ministry of Health subdivides its figures into: public hospitals (the vast majority of the system), private hospitals, federal hospitals and nursing stations, and nursing homes temporarily approved for chronic care. Private hospitals are in turn divided into active and chronic hospitals; public hospitals are divided into active treatment (which includes public general hospitals and about 10 Red Cross Outposts with a combined total of fewer than 200 beds), psychiatric hospitals, alcohol and drug addiction hospitals, general rehabilitation hospitals, special rehabilitation hospitals, and chronic hospitals. Each of the last three categories is further subdivided into hospitals and units within hospitals. As such divisions tend to be arbitrary, the Ministry has often re-grouped categories. Thus, seeming changes in the number of active treatment beds between 1976 and 1977–78 were instead, in large part, artifacts of changes in the way general rehabilitation, special rehabilitation, and chronic units within hospitals were categorized. Another increase in the number of beds in the system in 1980–81 was an artefact of the decision to begin including provincial psychiatric hospitals in the hospital statistics. Analysis of bed numbers must thus first address the question 'what beds?' – all hospitals, public hospitals, acute general hospitals, etc.

The definition of beds to be used must also be decided. The Ministry has employed three distinct ways of counting beds. 'Rated beds', which refer to the physical capacity of a given institution, are reported every year, but are not considered useful or reliable by the Ministry. 'Beds staffed and in operation' have been reported since 1974; however, these figures are provided by hospitals, vary from day to day, and are not subject to quality control checks from the Ministry. In addition, the Ministry's change from calendar years to fiscal years in 1977–78 confounds seasonal variations in utilization with time trends if figures before and after that year are compared. 'Approved beds' are the basis of the Ministry's official figures and of its planning exercises, but unfortunately this category has been defined and reported only since 1976, and therefore cannot be used to judge the success of the bed reduction programmes. In addition, since approved beds may not be in use, this figure may understate the impact of underfunding on bed availability, and hence understate the effectiveness of the programme. Not surprisingly, bed figures reported in *Annual reports* (Ontario Ministry of Health 1972–1981/82a), *Hospital statistics* (Ontario Ministry of Health 1972–1981/82b), and Minister's speeches often disagree. Other changes in data reporting limit the ability to make utilization comparisons. As the result of a change in the hospital statistics reporting system in 1976, one-day stays were excluded from in-patient care statistics, artefactually reducing days of care and increasing average length of stay. Thus, although the number of patients under care appears to have declined steadily, this decline may in part be an artefact of the change in the way 'day surgery' was counted. Accordingly, no tables of hospital bed or utilization data are presented, lest the numbers be given too much credence by the reader.

Similar difficulties are found when dealing with the question of how much money the Ministry spent on the institutional sector. No part of the Ministry has the responsibility for keeping internally consistent time series data on hospital payments. Figures in the Public Accounts tend not to match those given in the Budget, which may not always match those given in the *Annual report*, or in the Minister's speeches. In part, these discrepancies can be attributed to differences in how programmes which have been transferred from one Ministry to another are handled; some series will retrospectively reallocate spending by such programmes, and others will not. In addition, series differ as to the treatment of post-year budget adjustments which, as will be noted later, were often substantial. The Fiscal Resources Branch of the Ministry of Health was kind enough to construct a retrospective time series of hospital funding data (Table 29.1) and this demonstrates several of the points of our analysis. A high rate of expenditures for hospitals in 1974–77 was followed by three years where the increase in expenditure was below the rate of inflation, although in two of these years, the actual expenditures were greater than the estimates. In recent years, hospital expenditures have been climbing again, such that in 1981–82, adjusted hospital spending was nearly 21 per cent higher than in the previous year, with a similar increase projected for 1982–83.

It is probably safe to say that hospitals are giving roughly the same amount of service as before; the bed guidelines may have prevented more rapid increase, but did not result in substantial reductions. The number of 'approved beds' in Ontario hospitals has remained roughly constant, with minor reductions in acute beds and increases in chronic care beds. Some impact of spending constraints on bed availability may be reflected in the smaller number of hospital beds 'staffed and in operation', but this figure may also be a response to shortages in nursing staff.

However, examination of approved bed numbers understates the effect of the Ministry's policies. Instead of Ministry-directed closures, the major thrust of the Timbrell period was to encourage hospitals to make their own cuts by systematically constraining the growth of the hospital sector. It was felt that only the provision of less money would force institutions to economize. In effect, the attempt which had been made by Miller was inverted. Miller had allowed hospitals to make budget requests; the Ministry then analysed and tried to cut them on a line-by-line basis, using regression models to guide 'appropriate levels of expenditure'. Under the new policy, hospitals were to be provided with annual increases of less than inflation. Although the Ministry would be available to give advice if requested, determinations of how to economize would be made by the institutions. For three years (1977–78 to 1979–80) the hospitals received official increases below the rate of inflation. However, the fiscal discipline was uneven; many requests for additional funding were approved by the Ministry of Health. In particular, deficits, if incurred, were subsequently covered by the Ministry.

Other circumventions of the guidelines also occurred. In 1978–79, the Ministry had announced that hospitals would receive an average 4.5 per cent increase, although inflation was about 9 per cent. However, when the government's first quarter financial figures were released, the financial picture

**Table 29.1.** *Expenditures of the government of Ontario, the Ministry of Health, and payments to hospitals for the fiscal years 1972/73–1982/83*[1,2]

| Year | % incr total gov exp (act) | Provincial spending Ministry of Health | | | Provincial spending hospitals (corrected)[3] | | | | |
| | | % incr health exp (act) | % of prov budget (est) | % of prov budget (act) | % of health budget (act) | $ (est) | $ (act) | % incr (est) | % incr (act) |
|---|---|---|---|---|---|---|---|---|---|
| 1972–73 | n/a | n/a | n/a | 30.8 | 46.3 | 954.9 | 926.4 | n/a | n/a |
| 1973–74 | 12.7 | 7.9 | 30.1 | 29.5 | 45.6 | 1010.6 | 986.1 | 5.8 | 6.4 |
| 1974–75 | 20.8 | 17.3 | 27.7 | 28.7 | 49.6 | 1078.0 | 1256.5 | 6.7 | 27.4 |
| 1975–76 | 20.5 | 17.7 | 27.9 | 28.0 | 48.7 | 1377.9 | 1454.5 | 27.8 | 15.8 |
| 1976–77 | 12.1 | 13.8 | 27.9 | 28.5 | 50.9 | 1646.0 | 1730.7 | 19.5 | 19.0 |
| 1977–78 | 10.1 | 7.1 | 28.8 | 27.7 | 50.1 | 1887.2 | 1825.9 | 14.7 | 5.5 |
| 1978–79 | 7.8 | 8.6 | 27.6 | 27.9 | 49.0 | 1951.9 | 1938.0 | 3.4 | 6.1 |
| 1979–80 | 8.4 | 7.8 | 27.5 | 27.8 | 49.6 | 2072.6 | 2119.1 | 6.2 | 9.3 |
| 1980–81 | 9.7 | 13.7 | 28.0 | 28.8 | 48.5 | 2298.1 | 2355.3 | 10.9 | 11.1 |
| 1981–82 | 16.7 | 18.8 | 29.1 | 29.3 | 49.3 | 2641.2 | 2847.9 | 14.9 | 20.9 |
| 1982–83 | n/a | n/a | 29.6 | n/a | n/a | 3206.0 | n/a | 21.4 | n/a |

N/a data not available.
(act) actual expenditures as reported in Public Accounts.
(est) estimated expenditures as reported in Printed Estimates.
exp expenditures.
1. Prior to 1972, only net funding of hospitals was reported as expenditures by Ministry of Health; consistent series for earlier years are therefore not available.
2. All figures prior to 1978–79 are adjusted to reflect change from calendar year to fiscal year reporting.
3. Payments to hospitals during fiscal years 1972–73 to 1977–78 included payments for clinical education which were subsequently reported separately; from 1972–73 to 1979–80 included payments for Related Facilities; from 1972–73 to 1978–79 included payments for private physiotherapy and out of province care. Adjusted figures for hospital expenditures reflect these changes.
Source: Fiscal Resources Branch, Ontario Ministry of Health.

was more optimistic than projected. In consequence, a revised budget was produced by Cabinet, and spending targets were redistributed. As a result of strenuous lobbying by the Minister of Health and his Deputy, $65 million of the $81 million then added to all provincial spending was allocated to the Ministry of Health. All of this money went to hospitals; much of it was earmarked to extend hospital-based long-term care facilities. The effect of this bonus on hospital attitudes was unfortunate. Hospitals concluded with some accuracy that restraint was an 'exercise in futility', and that whatever they needed would, eventually, be provided.

Instead of cutting services, many hospitals thus chose to continue business as usual, and to budget for deficits in the expectation that the Ministry would pick up the bill. According to Ministry calculations, there had been no hospital deficits in Ontario prior to 1977–78. However, by 1981–82 the deficits reached over $50 million; between 1980–81 and 1981–82, to the dismay of the government, the number of hospitals incurring deficits had tripled. In 1981, the Ministry amended the Public Hospitals Act to give Cabinet the power to appoint a supervisor to oversee a hospital's internal operations whenever 'the quality of patient care is deemed by an impartial expert to be in jeopardy'. Although this Act has not yet been used to deal with the consequences of budgetary deficits, it may be so employed in the future.

The cost containment strategy also ran foul of public opinion. In 1979, the newspapers were filled with stories about the negative impact of 'underfunding' on hospitals. Typical front page headlines included 'Our hospital nightmare: You could die waiting'. The tone of letters (to the editors, to columnists, and presumably to the government) was critical of the government, and favourable to providers rather than to the critics of the health care system. It was therefore evident that the government would have to placate the public before the next election.

In 1980, the provincial government took out advertisements in 40 newspapers to list 58 communities whose hospitals would get over $360 million for over 144 capital construction projects; hospital budget increases reverted to above inflation. Although the government resumed its 'get tough' rhetoric after the 1981 election, in October 1982, it provided an additional $110 million to meet hospital deficits, raising its spending on hospitals to $3.3 billion in that fiscal year. It remains to be seen whether the government will carry out its stated policy that no future deficits would be accepted or paid for.

## Buffering

With the recognition that cuts were unpopular, the government also employed a time-honoured strategy – it attempted to shift the blame for unpopular decisions to other levels of government.

Public statements by provincial officials stressed the negative role being played by federal funding cut-backs. However, the greatest effort was employed in shifting the apparent responsibility for implementing budget cuts to a series of local advisory agencies, the District Health Councils (DHCs) (Dixon 1981).

These Councils were first established in 1975. They were descended from a number of initiatives in regionalization, including the establishment of planning and economic regions for the analysis of economic and social development and the implementation of regional municipal governments in some parts of the province. Public health services had long been delegated to local Boards of Health by the Ontario government.

District Health Councils differed in a number of ways from these previous regional entities. According to the government, the DHC mandate was to:

1. Identify district health needs and consider alternative methods of meeting those needs that are consistent with provincial guidelines.
2. Plan a comprehensive health programme and establish short-term priorities that are consistent with long-term goals.
3. Co-ordinate all health activities and ensure a balanced, effective and economical service, satisfactory to the people of the district.
4. Work toward co-operation in social development activities for the district.

The mandate included neither a role in service delivery, nor budgetary authority within the district. However, all proposed new and expanded programmes would have to be sent to the DHC for approval and 'priorization' before they would be considered by the Ministry. Thus, DHCs could serve as buffers for the Ministry of Health during a period of cost constraint, under the logical premise that local people would be better suited than more distant bureaucrats to determine where reductions should be made and what new programmes, if any, should be started.

New DHCs have been established gradually since 1975. In some districts, they had been preceded by (but superseded) voluntary local hospital councils. As of 1982, 25 DHCs existed in Ontario. All fall within, but are separate from, regional, county, or local government units, and contain at least 80 000 population. Six districts do not yet have Councils.

Councils exist in an ambiguous political and legal status, which hinders the accomplishment of their stated goals. They were established by Order-in-Council and do not have their own Act; thus, they could easily be abolished or changed by any future government. Their membership is roughly split among representatives of local government, providers, and consumers. Members are not elected, but appointed by the province on the basis of local recommendations. As a result, DHCs have no clear legitimacy and no accountability to their region. Although they serve as advisors to the Ministry of Health, they have no budgetary authority and their recommendations do not have to be followed. In recent years, negative recommendations made by DHCs have tended to be followed; low-rated or rejected programmes have not been funded. However, DHC approval has not guaranteed favourable government action under current cost constraints.

The DHCs have been effective in changing conventional lines of communication and fostering the resolution of priority conflicts at the local level. They have thus insulated the Ministry to some extent from local pressures. By including non-hospital members, they have also served to shift and broaden the health care planning base in some communities. However, the DHCs have small staffs and limited budgets. In 1976–77, the combined budget for the 15 then-existing DHCs was $2.3 million, whereas the average budget for one 300 bed community hospital without tertiary care was $15 million. As a result, many DHCs have been reluctant to confront the institutional sector.

Given the reluctance of the Ontario government to give up its statutory decision making responsibilities, the long-term future of DHCs may be in question. Their decisions have questionable local legitimacy. The medical associations and the opposition parties have called for their elimination. Although some have played a useful facilitating and co-ordinating role in rationalization of services, the effectiveness of shifting the blame to DHCs has been undercut by the recognition that few new programmes have been funded. Policy attention thus returned to the provincial government, which came under pressure to soften its cost containment policies.

### Demand reduction by shifting payment and resources outside the universal system

With the political unpopularity of expenditure reduction, the Ontario government considered policy alternatives. One alternative to decreasing expenditures is increasing revenues; if these revenues will not come from government, they must be sought elsewhere, by such measures as user fees. However, the ideology of the Canadian health system is that needed services should not be rationed by price. Thus, advocates of user fees must choose their arguments carefully. One favourite rationalization has been that free services are used frivolously; a user fee would thus serve to deter 'unnecessary' utilization. User-fee policies are thus generally coupled with exemptions and/or subsidies for the 'genuinely needy'.

The 'deterrent-fee' option was recommended by the Taylor committee (Joint Advisory Committee 1977), which the government had set up after the failure of its hospital closure policy. This recommendation had been favoured by the physicians who welcomed a source of 'private money' and by some bureaucrats within other Ministries who welcomed any non-government sources of revenue. It had been strongly opposed by some factions within the Ministry of Health, who were aware of a series of studies conducted on the impact of user fees which had concluded that such fees were not only ineffective in deterring 'unnecessary' utilization, but also served to discourage the poor and the elderly from seeking possibly necessary care (Badgley and Smith 1979; Barer et al. 1979). These studies revealed user fees to be purely sources of revenue, with a potentially detrimental impact on the universal system. As such, they would be politically risky unless levied only against 'luxury services'. Indeed, to the extent that user fees endangered access, their adoption might be in violation of the federal agreements and risk the forfeiture of federal funds. Accordingly, the Progressive Conservative government had consistently rejected adopting new user fees as revenue sources.

Following the failure of the hospital closure programme,

however, the government did attempt to increase the taxes paid to cover health care. Darcy McKeough, the Treasurer of Ontario, incorporated an increase in health insurance premiums into his 1978 budget. He stressed the importance of retaining a 'visible link' between citizen payments and the costs of medical care, and argued that Ontario Health Insurance Plan (OHIP) premiums should continue to meet a fixed proportion of health care costs. He announced that, as of 1 May 1978, OHIP premiums would rise by 37.5 per cent. The McKeough proposals failed for the same reason as the Miller hospital closures – there was still a minority government. Following opposition attacks in the legislature and the threat of an election, the government again backed off. The premium increase was cut to 18.75 per cent, and the question of health care financing was referred to a committee of the legislature. McKeough soon retired from active politics, lamenting his inability to make 'sound businesslike decisions' in the public sector.

In 1979, the government tried a somewhat different approach. The new Treasurer was Frank Miller who, as Minister of Health, had attempted to close hospitals. The government proposed a series of increases in selected user charges – for example for ambulance services and for semi-private and private hospital accommodation. Patients in chronic accommodations for more than 60 days would be charged a co-payment fee of $9.80 per day, in order to remove the financial disincentive to transfer such patients to other levels of institutional care, in which such co-payments already existed. Certain patients, such as those with low incomes, would be exempted from the charges. User fees were not imposed for acute hospitals or for physician services, which constituted the vast majority of health care spending.

These measures, in contrast to previous efforts, were successfully implemented; the opposition could do little to stop them. The entire package could be (and was) implemented bureaucratically by modifying existing regulations. The opposition leaders were also not eager for an election at that time. As the Liberal leader, a psychiatrist, commented, 'The Liberals will have no alternative but to oppose this part of the package, but I don't see this as something the whole province of Ontario should have to go to the polls over'.

After the 1981 election, the majority Progressive Conservative government convened seven policy review committees to examine various aspects of social service funding and to try yet again to limit costs. Their recommendations included a variation on the 'underfunding' policy which eliminated the government bail outs for hospital deficits which had undermined the previous effort. The plan, called BOND (the Business-Oriented New Development Plan), was announced December 1981, and would take effect 1 April 1982.

Under BOND, hospitals would be encouraged to be more 'businesslike', and would be given financial incentives to become more cost-efficient. They would be allowed to retain all savings in costs – which formerly had reverted to the Ministry – and would be able to keep all new revenue they could raise (which formerly had offset Ministry contributions). The Plan could thus increase hospital operating funds with no added cost to the Ministry. Instead of receiving the expected relief for their $100 million in deficits (a relief subsequently received in October 1982) hospitals thus were encouraged to adopt a 'free enterprise' approach. It was time for the hospitals to 'increase their motivation to function creatively with maximum efficiency'. The government spoke of this effort as an attempt to 'change the attitudes of hospital management' through incentives to increase revenues, cut expenditures, and improve organizational effectiveness. The government again hoped that innovative administration might lead to rationalization of services, multi-unit management, and even private sector involvement in financing and running health services.

Before BOND could be implemented, another cabinet shuffle occurred. The Minister of Health, Mr Timbrell, was shifted, at his request, into Agriculture. The new Minister of Health, Larry Grossman, who had helped to save Doctors Hospital, now had the responsibility of implementing BOND.

On balance, the attempts to 'turn the system around' during the Timbrell years have had an incremental impact. The costs of hospital care as a percentage of GNP and as a percentage of provincial spending have stayed roughly constant, although these figures did decrease temporarily. Little use was made of alternatives to traditional institutional care. The main innovations, such as chronic home care, had the potential to become add-ons because of the likelihood of an increased level of need for services. With the cautions concerning Ministry statistics mentioned earlier, the (corrected) total number of 'approved' beds in Ontario hospitals increased from 48 685 in 1976, to 49 035 in 1980–81 despite the 'de-institutionalization' policy (Ontario Ministry of Health 1972–1981/82b). In light of the population increase of approximately 300 000 during this period, the bed-constraint policy could thus be judged moderately successful.

The years of effort have had several other effects. Negatively, there is a public perception that the health care system is endangered, and some providers are now convinced that they will financially profit if they can sufficiently endanger the system. More positively, the concept of chronic care is now viewed by hospitals as a role which they can and should perform. There has been a small reallocation of institutional beds (both from acute to chronic care and regionally within the province – for example from the central city to the periphery).

Several factors have acted to limit the success of the policies described in this chapter (although it is too early to evaluate the ultimate success of BOND). Most importantly, external constraints have played an increasing role in limiting government actions.

Although the Progressive Conservative government had a stable minority (and, from 1981, a majority) in the legislature, public opinion has undermined both the cost-containment and the user-fee options. Universal health and hospital insurance is the most popular government programme, and visible cutbacks in it are unlikely to be viewed favourably. Both opposition parties have championed the needs of providers and consumers, as has much of the media coverage, although there has been increasing criticism of physicians' incomes. To accomplish meaningful reductions in the institutional care sector (and hence to realize any substantial

savings) the government will have to educate the public and the media about the costs of current programmes and the potentially beneficial nature of alternatives.

Further, provider groups who perceived that they were underfunded became antagonistic. The 'bail outs' of hospital deficits served to consolidate the belief that the only way to achieve results was through confrontation. Those administrators who had stayed within their budgets, often by making difficult cuts, resented the fact that hospitals that had not cut spending had been rewarded. Indeed, the 1982 addition of $110 million to meet hospital deficits is likely to have aggravated this problem. Similarly, labour actions have become more prevalent. Nurses, service employees, technicians, and internes and residents threatened or used both legal and illegal strike action, and received increased financial settlements. This pattern culminated, in 1982, in a series of day long 'study sessions' by practising physicians seeking (and receiving) substantial increases in the government fee schedule. In effect, the province's physicians conducted a successful series of rotating one day strikes.

Ultimately, some providers (especially physicians) have come to think that the best way to increase their funding is to attack the universal plan and push for a US-style health care system with the government as the insurer of last resort for those unable to afford private coverage. Such a system would increase provider incomes, because the total amount of money devoted to health care would be increased. However, from a societal perspective, an increased proportion of GNP would be devoted to health services without corresponding benefit. In addition, the universality of the system would be undermined. The primary attraction to government is that the increased costs would not appear in the public sector; however, they would remain as costs to the public, and to the national economy. To its credit, the Ontario government has refused to take this policy.

Ontario policy-making has been further constricted because the increasingly unpopular Liberal federal government has decided to change the rules of the jointly-financed health care and post-secondary education programmes. The federal deficit was large and growing and the government was seeking ways of reducing federal spending for non-federal programmes. The Prime Minister had announced, unilaterally, the death of 'co-operative federalism', while his government revealed an impending unilateral cut in transfer payments to the provinces for medical care and post-secondary education.

Ottawa also believes it politically advantageous to pose as the champions of universal insurance. Accordingly, they have issued a number of statements calling for the end of health-care premiums in those provinces employing them and for the prohibition (or at least limitation) of opting out, user charges and balanced billing. Although negotiations continue, the federal aim is to pay less money for shared programmes, gain more control over them, and ensure that they receive more political credit. The future federal role in and contributions to health and post-secondary education programmes is a matter of uncertainty, and thus limits provincial policy making and planning.

Finally, the downturn in the economy prevented new

money from being used to fund innovations. This lack of money for new services means that innovations must come from cuts in the most powerful sector of the health care system – institutional funds. Since the government remained committed to a high-quality health care system, the Ministry staff found it necessary to make continued compromises and add 'needed' money to hospital budgets. Each compromise, however, served to undermine the restraint programme, dissipate co-operation from other institutions, re-awaken public expectations for more spending, and necessitate cuts in other areas in order to keep down the deficit. New programmes and innovations prove most vulnerable in any such climate of restraint. The government's recent efforts to finance incremental costs by allowing limited increases in the role of the private sector in health care and the opening of additional sources of revenue to hospitals raises a new question – can this be managed without destroying the universal system itself?

## CONCLUSIONS

In setting health policy, the government of Ontario was confronted with two conflicting objectives. On the one hand, they wished to maintain a high-quality, universal health care system; on the other, they wished to constrain costs (and, in particular, to limit their own liability for costs). Marginal policy shifts have thus occurred according to whether 'maintaining quality' or 'controlling costs' was paramount at a given time. This emphasis, in turn, has varied as a function of the economic climate, the political security of the government, and the identity of key members of Cabinet. In making policy, the Ontario government has been constrained by the actions of others. The federal government, opposition parties, providers of health services, and the public have all advocated increasing the resources being directed to the hospital sector. To the extent that a policy of de-institutionalization meant that fewer resources would go to hospitals, the Ontario government could not count on external support. Its ability to enforce reductions to the hospital sector would thus depend on being insulated from accountability for its actions, as might only be the case in the early years of a majority government.

Given this dilemma, two alternative policies might be constructed. One would place the health care sector under greater government control, empowering the government to manage supply and demand to enforce its priorities. The other would shift much responsibility for health care away from government into the private sector. Both policies have attractions; both have risks.

Greater control implies increasing confrontation with provider groups and the need for a tough and consistent provincial stance; neither is easy for a government which must face re-election. Less control is superficially more attractive; it implies easier relationships with providers and a diminished provincial role (and budgetary responsibility) as private funding increases. However, this policy is likely to lead to greater total costs for health care, and potentially to a two-tier hospital and medical care system. This policy is also opposed by the federal government, which may withhold

funds if it considers the universal system to be endangered. As described previously, the middle-of-the-road Ontario government, reluctant to embrace either extreme, has, in turn, made tentative steps towards each policy.

Because of the popularity of the universal programme and the public support it enjoys, more private payment may not prove a viable option, particularly if the federal government retains its prohibition of private insurance. Ontario (like Quebec) could thus decide that greater control of the system (and its providers) will be the least costly political and economic decision, even given the likelihood of greater confrontation with providers. If the patterns of the last ten years which this review has described persist, the choice of policy direction may shift between greater and less governmental control, alternatively favouring providers and users. The pressure of the moment is likely to outweigh long-term considerations.

Even given its extraordinary advantages with respect to the ability to achieve its policy objectives, the government of Ontario was able to have, at best, an incremental impact on the size of the institutional sector. The desires of its planners to 'de-institutionalize' health care had mixed results. The direct attack on hospitals failed, while the indirect methods employed have had some impact. The 'alternatives' to institutional care have generally been additions rather than replacements, and the costs of hospitals have continued to grow. 'Get tough' policies have not been sustained over time. As one example, 'underfunded' hospitals were permitted to run deficits which the government eventually picked up, despite earlier vows not to do so. It remains to be seen whether current governmental determination to curb hospital spending will persist over time as a new election approaches.

In considering how the government might have been more successful, one recognizes that the successive policies described in this chapter have been modified because of public opposition to government goals. Even given political will and advantages, and a political system designed to permit governments to take actions they perceive as necessary, an accountable government cannot move too far ahead of the public. Greater success, then, will require communication with the public about the reasons for and alternatives to unpopular policies. The failure to implement plans in the absence of such public consent may be considered one of the inevitable consequences of democratic government.

### Acknowledgements

This chapter has benefitted from the comments of David Bogart, John Browne, Gary Chatfield, Allan Detsky, John Hastings, David Hoff, Peggy Leatt, A.I. Rands, G. Simpson, G. Turner, and Gail Thompson, and from the willingness of Susan Ironside to type, with accuracy, each new draft. However, no one other than the authors is responsible for the opinions, findings, and conclusions expressed herein.

## REFERENCES

Andreopoulos, S. (ed.) (1975). *National health insurance, can we learn from Canada?* Wiley, Toronto.

Badgley, R.F. and Smith, R.D. (1979). *User charges for health services.* Ontario Council of Health, Toronto.

Barer, M.L., Evans, R.G., and Stoddart, G.L. (1979). *Controlling health care costs by direct charges to patients: snare or delusion.* Occasional Paper No. 10, Ontario Economic Council, Toronto.

Boivin-Lesage, M. (1982). Quebec marches toward state medicine. *Can. Med. Assoc. J.* **127**, 314.

*Canada yearbook, 1978–79.* Statistics Canada, Ottawa.

Commission of Inquiry on Health and Social Service (1970). *Report Part Two, Tome II, Second title: The Health Plan.* (Castonguay Report.) Government of Quebec, Quebec City.

Committee on the Healing Arts (1970). *Report,* Vol. I. Queen's Printer, Toronto.

Department of Health and Social Development (1972). *White Paper on Health Policy.* Department of Health and Social Development, Manitoba.

Detsky, A.S., Stacey, S.R., and Bombardier, C. (1983). The effectiveness of a regulatory strategy in containing hospital costs. *N. Eng. J. Med.* **309**, 151.

Dixon, M. (1981). *The organization of district health councils in Ontario.* Ontario Ministry of Health, Toronto.

Evans, R.G. (1982). Health care in Canada: patterns of funding and regulation. In *The public/private mix for health* (ed. G. McLachlan and A. Maynard) p. 369. Nuffield Provincial Hospitals Trust, London.

Foulkes, R. (1973). *Health security for British Columbians,* Vol. 1. Government of British Columbia, Vancouver.

Fuchs, V.R. (1974). *Who shall live: health, economics and social policy.* Basic Books, New York.

Gross, M.J. and Schwenger, C. (1981). *Health care costs for the elderly in Ontario: 1976–2026.* Ontario Economic Council, Toronto.

Hall, E.M. (1980). *Canada's National-Provincial Health Program for the 1980s (Health services review '79).* Craft Litho, Saskatoon.

Hastings, J.E.F. (Chairman) (1973). *The Community Health Centre in Canada,* Vol. 1. Information Canada, Ottawa.

Hatcher, G.H. (1981). *Universal free health care in Canada. 1947–77.* NIH Pub. No. 81-2052. US Department of Health and Human Services, Washington.

Health and Welfare (1979). *National health expenditures in Canada, 1960–1975.* Health and Welfare Canada, Ottawa.

Health Planning Task Force (1974). *Report* (Mustard Report). Ontario Ministry of Health, Toronto.

Illich, I. (1975). *Limits to medicine: medical nemesis, the expropriation of health.* McClelland and Stewart, in association with Marion Boyers, London.

Joint Advisory Committee (1977). *Report of the Joint Advisory Committee of the Government of Ontario and the Medical Association on methods to control health care costs* (Taylor Report). Queen's Printer, Toronto.

Lalonde, M. (1975). *A new perspective on the health of Canadians.* Information Canada, Ottawa.

MacDonald, D.C. (ed.) (1980). *The government and politics of Ontario* (revised edition). Van Nostrand Reinhold, Toronto.

McKeown, T. (1979). *The role of medicine.* Blackwell, Oxford.

Ontario Economic Council (1976). *Issues and alternatives 1976: health.* Ontario Economic Council, Toronto.

Ontario Ministry of Health (1972 to 1981/82a). *Annual Reports.* Ontario Ministry of Health, Toronto.

Ontario Ministry of Health (1972 to 1981/82b). *Hospital Statistics* (formerly *Ontario hospital services commission, statistical supplement*). Ontario Ministry of Health, Toronto.

Ontario Ministry of Treasury and Economics (1981). *Expenditures of the health care system in Ontario, 1970/71 to 1977/78.* Ontario Ministry of Treasury and Economics, Toronto.

Roemer, M. (1961). Bed supply and hospital utilization. *Hospitals* **35**, 36.

Royal Commission on Health Services (1964 and 1965). *Summary, Vols 1 and 2* (Hall Report). Queen's Printer, Ottawa.

Simeon, R. (1972). *Federal-provincial diplomacy: the making of recent policy in Canada.* University of Toronto Press.

Soderstrom, L. (1978). *The Canadian health care system.* Croom Helm, London.

Task Force (1969). *Reports on the cost of health services in Canada.* Queen's Printer, Ottawa.

Taylor, M. (1978). *Health insurance and Canadian public policy.* McGill-Queen's University Press, Montreal.

VanLoon, R.J. and Wittington, M.S. (1981). *The Canadian political system: environment, structure and process.* McGraw-Hill Ryerson, Toronto.

Vayda, E., Evans, R.G., and Mindell, W. (1979). Universal health insurance in Canada: history, problems, trends. *J. Community Health* **4**, 217.

Wolfson, A.D. and Tuohy, C.J. (1980). *Opting out of medicare: private medical markets in Ontario.* Ontario Economic Council Research Study No. 19. University of Toronto Press.

# 30 Research and the delivery of primary care – the United Kingdom

David C. Morrell

## INTRODUCTION

It is only within the last 30 years that primary care has been identified as a separate discipline within medicine which demands special knowledge and skills. The emergence of the discipline was closely linked to the increasing specialization within medicine which arose from the rapid increase in medical knowledge in the years following the Second World War. This led many physicians and surgeons to specialize, so that they could study their subjects in depth and apply the new technology and skills. In order to use their time economically, it was sensible for patients requiring their specialized knowledge to be selected to consult them.

In many countries, particularly the UK, the Netherlands, parts of Scandinavia, and Canada, this fact was recognized in shaping the national systems of health care which were being developed at the time. In the UK the service was so organized that the general practitioner (GP) should be directly accessible to the population for consultation about any problem within the whole field of medicine. The specialist, in contrast, would usually only see those patients referred on to him or her by the generalist. As the system of specialization and sub-specialization became more complex the role of the GP as the point of entry to the system, became more important. He was responsible for identifying his patients' needs for care and directing those who required specialist care to the appropriate resources. More often, however, he was satisfying their day to day needs for care and was providing continuity of care, usually over a long period of time during which short episodes of specialist care might be required.

It soon became clear that the GP was, in fact, able to deal with most of the medical needs of his patients. It was for instance demonstrated by Morrell et al. (1971), that at less than 3 per cent of consultations was a patient referred to a specialist, and that while over 70 per cent consulted the GP in one year, only 10 per cent had any contact with a specialist. One result of this is that the sort of illness seen in general practice is inevitably very different from the selected illnesses seen by specialists. The decision to seek primary care is made by the patient and is influenced by a wide variety of factors. The decision to seek secondary care is a medical one, usually made by a GP who concludes that the patient needs the skills of a specialist. It is not difficult to imagine that the diagnostic method of the GP may differ from that employed by the specialist and this has been described by Wright and McAdam (1979).

In those countries which developed national systems of care which divided doctors into providers of primary and providers of secondary care, it soon became apparent that the knowledge, skills, and indeed attitudes of the doctors working in different fields must necessarily be different. In addition, the increasing recognition of the importance of prevention and health education which could most easily be practised by GPs who are in frequent contact with their patients, as Russell et al. (1979) have commented, opened up new areas of importance in primary care. The discipline of primary care can be defined and must be submitted to research and placed on a scientific foundation.

In countries where the system of care did not separate primary from secondary care, it was less easy to identify the training required by a doctor specializing in primary care. Gradually, however, this has become apparent in most countries and there are now doctors throughout the world providing primary care who are variously named primary physicians, family physicians, or general practitioners. In this chapter the term general practitioner (GP) will be used and should be translated by the reader into the local vernacular.

## THE CHARACTERISTICS OF PRIMARY CARE

Before describing the research and development which is needed to provide a scientific foundation for the work of the GP, it may be useful to identify the special characteristics of primary care.

### The population for whom the primary physician is responsible

In some systems of primary care the physician is responsible for a definable population. In the British National Health Service (NHS) this population consists of the patients who register with a particular GP. They can be defined in terms of name, address, age, and sex. In other systems the population may be defined in terms of those who live in a particular geographical area or who consult the doctor over a particular period of time.

The concept of a defined population for whom the GP accepts responsibility carries with it, the role of not simply responding to new requests for medical care, but also of identifying the needs of that population and where necessary initiating education, prevention, and treatment. The knowledge and skills required to identify the medical needs of a defined population and the medical organization necessary to respond to these needs are essential for good primary care.

### The presentation of illness in primary care

The decision to seek primary medical care is a lay decision. Patients consult because the anxiety engendered by the symptoms of illness which they experience is such as to provoke a consultation. The factors which determine when an individual experiencing symptoms of illness will seek medical care are not concerned simply with the nature of the symptoms experienced, but with many other factors including the personality of the patient, the support which is available to him in the community, and his expectations and access to the medical care system. To function effectively in the community, the GP must be aware of the factors which influence patients to seek medical care. The GP must have the skill to obtain the information necessary to identify the patient's problems and the knowledge to provide appropriate management.

### The doctor-patient relationship

In primary care, the doctor usually relates to his patients over a period of time measured in years rather than weeks or months. In the course of time, each develops expectations of the other. This influences the way the patients use their doctor and the way in which doctors respond to their patients. It affects communications, and the mutual trust which is built up between doctor and patient, can influence the management of the early symptoms of illness, the management of serious, even life-threatening disease and terminal care. The GP needs to know how to enhance and use this relationship for the benefit of the patient.

### Continuing care

Many patients for whom the GP is providing care will be suffering from chronic and incurable disease. The GP must develop methods of ensuring that these patients are reviewed at appropriate intervals and that when necessary, they are referred for specialist care. Chronic disease causes disability and it is in helping these patients to adapt to their disabilities by drug therapy and other means, that the GP is particularly concerned. This normally demands a team approach in which doctor, nurse, social worker, and a variety of other health professionals are involved. The GP must therefore, possess the necessary management skills to work with the team to achieve their therapeutic goals.

## RESEARCH IN PRIMARY CARE

The characteristics of primary care which have been identified indicate the areas of research which are needed to develop this branch of medicine.

### Illness behaviour

This may be seen as particularly important to the research activities of social scientists and chapters in this book are devoted to the type of work which they carry out. In interpreting new requests for medical care the results of their work are, however, highly relevant to the primary physician. There is a need for multidisciplinary studies in which the research of social scientists is linked with that of primary physicians seeking a better understanding of the factors influencing their patients to seek care and the factors which affect the way individuals adapt to disease and disability.

### The delivery of care

The method of delivering primary care is likely to influence the care provided. This is concerned with such subjects as ease of access; economic barriers to care; care provided in a pre-paid system as opposed to payment for each item of service; care provided from the physician's home as opposed to a health centre or polyclinic; care provided by one physician for the whole family as opposed to different physicians caring for different age groups. This area of research is also concerned with the role of the primary physician in the home and in the hospital. Studies in this field are likely to measure work load, outcome, and costs.

### The natural history of disease

The GP needs to be aware of the significance and the outcome of the common symptoms presented to him. It is also important for him to know how the outcome can be influenced by treatment. There is a need here for simple descriptive studies of outcome with and without treatment. A great deal of ignorance still exists about the long-term effects of common diseases, such as, asthma, hay fever, and hypertension and how these can be modified. The GP is ideally placed to clarify these issues.

### The management of illness

Studies in this area of primary care develop inevitably from the studies of the natural history of disease. Management strategies in primary care however, embrace not just therapeutic trials of treatment, but also alternative methods of management in a wider sense. This includes strategies for health education and prevention; the role of different members of the primary care team; the use of laboratory and radiological facilities and the interface between primary physicians and specialists. Many different systems of care have been developed, few have been subjected to careful measurement in terms of outcome and costs.

Research methods which may be applied in primary care have been described in earlier chapters in this volume. This chapter describes the special problems which may be encountered when these methods are applied in the primary care setting. It then goes on to consider how the techniques used to investigate the work of the GP may be modified and developed to improve the day to day care GPs provide for their patients.

## SOME PROBLEMS IN PRIMARY CARE RESEARCH

### Recording events in primary care

The primary physician who is concerned with carrying out a research project or simply studying critically his own performance will need to measure the frequency with which certain events occur in his practice. These events may be the number of consultations conducted over a particular period of time; the number of individuals who consulted with a particular diagnosis or disability; or the number of times a particular form of management was prescribed. Sometimes the measurement of non-events may be of interest, such as the number of children in the community who have failed to attend for immunization, or the number of elderly patients who have not consulted him in the last year. The accurate recording of events in primary care, be they for service or research purposes is beset with difficulties.

### Defining events

If a doctor wishes to record particular events occuring in his practice, he must first define these events and subsequently adhere strictly to that definition. To know how many consultations he carries out, for instance, he must define a consultation. Clearly this will include face-to-face consultations in the office. Does it also include telephone consultations, requests for 'repeat prescriptions', and home visits? He may alternatively just wish to study all patients who come to him with a particular complaint, such as urinary tract infection. The purpose may either be research into the aetiology of these infections or simply to 'audit' the care provided. How then does he define a urinary tract infection on the occasion it first presents? What combination of symptoms and signs will determine whether or not a patient is entered in this study? He may conclude that this is too difficult and decide to look instead at all patients presenting with dysuria. Does this mean dysuria as the primary symptom or dysuria associated with other symptoms? Is he interested in studying elderly males with prostatic problems or only females in the reproductive age groups? This simple example demonstrates that to look critically at even the simplest aspects of care and subsequently compare and discuss these results with others the physician must define precisely what he is studying and adhere to this definition.

The first stage in defining events in primary care is to organize a discussion between those who are going to take part in the study. The next stage is to test how well the doctors are able to interpret the definitions which have been agreed upon. One method which has proved useful in testing definitions, in terms of the variation between doctors in their interpretations, is to prepare a series of fictional case histories (Morrell *et al.* 1970). The doctors who are going to take part in the recording can complete the research record in response to these case histories. Subsequent discussion on the responses they have made will often reveal special areas of difficulty and lead to modifications of the definitions used or the design of the research record which is being planned. Theoretical definitions prepared in group discussion, however, may in practice prove too rigorous or too permissive. It is difficult to predict how a definition will work in practice. The only answer is to test it and modify it as a result of a pilot trial.

A common mistake is to assume that a definition that has worked in one setting can automatically be applied in a different setting. Definitions used by research assistants in administering questionnaires in population surveys, or by hospital specialists in the out-patient department may not be applicable in primary care where the pattern, content, and tempo of work is so different. They must always be tested. Those who wish to do research in primary care are often tempted to get on with the project and not waste time on a pilot trial. Such haste will always lead to disappointments and very commonly to disasters in terms of the definitive study.

### The problems of diagnosis

An example has been provided of the difficulty of defining a urinary tract infection at the time it presents at primary care level. Many would regard this as a relatively clear-cut disease. Problems such as anxiety, or depression, or back strain are much more difficult to define. One of the difficulties peculiar to primary care is that many of the diseases are seen at a very early stage in their natural history. Some of the characteristics of these diseases described in textbooks are absent at this time and a large proportion of the patients will recover before the full clinical picture has evolved. It has been estimated that for about 50 per cent of the new illnesses presented in primary care, a definitive diagnosis is never reached.

This presents a difficulty for doctors who wish to study the incidence or management of particular diseases and to monitor the care which they are providing. Because they have decided to take part in a study they may feel under some obligation to reach a diagnosis at each consultation. This may lead them to record a spurious diagnosis when it would be more accurate simply to record the presenting symptom. The pressure on the doctor to record a diagnosis is also influenced by his training and by the therapeutic options open to him in response to different diagnoses. Doctors are trained in a diagnostic model which may be appropriate in a secondary care setting in which history taking, examination of the patient, and laboratory or X-ray investigations lead to a diagnosis. The diagnosis is a prerequisite for determining the management of the patient. This model does not stand up to critical evaluation in primary care (Wright and McAdam 1979). In this situation symptomatic treatment is often appropriate once the doctor has established that the patient's symptoms do not indicate serious disease, and that the current illness is likely to respond spontaneously. Doctors in their early years in primary care may feel constrained to fit their patient into a particular diagnostic category. A patient for instance, presenting with vague symptoms of fatigue may be interrogated aggressivly about sleep disturbance, appetite, and mood change. If appropriate answers can be obtained, the patient can be categorized as suffering from depression and on the basis of this diagnosis, specific therapy may be prescribed.

Much more serious problems occur in carrying out international comparisons of morbidity in primary care. Diagnostic habits vary in different countries and different cultures. The story of chronic bronchitis and emphysema is the classic example where the differing prevalence of the disease chronic bronchitis in the US and the UK was shown to be due, not to a real difference in disease experience, but to the application of different diagnostic criteria (Meneely *et al.* 1960).

The difficulty of making a precise diagnosis when illness is seen at an early stage in its natural history, has been tackled by using a problem-orientated approach to illness in primary care rather than a disease-orientated approach. This was first described by Weed (1969) in the US. It has been usefully applied in hospital care but is particularly relevant in primary care. In this system of recording, the symptoms presented by the patient and the objective findings of the physician are integrated to define the patient's main problem. This may or may not be a diagnosis in pathological terms. Over the course of time the problem may be advanced to a point at which a precise diagnosis is admissable and a diagnostic label can be applied. In many instances, however, the problem will resolve before a diagnosis is reached. This approach reflects much more accurately the morbidity patterns encountered by the primary physician than a system which is linked to a diagnostic index related to diseases.

### Methods of collecting information in primary care

Many doctors anxious to carry out research or to look critically at the care that they are providing have attempted to obtain useful information by a retrospective analysis of their records. This very frequently leads to disappointment. The reason for this can be appreciated when the many roles which GPs' records are expected to fulfill are considered. It may be useful for those planning to use routine records for evaluating care or carrying out research to consider the content and reliability of different aspects of the routine record.

1. The date of the consultation and the problem presented are usually recorded in the routine records but may not be. If the consultation concerns some trivial incident or takes place in the street or incidently when a consultation with one member of the family leads to a consultation with another, the doctor may not have the patients records available and may record no information.

2. The symptom presented at the consultation may be recorded. But in many cases it is not because the presenting symptom is seen in retrospect to be irrelevant to the patient's main problem. A patient may, for instance, present with chest pain. In the course of consultation it may transpire that the real problem is that the patient has noticed a lump in the breast, palpitations thought to be due to heart disease or received a blow on the chest by her husband. Unless specifically designed to do so, routine records cannot be depended on to reflect the spectrum of the symptoms presented in primary care.

3. The diagnosis recorded has already been discussed in this chapter. It may or may not reflect the patients real problem which has led to the consultation.

4. Apart from the date of the consultation, the treatment prescribed is the item of information most likely to be included in the routine primary care record. The drugs recorded in the medical record may not, however, accurately reflect the medications being consumed by the patient.

5. The primary physician's notes are frequently used as 'an *aide-mémoire*'. The doctor is concerned not just with the reason for the consultation and the treatment prescribed, but also with maintaining a relationship with his patient. The note which reads 'budgie died last week' or 'visited daughter in Australia', may be important information to the doctor in his continuing relationship, but is of doubtful value in research or in auditing GP care.

6. Certified sickness absence is often recorded in primary care records. This information is usually reliable for males who, in the UK, need national insurance certificates in order to obtain sickness benefit, but may be less reliable for females who are not always entitled to this benefit.

The routine records of primary physicians are used for a variety of purposes, each of which may be very relevant to the doctor providing care. The record is, however, very rarely valuable for retrospective research or audit unless it has been specifically designed for this purpose.

### Coding information in primary care

If information collected in primary care is to be used for research purposes, then it is necessary to be able to classify or group the information collected in such a way that it can subsequently be analysed. At the simplest level, consultations may be divided into those initiated by the doctor or those initiated by the patient and each can be allotted a code. It may be desirable to develop a code to represent the place of consultation or to reflect referral procedures or investigations. Most of these codes can be encompassed in a range from numbers 1 to 9, and it is not difficult in these cases for the doctor to carry out coding at the time of consultation.

More difficult problems are encountered in coding morbidity data. It has already been pointed out that many of the problems encountered in general practice cannot easily be ascribed a particular diagnosis. The International Classification of Diseases (1977) has been built up from data derived from post-mortem material and hospital medicine, and is not therefore, very satisfactory as a means of coding illness recorded in general practice. A modification of this index which greatly simplifies coding morbidity in general practice was developed by the College of General Practitioners in the UK (1963).

More recently an International Classification of Health Problems in Primary Care (ICHPCC) has been developed by the World Organization of National Colleges and Academic Associations of General Practitioners/Family Physicians (1979). Readers interested in this problem should refer to this monograph. It should, however, be pointed out that a satisfactory system for coding morbidity in general practice should have certain qualities:

1. It should be easy to use, i.e. it should be possible for a clerical assistant with some supervision to code the problems recorded at each consultation.

2. It should be able to accept problems at a symptomatic level as well as diagnoses and classify them under the appropriate broad rubrics of the system; such problems as coryza, diarrhoea, or rash should be classified respectively as respiratory disease, gastro-intestinal disease, or skin disease and not presumed to be of infective origin and classified as infectious diseases.

3. There should be facilities for coding social problems rather than forcing them into a rubric which describes the effects of these problems on the behaviour of the patient which may or may not be pathological.

4. It should be possible to relate the coding system used in primary care to the International Classification of Diseases.

Some doctors working in primary care may be interested in studying not the problems or disease presented to them, but the symptoms of which their patients complain. No widely accepted method of symptom coding has been evolved. The ICHPCC probably offers the most useful method of coding such information at present available, but was not designed specifically for this purpose.

Coding information about presenting symptoms and morbidity can rarely be carried out at the time of the consultation. If a doctor wishes to do research in these areas, it is usually necessary for him to train a clerical assistant who can undertake this work. The assistant will need, either to scan the practice record to obtain the information to be coded, or to extract information from a specially designed encounter sheet prepared for each consulting session. It is essential in such cases to ensure that this information is recorded in a legible fashion and many doctors underline or 'box' the data to be coded. The accuracy of coding should be checked at regular intervals.

### Seasonal variations in morbidity in primary care

In recording events in primary care it is important to realize how these events may be influenced by climatic factors and epidemics of infectious diseases from one year to another. It is not uncommon for doctors to wish to measure the effect of a change in the method of delivering care by measuring the events in the practice before and after change is carried out. In designing such studies it is essential to ensure that the periods being studied are influenced as little as possible by seasonal factors. The same months in successive years should, for instance, be studied. Even this precaution however, is not always sufficient. Such a large proportion of the demand for primary care is generated by respiratory illness that an influenza epidemic or a prolonged period of cold weather can markedly influence demand from one year to another. In order to cope with the demand produced by an epidemic of influenza, the primary physician will usually cut back on the time he gives to continuing care of chronic disease or anticipatory care. In such a year his whole pattern of work may be grossly distorted.

This can totally sabotage studies designed to compare the effect of changing the method of delivering care on the pattern of care provided from one year to another. In designing such studies it is essential to have a control practice which is not subjected to any changes in the method of delivering care, but is sensitive to seasonal variations in demand and morbidity (Morrell and Nicholson 1973).

### The primary care team

The sort of problems resulting from seasonal variations in morbidity in primary care are equally liable to occur due to variations in the staffing of the establishment delivering care. To relate events occurring in a practice to the care provided requires an awareness on the part of the doctor that he is just one member of a team which provides primary care services in the community. This community is subject to continual changes which may influence its demands for the GP's services. Such factors as unemployment, the cost of prescriptions or a change in social services may all influence demands and more immediately the availability of nurses, health visitors or hospital accident and emergency services will influence the way patients use the GP. Keeping these factors stable while studying a practice often presents insuperable problems.

## The population at risk

Recording events in primary care is of little value unless they can be related to the population at risk. Comparisons of data between one study and another are likely to be meaningless unless the populations in which the studies took place can be compared.

In the UK individuals are constrained to register for primary care with the GP of their choice and must obtain all their primary care services from him or his partners, if he is in group practice. As a result the population for whom a doctor accepts responsibility for providing care can be defined and described in terms of age and sex. To this information may be added data about marital status and occupation, but because these data are subject to change over time they tend to be rather inaccurate and may frequently be missing from the routine records. In the situation existing in the UK, it is relatively easy for a doctor to construct an age-sex register of the patients for whom he is responsible. It is less easy to keep this up-to-date. A system can be developed which ensures that each new patient registering with the doctor is added to the register. It is more difficult to identify and delete from the register those patients who leave the practice. Doctors should be informed when patients die, but will not be informed that a patient has left his practice until that patient registers with a new doctor. If this occurs the patient's records will, in due course, be withdrawn from the practice and the patient can be deleted from the register. There is, however, a tendency among patients who move from one area to another, not to register with a new doctor until they become ill and need a doctor's services. The practice register will therefore, contain information about patients who have left the area but not re-registered because they have not become ill. It will fail to contain information about patients who have moved into the area, for whom the doctor will provide services, but who have not yet become ill and registered. The level of inaccuracy created by this process of registration depends on the mobility of the population. In most cases this does not distort the age-sex distribution of the practice population, assuming that those moving out are replaced by those moving in. In areas in which there is selective migration of particular age groups, it can confuse the situation. There is an additional factor which operates in determining which individuals are included on the age-sex register. Those people who are chronically ill are more likely to register with a doctor when they arrive in an area as compared with those who are healthy and the same applies to those leaving the area. The register is therefore, more likely to be sensitive to the movement of ill individuals than those in good health. Again this tendency will balance out in most areas, but in those areas where there is selective migration in terms of age or morbidiy it may have an important influence on the age-sex register. Finally, individuals who re-register or emigrate, and representatives of individuals who have died are expected, in the UK to hand in their 'medical cards' to the new doctor, the customs or the registrar of deaths respectively. This does not always take place because in an important number of cases, the individual has lost his medical card. In these instances, individuals may remain for many years registered with one doctor, when they have left the area and re-registered with another. As a result of all these problems, many age-sex registers are inflated. In some cases up to 20 per cent of the individuals apparently registered are no longer living in the doctor's area of practice. This produces serious problems for workers who wish to use the register as a sampling frame.

In countries where patients do not have to register for primary care and can have more than one primary physician, the problems of describing the population for whom the doctor is responsible are more complex. In this situation the doctor can only describe his population in terms of the patients who consult him. This population can be described in terms of age, sex, social class, marital status, or whatever variables that may be chosen and events occurring in the practice can be related to this population. It cannot be assumed that the doctor is 'at risk' to these patients at all times nor that he is the only primary physician they consult. And the population who do not consult him cannot be described.

To overcome this problem many countries have measured demand for primary care services by carrying out surveys of random samples of the population, for example, Office of Population Censuses and Surveys (1973) and US Department of Health Education and Welfare (1979). In these surveys, individuals are usually asked to respond to a questionnaire about their illness experience and the use of services over a period of time (usually two weeks prior to the interview). The weakness in such surveys is that they are dependent on the individual's ability to recall symptoms of illness and their use of services.

## Quality control

Collecting data at the primary care consultation is never easy because of the time constraints under which most GPs work, and because, as the first contact for medical care in the com-

munity the doctor is exposed to an unpredictable work load. If accurate and complete data are to be collected in this setting, it is necessary to ensure some form of supervision. This must ascertain that events which should be recorded are in fact recorded and that all the data which should be collected about these events are in fact collected. If direct supervision of the recording is not possible, there must be at least built into the study design, some method of estimating the events and the data which have been omitted. Three aspects of this problem must be considered:

1. If a study is designed to collect information about a sample of patients exhibiting certain characteristics or suffering from specified diseases, it is necessary to ensure that every patient described in the research protocol as admissible to the study, is admitted. This may be difficult to achieve in a busy consulting session and in general the greater the task in data collection demanded of the doctor, the more likely is the patient to be omitted from the study.

2. Once a patient is entered into a study it is important to ensure that all the information described in the protocol is collected. The completeness of data recording is likely to be related inversely to the amount of data required and the ease in both logistic and emotional terms with which the doctor can elicit the information.

3. When a study is designed to elicit certain facts from the medical history and certain findings from a physical examination of the patient, it is important to ensure that the doctor adheres to the history taking and physical examination as defined in the research protocol.

A number of methods have been devised for use in primary care to ensure that studies measure up to these criteria:

1. At the end of each consulting session, medical records are checked by an independent assessor. The object is to identify all those patients who should have been included in the study and to ensure that they have been included and that a complete set of data has been recorded for each. If possible the check should take place within 24 hours of the consultation, because at this stage the doctor may still be able to recall the consultation and missing information may be retrieved. If patients have been wrongly excluded from a study it is at least possible to identify them in terms of age, sex, etc., so that they can subsequently be compared with those entering the study and in some cases it may be possible to recruit them. The identification and rapid feedback of missing data to the doctors in a study helps them to be aware of their errors and improve their performance. In some situations where a number of doctors in a single practice are carrying out a study, the assessor may be able to display, at regular intervals, the error rate of the different participants and introduce a competititve spirit. A prize may even be awarded at regular intervals for the best performance. To those unaccustomed to working in research departments this may seem an expensive and somewhat childish way to undertake data collection. Those with experience of data collection in primary care are aware of the difficulties of accurately completing records in this setting and recognize the need to establish and maintain, often over many months, enthusiasm to complete the project. The work of an assessor is usually best undertaken by a

clerical worker of obsessional personality, who possesses qualities which will convince the doctors taking part in the work that they can do better. It is not always necessary to employ someone specifically for this task. It may be undertaken part-time by a receptionist or record clerk who has the right personality and skills.

In some situations, regular checking of records and feedback of information may not be possible. In such cases spot checks may be carried out at intervals. This must always be followed by immediate feedback and measurement of the levels of error. If the spot checks are unpredictable, it offers a useful deterant to sloppy data collection, but it is rarely possible to retrieve missing data in this way, and it is less easy to develop the team spirit which can be engendered by regular supervision.

2. Where it is not possible to provide regular supervision of data recording, other strategies are necessary. These depend on obtaining independent evidence that a particular event has occurred, and confirming that this has also been recorded. Doctors may, for instance, agree to record every occasion on which a patient is referred to hospital, or an X-ray carried out, or a prescription issued. In such cases it is usually possible by reference to the hospital, the X-ray department or, in the UK, the Prescription Pricing Bureau, to check that these events have occurred. Data obtained from these sources may then be compared with the data recorded in primary care (Morrell *et al.* 1970).

3. Where the day-to-day monitoring of data collection is not possible, an attempt should be made to analyse the data collected at regular intervals as the study proceeds. In most cases, events occur with a consistent frequency over time. A fall off in the frequency with which events are recorded in a study may therefore indicate a loss of interest among those taking part. In studies which span a long period of time, it is essential that regular meetings take place at which the progress of the study is reported. This has implications for those concerned with extracting, coding, and analysing the information in that they must organize their work in such a way that they are continually able to provide updated information to those who are collecting the data.

4. In many epidemiological studies research assistants are used to collect data. In such work, they are trained, their methods are, as far as possible, standardized· and inter-observer variation is carefully measured. Research assistants may also be employed in some studies carried out in primary care, but in many, the data are collected by the doctors themselves. It is often forgotten that they also need training if the quality of the information they collect is to be high.

An important part of this training is to ensure that those taking part in the study have been involved in the planning stage and fully comprehend the objectives and the way these are to be achieved. They must be motivated to co-operate and be convinced that the questions to be answered by the work are not just important in general terms but important to them and their patients in the care they provide. A method of training the doctors in the use of definitions and completing research records has been described earlier in this chapter.

In studies where the doctors have to conduct a specific examination, it is desirable to observe the technique used in order to ensure that those taking part are carrying out the examination in the same way. By use of videotape (Roland 1981), it is possible to compare several doctors examining the same patient. This is not only valuable in training, but also allows an estimate of inter-observer error to be made and the error attributable to the patient performing differently at successive examinations.

Many studies over the last two decades have claimed to show wide differences between doctors in such variables as consultation rates, morbidity experiences, and use of hospital and laboratory services. Very few have been sufficiently stringent in their design to ensure that the differences observed are real and not an artefact introduced by different levels of accuracy in interpreting definitions and completing research records.

In ensuring good quality research in primary care, special problems may be encountered if it is necessary to collect specimens from the patient for laboratory examination. The GP is not so well placed in terms of facilities as the hospital physician. In addition, he has problems of transporting specimens to the laboratory which may be at some distance. Some specimens are affected by the lapse of time between collection and examination, e.g. urine, swabs, and some blood values. These difficulties should be anticipated in planning studies and expert advice obtained. The use of special transport media or special methods of storage can overcome many problems but need careful planning.

Similar problems occur in clinical trials when tests of compliance depend on measuring tracer substances in the urine or blood. Special arrangements may solve these problems. The most important resources in these cases is, however, the physician's time to carry out the tests prescribed, and it is lack of time which so often causes physicians to fail to comply with the study design.

## THE RANGE OF RESEARCH IN PRIMARY CARE

Research in primary care covers a very wide field. The primary physician is concerned with such issues as the perception of illness in the community, the factors which influence patients in seeking care, the acceptability of the care provided, the work load of the primary care team, the morbidity presented in primary care, methods of delivering primary care, the natural history of disease, clinical trials, and education. Some examples are described in the following sections:

### The perception of illness in the community

Two methods have been used to measure illness in the community. The first depends on questionnaires in which individuals are asked to respond to a series of questions concerning symptoms or disabilities which they have experienced in the preceding two weeks. The second is concerned with keeping diaries of their health over the period of enquiry. In the former, the patient is asked to recall his use of primary care services. In the latter, demands for care may be directly recorded by the GP. The results of such studies produce widely differing results. From the former (Horder and Horder 1954; Wadsworth *et al.* 1971) it would appear that about one perceived symptom in four leads to a consultation with a primary physician, while for the latter (Banks *et al.* 1975), it appears that only about one symptom in 40 leads to a consultation. There is no doubt that the use of health diaries opens up new possibilities in studying the perception of illness in the community. The diary is maintained by the patient who is invited, at the end of each day, to record any symptoms of illness experienced during the day and the action that they took in response to these symptoms. Although the maintenance of such diaries in the study by Banks *et al.* revealed that only one symptom in 40 led to a consultation, over 50 per cent of symptoms led to self-medication. This presents a new area of enquiry. In experiments conducted so far, health diaries have been well accepted by patients. If they are to be completed regularly they do, however, need regular surveillance and reinforcement. A telephone call at one or two weekly intervals or better still a visit from a research worker is the minimum required to ensure good data collection.

If accurate information is available about patients' use of services provided and particularly if this can be linked to some measure of the individual's perception of their health, it is possible to set up studies which compare the behaviour of different individuals in response to symptoms of illness. This area of enquiry provides opportunities for social scientists to work with primary physicians in mounting research in primary care. Many such studies have been conducted in the last decade which have related the level of demand for primary care to such variables as, objective measures of anxiety (Banks *et al.* 1975), social and community resources (Beresford *et al.* 1977) and disturbed family and community relationships (Rahe *et al.* 1970). This type of research is difficult and expensive, and demands a multidisciplinary approach, but it is necessary if the primary physician is to learn more about the many factors which influence demands for primary care. The reader interested in this field can consult the references given above to find out more about the methods employed to obtain this information.

## Attitudes to care

A lot of interest is focused on the attitudes of the community to different systems of primary care. These have mainly been carried out by social scientists. The methods most commonly employed involve the use of questionnaires, administered to random samples of the population. In some studies, it has been possible to link the individual's answers to the questionnaires to similar questionnaires submitted to the primary physicians providing care (Cartwright 1967). In one study it was possible to repeat the investigation after a period of ten years and thus to measure changes in attitudes over this period of time (Cartwright and Anderson 1981).

## The content of primary care

Many descriptive studies have been carried out of the work load of the primary physician throughout the world. Wide differences in work load have been demonstrated both between physicians in one country (Wright 1968), and between physicians in different countries (Marsh and Sweeney 1971). In carrying out this type of research, it is usual to develop a standard record which can be completed at the time of each consultation. Most of the data can be recorded in a pre-coded form and subsequently extracted by a research assistant.

Studies of this type have demonstrated clearly the need to define the events to be recorded and to develop ways of checking the completeness and accuracy of the research record. In many of the studies which have been conducted these precautions have not been taken and the differences demonstrated between different doctor's work load could easily have been spurious. Carefully designed studies, however, have been conducted that demonstrate real differences between doctors and numerous attempts have been made to explain these findings. Differences in the use of the GP by individuals in different age, sex, and socio-economic groups, and with different educational backgrounds have been demonstrated (Ashford and Pearson 1970), but these account for only a small part of the variance. Professional characteristics of the doctors and their methods of delivering care have also been examined, but the evidence that they play a major part in determining work load is minimal and confusing.

One way of examining the effect of the mode of delivery of primary care on work load is to devise experiments in which the method of delivery is changed and to measure the effect of this on the pattern and content of the work. It is often difficult to use a randomized controlled trial design and there are few examples (Spitzer *et al.* 1974; San Augustin *et al.* 1981) of this type of trial in this particular field. Most studies have been designed to measure work load before and after a change has been introduced in the method of delivering care. The problems encountered in this type of study design have already been discussed.

There are, however, major drawbacks to allocating patients within a single establishment to different patterns of medical care provision. Some contamination of the control group is almost inevitable and resentment may be created if the change in care is perceived by the control group as beneficial. An alternative strategy is to introduce changes in one practice and use other practices as controls. The organization of such experiments presents formidable difficulties.

Many studies of the content of primary care have focused on recording morbidity, of which perhaps the best known is that of the Office of Population Censuses and Surveys (1974). Such a study depends on regular returns from practices which agree to collect information at every consultation and feed this into a research unit which analyses the data. In interpreting these data, however, it is important to bear in mind their limitations. They must necessarily be collected from self-selected practices and while those working in this field try to ensure that the 'sentinel' practices are evenly distributed, both geographically and between urban and rural populations, this is not easy to achieve and inevitably those doctors prepared to take part in this onerous discipline of recording at every consultation cannot be representative of the profession. Morbidity statistics also depend on the diagnosis recorded at each consultation. The difficulties of recording a precise diagnosis in primary care where illness is seen very early in its natural history have already been described and the diagnosis recorded can sometimes be spurious. Finally, it is important to bear in mind that diagnosis is influenced by medical 'fashions', the treatment available, and the time which the doctor can devote to different types of problem. Changes in morbidity statistics over a period of time must be interpreted with great care. Morbidity statistics from primary care may be useful both in planning care and in planning the education of primary physicians. It is important that those who quote the statistics understand the contraints imposed on those who collect them.

### Trials of management in primary care

There are many illnesses which are seen only or mainly in primary care. Trials of treatment for these conditions must necessarily take place in this setting. There are numerous examples, such as, otitis media, urinary tract infection, mild hypertension, and acute respiratory illness, to mention but a few. Theoretically, there should be no difficulty in carrying out randomized controlled trials of treatment for these conditions and in practice this is generally true. It should, however, be recognized that GPs usually enjoy a continuing relationship with their patients over a period of years. If they are invited to take part in a randomized controlled trial in which they believe that one of the alternative treatments holds special advantages for their patients or perhaps more importantly, some special risk for their patients, they may be influenced emotionally in entering the patient in the trial and be too ready to apply escape clauses. Such problems should be clearly recognized and openly discussed. Demand for care from the GP is also unpredictable and in some settings he may see a new patient every five to seven minutes. Complex data sets should therefore be avoided in planning controlled trials in primary care.

The problems of applying the randomized controlled trial design in organizational studies in general practice have already been identified. This does not mean that this design cannot be applied in studying specific forms of management, prevention or health education. This design has indeed been applied successfully in the field of health education (Russell et al. 1979; Morrell et al. 1980) and in a major evaluation of screening in primary care (South-east London Screening Study Group 1977).

### The natural history of disease and long-term surveillance

The fact that patients are seen early in the natural history of illness and the continuing relationship which exists between patient and GP over long periods of time, makes primary care, potentially, an ideal setting for long-term surveillance of disease and its management. During the last two decades, however, there have been very few studies carried out in individual general practices (Fry 1979). The more successful studies of this subject have been multi-centre studies, organized either at a national level such as those by the Royal College of General Practitioners in the UK and by depart-

ments of community medicine. The work of Gillum et al. (1976) and The Royal College of General Practitioners (1974), demonstrate, in different ways, the types of problems likely to be encountered in research of this type. Examples have also been described in detail elsewhere in this volume. Most of the literature describing the probabilities of illness when individual symptoms are presented in primary care is still based on research undertaken at the level of secondary care and therefore in highly selected samples. Proper education for primary care, logical management of illness and trials of treatment depend on a clear understanding of the natural history and outcome of the common symptoms presenting at this level of care. Some of the difficulties encountered in studies of this kind have been described earlier in this chapter.

## PRIMARY CARE AND PUBLIC HEALTH

This chapter has so far been concerned with identifying the content of primary care, with the knowledge and skills required to deliver primary care and with the broad areas of research which are currently being undertaken.

If primary care is to play its full role in improving health, then it must be developed on a scientific basis in which the new knowledge obtained from research is applied in the field. To achieve this it is necessary to convince GPs that an experimental approach to primary care is important and that care must be organized in such a way that it can be constantly evaluated.

There are many ways in which this approach can be encouraged. It is possible for all GPs to keep registers of the patients for whom they provide care. All may develop records which focus attention on the special needs of their patients and facilitate a critical review of the care provided. Unfortunately there are few financial incentives in most systems of primary care to encourage this approach. More importantly, few GPs are educated to organize their practices in this way or possess the skills critically to evaluate their work. New methods of collecting and handling information and new ways of developing the primary care team are becoming available, so the time is ripe for new initiatives.

### Registers in primary care

The development and maintenance of age-sex registers in general practice makes it possible to identify individuals who, on the basis of these two variables, are particularly vulnerable to illness. The value of these registers may be enhanced if morbidity data are added and if specific items of the services provided are included on the register.

The development and maintenance of registers in general practice depend on obtaining the information which is to be recorded. There are a number of sources of information. Patients may be asked to complete questionnaires about their past medical history at the time they register with the practice. Past medical records received by the practice may be examined for relevant information. Data may be retrieved from the day-to-day medical records if a system is introduced in the practice whereby the records are scanned after each consultation. All these methods have been described by

Zander *et al.* (1978). It is important to bear in mind that this is a service function and not a research project. The morbidity data on the register will never be complete because of the limitations of the methods of data collection, but if all the methods proposed are carefully applied, they may well reflect 70–80 per cent of the chronic disease in the practice.

Items of care provided may be added to the register, such as, immunizations, cervical cytology, or opportunistic measurements of blood pressure which have been carried out. This makes it possible to use the register to review the preventive services provided.

Collections of data are of little value unless they can be made easily available to the practising physician. New developments in computer technology which make micro-computers available at a price within the budget of the GP present enormous opportunities in this field. It is vitally important that these developments should not be seen simply as a way of collecting large quantities of data. The relevance of these data to the outcome of medical care must constantly be challenged.

### Screening in primary care

One of the first examples of screening for asymptomatic disease was the use of mass miniature radiography in the diagnosis of asymptomatic pulmonary tuberculosis. When tuberculosis was common and as effective treatment became available, the value of this screening programme was quickly appreciated. It was hoped that population screening for other diseases would be equally effective and that by detecting disease at an asymptomatic stage, ill-health and disability could be prevented. As pointed out by Wilson and Jungner (1968), screening for asymptomatic diseases is likely to be of value only in those diseases where early treatment influences the outcome and where the disease is sufficiently prevalent for benefits of early treatment to outweigh the costs.

Their advice was unfortunately ignored and in many countries, population screening developed on a wide scale before there was good evidence of its value. The 'annual physical examination', a form of screening for asymptomatic disease, became an important part of primary care in some countries (Marsh and Sweeney 1971).

The value of screening in general practice was tested in a randomized controlled trial in South-east London (South-east London Screening Study Group 1977). The outcome measures included a variety of parameters of health, such as, mortality, morbidity and the rates of hospital referral over a period of five years. Screening was not shown to confer any benefits on the screened population as compared with the controls. A comparable experiment in California by Cutler *et al.* (1973), provided similar evidence.

As a result of these experiments, routine screening for asymptomatic disease has been largely abandoned in the UK and attention has been concentrated on 'case-finding' a term coined by Sackett and Holland (1975). This concept is well illustrated by DeSouza *et al.* (1976), who showed that in the UK, 70 per cent of patients are seen by their GP at least once in any one year and 90 per cent in five years. They demonstrated that all the patients subjected to a screening programme in general practice who were found to have asymptomatic hypertension needing treatment, had in fact, consulted their GP in the preceding five years. They argued that if GPs were to take advantage of the opportunities presented to them by patients consulting them, to measure the patient's blood pressure, then all those patients with asymptomatic hypertension requiring treatment would be identified. This concept can be extended to other diseases. All patients in whom a pelvic examination is carried out could have a cervical smear. All patients in whom a physical examination of the chest takes place could have their breasts palpated. The concept could also be applied selectively so that patients with a family history of diabetes could regularly have a urinalysis performed, while patients using an intra-uterine device for contraception or taking anti-inflammatory drugs for arthritis or those who have had a gastrectomy, could have a haemoglobin estimation carried out at regular intervals.

Such a system of opportunistic case-finding is likely to be more productive and more cost-effective than population screening. Its success, however, depends on the GPs being constantly aware of the opportunities presented to them, and perhaps more importantly, developing a record system which prompts them to carry out relevant examinations at regular intervals. There must be a place in the record to prominently display the blood pressure, a place to present the family history and current treatment. A medical record system which incorporates this has been described in a monograph by Zander, referred to above.

### The organization of primary care

The effectiveness of primary medical care is concerned with obtaining the optimal outcome from the care provided. Efficiency introduces a consideration of costs. An efficient system should produce, over the whole range of services provided, the greatest overall benefit within the financial constraints of the system. This necessarily means identifying priorities in the care provided. A system which provides immediate access may satisfy the needs and expectations of patients suffering from new episodes of illness. By providing time to respond to these needs, however, the GP may be prevented from giving adequate time to continuing care and prevention.

The essential problem is that the GP has a limited amount of time to give to providing services for a population which normally has unlimited needs and must determine how best to use the time available. Answers to this question are at present difficult to arrive at, because so many of the tasks which the GP undertakes have not been evaluated in terms of outcome. A doctor may, for instance, spend many hours each week counselling patients with psychiatric disorders. Does this improve the prognosis? He may organize group therapy for the obese or anxious patient. Again, does this improve the outcome? At present, the doctor must usually plan the use of his time on the basis of 'hunches' or on small uncontrolled experiments on selected individuals.

Another aspect of this problem is concerned with determining how much of the work currently carried out by GPs could as effectively, be conducted by other health professionals, such as nurses. There is good evidence that they can provide effective surveillance for patients suffering from such conditions as hypertension, pernicious anaemia, schizophrenia, and diabetes, to mention but a few. They are also capable of dealing with many new acute episodes of illness, such as acute trauma, wax in the ears, and acute skin infections.

In cost-benefit terms the organization of primary care is crucial to the production of an efficient service. Establishing a well organized primary care service depends on a number of factors:

1. The doctors concerned must define their objectives in terms of the care they wish to provide.

2. The methods they develop to achieve these objectives must be based on good evidence about the relative advantages in terms of outcome of the alternative methods available to them.

3. They must have good information in terms of records and registers of the needs of their patients and of the care they are providing.

4. They must have the ability to identify those areas of care which should be reserved to the GP and those which may safely be delegated to other health professionals.

Primary care throughout the world lacks the skills and the information necessary to provide a truly efficient service. There is a need for experiments which will demonstrate the benefits of alternative methods of providing care. There is a need to train GPs in management skills and in the skills necessary to collect and interpret information which will help them to look critically at the care they are providing. There is a need for a much closer relationship between GPs and those working in public health.

## Auditing care

Medical audit implies that the medical care provided is compared with predetermined criteria of good care. Two major problems exist. The first is in determining the criteria of good quality care in general practice. These may be decided by consensus from the views of other GPs – 'peer review'. More appropriately, the criteria are based on the results of research in primary care. Unfortunately, consensus is often difficult to achieve and the appropriate research may be wanting. The problems of setting criteria for audit are well described by Watkins (1980). In the case of chronic disease the main problem is that medical care really has very little influence on the prognosis and this is further complicated by the fact that many patients suffering from one chronic disease have other diseases which influence both the management and the outcome. The problem presented by multiple pathology in the elderly makes auditing care in this age group very difficult.

In the case of acute illness there is still considerable ignorance about the natural history of those illnesses in the absence of care. The benefits of medical care in, for instance, the management of tonsillitis or acute otitis media is minimal. It is difficult to demonstrate that the application of procedures agreed by peer review is more than marginally beneficial.

Medical audit in primary care is difficult largely due to the fact that there has been inadequate research in this field. This should provide a constant stimulus to the GP to undertake research in order to develop policies for the optimal management of the acute illnesses with which he is presented (Howie 1974; Stott 1976).

The second major problem in carrying out medical audit is that of obtaining information from the medical records which makes it possible to compare the care provided with the criteria of optimal care agreed in the practice. As has already been pointed out in this chapter a retrospective analysis of medical records is of limited value because they rarely contain the relevant information. It should not, however, be abandoned. Within a group practice, a routine review of medical records taken at random from a consulting session can lead to useful discussion as described by Morrell (1981). More formal review of the care provided for specific symptoms or diseases can be made if the doctor is asked to complete an encounter sheet for each consulting session or if a structured medical record is used for providing care for patients suffering from specified chronic diseases. The encounter sheet may be prepared by the receptionist, listing the names, date of birth, and sex of the patients booked for a particular consulting session. The doctor is then asked to record his diagnosis and the action he takes in respect of each patient consulting. His response to each episode may then be compared with predetermined criteria in respect of specific symptoms or diagnoses. This comparison may be carried out on a manual basis. Information may equally well be fed into a micro-computer and programmes written to compare the performance recorded on the encounter sheet with predetermined criteria of good care.

Medical audit has so far been considered only within the context of the individual general practice. In those systems of medical care where payment for primary care depends on billing for individual items of service, it is possible to compare the management of different conditions by different doctors on the basis of the details included in the claims for the services provided. In this situation, the same difficulties exist in defining criteria of good and bad care, as have been described, but gross discrepancies between the care provided and a predetermined 'norm' may merit further investigation. 'Peer review' has been applied most widely in the US (Brook and Appel 1973).

In the UK a degree of central auditing is carried out for drug prescribing. The prescriptions issued by GPs are collected centrally and can be analysed. This is done routinely in terms of cost and related to the size of the doctors' practice. The individual doctor is provided annually with a record of his total prescribing costs and the mean cost per prescription issued. His costs are compared with other doctors nationally and with the costs of doctors working in the same area of the country. More detailed analysis of prescription data has been carried out experimentally (Cochrane and Moore 1971; Wade and Hood 1972).

## Environmental medicine in primary care

Most GPs in the UK live and work within the same community for most of their professional lives. As a result, they are able to build up a body of knowledge about the special environmental hazards in the community and to identify those patients particularly vulnerable to them. This knowledge may be enlarged when a close working relationship exists between GPs, occupational physicians, and managers of commercial organizations. The development of well-organized registers and methods of data handling may greatly facilitate this aspect of the doctors work. There is, however, the prerequisite that doctors should be trained to think in terms of their community and to develop methods of collecting and using information.

This approach has been extended to develop the concept of a 'community diagnosis'. This envisages the application of epidemiological methods at a community level. The community may comprise all those individuals who receive primary care from one institution or may be applied to a particular geographical area within which a number of facilities deliver care.

The concept is not dissimilar from that on the basis of which the 'district community physician' was developed when the NHS was reorganized in the UK in 1974. The fact that the methods and information systems necessary to make a community diagnosis have not been more fully developed reflects, perhaps, the current priority accorded to preventive services in the allocation of resources. In addition, there can be little doubt that obtaining comprehensive information about a community and acting on it in a prescribed way does raise all sorts of political issues which might be more easily solved in a totalitarian situation than the 'entrepreneural' approach to medical care which exists in most societies today. In this situation, it is probably sensible to try to advance public health at community level both through GPs and through the appropriate community services.

## CONCLUSION

In this chapter an attempt has been made to identify ways in which public health principles enunciated in this book, may be applied in the day to day work of the primary physician. Many opportunities exist in his work for research and experimentation and they demand the application of rigorous research methods with which many primary physicians are unfamiliar. Opportunities also exist for the primary physician to apply the principles described in this book in his approach to patient care in which the rigid disciplines of research may be modified to fit into the system of care provided and produce useful results, particularly in preventive medicine and anticipatory care.

It has been suggested in this chapter that the practice of public health in primary care is essential if the quality of care is to improve. This has implications for education and also for the working relationships between public health workers and primary physicians. If this is to be harmonious and productive, each must recognize the strengths and weaknesses of the other, both in terms of skills and resources and in terms of the constraints imposed by the environment in which primary care is delivered.

## REFERENCES

Ashford, J.R. and Pearson, N.G. (1970). Who uses the health services and why? *J.R. Statist. Soc. A* **133**, 295.

Banks, M.H., Beresford, S.A., Morrell, D.C., Watkins, C.J., and Waller, J. (1975). Factors influencing demand for primary medical care in women aged 20–44 years: a preliminary report. *Int. J. Epidemiol.* **4**, 189.

Beresford, S.A., Waller, J.J., and Banks, M.H. (1977). Why women consult doctors: social factors and the use of the general practitioner. *Br. J. Prev. Community Med.* **31**, 220.

Brook, R.H. and Appel, F.A. (1973). Quality of care assessment: choosing a method for peer review. *N. Engl. J. Med.* **288**, 1323.

Cartwright, A. (1967). *Patients and their doctors.* Routledge and Kegan Paul, London.

Cartwright, A. and Anderson, R. (1981). *General practice revisited: a second study of patients and their doctors.* Tavistock Publications, London.

Cochrane, A.L. and Moore, F. (1971). Expected and observed values for the prescription of vitamin $B_{12}$ in England and Wales. *Br. J. Prev. Soc. Med.* **25**, 147.

College of General Practitioners Research Committee (1963). A classification of diseases. *J. Coll. Gen. Practit.* **6**, 204.

Cutler, J.L., Ramcharan, S., Feldman, R. *et al.* (1973). Multiphasic check-up evaluation study 1–4. *Prev. Med.* **2**, 197.

D'Souza, M.F., Swan, A.V., and Shannon, D.J. (1976). A long-term controlled trial of screening in general practice. *Lancet* i, 1228.

Fry, J. (1979). *Common diseases: their nature, incidence and care,* 2nd edn. Hasting's Hilton, London.

Gillum, R.F., Feinleid, H., Margolis, J.R., Fabsity, R.R., and Brasch, R.C. (1976). Community surveillance for cardiovascular disease. The Framingham cardiovascular disease survey. *J. Chronic Dis.* **29**, 289.

Horder, J. and Horder, E. (1954). Illness in general practice. *Practitioner* **173**, 177.

Howie, J.G.R. (1974). Further observations on diagnosis and management of general practice respiratory illness using simulated patient consultation. *Br. Med. J.* ii, 540.

International Classification of Diseases (1977). *A manual of the international statistical classification of diseases, injuries and causes of death, 9th Revision.* World Health Organization, Geneva.

Marsh, S.N. and Sweeney, G.P. (1971). Anglo-Canadian exchange in general practice. *Br. Med. J.* i, 336.

Meneely, G., Oglesby, P., Dorn, H., and Harrison, T. (1960). Cardiopulmonary semantics. *JAMA* **174**, 1628.

Morrell, D.C. (1981). Sampling medical records. In *Teaching general practice* (ed. J.J.C. Cormack, M. Marinker, and D.C. Morrell) p. 221. Kluwer Medical, London.

Morrell, D.C. and Nicholson, S. (1974). Measuring the results of changes in the method of delivering primary medical care: a cautionary tale. *J. R. Coll. Gen. Practit.* **24**, 111–18.

Morrell, D.C., Avery, A.J., and Watkins, C.J. (1980). Management of minor illness. *Br. Med. J.* i, 769.

Morrell, D.C., Gage, H.G., and Robinson, N.R. (1970). Patterns of demand in general practice. *J. R. Coll. Gen. Practit.* **19**, 331.

Morrell, D.C., Gage, H.G., and Robinson, N.R. (1971). Referral to hospital by general practitioners. *J. R. Coll. Gen. Practit.* **21**, 77.

Office of Population Censuses and Surveys (1973). *The general household survey: introductory report.* HMSO, London.

Office of Population Censuses and Surveys (1974). *Morbidity statistics from general practice.* Studies of medical and population subjects. No. 26. HMSO, London.

Rahe, R.H., Gundersoon, E., and Ranson, J.A. (1970). Demographic and social factors in acute illness reporting. *J. Chronic Dis.* **23**, 245.

Roland, M.O. (1981). What else can we do with our videotape? *Proceedings of the ninth meeting of the IEA, Edinburgh,* August.

Royal College of General Practitioners (1974). *Oral contraceptives and health.* Pitman Medical, London.

Russell, M.A., Wilson, C., Taylor, C., and Baker, C.M. (1979). Effect of general practitioners advice against smoking. *Br. Med. J.* **ii**, 231.

Sackett, D.C. and Holland, W.W. (1975). Controversy in the detection of disease. *Lancet* **ii**, 359.

San Augustin, M., Sidel, V., Drosness, D., Kelman, H., Levine, H., and Stevens, E. (1981). A controlled trial of family care as opposed to child only care in the comprehensive primary care of children. *Med. Care* **19**, 202.

South-east London Screening Study Group (1977). A controlled trial of multiphasic screening in middle age: results of the South-east London Screening Study. *Int. J. Epidemiol.* **6**, 357.

Spitzer, W.O., Sackett, D.C., and Sibley, J.C. (1974). The Burlington randomized trial of the nurse practitioner. *N. Engl. J. Med.* **290**, 251.

Stott, N.C.H. and West, R.R. (1976). Randomized controlled trial of antibiotics in patients with cough and purulent sputum. *Br. Med. J.* **ii**, 556.

United States Department of Health, Education and Welfare (1979): *Vital Health Statistics. Series 10.* DHEW Publication, Washington, DC.

Wade, O.L. and Hood, H. (1972). Prescribing of drugs reported to cause adverse reactions. *Br. J. Prev. Soc. Med.* **26**, 205.

Wadsworth, M.E., Butterfield, W.J., and Blaney, R. (1971). *Health and sickness: the choice of treatment.* Tavistock Publications, London.

Watkins, C.J. (1981). The measurement of the quality of general practitioner care. *J. R. Coll. Gen. Practit.* Occasional Paper 15.

Weed, L. (1969). *Medical records, medical education and patient care; the problem orientated record as a basic tool.* The Press of Case Western Reserve University, Chicago.

Wilson, J.M. and Jungner, G. (1968). *Principles and practice of screening for disease.* Public Health Papers No. 34. World Health Organization, Geneva.

Wright, H.J. (1968). General practice in South-west England. *J. Roy. Coll. Gen. Practit.* Reports from General Practice No. 8.

Wright, H.J. and McAdam, D.B. (1979). *Clinical thinking and practice.* Churchill Livingstone, Edinburgh.

World Organization of National Colleges, Academics and Academic Associations of General Practitioners/Family Physicians (1979). *International classification of health problems in primary care.* Oxford University Press.

Zander, L.I., Beresford, S.A., and Thomas, P. (1978). Medical records in general practice. *J. R. Coll. Gen. Practit.* Occasional Paper 5.

# 31 Sexually transmitted diseases

Michael Adler

## INTRODUCTION

The types of disease spread by sexual contact will vary in their incidence and clinical manifestations throughout the world. Despite this all clinicians realize that the three traditional venereal diseases of chancroid, syphilis, and gonorrhoea only account for part of their practice and that more and more diseases are being recognized as spread by sexual intercourse or contact. In the UK the sexually transmitted diseases (STDs) are now the commonest group of infectious diseases. The number of cases attending specially designated clinics is just over 500 000, compared with 180 000, 15 years ago. Syphilis is no longer a major problem, gonorrhoea still is but non-specific and *Chlamydia* infections are the commonest conditions seen. Other sexually transmitted conditions such as trichomoniasis, scabies, pediculosis pubis, and genital warts are increasingly diagnosed. Also commonly diagnosed is vaginal candidosis, which is rarely spread by the sexual route. In the last few years some of the new generation of diseases are being seen more frequently. The incidence of herpes genitalis is rising, more sexually transmitted hepatitis B as well as A is seen, and even more recently physicians have become aware of enteric pathogens (*Entamoeba histolytica* and *Giardia lamblia*) being spread by sexual contact.

## INFORMATION SYSTEMS AND ROUTINE MONITORING

An appreciation of the size of the problem represented by the STDs in any country is essential if adequate control programmes are to be implemented and monitored. The ability of an information system to give a 'true' picture depends to some extent on the medical care system in a country. However sophisticated the information system, it will need to be evaluated.

Probably the most basic system of notification is to report the number of cases, individuals or clinical problems (e.g. urethral discharge/genital ulceration) presenting for treatment, without necessarily being able to classify them into specific disease categories. This approach of case counting and problem orientation can be supplemented and evaluated by occasional *ad hoc* surveys with full microbiological support, which could allow for all cases to be correctly classified. Thus, some idea of the proportion of cases due to various important aetiological agents would be obtained and be assumed to prevail until the next survey was conducted. This approach has been used successfully in Africa where

studies on patients presenting with urethral discharge has shown that 82–95 per cent of these cases were gonococcal (Meheus 1976; Nathan *et al.* 1977; Meheus *et al.*, in press). Meheus *et al.* (1980) have indicated that this type of work only provides a rough estimate since it is usually limited to those seeking care, with no reference to true population at risk or those treated elsewhere, the self-medicated and untreated.

A more sophisticated information system would allow for the counting of patients presenting with different diagnoses confirmed by microbiological and serological tests. An illustration of this can be found in the UK where the 120 physicians in charge of 230 clinics for STDs notify the Department of Health of the number of cases seen by various diagnostic categories. These are syphilis, gonorrhoea, non-specific genital infection, trichomoniasis, candidosis, scabies, pubic lice, herpes simplex, warts, chancroid, granuloma inguinale, lymphogranuloma venereum, and molluscum contagiosum. These are divided into male and female cases. Additional data are returned for cases of gonorrhoea and syphilis, namely the age of the patient, whether the infection was contracted within or outside the UK and the number of sexual contacts sought, how many attended and the number found to have a positive diagnosis.

Even though this information system is well developed, and probably the most sophisticated in the world for the STDs, it has two major drawbacks which have required epidemiological investigation.

### Figures relate to cases not patients

The fact that the notification system relates to the number of cases not patients can produce errors in the system and mean that a patient can appear several times in the published statistics for each year and can do so for a number of different reasons. First, they may have more than one disease diagnosed at any one consultation; secondly they may have one or more disease on different occasions during the year, and, finally, there may be difficulty in differentiating a reinfection, which should be counted as a new case, from a relapse which should not. The other major problem associated with a notification system that is based on diagnoses and not individual patients is that certain essential demographic data are ignored or lost. For example this approach ignores the sexual orientation of patients.

The effect of only counting cases in this fashion is that the number of diagnoses made and thus cases reported misrepresents the size of the problem and leads to an overestimation in terms of individuals involved. The implications of this for the organization of clinical services and health education for STDs, are that it is not known whether STDs are as common as supposed or whether they are limited to a smaller, well-defined group of the population.

In an attempt to investigate and solve these problems a number of studies have been conducted. The first group of studies were only concerned to differentiate patients from cases. A study of all new patients attending an STD clinic in Belfast showed that there were 2093 diagnoses among 1753 patients, a mean of 1.2 cases per patient (Pemberton et al. 1972). A further study carried out in a large London STD clinic on a sample of 1071 patients found that these contributed towards 1909 cases, 1.8 per patient (Woodcock 1975). Unfortunately, the sampling method used in this second study meant that the more often a patient attended the clinic, the more likely he or she was to be included in the sample, so that patients with more than one case were probably overrepresented.

A more recent study has attempted to describe and answer some of the drawbacks outlined earlier and unlike the two studies just described was based on a sample of all STD clinics in England and Wales, thus giving a representative picture of consulters (Belsey and Adler 1981 a,b). Even though also concerned with providing an estimate of the number of patients treated it did this over a one year period and in addition examined the distribution of diagnoses among the patients.

A sample of all patients treated in STD clinics in England and Wales during 1978 was drawn in two stages, clinics being selected at the first stage and patients within selected clinics at the second. Stratification of clinics was based on the total number of cases seen in each clinic for the year 1976 (last year for which complete statistics were available prior to the start of this study). Three strata were constructed on the basis of number of cases (500 or less, 501–1000, and more than 1000) seen, and depending on these numbers a proportion of the clinics were randomly selected. Clinics in the study were visited and a systematic sample of patient notes drawn in each. Since the proportion of clinics included differed between strata, the proportion of patient notes selected was also varied to ensure that every patient seen in an STD clinic during 1978 had an overall probability of inclusion in the sample of 1/40.

The study indicated that there were approximately 100 000 fewer patients than cases. Females were more likely than heterosexual males to have several diagnoses made concurrently, whereas multiple episodes of disease were more common amongst homosexual males then heterosexual males or females. It was found that 9 per cent of male patients attending clinics in England and Wales were homosexual, and this group of patients contributed 10 per cent of all cases seen in males but 15 per cent of gonococcal infections. In heterosexual and homosexual males only 6 per cent of disease episodes involved more than one positive diagnosis as compared with 16 per cent of disease episodes in female patients.

This study has, for the first time, described the number and types of individuals consulting as well as their contribution towards disease and the different conditions suffered at one point in time by an individual. This type of quantification and categorization of patients, if collected routinely, would be useful in analysing the trends for the STDs and help to explain the rising incidence of most of the diseases.

## Lack of uniform criteria

The second major drawback associated with clinic statistics is that there is no guarantee that all the clinicians use the same criteria to diagnose or notify specific diseases. Unless these two steps are standardized or, at the very least, described so that allowances can be made for the variation, the changes in incidence of various STDs is difficult to assess. Are the changes real or due to changes in individual clinicians diagnostic and notification procedures, and likewise, are the differences in different parts of the country real or apparent for the same two reasons?

A recent study in the UK has attempted to examine these problems in greater detail (Adler et al. 1978; Adler 1978a–d; Belsey and Adler 1978; O'Connor and Adler 1979). The study was designed to collect information on the diagnostic and reporting criteria used by doctors in charge of clinics and to compare current treatment and management policies. It was hoped that the survey findings would allow individual clinicians to judge their own practices and standards against those of their peers, and provide the basis for the development of an improved and, possibly, a more rational basis for diagnosis, patient management and notification.

All consultant venereologists in charge of STD clinics in England and Wales were approached during the course of the study. A standard questionnaire was administered by personal interview. Information was sought on clinic facilities and on the diagnostic, treatment and reporting criteria in use for five diseases (gonorrhoea, non-specific genital infection, trichomoniasis, candidosis, and herpes genitalis).

An example of variation in diagnostic criteria is provided in relation to non-specific urethritis (NSU) – the most common disease seen in male patients in STD clinics. No agent can be isolated and the diagnosis is by exclusion of other known causes of urethritis such as gonorrhoea and Chlamydia trachomatis, and on the indrect basis of inflammation as witnessed by the presence of polymorphonuclear leucocytes on the Gram-stained smear. Consultants were asked to indicate the microscopic criteria that they used to make a diagnosis of NSU in male patients. The most frequently used criterion was between one and five leucocytes per high-power field (HPF) which was applied in 66 per cent of clinics, followed by 10 or more leucocytes per HPF (16 per cent of clinics) and finally 5–10 in the remaining clinics. It is unsatisfactory that when diagnosing NSU no consistent criteria are accepted since this must affect our concept of the size of the problem with regard to NSU.

## EPIDEMIOLOGICAL TECHNIQUES AND PLANNED INVESTIGATIONS

### Descriptive studies

*Patient management*

Descriptive studies are often an essential first step in epidemiological investigations. They may provide basic information that allows for changes in clinical practice to be made or point the way to more complex investigations.

The survey of practices in STD clinics, as well as identifying variation in diagnostic and notification criteria affecting the notification system, showed variation in clinical approach. For example, in some clinics serological tests for syphilis were carried out singly or in inappropriate combinations, were not repeated at all, or were repeated too early in the incubation period before they could possibly become positive. Some physicians were not sampling the correct anatomical sites or carrying out the appropriate tests to establish a diagnosis, whereas others were carrying out unnecessary tests. For instance, not all physicians would take urethral specimens from symptomless male gonorrhoea contacts, while those taking tests from female contacts would not necessarily repeat them if the initial tests were negative. Both of these approaches would result in cases of gonorrhoea being missed since it is known that 5–10 per cent of male cases can be asymptomatic (Handsfield et al. 1974; Perara and Lim 1975). Work carried out in the UK has shown that in a series of female patients who were eventually diagnosed as suffering from gonorrhoea one set of cultures missed 9 per cent of patients and 2 per cent were missed after two tests (Chipperfield and Catterall 1976) and this has been confirmed by the work of others (Evans 1976; Barlow et al. 1976). Thus, the failure of some clinicians to take more than one set of tests in women exposed to gonorrhoea will result in cases being missed.

As expected, the treatment of patients for a given disease varied throughout England and Wales and were often inappropriate. There were 17 different routine treatment schedules in use for male patients with gonorrhoea, and 15 for female patients. Some of the antibiotics were not appropriate and the dosage for some of the more efficacious preparations was inadequate. Physicians working in 22 per cent of clinics used idoxuridine for the treatment of herpes genitalis – an expensive substance of no proven value in this condition.

Even though the study outlined was a basic descriptive study it allowed individual clinicians to judge their own practices and standards against those of their peers and furnished information that provided the basis for the development of an improved and, possibly, a more rational service.

In clinical work, as in other fields, unless information is available about the results of our actions, we do not have the option to make material adjustments to these actions in the future (Acheson, E.D. – unpublished observation).

### Clinical diagnosis

Other descriptive studies in the field of STDs have made clinicians realize the difficulties of achieving the correct diagnosis, both, at the bedside and in the laboratory. The former is illustrated with regard to pelvic inflammatory disease or salpingitis. Studies comparing the use of clinical and laparoscopic criteria indicate that the use of the former gives a correct diagnosis in only 65 per cent of cases, with a false positive diagnosis rate of 23 per cent. In the remaining 12 per cent of cases other conditions such as ectopic pregnancy, appendicitis and endometriosis were found by the use of the laparoscope (Jacobson and Westrom 1969).

Laboratory variation and its affect on diagnosis can be illustrated by a study on observer variation in the interpretation of Gram-stained urethral smears (Willcox et al. 1981). The study was carried out to determine whether the diagnosis of NSU was affected by differences in the microscopical interpretation of urethral smears between individual observers (inter-observer variation) and the same observer on separate occasions (intra-observer variation). The study showed that even an experienced observer is surprisingly inconsistent in reporting on the same slide on two consecutive occasions, and the opinion of different observers looking at the same slide is even more variable. In approximately one third of instances variation was of such a degree that this would have affected whether to treat patients or not.

### Disease complications

The major cost of the STDs no longer lies with the acute diseases but with the chronic morbidity associated with them. For example, recent descriptive studies have highlighted the economic and human costs of pelvic inflammatory disease (PID). The incidence and prevalence varies throughout the world but in most developed and developing countries is rapidly increasing. In England and Wales the number of cases of acute PID admitted to hospital had doubled in the last 20 years. These figures, obtained from the Hospital In Patient Enquiry (HIPE) are an underestimate since they do not take into account non-hospitalized patients. Many of the patients with this condition and seen in STD clinics are managed on an out-patient basis. At one busy central London clinic, 92 per cent of women with PID are not admitted to hospital (Adler 1980). These patients do not appear in routinely published figures, thus the problem is substantially larger than suggested by the number of cases hospitalized per year. This shortfall was discovered by a descriptive study of clinical practice in one clinic. Naturally this finding needs to be tested in further large clinics to establish that the finding is not atypical. Likewise the management of PID by other groups, particularly gynaecologists, needs to be quantified.

Descriptive studies in other countries have itemized the important financial costs of PID. It has been calculated that over 850 000 episodes occur annually in the US, that these account for 212 000 hospital admissions, 115 000 surgical procedures and 2 500 000 physician visits (Curran 1980). The direct costs alone of these is calculated at 645 million dollars, and this does not take into consideration the direct costs of ectopic pregnancy or the indirect costs associated with PID.

A particularly disastrous consequence of PID is infertility. This long term sequelae is costly both in terms of hospitalization and related investigation and also in human suffering, the latter being particularly difficult to quantify in monetary terms. Arya and Taber (1975), working in Zambia described a relationship between gonorrhoea and infertility. This work was based on population surveys, which will give a clearer picture than case finding studies in specific clinical settings. By necessity, most other African studies have been of the latter type. Amongst hospitalized patients with PID in Uganda, one-third were suffering from a gonococcal infection and 25 per cent of all patients were infertile (Grech et al. 1972). In the Western Pacific descriptive studies have shown combined primary and secondary infertility rates of 40 per cent and in certain tribes 74 per cent of named couples were infertile (Scragg, unpublished observation 1957).

## Prevalence studies

The routine published statistics for the STDs for the UK are derived from the returns of cases made from STD clinics each year. These figures omit three categories of patients; those treated in general or private practice, or in antenatal and gynaecology clinics, symptomless patients who may never be treated; and symptomatic patients who decide to ignore their symptoms.

In the past, surveys have been carried out in gynaecology, antenatal and family planning clinics, to provide fairly crude estimates of the prevalence of certain STDs. These studies were limited to specific age groups and those who had opted to seek medical care. To some extent the varying rates reported in these types of studies reflect these demographic and consulting differences and not 'true' differences in disease prevalence. Since the women studied only represented one part of the total population at risk of contracting an STD, the findings could not be related to a defined population at risk and correct incidence or prevalence rates could not therefore be obtained.

'Accurate estimates of the incidence or prevalence of most of the agents or clinical syndromes of sexually transmitted diseases are not available ... To develop effective control programmes, these data need to be obtained' (WHO 1981).

In view of the potential shortfall in the current statistics, as outlined, and the *ad hoc* nature of past surveys, a study of gonorrhoea, trichomoniasis, and candidosis in a defined population of women (209 100) was carried out (Adler *et al.* 1981). The study was designed to identify patients both with and without symptoms seeking care or failing to seek care at all. Those patients who ignore their symptoms were identified by screening carried out in general practice, antenatal and family planning clinics. Likewise the symptomless women, unaware of disease, will not consult but were picked up by screening in these three agencies. The divisions between symptomatic and symptomless patients and where they may seek care are arbitary. Obviously overlap does occur and the theoretical division was only created in an attempt to construct a way of identifying the different agencies that need to be sampled if a total picture of STD is to be obtained.

Since the study was carried out in a defined population sampling symptomatic, asymptomatic, consulters and non-consulters, it was possible to calculate prevalence rates. This composite and total approach illustrates how false *ad hoc* surveys limited to one agency will be in telling us anything of the total picture of disease in the community. The results of this type of total screening suggest, for the first time, that the proportion of women with gonococcal infections not receiving care in the UK is low. The clinic service for STDs is effective in controlling disease and only small amounts of serious disease remain undetected.

The major criticism of this type of work is that it was carried out in one part of the country, and those studied are not necessarily representative of patients of similar ages in the rest of the UK. Studies in other parts of the country would be required to estimate national incidence and prevalence figures.

The same problems occurring in the UK with regard to establishing the 'true' size of the problem of STDs are seen and magnified in other countries, particularly since they do not have uniform notification and clinical systems of control. In America, for example, 80 per cent of cases of syphilis and gonorrhoea are treated by physicians in private practice and they notify only just over 10 per cent of those treated cases to the health authorities (McKenzie-Pollock 1970; Fleming *et al.* 1970). The reporting system within the US has improved considerably over the last decade but there is still some under reporting. For example, in 1980 there were just over one million cases of gonorrhoea reported, but the estimated number is thought to be nearer 1.6 to 2.0 million cases.

## Studies of incidence and longitudinal studies

### Transmission of infection

The infectivity of virtually all the sexually acquired diseases remains unknown. This is not altogether surprising when it is realized that some of the diseases can be asymptomatic. For example, 5–10 per cent of men and 50 per cent of women attending STD clinics in whom gonorrhoea is diagnosed are found to be asymptomatic. In these situations the patients may have had their disease for variable times and experienced intercourse with any number of contacts. Thus the probability of acquiring a sexually transmitted infection following intercourse with an infected person has been difficult to ascertain. Most of the work has involved the use of 'captive' populations. Holmes and his colleagues (1970) calculated that the risk of a male acquiring gonorrhoea by contact with an infected female is 22 per cent. This figure was derived by identifying infection among 2191 crew members of an aircraft carrier, who admitted to intercourse during shore leave with prostitutes in whom the prevalence of gonorrhoea had been previously calculated in a sub-sample of 4800 licensed hostesses with whom the men admitted having sexual intercourse. The limitations of such an approach are freely recognized by the authors of the study who point out that the possibility of self-medication by the men, the honesty with which they filled in the post-exposure questionnaire and the possibility that the way the couples paired off may not have been truly random, could all affect the ultimate figure for infectivity. Certainly other workers suggest anything from 5–80 per cent as being the risk of contracting gonorrhoea per sexual exposure (Marcussen 1953; Cutler 1969; Felton 1979). The correct figure will probably be most accurately calculated through the use of mathematical models (Reynolds 1973). Felton (1972) has maintained that it is important to have accurate knowledge of the rate of infection if any sensible control programme is to be developed. He suggests that a low rate implies a large number of infectious cases are to be found in the general population and that control should be through screening and contact tracing. In contrast, if the infectivity rate were high this would suggest that infection is passing rapidly in the community and that screening and contact tracing would be inappropriate control procedures.

## Sequelae of infection

The association of PID with certain of the STDs, and in particular gonococcal, chlamydial and non-specific infections has been mentioned previously (Descriptive Studies, pp. 476–8). Even though descriptive studies have proved valuable in highlighting this complication, it is only through longitudinal or prospective studies that the sequelae of PID can be assessed. Westrom (1975) followed up 415 women in Sweden with laparoscopically proven PID for 9.5 years and compared them with 282 women matched for age and parity who had also undergone laparoscopy but were found not to have PID. It was found that tubal occlusion had occurred in 13 per cent of Swedish women with one attack of salpingitis, in 35 per cent after two, rising to 75 per cent with three or more attacks. Holtz (1930) followed up patients for four years, after an acute attack of PID, and found 17 per cent to be involuntarily sterile, and Hedberg and Speyz (1958) followed up patients for the same length of time and found 40 per cent to be sterile.

Even though infertility is the most dramatic sequela of PID, others exist. Westrom, in the study just mentioned, also noted that 18 per cent of the patients had pain lasting longer than six months causing them to seek medical advice. Another prospective controlled study, this time in the UK, reported higher figures. Over a two year follow up period 74 per cent of patients had complained of abdominal pain, and even though this decreased over time, 20 per cent still reported this two years after the initial attack of PID (Adler et al. 1982). The differences between the Swedish and British studies in the proportion of patients experiencing abdominal pain may be accounted for by the different design of the two studies. Westrom carried out a hospital based study whereas Adler's was community based. Thus in the latter situation patients were interviewed in their homes and the abdominal pain that they admitted to was not necessarily taken to a doctor and could have been less severe. Pain was also experienced during menstruation and sexual intercourse and at the end of a two-year follow up, Adler found that 80 per cent of patients had noticed some change in their periods in that they tended to be longer and more painful and 40 per cent had experienced dyspareunia over the two years. These differences were statistically significant when compared to a control group of women followed up and then interviewed in a similar fashion.

## Intervention and experimental studies

The main emphasis of intervention and experimental studies with regard to the STDs has been either in relation to drug trials or the testing of vaccines. Modifying risk by health education or the use of the condom have also been attempted but are difficult to evaluate.

### Drug trials

Treatment trials in this field of medicine have either attempted to test a newly introduced antibiotic for a disease that is already well treated with good cure rates (e.g. NSU, gonorrhoea and candidosis) or to test new agents for disease for which, as yet, no treatment is available (e.g. genital herpes). In the UK trials belonging to the former category have tended to concentrate on treatment for non-specific urethritis (NSU). Many of these trials illustrate how not to conduct experimental work. Often those carrying out the studies do not use or state their diagnostic criteria, do not use controls or double blind assessment, and some count those patients who do not return for assessment after treatment as being cured whereas others proclaim them all as failures. Finally, the periods of assessment following treatment vary, some authors only following patients up for one week others for as long as four weeks, which allows a generous interval to assess treatment failures or relapses. Such variation in design and measurement of outcome makes it difficult to compare different drug trials.

### Testing of vaccines

In contrast to the rather poorly designed drug trials, a recent study that tested the efficacy of a vaccine against hepatitis B illustrates a carefully constructed and executed study (Szmuness et al. 1980). The efficacy of the vaccine was tested in a double-blind placebo randomized controlled trial on a group of homosexuals in the US. The two groups were followed up for 18 months and hepatitis B or subclinical infection developed in 1.4–3.4 per cent of those vaccinated as compared with 18–27 per cent of those receiving a placebo. The drop out rate in the two groups over the follow up period was similar at approximately 15 per cent.

### Testing health education and prevention

It has always proved extremely difficult to evaluate how effective education through the media and by specially mounted campaigns is in altering behaviour (Dalzell-Ward 1970, 1973; Rowntree 1975). This is illustrated by a study that measured the effect on the workload of an STD clinic featured in a television programme devoted to these conditions (Adler 1982). All new patients' source of referral was recorded before and after the programme. For the two weeks after the programme, just under a fifth of the male patients and one-eighth of the female patients, coming to the clinic, consulted as a result of watching it. A STD was diagnosed in less than a third of the males and a quarter of the females. This proportion of positive diagnoses was lower than for other sources of referral not related to watching the programme. It could be suggested from this that the programme resulted in only the anxious and hypochonidriacal seeking care, since most of those coming as a result of the programme had no disease, and thus the programme was no use as a form of health education. This would probably not be true since it would require a very elaborate prospective research project to answer accurately the true effect of a programme, media or health education campaign, with samples of non-attenders as well as attenders, and of those who had modified their chances of contracting disease as a result of the new information on STDs.

Many of those working with the STDs are sceptical about the role of health education in altering behaviour and feel that it is unrealistic to preach prevention through chastity but more appropriate to suggest to individuals ways in which risk can be reduced. For example, the Swedish campaign to persuade people to alter their method of contraception from non-barrier to barrier techniques is given as the major reason for the decline in gonorrhoea since the early 1970s. Little scientific evidence exists to support this contention but Barlow (1977) studied the use of the condom in men attending an STD clinic. He found that the correct use of this type of contraception was associated with a significantly reduced chance of acquiring gonorrhoea but this was not so for non-specific urethritis.

## Case-control studies

### Carcinoma of the cervix

Carcinoma of the bronchus and cervix have provided two of the most fascinating modern epidemiological problems. Unfortunately, the multi-factional nature of the latter has made it hard to be certain of the contribution played by sexually transmitted agents. The role and age of first intercourse have been described in numerous studies (Terris and Oalmann 1960; Martin 1967; Rotkin 1967). Case-control studies indicate that women with cervical cancer experience intercourse at a younger age and have more life time sexual partners than controls without cancer.

Original studies attempting to explore the association between sexually transmitted agents and carcinoma of the cervix concentrated on syphilis and trichomoniasis. Case studies showed that women with carcinoma had a higher rate of syphilis than controls (Levin et al. 1942; Terris and Oalmann 1960). Other infections described as contributing an increased risk are trichomoniasis (Naguib et al. 1966; Norin 1966) and gonorrhoea (Rotkin and King 1962). Other factors relating to religion, circumcision, type of contraception, race, parity and role of spermatozoa have also been explored.

The association of cervical carcinoma with the viral STDs has also provided interesting aetiological case-control studies. The possibility of an association has been the subject of controversy for nearly two decades. Evidence supporting the existence of a relationship has been mainly provided by a series of sero-epidemiological studies comparing the prevalence of antibodies to herpes virus type 2 (HSV-2) among women with dysplasia, carcinoma in situ, and invasive carcinoma with that found in control groups (Rawls et al. 1969; Nahmias et al. 1970; Royston and Aurelian 1970; Catalano and Johnson 1971). These studies have shown that positive antibodies are more common among women with dysplasia, carcinoma in situ, and invasive carcinoma than among their respective controls, and furthermore that there is a graded effect. Thus, positive antibodies are less common among women with dysplasia than among those with carcinoma in situ, and most prevalent among women with invasive carcinoma. However, the control groups in these studies were not matched for age at first intercourse or number of sexual partners. As previously mentioned, both of these factors have been shown to be related to the possible development of carcinoma of the cervix. In view of this it is possible that sexual promiscuity is an associated variable affecting both the risk of developing cervical cancer and the risk of exposure to herpes genitalis.

Nahmias and colleagues (1973) reported on a prospective study and found that the rate of cervical dysplasia was twice as great, and that of carcinoma in situ eight times higher in patients with herpes than in a control group in whom no type 2 antibodies could be detected. If this is so and the sexual transmission of HSV-2 is accepted then the exact role of the virus in the neoplastic process has to be explained. Recently, Aurelian (1976) reviewing the evidence linking carcinoma and herpes indicated that evidence now exists to show that cervical tumour cells 'contain a fragment of the viral genome, messenger RNA and some viral proteins'. Further work suggests a tumour specific antigen (AG-4) which could account for the role of HSV-2 in tumour growth and act as the mechanism for HSV-2 induced oncogenesis (Aurelian et al. 1973). The whole issue of cervical cancer and the association with HSV-2 infection is still open but the body of evidence does support the link. Aurelian (1976) fairly summarizes the situation '. . . even if HSV-2 causes cervical cancer it cannot do so alone, as a relatively high proportion of women with HSV-2 infections do not develop cervical cancer. The role of physiological and environmental factors as well as that of the host immune responses in the control or progression of the neoplasma should be given serious consideration'.

1981 also saw the first reports linking HSV-2 with squamous cell carcinoma in situ of the vulva. Kaufman and his colleagues (1981) demonstrated the presence of HSV-2 induced non-structural protein antigens in association with carcinoma in situ of the vulva in nine out of ten cases. They suggest that these observations in association with the increase in both HSV-2 infections and vulvar carcinoma in situ, suggest a link between the virus and the carcinoma. It is too early to say whether HSV-2 is aetiologically important in this situation or represents an opportunistic infection. Clearly the answer to this will need to be sought initially by good case-control studies, possibly followed by prospective longitudinal studies.

Even though much attention has been paid to the HSV-2 virus, other potentially oncogenic viruses should not be overlooked, for example papilloma and cytomegalovirus viruses. The papilloma virus is a small DNA papovirus that can cause genital and skin warts. Malignant transformation of vulval cervical and penile warts has been described clinically. As yet no case control studies confirming this possible association have been undertaken in humans.

Cytomegalovirus (CMV) has been at the centre of one of the most fascinating recent 'outbreaks' of a possibly sexually transmitted cancer, Kaposi's sarcoma. During the second half of 1981 a series of case reports started to appear describing outbreaks of this rare condition, often in association with Pneumocystis carinii and in most instances in homosexuals (e.g. Gottlieb et al. 1981; Hymes et al. 1981). Most cases occurred in urban areas, particularly New York State and California. Kaposi's sarcoma usually occurs amongst elderly men (mean age, mid-sixties) and runs a chronic, and rarely fatal, course (mean survival time 8–13 years). Most of the patients described in the case reports itemized above were young (95 per cent aged less than 50), most homosexual or bisexual (94 per cent) and experienced a particular high case-fatality rate.

The final intriguing factor about these homosexual men was that virtually all of them showed evidence of past or present infection with CMV. It has been postulated that this infection with CMV alters the normal ratio of T-helper to T-suppressor cells so that the patient is, in effect, immuno-compromised. However, CMV is particularly common amongst 'healthy' homosexuals and other factors that could give rise to such a profound depression of cell mediated immunity have been sought. Case-control studies have suggested that the long-term use of amyl nitrate as a sexual stimulant maybe such an agent (Goedert *et al.* 1982).

Even though case-control and prospective studies are often required to confirm the contribution of an aetiological factor in the subsequent development of carcinoma, a great deal can also be learnt by well conducted descriptive studies. This is illustrated by Beral (1974) who compared the mortality patterns for cancer of the cervix with the trends for STDs in England, Wales, and Scotland. She calculated cohort mortality due to cervical cancer in relationship to incidence of gonorrhoea. By this she explored the hypothesis that cervical cancer is causally related to a venereally transmitted agent and showed such an agent(s) is an important determinant of cervical cancer.

## SOCIAL SCIENCE TECHNIQUES

It is sad that there is very little information available on the behavioural factors that affect patterns of infection and utilization of medical services for these important diseases. In Glasgow a study was undertaken to describe demographic factors amongst patients attending the clinic for gonorrhoea and how these had altered over time from 1967 to 1976 (Schofield 1979). These were compared with the total population of Glasgow. Over the nine-year period, there had been a steady increase in the proportion of unmarried men and women in social class II, in excess of that expected, while the proportion of married patients had remained at the expected rate. During the whole period there had always been a lower proportion than expected in both sexes of social class III individuals. The investigators maintained that 'middle class morality' still exerted some effect in the control of gonorrhoea. American workers have also examined the effect of social class or socio-economic status on disease. Morton and his colleagues (1979) examined the effects of socio-economic status on the incidence of cervical cancer, gonorrhoea, and syphilis. Cases were identified for the latter two conditions by examining cases reported to the Venereal Disease Program of the State Health Division of Oregon. For these cases, area of residence was then fitted to one of the three census tracts for Metropolitan Oregon, all of which had been previously given a socio-economic score (this included income, education and crowding). There was a strong socio-economic effect on the incidence of gonorrhoea and syphilis, namely the lower the score the higher the incidence.

These two studies illustrate the major methodological problems associated with research in this field of medicine and social science, that of obtaining representative samples and making judgments about behaviour on the basis of crude demographic measurements. Both research projects only studied patients who had sought care. In the UK most patients who consult with an STD do so at clinics and few are treated within general or private practice. Even so, those consulting are not representative of the diseased population. Firstly, because non-consulters may be totally different in demographic and behavioural terms to those attending and studied. Secondly, the consulters may not be representative of other consulters in other clinics in the same country or even city. It is well established that the clientele of different London clinics vary considerably, and a study conducted in one would give a false and unrepresentative picture. In the US most patients are treated within the private sector and are never notified. Those patients seen in public health clinics are bound to be different, as are those who appear on the files of the State Venereal Disease Program and possibly consult at public clinics since they are poorer and the service is free. Thus, it is unreasonable and dangerous to extrapolate from these findings and make statements about social class or socio-economic scores and STD.

The other fallacy of using demographic labels or handles in relation to behaviour is the belief that they are fine measures of how people behave. Darrow (1979) rightly criticizes this approach, since bland measurements of social standing indicate very little about sexual behaviour and treatment seeking patterns, both of which are the important variables if adequate control strategies are to be developed. He makes the point that susceptibles of whatever social class will behave differently in relation to sexual behaviour. Some behaviour could be viewed as potentially increasing the risk of infection, whereas other types of behaviour will lower the risk while the individual may remain as sexually active as the high-risk group.

As indicated, not only are these problems related to the representativeness of different groups of consulting patients, but also in relation to non-consulters. To make statements about demographic variables in relation to STD it is important that one should not forget that non-consulters may be essentially different with regard to these variables, and by definition are bound to be different in behavioural terms, not least of all, in consulting terms, but possibly also in sexual behaviour.

Attempts have been made to understand why patients who have symptoms that could be attributable to an STD do not consult. Harrison (1982) studied women with genital symptoms in an attempt to understand the ways in which these women reached a decision on whether or not to seek treatment. Three groups were studied, first those women with symptoms potentially attributable to an STD who had not sought care for these, secondly, those with such symptoms who had taken them to their GP, family planning clinic or other medical agencies, and thirdly, those who had sought care with their symptoms in an STD clinic. Harrison found that a quarter of the women who did not seek care did not perceive that their symptoms were abnormal, and even those who did go did so after a delay, a factor which maybe as important in disease transmission as not seeking cure at all. He commented 'women are only confident about the possibility of STD when the symptoms are very pronounced or they arise in a stereo-typical behavioural context . . . Women harbouring STDs may fail to seek treatment primarily because the range, both in intensity and type, of STD symptoms combined with their similarity to many common complaints (which women regard as part of their lot or trivial) make self-diagnosis extremely difficult'. He points out that this on its own will make it difficult to change patterns of illness behaviour in women. Even though this is true it should be possible to offer certain guide lines which will allow individuals to gauge their own 'risk' of contracting or suffering from an STD. Thus, if a person develops symptoms after a recent partner change, is having multiple partners, her partner develops or suffers from symptoms or she has recurrent or persistent symptoms after previous treatment, she should consider herself at high risk and attend an STD clinic.

## CONCLUSIONS

The sexually transmitted diseases represent a major and growing public health problem in most countries. Unfortunately, these diseases have not been considered as priorities by either health care administrators or research workers and funding agencies.

'Information on the size of the problem, infectivity, behavioural determinants and long-term sequelae are central to understanding the STDs as an epidemic phenomenon, planning appropriate medical and other facilities required for clinical care and control and monitoring changes. These are exactly the type of problems that behavioural scientists and epidemiologists have been trained to describe and solve' (*International Journal of Epidemiology* 1979).

## REFERENCES

Adler, M.W. (1978a). Diagnostic, treatment and reporting criteria for gonorrhoea in sexually transmitted disease clinics in England and Wales. 1: Diagnosis. *Br. J. Vener. Dis.* **54**, 10.

Adler, M.W. (1978b). Diagnostic, treatment and reporting criteria for gonorrhoea in sexually transmitted disease clinics in England and Wales. 2: Treatment and reporting criteria. *Br. J. Ven. Dis.* **54**, 15.

Adler, M.W. (1978c). Diagnostic, treatment and reporting criteria for non-specific genital infection in sexually transmitted disease clinics in England and Wales. 1: Diagnosis. *Br. J. Vener. Dis.* **54**, 422.

Adler, M.W. (1978d). Diagnostic, treatment and reporting criteria for non-specific genital infection in sexually transmitted disease clinics in England and Wales. 2: Treatment and reporting criteria. *Br. J. Vener. Dis.* **54**, 428.

Adler, M.W. (1980). Trends for gonorrhoea and pelvic inflammatory disease in England and Wales and gonorrhoea in a defined population. *Am. J. Obstet. Gynecol.* **138** (2), 901.

Adler, M.W. (1982). Consulting patterns after a television programme on sexually transmitted diseases. *Br. J. Vener. Dis.* **58**, 259.

Adler, M.W., Belsey, E.M., and O'Connor, B.H. (1982). Morbidity associated with pelvic inflammatory disease. *Br. J. Vener. Dis.* **58**, 151.

Adler, M.W., Belsey, E.M., and Rogers, J.S. (1981). Sexually transmitted diseases in a defined population of women. *Br. Med. J.* **283**, 29.

Adler, M.W., Belsey, E.M., O'Connor, B.H., Catterall, R.D., and Miller, D.L. (1978). Facilities and diagnostic criteria in sexually transmitted disease clinics in England and Wales. *Br. J. Vener. Dis.* **54**, 2.

Arya, O.P. and Taber, J.R. (1975). *Correlates of veneral diseases and fertility in rural Uganda.* WHO/VDT/Res 75, 339. WHO, Geneva.

Aurelian, L. (1976). Sexually transmitted cancers? The case for genital herpes. *Am. J. Vener. Dis. Assoc.* **2**, 10.

Aurelian, L., Davis, H.J., and Julian, C.G. (1975). Herpes virus type 2 induced tumour specific antigens in cervical carcinoma. *Am. J. Epidemiol.* **98**, 1.

Barlow, D. (1977). The condom and gonorrhoea. *Lancet* **ii**, 811.

Barlow, D., Nayyar, K., Phillips, I., and Barrow, J. (1976). Diagnosis of gonorrhoea in women. *Br. J. Vener. Dis.* **52**, 326.

Belsey, E.M. and Adler, M.W. (1978). Current approaches to the diagnosis of herpes genitalis. *Br. J. Vener. Dis.* **54**, 115.

Belsey, E.M. and Adler, M.W. (1981a). Study of S.T.D. clinic attenders in England and Wales 1978. 1: Patients versus cases. *Br. J. Vener. Dis.* **57**, 285.

Belsey, E.M. and Adler, M.W. (1981b). Study of S.T.D. clinic attenders in England and Wales 1978. 2: Patterns of diagnosis. *Br. J. Vener. Dis.* **57**, 290.

Beral, V. (1974). Cancer of the cervix: a sexually transmitted infection? *Lancet* **i**, 1037.

Catalano, L.W. and Johnson, L.D. (1971). Herpes virus antibody and carcinoma in situ of the cervix. *JAMA* **217**, 447.

Chipperfield, E.J. and Catterall, R.D. (1976). Reappraisal of Gram-staining and cultural techniques for the diagnosis of gonorrhoea in women. *Br. J. Vener. Dis.* **52**, 36.

Curran, J.W. (1980). Economic consequences of pelvic inflammatory disease in the United States. *Am. J. Obstet. Gynecol.* **138**, 848.

Cutler, J.C. (1969). *In VD. The challenge to man.* New York American Social Health Association, Social Health Paper 4.

Dalzell-Ward, A.J. (1970). Forward planning in the United Kingdom for anti V.D. education. *Brit. J. Vener. Dis.* **46**, 159.

Dalzell-Ward, A.J. (1973). The design of action research experimental campaigns. *Br. J. Vener. Dis.* **49**, 171.

Darrow, W.W. (1979). Social stratification, sexual behaviour and the sexually transmitted diseases. (Editorial.) *Sex. Transm. Dis.* July–September, 228.

Evans, B.A. (1976). Detection of gonorrhoea in women. *Br. J. Vener. Dis.* **52**, 40.

Felton, W.F. (1972). How infectious is gonorrhoea? (Letter.) *Br. Med. J.* **ii**, 431.

Felton, W.F. (1979). A theory of the epidemiology of gonorrhoea. *Br. J. Vener. Dis.* **55**, 58.

Fleming, W.L., Brown, W.S., Donohue, J.F., and Branigan, P.W. (1970). National Survey of Venereal Disease treated by physicians in 1968. *JAMA* **211**, 1827.

Goedert, J.J., Wallen, W.C., Mann, D.L. *et al.* (1982). Amyl nitrite may alter T. lymphocytes in homosexual men. *Lancet* **i**, 412.

Gottlieb, M.S., Schauker, H.N., Fan, P.T., Saxon, A., Weisman, J.D., and Pozalski, I. (1981). Pneumocystis pneumonia – Los Angeles. *Morbid. Mortal. Weekly Rep.* **30**, 250.

Grech, E.J., Everett, J.V., and Mukasa, F. 61972). Epidemiological aspects of acute pelvic inflammatory disease in Uganda. *Trop. Doct.* **3**, 123.

Handsfield, H.H., Lipman, T.O., Harnisch, J.P., Tronca, E., and Holmes, K.K. (1974). Asymptomatic gonorrhoea in men. Diagnosis, natural course, prevalence and significance. *N. Engl. J. Med.* **290**, 117.

Harrison, R.M. (1982). Women's treatment decisions for genital symptoms. *J. R. Soc. Med.* **75**, 23.

Hedberg, E. and Speyz, S.O. (1958). Acute salpingitis. View on prognosis and treatment. *Acta Obstet. Gynecol. Scand.* **73**, 131.

Holmes, K.K., Johnson, D.W., and Trostle, H.J. (1970). An estimate of men acquiring gonorrhoea by sexual contact with infected females. *Am. J. Epidemiol.* **91**, 170.

Holtz, F. (1930). Klinische studien uber die nicht tuberkulose salpingoophritis. *Acta Obstet. Gynecol. Scand.* **10**, Suppl. 1.

Hymes, K.B., Greene, J.B., and Marcus, A. (1981). Kaposi's sarcoma in homosexual men – a report of eight cases. *Lancet* **ii**, 598.

*International Journal of Epidemiology* (1979). Comment: Sexually transmitted diseases. *Int. J. Epidemiol.* **8**, 3.

Jacobson, L. and Westrom, L. (1969). Objectivized diagnosis of pelvic inflammatory disease. *Am. J. Obstet. Gynecol.* **105**, 1088.

Kaufman, R.H., Dressman, G.R., Burek, B.S. *et al.* (1981). Herpes virus induced antigens in squamous cell carcinoma in situ of the vulva. *N. Engl. J. Med.* **305**, 483.

Levin, M.L., Dress, L.C., and Goldstein, H. (1942). Syphilis and cancer. *N. Y. State Med. J.* **42**, 1737.

McKenzie-Pollock, J.S. (1970). Physician reporting of venereal disease in the U.S.A. *Br. J. Vener. Dis.* **46**, 114.

Marcussen, P.V. (1953). Variations in stability of sexual relations as explanations of differences in spread of syphilis and gonorrhoea. *Am. J. Syph.* **37**, 355.

Martin, C.E. (1967). marital and coital factors in cervical cancer. *Am. J. Public Health* **57**, 803.

Meheus, A. (1976). Epidemiologie en bestrijding van geslachtszlekten in Rwanda. PhD Thesis. University of Antwerp.

Meheus, A., Van Dyck, E., and Friedman, F. (in press). *Importance of genital infections in Swaziland. Proceedings First African Regional Conference on Sexually Transmitted Diseases, Yaba, Nigeria, 1979.* National Institute for Medical Research, Lagos.

Meheus, A., Ballard, R., Dlamini, M., Ursi, J.P., Van Dyck, E., and Piot, P. (1980). Epidemiology and aetiology of urethritis in Swaziland. *Int. J. Epidemiol.* **9**, 239–45.

Morton, W.E., Horton, H.B., and Baker, H.W. (1979). Effects of socio-economic status on incidences of three sexually transmitted diseases. *Sex. Transm. Dis.* July–Sept., 206.

Naguib, S.M., Lundin, F.E., and Davies, J.H. (1966). Relation of various epidemiological factors to cervical cancer as determined by a screening programme. *Obstet. Gynaecol.* **28**, 451.

Nahmias, A.J., Josey, W.E., Naib, Z.M., Luce, C.F., and Guest, B.A. (1970). Antibodies to herpesvirus hominis type 1 and 2 in humans; woman with cervical cancer. *Am. J. Epidemiol.* **91**, 547.

Nahmias, A.J., Naib, Z.M., Josey, W.E., Franklin, E., and Jenkins, R. (1973). Prospective studies of the associating of genital herpes simplex infection and cervical anaplasia. *Cancer Res.* **33**, 1491.

Nathan, P.S., Jegathsan, M., and Ramalingan, S. (1977). Prompt points to the aetiology of male urethritis. *Med. J. Malaysia* **32**, 82.

Norin, L.C. (1966). Current serodiagnosis and treatment of syphilis. *JAMA* **198**, 37.

O'Connor, B.H. and Adler, M.W. (1979). Current approaches to the diagnosis, treatment and reporting of trichomoniasis and candidosis. *Br. J. Vener. Dis.* **55**, 52.

Pemberton, J., McCann, J.S., Mahony, J.D.H., Mackenzie, G., Dougan, H., and Hay, I. (1972). Socio-medical characteristics of patients attending a V.D. clinic and the circumstances of infection. *Br. J. Vener. Dis.* **48**, 391.

Perera, P. and Lim, K.S. (1975). Asymptomatic urethral gonorrhoea in men. *Br. Med. J.* **iii**, 415.

Rawls, W.E., Tompkins, W.A.F., and Melnick, J.L. (1969). The association of herpes virus type 2 and carcinoma of the uterine cervix. *Am. J. Epidemiol.* **89**, 547.

Reynolds, G.H. (1973). *A control model for gonorrhoea.* PhD thesis. Emory University, Atlanta, America.

Rotkin, I.D. and King, I.W. (1962). Environmental variables related to cervical cancer. *Am. J. Obstet. Gynecol.* **83**, 720.

Rotkin, F.H.D. (1967). Adolescent coitus and cervical cancer: associations of related events with increased risk. *Cancer Res.* **27**, 603.

Rowntree, F.H.D. (1973). Health education. In *Recent advances in sexually transmitted diseases* (ed. R.S. Morton and J.R.W. Harris) p. 388. Churchill Livingstone, Edinburgh.

Royston, I. and Aurelian, L. (1970). The association of genital herpes virus with cervical atypia and carcinoma *in situ. Am. J. Epidmiol.* **91**, 531.

Schofield, C.B.S. (1979). *Secually transmitted diseases.* Churchill Livingstone, Edinburgh.

Szmuness, W., Stevens, C.E., Harley, E.J. *et al.* (1980). Hepatitis B vaccine. Demonstration of efficacy in a controlled clinical trial in a high risk population in the United States. *N. Engl. J. Med.* **303**, 833.

Terris, M. and Oalmann, M.C. (1960). Carcinoma of the cervix – an epidemiological study. *JAMA* **174**, 1847.

Westrom, L. (1975). Effect of acute pelvic inflammatory disease on fertility. *Am. J. Obstet. Gynecol.* **121**, 707.

Willcox, J.R., Adler, M.W., and Belsey, E.M. (1981). Observer variation in ths interpretation of Gram-stained urethral smears. *Br. J. Vener. Dis.* **57**, 134.

Woodcock, K. (1975). How useful are our present statistics on sexually transmitted diseases? *Br. J. Vener. Dis.* **51**, 153.

WHO (1981). *Report of a WHO Scientific Group. Non gonococcal urethritis and other selected sexually transmitted diseases of public health importance.* Technical report series 660. World Health Organization, Geneva.

# Index